NUCLEAR ONCOLOGY

DIAGNOSIS AND THERAPY

NUCLEAR ONCOLOGY

DIAGNOSIS AND THERAPY

Editors

IRAJ KHALKHALI, M.D., F.A.C.R.

Professor of Radiological Sciences
University of California, Los Angeles School of Medicine
Chief of Breast Imaging
Director of Outpatient Radiology Services
Harbor-UCLA Medical Center
Torrance, California

JEAN C. MAUBLANT, M.D., Ph.D.

Professor of Biophysics
Auvergne University
Chief of Nuclear Medicine
Anticancer Centre Jean Perrin
Clermont-Ferrand, France

STANLEY J. GOLDSMITH, M.D., F.A.C.P., F.A.C.N.P.

Professor of Radiology and Medicine
Weill Medical College of Cornell University
Director of Nuclear Medicine
New York Presbyterian Hospital—Weill Cornell Medical Center
New York, New York

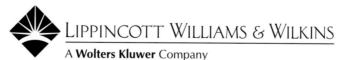

LIPPINCOTT WILLIAMS & WILKINS
A **Wolters Kluwer** Company

Philadelphia · Baltimore · New York · London
Buenos Aires · Hong Kong · Sydney · Tokyo

Acquisitions Editor: Joyce-Rachel John
Developmental Editor: Alexandra T. Anderson
Production Editor: Deirdre Marino
Manufacturing Manager: Benjamin Rivera
Cover Designer: Christine Jenny
Compositor: Lippincott Williams & Wilkins Desktop Division
Printer: Edwards Brothers

© 2001 by LIPPINCOTT WILLIAMS & WILKINS
530 Walnut Street
Philadelphia, PA 19106 USA
LWW.com

Library of Congress Cataloging-in-Publication Data

Nuclear oncology : diagnosis and therapy / editors, Iraj Khalkhali, Jean Maublant, Stanley J. Goldsmith.
    p. cm.
    Includes index.
    ISBN 0-7817-1990-9
    1. Cancer—Radionuclide imaging. 2. Cancer—Radiotherapy. 3. Cancer—Tomography.
  I. Khalkhali, Iraj. II. Maublant, Jean. III. Goldsmith, Stanley J.

RC270.3.R35 N83 2000
616.99'407575—dc21   00-048746

Care has been taken to confirm the accuracy of the information presented and to describe generally accepted practices. However, the authors, editors, and publisher are not responsible for errors or omissions or for any consequences from application of the information in this book and make no warranty, expressed or implied, with respect to the currency, completeness, or accuracy of the contents of the publication. Application of this information in a particular situation remains the professional responsibility of the practitioner.

The authors, editors, and publisher have exerted every effort to ensure that drug selection and dosage set forth in this text are in accordance with current recommendations and practice at the time of publication. However, in view of ongoing research, changes in government regulations, and the constant flow of information relating to drug therapy and drug reactions, the reader is urged to check the package insert for each drug for any change in indications and dosage and for added warnings and precautions. This is particularly important when the recommended agent is a new or infrequently employed drug.

Some drugs and medical devices presented in this publication have Food and Drug Administration (FDA) clearance for limited use in restricted research settings. It is the responsibility of the health care provider to ascertain the FDA status of each drug or device planned for use in their clinical practice.

10 9 8 7 6 5 4 3 2 1

CONTENTS

CONTRIBUTING AUTHORS

Hussein M. Abdel-Dayem, M.D. Professor, Department of Radiology, Division of Nuclear Medicine, New York Medical College, Valhalla, New York; Director of Nuclear Medicine, Saint Vincent's Hospital and Medical Center, New York, New York 10011

Lee P. Adler, M.D. Professor, Section of Nuclear Medicine, Division of Radiologic Sciences, The Wake Forest University Baptist Medical Center, Medical Center Boulevard, Winston-Salem, North Carolina 27157

Abdulaziz A. Al Sugair, M.D. Department of Radiology, King Faisal Specialist Hospital and Research Center, Riyadh 11211, Saudi Arabia

George Bakale, Ph.D. Department of Radiology, Case Western Reserve University, University Hospitals of Cleveland, Cleveland, Ohio 44106

Willem H. Bakker, Ph.D. Department of Nuclear Medicine, Erasmus Medical Center Rotterdam, 3015 GDRotterdam, The Netherlands

Neil H. Bander, M.D. Bernard & Josephine Chaus Professor of Urology, Department of Urology, Weill Medical College of Cornell University; Surgeon, Department of Urology, New York Presbyterian Hospital—Weill Cornell Medical Center, New York, New York 10021

Bruce J. Barron, M.D. Associate Professor, Department of Radiology, The University of Texas—Houston Medical School; Division of Nuclear Medicine, Memorial Hermann Hospital, Houston, Texas 77030

Catherine Beckers, M.D. Department of Nuclear Medicine, University Hospital Sart Tilman, 4000 Liege, Belgium

Tarik Z. Belhocine, M.D. Fellow, Department of Nuclear Medicine, University Hospital of Liege, 4000 Liege, Belgium

Claudia G. Berman, M.D. Professor, Department of Radiology, University of South Florida; Attending Radiologist, H. Lee Moffitt Cancer Center and Research Institute, Tampa, Florida 33612

Jay E. Blum, M.D. Director of Pulmonary Medicine, CIGNA HealthCare of Arizona, Phoenix, Arizona 85006; Associate Professor, Department of Medicine, University of Arizona College of Medicine, Tucson, Arizona 85724

Wout A. P. Breeman, Ph.D. Department of Nuclear Medicine, Erasmus Medical Center Rotterdam, 3015 GD Rotterdam, The Netherlands

Norman J. Brodsky, M.D. Clinical Assistant Professor, Department of Radiology, University of South Florida, Tampa, Florida 33612; Attending Physician, Department of Radiation Oncology, Lykes Cancer Center, Clearwater, Florida 34616

Inga Buchmann, M.D. Physician, Division of Nuclear Medicine, University Hospital Ulm, D-89081 Ulm, Germany

John R. Buscombe, M.B.B.S., M.Sc. , M.D. Consultant, Department of Nuclear Medicine, Royal Free Hospital, London NW 2QG, United Kingdom

Pablo J. Cagnoni, M.D. Assistant Professor of Medicine, Bone Marrow Transplant Program, University of Colorado, Denver, Colorado 80220

R. Edward Coleman, M.D. Professor and Vice-Chairman, Department of Radiology, Duke University Medical Center, Durham, North Carolina 27710

Leonard P. Connolly, M.D. Assistant Professor, Department of Radiology, Harvard Medical School; Division of Nuclear Medicine, Children's Hospital, Boston, Massachusetts 02115

Peter S. Conti, M.D., Ph.D. Associate Professor, Department of Radiology, Director, PET Imaging Science Center, University of Southern California, Los Angeles, California 90033

Frédéric Daenen, M.D. Department of Nuclear Medicine University Hospital Sart Tilman, 4000 Liege, Belgium

Marion de Jong, Ph.D. Associate Professor, Department of Nuclear Medicine, Erasmus Medical Center Rotterdam, 3015 GD Rotterdam, The Netherlands

Dominique Delbeke, M.D., Ph.D. Associate Professor, Department of Radiology and Radiological Sciences, Director, Nuclear Medicine and Positron Emission Tomography, Vanderbilt University, Nashville, Tennessee 37232

Sally J. DeNardo, M.D. Professor, Department of Internal Medicine and Radiology, Division of Radiodiagnosis and Therapy, University of California Davis, Sacramento, California 95816

Anne Devillers, M.D.   Department of Nuclear Medicine, University Hospital Rennes, 3500 Rennes, France

Chaitanya R. Divgi, M.B.B.S.   Associate Professor, Department of Radiology, Weill Medical College of Cornell University; Associate Member, Department of Radiology and Medicine, Memorial Sloan-Kettering Cancer Center, New York, New York 10021

Laura A. Drubach, M.D.   Instructor, Department of Radiology, Harvard Medical School; Physician, Division of Nuclear Medicine, Children's Hospital, Boston, Massachusetts 02115

Marc Ferriere, M.D.   Physician, Department of Cardiology, University Hospital Arnaud de Villeneuve, 34295 Montpellier, France

Paula M. Fracasso, M.D., Ph.D.   Associate Professor, Department of Internal Medicine, Division of Oncology, Washington University Medical School; Attending Physician, Department of Medical Oncology, Barnes-Jewish Hospital, St. Louis, Missouri 63110

Leonard M. Freeman, M.D.   Professor, Department of Nuclear Medicine and Radiology, Albert Einstein College of Medicine; Director, Department of Nuclear Medicine, Montefiore Hospital, Moses Division, Bronx, New York 10467

†Dov Front, M.D., Ph.D.   The Dr. Paul and Rose N. Geyser Chair in Clinical Radiology, Department of Nuclear Medicine, Rambam Medical Center and Faculty of Medicine, Haifa 35254, Israel

Gary F. Gates, M.D.   Clinical Professor, Department of Diagnostic Radiology, Oregon Health Science University School of Medicine; Director, Department of Nuclear Medicine, Providence St. Vincent Medical Center, Portland, Oregon 97225

Francesco Giammarile, M.D.   Physician, Division of Nuclear Medicine, Centre Leon Berard, 69373 Lyon, France

David M. Goldenberg, Sc.D., M.D.   Adjunct Professor, Department of Microbiology and Immunology, New York Medical College, Valhalla, New York 10595; President, Garden State Cancer Center, Belleville, New Jersey 07109

Stanley J. Goldsmith, M.D., F.A.C.P., F.A.C.N.P.   Professor, Department of Radiology and Medicine, Weill Medical College of Cornell University; Director, Department of Nuclear Medicine, New York Presbyterian Hospital—Weill Cornell Medical Center, New York, New York 10021

Milton D. Gross, M.D.   Professor, Division of Nuclear Medicine, Department of Radiology and Internal Medicine, University of Michigan; Chief and Director, Nuclear Medicine Service, Department of Veterans Affairs Health System, Ann Arbor, Michigan 48105

Hirsch Handmaker, M.D.   President, Healthcare Technology Group, Phoenix, Arizona 85016

Michael K. Haseman, M.D., F.A.C.N.P.   Clinical Associate Professor, Department of Nuclear Medicine, University of California Davis; Medical Director, Department of Nuclear Medicine, Sutter Medical Center, Sacramento, California 95816

Horace H. Hines, Ph.D.   Chief Technical Officer, ADAC Laboratories, Milpitas, California 93035

Carl K. Hoh, M.D.   Associate Professor, Department of Radiology, University of California San Diego; Division Chief, Department of Nuclear Medicine, University of California San Diego Medical Center, San Diego, California 92103

Roland Hustinx, M.D.   Department of Nuclear Medicine, University Hospital Sart Tilman, 4000 Liege, Belgium

Ora Israel, M.D.   Department of Nuclear Medicine, Rambam Medical Center, Haifa 35254, Israel

Denise L. Johnson, M.D., F.A.C.S.   Assistant Professor of Surgery, Stanford University School of Medicine, Stanford, California 94305

Malik E. Juweid, M.D.   Associate Professor, Department of Radiology, University of Iowa College of Medicine; Physician, Division of Nuclear Medicine, University of Iowa Hospital and Clinics, Iowa City, Iowa 52242

Iraj Khalkhali, M.D., F.A.C.R.   Professor of Radiological Sciences, University of California, Los Angeles School of Medicine, Los Angeles, California 90095; Chief of Breast Imaging, Director, Outpatient Radiology Services, Harbor-UCLA Medical Center, Torrance, California 90502

Peter P. M. Kooij   Department of Nuclear Medicine, Erasmus Medical Center Rotterdam, 3015 GD Rotterdam, The Netherlands

Lale Kostakoglu, M.D.   Assistant Professor, Department of Radiology, Division of Nuclear Medicine, Weill Medical College of Cornell University, New York, New York 10021

Eric P. Krenning, M.D., Ph.D.   Department of Nuclear Medicine, University Hospital Dijkzigt and Erasmus University Rotterdam, 3015 GD Rotterdam, The Netherlands

---

†deceased

Amir Kurtaran, M.D.   Professor, Department of Nuclear Medicine, Vienna University Hospital, A-1090 Vienna, Austria

Lamk M. Lamki, M.D.   Professor, Department of Radiology, The University of Texas—Houston Medical School; Chief, Division of Nuclear Medicine, Memorial-Hermann Hospital, Houston, Texas 77030

Steven M. Larson, M.D.   Professor, Weill Medical College of Cornell University; Chief, Nuclear Medicine Service, Memorial Sloan-Kettering Cancer Center, New York, New York 10021

Gidon Lieberman, M.B.Ch.B.   Research Registrar, Department of Obstetrics and Gynecology, Royal Free and University College Medical School, London NW3 2PF, United Kingdom

Jonathan M. Links, Ph.D.   Professor, Department of Environmental Sciences, Johns Hopkins School of Public Health, Baltimore, Maryland 21205

Val J. Lowe, M.D   Associate Professor, Department of Radiology, Mayo Medical School; Senior Associate Consultant, Department of Radiology, Mayo Clinic, Rochester, Minnesota 55905

Kathryn E. Luker, Ph.D.   Research Associate, Department of Radiology, Washington University School of Medicine, St. Louis, Missouri 63110

Daniel J. Macey, Ph.D.   Associate Professor of Radiation Oncology, University of Alabama at Birmingham, Birmingham, Alabama

Homer Macapinlac, M.D.   Department of Radiology, Memorial Sloan-Kettering Cancer Center, New York, New York 10021

Jean C. Maublant, M.D., Ph.D.   Professor, Department of Biophysics, Auvergne University; Chief, Division of Nuclear Medicine, Anticancer Centre Jean Perrin, 63011 Clermont-Ferrand, France

Ruby F. Meredith, M.D., Ph.D.   Professor, Department of Radiation Oncology, University of Alabama at Birmingham, Birmingham, Alabama 35233

Renee M. Moadel-Sernick, M.D.   Resident, Department of Nuclear Medicine, Albert Einstein College of Medicine and Montefiore Medical Center, Bronx, New York 10467

Lloyd Old, M.D.   Chief Executive Officer, Ludwig Institute for Cancer Research, New York, New York 10021

Egbert Oosterwijk, Ph.D.   Associate Professor, Department of Urology, University Medical Center Nijmegen, 6500 Nijmegen, The Netherlands

Patrick Paulus, M.D.   Department of Nuclear Medicine, University Hospital Sart Tilman, 4000 Liege, Belgium

Stan Pauwels, M.D., Ph.D.   Professor, Department of Internal Medicine, Catholic University of Louvain, Department of Nuclear Medicine, University Clinic Saint-Luc, 10200 Brussels, Belgium

David R. Piwnica-Worms, M.D., Ph.D.   Professor and Radiologist, Mallinckrodt Institute of Radiology, Washington University School of Medicine, St. Louis, Missouri 63110

Donald A. Podoloff, M.D.   Professor and Chair, Department of Nuclear Medicine, University of Texas M.D. Anderson Cancer Center, Houston, Texas 77030

Sven N. Reske, M.D.   Professor, Department of Nuclear Medicine, University of Ulm; Chief, Department of Nuclear Medicine, University Clinic, D-89081 Ulm, Germany

Carol Richman, M.D.   Professor, Department of Internal Medicine, Division of Hematology and Oncology, University of California Davis, Sacramento, California 95817

Pierre Rigo, M.D.   Department of Nuclear Medicine, University Hospital Sart Tilman, 4000 Liege, Belgium

George Segall, M.D.   Associate Professor, Department of Radiology, Stanford University, Stanford, California 94305; Chief, Division of Nuclear Medicine, VA Palo Alto Health Care Center, Palo Alto, California 94304

Brahm Shapiro, M.B., Ch.B., Ph.D.   Professor, Division of Internal Medicine, University of Michigan Medical Center; Attending Physician, Department of Nuclear Medicine, Ann Arbor VA Medical Center, Ann Arbor, Michigan 48109

Edward B. Silberstein, M.D.   Eugene L. and Sue R. Saenger Professor of Radiological Health and Professor of Medicine, University of Cincinnati Medical Center; Associate Director of Nuclear Medicine, University Hospital, Cincinnati, Ohio 45219

Partha Sinha, M.B.B.S., D.R.M.   Fellow, Department of Radiology, Hospital of the University of Pennsylvania, Philadelphia, Pennsylvania 19104

Brendan C. Stack, M.D. Associate Professor, Department of Surgery, Director, Head and Neck Oncology, Penn State Milton S. Hershey Medical Center, College of Medicine, Hershey, Pennsylvania 17033

Raymond Taillefer, M.D., F.R.C.P. Professor, Department of Radiology, Université de Montréal; Chief, Department of Nuclear Medicine, Hôtel-Dieu du Centre Hospitalier de Université de Montréal, Montreal, H2W IT8 Quebec, Canada

S. Ted Treves, M.D. Professor, Department of Radiology, Harvard Medical School; Chief, Division of Nuclear Medicine, Children's Hospital, Boston, Massachusetts 02115

Peter E. Valk, M.B., B.S. Professor, Department of Molecular and Medical Pharmacology, University of California—Los Angeles School of Medicine, Los Angeles California 90095; Medical Director, Northern California PET Imaging Center, Sacramento, California 95816

Roelf Valkema, M.D., Ph.D. Department of Nuclear Medicine, University Hospital Dijkzigt and Erasmus University Rotterdam, 3015 GD Rotterdam, The Netherlands

Shankar Vallabhajosula, Ph.D. Director of Research, Division of Nuclear Medicine, The New York Presbyterian Hospital—Weill Cornell Medical Center, New York, New York 10021

Irene J. Virgolini, M.D. Professor, Department of Experimental Nuclear Medicine and Internal Medicine, Director, Institute of Nuclear Medicine, Lainz Hospital of the City of Vienna, A-1130 Vienna, Austria

Theo J. Visser, Ph.D. Department of Internal Medicine, Erasmus Medical Center Rotterdam, 3015 GD Rotterdam, The Netherlands

Richard L. Wahl, M.D. Professor of Internal Medicine and Radiology Director, Division of General Nuclear Medicine University of Michigan 1500 East Medical Center Drive Ann Arbor, Michigan 48109

Alan D. Waxman, M.D. Clinical Professor of Radiology, University of Southern California School of Medicine, Co-Chair, Department of Imaging, Director of Nuclear Medicine, Cedars-Sinai Medical Center, Los Angeles, California 90048

Sydney Welt, M.D. Nuclear Medicine Service, Memorial Sloan-Kettering Cancer Center, New York, New York 10021

Franklin C. L. Wong, M.D., Ph.D., J.D. Associate Professor, Department of Nuclear Medicine, University of Texas M.D. Anderson Cancer Center, Houston, Texas 77030

Jeffrey Y.C. Wong, M.D. Chair, Division of Radiation Oncology, City of Hope National Medical Center, Duarte, California 91010

Lionel S. Zuckier, M.D. Associate Professor, Departments of Nuclear Medicine and Radiology, Albert Einstein College of Medicine; Attending Physician, Department of Nuclear Medicine, Jacobi Hospital, Bronx, New York 10461

FOREWORD

Nuclear oncology came of age, cheek by jowl, with medical oncology. Surgery and radiation oncology, which had pre-existed, dealt primarily with local and regional disease. The demonstration that a few disseminated cancers and some instances of micrometastatic disease could be curable by chemotherapy, evidenced by the change in survival rates of patients with choriocarcinoma, acute lymphocytic leukemia, or osteosarcoma, opened a new horizon. More recently breast, colon, and some lung cancers, all of which can show augmented survival rates with adjuvant chemotherapy, broadened this new era. Thus, the need to search for micrometastatic, minimetastatic, and macrometastatic disease became more pressing. Advances in imaging techniques, notably computerized tomography and magnetic resonance imaging, dominated the discovery of minimetastatic and macrometastatic disease. Precise anatomic staging of cancers using these new modalities produced stage migration analogous to what has been called the "Will Rogers effect." This great American humorist stated that in the great drought of the 1930s, when the Oklahoma dust bowl farmers migrated to California, they improved the intellect of both states. Similarly the survival of true stage 1 patients was improved by exclusion of metastatic disease, discoverable only by these new techniques, as was the survival of patients with metastatic disease, now including cases with hitherto undiscovered minimetastases.

Nuclear oncology has made unique and major strides in functional imaging, an approach clearly able to visualize not only macro- and minimetastatic disease, but in some instances, micrometastatic disease. Bone scans are indispensable for staging neoplasms that frequently metastasize to bone: carcinomas of the breast, lung, prostate, kidney, and thyroid. Although other abnormalities of osseous tissue can also give rise to increased osteoblastic activity on bone scan, requiring differential diagnosis, metastatic disease below the threshold of detection by conventional radiology can readily be indicated by this nuclear oncologic test.

The clever use of metabolic characteristics of tumors, including their nearly universal increased metabolism of glucose, have made radioisotopic fluorinated deoxyglucose (FDG) and positron emission tomography (PET) major new branches of nuclear oncology. Small opacities in pulmonary roentgenograms, indefinite by computerized tomography and poorly visualized by magnetic resonance, may be characteristic on PET scanning, both in the sensitivity and specificity of diagnosing malignant or benign lesions. Furthermore, the ability of computerized tomography to diagnose lymph node metastasis, based entirely on abnormal enlargement, can be substantially improved by the metabolic characteristics of tumor cells in lymph nodes visualized by FDG and PET scanning. Many tumor entities remain to be characterized in prospective studies of this important technique. Using radioactive nitrogen compounds or radiofluorine-substituted amino acids and nucleosides, other quantitative metabolic differences from normal tissues can confidently be anticipated, with additional functional nuclear oncologic applications.

Qualitative differences between cancer cells and normal cells, the Holy Grail of decades of cancer research, have now been described. Oncogenes, if not dichotomizing cancer cells from normal cells absolutely, may nonetheless be present in cancer cells and not in any other normal cells of the adult individual. Some oncogenes are receptor proteins; their ligands, when properly tagged, could localize tumors. Other oncogenes impart epitopes to the cancer cell to which monoclonal antibodies are already raised and labeled to detect tumor sites. Mutated p53 is present in nearly half of all cancers, and the FHIT gene and its unique protein product are even more common in cancers. Telomerase is an enzyme present in nearly every neoplastic cell, and in only a few stem cells. These several qualitatively unique molecules offer attractive targets for imaging.

The vast amount of information that recognizes neoangiogenesis as an essential characteristic of malignant neoplasia has not been fully incorporated into nuclear oncology. The permeability of these new vessels can be increased by vascular endothelial growth factor (VEGF), also previously known as vascular permeability factor. Such augmentative techniques to increase antibody or ligand access to tumors have not been fully exploited. Use of labeled small molecular fragments of antibodies is a step in the right direction. In addition, antibodies against VEGF receptors might visualize characteristic neovasculature at the stage of micrometastatic disease. Similarly, reticuloendothelial blockade with macromolecules, such as aggregated albumin or particulate carbon, might improve tumor imaging by decreasing background.

Functional nuclear oncology, as distinct from anatomic nuclear oncology, has two vast arenas in which it can change the practice of all the other oncologic specialties. Real-time functional change visualized by altered metabolic pathways could predict early recognition of therapeutic sensitivity. Instead of waiting months or weeks after the initiation of hormones, chemotherapy, radiotherapy, or immunotherapy to determine if there had been anatomic regression, functional studies, perhaps within days or even hours of therapy, might confirm sensitivity, or reveal insensitivity so that a more appropriate approach could be employed. Controlled trials are imperative and urgently needed. Secondly, increased specificity may carve a major role for nuclear oncology in the field of preventive oncology. Immunologists have been developing better antibodies with high specificity for molecular changes in the cells of carcinomas in situ. It is therefore not beyond imagination that mucosal changes in bronchi, pancreas, bladder, and endometrium, for example, could be visualized with sufficient specificity to decrease the need for highly invasive and less specific procedures. Such initiated cells might have biochemical characteristics of early cancer in common, so that a few reagents could cover the breadth of most aspects of the cancer process. Intervention at this stage might prevent cancer progression.

The purview of surgery and radiotherapy will likely change in the course of the evolving oncologic specialties.

Certain cancers will be cured without surgical intervention, and others where regional therapy once seemed fruitless will be encompassed in multimodality therapies where surgery and/or radiation will play indispensable roles. Since the real impediment to cancer cure is usually the metastatic process, nuclear oncology, in its exquisite sensitivity in bone and emerging sensitivity and specificity in other tissues, will be a central part of the imaging specialties. High sensitivity and high specificity are the sine qua non for therapeutic nuclear oncology, a promising universe outside the thyroid still to be realized.

Those who thought cancers were intrinsically incurable have suffered successive defeats with the advances in the therapy of choriocarcinoma, acute leukemia, Burkitt's lymphoma, Wilms' tumor, and embryonal rhabdomyosarcoma. Lesser, but nonetheless significant, increments in the survival of the common adult carcinomas, because of improvement in multimodality therapy, demonstrate that cures are possible, and that research pays off. Improvements in instrumentation, specificity of targeting, and characterization of tumor metabolism augur well for future therapeutic and preventive strategies by nuclear oncology. This book makes a seminal contribution to opening that future. The editors and authors deserve accolades for critical assessment of the present, and thoughtful speculation on what is yet to come.

James F. Holland, M.D.
Distinguished Professor of Neoplastic Diseases
Director Emeritus, Derald H. Ruttenberg Cancer Center
Mount Sinai Medical Center
New York, New York

FOREWORD

The editors of *Nuclear Oncology: Diagnosis and Therapy* have assembled an impressive group of authors to present information on this important topic. The main purpose of this text is to review the role of the radioactive tracer method in the diagnosis and management of patients with cancer. Following an overview, the main subjects in oncology are covered, both from a diagnostic and a therapeutic point of view. Up-to-date chapters cover the significant areas of practice, and there are some additional contributions describing lesser-known topics (such as the therapy of primary tumors of the liver, intraperitoneal radionuclide therapy, and multidrug resistance). Perhaps not surprisingly, chapters vary significantly in length, and some indeed present a very comprehensive review of their topic.

There is, no doubt, something for everyone in this textbook. Physicians, therapists, radiologists, and nuclear medicine practitioners will all find something relevant to their practice. This is a useful and up-to-date reference text that addresses nuclear medicine in pediatric oncology and the effects of cancer therapy in regard to cardiac and renal function. I am pleased to see that not only is the more advanced technology appropriately described (e.g., PET, SPECT, labeled peptides, and MoABs), but also that the authors found it necessary to cover the renewed interest in lymphoscintigraphy and sentinel node technology. There are two good contributions describing this approach in breast cancer and melanoma.

The application of nuclear medicine in oncology is no doubt a growing and exciting area of endeavor. Rich pickings are to be made, and even the larger pharmaceutical industries have, of late, appreciated the potential and committed themselves to significant investments. This underlines the clear clinical impact of nuclear medicine practice in the diagnosis and treatment of patients with cancer. The challenge is to disseminate this growing field to those who are finally responsible for delivering health care in oncology. This book will have its contribution to make.

Peter Josef Ell, M.D., M.Sc., P.D., F.R.C.R., F.R.C.P.
Director, Institute of Nuclear Medicine
University College London
United Kingdom

PREFACE

Nuclear Oncology: Diagnosis and Therapy is intended to serve clinical nuclear medicine practitioners, and physicians such as oncologists and radiologists, in understanding the utility and practice of nuclear procedures in oncology. It also serves as an introduction and guide for residents in any of these specialties, introducing them to the practice of nuclear oncology and providing a basis for the understanding of future developments as they evolve into clinically useful procedures.

The editors conceived this text as an up-to-date compilation of the current practice of nuclear oncology; that is, of the role of nuclear medicine in the diagnosis, management, and therapy of patients with tumors. This area of nuclear medicine has undergone profound changes in the past decade, and it was clear there was a need for a comprehensive text that balanced practical clinical insights with an assessment of the scientific literature on which clinical applications are based. Drs. Khalkhali, Maublant, and I were delighted when so many leading nuclear medicine physicians and scientists accepted our invitation to participate in this enterprise.

In the first part of the text, we provide overview chapters that review the current status of broad concepts and areas of nuclear oncology. This includes an instructive treatise on current instrumentation, and a remarkable, clear, and comprehensive chapter on radiopharmaceuticals in nuclear oncology by Shankar Vallabhajosula. This part features two sections on the phenomenon of multiple drug resistance assessed by nuclear imaging in breast carcinoma and other tumors. There is also a chapter on the factors that influence the choices investigators face in developing radiolabeled monoclonal antibodies for diagnosis and therapy. Leonard Connolly provides a comprehensive summary of pediatric nuclear oncology. This part ends with chapters on radiopharmaceutical therapy of painful bone metastases and an introduction to understanding the impact of chemotherapy on cardiac and renal functions.

In the second part, there is an organ-system-by-organ-system review of the traditional nuclear medicine techniques: positron emission tomography, monoclonal antibody, and peptide imaging and therapy of tumors affecting these systems. These are compared with traditional imaging and therapy methods. All of the subjects are presented with authority and firsthand knowledge by experienced nuclear medicine practitioners.

Some chapters are so remarkably comprehensive that they could stand alone as monographs; in particular, Chapter 10 on PET imaging of central nervous system tumors by Peter Conti; Chapter 14 on parathyroid scintigraphy by Raymond Taillefer; Chapter 28 on monoclonal antibody therapy of lymphoma and Hodgkin's disease by Richard Wahl; and Chapter 36 presenting the Rotterdam group's update on neuroendocrine tumor scintigraphy. Claudia Berman and Norman Brodsky's remarkable reviews of lymphoscintigraphy of the breast and melanomas provide the nuclear medicine community with a comprehensive survey of all of the medical science involved in assessing nodal involvement of these tumors. The chapter on scintigraphy of osseous metastases by Leonard Freeman and his young colleague is an example of a master teacher at work, presenting well-established observations in an organized format. My co-editor, Iraj Khalkhali, and his co-author, John Buscombe, provide a similar masterful approach to scintimammography. On a personal note, I am grateful to have had the opportunity to review the role of nuclear medicine in thyroid carcinoma management, a subject that has fascinated me for more than 30 years.

In planning *Nuclear Oncology,* the editors intended that it would present the practice of nuclear oncology, rather than just a review of the literature compiled during the past 10 to 20 years. Initially, we invited authors to describe technical details and to compare the utility of nuclear medicine techniques with the results obtained with traditional imaging or therapeutic methods. To a great degree, these expectations have been met. The pace of development and transition from the laboratory to the clinic of both radionuclide imaging and therapy has accelerated so much that any text describing nuclear oncology practice has faced the possibility that procedures that had been available only to research centers might transition into routine practice as the result of the completion of a pivotal trial. Thus, there could be serious omissions in the description of current practice. Accordingly, despite the emphasis on the practical, the editors expanded the scope of the text to include descriptions of innovative investigations that appear poised to transition to clinical practice. In doing so, we hope that the utility of the text as a description of the clinical practice of nuclear oncology has been extended.

Stanley J. Goldsmith, M.D., Ph.D.

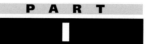

PART

I

OVERVIEW

NUCLEAR ONCOLOGY IMAGING AND THERAPY: AN OVERVIEW

STANLEY J. GOLDSMITH

Despite advances in medical science throughout the 20th century, the incidence and mortality of cancer continue to increase throughout the world. In developed countries, cancer is the second leading cause of death. During the past several decades, remarkable insight into the cell and the molecular biology of malignancy has been acquired. Nevertheless, changes in the geographic distribution of tumor types and the incidence of various tumors remain largely unexplained. Some of these changes appear to be related to environmental factors. A disease like non-small cell lung carcinoma is now the most common malignant tumor in both men and women in the United States and throughout Europe, whereas formerly it was uncommon among women. This change is probably related to increased cigarette smoking among women in the later half of the century. Other apparent increases in the incidence of particular tumors may be related to earlier detection and other improvements in medical care. Cancer is now identified in people who formerly might have died of other causes before detection. Malignancies such as breast or prostate carcinoma are currently detected at an earlier stage as a result of mammography to screen for breast cancer and determination of serum prostate-specific antigen to screen for prostate cancer. These changes in the frequency and stage of presentation of tumors present challenges and opportunities for nuclear oncology.

IMPACT OF ADVANCES IN NUCLEAR ONCOLOGY

Nuclear oncology, the application of nuclear medicine to the study and management of patients with malignant disease, has progressed with increases in the understanding of neoplastic disease. Newly acquired information has led

S. J. Goldsmith: Departments of Radiology and Medicine, Weill Medical College of Cornell University; Department of Nuclear Medicine, New York Presbyterian Hospital—Weill Cornell Medical Center, New York, New York 10021.

to better diagnostic and therapeutic uses of nuclear medicine, as has the greater availability of tracers to identify special or unique features of malignant tissue and instrumentation to detect tracers with ever improving sensitivity and accuracy. Many advances in nuclear medicine have evolved from efforts or quests to improve the management of a particular type of tumor-related problem. For example, in the era before computed tomography (CT) and magnetic resonance imaging (MRI), when even contrast angiography was not yet fully developed, neurosurgeons sought help in defining the extent of brain tumors. This problem was challenging even when a tumor had been localized clinically. Although tumors were exposed at surgery, the precise extent of involvement remained unknown. Given the special function of the brain, excision of a wider volume than necessary carried a big price in terms of permanent neurologic deficit and associated morbidity. Initially, fluorescent dyes were used that could be seen under ultraviolet light. This technique provided some guidance; direct visualization of fluorescence at the operating table was based on increased tumor vascularity and leakage of dye into the extracellular fluid of the tumor. It was soon appreciated that a radiolabeled dye and hand-held probe might provide a more sensitive method to estimate the extent of tumor involvement. Use of the probe permitted evaluation through the intact skull. It was not long before a multiprobe "helmut" device was developed that allowed spatial "visualization" of the distribution of the radiolabeled indicator, a short step from imaging (1) (Fig. 1.1). Initially, fluorescein labeled with radioactive iodine (^{131}I) was used. This was replaced by human serum albumin (hSA) labeled with ^{131}I, then chlormeridrin (a mercurial diuretic) labeled with radioactive mercury (^{203}Hg, ^{197}Hg), and subsequently ^{99m}Tc-pertechnetate in the late 1960s and ^{99m}Tc-DTPA (diethylenetriamine pentaacetic acid) in the 1970s, up to the introduction of CT (2). The use of all these compounds was based on the vascularity of tumor tissue in comparison with white matter, and on the characteristics of tumor

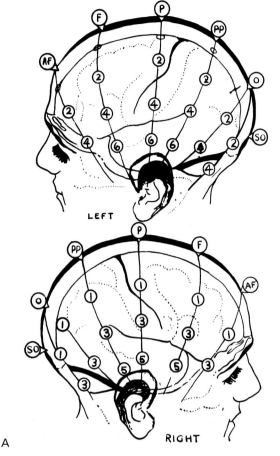

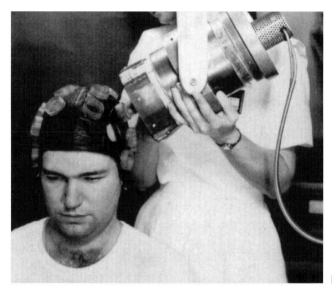

FIGURE 1.1. Early detection of brain tumors with radiopharmaceuticals. A diagram is used to designate the positions of standard electroencephalography ports, with holes to facilitate positioning of a collimated sodium iodide crystal—photomultiplier tube assembly. Twenty-four hours after intravenous injection of 150 to 250 µCi of human serum albumin tagged with ^{131}I, each site is counted individually. A minimum of 1,000 counts is obtained, expressed as counts per minute, and compared with the value obtained over the contralateral side. An increase of 20% or more is considered a positive result, although it is recognized that differences may be smaller in patients with deep or slow-growing tumors (From Blahd WH, Bauer FK, Cassen BF. Tumor localizing procedures. In: *The practice of nuclear medicine*. Philadelphia: Charles C Thomas Publisher, 1958:85–115, with permission.)

vasculature, which does not exclude tracers from the tumor, unlike normal brain vasculature and the blood–brain barrier, which exclude many substances from interstitial spaces in the brain. In addition, the increased extracellular fluid content of tumors resulted in the prolonged retention of tracer in the tumor.

These findings, initially observed more than 40 years ago with early nuclear tracers and instrumentation, are the basis for contemporary techniques of tumor visualization with contrast CT and MRI. Although CT and MRI provide a more exact anatomic definition and hence frequently make possible earlier detection and a better differential diagnosis in patients with symptoms suggestive of brain tumor, the problem of precise delineation between

malignant tumor and normal tissue remains. Currently, positron emission tomography (PET) with ^{18}F-fluorodeoxyglucose (FDG) provides a means to identify tumor in patients with progressive symptoms following surgery or radiation therapy. In these cases, the normal brain architecture is so disrupted that CT and MRI are unable to differentiate between recurrent tumor and scar or radiation necrosis. Recurrent tumor usually develops at the margin of the surgical resection or radiotherapy field. As tumor-specific tracers improve, along with our understanding of guided radionuclide therapy, combined therapeutic approaches will be developed; debulking of tumor by surgery or external radiotherapy will be followed by the administration of adjuvant radiolabeled tumor-seeking compounds, so that additional therapy can be delivered with precision to microscopic foci of residual tumor.

IMPACT OF ADVANCES IN CLINICAL ONCOLOGY

As the frequency and presentation of tumors have changed during the past 30 years, so have the type and role of nuclear medicine procedures. These changes are exemplified by the current presentation of prostate and breast carcinoma.

Prostate Carcinoma

Before the measurement of serum prostate-specific antigen (PSA) was developed and became widely available, prostate carcinoma was often discovered as an incidental finding in tissue removed during treatment for benign prostatic hypertrophy, during rectal examination in patients with more advanced disease, or late in the course of disease, when symptoms of metastases developed. Seventy percent to ninety percent of patients with advanced disease have bone metastases. The bone scan, performed for the past 30 years with ^{99m}Tc phosphate or ^{99m}Tc phosphonate compounds, was used to detect skeletal metastases, and bone scanning became common in the management of patients with prostate carcinoma. Presently, with widespread availability of serum PSA measurement, prostate carcinoma is detected and treated earlier. In many instances, the initial therapy is curative. Unsuspected metastases are found less frequently. Moreover, because the level of PSA correlates with tumor burden, bone scintigraphy is no longer performed in asymptomatic patients with serum PSA values below 10 ng/mL because the procedure has such a low yield in these circumstances. Although bone scintigraphy remains useful in patients with elevated PSA to confirm osseous involvement, the number of bone scans performed to monitor patients with prostate carcinoma has decreased. Other techniques are being evaluated to identify soft-tissue involvement not specifically detected by CT or MRI. A radiolabeled antibody, ProstaScint (Cytogen) is available to detect soft-tissue metastases (see Chapter 31). Various PET tracers are being evaluated for their utility in determining the extent of disease or other biologic features of this tumor. Beta-emitting bone-seeking radionuclides, such as ^{89}Sr diphosphonate and ^{153}Sm diphosphonate, are being used in the management of painful bone metastases (see Chapter 6). Because advanced prostate carcinoma is frequently unresponsive to available forms of chemotherapy, a number of strategies are being evaluated to deliver targeted radionuclide therapy with monoclonal antibodies or other high-affinity ligands (see Chapters 32 and 24).

Breast Carcinoma

The type and use of nuclear medicine procedures in the management of patients with breast carcinoma have also undergone considerable evolution. In the early 1970s, when the ^{99m}Tc phosphates and subsequently ^{99m}Tc phosphonates were introduced, bone scintigraphy to detect and monitor bone metastases became commonplace in oncology in general and in the management of patients with breast cancer in particular despite the sometimes nonspecific nature of increased bone turnover detected with this procedure (see Chapter 40). In the mid-1980s, whole-body ^{18}F-FDG imaging was introduced. This procedure is more specific than bone scintigraphy in determining whether focal areas of increased bone turnover are secondary to degenerative changes or to metastatic tumor (3) (Fig. 1.2). Although this technique is still not yet widely available, commercial distribution of ^{18}F-FDG with a 2-hour half-life is a reality in and near many urban centers, and coincident imaging devices are more widely available. FDG imaging to detect metastases in patients with breast carcinoma or other tumors is likely to be performed more frequently in clinical oncology practice. Direct imaging of breast carcinoma with the single-photon emitter ^{99m}Tc-MIBI (methoxyisobutylisonitrile), an agent introduced to assess myocardial perfusion, is now performed to assess dense breasts that are not evaluated thoroughly with mammography. In some centers, the technique is being applied to detect nonpalpable tumors and to provide differential diagnostic information for tumors identified by palpation or mammography (see Chapter 18).

During the past few years, radionuclide lymphoscintigraphy and identification of the sentinel lymph node have become a significant component of the management of patients with breast carcinoma (see Chapter 20). When a small amount of ^{99m}Tc-labeled colloid is injected interstitially, lymphatic drainage from the involved breast to specific lymph nodes can be identified. The sentinel node concept was developed earlier, in the management of patients with malignant melanoma. With identification and removal of the sentinel node, rather than the entire regional lymph node complex, more effort and resources can be applied to examination of the sentinel node. Currently, this procedure is believed to be the most sensitive and accurate means to detect or exclude lymphatic spread of tumor. In addition to its current widespread use in the surgical management of patients with melanoma and breast carcinoma, lymphoscintigraphy is used to assess lymph node involvement in melanoma (see Chapter 41) and is being evaluated in other malignant tumors.

A positron-emitting radiolabeled estrogen, ^{18}F-estradiol, has been demonstrated to identify estrogen receptors in breast carcinoma (4) (Fig. 1.3). Although this technique has been used only in a research setting to date, it has the

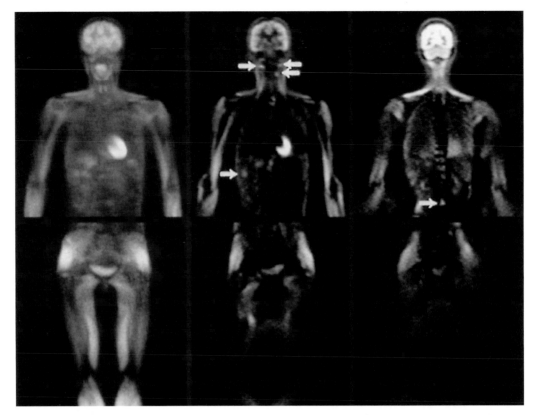

FIGURE 1.2. Imaging with ^{18}F-fluorodeoxyglucose in 1991. Whole-body coronal and volume display in a 42-year-old woman with the diagnosis of breast carcinoma. At the time of the study, no evidence of hepatic involvement had been noted, nor was it suspected clinically. Coronal slices reveal cervical lymph node involvement, focal hepatic metastases, and a lumbar spine lesion. (From Hoh CK, Hawkins RA, Dahlbom M, et al. Two-dimensional FDG total body distribution. *J Nucl Med* 1991;32:578, with permission.)

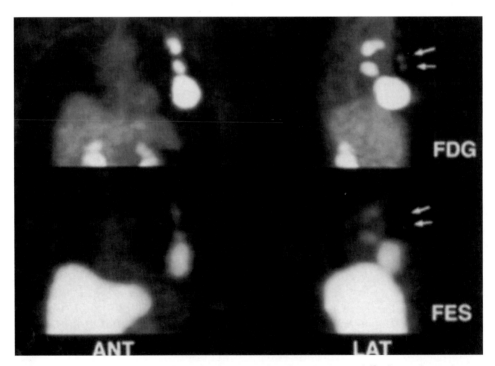

FIGURE 1.3. Anterior and left lateral volume rendered projections of ^{18}F-fluorodeoxyglucose and ^{18}F-fluoroestradiol from a patient with locally advanced breast cancer. Concordant tracer localization is demonstrated in an estrogen receptor-positive tumor in the primary left breast mass and in left axillary lymph node and internal mammary lymph node (*arrows*) metastases. (From Dehdashti F, Mortimer JE, Siegel BA, et al. Positron tomographic assessment of estrogen receptor in breast cancer: comparison with FDG-PET and *in vitro* receptor assays. *J Nucl Med* 1995;36:1766–1774, with permission.)

potential to provide important information about tumor biology that is valuable in guiding patient therapy.

TRACER PRINCIPLE

In nuclear medicine, radioactive elements in compounds that localize in tissues and organs are used to diagnose and treat disease and to evaluate the response to therapy. The use of radioactive material is based on the tracer principle, which is that radioactive forms of an element can be substituted for their naturally occurring counterparts in compounds without affecting the underlying processes in which the compounds are involved. Hence, depending on the type of emission from the radionuclide incorporated into a compound, the labeled compound can be used either to trace the distribution of the naturally occurring material (kinetics, biodistribution, diagnostic imaging) or to deliver a therapeutic dose of radioactivity (targeted radiotherapy). Nuclear medicine procedures have played a significant role in the diagnosis and treatment of patients with tumors since the earliest development of the specialty. Indeed, many of the advances in nuclear medicine

in general have arisen from efforts to improve the detection or treatment of tumors.

RADIOPHARMACEUTICALS
Diagnostic Imaging

Because the tracer principle is inherent in nuclear medicine procedures, it follows that these procedures can provide a noninvasive means to monitor physiologic and biochemical processes and potentially detect aberrations therein at the time of initial diagnosis and during follow-up, before anatomic changes develop (Fig. 1.4). Hence, nuclear imaging with radiolabeled peptide ligands, monoclonal antibodies, or ^{18}F-FDG identifies tumor foci in organs and lymph nodes that are not apparent on anatomic imaging with CT or MRI in lung, breast, colorectal, or ovarian carcinomas and in neuroendocrine tumors (Fig. 1.5).

The use of radionuclides or labeled compounds as tracers to identify and characterize tumors depends on the differential localization of the tracer within and around them. Accordingly, it would seem that selection of a tracer is based on a recognition that the tumor is different from

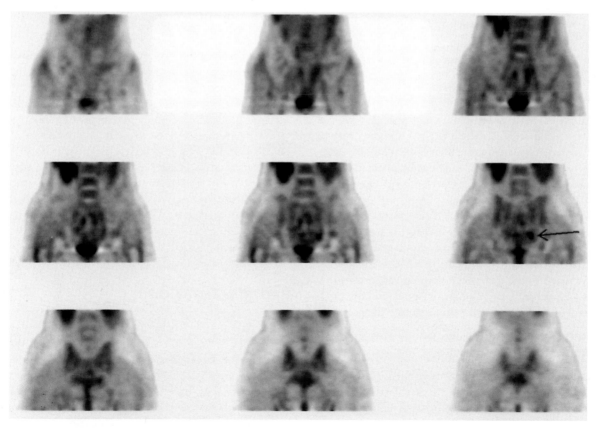

FIGURE 1.4. Coronal images of the pelvis of a 46-year-old woman with a history of ovarian carcinoma resected 2 years earlier demonstrate small foci of increased uptake of ^{18}F-fluorodeoxyglucose (*FDG*) in an area that appeared normal on computed tomography. Prior ^{18}F-FDG images of this area had been negative.

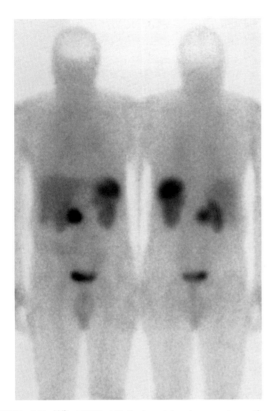

FIGURE 1.5. ^{111}In-DTPA (diethylenetriamine pentaacetic acid) pentetreotide (Octreoscan) whole-body planar images at 4 hours identify a primary bowel carcinoid in a 73-year-old man who had recently undergone a thoracotomy to remove a mediastinal mass subsequently found to be carcinoid. The abdominal mass had not been detected during preoperative evaluation with computed tomography.

surrounding tissue. In some cases, this insight has evolved from advances in tumor biology, such as the discovery of unique (or relatively unique) surface markers, like carcinoembryonic antigen (CEA), to the subsequent development, over many years, of radiolabeled monoclonal antibodies for tumor localization. One such product, CEA-Scan (Immunomedics), a ^{99m}Tc-labeled Fab′ fragment of a monoclonal antibody to CEA, has been used to stage patients with colon carcinoma with a greater overall accuracy than that of CT (see Chapter 24). It is currently being evaluated in the identification of other CEA-bearing tumors, such as breast carcinoma, non-small cell lung carcinoma, and medullary thyroid carcinoma (see Chapter 15).

Response to Therapy

Nuclear imaging procedures can be used to confirm restoration of normal physiology during or after treatment before the resolution of altered anatomy because radiotracers are indicators of tissue physiology and biochemistry. Scintigraphy with ^{67}Ga (see Chapter 36) and more recently ^{18}F-FDG (see Chapter 37) demonstrates the presence or absence of tumor activity in enlarged lymph nodes or frank tumor masses, although the enlarged node or mass may not disappear on anatomic imaging even after successful therapy. Finally, the procedures can be used to differentiate between recurrent disease and alterations that occur as a consequence of therapy. Following excision or radiotherapy of a brain tumor, it is difficult, if not impossible, to distinguish with anatomic imaging (CT or MRI) between altered anatomic features and associated tissue edema on the one hand and tumor recurrence on the other. ^{18}F-FDG imaging identifies highly metabolic tumor foci despite disruption of the normal anatomy.

Radionuclide Therapy

The knowledge and skill involved in the preparation of radiolabeled molecules that localize in tumor can be used to design agents intended to deliver a therapeutic dose of radiation. Radioablation of tissue depends on the delivery of emitted charged particles (conversion or Auger electrons, beta or alpha particles) that deposit radiation in tissue, whereas imaging utilizes gamma emissions, x-rays, or photons produced during positron annihilation. These forms of radiation penetrate tissue with little deposition of energy and are recorded externally. Nevertheless, during the development and monitoring of therapeutic radiolabeled compounds, it is necessary to track their distribution and turnover. Some radionuclides, such as ^{131}I, ^{153}Sm, and ^{186}Re, decay with the emission of useful beta particles in addition to gamma photons. In these instances, the radionuclide can be used both as a therapeutic agent and as a means to evaluate the biodistribution and effective half-life of the proposed or actual therapeutic dose. Other therapeutic applications employ pure beta emitters, such as ^{90}Y and ^{89}Sr. In these instances, other isotopes of the element, such as ^{86}Y and ^{85}Sr, respectively, or proxy isotopes, such as ^{111}In, are used to assess the biodistribution and pharmacokinetics of the labeled compounds. Differences in physical decay alter the use and role of a radiolabeled compound but do not influence its biodistribution. Nuclear oncology depends on an awareness of these variables and their utilization for the benefit of patients with malignant tumors.

INSTRUMENTATION

The application of nuclear medicine to oncology during the past 30 to 50 years has depended on advances in the development of radiopharmaceuticals (see Chapter 2) and instrumentation (see Chapter 4). Initially, it might appear that far greater changes have occurred in radiopharmaceuticals. Although these have been significant, many of the successes would not have been realized without concomitant advances in instrumentation. Thirty-five years ago, the development of the ^{99m}Tc generator marked a milestone in nuclear medicine and nuclear oncology. However, the nearly concomitant development of the gamma camera by Hal Anger made possible the numerous successful applications that depend on the exquisite resolution of high-count static images and rapid sequential images of an entire field of view. Whole-body scanning, dual-detector devices. and single-photon emission tomography (SPECT) represent further developments without which current advances in nuclear oncology could not have been realized. SPECT imaging of ^{67}Ga and the newer radiolabeled peptides and antibodies has a greater sensitivity and overall accuracy than planar imaging of the same radiopharmaceuticals.

Coincident Imaging

Although glucose metabolism is not unique to tumors, the recognition that glycolytic metabolism is increased in many tumors in comparison with surrounding tissues provides a basis for the use of ^{18}F-FDG as a tracer to identify tumor. The success of ^{18}F-FDG imaging is related not only to the biologic qualities of the tracer but also to its physical qualities. Because ^{18}F decays by positron emission, resulting in the production of two 511-keV photons with pathways 180 degrees in opposition, it provides a signal that is inherently tomographic and capable of being localized in a three-dimensional volume without collimation in coincident imaging. This feature, combined with a high rate of photon flux resulting from a short half-life and the lack of collimation, allows images to be produced that are usually of high quality, so that tumors can be detected and images interpreted with greater certainty and confidence.

Coincident imaging with positron-emitting radiotracers (positron emission tomography, or PET) represents a tremendous contribution of electronics and instrumentation to the needs of the nuclear medicine community to optimize imaging and quantification of radionuclide distribution. Even after the development of PET, the upgrade of computer processing and display capability to provide coronal and sagittal tomographic slices, in addition to whole-body imaging with a display of contiguous segments "knitted" or "zippered" together, has contributed significantly to the success of PET in clinical nuclear oncology (Fig. 1.2). Fusion imaging, the superimposition of two types of images, either complementary radionuclide distribution or a nuclear medicine tomographic image superimposed on a corresponding slice from an anatomic imaging study (Figs. 1.6 and 1.7, see also Color Plates 1 and 2 following p. 350), is likely to be the next contribution of instrumentation to the practice of nuclear oncology.

TUMOR-TO-BACKGROUND CONTRAST
Detection

The ability to detect tumor depends on achieving tracer contrast between tumor and normal tissue. Such contrast may in turn depend on the tumor being more metabolically active than the surrounding tissue, as when ^{18}F-FDG is used as a tracer. Nevertheless, this is a rather nonspecific mechanism that works well for the purpose of identifying tumor in a suspect population. Although the sensitivity of this tracer for the detection of tumor is likely to remain high because so many tumors are hypermetabolic, other hypermetabolic lesions will also be identified, particularly as the technique is applied more broadly. Hence, the specificity of ^{18}F-FDG imaging for tumor detection is likely to decrease from the values reported currently in selected populations. Positron-emitting radiolabeled amino acids and nucleotides demonstrate differences in protein synthesis and RNA turnover. These tracers may be more specific for tumor identification than ^{18}F-FDG, but their clinical use will depend on the demonstration that these metabolic mechanisms offer an advantage in characterizing clinically meaningful features of neoplastic disease (i.e., detection of tumors and identification of changes following therapy).

Contrast between tumor and normal or treated tissue may be a result of unique or relatively unique markers or mechanisms, such as an increase in surface receptors, detected with OctreoScan (Mallinckrodt), Neotec (Diatide), and MIBG (metaiodobenzylguanidine); an increase in surface or exposed epitopes, detected with ProstaScint (Cytogen) and CEA-Scan (Immunomedics); or increase in intracellular binding of a diffused or nonspecifically transported tracer, such as ^{99m}Tc-MIBI (Miraluma) or ^{67}Ga citrate (see Chapter 2). ^{67}Ga has been shown to enter tumor cells by two different mechanisms. In lymphoma and hepatoma, cellular uptake is mediated by transferrin receptors. In other tumors, it has been demonstrated that Ga species dissociate from the circulating Ga-transferrin complex in a reduced pH environment. Intracellular pH is reduced in tumors with increased anaerobic metabolism. The dissociated Ga freely diffuses into the cell and binds to intracellular components.

Therapy

Differentiated thyroid tumors trap and organify iodide (thus increasing the intracellular retention time). This relatively unique mechanism of delivery and localization accounts for the use of ^{131}I to identify and treat (ablate) thyroid remnants left after thyroidectomy and metastatic lesions of differentiated thyroid carcinoma.

The use of a radioactive form of an essential component of specialized tissue for diagnosis and therapy is mimicked to a certain extent by the the use of bone-seeking radionuclides that localize at the tumor–bone interface to deliver targeted radiotherapy. When ligands are used to deliver radionuclides, the ligand and its biology influence the contrast achieved and the choice of tracer. Internalization of the ligand may lead to hydrolysis of the tracer. In targeted radionuclide therapy, these conditions favor a nonsoluble tracer, such as a radiometal, rather than a soluble tracer.

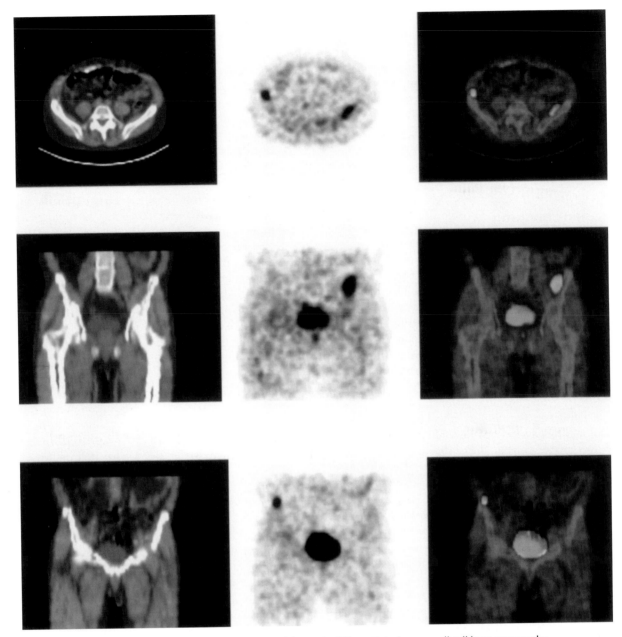

FIGURE 1.6. In this 51-year-old patient with poorly differentiated non-small cell lung cancer who had previously undergone chemotherapy and radiotherapy, computed tomography of the chest detected a new lesion in the lower lobe of the left lung. The patient was referred for an ^{18}F-flu-orodeoxygluclose (*FDG*) coincidence study for restaging. Transmission and emission tomographic images (first and second columns) are displayed. The third column represents "fusion" images of the simultaneously displayed first and second columns. On the ^{18}F-FDG images, two areas of abnormal uptake are apparent, one on either side of the pelvis. The combined image localizes one area in the right ilium. This finding was confirmed on bone scintigraphy. The other area of increased uptake is localized in the soft tissues adjacent to the left ilium. Magnetic resonance imaging confirmed the presence of a mass in the left iliac muscle. (See also Color Plate 1 following p. 350.) (Images courtesy of Dr. Ora Israel, Rambam Medical Center, Haifa, Israel.)

Targeted radiation therapy is achieved by increasing the administered dose of the radiolabeled compound that is used diagnostically (as in the treatment of thyroid carcinoma) or by replacing the diagnostic gamma-emitting radionuclide with one that is more suitable for therapy; for example, ^{153}Sm or ^{186}Re is substituted as a therapeutic bone-seeking agent in place of the diagnostic tracer, ^{99m}Tc diphosphonate. This usually means replacing a gamma-emitting radionuclide with a beta emitter. In the case of ^{111}In-labeled compounds, it is necessary to decide whether the Auger electron emission of ^{111}In is more or less suitable for therapeutic purposes that the beta emission of ^{90}Y.

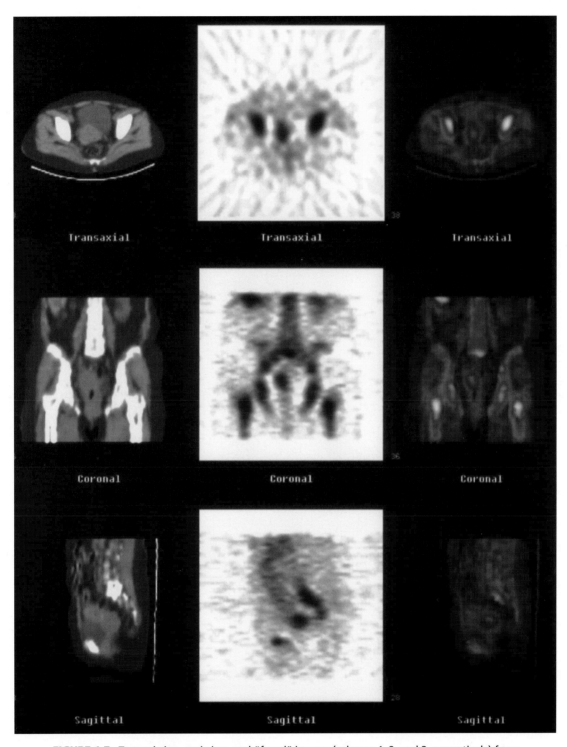

FIGURE 1.7. Transmission, emission, and "fused" images (columns 1, 2, and 3, respectively) from a patient who underwent ^{67}Ga scintigraphy after resection of the uterine cervix with the unexpected histopathologic finding of diffuse mixed large and small cell non-Hodgkin's lymphoma. Pelvic activity in residual tumor in the uterus is demonstrated to be distinct from bladder and rectal activity. It is likely that the ^{67}Ga activity in the pelvis would have been interpreted as physiologic without the improved anatomic localization available with fusion imaging. (See also Color Plate 2 following p. 350.) (Images courtesy of Dr. Ora Israel, Rambam Medical Center, Haifa, Israel.)

The relationship between the path length of the emitted radiation in tissue and the therapeutic response probably varies depending on tumor perfusion and other factors that influence microdosimetry. No consensus has been reached regarding the optimal physical characteristics of emitted radiation for therapy. Indeed, it is probably not possible to identify a single set of characteristics because the requirements change depending on the distribution of target sites and whether or not these sites are on the cell surface or internalized. The physical characteristics of the radiolabel affect the external detection of the radiolabeled therapeutic compound. External detection is necessary to quantify distribution and to provide dosimetry estimates of the radiation absorbed dose delivered to the tumor and surrounding tissue, in addition to the radiation absorbed dose delivered to other tissues that localize the radiolabeled compound.

CONCLUSIONS

The term *nuclear oncology* encompasses the numerous diagnostic (predominantly imaging) and therapeutic procedures used to assess and treat patients with known or suspected malignant disease. The current state of nuclear oncology rests on 50 years of development of the radiolabeled compounds in use today and on parallel timely advances in the equipment available to characterize the distribution of radioactive tracers. Future progress depends on further advances in radiation physics, radiochemistry, radiopharmacy, and radiopharmacology; on the availability of improved instruments to characterize the distribution of radiotracers; and on a better understanding of the interaction of radiation and biologic systems and the nature of the neoplastic process.

REFERENCES

1. Blahd WH, Bauer FK, Cassen BF. Tumor localizing procedures. In: Blahd, Bauer, and Larsen, eds: *The practice of nuclear medicine.* Philadelphia: Charles C Thomas Publisher, 1958:85–115.
2. Oldendorf WH. Detection of brain tumors using radioisotopes. *Bull Los Angeles Neurol Soc* 1967;32:220–233.
3. Hoh CK, Hawkins RA, Dahlbom M, et al. Two-dimensional FDG total body distribution. *J Nucl Med* 1991;32:578.
4. Dehdashti F, Mortimer JE, Siegel BA, et al. Positron tomographic assessment of estrogen receptor in breast cancer: comparison with FDG-PET and *in vitro* receptor assays. *J Nucl Med* 1995;36: 1766–1774.

2

INSTRUMENTATION

JONATHAN M. LINKS
HORACE H. HINES

Nuclear medicine is a vibrant and dynamic medical specialty because it combines advances in basic science, technology, and medical practice to solve patients' problems. The goal of clinical nuclear medicine imaging is to aid the physician in diagnosis, prognosis, treatment planning, and monitoring of response. These goals are particularly well suited to oncology. Nuclear medicine images must be of high diagnostic and quantitative accuracy, and they must provide cost-effective (i.e., conducive to reducing the total cost of patient management) solutions to clinical problems. Advances in nuclear medicine instrumentation should increase the diagnostic and quantitative accuracy of images and decrease study costs. To increase accuracy, advances in instrumentation must improve resolution and sensitivity, incorporate appropriate corrections for physical effects that reduce accuracy, and increase the ability to perform technically demanding studies (e.g., studies with dual radionuclides). To decrease study costs, advances in instrumentation must provide faster acquisitions, automated processing, and shorter interpretation times (and increased confidence in interpreting results). Acquisition, processing, and interpretation time affect clinical throughput, which ultimately is measured by the number of patients a center is able to study per day.

This chapter presents a review of recent advances in nuclear medicine instrumentation, with particular emphasis on emission computed tomography, including both single-photon emission computed tomography (SPECT) and positron emission tomography (PET). The chapter assumes some background in nuclear medicine and nuclear medicine instrumentation; for a general introduction to nuclear medicine instrumentation, the reader is referred to the classic text by Sorenson and Phelps (1).

FUNDAMENTALS OF ANGER SCINTILLATION CAMERAS

The Anger scintillation camera was invented by Hal Anger of the Donner Laboratory, University of California at Berkeley, in the late 1950s. The scintillation (or "gamma") camera is the most commonly used imaging instrument in nuclear medicine today. The complete camera system consists of a lead collimator; a 10- to 25-in circular, square, or rectangular sodium iodide scintillation crystal; an array of photomultiplier tubes on the crystal; a positioning logic network; a pulse height analyzer; and an image recording and display device, which is typically a computer system.

The collimator is typically a honeycomb array of holes, 0.5 to 2 in thick, with lead septa. It has the same dimensions as the scintillation crystal. The pinhole collimator, discussed below, is the exception to this general description. The collimator acts to select the photons emitted from the patient by allowing only those photons traveling in an appropriate direction to pass through the collimator holes. Photons passing through the holes are transmitted to the crystal, whereas those that encounter the septa are attenuated. Collimators thus discriminate based on direction of flight, and not on whether the photons have been scattered or not. Several types of collimators are used with Anger cameras: parallel hole, converging, diverging, and pinhole. Most collimators transmit only one of 10,000 photons emitted from the patient. The collimator is a major factor limiting the number of counts acquired in a nuclear medicine image.

The most commonly used collimator is the parallel hole type. It consists of an array of parallel holes that are perpendicular to the crystal face, and thus presents a real-size image to the crystal face. The spatial resolution of a parallel hole collimator is best at the collimator surface and degrades approximately linearly as the collimator-to-source distance increases. However, the sensitivity (counts per unit of radioactivity) of the collimator is independent of the distance between the source and the collimator. The reason for this constant sensitivity is that the field of view of each hole increases with increasing distance. This means that each hole "sees" a larger area at a greater distance from the collimator. In other words, more holes see the same source farther from the collimator. As a radioactive source is moved away from the face of the collimator, the count rate through each hole decreases because of the inverse-square law. However, more and more holes "see" the source, and the total count rate remains constant. Because more holes "see" the

J.M. Links: Department of Environmental Sciences, Johns Hopkins School of Public Health, Baltimore, Maryland 21205.
H.H. Hines: ADAC Laboratories, Milpitas, California 95035.

source, the image is spread over a larger area of the crystal face (i.e., the image is progressively smeared or blurred). Thus, resolution decreases with increasing distance.

Converging, diverging, and pinhole collimators affect resolution and sensitivity by geometrically changing the size of the image presented to the detector as the collimator-to-source distance is increased. Converging collimators have an array of tapered holes that aim at a point at some distance in front of the collimator; this point is called the *focal point*. The image that is presented to the crystal is a magnified version of the real object. The best resolution of converging collimators is at the surface of the collimator. The sensitivity of a converging collimator slowly increases as the source is moved from the collimator face back to the focal plane (the plane parallel to the collimator face that passes through the focal point), and then decreases. The trade-off for this increasing sensitivity is a decreasing field of view.

Diverging collimators are essentially upside-down converging collimators. They have an array of tapered holes that diverge from a hypothetical focal point behind the crystal. The image presented to the crystal face is a reduced image of the real object. The field of view of this collimator increases with collimator-to-source distance. Because converging and diverging collimators are simply flipped versions of each other, some collimators may have an insert that can be flipped either way, in effect producing two collimators in one. This combination collimator is sometimes called a *div/con collimator.*

Pinhole collimators are thick conical collimators with a single 2- to 5-mm hole at the apex of the cone (focal point). As a source is moved away from the focal point of a pinhole collimator, the camera image becomes smaller. Furthermore, the camera image is magnified (i.e., appears larger than the real size) when the source-to-focal point distance is less than the focal point-to-detector distance. The camera image is progressively reduced at larger distances. The sensitivity of a pinhole collimator decreases as one over the square of the distance between the source and the focal point.

Spatial resolution can be defined in terms of the amount by which a system blurs the image of a very small point source or a very thin line source of radioactivity. A profile of counts is generated along a line through the point source image (which is called the *point spread function*) or through the line source image (perpendicular to the line, which is called the *line spread function*), usually with computer-aided analysis. Resolution is quantified as the full-width at half-maximum (FWHM) of the point or line spread function and is generally expressed in millimeters. In practice, the FWHM in millimeters is nearly identical to the minimum distance by which two point sources must be separated in space to be distinguished as separate in an image. Sensitivity, on the other hand, is the overall ability of the system to detect the radioactive emissions from the source. The higher the sensitivity, the greater the fraction of emissions that is detected. In practical terms, a system with higher

sensitivity detects more x-rays or gamma rays when the same radioactive source is viewed. In practice, there is a trade-off between resolution and sensitivity.

Because of this trade-off, a collimator is not completely described by its geometric type (e.g., parallel hole, pinhole). For multihole collimators, sensitivity can be increased (at the expense of resolution) by increasing the diameter of each hole or shortening the length of the septa. This reduces the amount of lead in the path of the x-rays or gamma rays, so that a larger fraction can reach the crystal. Conversely, resolution can be improved by using many more, smaller holes or by making the collimator septa longer, thus increasing the hole length. This reduces the sensitivity because of a net increase in the amount of lead in the collimator. These relationships are illustrated in the following simplified equations for a parallel hole collimator:

$$\text{Resolution} = \text{Diameter}\left(\frac{\text{Length} + \text{Distance}}{\text{Length}}\right)$$

$$\text{Sensitivity} = \left(\frac{\text{Diameter}}{\text{Length}}\right)^2 \left(\frac{\text{Diameter}}{\text{Diameter} + \text{Thickness}}\right)^2$$

Here, *resolution* is the geometric resolution of the collimator (the smaller the number, the better), *diameter* is the diameter of each hole, *length* is the length of the septa, and *distance* is the distance between the face of the collimator and the patient or point in the organ of interest. Note that increasing the hole diameter or distance increases the resolution value (i.e., makes it worse), whereas increasing the hole length decreases the resolution value. *Sensitivity* is the geometric sensitivity of the collimator (the larger the number, the better), and *thickness* is septal thickness. Note that increasing the hole diameter increases the sensitivity value (i.e., makes it better), whereas increasing the septal thickness decreases the sensitivity value.

It is important to note that the geometric spatial resolution of a collimator is only one of several factors that influences the actual spatial resolution in an image. In planar imaging, intrinsic camera resolution, collimator resolution, scatter, and "patient resolution" effects caused by patient or organ movement all influence the actual resolution in the image. A simple way to estimate total resolution (R_T) from intrinsic (R_I), collimator (R_C), scatter (R_S), and patient (R_P) resolution is the following:

$$R_T = \sqrt{R_I^2 + R_C^2 + R_S^2 + R_P^2}$$

Note that the total resolution cannot be better (i.e., have a smaller value) than the largest term in the equation. Thus, changes in intrinsic resolution (e.g., < 1 mm) rarely, if ever, influence image resolution.

The crystal used in Anger cameras is a large flat plate of "thallium-activated" sodium iodide measuring from 7 to more than 25 in across. In the past, virtually all crystals had circular cross sections. Today, rectangular crystals are very popular, as these typically provide an increased field of view. Crystals are typically 1/4- to 1/2- in thick, with a 3/8-in thickness the most popular, although crystals up to 1 in thick are now emerging for coincidence imaging (as described below). As the crystal thickness increases, the probability that an incoming photon will interact by the photoelectric effect increases. This effect absorbs all the photon energy in the crystal, which permits the separation of primary and scattered photons (because in scatter only a portion of the photon's energy is absorbed). In practice, therefore, a thicker crystal increases the sensitivity of the camera. With increasing crystal thickness, however, the spatial resolution degrades. This is a consequence of the complex (geometric optics) interaction between the crystal, photomultiplier tubes, and the light pipe that is generally used to couple the two optically. The intrinsic resolution of crystals with a thickness of 1/4 in is about 1 mm better than that of crystals with a thickness of 1/2 in. When low-energy radionuclides such as thallium 201 are counted, no difference in sensitivity occurs. However, when technetium 99m is counted, the sensitivity of 1/4-in-thick crystals is 15% less than that of 1/2-in-thick crystals. At higher energies, the difference in sensitivity is even more significant. Crystals with a thickness of 3/8 to as much as 1 in are required to detect gamma rays above 200 keV efficiently (see below).

Anger cameras have an array of photomultiplier tubes optically coupled to the back of the scintillation crystal. The actual number of tubes depends on the size and shape of the crystal and each individual photomultiplier tube. For example, early cameras had 7 or 19 photomultiplier tubes. Today, it is common for cameras to have 37, 55, or 61 tubes. In general, the more photomultiplier tubes, the better the spatial resolution and linearity. Early photomultiplier tubes had a round cross section. Current tubes often have a hexagonal cross section to cover more of the crystal area for more efficient detection of scintillation photons. When a scintillation event occurs, each photomultiplier tube produces an output pulse. The amplitude of the pulse from a given photomultiplier tube is directly proportional to the amount of light (number of scintillation photons) its photocathode has received. Those photomultiplier tubes closest to the scintillation event produce the largest output pulses. By combining the pulses from each photomultiplier tube, a high-resolution x-, y-coordinate of the gamma ray location can be generated, based on a centroid or center-of-mass approach (often called *Anger positioning logic*).

In current, so-called digital cameras, the output of each photomultiplier tube is digitized with an analogue-to-digital converter. The resulting digital signals are then used with a software-based positioning algorithm. In many cases, this algorithm is simply a "digital version" of Anger positioning logic. In some cases, more sophisticated algorithms are used. This highlights the theoretical advantage of a digital camera, which is the ability to change and upgrade positioning algorithms more easily. It should be noted, however, that the term *digital camera* does not have a universally accepted definition, and different vendors use the term to denote digitization of the signals at different stages. Although it is tempting automatically to consider a digital camera superior to an analogue camera, in practice, the functional performance, flexibility, and reliability of a camera determine its value. Thus, excellent analogue and digital cameras both exist.

The desired goal of the Anger camera is to create an image that portrays the spatial distribution (i.e., positions and numbers of radioactive atoms) of radioactivity within the patient. If it is assumed that the collimator allows only those photons traveling in predetermined directions to interact in the crystal, a line may be drawn from the scintillation event in the crystal through the nearest collimator hole. This is presumed to intersect with the site of origin in the patient. If the photon has been scattered in the patient, a line drawn through its direction of flight will not intersect with its site of origin but will pass through the site of the Compton scattering interaction. Thus, photons scattered into the field of view can be falsely attributed to activity at the sites of Compton interactions in the patient. It is not desirable to have these scattered photons contribute to the final image because they can significantly degrade resolution and contrast. It is important to note that a large percentage of photons striking the crystal have been scattered in the patient. A pulse height analyzer is used to discriminate against these scattered photons, by analyzing the amount of energy deposited in the crystal by a detected photon. The pulse height analyzer is used to set a window around the photopeak(s). Because the window has a finite width, some scattered photons may still be accepted (i.e., those that are scattered through a small angle, and thus retain most of their energy). For example, 140-keV photons can scatter by as much as 55 degrees and still be accepted by the often-used 20% window.

FUNDAMENTALS OF SINGLE-PHOTON EMISSION COMPUTED TOMOGRAPHY

The term *single-photon emission computed tomography* is generally used today to refer to true transaxial tomography performed with standard nuclear medicine radiotracers (i.e., those that emit a single photon on decay, as opposed to positron emitters, with emissions that result in two coincident annihilation photons). SPECT is performed with either specialized ring detector systems or rotating Anger scintillation cameras. The ring systems consist of an array of individual detectors (usually sodium iodide crystals) that surround the patient. These systems, which produce excellent tomograms, tend to be very expensive and are limited in their ability to perform general nuclear medicine procedures. By far the most popular method of performing SPECT is with a rotating Anger camera (or multiple detectors; see below) mounted on a special gantry that allows 360-degree rotation around the patient.

The essence of emission transaxial tomography is similar to that of x-ray computed tomography (CT); two-dimensional (2D) images of an object are produced by combining data obtained from several different views of the object at a number of angles. The data are acquired at many angles, each representing one "projection" of the object. In general, a parallel hole collimator is used, and the projections therefore have "parallel beam geometry." In some cases, a "fan beam" collimator is used; this collimator has holes that converge in the plane of the slice but are parallel from slice to slice (2). In other cases, a "cone beam" collimator is used, in which the field of view converges in both dimensions (3). A well-designed parallel, fan, or cone beam collimator optimizes the trade-off between spatial resolution, field of view, and system sensitivity in SPECT (4). To reconstruct a 2D image or slice through an object, each projection needs to be only a 1D linear scan of the object. When an Anger camera is used for acquisition, 2D projection data are produced, allowing simultaneous acquisition of data for a number of contiguous transaxial slices. Note, however, that the data used to reconstruct a given slice come only from the corresponding projection data. The contiguous slices are combined into a 3D representation of the radionuclide. As in CT, a filtered back projection algorithm is typically used for slice reconstruction. An alternative, so-called iterative reconstruction can be used; this represents a significant advance, and will be discussed in detail.

FUNDAMENTALS OF POSITRON EMISSION TOMOGRAPHY

One of the most exciting emission tomographic techniques is PET. Positron-emitting radionuclides distributed in a patient are imaged with this technique. Recall that a positron is an antimatter electron. After a positron is emitted, it travels several millimeters in tissue and deposits its kinetic energy along the way. After it loses its kinetic energy, the positron combines with a free electron in the tissue, and mutual annihilation occurs. From conservation of energy, two 511-keV annihilation photons appear (because 511 keV is the energy equivalent to the rest mass of an electron and a positron). Because of conservation of momentum, the two photons are emitted simultaneously 180 degrees apart, back to back. An Anger camera could be used to detect these 511-keV gamma rays individually (i.e., without explicitly considering the other photon in the pair). However, more photons can be detected if the patient is surrounded with a ring of detectors. The detectors on opposing sides in the ring are electronically coupled to simultaneously identify the pair of gamma rays.

When two 511-keV gamma rays are detected by opposing detectors in coincidence, an annihilation event must have occurred along the line joining the two detectors. The direction of travel of the photons is thus determined without the need for a collimator. Conceptually, the raw PET scan data consist of a number of these coincidence lines. Reconstruction could simply be the drawing of these lines; they would cross and superimpose wherever activity occurred in the patient. In practice, the data set is reorganized into projections, and either filtered back projection or iterative reconstruction methods are used. In some PET scanners, the difference in arrival times of the two photons is used to position the event along the coincidence line. In practice, this "time-of-flight" spatial resolution is limited to several centimeters along the coincidence line because of temporal resolution limitations (hundreds of picoseconds). These limitations are a consequence of both the electronics and the decay time of the scintillation detectors used. (*Decay time* refers to the amount of time required for light to be emitted following deposition of energy in the crystal.) Thus, time-of-flight is used in combination with back projection reconstruction. Even without time-of-flight, PET differs from SPECT in that the "electronic collimation" of coincidence counting reduces the need for actual lead collimation, so that sensitivity is dramatically increased.

PARAMETERS TO OPTIMIZE IN EQUIPMENT DESIGN AND SELECTION

In general, the "quality" of an image can be described (quantitatively) by its signal-to-noise ratio (5). The signal-to-noise ratio directly relates to diagnostic and quantitative accuracy. In essence, then, a major goal of nuclear medicine imaging equipment is to maximize the signal-to-noise ratio of an image. The signal-to-noise ratio describes the relative "strength" of the desired information relative to the noise in the image. To achieve a high signal-to-noise ratio, high resolution and high sensitivity are required. Nuclear medicine imaging forces a compromise between resolution and sensitivity. In 1985, Muehllehner published an important study relating these two factors to perceived image quality (6). Observers viewed computer simulations of the Derenzo phantom and were asked to match images of similar image quality. Muehllehner found that an improvement in resolution of 2 mm (e.g., from 10 mm to 8 mm) resulted in comparable image quality with only about one-fourth as many counts. Fahey and co-workers (7) confirmed and extended Muehllehner's findings in a phantom study with a multicamera SPECT system. Thus, the signal-to-noise ratio may be increased by either increasing contrast (through improved spatial resolution) or decreasing noise (through increased sensitivity). Accordingly, appropriate system design must consider both resolution and sensitivity.

EFFECTS OF RESOLUTION, SCATTER, AND ATTENUATION

From the perspective of physical principles, five major factors affect the ability to detect small lesions and quantify absolute radioactivity. These include attenuation of photons by tissue (8,9); finite spatial resolution (e.g., the transaxial spatial resolution and effective slice thickness of a SPECT or PET scanner) (10–15); detection of scattered photons (16,17); accidental counting of "random" (nonpaired) photons in the coincidence window (18) (applicable only to coincidence imaging); and "noise" resulting from the statistical nature of radioactive decay (19,20).

All imaging systems have a limited ability to depict small objects as separate from each other. The spatial resolution of a system can be thought of as the distance over which two small point sources of radioactivity must be separated for them to be distinguished as different objects in the image. Finite spatial resolution of the imaging system results in two important effects. First, the image is blurred, and the degree of blurring depends on the spatial resolution. Blurring prevents the delineation of edges of larger structures and may prevent the distinct visualization of smaller objects. Furthermore, smearing and averaging together of neighboring areas reduce the measured value in the areas with greater radioactivity and increases it in areas with lesser radioactivity (i.e., reducing contrast). Finite spatial resolution produces an underestimation of radioactivity in small structures, with progressively greater underestimation as the structures get smaller (21). This underestimation ceases to be a problem when the size of the structure is approximately three times the resolution of the imaging system. These effects are sometimes referred to as *partial volume effects.* They also apply to the axial resolution of a tomographic scanner. Note that axial resolution is sometimes mistakenly called *slice thickness.*

The partial volume effect also depends on the contrast between the "target" (i.e., the structure or lesion of interest) and the surrounding or "background" activity in the patient (14,21,22). For example, Raylman and colleagues (22) found that lesions greater than 9 mm in diameter were detectable with fluorodeoxyglucose (FDG)-PET essentially independently of contrast (lesion-to-background ratio), but that for lesions smaller than 9 mm, a contrast greater than 18:1 was required. To characterize their results, they compared visual lesion detection with the quantitative recovery coefficient. The recovery coefficient (*RC*) is the ratio of measured to true lesion activity and was first described by Hoffman et al. (10). In doing so, they used both the measured *RC* and that calculated from Kessler et al. (14). The equation from Kessler et al. used to calculate *RC* is valid when no background activity is present (i.e., for an infinite lesion-to-background contrast). Following the nomenclature of Kessler et al., this *RC* is known as the *hot spot RC* (*HSRC*). A corresponding *cold spot RC* (*CSRC*) can be measured or calculated when the lesion-to-background contrast is zero. Of importance, *HSRC* and *CSRC* always sum to 1. Thus, the observed counts in the lesion may always be calculated as follows:

Observed Lesion Counts = (*HSRC* x True Lesion Counts) + (*CSRC* x True Background Counts)

This equation emphasizes that the observed lesion counts differ from the true lesion counts because of both "spill out" of lesion counts from the lesion (represented by *HSRC*) and "spill in" of counts from the background (represented by *CSRC*). To emphasize further the importance of background contribution to the observed lesion counts, the equation may be rewritten as follows:

Observed Lesion Counts = Background Counts [*HSRC* x Contrast + *CSRC*]

From this formulation, it is obvious that the observed counts, and thus the "effective" RC in the case of a lesion-to-background contrast other than infinity or zero, will depend on the contrast. This finding, first described by Kessler and colleagues (14), represents an important contribution to our understanding of resolution effects. Table 2.1 presents observed lesion contrasts for different lesion sizes (expressed as the ratio of lesion diameter to system spatial resolution) and true contrasts (i.e., true lesion-to-background ratios) of 0.5, 1, 2, 4, and 8; the data in Table 2.1 result from a simple recasting of data published previously (21). As the data indicate, for contrasts greater than 1 (i.e., when the lesion is relatively "hot"), the observed contrast is less than the true contrast, with progressively greater underestimation at smaller lesion sizes. Thus, for a small lesion to be detectable visually (i.e., look "hot" in comparison with its surroundings), it must start with a high enough true contrast to have sufficient "remaining" contrast in the image to be distinguishable from background. Whether or not the image contrast is "sufficient" depends on a number of factors, including noise and observer training and acuity. When the true contrast is less than 1 (i.e., when the lesion is relatively "cold"), the observed

TABLE 2.1. OBSERVED LESION CONTRAST AS A FUNCTION OF LESION SIZE AND TRUE CONTRAST

Lesion size/system resolution	Observed lesion contrast				
	C = 0.5	C = 1	C = 2	C = 4	C = 8
1	0.84	1.00	1.33	1.99	3.31
2	0.57	1.00	1.86	3.58	7.02
3	0.53	1.00	1.94	3.82	7.58
4	0.52	1.00	1.97	3.91	7.79

contrast is closer to 1 than the true contrast, with progressively larger observed contrast at smaller lesion sizes. In this case, for a small lesion to be detectable visually (i.e., look "cold" compared with its surroundings), it must start with a low enough true contrast to have sufficient contrast in the image to be distinguishable from background. When the lesion contrast is 1, quantitative recovery is perfect but the lesion is absolutely not detectable because it has the same count value as its surroundings.

The photons detected in nuclear medicine imaging are electromagnetic radiation. As such, they undergo two major types of interactions in tissue: photoelectric effect and Compton scattering. The photoelectric effect results in complete absorption of the photon, which reduces the observed count rate, whereas scattered photons are still detected. Because attenuation is a combination of absorption (by photoelectric effect) and scatter (by Compton scattering), correction schemes can treat these processes either independently or jointly. Large-angle scatter produces a low-level background "haze" in the image, which reduces contrast. Absorption produces a gradual, progressive underestimation of radioactivity from the edge to the center of the body by a factor of about 5 to as much as 50, depending on body habitus, photon energy, and single-photon versus coincidence detection. Both attenuation and scatter influence the apparent relative and absolute distribution of activity within the image. Therefore, it is important to try to correct or consider these effects during subjective visual interpretation or relative quantification (i.e., a comparison of the counts in one region with those in another). These effects must be accounted for and corrected to achieve accurate absolute quantification (i.e., determination of the radioactivity concentration in μCi/cc).

It is important to remember that these "deterministic" effects influence only the "signal" component of an image's signal-to-noise ratio; in other words, they influence only quantitative accuracy. Noise arises from the random statistical nature of radioactive decay, and potentially from inaccuracies or assumptions in the imaging hardware and certain image-processing operations. These influence the "noise" component of the signal-to-noise ratio—in other words, precision. Ultimately, key performance parameters such as lesion detectability and quantitative accuracy and precision depend on the signal-to-noise ratio or total error. Obviously, a focus on signal-to-noise ratio implies equal weighting to both components, and factors that influence noise must be given sufficient attention. These factors include the sensitivity of the system and the effects of software corrections (see below) on the propagation of noise through the image-processing chain.

NEW RECONSTRUCTION ALGORITHMS AND CORRECTION SCHEMES

Filtered back projection is the most commonly used reconstruction algorithm in SPECT. Filtered back projection is typically implemented with a "pixel-driven" approach. In this approach, all the pixels in the reconstruction matrix (image matrix) are initially set to zero. The value of each pixel in the projection data is back-projected into the reconstruction matrix. This is done by adding counts to the pixels in the reconstruction matrix that lie along a line corresponding to the projection pixel. By adding the values from multiple projection angles, a 2D image is produced from the projection data. This method assumes that each projection pixel value is the sum (or average) of the counts along a line in the reconstruction matrix. More accurate reconstructions are achieved when the projection data are interpolated and filtered before this pixel-driven back projection. This algorithm can be implemented efficiently and is relatively robust to those physical factors present in SPECT imaging that corrupt the imaging process (i.e., finite resolution, scatter, attenuation, and noise).

A number of investigators have proposed alternative reconstruction algorithms, many of which utilize iterative approaches (23). In iterative reconstruction, forward projection of the reconstructed images is used to create new estimated projection data that can be compared with the original projection data. If the acquisition and reconstruction process is correctly modeled, and if the reconstructed images are "perfect," the forward projection data should match the actual acquired projection data. The extent and manner in which they do not match reflect errors. These errors can be incorporated into an iterative back project-reproject-back project process. An important feature of many of these algorithms is an attempt to "unify" compensation for attenuation, scatter, and depth-dependent blurring (24–26). These approaches include the general class of algorithms known as *maximum likelihood by expectation maximization* (ML-EM). This class of algorithms permits the incorporation of models of depth-dependent blur, scatter, and attenuation effects into the projection-back projection process. The ability to account approximately for these three main physical effects has resulted in very accurate reconstructions. However, such approaches have suffered from increased reconstruction times, perhaps the main problem (26), and difficulty in converging to a useful solution, particularly in the presence of significant noise.

A particularly promising algorithm utilizes "ordered subsets" to accelerate iterative reconstruction (27). In this approach, projection data are grouped into an ordered sequence of subsets or blocks. Of major importance, these subsets represent mutually exclusive and exhaustive use of the projection data and are treated independently in parallel. One iteration of the algorithm is a single pass through all the subsets. Ordered subsets are an extension of iterative reconstruction. In the original implementation of Hudson and Larkin (27), they used the expectation maximization approach of Shepp and Vardi. Like any standard EM algorithm, this consists of a back projection-projection-back projection sequence. At each iteration, the reconstruction from the previous iteration is the starting point. In ordered-subsets EM (OS-EM), the standard EM algorithm is applied to each of the subsets in turn. In SPECT, the subsets may correspond to natural groupings of projections—for example, each head in a triple-head system. In PET, projection data may be reorganized after acquisition to define blocks or subsets in a similar fashion. OS-EM is rapidly becoming the preferred approach to reconstruction in emission tomography.

The two main approaches to attenuation correction may be used with either filtered back projection or iterative reconstruction algorithms. In the first, attenuation is measured before SPECT or PET begins. Photons from a point, line, sheet, or ring source of single-photon or positron-emitting activity are transmitted through the patient's body to produce a transmission projection. These data are divided by the corresponding projection data acquired in a second measurement without the patient present. From the natural logarithm of this ratio, the attenuation experienced by radioactivity at each point within the body can be estimated. This approach has been routinely used in PET for many years but has only relatively recently been extended to SPECT (28,29).

The second approach to attenuation correction does not require any additional measurements. After the uncorrected image is reconstructed, the computer operator defines the body with either an ellipse or body-following outline. A constant average value for attenuation is assumed for each point inside this outline of the body. (This average value depends on both the tissues involved and the characteristics of the particular SPECT or PET scanner.) It is important to define the outline of the entire body, not just the organ of interest. This approach works well for the brain but is not widely used in the torso. In more sophisticated approaches, internal structures or areas with significantly different attenuation values are separately identified, either manually or automatically (perhaps with use of a scatter image). The distinction between the two approaches is shown in Fig. 2.1.

It is important to note that the effects of attenuation at the projection level are not the same for SPECT and PET. In one dimension, a simplified SPECT projection ray integral is written as follows:

$$P_{SPECT} = \int_0^Z a(x,y,z)[\exp - \int_z^Z \mu(w)dw]dz$$

where a is the activity term and the bracketed portion is the attenuation term. It is important to note that the activity term [i.e., $a(x,y,z)$] and the attenuation term (in the brackets) are not mathematically separable because it is necessary to know z, the position or depth of the activity. Therefore, we cannot mathematically correct perfectly for attenuation in SPECT, even if the attenuation coefficient distribution is known. In PET, the situation is different because two photons must leave the patient for them to be in coincidence. This means that the attenuation is independent of where a source is along a line. The corresponding simplified PET projection ray integral can be written as follows:

$$P_{PET} = \int_0^Z a(x,y,z)[\exp - \int_z^Z \mu(w)dw][\exp - \int_0^Z \mu(w)dw]dz$$
$$= \int_0^Z a(x,y,z)[\exp - \int_0^Z \mu(w)dw]dz$$

Note that the activity and attenuation terms here are separable. Thus, if we exactly know the attenuation coefficient distribution in PET, we can exactly correct for attenuation.

The same physics and mathematics that make "perfect" attenuation correction at least theoretically achievable in PET, but not in SPECT, make the effects of attenuation itself more dramatic in PET than in SPECT. The underlying basis is the fact that both photons must escape the subject and be detected in PET, which means that the total attenuation path length is longer for PET than for SPECT, as illustrated in Fig. 2.2. This distinction increases exponentially with patient size. For example, with PET, a 30-cm-diameter patient requires an average attenuation correction factor of 16, whereas a 40-cm-diameter patient requires a correction factor of 50.

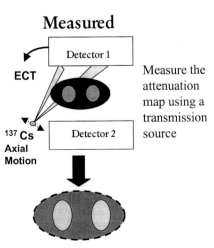

Calculated

Image of body with ROI

Uniform attenuation map

Measured

Detector 1

ECT

^{137}Cs
Axial
Motion

Detector 2

Measure the attenuation map using a transmission source

Measured attenuation map

FIGURE 2.1. In calculated attenuation correction, an image of the body is acquired (e.g., the emission image is directly used), and an outline is drawn around the body. This outline is then used to estimate the attenuation map by assuming the body has a uniform density or attenuation coefficient. In measured attenuation correction, a source is used to determine the attenuation coefficients on a pixel-by-pixel basis.

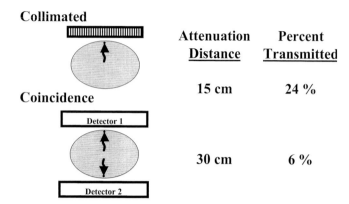

	Attenuation Distance	Percent Transmitted
	15 cm	24 %
	30 cm	6 %

FIGURE 2.2. A higher percentage of the emitted photons are attenuated in coincidence imaging than in single-photon imaging. This is a consequence of the increased path length in coincidence imaging, as both photons must escape for them to be detected in coincidence. The figure shows a situation in which the source is at the center of a small object. If the source had been closer to the anterior surface, the differences would have been even greater because the coincidence path length would have remained the same but the single-photon (anterior) attenuation distance would have decreased.

If scatter is to be corrected independently, large-angle scatter can be estimated through the use of a second "scatter" pulse height window (30), or through the use of two or three windows around the photopeak (31). If a separate scatter correction is used, this must be taken into account when either the transmission-based or calculated attenuation correction schemes above are utilized. It is important to note that scattered photons may either be "eliminated" via subtraction or "repositioned" via deconvolution (e.g., during deblurring by Wiener or Metz filtering) (32). If scatter is not corrected, less accurate reconstructions are the result. Data can be either overcorrected or undercorrected, depending on the attenuation coefficient that is used to calculate the correction factor.

Early attempts to reduce effects of partial volume concentrated on improving the spatial resolution in the image—for example, through the use of higher-resolution collimation (and unique collimator designs) in SPECT (33), smaller detectors in PET (34), and a reconstruction filter with a higher-frequency cutoff. Newer approaches incorporate the effects of depth-dependent blurring into the reconstruction algorithm (see above). The latest attempts have utilized co-registered anatomic images from CT or magnetic resonance imaging (MRI) (35). In this approach, currently best applicable to brain studies, anatomic images are segmented into tissue classes and blurred to the resolution of the SPECT or PET imaging system. The blurring process identifies the degree of "spill in" and "spill out" of counts from and to the structures of interest, which can then be corrected.

This approach is also an example of a more general advance: the use of co-registered anatomic images. Multimodality display and analysis software will significantly enhance diagnostic interpretation and quantitative analysis, but only if reliable and accurate fully automated approaches are available. Such is already the case for the brain, either with a head holder (36–39) or solely with software (40–42), but the torso presents a much more difficult situation, although some recent success has been reported (43). It is interesting to note that co-registered anatomic images have already been used in image reconstruction itself (44).

NEW DETECTOR MATERIALS AND CAMERA DESIGNS

A number of exciting new detector materials are being vigorously investigated by industry and academia. These include cerium-doped lutetium oxyorthosilicate (LSO), yttrium oxyorthosilicate (YSO), germanium oxyorthosilicate (GSO), which are single-crystal inorganic scintillators, and cadmium zinc telluride (CZT), which is an extension of the semiconductor cadmium telluride (CdTe). The interest in LSO, GSO, and YSO is based on their physical properties, which offer potential improvements over either sodium iodide (NaI) or bismuth germanate (BGO).

As the data in Table 2.2 demonstrate, LSO, BGO, and GSO have a higher density and more effective Z than NaI, which results in a lower mean free path ($1/\mu$, or equivalently a higher stopping power) at both 140 and 511 keV. LSO, GSO, and YSO have a significantly shorter decay time than either NaI or BGO. Shorter decay times should lead to systems with much higher count rate capability (and decreased random events in coincidence imaging). The high light output of YSO produces very good energy resolution. Unfortunately, LSO is intrinsically radioactive (because of the isotope lutetium 176), so it must be used with care in single-photon counting applications.

Taken together, these data imply that LSO and GSO may be significantly better detectors for PET than the current standard, BGO. Further, they suggest that a "sandwich" of LSO and YSO or NaI (a so-called phoswich detector) could have interesting properties for dual SPECT/PET imaging. In such a detector, a front layer (e.g., 1.5 to 2 cm) of YSO or NaI is used as the entrance material for detection of low-energy photons (e.g., 140 keV), with a second layer (e.g., 1 to 2 cm) of LSO used for higher-energy photons (e.g., 511 keV). In this arrangement, the stopping power of YSO or NaI is sufficient for the lower-energy photons, and the LSO acts as a light pipe for the scintillation photons produced in the YSO or NaI. The stopping power of YSO or NaI is not sufficient for the higher-energy photons, which thus mainly pass through the YSO or NaI and interact in the LSO. The signals from the two detector materials would be separated

TABLE 2.2. PHYSICAL PROPERTIES OF SCINTILLATION DETECTORS OF INTEREST IN NUCLEAR MEDICINE

	Detector material				
	NaI	BGO	LSO	YSO	GSO
Density (g/cc)	3.67	7.13	7.40	4.54	6.71
Effective *Z*	51	74	66	34	59
Decay time (ns)	230	300	40	70	60
Relative light output	100	15	75	120	25
Energy resolution	7.8%	10%	<10%	<7.5%	9%
$1/\mu$ @140 keV (mm)	4.2	0.82	1.0	7.7	
$1/\mu$ @ 511 keV (mm)	30	11	12	26	14

NaI, sodium iodide; BGO, bismuth germanate; LSO, lutetium oxyorthosilicate; YSO, yttrium oxyorthosilicate; GSO, germanium oxyorthosilicate.

by time-based pulse-shape discrimination because the decay times are so different. The single-photon image quality from a phoswich system remains unproven because of the limited energy resolution in these detectors.

There is particular emphasis on the use of new detectors in systems built specifically for scintimammography. It is highly desirable to design these systems so that they are physically small and easily positioned and have very high spatial and energy resolution. A good example of the current state of the art is a system based on a cesium iodide (CsI) scintillation detector with a position-sensitive photomultiplier tube (PMT) (45). As an alternative to scintillator PMT-based detectors, semiconductors have been investigated. The motivation for using semiconductors is that scintillation detectors have poor energy resolution because of their design, which requires the conversion of incident radiation energy to light and then into charge. The subsequent generation of an electrical signal involves many inefficient steps. Thus, the energy required to produce one photoelectron at the photocathode of the photomultiplier tube is about 100 eV, so a typical radiation–crystal interaction results in only a few thousand photoelectrons representing the "signal." For this reason, the statistical fluctuation is relatively high. Semiconductor materials offer the promise of producing more signal per radiation interaction, thereby reducing statistical noise and increasing energy resolution. Of major importance, the statistical uncertainty in the signal of each detector element also ultimately limits spatial resolution, so decreasing the statistical fluctuations improves intrinsic spatial resolution.

The basic signal in a semiconductor detector is produced by "electron hole pairs" created along the path as radiation passes through the detector and produces ionization. Each electron hole pair is somewhat analogous to an ion pair formed in a gas-filled detector. Like ion pairs in a gas-filled detector, the motion of electron hole pairs in an applied electric field generates the electrical signal. Although many semiconductors have been studied, CZT, which is an extension

of the semiconductor CdTe, has generated the most interest. CZT has a relatively high effective atomic number and exceptionally good energy resolution. For example, a CZT detector 7 mm thick has the equivalent stopping power of 1 cm of NaI (at 140 keV). The theoretically achievable energy resolution of CZT is well under 1% (at 140 keV), based solely on the statistical variation in the number of electron hole pairs created. Actual energy resolutions are currently in the 3% to 6% range and are probably limited because of problems with hole trapping and electronic noise. It is hoped that the energy resolution will be improved to 2% in a real-world system; this is in contrast to the energy resolution of CdTe, which is very poor (Dr. John Engdahl, *personal communication*). The detector is intrinsically "digital," which means that each detector is a pixel. The signal produced in the semiconductor is processed by ASIC-based (application-specific integrated circuits) read-out electronics. Therefore, any pixel size (and therefore intrinsic resolution) is possible, with cost the major limitation. In a solid-state camera, the system spatial resolution would be limited primarily by the resolution of the collimator.

It is not clear that any of the scintillators or solid-state (semiconductor) detectors now being investigated will ever make it to market, or be a significant advance if they do. Of importance, it is not obvious how improvements in one performance parameter (e.g., energy resolution) will quantitatively translate into improvements in another (e.g., intrinsic spatial resolution) or into system-level performance. As an example, consider a "system" consisting of a series of factors that influence spatial resolution. The point spread function of the system (h_T) can be modeled as the convolution of the factors' own impulse response functions or point spread functions ($h_T = h_1 \otimes h_2 \otimes \ldots h_n$). In practice, if we assume a series of gaussian-like point spread functions, total system resolution, R_T, can be estimated from the series of independent resolutions of all components, as given above. For example, if the factors or components are

TABLE 2.3. COMPARISON OF RELATIVE SENSITIVITIES FOR SINGLE-HEAD AND MULTIHEAD SYSTEMS WITH IDENTICAL CAMERA HEADS AND COLLIMATION

	Acquisition of 360 degrees		Acquisition of 180 degrees	
	Acquisition time	Relative sensitivity	Acquisition time	Relative sensitivity
Single	30	1	30	1
Double (heads at 180 degrees)	15	2	30	1
Double (heads at 90 degrees)	15	2	15	2
Triple	10	3	20	1.5

intrinsic resolution (R_I), collimator resolution (R_C), processing resolution such as filtering (R_P), and patient or organ motion (R_M), then R_T is given by the following:

$$R_T = \sqrt{R_I^2 + R_C^2 + R_P^2 + R_M^2}$$

If we assume that only intrinsic resolution and collimator resolution are at play, and that R_C is 1 cm, then intrinsic resolutions of 1, 2, 3, and 4 mm would result in R_T values of 10.05, 10.20, 10.44, and 10.77 mm, respectively. In other words, if factors other than intrinsic resolution limit R_T, changes in R_I have minimal effect on R_T. On the other hand, if R_C is reduced to 5 mm, then intrinsic resolutions of 1, 2, 3, and 4 mm would result in R_T values of 5.10, 5.39, 5.83, and 6.40 mm, respectively. In this situation, a decrease in R_I from 4 to 2 mm would produce a 1-mm (i.e., useful) improvement in R_T.

Perhaps the biggest actual advance in SPECT systems has been the use of multiple detectors (46). As shown in Table 2.3, adding camera heads increases sensitivity. Dual-head variable-angle systems that are capable of orienting the heads at both 90 and 180 degrees are particularly popular, as this feature optimizes the acquisition geometry for the two most commonly performed nuclear medicine procedures, cardiac SPECT and whole-body bone scans. These two studies account for at least 70% of all nuclear medicine imaging procedures. The increased sensitivity provided by multihead systems can be used primarily in three ways: It can be used to decrease noise (when the same acquisition time is used as with a single-head system). Second, it can be used to decrease acquisition time (to obtain the same counts as with a single-head system or decrease tracer washout effects). Third, it may be "traded" for higher resolution through the use of collimators with higher resolution and lower sensitivity.

In PET, one of the biggest advances of the past several years is the strong trend to fully 3D ("septa-less") acquisition and reconstruction. The use of a scanner with retractable septa for 3D operation provides an increase in sensitivity by a factor of about 5. (Note that the count rate capability does not change, so activity must be adjusted to minimize dead time.) This increase in sensitivity comes with a cost, significantly higher scatter, but accurate algorithms now exist for scatter correction in 3D PET. As nuclear medicine moves more and more toward more "specific" biochemical studies, such as receptor binding, the fraction of the injected dose that goes to the target organ will likely decrease, so that the importance of a high degree of sensitivity is further increased.

A second important advance in PET is the use of whole-body imaging in oncology (47). In this approach, coronal whole-body images are created by using transaxial reconstructed data from serial acquisitions of multiple axial fields of view as the patient's bed is indexed through the PET scanner.

ULTRA-HIGH–ENERGY COLLIMATORS FOR SINGLE-PHOTON EMISSION COMPUTED TOMOGRAPHY

Positron-emitting radionuclides can be imaged with a gamma camera by using either collimators or coincidence methods. In collimated detection, one or both of the two photons are detected in noncoincidence mode (i.e., by one or more collimated heads in a conventional SPECT system) (48). Alternatively, imaging can be performed with collimator-less coincidence detection of both photons by opposing detectors (i.e., by a dual-head, uncollimated, 180-degree SPECT system) (49). Most manufacturers have now developed 511-keV collimators. Two main issues regarding the use of such collimators are the following: (a) the design tradeoffs between collimator resolution and sensitivity (see equations above) and (b) appropriate "tuning" and "correction" of the intrinsic spatially varying energy response, linearity, and uniformity of the camera head.

With respect to the tradeoff between resolution and sensitivity, the "optimum" design would be one producing the highest signal-to-noise ratio in a given situation. For cardiac imaging with FDG, an abnormality is a decrease in FDG concentration in comparison with the surrounding normal myocardium. Given the relatively large vascular territories, abnormalities, such as perfusion abnormalities, might commonly represent relatively large areas of myocardium. The interpretation of the images is also aided by the known normal distribution of the tracer. In tumor imaging with FDG, an abnormality is an increase in FDG concentration in comparison with surrounding normal tissues. These lesions can be very small (measured in units smaller than centimeters) and develop at random locations. Consequently, it is conceivable that the optimum collimator for FDG myocardial viability studies would have sufficiently good sensitivity, even at the expense of resolution, to produce low-noise images depicting a small reduction in FDG in a relatively large area. Alternatively, the optimum collimator for FDG tumor detection and localization studies would have sufficiently good resolution, even at the expense of sensitivity, to produce images with few partial volume effects and adequate quantitative recovery for small, hot lesions to be visible. Thus, the optimum designs for these two applications might be significantly different. The resolution and sensitivity of current ultra–high-energy collimators are relatively poor in comparison with those of low-energy collimators; their resolution is particularly bad. Consequently, ultra–high-energy collimators have not been recommended for use in nuclear oncology.

DUAL-DETECTOR COINCIDENCE IMAGING

As an alternative to the use of 511-keV collimators with "conventional" SPECT, dual-head SPECT systems may be used without collimators in a coincidence mode (49). In this mode, the opposing cameras are electronically config-

ured in coincidence (Fig. 2.3), and the coincident detection of the two 511-keV annihilation photons is used to define a "coincidence line" that passes through the annihilation site. This annihilation site differs from the positron emission site by about 1 mm, which fundamentally limits the achievable resolution in coincidence imaging. The absence of collimation, coupled with high-speed electronics, permits spatial resolution only slightly degraded relative to the intrinsic resolution of the camera (i.e., about 4 to 5 mm).

The lack of collimation in coincidence imaging also means that the sensitivity is considerably higher (higher per head by at least a factor of 10^4 or so) than with collimated SPECT. However, because both photons must be detected, the effective gain in sensitivity is about 100. Furthermore, because both photons must exit the body, the overall attenuation is actually greater than at 140 keV, as mentioned above. Consequently, overall sensitivity is higher than in collimated imaging by a factor of only about 10. In coincidence imaging, the actual number of counts in the image depends on both sensitivity and high count rate capability. The sensitivity is primarily set by the crystal thickness and is measured at low count rates. As the amount of activity in the patient is increased, the "effective" sensitivity decreases at high count rates because of the dead time of the system. When no collimator is present, the same activity causes many more photons to strike the crystal, and the camera operates at a significantly higher count rate than in collimated operation. This can drive operation into the paralyzable region. Thus, the administered dose must be decreased in comparison with the dose in collimated operation. Typical administered doses of FDG are 10 mCi for collimated

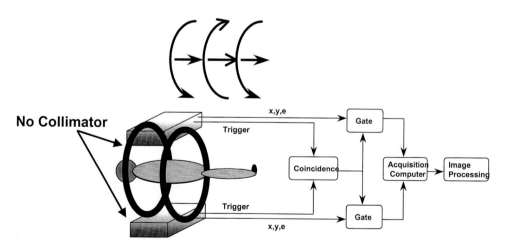

FIGURE 2.3. In coincidence imaging with a scintillation camera, high-speed trigger signals are sent to a coincidence circuit within the first 10 ns of the photon interactions. When the two trigger signals are within the coincidence time window, a gate is opened that allows the x, y, and z signals to be transmitted so that energy window analysis may be performed. Because the collimators are removed, the detectors must be able to handle very high counting rates. Images are acquired from multiple bed positions with tomographic motion (as in single-photon emission computed tomography), followed by a translate to the next bed position for whole-body imaging.

systems and 3 to 5 mCi for cameras in coincidence mode, depending on the specific manufacturer.

The counting rate limitation is particularly important because only about 1% to 2% of the so-called singles count rate at each head produces coincidence counts. (The singles counting rate is the counting rate in a single detector.) Therefore, to achieve a coincidence count rate of 1,000 counts per second, the expected singles count rate is about 100,000 counts per second. To achieve a clinically useful coincidence count rate, the count rate capability of each camera (singles) must be exceptionally good (e.g., > 500,000 counts per second). This is the reason why a high singles count rate capability is so important. To achieve these count rate capabilities, several methods are used: multiple trigger channels, lower dead time through pulse shortening, and local centroid calculation (Fig. 2.4). These approaches are fully possible only with today's digital detectors.

To improve the performance of dual-head coincidence imaging, several manufacturers have begun to offer thicker crystals. The efficiencies for 511-keV photons are shown in Table 2.4 for different thicknesses of NaI. Here, single-crystal efficiency is shown both for the full spectrum (unweighted sum of the probability of interaction from 50 to 511 keV) and for the photopeak (511 keV) only. Of importance, the coincidence efficiency is the square of the single-crystal photopeak efficiency, so changing the crystal thickness has a greater effect on coincidence efficiency than on photopeak efficiency. (The photopeak efficiency must be squared to estimate coincidence efficiency because both detectors must register 511-keV events to generate a coincidence count.) The use of a thicker crystal degrades intrinsic spatial resolution, but the effect on system resolution is much less pronounced, as discussed above. For example, with a representative digital detector, intrinsic resolution degrades from 3.5 mm to 3.9 mm when the thickness is increased from 3/8 to 5/8 in. A critical issue is whether this reduced intrinsic spatial resolution significantly degrades system resolution in either single-photon counting or coincidence mode. The change in intrinsic resolution is typically less than 0.5 mm; given the arguments above, thicker crystals do not influence system resolution in either mode, and they should be considered if the system will be used frequently for coincidence imaging.

Another innovative approach to increasing sensitivity is the use of photopeak-to-Compton coincidences. Each head

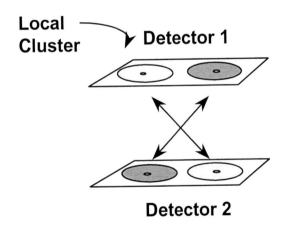

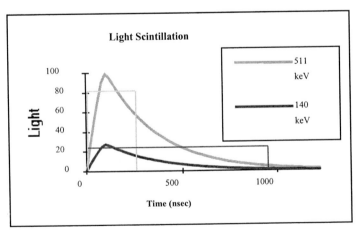

FIGURE 2.4. Digital detectors are used in scintillation cameras to increase the counting rate capabilities. The ability to process multiple events virtually simultaneously (> 40 ns apart) can almost double the count rate capabilities. To process multiple events, the detector must output separate trigger signals and be able to develop x, y, and z signals separately for each interaction. Multiple trigger channels enable separate triggers and start local centroid calculations (x, y, z). By decreasing the pulse integration time for the 511-keV interactions, the dead time can be dramatically reduced relative to single-photon counting (e.g., at 140 keV). The digital detector also enables pulse shortening.

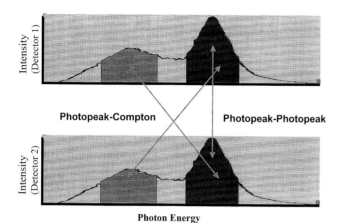

FIGURE 2.5. Allowing coincidences between different types of interactions in the crystal can increase the counting efficiency of a scintillation camera in coincidence mode. The *vertical arrow line* shows the photopeak-to-photopeak coincidence events that are allowed between detector 1 and detector 2. The *crossed arrow lines* show the photopeak-to-Compton coincidence events that are also allowed in many systems. The Compton energy window is set at a lower energy to avoid those photons that are Compton-scattered in the patient. These photons are predominantly forward scatters and are therefore close to 511 keV and undesirable.

is set up with dual energy windows—one for the photopeak and another for a broad part of the Compton region (about 100 keV wide). Coincidences are allowed when one of the heads registers a photopeak event and the other head registers either a photopeak or a Compton event (Fig. 2.5). This approach can significantly increase sensitivity while only modestly increasing the acquisition of scattered events. In this regard, it is important to note that the efficiency of NaI detectors for photoelectric interactions at 511 keV is low (Table 2.4). Many of the photons that are not scattered in the patient may interact with the detector by Compton scattering. Requiring this "Compton window" event to be in coincidence with a photopeak event increases the probability that a true annihilation took place on a line between the two detected locations. The increase in sensitivity is by a factor of about 2. For example, with a 3/8-in crystal and the National Electrical

TABLE 2.4. EFFICIENCIES OF CRYSTALS OF DIFFERENT THICKNESS USED IN DUAL-HEAD IMAGING

Thickness (in)	Full spectrum	Photopeak	Coincidence
3/8	0.275	0.104	0.011
1/2	0.346	0.145	0.021
5/8	0.413	0.189	0.036
3/4	0.472	0.228	0.052

Manufacturers Association (NEMA) 3D phantom on a representative dual-head coincidence imaging system, the sensitivity for photopeak-only counting is 21.5 kcps/µCi per cubic centimeter, whereas for photopeak–photopeak and photopeak–Compton counting, it is 50.4 kcps/µCi per cubic centimeter. The scatter fraction rises from 23% to 37% in the change from photopeak-only to photopeak–photopeak and photopeak–Compton counting. Although the increase in scatter obviously represents a decrease in quantitative accuracy, this may be an example of a situation in which an increase in sensitivity justifies its use, in terms of both noise and throughput.

Another important issue that is related to both apparent system sensitivity and image contrast is the (unwanted) acquisition of scattered and random coincidence events. As described above, scattered events introduce a background "haze" that reduces contrast. In general, random events can also produce the same effect (Fig. 2.6). The random coincidence count rate is given by the product of the coincidence time window and the singles count rates from the two detectors. As the activity in the field of view increases, the true coincidence rate increases linearly (ignoring effects of dead time), but the random coincidence rate increases as the square of the increase in activity. Sensitivity may be increased by increasing the width of the coincidence time window (up to the point at which the full coincidence time spectrum has been included), but only at the expense of acquisition of more random coincidences. A great challenge in dual-head coincidence imaging is to balance sensitivity with randoms in optimizing the time window setting. Some manufacturers specify the window in terms of the time resolution of the system; others do so in terms of twice the time resolution, which is usually the actual window width, and therefore the more traditional specification.

An important recent advance in dual-head coincidence imaging is attenuation correction, which is often coupled with randoms and scatter corrections. Performing these corrections leads to more accurate reconstructions, which can improve image quality. The improvement in image quality is shown in Fig. 2.7. Attenuation correction can dramatically change the appearance of the images, particularly for whole-body imaging (e.g., the lungs go from relatively hot to relatively cold). Figure 2.8 shows a system for acquiring the attenuation correction data. In the implementation of the dual-head coincidence system, the approach borrows from that used in cardiac SPECT, with scanning point or line sources and with a scanning spatial window (Fig. 2.9). A problem with attenuation correction is that noise in the transmission data propagates into the emission data; this can also be a problem with dedicated PET. To decrease the transmission noise, the use of a single-photon radionuclide, cesium 137, has been described for PET (50–52) and has now been extended for dual-head coincidence imaging.

Acquisition Geometry

Reconstructed Transverse slice

Transverse Image

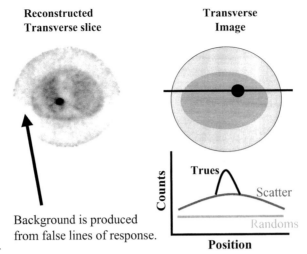

Randoms and scattered events (solid lines) produce falsely reconstructed lines of response (dotted lines).

Background is produced from false lines of response.

FIGURE 2.6. Random and scattered events reduce the contrast in coincidence images by producing false coincidence counts. Randoms (events in the coincidence window from separate disintegrations) produce a flat background. Events that are Compton-scattered produce a background peaked around the scattering material and the source distribution.

With Corrections:
- **Randoms**
- **Scatter &**
- **Attenuation correction**

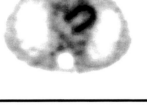

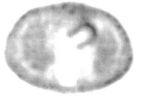

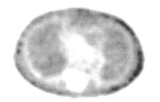

Without Corrections

FIGURE 2.7. Images of an anthropomorphic phantom that were reconstructed with and without corrections for randoms, scatter, and attenuation. The heart and body portions of the phantom were filled with fluorine 18. The lung regions contained no fluorine 18. Note in the uncorrected images the buildup of counts at the edge of the body and the low counts in the center. This is caused by attenuation. Also note the false counts in the lungs, not present in the corrected images. The counts are also distorted in the walls of the heart. In the corrected images, one can see the tumors located near the spine and the plastic insert supporting the heart.

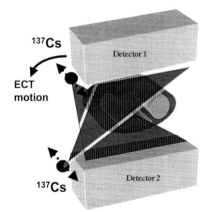

Transmission Acquisition:

- **Patient contains FDG** (511 keV)

- **TX acquired at 662 keV** (Singles mode)

- **TX continuous 360° ECT**

- **TX sources translate axially**

- **Scanning window synchronized with source**

FIGURE 2.8. Two transmission sources are lateral to the detectors and move axially down the detectors. They emit a fan beam of 662-keV photons that are used to measure the attenuation through the patient. The transmission sources translate axially. Sufficient projection data are acquired for reconstruction of attenuation coefficients at a given bed position by rotating in tomographic angular motion through 360 degrees around the patient.

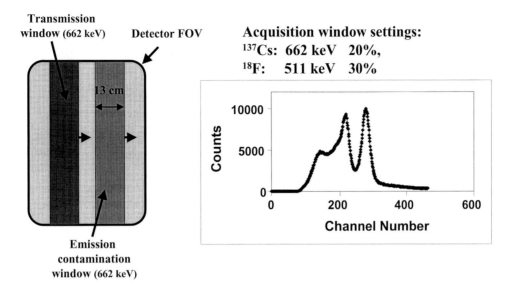

Transmission window (662 keV)   Detector FOV

13 cm

Emission contamination window (662 keV)

Acquisition window settings:
^{137}Cs: 662 keV 20%,
^{18}F: 511 keV 30%

FIGURE 2.9. To reconstruct the transmission map accurately, it is necessary to correct the 662-keV data for 511-keV crossover, or "cross talk." As seen in the energy spectra, a small number of the 511-keV photons will "tail" into the 662-keV photopeak. A correction for these crossover photons is acquired with the use of spatially scanning energy windows—one for the 662-keV transmission data and one for emission crossover data.

With either PET or dual-head coincidence, all the singles counts contribute toward the transmission images, thus providing low noise. The clinical impact of attenuation correction in dual-head coincidence imaging and dedicated PET whole-body imaging is still a subject of debate for oncology (53,54). In this debate, it is important also to consider the methods used to reconstruct the images. Iterative methods provide significantly improved image quality in comparison with filtered back projection when both use attenuation correction.

One other factor that stills seems somewhat controversial is the use of axial collimation (sometimes referred to as *axial filters*, *scatter shields*, *axial septa*, or *slats*) in dual-head coincidence imaging. A fully 3D acquisition, without lead collimation of any kind, provides a higher geometric efficiency in comparison with 2D acquisition (Fig. 2.10). However,

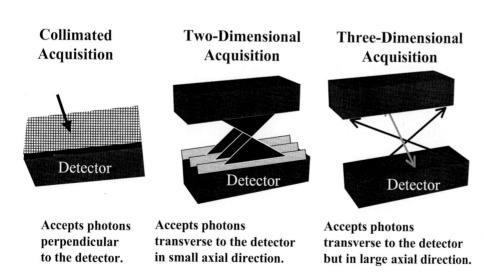

Collimated Acquisition

Accepts photons perpendicular to the detector.

Relative efficiency:
0.3X

Two-Dimensional Acquisition

Accepts photons transverse to the detector in small axial direction.

1X

Three-Dimensional Acquisition

Accepts photons transverse to the detector but in large axial direction.

5X

FIGURE 2.10. The final counting efficiency of a gamma camera system is related to its geometric efficiency or the solid angles the detector accepts. Collimated systems limit the acceptance angle through a grid of lead holes. Two-dimensional systems limit the acceptance angles through the use of thick septa positioned axially across the detector. Three-dimensional systems accept photons in both the transaxial and caudal–cephalic directions.

3-D acquisition
- **Accepts caudal/cephalic events**
- **4-5 times higher trues**
- **More scatter than 2-D systems**

2-D acquisition
- **Limited to transaxial events**
- **Lower trues**
- **Less scatter**
- **Limits events out of FOV**

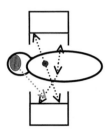
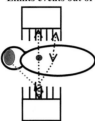

FIGURE 2.11. The higher geometric efficiency of three-dimensional acquisition is somewhat offset by the lower scatter and decreased influence of activity outside of the field of view for two-dimensional acquisition. Note that the septa in the two-dimensional acquisition reduce the scatter in the field of view and the contribution from activity in the brain.

3D acquisition also yields higher scatter (Fig. 2.11). Axial collimation is therefore used on some systems to reduce the influence of "out-of-plane" scatter.

COMPARISON OF PERFORMANCE OF DIFFERENT TYPES OF IMAGING SYSTEMS

The performance characteristics of ultra–high-energy collimators and SPECT imaging may be compared with those of dual-head coincidence imaging and dedicated PET scanners. In general, the resolution and sensitivity measurements of collimators are based on planar imaging of point sources, whereas those of coincidence imaging systems and dedicated PET scanners are based on reconstructed point sources for resolution and cylindric phantoms for sensitivity. For example, collimator sensitivity is specified in units of cpm/μCi from a point source or Petri dish source, whereas PET sensitivity is specified in units of cps or cpm/μCi per cubic centimeter from a 20-cm-diameter cylindric phantom. This means that the resolution and sensitivity figures from single-photon and coincidence imaging are not generally directly comparable. Nonetheless, it is worthwhile to try to put parameter values into a standardized context and draw conclusions. The ADAC MCD system is cited as representative of a current dual-head coincidence imaging system, the GE 4096 as representative of an "older"-generation dedicated PET scanner, the ADAC C-PET and Siemens ART as representative of current "lower-cost" dedicated PET scanners, and the GE Advance and Siemens EXACT HR+ as representative of current state-of-the-art dedicated PET scanners. In practice, dedicated PET scanners are typically operated in 3D mode for brain imaging and in 2D mode for whole-body imaging. Dual-head coincidence imaging systems are typically operated in either full 3D mode or in a pseudo-2D mode via axial collimation, as described above. Thus, the system sensitivities for whole-body studies, the most commonly performed in clinical nuclear oncology, should be compared for 2D operation. Table 2.5 indicates that the volume or system sensitivity of dual-head coincidence systems (operating in 3D mode) approaches that of a dedicated PET scanner operating in 2D mode. (Although a PET scanner has higher slice sensitivity, even in 2D mode, dual-head coincidence imaging systems have a larger axial field of view, which somewhat compensates when the parameter is system sensitivity.) The system sensitivity of the dual-head coincidence imaging system given in Table 4.5 is greater by a factor of about 8 than the system sensitivity of the same dual-head system operated with 511 keV collimators. Dual-head coincidence imaging systems are here to stay and represent an important instrumentation advance that permits many nuclear medicine practitioners to utilize FDG.

CONCLUSIONS

Nuclear medicine remains a vibrant technique and specialty as a result of advances in both instruments and tracers.

TABLE 2.5. COMPARISON OF SPECIFICATIONS FOR CAMERA AND DEDICATED POSITRON EMISSION TOMOGRAPHY SYSTEMS

	Model					
Specification	ADAC MCD	GE 4096	ADAC C-PET	GE Advance	Siemens ART	Siemens Exact HR+
Axial FOV (cm)	38	10	25	15	16	16
Number of slices	95	15	125	35	47	63
In-plane resolution (mm)	4.8	6.0	5.0	4.8	6.3	4.6
Axial resolution (mm)	5.5	6.0	5.5	4.0	5.9	4.2
System sensitivity (kcps)—2D	n/a	91	n/a	220	n/a	200
System sensitivity (kcps)—3D	100	n/a	400	1,225	240	900

FOV, field of view; 2D, two-dimensional; 3D, three-dimensional.

These advances, which go hand in hand, permit the imaging of physiologic and biochemical processes with ever-increasing sensitivity and specificity. To maximize diagnostic and quantitative accuracy, appropriate attention must be paid to instrument selection, instrument setup, and digital processing. Ultimately, the choice of instrument and its operational parameters depends on the specific clinical study. The practical performance requirements that arise from such considerations should be kept in mind when new equipment is purchased and when existing equipment is operated. Often, improvements in performance can be realized by more careful attention to optimizing subtle details in acquisition and processing protocols, and readers are encouraged to do so with the aid of the manufacturer.

REFERENCES

1. Sorenson JA, Phelps ME. *Physics in nuclear medicine*, 2nd ed. Orlando, FL: Grune & Stratton, 1987.
2. Tsui BMW, Gullberg GT, Edgerton ER, et al. Design and clinical utility of a fan beam collimator for SPECT imaging of the head. *J Nucl Med* 1986;27:810–819.
3. Jaszczak RJ, Greer KL, Coleman RE. SPECT using a specially designed cone beam collimator. *J Nucl Med* 1988;29:1398–1405.
4. Moore SC, Kouris K, Cullum I. Collimator design for single photon emission tomography. *Eur J Nucl Med* 1992;19:138–150.
5. Shosa D, Kaufman L. Methods for evaluation of diagnostic imaging instrumentation. *Phys Med Biol* 1981;26:101–112.
6. Muehllehner G. Effect of resolution on required count density in ECT imaging: a computer simulation. *Phys Med Biol* 1985;30:163–173.
7. Fahey FH, Harkness BA, Keyes JW, et al. Sensitivity, resolution and image quality with a multi-head SPECT camera. *J Nucl Med* 1992;33:1859–1863.
8. Huang SC, Hoffman EJ, Phelps ME, et al. Quantification in positron emission computed tomography: 2. Effects of inaccurate attenuation correction. *J Comput Assist Tomogr* 1979;3:304–314.
9. King MA, Tsui BMW, Pan TS. Attenuation compensation for cardiac single-photon emission computed tomographic imaging: part 1. Impact of attenuation and methods of estimating attenuation maps. *J Nucl Cardiol* 1995;2:513–524.
10. Hoffman EJ, Huang SC, Phelps ME. Quantification in positron emission computed tomography: 1. Effect of object size. *J Comput Assist Tomogr* 1979;3:299–308.
11. Huang SC, Hoffman EJ, Phelps ME, et al. Quantification in positron emission computed tomography: 3. Effect of sampling. *J Comput Assist Tomogr* 1980;4:819–826.
12. Mazziotta JC, Phelps ME, Plummer D, et al. Quantification in positron emission computed tomography: 5. Physical-anatomical effects. *J Comput Assist Tomogr* 1981;5:734–743.
13. Hoffman EJ, Huang SC, Plummer D, et al. Quantification in positron emission computed tomography: 6. Effect of nonuniform resolution. *J Comput Assist Tomogr* 1982;6:987–999.
14. Kessler RM, Ellis JR, Eden M. Analysis of emission tomographic scan data: limitations imposed by resolution and background. *J Comput Assist Tomogr* 1984;8:514–522.
15. Kojima A, Matsumoto M, Takahashi M, et al. Effect of spatial resolution on SPECT quantification values. *J Nucl Med* 1989;30:508–514.
16. Bergstrom M, Eriksson L, Bohm C, et al. Correction for scattered radiation in a ring detector positron camera by integral transformation of the projections. *J Comput Assist Tomogr* 1983;7:42–50.
17. Logan J, Bernstein HJ. A Monte Carlo simulation of Compton scattering in positron emission tomography. *J Comput Assist Tomogr* 1983;7:316–320.
18. Hoffman EJ, Huang SC, Phelps ME, et al. Quantification in positron emission computed tomography: 4. Effect of accidental coincidences. *J Comput Assist Tomogr* 1981;5:391–400.
19. Budinger TF, Derenzo SE, Greenberg WL, et al. Quantitative potentials of dynamic emission computed tomography. *J Nucl Med* 1978;19:309–315.
20. Hoffman EJ, van der Stee M, Ricci AR, et al. Prospects for both precision and accuracy in positron emission tomography. *Ann Neurol* 1984;15:S25–S34.
21. Links JM, Zubieta JK, Meltzer CC, et al. Influence of spatially heterogeneous background activity on "hot object" quantitation in brain emission computed tomography. *J Comput Assist Tomogr* 1996;20:680–687.
22. Raylman RR, Kison PV, Wahl RL. Capabilities of two- and three-dimensional FDG-PET for detecting small lesions and lymph nodes in the upper torso: a dynamic phantom study. *Eur J Nucl Med* 1999;26:39–45.
23. Hutton BF, Hudson HM, Beekman FJ. A clinical perspective of accelerated statistical reconstruction. *Eur J Nucl Med* 1997;24:797–808.
24. Liang Z, Turkington TG, Gilland DR, et al. Simultaneous compensation for attenuation, scatter and detector response for SPECT reconstruction in three dimensions. *Phys Med Biol* 1992;37:587–603.
25. Zeng GL, Gullberg GT, Tsui BMW, et al. 3D iterative reconstruction algorithm with attenuation and geometric point response corrections. *IEEE Trans Nucl Sci* 1991;38:693–702.
26. Tsui BMW, Frey EC, Zhao X, et al. The importance of accurate 3D compensation methods for quantitative SPECT. *Phys Med Biol* 1994;39:509–530.
27. Hudson HM, Larkin RS. Accelerated image reconstruction using ordered subsets of projection data. *IEEE Trans Med Imag* 1994;13:601–609.
28. Bailey DL, Hutton BF, Walker PJ. Improved SPECT using simultaneous emission and transmission tomography. *J Nucl Med* 1987;28:844–851.
29. Ficaro EP, Fessler JA, Shreve PD, et al. Simultaneous transmission/emission myocardial perfusion tomography. *Circulation* 1996;93:463–473.
30. Jaszczak RJ, Greer KL, Floyd CE, et al. Improved SPECT quantification using compensation for scattered photons. *J Nucl Med* 1984;25:893–900.
31. King MA, Hademenos GJ, Glick SJ. A dual-photopeak window method for scatter correction. *J Nucl Med* 1992;33:605–612.
32. Links JM. Scattered photons as "good counts gone bad": are they reformable, or should they be permanently removed from society? [Invited Editorial]. *J Nucl Med* 1995;36:130–132.
33. Mueller SP, Polak JF, Kijewski MF, et al. Collimator selection for SPECT brain imaging: the advantage of high resolution. *J Nucl Med* 1986;27:1729–1738.
34. Phelps ME, Huang SC, Hoffman EJ, et al. An analysis of signal amplification using small detectors in positron emission tomography. *J Comput Assist Tomogr* 1982;6:551–565.
35. Meltzer CC, Zubieta JK, Links JM, et al. MR-based correction of brain PET measurements for heterogeneous gray matter radioactivity distribution. *J Cereb Blood Flow Metab* 1996;16:650–658.
36. Bergstrom M, Boethius J, Eriksson L, et al. Head fixation device for reproducible position alignment in transmission CT and

positron emission tomography. *J Comput Assist Tomogr* 1981;5: 136–141.

37. Mazziotta JC, Phelps ME, Meadors AK, et al. Anatomical localization schemes for use in positron computed tomography using a specially designed headholder. *J Comput Assist Tomogr* 1982;6: 848–853.

38. Kearfott KJ, Rottenberg DA, Knowles RJR. A new headholder for PET, CT, and NMR imaging. *J Comput Assist Tomogr* 1984; 8:1217–1220.

39. Meltzer CC, Bryan RN, Holcomb HH, et al. Anatomical localization for PET using MR imaging. *J Comput Assist Tomogr* 1990; 14:418–426.

40. Dann R, Hoford J, Kovacic S, et al. Evaluation of elastic matching system for anatomic (CT, MR) and functional (PET) cerebral images. *J Comput Assist Tomogr* 1989;13:603–611.

41. Fox PT, Perlmutter JS, Raichle ME. A stereotactic method of anatomical localization for positron emission tomography. *J Comput Assist Tomogr* 1985;9:141–153.

42. Pelizzari CA, Chen GTY, Spelbring DR, et al. Accurate three-dimensional registration of CT, PET, and/or MR images of the brain. *J Comput Assist Tomogr* 1989;13:20–26.

43. Hamilton RJ, Blend MJ, Pelizzari CA, et al. Using vascular structure for CT-SPECT registration in the pelvis. *J Nucl Med* 1999;40: 347–351.

44. Bowsher JE, Johnson VE, Turkington TG, et al. Bayesian reconstruction and use of anatomical *a priori* information for emission tomography. *IEEE Trans Med Imag* 1996;15:673–686.

45. Maini CL, de Notaristefani F, Tofani A, et al. Tc-MIBI scintimammography using a dedicated nuclear mammograph. *J Nucl Med* 1999;40:46–51.

46. Links JM. Multidetector single-photon emission tomography: are two (or three or four) heads really better than one? [Review Article]. *Eur J Nucl Med* 1993;20:440–447.

47. Dahlbom M, Hoffman EJ, Hoh CK, Schiepers C, et al. Whole-body positron emission tomography: part I. Methods and performance characteristics. *J Nucl Med* 1992;33:1191–1199.

48. Martin WH, Delbeke D, Patton JA, et al. FDG-SPECT: correlation with FDG-PET. *J Nucl Med* 1995;36:988–995.

49. Delbeke D, Patton JA, Martin WH, et al. FDG PET and dual-head gamma camera positron coincidence detection imaging of suspected malignancies and brain disorders. *J Nucl Med* 1999;40: 110–117.

50. Yu SK, Nahmias C. Single-photon transmission measurements in positron tomography using Cs-137. *Phys Med Biol* 1995;40: 1255–1266.

51. Karp JS, Muehllehner G, Qu H, et al. Singles transmission in volume-imaging PET with a Cs-137 source. *Phys Med Biol* 1995;40: 929–944.

52. Benard F, Smith RJ, Hustinx R, et al. Clinical evaluation of processing techniques for attenuation correction with Cs-137 in whole-body PET imaging. *J Nucl Med* 1999;40: 1257–1263.

53. Bengel FM, Ziegler SI, Avril N, et al. Whole-body positron emission tomography in clinical oncology: comparison between attenuation-corrected and uncorrected images. *Eur J Nucl Med* 1997; 24:1091–1098.

54. Zimny M, Kaiser HJ, Cremerius U, et al. Dual-head gamma camera FDG positron emission tomography in oncological patients: effects of non-uniform attenuation correction on lesion detection. *Eur J Nucl Med* 1999;26:818–823.

3

RADIOPHARMACEUTICALS IN ONCOLOGY

SHANKAR VALLABHAJOSULA

ONCOLOGY AND NUCLEAR MEDICINE

Cancer is a group of diseases in which a variety of disorders with different pathophysiologic mechanisms result from a series of changes in genes that control cell growth and behavior. Cancerous growth often depends on complete or partial block of the differentiation pathway, so that the transformed cell is trapped in a relatively undifferentiated, highly proliferated cell compartment. In general, a cancer cell has lost its ability to function normally and control its growth and division. Tumor grading, which estimates differentiation, is thus an indicator of the degree of malignancy. In addition, the vascularity and perfusion of tumors are different from those of normal tissues. As tumors grow, their own blood supply develops. However, as the tumor enlarges, cells in the periphery are well perfused, while the core of the tumor is relatively avascular and hypoxic. An exponential inverse relationship exists between blood flow and tumor mass (1).

By the time a human tumor is clinically recognizable, it has gone through the greater part of its growth. By the time a tumor is palpable or visible on a radiograph, it has a mass of 1 g and 10^9 cells (2). In general, the smaller the tumor at the time of diagnosis, the better the prognosis. The majority of the tumors, however, go undetected until patients present with clinical symptoms.

Noninvasive Imaging

The challenge of an imaging technique is to demonstrate the morphology (structure and tissue characterization) and functional status of tumor tissue. Tumors are classified on the basis of tissue of origin, cell type, whether they are benign or malignant, degree of differentiation, anatomic site, and function. Because of this diversity, no single imaging technique is capable of detecting all tumors. Although radiologic techniques (roentgenography, computed tomography, magnetic resonance imaging, ultrasonography) can delineate the location and size of a tumor and provide better resolution than nuclear imaging techniques, they lack specificity and sometimes cannot even distinguish residual, viable disease from fibrosis. Nuclear medicine techniques, on the other hand, have the potential to indicate the functional status of tumor tissue (metabolism, receptor expression) and are more specific, but with limited resolution. A number of radiopharmaceuticals (Table 3.1) have been designed and developed during the last three decades to image and identify unique biochemical characteristics of tumor tissue. However, most of the radiopharmaceuticals used in oncology are either organ-, tissue-, or receptor-specific, but not necessarily tumor-specific (3). Despite this lack of absolute tumor specificity, nuclear techniques can still provide important information regarding diagnosis and staging, detection of relapse or residual disease, response to therapy, and prognosis for a variety of tumors.

Radionuclide Therapy

Since 1936, when Dougherty and Lawrence first introduced ^{32}P for the treatment of leukemia, the use of radiopharmaceuticals to deliver therapeutic doses of ionizing radiation has been extensively investigated. Conventional radiotherapy plays a major role in the treatment of cancer in a specific region in the body, but it is not useful for the treatment of widespread metastases. In addition, conventional radiotherapy or brachytherapy has no role in the treatment of micrometastases. In contrast, targeted radionuclide therapy by systemic administration of a radiopharmaceutical has the potential to treat widely disseminated cancer tissue. A number of radiopharmaceuticals (Table 3.2) are now available to treat various malignancies or palliate the pain caused by bony metastases. Monoclonal antibodies and peptide ligands labeled with a variety of radionuclides emitting either β or α particles having different energies and ranges in tissue are being developed for the treatment of bulky disease or micrometastases. The most important factors that influence the tumor localization of therapeutic radiopharmaceuticals include the chemical and biochemical nature of the carrier molecule transporting the radionuclide of choice to the tar-

S. Vallabhajosula: Division of Nuclear Medicine, Department of Radiology, New York Presbyterian Hospital–Weill Cornell Medical Center, New York, New York 10021.

TABLE 3.1. RADIOPHARMACEUTICALS FOR DIAGNOSTIC IMAGING STUDIES IN ONCOLOGY

Radiopharmaceutical	Application	Specific tumors
^{123}I- or ^{131}I-sodium iodide	Thyroid function	Differentiated thyroid cancer
^{123}I- or ^{131}I-MIBG	Adrenergic tissue	Pheochromocytoma, Neuroendocrine tumors and APUDomas, neuroblastomas
^{131}I-NP-59	Cholesterol metabolism	Adrenal carcinoma, adenoma, Cushing's syndrome
^{123}I-IBZM	Dopamine D_2 receptors	Malignant melanoma
^{123}I-VIP	VIP receptors	Gastrointestinal tumors
^{67}Ga citrate	Tumor viability and Infection	Lymphoma, hepatoma, lung cancer, melanoma
^{111}In-OncoScint	Colorectal	Colorectal and ovarian cancer
^{111}In-ProstaScint	Anti-PSMA antibody	Prostate cancer
^{111}In-pentetreotide	Somatostatin receptors	Neuroendocrine tumors, medullary thyroid cancer
^{201}Tl-thallous chloride	Tumor viability	Brain tumors, osteosarcoma, parathyroid and thyroid metastases
^{99m}Tc-CEA scan	Anti-CEA antibody	Colorectal cancer
^{99m}Tc-P829 peptide	Somatostatin receptors	Lung cancer, neuroendocrine tumors
^{99m}Tc-sestamibi, -tetrafosmin	Tumor viability and MDR (Pgp expression)	Breast cancer, parathyroid adenoma, brain tumor
^{18}F-FDG	Glucose metabolism	Head and neck cancers, lymphoma, lung cancer
^{11}C-thymidine	DNA synthesis	Brain tumors
^{11}C-methionine	Amino acid transport	Brain tumors, pancreas
^{18}F-fluoromisonidazole	Hypoxia and oxidative metabolism	Tumors selected for radiotherapy

MIBG, metaiodobenzyguanidine; NP-59, 6B-iodomethyl-19-norcholesterol; IBZM, iodobenzamide; VIP, vasoactive intestinal peptide; CEA, carcinoembryonic antigen; FDG, fluorodeoxyglucose; PSMA, prostate-specific membrane antigen; MDR, multidrug resistance; Pgp, P-glycoprotein; APUD, amine precursor uptake and decarboxylation.

geted area. Tumor-specific radiopharmaceuticals that are clinically useful in the noninvasive imaging of tumors are being modified to treat tumors.

RADIOPHARMACEUTICALS

Radionuclides

Physical Characteristics

Various radionuclides used for diagnostic and therapeutic application in oncology are listed in Tables 3.3, 3.4, and 3.5.

Radionuclides that decay by isomeric transition (IT), electron capture (EC), or positron emission are used for diagnostic imaging studies, whereas radionuclides that decay by emission of β and α particles are used for therapy. Among the radioisotopes of iodine, ^{123}I, with a short half-life and 159-keV gamma photon, is ideal for diagnostic studies. Recently, ^{124}I, with β⁺ emission (Table 3.4),has been explored in positron emission tomography (PET) with radioiodinated antibodies and DNA substrates. ^{111}In is the most suitable nuclide to label antibodies and proteins because its physical half-life is close to the biologic half-life of antibodies, whereas

TABLE 3.2. RADIOPHARMACEUTICALS FOR THERAPY

Radiopharmaceutical	Application	Specific tumors
^{131}I-sodium iodide	Thyroid function	Differentiated thyroid carcinoma
^{131}I-MIBG	Adrenergic tissue	Pheochromocytoma and other neuroendocrine tumors
^{125}I-5-iodo-2'-deoxyuridine	Cell proliferation	Colorectal cancer metastatic to liver and bladder cancer
^{131}I-anti-B1 antibody	anti-CD22 antigen	Lymphoma
^{90}Y-MX-DTPA-anti-B1 antibody	anti-CD22 antigen	Lymphoma
^{32}P-chromic phosphate (colloid)	Cell proliferation and protein synthesis	Peritoneal metastases, recurrent malignant ascites
^{32}P-orthophosphate	Cell proliferation and protein synthesis	Polycythemia vera
^{89}Sr chloride	Exchanges with Ca in bone	Palliation of pain of bony metastases
^{153}Sm-EDTMP	Binds to hydroxyapatite	Palliation of pain of bony metastases
^{117m}Sn-DTPA	Binds to hydroxyapatite	Palliation of pain of bony metastases
^{186}Re-HEDP	Binds to hydroxyapatite	Palliation of pain of bony metastases
^{90}Y-DOTA-Tyr^3-octrotide	Somatostatin receptor	Neuroendocrine tumors
^{90}Y-DOTA-lanreotide	Somatostatin receptor	Neuroendocrine tumors

MIBG, metaiodobenzyguanidine; DTPA, diethylenetriaminepentaacetic acid; HEDP, hydroxyethylidene diphosphoric acid; DOTA, 1,4,7,10-tetraazacyclododecane-*N,N',N'',N'''*-tetraacetic acid; EDTMP, ethylenediaminetetramethyl phosphonate.

TABLE 3.3. RADIONUCLIDES FOR DIAGNOSTIC STUDIES IN NUCLEAR ONCOLOGY

Nuclide	Half-life (h)	Decay mode	Photon energy (keV)	Abundance τ emission (%)
^{99m}Tc	6	IT	140	89
^{131}I	193	β⁻, τ	364	81
^{123}I	13	EC	159	83
			33 (Te x-rays)	
^{67}Ga	78	EC	93, 185, 300, 394	37, 20, 17,5
			10 (Zn x-rays)	
^{111}In	67	EC	171, 245	90, 94
			26 (Cd x-rays)	
^{201}Tl	73	EC	135, 167	3, 20
			80 (Hg x-rays)	100 (x-rays)

EC, electron capture.

TABLE 3.4. POSITRON-EMITTING RADIONUCLIDES USED IN ONCOLOGY

Nuclide	Half-life (min)	β⁺ Decay (%)	Energy of particles (MeV) β⁺ E$_{max}$	Photon	β⁺ Range (mm)
^{11}C	20.4	99.8	0.96	0.511	4.1
^{13}N	10	100	1.2	0.511	5.1
^{15}O	2.07	99.9	1.7	0.511	7.3
^{18}F	110	96.9	0.63	0.511	2.4
^{124}I	4.2 d	25	1.6, 2.2	0.511	
^{64}Cu	0.54 d	39, 19	0.578, 0.65	0.511	
^{68}Ga	68.3	90	1.9	0.511	

TABLE 3.5. RADIONUCLIDES FOR THERAPY IN ONCOLOGY

Nuclide	Half-life (d)	Decay mode	Energy (MeV) Max	Average	Range in tissue (mm) Max	Mean	τ Photon (MeV)	Abundance (%)
^{90}Y	2.67	β⁻	2.28	0.935	12.0	2.76	None	
^{188}Re	0.71	β⁻	2.12	—	10.8	2.43	155	15
^{32}P	14.3	β⁻	1.71	0.695	8.7	1.85	None	
^{89}Sr	50.5	β⁻	1.49	0.58	8.0	—	None	
^{186}Re	3.77	β⁻	1.08	0.35	5.0	0.92	137	9
^{153}Sm	1.95	β⁻	0.81	0.225	3.0	0.53	103	29
^{131}I	8.04	β⁻	0.61	0.20	2.4	0.4	364	81
^{67}Cu	2.58	β⁻	0.57	—	—	0.27	92, 185	11 and 49
^{177}Lu	6.7	β⁻	0.497	0.133	—	—	208	11
^{117m}Sn	13.6	β⁻	0.16	—	—	—	159	87
^{213}Bi	45.6 min	α	8.0 (98%)		< 0.1	—	440	17
^{212}Bi	60.6 min	α	6.0 (36%)		70.0 μm	—	727	7
			9.0 (64%)					
^{211}At	0.30	α	6.0 (42%)		65.0 μm	—	670	0.3
		α	7.5 (58%)					
^{125}I	60.3	EC	0.4 keV (Auger e⁻)		10.0 nm		25–35 keV	

Ec, electron capture.

^{99m}Tc is the nuclide of choice for imaging studies with molecules that have a faster blood clearance, such as chelates, peptides, and antibody fragments.

^{131}I, with an 8-day half-life and β⁻ emission, is the isotope of choice for therapy; ^{125}I, with a longer half-life ($t_{1/2}$, 60 days), EC decay mode, and low-energy (25 to 35 keV) photons, also may be useful for therapy. A number of β-emitting nuclides with varying β particle energies and path lengths are available for therapy, and the choice of a specific nuclide depends on the molecule being labeled and the size and location of tumor tissue. Among these radionuclides, ^{90}Y and ^{186}Re are currently being investigated for radioimmunotherapy.

Production of Radionuclides

All the radionuclides used in nuclear medicine for diagnosis and therapy are produced artificially, either in reactors or accelerators (Table 3.6). Radionuclide generators are designed to separate daughter radionuclides with a shorter half-life from a parent with a longer half-life that was originally produced in a reactor or cyclotron. Radionuclides decaying by β- emission are generally produced in a reactor either by fission of ^{235}U or by neutron capture reactions (n,τ or n,p) involving the absorption of a thermal neutron by a stable element. Radionuclides decaying by EC or β⁺ are produced in an accelerator such as cyclotron, where accelerated protons with high energies (projectiles) interact with a stable nuclide (target). When a stable atom absorbs a proton, the resulting radionuclide decays by EC or positron emission. The production of radionuclides with a high atomic number, such as ^{123}I, ^{67}Ga, ^{111}In, and ^{201}Tl, requires cyclotrons with high-energy protons (> 30 MeV), whereas nuclides with a low atomic number, such as ^{11}C, 13N, ^{15}O, and ^{18}F, can be produced with low- or medium-energy protons (10 to 20 MeV).

Chemistry

A number of radiopharmaceuticals with different physical and chemical properties that are routinely used for diagnosis and therapy of tumors are summarized in Tables 3.1 and

TABLE 3.6. PRODUCTION OF RADIONUCLIDES

Source	Radionuclide	Nuclear reaction	
Reactor			
	^{131}I	^{235}U(n, fission)^{131}I, *or* ^{130}Te(n, τ)^{131}Te $\xrightarrow{\beta-}$ ^{131}I	
	^{32}P	^{31}P(n,τ)^{32}P, *or* ^{32}S(n,p)^{32}P	
	^{67}Cu	^{67}Zn(n,p)^{67}Cu	
	^{177}Lu	^{176}Lu(n,τ)^{177}Lu	
	^{89}Sr	^{88}Sr(n,τ)^{89}Sr	
	^{186}Re	^{185}Re(n,τ)^{186}Re	
	^{153}Sm	^{152}Sm(n,τ)^{153}Sm	
	^{117m}Sn	^{117}Sn(n,n'τ)^{117m}Sn	
Accelerator/ cyclotron			
	^{123}I	^{124}Xe(p,2n)^{123}Cs $\xrightarrow[5.9 \text{ min}]{EC}$ ^{123}Xe $\xrightarrow[2.08 \text{ h}]{EC}$ ^{123}I ^{127}I (p,5n) ^{123}Xe $\xrightarrow[2.08 \text{ h}]{EC}$ ^{123}I	
	^{67}Ga	^{67}Zn(p,n)^{67}Ga	
	^{111}In	^{111}Cd(p,n)^{111}In	
	^{201}Tl	^{203}Tl (p,3n)^{201}Pb→^{201}Tl	
	^{11}C	^{14}N(p,α)^{11}C	
	^{13}N	^{16}O(p,α)^{13}N, *or* ^{13}C(p,n)^{13}N	
	^{15}O	^{14}N(d,n)^{15}O, *or* ^{15}N(p,n)^{15}N	
	^{18}F	^{20}Ne(d,α)^{18}F, *or* ^{18}O(p,n)^{18}F	
	^{124}I	^{124}Te(d,2n)^{124}I	
	^{211}At	^{207}Bi(α,2n)^{211}At	
	^{64}Cu	^{64}Ni(p,n)^{64}Cu	
Generator			
	^{99m}Tc	^{235}U(n, fission)^{99}Mo $\xrightarrow[66 \text{ hr}]{\beta-}$ ^{99m}Tc	^{99}Mo generator
	^{68}Ga	^{68}Ge $\xrightarrow[271 \text{ d}]{EC}$ ^{68}Ga	^{68}Ge generator
	^{90}Y	^{235}U(n, fission)^{90}Sr $\xrightarrow[28.8 \text{ y}]{\beta-}$ ^{90}Y	^{90}Sr generator
	^{188}Re	^{187}W(n,τ)^{188}W $\xrightarrow[69.4 \text{ d}]{\beta-}$ ^{188}Re	^{188}W generator
	^{212}Bi	^{228}Th$\xrightarrow{\text{decay chain}}$ ^{224}Ra → ^{212}Pb $\xrightarrow[10.64 \text{ h}]{\beta-}$ ^{212}Bi	^{224}Ra generator
	^{213}Bi	^{229}Th$\xrightarrow{\text{decay chain}}$ ^{225}Ac $\xrightarrow[10 \text{ d}]{\alpha}$ ^{221}Fr $\xrightarrow{\alpha}$ ^{217}At $\xrightarrow{\alpha}$ ^{213}Bi	^{225}Ac generator

3.2. The clinical utility of a particular radiopharmaceutical, however, depends on the specific application and tumor type. To understand the specific mechanisms involved in the tumor localization of these radiopharmaceuticals, it is important to appreciate both the similarities and the differences in the chemistry of many of these agents. Basically, the radiopharmaceuticals can be grouped into three major categories: (a) radioiodine and iodinated agents, (b) radiometals and metal–chelate complexes, and (c) positron radiopharmaceuticals.

Radioiodine and Radioiodinated Compounds

Iodine belongs to group VIIA of the periodic table of elements. Stable iodine 127, with atomic number 53, has 74 neutrons and occurs with 100% natural abundance. Radioisotopes of iodine have been extensively used in a number of radiopharmaceuticals for diagnosis and therapy. As a halogen, iodine has a valence of 1. Radionuclides of iodine are usually supplied as a salt, sodium iodide (I^-). ^{123}I- or ^{131}I-sodium iodide is supplied as a solution or in the form of capsules. Air and radiolytic free radicals oxidize iodide to volatile iodine. To prevent these reactions, radioiodide solutions are mixed with sodium ascorbate or thiosulfate and maintained at an alkaline pH of between 7.5 and 9.0. ^{123}I as sodium iodide is used mainly for imaging studies of the thyroid, but ^{131}I is the radionuclide of choice for the treatment of hyperthyroidism and thyroid cancer.

Because iodine can form strong covalent bonds with carbon, it is relatively easy to prepare radiopharmaceuticals with radioiodine. For radioiodination methods involving nucleophilic reactions, radioiodide can be used without any modification. However, electrophilic radioiodination requires oxidation of iodide to molecular iodine (I_2). The choice of an appropriate method for radioiodination depends on the type of molecule to be iodinated and the desired specific activity (MBq/μmol).

1. Isotope exchange is the method of choice for the routine preparation of many radiopharmaceuticals. In a nucleophilic reaction, radioiodination is performed by substituting a radioactive iodine atom for an iodine atom of the nonradioactive analogue. ^{123}I- or ^{131}I-MIBG (metaiodobenzylguanidine) and ^{131}I-NP-59 (^{131}I-6β-iodomethyl-19-norcholesterol) are prepared by means of this technique (4,5). Exchange labeling is generally preferred when very high specific activities are not required and these reactions can be carried out in an aqueous solvent or in a solid phase.

2. In electrophilic substitution reactions, radioiodination is performed by using molecular iodine ($I_2 = I^+ + I^-$), which is generated by mild oxidation of radioiodide with oxidizing agents such as peracetic acid (obtained by mixing hydrogen peroxide and acetic acid), chloramine T, iodogen, or lactoperoxidase enzyme. A number of peptides (^{123}I-Tyr-octreotide, ^{123}I-vasoactive intestinal peptide) (6) and mon-

oclonal antibodies (^{131}I-labeled B1 antibody) (7) are labeled with radioiodine for both diagnostic and therapeutic applications. This technique was originally developed to radioiodinate tyrosine residues in proteins and peptides, in which the radioiodine atom is attached at an *ortho* position relative to the hydroxyl group on the aromatic ring. As a result, the radioiodinated peptides and proteins are unstable *in vivo*, and more than 50% of radioiodine is dehalogenated and excreted as free radioiodide or as a low-molecular-weight radioiodinated antibody fragment. To minimize *in vivo* dehalogenation, an indirect radioiodination technique can be used in which the radioiodine is attached to the lysine residues in proteins. In the most common method, either the *N*-succimidyl-3-(4-hydoxyphenyl)-propionate (Bolton-Hunter) reagent or *N*-succimidylbenzoate reagent is used after being labeled with radioiodine by means of chloramine T, which results in a *meta* substitution of radioiodine in the aromatic ring. The radioiodinated succinimide ester is then conjugated to amino groups of lysine residues of proteins, such as antibodies (8).

Radiometals and Their Chelates

A number of ligands and chelates are labeled with radionuclides of various metals (Tables 2.1 and 2.2). To understand the chemistry of these agents, the similarities among these metals must be understood. In the periodic table of elements, technetium and rhenium belong to group VIIA; gallium, indium, and thallium belong to group IIIB; and yttrium belongs to group IIIA.

Chemistry of Technetium 99m Radiopharmaceuticals

^{99m}Tc, generated by the decay of ^{99}Mo, is isolated from the fission fragments of ^{235}U in a reactor. Following elution of $^{99}Mo \rightarrow \, ^{99m}Tc$ generator with physiologic saline solution, ^{99m}Tc is obtained in chemical form as an anion, pertechnetate ($^{99m}TcO_4^-$), with a highest possible oxidation state of +7. The specific activity of ^{99m}Tc is very high, and typically, 10 to 20 mCi represents only a few nanograms.

As pertechnetate, ^{99m}Tc is chemically stable and does not bind to any ligand directly. However, because technetium is a transition metal, it is capable of existing in multiple oxidation states and forms stable complexes with a number of chelating agents. Complexing of ^{99m}Tc with ligands and chelating agents requires reduction of ^{99m}Tc to a lower oxidation state with reducing agents such as stannous chloride, which can provide electrons to pertechnetate. The reduced ^{99m}Tc (+1 to +6 oxidation level) can then form a complex with molecules (ligand or chelating agent) containing nitrogen (amine), oxygen (carboxyl or hydroxyl), or sulfur (thiol) atoms. The most common chelating agents are methylene diphosphonate (MDP), diethylenetriamine pentaacetic acid (DTPA), and dimercaptosuccinic acid (DMSA) (Fig. 3.1).

The preparation of a ^{99m}Tc complex can be one- or two-step process. In a direct labeling technique, the reduced

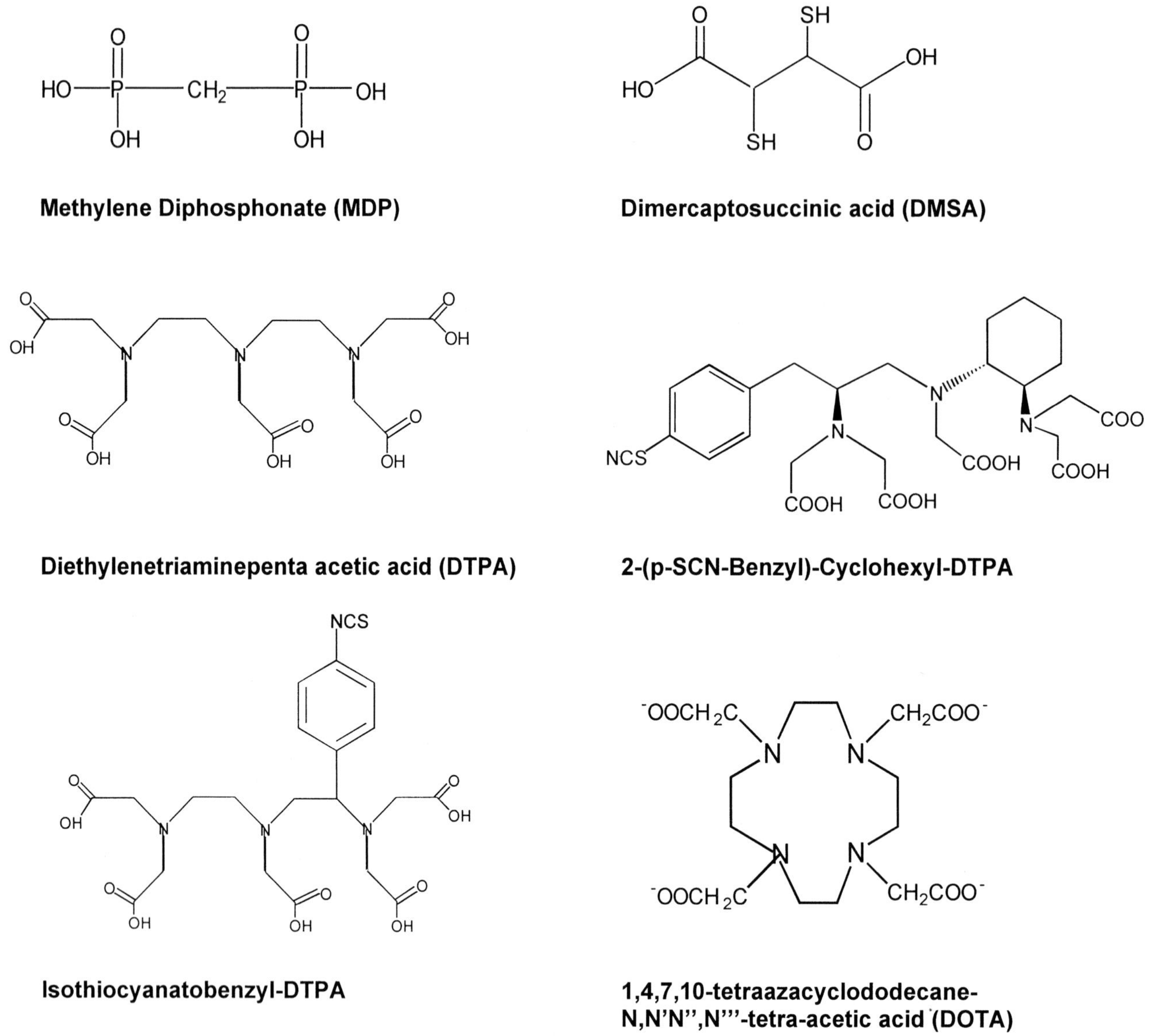

Methylene Diphosphonate (MDP)

Dimercaptosuccinic acid (DMSA)

Diethylenetriaminepenta acetic acid (DTPA)

2-(p-SCN-Benzyl)-Cyclohexyl-DTPA

Isothiocyanatobenzyl-DTPA

**1,4,7,10-tetraazacyclododecane-
N,N'N'',N'''-tetra-acetic acid (DOTA)**

FIGURE 3.1. Chelating agents used to complex a number of radiometals.

^{99m}Tc complexes with strong coordinating chelating agents such as MDP, DMSA, or DTPA in the presence of a reducing agent. ^{99m}Tc-MDP is a neutral complex, and ^{99m}Tc-DTPA is a polar molecule with a net negative charge. ^{99m}Tc can form a complex with DMSA either in a trivalent state (renal agent) or in a pentavalent form (tumor-imaging agent). In an exchange labeling technique, the reduced ^{99m}Tc forms a complex with a weak coordinating ligand (such as citrate) first, and then the ^{99m}Tc transchelates to a strong coordinating ligand, such as MAG-3 (mercaptoacetyl glycl glycl glycine), MIBI (methoxyisobutylisonitrile), or tetrofosmin. The exchange labeling technique requires less stannous ion; the mixture is heated in a boiling water bath for 10 to 15 minutes.

To label antibodies with ^{99m}Tc, the direct labeling technique is used, in which ^{99m}Tc forms stable complexes with sulfur-containing amino acids. In an antibody molecule, the thiol groups are in the oxidized, disulfide form and are not available for labeling with ^{99m}Tc. In the presence of mild reducing agents, such as stannous ion or mercaptoethanol, free thiols can be exposed to form a stable complex with ^{99m}Tc. Arcitumomab (CEA-Scan) is a ^{99m}Tc-labeled Fab' fragment of IMMU-4, an anti-CEA (carcinoembryonic antigen) antibody of the IgG1 class specific for CEA. The reduction of the F(ab')$_2$ to Fab' fragment exposes the disulfide groups in such a manner as to enhance direct and stable binding with ^{99m}Tc in the presence of stannous chloride (9).

Because the chemistry of rhenium is similar to that of technetium, a number of radiopharmaceuticals of ^{186}Re and ^{188}Re are being developed for therapy. ^{186}Re-labeled antibodies and peptides and ^{186}Re-HEDP for the treatment of bone pain caused by metastases are under clinical investigation.

Chemistry of Group III Metal Complexes

Radionuclides of gallium (^{67}Ga, ^{68}Ga), ^{111}In, ^{201}Tl, and ^{90}Y are extensively used in diagnostic and therapeutic studies in oncology. As members of group III, these four metals have a valence of 3 and three possible oxidation states (+1, +2, +3). However, for gallium, indium, and yttrium, the trivalent ion is most stable in aqueous solution. These metal ions form insoluble hydroxides in aqueous medium, depending on the pH. At acidic pH, the +3 oxidation state is more important for indium and gallium, which exist in the hexacoordinated form with water and are soluble. As the pH is increased, they tend to precipitate as insoluble hydroxides, such as $In(OH)_3$ and $Ga(OH)_3$. At pH 8, gallium even forms a gallate ion, $Ga(OH)_4^-$. The precipitation of these metals in aqueous media can be prevented if they first form complexes with ligands such as citrate, acetate, and tartrate at acidic pH and then the pH is slowly increased to physiologic levels. The radiopharmaceutical ^{67}Ga citrate contains citrate ligand that can keep the gallium in solution even at pH 8. Similarly, ^{111}In acetate and ^{90}Y acetate are the preferred radiochemical forms used for labeling with peptides and antibodies conjugated with bifunctional chelating agents. In the presence of strong chelating agents with a higher affinity for metals, the radionuclides leave the weak ligands and bind to the strong chelates, which can provide higher coordination sites. Hexadentate polycarboxylic acids such as DTPA and EDTA (ethylenediaminetetraacetic acid) chelates have been successful with gallium and indium.

For the preparation of ^{111}In-pentetreotide (Octreoscan), the carboxyl group of the DTPA molecule is first conjugated to the amine group of the amino acid D-phenylalanine of the octreotide molecule (10). Subsequently, radiolabeling with ^{111}In is accomplished following the addition of ^{111}In chloride in acetate buffer to DTPA-octreotide conjugate (10 μg). To develop ^{111}In-labeled monoclonal antibodies (OncoScint and ProstaScint), Cytogen has developed a site-specific conjugation technique with use of a glycyl-tyrosyl-lysyl (GYK)-DTPA linker, which is attached to the antibody sugars through the glycine amine group (11,12).

For the preparation of ^{90}Y-labeled therapeutic peptides and antibodies, DTPA is not an ideal chelating agent. Yttrium is better bound by octadentate coordinating ligands such as 1,4,7,10-tetraazacyclododecane-*N,N′,N″,N‴*-tetraacetic acid (DOTA), a macrocyclic agent (13). A number of DTPA and DOTA analogues have been developed (Fig. 3.1) to label peptides and proteins with different radiometals.

Positron Radiotracers

The most common positron-emitting radionuclides useful for the preparation of radiopharmaceuticals for PET imaging studies are listed in Table 3.4. One major advantage of the PET technique, in comparison with conventional nuclear medicine imaging techniques, is that the positron-emitting radionuclides, such as ^{11}C, ^{13}N, and ^{15}O, can replace natural carbon, nitrogen, and oxygen in biologically active biochemicals. In particular, ^{11}C can be used to label any organic molecule, but the 20-minute half-life is suboptimal for the synthesis of radiotracers. By comparison, the relatively longer half-life of ^{18}F (110 minutes) is adequate for the synthesis of many ^{18}F radiotracers. Unlike the resolution of planar and single-photon emission computed tomography (SPECT) imaging techniques, that of PET imaging technology is inversely dependent on the energy of the positron. Therefore, ^{18}F can provide the best resolution (2.4 mm) among the positron radiotracers. In addition, ^{18}F is also very useful to label many biochemicals because fluorine can readily be substituted for a hydrogen atom or hydroxyl group in a molecule without the loss of biologic activity. ^{18}F-Fluorodeoxyglucose (FDG) and ^{18}F- or ^{11}C-labeled amino acids are the most frequently used radiotracers for PET imaging studies in oncology.

The nuclear reactions commonly used to produce positron emitters in a cyclotron are shown in Table 3.6. ^{18}F as fluoride ion is most commonly produced in a cyclotron with use of a proton beam and a water target containing the enriched ^{18}O stable isotope ($H_2{}^{18}O$). ^{18}F$^-$ fluoride ion is incorporated into an organic molecule via nucleophilic substitution reactions. In the preparation of FDG, ^{18}F$^-$ ion interacts with tetraacetylmannose triflate and replaces the triflate group. Following acid hydrolysis, removal of the protective acetyl groups results in the formation of FDG (14). ^{18}F can also be produced as elemental fluorine gas with use of a deuteron beam and neon gas (^{20}Ne) containing a trace of F_2. The product, $^{18}F_2$, can be used to prepare electrophilic ^{18}F fluorinating agents to label a number of aliphatic and aromatic compounds. The other ^{18}F-labeled radiotracers commonly used include amino acids, estradiol, and imidazole analogs.

^{11}C as carbon dioxide or methane is produced in a cyclotron with a proton beam and natural nitrogen gas or a mixture of nitrogen and hydrogen as the target material. ^{11}C-carbon dioxide can be used to label organic molecules via Grignard reactions, or it can be quickly converted to $^{11}CH_3I$ (methyl iodide), which is commonly used to attach $^{11}CH_3$ (methyl) groups to either a nitrogen (*N*-alkyl) or an oxygen (*O*-alkyl) atom in an organic molecule (15). For example, L-[*S*-methyl-^{11}C]methionine is prepared by alkylation of the sulfide anion of L-homocysteine with ^{11}C-iodomethane (16). The preparation of L-[1-^{11}C]methionine involves a reaction of ^{11}C as hydrogen cyanide (HCN) with 3-*S*-methyl-propylaldehyde, followed by hydrolysis under basic conditions and subsequent purification of the racemic mixture by means of reverse-phase high-performance liquid chromatography with a chiral eluent (17). ^{11}C-labeled amino acids and thymidine are the most commonly used positron radiotracers in oncology.

MECHANISM(S) OF RADIOPHARMACEUTICAL LOCALIZATION

The uptake and retention of radiopharmaceuticals by tumors involve many different mechanisms, which are summarized in Table 3.7. In comparison with normal cells, tumor cells have very distinct characteristics. These include (a) an increased rate of cell proliferation, (b) altered membrane transport features associated with blood vessels and tumor cells, (c) altered perfusion within the tumor, (d) altered metabolism, (e) altered expression of specific receptors for hormones, and (f) expression of specific tumor-associated antigens. Because most of the radiopharmaceuticals used in nuclear oncology are not tumor-specific, the uptake any particular tracer might include a combination of different mechanisms, as in the case of ^{67}Ga citrate. However, the unique chemistry of each radiopharmaceutical determines the manner in which it is transported and retained within the tumor. The many different mechanisms associated with tumor localization of clinically useful diagnostic and therapeutic radiopharmaceuticals have been discussed in several recent reviews (3,18).

Membrane Transport

Biologic membranes are an organized sea of lipids in a fluid state. They control the composition of the space they enclose by excluding a variety of molecules and allowing the movement of specific molecules from one side to the other by selective transport systems. The basic mechanisms by which molecules are transported across cellular membranes

TABLE 3.7. MECHANISMS OF RADIOPHARMACEUTICAL LOCALIZATION IN TUMORS

Mechanism	Radiopharmaceutical
Increased membrane transport	
Active cellular transport	Radioiodide, [99m]TcO$_4^-$, ^{201}Tl-thallous cation ^{18}F-FDG, radiolabeled amino acids
Na$^+$-K$^+$ ATPase pump	^{201}Tl-thallous cation
Simple diffusion	[67]Ga citrate, ^{99m}Tc-sestamibi and tetrafosmin
Diffusion and mitochondrial binding	^{99m}Tc-sestamibi and tetrafosmin
Facilitated diffusion	^{18}F-FDG
Increased vascular permeability within the tumor	[67]Ga citrate, radiolabeled proteins
Transport protein upregulation	^{18}F-FDG, ^{11}C-methyltyrosine, methionine
Increased cell proliferation	^{11}C-thymidine, [124]I-iododeoxyuridine
Increased tumor metabolism	^{18}F-FDG, radiolabeled amino acids
Specific receptor binding	
Somatostatin receptors	^{111}In-pentetreotide (OctreoScan), ^{99m}Tc-P829 peptide (NeoTect)
VIP receptors	^{123}I-VIP
Transferrin receptors	^{67}Ga-citrate
Estrogen receptors	16α-^{18}F-fluoro-17β-estradiol (FES)
Dopamine D$_2$ receptors	^{123}I-IBZM
LDL receptors	[131]I-6β-iodomethyl-19-norcholesterol (NP-59)
Presynaptic adrenergic reuptake	[131]I- or ^{123}I-MIBG
Specific binding to tumor antigens	
PSMA	ProstaScint
CEA	CEA-Scan
TAG-72	OncoScint
Cell surface 40-kd glycoprotein	Verluma
Tumor acidic pH	[67]Ga citrate,
Tumor hypoxia	^{18}F-fluoromisonidazole,
Physicochemical adsorption	^{99m}Tc-MDP, HDP
Phagocytosis	^{99m}Tc-colloids in RES and lymph nodes
Altered perfusion/metabolism around tumor	^{99m}Tc-MDP, HDP

LDL, low-density lipoprotein; PSMA, prostate-specific membrane antigen; CEA, carcinomembryonic antigen; TAG-72, tumor-associated glycoprotein 72; FDG, fluorodeoxyglucose; VIP, vasoactive intestinal peptide; IBZM, iodobenzamide; MIBG, metaiodobenzylguanidine; MDP, methylene diphosphonate; HDP, hydroxydiphosphonate; RES, reticuloendothelial system.

include simple diffusion, facilitated diffusion, and active mediated transport.

Active Transport

Plasma membranes contain transport systems (transporters) that involve intrinsic membrane proteins and actually translocate a molecule or ion across the membrane by binding and physically moving it. Transporters are classified on the basis of their mechanism of translocation of the substance and the energetics of the system. Transporters are specific for the substance to be transported, have defined reaction kinetics, and can be inhibited by both competitive and noncompetitive mechanisms. Active transport involves translocating a solute through a cell membrane against its concentration gradient and requires the expenditure of some form of energy. Active transport is driven either by hydrolysis of adenosine triphosphate (ATP) to adenosine diphosphate (ADP) (primary active transporters) or by utilization of an electrochemical gradient of Na^+ or H^+ (secondary active transporters) across the membrane. If the energy source is inhibited or removed, the transport system will not function.

Radioiodide and ^{99m}Tc-Pertechnetate

Thyroid tissue selectively traps certain anions, such as I^-, TcO_4^-, Br^-, and ClO_4^-, by an active transport mechanism. However, only iodide is organified by the thyroid gland to synthesize thyroid hormones; the other anions diffuse out of the gland. In addition to thyroid tissue, salivary glands, stomach, bowel, and genitourinary tract show significant uptake (secretion) of radioiodide and pertechnetate. Radioiodide is rapidly absorbed from the gastrointestinal tract after oral administration and is accumulated in thyroid tissue during the next 24 hours. This uptake may be affected by levels of thyroid-stimulating hormone, thyroid and nonthyroid medications, and the total-body pool of iodine. Normal thyroid tissue has a very high avidity for iodide, whereas thyroid cancer and metastases accumulate iodide less avidly than normal thyroid. Papillary and follicular cancers arise from the thyroid follicular cells and retain to a certain extent the ability to trap iodide. By contrast, medullary carcinoma of the thyroid arises from the parafollicular or C cells of the thyroid and does not accumulate radioiodide.

Thallous Tl 201 Chloride

Because of the similarity of thallium to alkaline earth metals, ^{201}Tl was suggested as a potential tumor-imaging agent by Lebowitz et al. in 1975 (19). The clinical utility of ^{201}Tl to image lung and thyroid malignancies was first reported in 1977 by Tonami and Hisada (20). Subsequently, the diagnostic value of ^{201}Tl imaging was established in the evaluation of brain tumors, osteosarcoma, low-grade lymphoma, Kaposi's sarcoma, and parathyroid tumors (21).

After intravenous administration, the accumulation of ^{201}Tl in the tumor is a function of tumor blood flow and increased cell membrane permeability. Based on biodistribution studies in tumor-bearing animals, Ando et al. (22) observed that ^{201}Tl is accumulated mainly by viable tumor tissue, less in connective tissue containing inflammatory cells, and minimally in necrotic tissue. These findings suggest that in comparison with ^{67}Ga, ^{201}Tl is more specific for differentiating tumors from acute inflammatory lesions. ^{201}Tl is handled by cells similarly to potassium and is concentrated in the cells by an active transport system involving the Na^+-K^+ ATPase pump within cell membranes. However, results of *in vitro* studies with erythrocytes (23) and kidney cells (24) suggest that ^{201}Tl ions substitute with a higher affinity for potassium in the activation of the ATPase-dependent Na^+-K^+ pump. In addition, the uptake of these two ions is not identical; ^{201}Tl appears to bind to two sites on ATPase, whereas potassium binds only to one site. In studies with murine Ehrlich ascites tumor cells, Sessler et al. (25) demonstrated that the cellular uptake of ^{201}Tl is inhibited by ouabain, digitalis, and furosemide, which block the Na+-K+ pump. The drug ouabain blocks only the ATPase-dependent Na^+-K^+ pump, whereas furosemide also blocks a chloride co-transport system. Sessler et al. (26) observed that the inhibition of ^{201}Tl uptake by ouabain and furosemide is additive and suggested that ^{201}Tl uptake into the cell may involve two separate transport mechanisms. In addition, even after blockade of the Na^+-K^+ ATPase and chloride transport systems, a minimal amount of ^{201}Tl is taken up by the cells, and this transport mechanism may be mediated by a calcium-dependent ion channel (26).

Diffusion and Facilitated Diffusion

The direction of movement of solutes by diffusion is always from a higher to a lower concentration; the rate is described by Fick's first law of diffusion. The initial rate of diffusion is directly proportional to the concentration of the solute. A net movement of molecules from one side to the other will continue until the concentration at each side is at chemical equilibrium. Diffusion of gases such as oxygen and carbon dioxide occurs rapidly and depends entirely on the concentration gradient. The rate of diffusion of a lipophilic substance is directly proportional to its lipid solubility and diffusion coefficient in lipids. Uncharged lipophilic molecules (fatty acids, steroids) diffuse relatively rapidly, but water-soluble substance (sugars, inorganic ions) diffuse very slowly. Passive transport or facilitated diffusion involves translocating a solute through a cell membrane down the concentration gradient, as in simple diffusion without expenditure of metabolic energy. The transport of D-glucose is facilitated, and a family of transporters (glucose permeases, or GLUT1–6) has been identified.

⁹⁹ᵐTc-Sestamibi and Tetrofosmin

A number of lipophilic, cationic ⁹⁹ᵐTc radiopharmaceuticals (sestamibi, tetrofosmin, furifosmin) were initially developed for imaging myocardial perfusion (Fig. 3.2). During cardiac imaging studies, Muller et al. (27) first observed in 1987 that ⁹⁹ᵐTc-*hexakis*-2-methoxyisobutylisonitrile (sestamibi, or MIBI) accumulates in lung tumors. Subsequently, a number of investigators reported the potential diagnostic potential of ⁹⁹ᵐTc lipophilic cationic complexes to image parathyroid adenomas, osteosarcoma, and tumors of brain, breast, lung, and thyroid.

Although ⁹⁹ᵐTc-sestamibi is cationic, similar to ²⁰¹Tl+, the transport of this agent through the cell membrane involves only passive diffusion because the transport process is temperature-dependent and nonsaturable (28). The myocardial cell uptake of ⁹⁹ᵐTc-sestamibi was initially considered to be a consequence of binding to lipid components of the cell membrane. Subsequently, it was shown that intracellular binding of ⁹⁹ᵐTc-sestamibi is mainly associated with mitochondria (29). Using cultured chicken myocytes, Piwnica-Worms et al. (30) observed that the cellular entry of ⁹⁹ᵐTc-sestamibi is related to mitochondrial metabolism and the negative inner membrane potential of the mitochondria.

The mechanisms of uptake of sestamibi, tetrofosmin, and furifosmin have been compared with that of ²⁰¹Tl in tumor cell lines (31,32). The uptake of sestamibi and tetrofosmin is temperature-dependent, and furifosmin uptake shows a slight temperature dependence. Although the ⁹⁹ᵐTc agents are associated with mitochondria, ²⁰¹Tl remains in the cytoplasmic compartment (33). Significant differences were noted between sestamibi and tetrofosmin regarding membrane transport and intracellular localization in studies performed *in vitro*. Ouabain, a cell membrane Na⁺-K⁺ ATPase inhibitor, either had no effect or increased the cellular uptake of sestamibi, whereas the cellular uptake of tetrofosmin was reduced significantly, which suggests that 20% to 30% of the uptake of tetrofosmin is mediated

by an active transport process. By contrast, more than 70% of ²⁰¹Tl uptake by the cells is inhibited by ouabain. Nigericin, a drug that causes disruption of the cell membrane and results in a secondary increase of mitochondrial inner membrane, significantly decreased the cellular uptake of ²⁰¹Tl and increased the accumulation of both sestamibi and tetrofosmin. Preincubation studies with carbonyl cyanide *m*-chlorophenylhydrazine (CCCP), an uncoupler of oxidative phosphorylation that depolarizes the mitochondrial membrane potential, suggest that whereas 90% of total sestamibi is associated with mitochondria, most of the tetrofosmin accumulates in the cytosolic fraction (32). In addition, the intracellular localization and back-diffusion or efflux of ⁹⁹ᵐTc agents differ significantly in comparison with ²⁰¹Tl⁺ intracellular retention mechanisms (32).

Dead cells do not accumulate any of these tracers, which indicates that tumor uptake of these ⁹⁹ᵐTc agents, like the uptake of ²⁰¹Tl, represents only viable and metabolically active cells. The mitochondrial retention of ⁹⁹ᵐTc-sestamibi, however, is not organ-specific or tumor-specific but appears to be a mechanism common to most tissue. The intracellular levels of Ca²⁺ in normal cells are significantly low. However, with irreversible ischemia, extracellular calcium enters the cell and is sequestered in the mitochondria, which results in mitochondrial destruction. The increased calcium concentration in mitochondria blocks the binding of ⁹⁹ᵐTc-sestamibi to mitochondria.

Multidrug Resistance and P-glycoprotein. The uptake and retention of lipophilic ⁹⁹ᵐTc cationic agents by tumor cells appear to be related to the back-diffusion or efflux of the tracer from the cell. Extensive evidence now suggests that transport of the tracer out of the tumor cell is mediated by P-glycoprotein (Pgp) (34), a 17-kd plasma membrane lipoprotein encoded by the human multidrug resistance (MDR) gene (35). In addition, mutation of p53 suppressor and p21 ras oncogenes results in an increased expression of

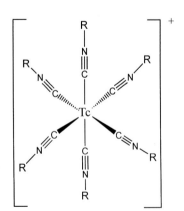

R = CH₂C(CH₃)₂OCH₃

⁹⁹ᵐTc-Sestamibi (Cardiolyte®)   ⁹⁹ᵐTc-Tetrophosmin (Myoview®)

FIGURE 3.2. ⁹⁹ᵐTc-Cationic complexes (myocardial perfusion agents) useful to image tumor tissue and P-glycoprotein expression.

MDR1 gene. Pgp is present in the cells of many normal tissues and has the ability to pump cationic and lipophilic cytotoxic and harmful agents out of the cell by an ATP-dependent process. MDR tumors often overexpress Pgp, and as result, certain chemotherapeutic agents, such as anthracyclines, taxanes, and vinca alkaloids, are pumped out of the cell (35). Piwnica-Worms et al. (36) demonstrated that sestamibi is a transport substrate for Pgp and that drugs such as cyclosporin A and verapamil, which inhibit Pgp function, enhance sestamibi accumulation to levels 8 to 10 times greater than normal. In addition, they also reported that depletion of cellular ATP increases sestamibi accumulation by tumor cells. Subsequently, several investigators (37–40) showed that tetrofosmin and furifosmin are also substrates for Pgp and compared the uptake of these tracers in several non-MDR and MDR tumor cell lines. These studies clearly suggest that sestamibi is a superior tracer to image Pgp expression and that tumor uptake of tetrofosmin is about 30% to 70% of sestamibi levels, whereas uptake of furifosmin is only about 5% to 25% of sestamibi levels. These studies also clearly suggest that the ^{99m}Tc radiopharmaceuticals may have a clinical role in imaging Pgp expression in MDR tumors and in assessing the effectiveness of chemotherapy and MDR modulators.

Gallium Ga 67 Citrate

Dudley et al. (41) first observed in the 1950s that reactor-produced ^{72}Ga citrate with low specific activity localized in osteogenic sarcoma tissue of rabbits and dogs. Subsequently, in 1969, Edwards and Hayes (42) made a serendipitous discovery that cyclotron-produced ^{67}Ga citrate with high specific activity (> 10 mCi/μg) localized in soft-tissue tumor of involved lymph nodes in a patient with Hodgkin's disease who was being evaluated for possible bone metastases. Since then, ^{67}Ga has been shown to localize in a variety of tumors and inflammatory lesions. During the last three decades, a number of investigators have reported various physical and biochemical factors responsible for the tumor uptake of ^{67}Ga citrate. However, there is still no general agreement regarding the exact mechanisms of localization in tumors, as indicated by many review articles (43–47).

Although many factors affect the biodistribution and accumulation of ^{67}Ga in tumors, its localization in tumors basically involves four major steps: (a) transport in circulation, (b) transport across vascular endothelium, (c) transport across the tumor cell membrane, and finally (d) ^{67}Ga intracellular binding and localization.

1. Transport of ^{67}Ga in circulation. Following intravenous administration of 5 to 10 mCi of carrier-free ^{67}Ga (< 3 nM) as gallium citrate, ^{67}Ga is bound exclusively to the two specific metal-binding sites of the iron-transport glycoprotein transferrin in normal plasma and is transported to normal tissues and tumor sites predominantly as ^{67}Ga–transferrin complex (48,49). Other iron-binding proteins, like lactoferrin and ferritin, can also bind ^{67}Ga with equal or higher affinity. However, because the plasma concentration of these proteins is much lower (< 2 μg/mL) than that of transferrin (2 mg/mL), ^{67}Ga is exclusively bound to transferrin in blood. The degree of ^{67}Ga binding to transferrin, however, depends on several factors. Even though gallium is regarded as an iron analogue in terms of binding to transferrin, the biodistribution and tissue localization of ^{67}Ga and ^{59}Fe are significantly different because of differences in the solubility and oxidation–reduction properties of these two metals (47). Under physiologic conditions, gallium has only one stable valence state, Ga^{3+}, whereas iron can cycle between two stable valence states, Fe^{2+} and Fe^{3+}. At the physiologic pH of 7.4, gallium exists mostly as gallate ion, $Ga(OH)_4^-$, which is very soluble, whereas Fe^{3+} tends to form insoluble polymers of iron hydroxides. Therefore, in the circulation, it is absolutely essential that iron bind to transferrin, whereas gallium can be transported as a free soluble species. The affinity of transferrin for iron is higher than that for gallium. As a result, increased iron levels in plasma can easily displace gallium from transferrin (47).

2. Transport of ^{67}Ga across vascular endothelium. The volume of distribution of ^{67}Ga in patients is about 23 L, compared with 4 L for ^{59}Fe, which suggests that gallium is extensively distributed in the extravascular space (50). While the ^{67}Ga–transferrin complex is slowly transported through the capillary vessel wall, the non–transferrin-bound free gallium rapidly leaves the blood compartment and equilibrates with the interstitial fluid of normal and tumor tissue. The increased capillary permeability and expanded extracellular space of tumor tissue would also augment the transport of macromolecules such as transferrin (80 kd) across the leakier tumor blood vessels (51). The increased transferrin concentration within the interstitial fluid of tumors (52) would also lend support to the role of increased capillary permeability in ^{67}Ga tumor localization.

3. Transport of ^{67}Ga across the tumor cell membrane. The mechanisms involved in the uptake of ^{67}Ga by tumor cells are very complex because a variety of factors appear to affect transport and retention of ^{67}Ga within the tumor tissue. However, extensive investigations during the last three decades provide evidence of two different mechanisms of ^{67}Ga transport into tumor cells.

Receptor-mediated uptake. Several investigators initially proposed that a common pathway exists for tumor cell uptake of ^{67}Ga and ^{59}Fe via a transferrin receptor, and that ^{67}Ga localization in tumors involves endocytosis of ^{67}Ga–transferrin receptor complex (53). *In vitro* studies clearly demonstrated that transferrin, at low concentrations (< 0.1 mg/mL), stimulated and increased ^{67}Ga uptake by tumor cells. However, *in vivo* studies with animal tumor models provided conflicting results regarding the role of transferrin receptors in ^{67}Ga localization (46). In addition, ^{67}Ga tumor uptake was also observed in tumor-bearing mice with a congenital absence of transferrin (hypotransferrinemia) (54). Although some evidence suggests that the number of transferrin receptors in tumor cells may be increased 10-fold in comparison with the number in normal cells (47), the exact connection between transferrin receptors and ^{67}Ga tumor uptake *in vivo* has not been established. Even the role of transferrin receptors in iron uptake by normal and neoplastic cells is not clearly understood. In a recent review summarizing the mechanisms of iron uptake by normal and neoplastic cells, Richardson and Ponka (55) reported that in addition to receptor-mediated endocytosis of Fe–transferrin, nonspecific processes such as adsorptive or fluid-phase endocytosis (pinocytosis) cause iron to accumulate in certain cells (hepatocytes, melanoma cells) by.

Simple diffusion. Based on *in vivo* studies, Hayes et al. (56) concluded that the initial entry of ^{67}Ga into tumor tissue involves mainly an unbound or loosely bound form of ^{67}Ga, whereas its uptake by normal soft tissues is strongly promoted by its binding to transferrin. Many factors that might augment the amount of free gallium species in tumor tissue would increase the transport of ^{67}Ga across tumor cell membranes by simple diffusion. The increased permeability of the tumor cell membrane in comparison with normal cells may also account for increased diffusion of non–transferrin-bound gallium species into cells. Administration of iron or scandium, which compete with ^{67}Ga for transferrin binding, increases ^{67}Ga uptake by tumor cells (56). The stability of the ^{67}Ga–transferrin complex is very much dependent on bicarbonate concentration and pH; decreasing either bicarbonate or pH would cause more ^{67}Ga to dissociate from transferrin (57) and help generate more free gallium species. The pH of the interstitial fluid of tumors is slightly acidic in comparison with that of normal tissue, and reducing tumor pH by enhancing anaerobic glycolysis in tumor-bearing rats actually increased ^{67}Ga uptake by tumors (58). In contrast, increasing ^{67}Ga binding to transferrin in blood decreased tumor uptake by indirectly decreasing the amount of free gallium available for diffusion (56).

4. Intracellular binding and localization of [67]Ga. The accumulation of ^{67}Ga within tumor cells is very much dependent on the intracellular binding of ^{67}Ga to iron-binding proteins, such as lactoferrin and ferritin, or other, higher-molecular-weight molecules that can form chelates with gallium with greater affinity and thereby prevent back-diffusion of free gallium species. The intracellular glycoprotein lactoferrin (90 kd), with a structure similar to that of transferrin, has a greater affinity for iron and gallium at acidic pH (59). Within the tumor cell, at an acidic pH environment, free ^{67}Ga species transported into the cell or generated as a result of lysosomal digestion of ^{67}Ga–transferrin complex may be bound to lactoferrin. Similarly, ferritin (450 kd), an intracellular iron storage protein, has a greater affinity for ^{67}Ga than either transferrin or lactoferrin and might act as a repository for ^{67}Ga in the tumor cell (47).

The localization of ^{67}Ga varies significantly with tumor type and is related to the degree of malignancy and the metabolic activity of cells. Clinically, certain malignancies, such as lymphoma, hepatoma, and lung cancer, are more gallium-avid than other tumor types. Although ^{67}Ga binds to transferrin, like iron, the mechanisms involved in ^{67}Ga tumor localization may include both transferrin-mediated and transferrin-independent pathways, depending on specific tumor type, metabolic rate, and relative concentrations of iron-binding proteins within the tumor (60,61).

Metabolic Substrates and Precursors

The metabolism of cancer cells is different from that of normal cells. As a result, cancer cells use more glucose than normal cells. Because of an increased rate of cell proliferation, protein and DNA synthesis is augmented, and the cancer cells must transport increased amounts of precursors, such as amino acids and nucleotides. A number of radiopharmaceuticals were developed based on the increased demand for metabolic substrates of tumor cells.

Glucose Metabolism

The increased glucose metabolism of tumor cells was initially recognized in 1925 by Warburg (62), who observed that tumor cells have increased rates of anaerobic and aerobic glycolysis in comparison with most normal tissues. Hatanaka (63) subsequently demonstrated that an increase in sugar transport occurs simultaneously with the appearance of morphologic changes in transforming cells. All cells use glucose to generate metabolic energy; glucose is transported into the cell across the plasma membrane by facilitated diffusion mediated by members of the GLUT protein family (GLUT1–6) (64). Although GLUT1 and GLUT3 are the most frequent, activation of the gene coding for the synthesis of GLUT1 is regarded as a major early marker of cellular malignant transformation (65). The oxidation of glucose is a complex process that requires reactions in both cytoplasm and mitochondria.

The initial reaction sequence, glycolysis, takes place in cytoplasm, where glucose is converted to two molecules of pyruvate. Under aerobic conditions, pyruvate enters the mitochondrion, where it is converted to actyl-CoA, which then enters the tricarboxylic acid cycle and is oxidized to carbon dioxide, effectively generating ATP molecules. However, under anaerobic conditions, this mechanism is unavailable; pyruvate is converted to lactic acid by lactate dehydrogenase and accumulates. Consequently, the pH of the tumor tissue is lightly acidic in comparison with the normal tissue pH of 7.4. Glycolysis is useful for cells with low energy requirements and as a temporary device to survive episodes of hypoxia or cope with increased energy demands. Poorly differentiated and rapidly growing tumors exhibit high rates of aerobic and anaerobic glycolysis and exhibit an increase in hexokinase activity. The highly active hexokinase bound to tumor mitochondria is in large part responsible for the increased glycolytic rate of tumors (66).

[18]F-Fluorodeoxyglucose

Many glucose analogues were investigated as potential glucose antimetabolites to inhibit glycolysis and tumor growth. In 1954, Solos and Crane (67) first used 2-deoxy-D-glucose, an analogue of D-glucose, as a substrate for the enzyme hexokinase and observed that the hexose phosphate formed is metabolically trapped and does not enter into the subsequent metabolic steps of glycolysis. Subsequently, in 1972, Coe (68) reported that 2-FDG significantly inhibits glycolysis in ascitic tumor cells. In 1977, ^{18}F-2-deoxy-2-fluoro-D-glucose (Fig. 3.3) was developed to measure local cerebral glucose utilization with PET (69). In 1980, Som et al. (70) demonstrated that FDG accumulates in a variety of transplanted and spontaneous tumors in animals. FDG-PET is now extensively used for an increasing number of clinical indications in cancer diagnosis and staging, monitoring of response to therapy, and detection of recurrence.

Like D-glucose, FDG is transported into the cell by facilitated diffusion and is phophorylated by hexokinase to FDG-6-phosphate. The enzyme glucose-6-phosphate isomerase in the next step of glycolysis does not react with FDG-6-phosphate because of very strict structural and geometric demands. As a result, the very polar FDG-6-phosphate is trapped in the cytoplasm (71). Although FDG-6-phosphate may be converted back to FDG, the enzyme glucose-6-phosphatase, responsible for this reaction, is either very scarce or absent in cancer tissue. Therefore, the cellular concentration of FDG in tumor closely represents the glycolytic activity of exogenous glucose. Hyperglycemia significantly reduces FDG uptake in tumors because high glucose levels can competitively inhibit FDG uptake by tumors. Because all cells metabolize glucose to some degree, FDG is not a tumor-specific radiotracer, and tumor uptake of FDG may not correlate strongly with the proliferation rate of all tumor types. FDG uptake is seen only in the viable part of the tumor and not in the necrotic mass. FDG accumulates in granulomatous tissue and in macrophages infiltrating the areas surrounding necrotic tumor tissue (72).

Cell Proliferation

In normal tissue, cell growth and cell death are balanced. Within tumor, growth is favored. Until recently, an increased mitotic rate, cell proliferation, and a lack of differentiation were regarded as the main factors responsible for the accelerated growth of malignant tissue. Recently, it has been shown that in most malignant tumors, apoptosis (programmed cell death) is inhibited, so that tissue homeostasis is altered (73). In addition, a great deal of evidence suggests that growth of solid tumors depends on angiogenesis, which is mediated by several angiogenic factors, such as vascular endothelial growth factor, platelet-derived growth factor, and fibroblast growth factor (74).

Most benign tumors grow slowly over a period of years, but most malignant tumors grow rapidly, sometimes at an erratic pace. In general, the growth rate of tumors correlates with their level of differentiation, and so most malignant tumors grow more rapidly than do benign tumors. Therefore, in tumor tissue, mitotic activity is increased. The number of cells in the S phase of the cell cycle is also higher in tumors than in normal tissue. As a result, the requirement for substrates (nucleotides) for DNA synthesis is increased. The measurement of nucleotide incorporation into DNA in tumor tissue *in vitro* with ^{3}H-thymidine (thymidine labeling index) indicates the rate of tumor proliferation (75).

[11]C-Thymidine and Analogues

[11]C-Thymidine (Fig. 3.4) has been used for many years as a PET tracer to image tumors of the head and neck (76). Because of the rapid metabolism of this tracer in blood, however, the tumor uptake of ^{11}C-thymidine is not optimal for imaging studies, and quantification is difficult. An analogue of thymidine, ^{125}I-5-iodo-2′-deoxyuridine (Fig. 3.4), has been developed recently by replacing the 5-methyl group with an iodine atom (77). Within the tumor cell, ^{125}I-5-iodo-2′-deoxyuridine is phosphorylated and incorporated in DNA. The tracer is stable *in vitro*, but the half-life in circulation is less than 5 minutes. The therapeutic potential of 5-iodo-2′-deoxyuridine labeled with either [123]I

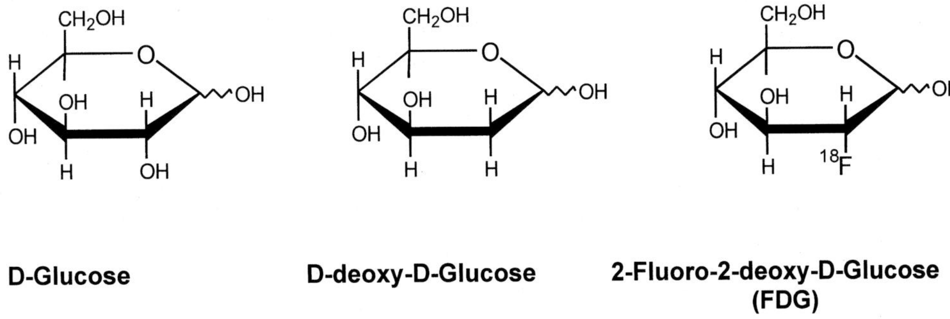

D-Glucose   **D-deoxy-D-Glucose**   **2-Fluoro-2-deoxy-D-Glucose (FDG)**

FIGURE 3.3. D-Glucose and synthetic analogues.

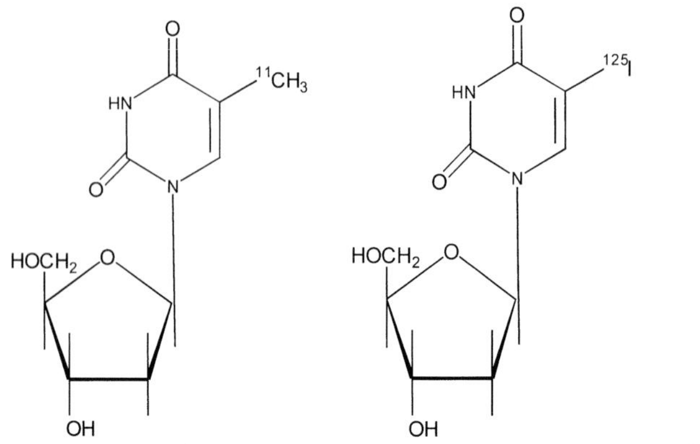

FIGURE 3.4. Radiolabeled thymidine analogues used for diagnosis and therapy.

or ^{125}I has been attributed to the Auger electron emission from these radionuclides (78).

Precursors

Radiolabeled Amino Acids

Because amino acids are the biologic building blocks of proteins, the uptake of radiolabeled amino acids within tumors may reflect the increased protein synthesis rate of proliferating tumor cells or simply an increased rate of amino acid transport across the tumor cell membrane (79). Features of an ideal radiolabeled amino acid tracer to study protein synthesis would include a rapid incorporation rate and retention in proteins, insignificant alternative metabolic pathways to nonproteins, rapid plasma clearance, a high degree of blood–brain barrier permeability in case of brain tumors, and availability of a convenient labeling procedure (80). In the last three decades, the potential clinical diagnostic utility of a number of natural amino acids, such as leucine, methionine, tyrosine, phenylalanine, and aspartate, radiolabeled with either positron-emitting radionuclides or radioiodine has been investigated (Fig. 3.5). Despite its complex biochemistry and *in vivo* metabolism, methionine has been the most widely used amino acid tracer as L-methyl-[^{11}C]methionine (81). Accumulation of this tracer much more tumor cell-specific than that of FDG, which is taken up by macrophages as well as tumor cells. The predominant mechanism of methionine uptake by tumor reflects an increased rate of active membrane transport rather than an increased rate of protein synthesis (82). Because tyrosine reflects the protein synthesis rate, a number of radiolabeled tyrosine and tyrosine analogues have been evaluated (83–85). These include L-[1-^{11}C]tyrosine, L-[2-^{18}F]fluorotyrosine, L-[4-^{18}F]fluoro-*m*-tyrosine, and L-[3-^{18}F]α-methyltyrosine. Among these tracers, L-[3-^{18}F]α-methyltyrosine is relatively easy to synthesize and displays high *in vivo* stability, with 75% of the injected dose

appearing in the unmetabolized form in the circulation (86). Recently, a tyrosine analogue, L-*O*-[2-^{18}F]fluorethyltyrosine, which is not incorporated into proteins but nevertheless is transported by an active transport mechanism, has been developed (80). ^{18}F-Fluoroalkylation with the formation of an ether bond is relatively easy to perform when starting with nucleophilic ^{18}F-fluoride. This compound is stable *in vivo*, with fast brain and tumor uptake kinetics, and the biodistribution is that of an unnatural amino acid (80). Radiolabeled natural amino acids and analogues also exhibit high uptake in normal brain tissue. A number of unnatural nonmetabolized amino acids can be used as substrates for active transport, with minimal accumulation in normal brain tissue. Labeled with positron emitters, these compounds have been investigated as tumor-imaging agents. Among them, [^{11}C]α-aminocyclobutane carboxylic acid and an ^{18}F analogue showed intense uptake in brain tumors such as astrocytomas and glioblastomas (86).

Radiolabeled Cholesterol

Plasma low-density lipoprotein (LDL) carries cholesterol to the adrenal glands. Cholesterol is the substrate for adrenal steroid hormone (cortisol and aldosterone) synthesis. In the last two decades, ^{131}I- and ^{75}Se-labeled cholesterol agents (Fig. 3.6) have been evaluated as tracers to image the adrenal cortex. In 1970, ^{131}I-19-iodocholesterol (NM-145) was first used to image a patient with Cushing's syndrome (87). Subsequently, it was discovered that the adrenal uptake of ^{131}I-6β-iodomethyl-19-norcholesterol (NP-59), a contaminant of the NM-145 preparation, was even higher (88). NP-59 soon became the agent of choice to image patients with adrenal cortical diseases. Two other analogues, ^{131}I-6-iodocholesterol (Ioderin) and ^{75}Se-β-iodomethyl-19-norcholesterol (Scintadren), have also proved clinically useful in imaging adrenal glands (89). At this time, NP-59 is available in the United States only as an investigational new drug. Typically, 18.5 to 37 MBq (0.5 to 1.0 mCi) is injected intravenously following appropriate preparation of the patient.

^{131}I-NP-59 is transported by plasma LDL and accumulates in the adrenal cortex via LDL receptors. Subsequently, it is esterified, like cholesterol, and stored intracellularly without further metabolism or incorporation into adrenocortical steroid hormones. Normal adrenal glands show bilateral symmetric uptake of NP-59. Bilateral increased adrenal uptake of NP-59 may reflect Cushing's disease [excess production of adrenocorticotropin (ACTH) by a pituitary adenoma] or ectopic secretion of ACTH. Adrenal adenoma is identified as intense unilateral uptake (90). On the other hand, adrenal carcinoma shows no uptake of NP-59. Dexamethasone, which suppresses pituitary ACTH secretion, decreases the uptake of NP-59 by the adrenal cortex, whereas intramuscular administration of ACTH increases NP-59 accumulation by the adrenal cortex. Hyperfunctioning adrenal adenoma can be imaged following dexmethasone to suppress the uptake of normal adrenal cortex.

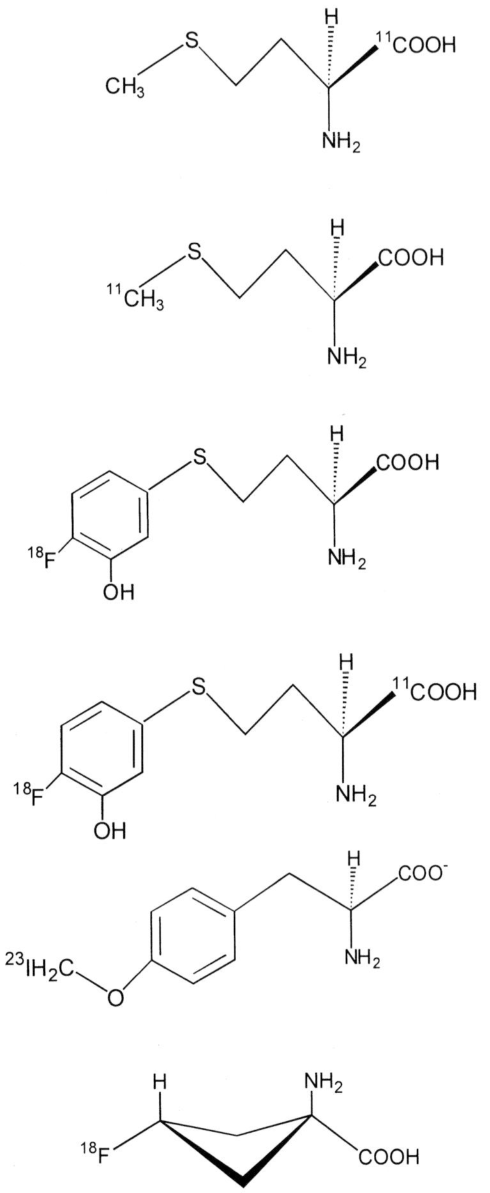

FIGURE 3.5. Radiolabeled amino acids.

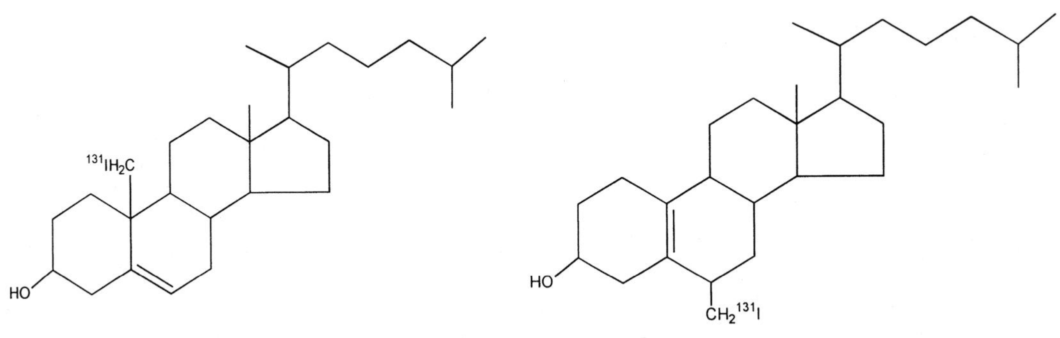

L-[^{11}C]methionine

L-[methyl-^{11}C]methionine

[1-^{11}C]tyrosine

L-[2-^{18}F]fluorotyrosine

^{123}I-α-methyl-Tyrosine

[^{18}F]-1-Amino-3-fluorocyclobutane-
1-carboxilic acid (FACBC)

[^{131}I]-19-Iodocholesterol

6β-[^{131}I]-Iodomethyl-19-Nor Cholesterol
(^{131}I-NP-59)

FIGURE 3.6. Radioiodinated cholesterol analogues.

Specific Binding to Hormone Receptors and Tumor Antigens

Two different classes of radiopharmaceuticals that are relatively more tumor-specific for imaging studies have been developed. These agents include radiolabeled peptides and antibodies with specific binding to cellular receptors or tumor-associated antigens. Although some of these radiotracers are available for routine clinical use, many other potential agents are under clinical investigation.

In 1907, J. N. Langley (91) introduced the term *receptive substance* to designate the hypothetical material in or on an effector cell with which a given agent (nicotine or adrenaline) had to react to evoke its characteristic biological response. Subsequently, Paul Ehrlich introduced the term *receptor* to describe the interaction of tetanus toxin with a specific protoplasmic site (92). The term *receptor*, however, is generally used to denote a specific cellular binding site for a small ligand, such as peptide hormones and neurotransmitters. In the case of antigen–antibody interactions, antigen expressed on a cell may be regarded as a receptor for a specific antibody. Antigen molecules may be present in or on cells and may also be secreted into the extracellular fluid and circulation.

Kinetics of "Hormone–Receptor" or "Antigen–Antibody" Interaction

The kinetics of interaction between hormone (or drug) and receptor have been well characterized. The interaction of an antibody molecule with an antigen is qualitatively and quantitatively similar to a hormone–receptor interaction. To describe the kinetics, therefore, the term *ligand* would imply hormone or antibody, and the term *receptor* could also imply antigen. Based on these interactions, major parameters have been identified that quantify receptor expression in tissue and the affinity of a ligand to a specific receptor.

Basically, the ligand (L) and receptor (R) interact to form a ligand–receptor (LR) complex, and this interaction is reversible. Based on the law of mass action, the ligand–receptor interaction is described by the following equations:

$$L + R \underset{K_2}{\overset{K_1}{\rightleftharpoons}} LR$$

1. Affinity. The strength of the bond between ligand and receptor is known as *ligand affinity*, which can be measured for any ligand–receptor interaction. The rate of association, K_1 (mol^{-1}s^{-1}), is proportional to the concentration of unreacted L and R, whereas the rate of dissociation, K_2 (s^{-1}), is proportional to the concentration of LR complex. At equilibrium, the rate of association is equal to the rate of dissociation:

$$K_1(L)(R) = K_2(LR)$$

The ratio of the two constants gives the equilibrium constant, K_a, or overall affinity of the ligand for the receptor:

$$K_a = \frac{K_1}{K_2} = \frac{(LR)}{(L)(R)}$$

The equilibrium dissociation constant, K_d, is the reciprocal of K_a ($K_d = 1/K_a$) and has units of moles or moles per liter. The K_d is a useful parameter to compare the overall affinity of different ligands for the same receptor.

2. B_{max}. The number of receptors per cell or milligrams of cellular protein is described by B_{max}, which can be calculated with the measured concentrations of L, R, and LR complex. Typically, Scatchard analysis of the data shows that the ratio of bound ligand to free ligand (B/F) decreases linearly with increasing concentration of free ligand (F), where the slope of the line represents the affinity constant (K_a). When the B/F ratio equals zero, the x-intercept represents the total receptor-binding capacity, or B_{max}.

Factors Influencing the Uptake of Receptor-binding Radiopharmaceuticals

Because the mechanism of tumor localization of receptor-binding radiopharmaceuticals is specific and depends on receptor or antigen expression of the tumor tissue, multiple factors representing many characteristics of the radiopharmaceutical influence the uptake of radiotracer in the tumor, image quality, and ultimately the clinical utility of these agents.

1. Blood clearance. Receptor-binding radiopharmaceuticals are radiolabeled synthetic analogues of peptide hormones, steroids, neurotransmitters, and drug molecules. In general, these tracers are small in size (< 5,000 d) and clear from the circulation quite rapidly, with very short plasma half-lives. In contrast, radiolabeled antibodies (150,000 d) remain in circulation for a longer period of time. The IgG class of antibodies have a relatively long plasma half-life of 20 days. Antibody fragments (Fab′) are relatively small in size (25,000 d) and have shorter plasma half-lives.

2. Specific activity. Specific activity is the amount of radioactivity per unit mass of radiopharmaceutical (mCi/mg or mCi/μg). Very high specific activity of the tracer is required for binding to receptors that are very specific for the tracer but low in concentration (high-affinity receptors) in the tumor tissue. In general, an agent with higher specific activity can be developed by radiolabeling a tracer molecule with a radionuclide having a shorter physical half-life. A more important requirement is the number of molecules of the agent (both radiolabeled and unlabeled carrier) in relation to the number of receptors or antigens in the tumor tissue. For example, the specific activity of Octreoscan (5 to 6 mCi of ^{111}In/10 μg of peptide) is higher than that of ProstaScint (5 to 6 mCi of ^{111}In/500 μg of IgG antibody molecule). However, because of differences in their molecu-

lar weights, the total number of molecules are approximately similar for both tracers.

3. Affinity of the tracer. A radiotracer may have a very high K_a (high affinity) for one receptor and a very low K_a (low affinity) for a different receptor. It is very important to understand that at very low concentrations of both radiotracer and receptor, as in the case of hormone–receptor interactions, the K_a of the radiotracer must be very high to provide sufficient binding. The higher the K_a and/or the B_{max}, the higher the B/F ratio and the greater the chance to visualize the tumor by noninvasive imaging.

4. Immunoreactivity or relative biologic potency. The ability of a tracer molecule to bind to a specific antigen or receptor in tumor tissue may be drastically affected by the type of radionuclide or by the technique of radiolabeling. For example, a peptide or an antibody molecule labeled with ^{111}In may have a higher receptor affinity than an ^{131}I-labeled agent. Similarly, radioiodination by the iodogen technique may preserve the immunoreactivity of an antibody molecule better than the chloramine T-labeling technique.

5. *In vivo* stability. Radioiodinated tracer molecules may be less stable *in vivo* than ^{111}In-labeled DTPA- or DOTA-conjugated antibodies because of dehalogenation by iodinases in tissues. In contrast, ^{111}In complexes are more stable *in vivo*. In addition, following transport into the tumor cell, ^{111}In atoms bind to intracellular proteins and are trapped within the cells.

6. Nonspecific binding. With hormone receptor-binding radiotracers, nonspecific binding is much less of a concern than with radiolabeled antibodies, which may also bind to tumor-associated antigens that have been secreted into the circulation (as in the case of CEA). In nonspecific uptake, normal tissues expressing receptors or antigens compete with specific sites in tumor tissue. Nonspecific uptake, in general, is characterized as a low-affinity, high-capacity interaction. In addition, cross-reactivity of the radiotracer with non–target-binding sites increases nonspecific uptake and decreases tumor localization of the radiotracer.

7. Blood flow and perfusion of tumor tissue. The absolute total amount of radiotracer uptake within the tumor (percentage of injected dose per gram of tissue) depends on blood flow to the tumor, tissue perfusion, capillary permeability, and diffusion of the agent within the tumor. Because of increased intratumoral pressure, diffusion of molecules within tumor tissue is more dependent on molecular size; antibody molecules have greater difficulty in penetrating into tumor tissue than do small peptides and substrate molecules.

Radiolabeled Peptides

Cells are regulated by the transmission of chemical signals or messenger molecules (endocrine, paracrine, or autocrine hormones and growth factors) that bind to a specific receptor protein on the cell membrane or to an intracellular receptor and initiate a physiologic response. In tumor cells, the expression of receptors for some of these ligands is altered significantly by cellular dedifferentiation. For example, in many neuroendocrine tumors, increased expression of receptors for somatostatin (SST) and vasoactive intestinal peptide (VIP) has been well documented (93,94). A number of receptor-binding radiopharmaceuticals have been developed to target specific receptors in tumor tissue.

Somatostatin Receptors

There are two naturally occurring bioactive somatostatin (SST) products: a 14-amino acid form (SST_{14}) and a 28-amino acid form (SST_{28}). SST is secreted throughout the body and has multiple physiologic functions, including inhibition of secretion of growth hormone, glucagon, insulin, gastrin, and other hormones secreted by the pituitary and gastrointestinal tract. The diverse biologic effects of SST are mediated through a family of G protein-coupled receptors, of which five subtypes have been identified by molecular cloning (95). Human SST receptors (SSTRs) have been identified on many cells of neuroendocrine origin (95) and on lymphocytes (96). In addition, most neuroendocrine tumors, small cell lung cancers, and medullary thyroid carcinomas express SSTRs in high densities (93,97). The expression of SSTR subtypes in human tumor tissues, however, seems to vary among different tumor types (98). Initial studies suggested that SSTR2 is the most common receptor subtype, expressed in most primary human neuroendocrine tumors. However, recent studies (98) suggest that SSTR3 and SSTR5 are also expressed by many tumors.

Somatostatin exerts an antiproliferative effect on neuroendocrine tumors by several different mechanisms, and also inhibits the release of other regulatory peptides from pituitary, intestinal, pancreatic, and other somatostatin-sensitive endocrine tissues. In addition, somatostatin displays a direct antagonism to the effect of growth factors on tumor cells (99). To improve the therapeutic effectiveness of somatostatin, a number of analogues (seglitide, octreotide, somatuline, and lanreotide) have been synthesized that have a greater biologic stability than SST_{14}. These derivatives consist of hexapeptide and octapeptide molecules (Fig. 3.7) that incorporate the biologically active core of SST_{14} (100). Structure–function studies have shown that amino acid residues Phe^7, Trp_8, Lys^9, and Thr^{10} in SST_{14} are necessary for biologic activity; residues Trp and Lys are essential, whereas Phe and Thr can undergo minor substitutions (95). The octapeptide analogues octreotide and lanreotide are used clinically as long-acting SST analogues for the treatment of neuroendocrine tumors and gastrointestinal disorders. The selectivity or relative affinity of different synthetic peptides in comparison with natural SST for different SSTRs is summarized in Table 3.8. It is important to recognize that SST_{14} binds to all five SSTR subtypes with comparable affinity. In contrast, octreotide binds with higher affinity to SSTR2, SSTR3, and SSTR5, whereas lan-

SST₁₄ $\text{Ala}^1 - \text{Gly}^2 - \text{Cys}^3 - \text{Lys}^4 - \text{Asn}^5 - \text{Phe}^6 - \textbf{\textit{Phe}}^7 - \textbf{\textit{Trp}}^8 - \textbf{\textit{Lys}}^9 - \textbf{\textit{Thr}}^{10} - \text{Phe}^{11} - \text{Thr}^{12} - \text{Ser}^{14} - \text{Cys}^{14}$
(somatostatin)

Octreotide $\text{D-Phe}^1 - \text{Cys}^2 - \textbf{\textit{Phe}}^3 - \textbf{\textit{D-Trp}}^4 - \textbf{\textit{Lys}}^5 - \textbf{\textit{Thr}}^6 - \text{Cys}^7 - \text{Thr}^8(\text{ol})$

Tyr³-Octreotide $\text{D-Phe} - \text{Cys} - \textbf{\textit{Tyr}}^3 - \textbf{\textit{D-Trp}} - \textbf{\textit{Lys}} - \textbf{\textit{Thr}} - \text{Cys} - \text{Thr}(\text{ol})$

Vapreotide $\text{D-Phe} - \text{Cys} - \textbf{\textit{Tyr}} - \textbf{\textit{D-Trp}} - \textbf{\textit{Lys}} - \textbf{\textit{Val}} - \text{Cys} - \text{Trp}$
(RC-160)

lanreotide $\text{D-}\beta\text{Nal} - \text{Cys} - \textbf{\textit{Tyr}} - \textbf{\textit{D-Trp}} - \textbf{\textit{Lys}} - \textbf{\textit{Val}} - \text{Cys} - \text{Thr}$
(Somatuline)

P829 $\text{cyclo-(N-}\alpha\text{-CH}_3)\text{Phe} - \textbf{\textit{Tyr}} - \textbf{\textit{D-Trp}} - \textbf{\textit{Lys}} - \textbf{\textit{Val}} - \text{Hcy(CH}_2\text{CO-(}\beta\text{-Dap)} - \text{Lys} - \text{Cys} - \text{Lys-NH}_2$

FIGURE 3.7. Somatostatin receptor-binding peptides.

reotide and RC-160 bind to SSTR1 through SSTR4 with comparable affinity. None of the synthetic peptides shows high-affinity binding to SSTR1.

Radiolabeled Somatostatin Peptide Analogues

1. ^{123}I-Tyr³-octreotide. Tyr³-octreotide labeled with ^{123}I was the first radiotracer introduced to image SSTR-positive tumors (101). This tracer has several drawbacks for routine clinical use: (a) ^{123}I with high specific activity is not readily available; (b) radiolabeling and purification are time-consuming; (c) *in vivo* dehalogenation and biliary excretion cause a substantial accumulation of activity in the intestines and bladder, which makes image interpretation difficult.

2. ^{111}In-DTPA-D-Phe¹-pentetreotide. To label octreotide molecules with metals like ^{111}In, octreotide is first conjugated with a DTPA molecule coupled to the α-NH₂ group of the amine terminal D-Phe¹ residue of octreotide (10). Radiotracer with high specific activity was developed by labeling DTPA-D-Phe¹-octreotide (10 μg) efficiently with 5 to 6 mCi of ^{111}In chloride in an acetate buffer. ^{111}In-DTPA-D-Phe¹-pentetreotide, or Octreoscan (Mallinckrodt, St. Louis) (Fig.

3.8), which has a high specificity for SSTRs, was the first radiolabeled peptide successfully developed to image human neuroendocrine tumors.

After intravenous administration, Octreoscan is rapidly cleared from the circulation via the kidneys (about 50% within 5 hours), so that an image with less intestinal activity is obtained than with ^{123}I-Tyr³-octreotide. Analysis of plasma and urine samples suggests that most Octreoscan activity is excreted in an unmetabolized form. The prolonged residence time of ^{111}In activity in kidneys suggests that following glomerular filtration, part of the radiolabeled peptide is actively reabsorbed in the renal tubules (97).

3. Novel peptides. Biologically active synthetic octreotide analogues have a disulfide bridge between the two cysteine amino acid residues (Fig. 3.7). Labeling these peptide analogues with ^{99m}Tc is problematic because the reducing agent (stannous ion) used in ^{99m}Tc labeling can reduce (open) the disulfide bond, which result in considerable loss of SSTR-binding affinity. To avoid the problem of a disulfide residue in a molecule, a peptide known as P-829 has been developed (Diatide, Londonderry, New Hampshire) to hold the phar-

TABLE 3.8. PEPTIDE SELECTIVITY (AFFINITY) OF CLONED HUMAN SOMATOSTATIN RECEPTORS

Peptide	Inhibition constant, K_1 or IC_{50} (nM)[a] of peptide for				
	SSTR1	SSTR2	SSTR3	SSTR4	SSTR5
Somatostatin (SST₁₄)	1.1	1.3	1.6	0.53	0.9
Octreotide	>1,000	2.1	4.4	>1,000	5.6
Lanreotide	>1,000	1.8	43	66	0.62
RC-160	>1,000	5.4	31	45	0.7

[a]Cell lines (COS-7, COS-1) transfected with hSSTR1 through 5 were incubated with ^{125}I-SST₁₄ and increasing amounts of the competing cold peptides. All SSTR subtypes bind the SST₁₄ with comparable affinity, while the affinity of synthetic SST peptide analogues differs considerably between the receptor subtypes.
SSTR, somatostatin receptor.
From Reubi JG. *In vitro* identification of vasoactive intestinal peptide receptors in human tumors: implications for tumor imaging. *J Nucl Med* 1995;36:1846–1853, with permission.

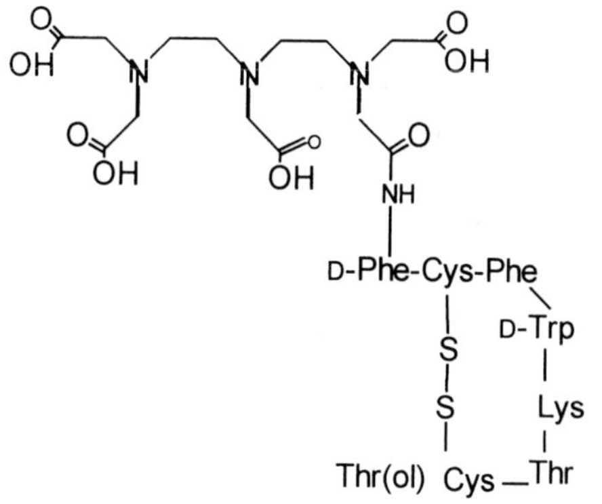

DTPA-Octreotide (OctroScan®)

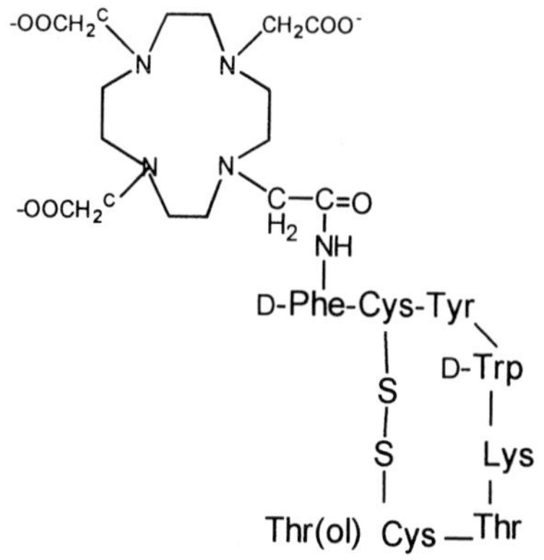

DOTA-Tyr^3-Octreotide (DOTATOC)

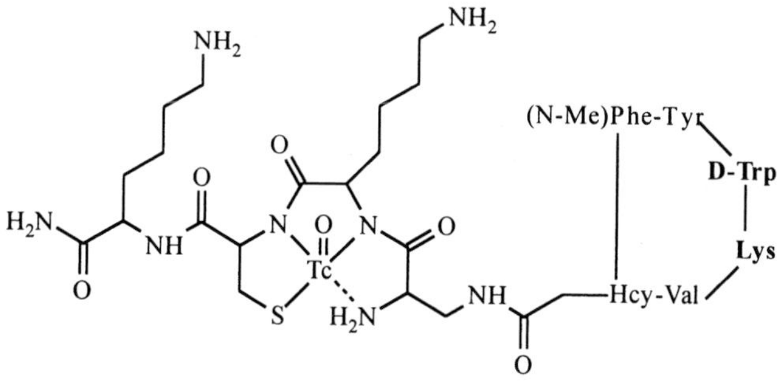

^{99m}Tc-P829 peptide (NeoTec®)

FIGURE 3.8. Somatostatin receptor-binding peptides.

macophore (the amino acid residues essential for SSTR binding) in a cyclic configuration that is not susceptible to reductive cleavage (102). In addition, a novel monoamine, bisamide, monothiol chelating sequence [(β-Dap)-Lys-Cys], was appended to the homocysteine side chain. The P-829 (Fig. 3.8) peptide can be efficiently labeled with 50 to 100 mCi of ^{99m}Tc by incubating in a boiling water bath for 15 minutes. In a rat pancreatic cell membrane assay, the inhibition constant, K_i, for P-829 peptide was 10 nM, compared with 1.6 nM for DTPA-octreotide. However, the metallocomplex, rhenium–P-829 (a molecular surrogate of technetium-P-829), has higher affinity than ^{111}In-DTPA-octreotide (0.32 vs. 1.2 nM). In preclinical studies, ^{99m}Tc-P-829 showed very high specificity for SSTR (102), and in particular specific binding to SSTR2 and SSTR3 subtypes (103). In a number of clinical studies, ^{99m}Tc-P-829 showed potential diagnostic utility to image a number of SSTR-expressing tumors (104). Recently, ^{99m}Tc-P-829 (NeoTec, Nycomed Amersham) was approved by the Food and Drug Administration to image lung tumors.

A number of other radiolabeled SSTR-binding peptides have been investigated as potential imaging agents (105–107). In addition, octreotide labeled with positron-emitting radionuclides such as ^{64}Cu, ^{68}Ga, ^{18}F, and ^{86}Y have been investigated as potential diagnostic imaging agents (108–110) and as agents to quantify biodistribution and pharmacokinetic properties related to the potential therapeutic use of appropriately labeled peptides.

Radiolabeled Octreotide Analogues for Therapy

Because of the very specific localization of octreotide analogues in neuroendocrine tumors, investigations have been undertaken of peptides coupled to radionuclides emitting low-energy x-rays (^{125}I), Auger or conversion electrons (^{111}In), or β particles (^{131}I, ^{90}Y, ^{188}Re) as therapy for neuroendocrine tumors (Table 3.5). Krenning et al. (111) reported that ^{111}In-DTPA-D-Phe^1-octreotide in high doses could be used as a therapeutic agent because of the potential antiproliferative effect of Auger and conversion electrons emitted by ^{111}In. Even though these initial studies have shown some therapeutic potential for this agent, ^{111}In emits significant τ photons that create radiation protection problems for personnel and increase the cost of patient management. In addition, for Auger electrons to deliver radiation damage that results in cell killing, the ^{111}In-labeled peptide must be internalized. Because SSTR expression is not very homogenous within tumor tissue, ^{111}In may not be an appropriate radionuclide for therapy of neuroendocrine tumors; radionuclides emitting β particles that can penetrate several millimeters in tissue may be more suitable for radiolabeled peptide therapy of neuroendocrine tumors.

1. ^{90}Y-DOTA-Tyr^3-octreotide. The peptide conjugate DTPA-D-Phe^1-octreotide can be efficiently labeled with both ^{111}In and ^{90}Y. It has been well documented that ^{90}Y-DTPA-protein complex is relatively less stable *in vivo* than ^{111}In-DTPA-protein complex, resulting in an increased accumulation of free ^{90}Y activity within bone marrow (112). By contrast, the macrocyclic DOTA chelate provides a much higher *in vivo* stability of radiolabeled proteins or peptides. Structure–activity studies suggest that substitution of the Tyr amino acid residue for the Phe^3 position in the octreotide molecule provides favorable SSTR-binding affinity of the octreotide molecule (95). Based on these chemical and pharmacologic advantages, DOTA-Tyr^3-octreotide (DOTATOC) was developed as an SST analogue for radionuclide therapy with ^{90}Y. DOTATOC (Fig. 2.8) can be labeled efficiently with ^{90}Y chloride in an acetate buffer by heating the mixture for 25 minutes at 100°C (113,114). Like Octreoscan, ^{90}Y-DOTATOC (^{90}Y-SMT-487) binds with nanomolar affinity to tumor cells *in vitro* expressing SSTR2 (Table 3.9). In animal studies, a single administration of ^{90}Y-DOTATOC (10 mCi/kg) resulted in complete remission of SSTR-positive tumors in five of seven rats bearing CA20948 pancreatic tumor (115). The potential therapeutic utility of ^{90}Y-DOTATOC is currently under clinical investigation.

2. ^{90}Y-DOTA-lanreotide. Because lanreotide binds to SSTR2 and five subtypes with equal or slightly higher affinity than octreotide, ^{90}Y-DOTA-lanreotide has been developed for the treatment of tumors expressing SSTR (116). Unlike Octreoscan, ^{111}In-DOTA-lanreotide binds to SSTR2, SSTR3, SSTR4, and SSTR5 subtypes with high affinity (K_d, 1 to 10 nM) and to SSTR1 with low affinity (K_d, 200 nM) (117), as shown in Table 3.9. The therapeutic potential of ^{90}Y-DOTA-lanreotide is also being investigated in a number of clinical trials.

Vasoactive Intestinal Peptide Receptors

Vasoactive intestinal peptide is a 28-amino acid neuroendocrine mediator with a broad range of biologic activity in diverse cells and tissues. In addition to being a vasodilator, VIP promotes growth and proliferation of normal and malignant cells (118). Cell membrane VIP receptors are widely distributed throughout the gastrointestinal tract and are also found on various other cell types. Increased VIP receptor expression has been seen in adenocarcinomas, breast cancers, melanomas, neuroblastomas, and pancreatic carcinomas (94).

^{123}I-VIP with high specific activity (150 to 200 MBq/μg) was prepared by Virgolini et al. with the iodogen method and preparative high-performance liquid chromatography (6). In clinical studies, they were able to visualize tumors in primary tumors and liver, lung, and lymph node metastases in pancreatic adenocarcinoma, colon adenocarcinoma, and gastrointestinal neuroendocrine tumors. *In vitro* receptor studies with cloned VIP receptors (transfected into COC-7 cells) clearly demonstrated that ^{123}I-VIP is bound to VIP receptors as well as unlabeled VIP (119). In addition, they observed interaction between VIP and SST on various cell types, including primary tumor cells. The high-affinity binding of ^{123}I-VIP to SSTR3 suggests that the SSTR3 receptor subtype may be the site of cross-competition between VIP and SST (119).

To label VIP with ^{99m}Tc, VIP$_{28}$ has been modified recently at the carboxyl terminus by the addition of four amino acids that provide an N$_4$ configuration. ^{99m}Tc-labeled modified VIP$_{28}$ receptor agonist showed tumor binding and VIP receptor specificity similar to that of ^{125}I-VIP (120). The tumor uptake of this tracer in nude mice bearing colorectal carcinoma was several times higher than uptake of radioiodinated VIP.

A number of other neuropeptides have been labeled with radionuclides to evaluate their potential utility as tumor-specific receptor-imaging agents. These peptides include substance P, bombesin, gastrin, cholecystokinin, calcitonin, gonadotropins, endothelin, and growth factors. Although preclinical studies have demonstrated receptor specificity of

TABLE 3.9. AFFINITY OF RADIOLABELED PEPTIDES TO CLONED HUMAN SOMATOSTATIN RECEPTORS

Peptide	Affinity, K_1 (nM)^a of peptide for				
	SSTR1	SSTR2	SSTR3	SSTR4	SSTR5
^{125}I-Tyr^{11}-SST$_{14}$	1.0	0.3	0.8	0.7	1.0
^{111}In-DTPA-octreotide	>1,000	1.5	32	>1,000	1.1
^{111}In-DOTA-lanreotide	215	4.3	5.1	3.8	10

^{a}Cell lines (COS-7) transfected with hSSTR1 through 5 were incubated with ^{125}I-SST$_{14}$, ^{111}In-DTPA-octreotide, ^{111}In-DOTA-lanreotide. Nonspecific binding was determined in the presence of 100 μM of SST$_{14}$. Control COS-7 (not transfected) cells did not show any binding of radiolabeled peptides. hSSTR, human somatostatin receptor; DTPA, diethylenetriaminepentaacetic acid; DOTA, 1,4,7,10-tetraazacyclododecane-*N*, *N'*, *N"*, *N'''*-tetraacetic acid.

some of these radiolabeled neuropeptides, their clinical utility has not yet been established.

Steroid Hormone Receptors

Sex steroid hormones (estrogen, progesterone, testosterone) bind with high affinity to intracellular receptors. The majority of breast cancers are hormone-dependent, as indicated by increased expression of intracellular estrogen or progesterone receptors. Noninvasive quantitative imaging of estrogen or progesterone receptor content in breast cancers may be useful in predicting responsiveness to hormonal therapy. Various steroidal and nonsteroidal estrogen analogues have been radiolabeled with the positron-emitting radionuclides [77]Br and [18]F. Among these tracers, 16α-[^{18}F]fluoro-17β-estradiol (Fig. 3.9) showed high affinity and selectivity for estrogen receptors *in vitro* (121). In clinical studies, PET with 16α-[^{18}F]fluoro-17β-estradiol has been shown to be highly sensitive for the detection of estrogen receptor-positive metastatic foci (122). Among several radiolabeled progesterone analogues, 21-[^{18}F]fluoro-16α-ethyl-19-norprogesterone has shown the potential to image progesterone receptors *in vivo* (121).

In the last decade, a number of radioiodinated analogues of estradiol have been evaluated for imaging estrogen receptors with planar and SPECT techniques. Recently, ^{123}I-labeled *cis*-11β-methoxy-17α-iodovinylestradiol (Z-[^{123}I]MIVE) was introduced as a radioligand to image estrogen receptor expression in breast cancers (123). Preliminary clinical studies clearly showed specific estrogen receptor-mediated accumulation of this tracer in primary and metastatic breast tumors (124). However, in previous clinical trials, the *trans* isomer (E-[^{123}I]MIVE)

was unsuccessful in detecting estrogen receptor-positive breast carcinoma.

Adrenergic Presynaptic Receptors and Storage: ^{131}I-Metaiodobenzylguanidine

Tumors arising from the neural crest share the characteristic of amine precursor uptake and decraboxylation (APUD) and contain large amounts of adrenaline, dopamine, and serotonin within secretary granules in cytoplasm. Tumors of the adrenergic system include pheochromocytomas (arising in adrenal medulla) and paragangliomas (arising in extraadrenal tissue). MIBG is an analogue of noradrenaline (Fig. 3.10) originally developed by Wieland et al. (125), who linked the benzyl portion of bretylium with the guanidine group of guanethidine. Among the three isomers of iodobenzylguanidine, the *meta* isomer (MIBG) shows less *in vivo* deiodination and liver uptake than the other two isomers (126). Specific activities for diagnostic studies are typically 107 to 148 MBq/mg (2.9 to 4.0 mCi/mg) for ^{131}I-MIBG and 111 to 259 MBq/mg (3.0 to 7.0 mCi/mg) for ^{123}I-MIBG. For therapeutic studies with ^{131}I-MIBG, higher specific activities of 15 to 40 mCi/mg are typically employed. After intravenous administration, the tracer is cleared mainly by excretion into the urine (127).

^{131}I-MIBG was initially used to image pheochromocytoma. Subsequently, ^{131}I-MIBG has been used for imaging neuroblastoma, medullary thyroid carcinoma, retinoblastoma, melanoma, and bronchial carcinoma (128). Jaques et al. (129) observed that ^{131}I-MIBG accumulates in the chromaffin cells of adrenal medulla. Because MIBG is structurally similar to noradrenaline, MIBG is believed to be transported into the cell by the reuptake pathways of the adrenergic presynaptic neurons (129,130). Within the cells, MIBG is transported into the catecholamine-storing granules by means of the ATPase-dependent proton pump. The

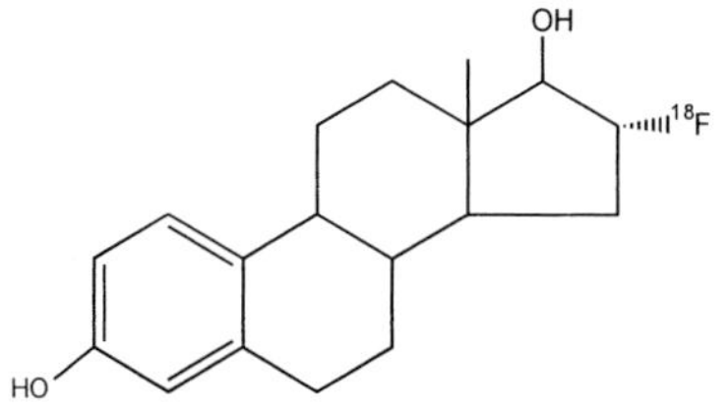

16α-[^{18}F]fluoro-17β-estradiol (FES)

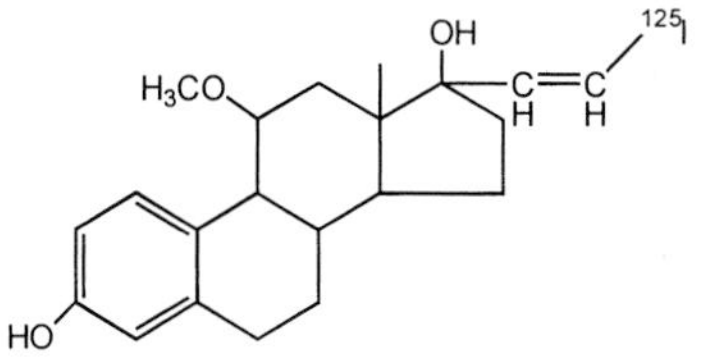

[^{123}I or ^{125}I] cis-11β-methoxy-17α-iodovinyloestradiol (Z-MIVE)

FIGURE 3.9. Steroid hormone receptor-binding radiopharmaceuticals.

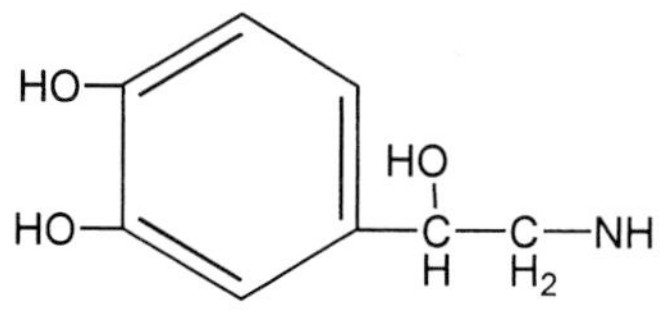

Norepinephrine

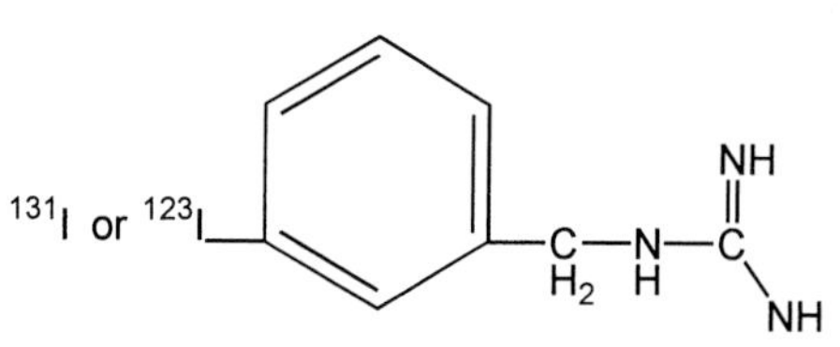

Metaiodobenzylguanidine (MIBG)

FIGURE 3.10. Adrenergic presynaptic localizing radiotracer metaiodobenzylguanidine (analogue of noradrenaline).

major difference between MIBG and noradrenaline is that MIBG does not bind to postsynaptic adrenergic receptors. Reduced ^{131}I-MIBG uptake by tumors is seen in patients using drugs like labetolol, calcium channel blockers, and antipsychotic and sympathomimetic agents (127).

Dopamine Receptors

It has been proposed that ^{123}I-IBZM (iodobenzamide), a dopamine D$_2$ receptor antagonist, is useful as a highly specific and sensitive ligand to image pituitary adenomas with SPECT (131). The presence of high-affinity dopamine D$_2$ receptors in prolactinomas and many pituitary adenomas is the rationale for the use of radiolabeled benzamide for tumor imaging. The sensitivity of ^{123}I-IBZM SPECT studies to image pituitary adenomas is rather poor because of a low target-to-background ratio. Recent clinical studies have demonstrated that another radiolabeled benzamide, ^{123}I-epidepride, provides high-quality images of pituitary adenomas (132). This may be partly a consequence of the fact that ^{123}I-epidepride is a high-affinity, irreversible dopamine D$_2$ receptor ligand (K_d, 20 to 30 pM) in comparison with IBZM (K_d, 0.3 to 1.2 nM).

Recently, radioiodinated benzamides have been proposed as highly specific and sensitive ligands for the detection of malignant melanoma (133). Dopaminergic neurons and melanoma cells are both of ectodermal origin. Melanocytes and dopaminergic neurons of the substantia nigra produce melanin. In addition, dopamine and melanin are biochemically derived from the amino acid tyrosine. The mechanism of radiolabeled benzamide localization, however, does not appear to be related to dopamine D$_2$ receptors because no evidence has been found that melanocytes exhibit dopamine receptors. It has been hypothesized that IBZM tumor uptake is the result of intracellular binding of IBZM to melanin (134). This hypothesis has been validated in a clinical study demonstrating differential accumulation of IBZM in melanotic and amelanotic melanoma metastases (134).

Radiolabeled Antibodies

Antibodies

Antibodies, also called *immunoglobulins*, are a group of glycoprotein molecules produced by B lymphocytes in response to antigenic stimulation. Each antibody binds to a restricted part of the antigen, called an *epitope*. A particular antigen can have several different epitopes. However, an antibody is specific for a particular epitope rather than the whole antigen molecule. Five distinct classes of immunoglobulins, IgG, IgA, IgM, IgD, and IgE, are recognized in most higher mammals. They differ in size, charge, amino acid composition, and carbohydrate content (135). IgG is the major immunoglobulin in human serum and may be thought of as a typical antibody. It has a molecular weight of 146,000 d and a plasma half-life of 21 days. It consists of two identical light polypeptide chains and two identical

heavy polypeptide chains linked together by disulfide bonds. The smaller (light) chain, common to all classes, is composed of a variable and a constant region with a molecular weight of 25,000 d, whereas the larger (heavy) chain has a molecular weight of 50,000 to 77,000 d and is structurally distinct for each class or subclass.

The enzyme pepsin cleaves the heavy chain of human IgG to yield the F(ab′)$_2$ and pFc′ fragments; the enzyme papain splits the IgG molecule into two Fab fragments and the Fc fragment. The Fab region binds to the antigen, and the Fc region mediates effector functions, such as complement fixation and monocyte binding (136). Almost all monoclonal antibodies used in nuclear medicine for diagnosis and therapy belong to IgG class. Monoclonal antibodies derived from mice are called *murine* monoclonal antibodies. Because the Fc portion of the murine antibody is antigenic in humans and induces the formation of human anti-mouse antibody (HAMA), chimeric antibodies are being developed in which murine variable regions of Fab′ are attached to constant regions of human IgG.

Tumor-associated Antigens

The most important requirement in developing radiolabeled antibodies for diagnosis and therapy is to identify an antigen or epitope specific to a particular type or class of cancer. Most tumor cells synthesize many proteins or glycoproteins that are antigenic in nature. These antigens may be intracellular, expressed on the cell surface, or shed or secreted from the cell into extracellular fluid or the circulation. Tumor-associated antigens, such as CEA, tumor-associated glycoprotein 72 (TAG-72), prostate-specific antigen (PSA), and prostate-specific membrane antigen (PSMA), may also be expressed in small amounts in normal cells, but typically tumor cells produce them in large amounts. Based on their source and origin, tumor-associated antigens can be categorized into five different groups (18,92).

1. Oncofetal antigens. These antigens are derived from epitopes that were expressed in fetal life and appear on tumor cells as a result of undifferentiated growth associated with the malignant process. They are not expressed in completely differentiated cells. Some of them, such as CEA and α-fetoprotein (AFP), are expressed on the cell surface and are also present in the circulation.

2. Epithelial surface antigens. These antigens are derived from cell surface structural components that are exposed because of an architectural disruption of malignant tissue. Antigens such as epithelial membrane antigen (EMA) and human milk fat globule (hMFG) are excluded from the blood by biologic barriers and are present in tumor tissue only.

3. Tumor-derived antigens. These epitopes are expressed mainly by tumor tissue, and in certain tumors, the expres-

sion of these epitopes is even increased. The antigen TAG-72 is expressed on the tumor cell surface in a variety of adenocarcinomas, such as those of colon, breast, and ovary. PSA and prostatic acid phosphatase (PAP) are secreted by prostate carcinoma cells and are present in tumor tissue and in circulation. PSMA is an integral transmembrane glycoprotein with intracellular and extracellular epitopes.

4. Receptor antigens. Tumor cells express regulator receptors that promote interaction with a number of growth factors. The receptor proteins with increased expression on tumor tissues may be regarded as receptor antigens. The human epidermal growth factor receptor (EGF-r) is a transmembrane glycoprotein that contains extracellular and cytoplasmic epitopes for EGF binding. EGF-r overexpression has been found in a variety of malignant epithelial tumors arising in breast, colon, lung, and bladder.

5. Viral antigens. These epitopes are present in certain tumor cell membranes in which the induction of malignancy is associated with the presence of transforming genes carried by DNA viruses. Congenital or acquired (as in AIDS) Epstein-Barr virus (EBV)-positive malignancies (such as Burkitt's lymphoma) are examples of receptor antigens.

Radiolabeled Antibodies

Monoclonal antibodies or antibody fragments have been labeled with a number of radionuclides for diagnostic and therapeutic applications. Several important characteristics of a number of radiolabeled antibodies (7,9,11,12,137,138) already approved by the Food and Drug Administration for diagnostic imaging studies or under clinical investigation for radioimmunotherapy are summarized in Table 3.10. Although ^{123}I, ^{99m}Tc, and ^{111}In are the preferred radionuclides for imaging studies, a number of β- and α-emitting radionuclides (Table 3.5), such as ^{131}I, ^{90}Y, and ^{188}Re, are attached to antibodies for targeted radioimmunotherapy of cancer. Radiolabeling techniques have been designed to produce radiolabeled antibodies with high specific activity while preserving the immunoreactivity of the labeled antibody. The selection of an appropriate radionuclide for diagnostic and therapeutic studies and the advantages and disadvantages of different radiolabeling techniques depend on many factors.

1. Selection of radionuclide. Because antibodies (IgG) have a long plasma half-life (21 days), it is appropriate to use radionuclides with a relatively longer half-life. ^{123}I and ^{99m}Tc are useful only when antibody fragments (such as CEA-Scan) are used for diagnostic studies. For therapeutic purposes, the choice of radionuclide depends on the size of tumor to be treated; for bulky tumors, radionuclides emitting high-energy β particles (^{90}Y, ^{186}Re, ^{131}I), which penetrate several millimeters into tumor tissue, are more appropriate than radionuclides emitting α or β particles (^{213}Bi, ^{67}Cu, ^{177}Lu) or Auger electrons (^{111}In), which have a short range and are more appropriate for treating micrometastases.

2. Radioiodination. ^{131}I is the most commonly used radionuclide for both diagnostic and therapeutic studies. Its physical half-life of 8 days is ideally suited for labeling the IgG molecule. Recently, ^{124}I, a positron emitter with a 4-day half-life, has shown diagnostic potential in tumor imaging with PET. Radioiodinated antibody with high specific activity (10 to 15 mCi/mg) can be easily prepared with the iodogen method. To avoid radiolysis, ascorbic acid, human serum albumin, or polyvinyl pyrrolidone (PVP) is added to the radioiodinated antibody and the mixture is kept frozen for several days until ready to use. Several problems are associated with radioiodination: (a) After intravenous administration, the radiotracer is not stable *in vivo* because of dehalogenation, and a major fraction of radionuclide is excreted as free radioiodide; (b) because radioiodide atoms label the tyrosine residues in the antibody molecule, it is quite possible that tyrosine residues of the variable region of the IgG molecule are labeled, which results in significant loss of immunoreactivity.

3. Labeling with radiometals. Antibody molecules can be labeled with ^{99m}Tc by either direct or indirect labeling techniques. Direct labeling involves reduction of the disulfide groups of the antibody molecule and subsequent labeling of reduced ^{99m}Tc to the sulfide moieties of antibody. This is the most common technique used to label antibody fragments, such as CEA-Scan and Verluma. Indirect labeling involves the conjugation of chelating agents, consisting of an N_2S_2 or N_2S_4 core, to complex the ^{99m}Tc atom. ^{186}Re, a chemical surrogate of ^{99m}Tc, is also attached to antibodies by indirect techniques.

Indirect labeling of antibodies with radiometals such as ^{111}In or ^{90}Y requires a bifunctional chelating agent, which is attached covalently to the antibody molecule. In developing a radiolabeled antibody that is stable *in vivo*, the choice of a chelating agent depends on the radiometal to be complexed. DTPA or isothiocyanatobenzyl-DTPA chelating agents provide high *in vivo* stability to ^{111}In-labeled antibodies. For radiometals like ^{90}Y and ^{76}Cu, however, macrocyclic bifunctional chelating agents such as DOTA and TETA (triethylenetetraamine) provide greater *in vivo* stability. To preserve the immunoreactivity of the antibody, the preferred site for conjugation of the chelating agent is the Fc segment (as in the case ProstaScint and OncoScint) of antibody because this region does not participate in antigen binding. Even random attachment of the chelating agent on the antibody appears to provide radiolabeled antibodies with high specific activity and immunoreactivity, as in the case of ^{90}Y-IDEC-Y2B8 (138). For antibodies that are internalized following binding to antigen on the cell surface, radiolabeling with ^{111}In and ^{90}Y provides greater intracellular retention of radioactivity than iodination.

4. Radiolabeling antibodies *in vivo* with biotin and streptavidin. The relatively long residence time of radiolabeled antibodies in the circulation increases the back-

TABLE 3.10. RADIOLABELED ANTIBODIES FOR DIAGNOSIS AND THERAPY

Tradename	Generic name	Epitope	Antibody	Description	Mass (mg)	Label	Activity (mCi)	Technique	Indication
OncoScint CR/OV	Satumomab pendetide	TAG-72	B72.3	Murine IgG1	1.0	^{111}In	5.0	Site-specific conjugation using DTPA	Colorectal carcinoma
ProstaScint	Capromab pendetide	PSMA (intracellular epitope)	7E-11-C5.3	Murine IgG1	0.5	^{111}In	5.0	Site-specific conjugation using DTPA	Prostate carcinoma
CEA-Scan	Arcitumomab	200-kd CEA	IMMU-4	Murine IgG1 Fab'	1.0	^{99m}Tc	20–25	Direct labeling of sulfide groups	Colorectal Carcinoma
Verluma	Nofetumomab	40-kd cell surface GP	NR-LU-10	Murine IgG2b, Fab'	5–10	^{99m}Tc	15–30	Direct labeling	Small cell lung cancer
Lympho-Scan		CD22	LL2	Murine IgG2a Fab'	0.6	^{99m}Tc	20	Direct labeling	Acute B-cell malignancy
BEXAR	Tositumomab	CD20	Anti-B1	Murine IgG2a	35	^{131}I	40–150	Iodogen labeling	Therapy of NHL
IDEC-Y2B8	Ibritumomab tiuxetan	CD20	Anti-B1	Murine IgG1	5–10	^{90}Y	32 (0.4 mCi/kg)	Random conjugation using MX-DTPA	Therapy of NHL

CEA, carcinoembryonic antigen; DTPA, diethylenetriaminepentaacetic acid; NHL, non-Hodgkin's lymphoma; MX-DTPA, 2-(4-isothiocyanatobenzyl)-6-methyl DTPA.

ground and decreases the target-to-background ratio and also increases the radiation dose to bone marrow. Antibody fragments facilitate faster clearance and decrease the residence time of radionuclide in the circulation. The increased uptake of radiolabeled fragments in the kidney, however, makes image interpretation more difficult, especially in the area of abdomen. To accelerate the clearance of radiolabeled antibodies from the circulation and improve the delivery of radionuclides to tumor tissue, biotin and streptavidin have been used in a two- or three-step process (137). Streptavidin and avidin are proteins (60 to 66 kd) with a very high affinity (K_d, 10^{-15} M) for biotin, a vitamin (244 d) (139). In a two-step method, patients are first injected with cold biotin-labeled antibodies (140). After 3 to 4 days, radiolabeled avidin is administered, which rapidly removes the circulating antibodies and binds to the pretargeted biotin–antibody complex at the tumor site. This is a very effective approach for both diagnosis and therapy. A three-step method designed specifically for imaging studies includes the following steps (141): (a) tumor pretargeting by cold biotin-labeled antibody; (b) subsequent (1 or 2 days later) administration of cold avidin to remove the circulating antibodies and avidinate the biotin–antibody complex at the tumor site; (c) administration of radiolabeled biotin, which clears rapidly from circulation and binds to the avidin–biotin–antibody complex at the tumor site. A number of clinical studies have demonstrated the advantage of this approach (142). However, because streptavidin and avidin are proteins of bacterial and plant origin, immunogenicity appears to be a major concern (141).

Tumor Hypoxia

In many tumors, oxygen-consuming tumor cell populations increase more rapidly than the oxygen-supplying functional microvasculature can expand. As a consequence, tumor hypoxia may result from either insufficient regional perfusion (acute or transient hypoxia) or insufficient oxygen diffusion (chronic hypoxia) (143). Hypoxia has a dramatic impact on malignant progression in terms of tumor spread and resistance to radiotherapy or chemotherapy. Because tumor hypoxia cannot be predicted, noninvasive techniques to identify the hypoxic fraction of tumors are being developed to optimize the planning of radiotherapy.

In 1955, Nakamura (144) discovered that 5-nitroimidazole (azomycin) is active against infections associated with anaerobic conditions. Subsequently, it was shown that changing the substitution pattern from the 5-nitro in nitroimidazole to the 2-nitro in misonidazole (MISO) increases the reduction of the molecule under slightly aerobic conditions. These compounds enter cells by diffusion. In the cytoplasm, the nitro group (NO_2) undergoes one-electron enzymatic reduction to the free radical anion. In

normoxic cells, this reaction step is reversed by intracellular oxygen, and the oxidized molecule diffuses out of the cell. In hypoxic tissue, the free radical is further reduced to a reactive species, hydroxylamine, and then to an amine (144). Free radicals are attached irreversibly to cellular macromolecules and are retained within the cell. Reduction of these molecules occurs in all tissues with viable enzymatic processes, but retention occurs only in those tissues with low oxygen tension.

A number of radiolabeled compounds incorporating a 2-nitroimidazole moiety to image tumor hypoxia have been developed (144) (Fig. 3.11). ^{77}Br-4-bromomisonidazole was the first radiotracer developed for imaging tumor hypoxia (145). ^{18}F-Fluoromisonidazole (FMISO) is probably the most extensively studied hypoxia-selective radiopharmaceutical (146). Because the blood clearance of FMISO is slow, imaging studies performed 90 minutes after the administration of the tracer provide images with limited contrast between normal and hypoxic tissue. To develop PET tracers for hypoxia imaging, radiolabeled agents of copper have been investigated because the coordination and electrochemistry are amenable to redox-mediated trapping in cells (147). One of these compounds, ^{64}Cu-ATSM (Cu-diacetyl-*bis*-N_4-methylthiosemicarbazone), has been shown to be selectively trapped in hypoxic tissue but rapidly washes out of normoxic cells (148).

Among the iodinated compounds, successful imaging of tumor hypoxia has been reported with the use of a sugar-containing MISO derivative, ^{123}I-iodoazomycin arabinoside (IAZA) (149). Significant *in vivo* deiodination, however, limits the clinical usefulness of this compound. A ^{99m}Tc-labeled hypoxic imaging agent, a propylene amine oxime derivative of 2-nitroimidazole, also known as BMS181321, showed hypoxia selectivity in tumor models but has slow clearance because of its high degree of lipophilicity (150). Recently, it has been reported that a complex of core ligands without the nitroimidazole group labeled with ^{99m}Tc also shows very high selectivity for hypoxic tumor. A prototype formulation of one of these compounds, ^{99m}Tc-HL91 (4,9-diaza-3,3,10,10-tetramethyldodecan-2,11-dione dioxime), has demonstrated uptake in a variety of tumors (151).

Miscellaneous Agents

A number of radiopharmaceuticals, such as ^{99m}Tc-sulfur colloid, ^{99m}Tc-MDP, DTPA, and MAG-3, are routinely used in nuclear medicine to assess a specific function of an organ or tissue (Table 3.11). The presence of tumor in that organ or an effect of cancer therapy may alter the normal function of the organ and, as a consequence, radiopharmaceutical uptake in that organ. The radiotracers used in these procedures may or may not actually accumulate within the tumor cells. Certain radiopharmaceuticals, such as pentavalent ^{99m}Tc-DMSA, are known to accumulate in thyroid

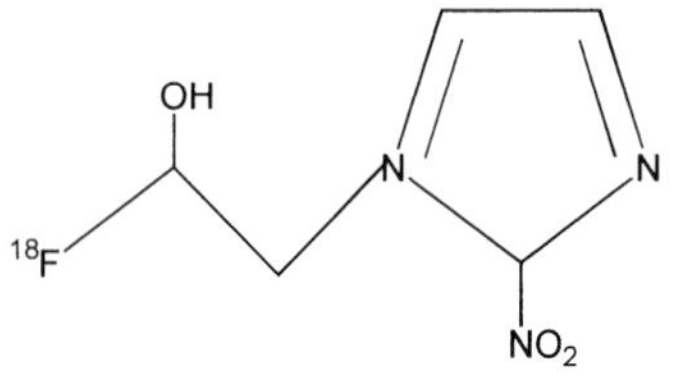

^{18}F-fluoromisonidazole (FMISO)

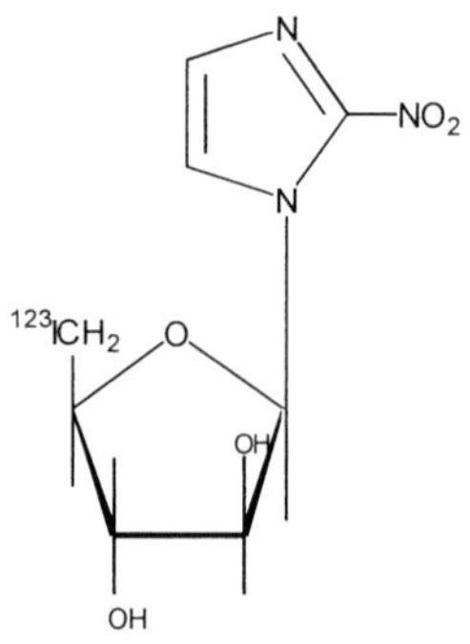

^{123}I-iodoazomycin arabinoside (IAZA)

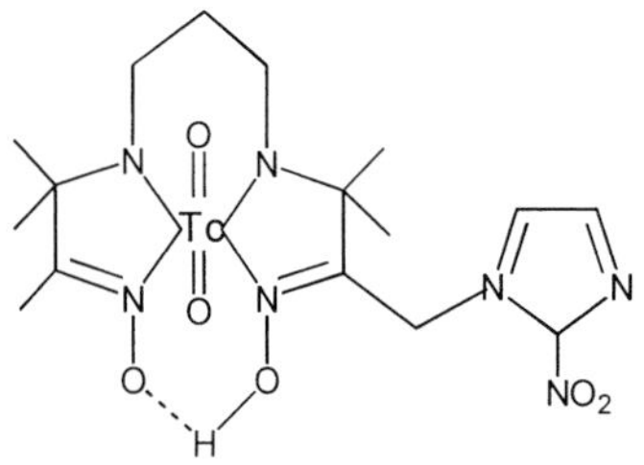

^{99m}Tc-labeled 2-nitroimidazole derivative of
propylene amine oxime chelator (BMS181321)

FIGURE 3.11. Radiolabeled hypoxia-localizing agents.

medullary carcinoma, lung cancers, and osseous metastatic tumors. The exact mechanism of uptake in the tumor, however, is not known.

^{99m}Tc-Sulfur Colloid

Particles of ^{99m}Tc-sulfur colloid are prepared by heating a mixture of sodium thiosulfate, hydrochloric acid, and ^{99m}Tc-pertechnetate for 5 minutes at 100°C. Most of the particles are in the range of 0.1 to 1.0 μm. Following intravenous administration, cells of the reticulendothelial system engulf colloidal particles and remove them from the circulation. Kupffer cells (macrophages in liver sinusoids) and reticular cells (macrophages in spleen) accumulate the particles by phagocytosis. Cold lesions identified on a liver scan with ^{99m}Tc-sulfur colloid may represent an intrahepatic tumor displacing the usual distribution of reticuloendothelial cells. Similarly, radiation damage in liver and bone mar-

TABLE 3.11 RADIOPHARMACEUTICALS FOR DIAGNOSTIC IMAGING STUDIES IN ONCOLOGY

Radiopharmaceutical	Application	Specific tumors
^{99m}Tc-colloid (SC, nanocolloid)	Reticuloendothelial function	Hepatic tumors and liver metastases
	Lymphatic drainage	Breast and melanoma
^{99m}Tc-MDP, HDP	Bone formation	Metastatic bone disease Neuroblastoma, osteosarcoma
^{99m}Tc-DTPA	Blood–brain barrier disruption	Brain tumors
^{99m}Tc-DMSA	Mechanism of uptake unknown	Medullary carcinoma of thyroid Osseous metastatic tumors
^{99m}Tc-DISIDA, Choletec	Hepatocellular function	Hepatic tumors and liver metastases
^{99m}Tc-RBC	Blood pool	Hemangioma
	Cardiotoxicity	Cancer therapy with Adriamycin

SC, sulfur colloid; MDP, methylene diphosphonate; HDP, hydroxymethylenediphosphonate; DTPA, diethylenetriaminepentaacetic acid; DMSA, dimercaptosuccinic acid; DISIDA, diisopropyliminodiacetic acid; RBC, red blood cell.

row is seen as cold areas resulting from decreased reticulendothelial system function.

Recently, ^{99m}Tc-sulfur colloid has been used extensively in lymphoscintigraphy to identify a "sentinel node" (first lymph node to receive lymphatic drainage from a tumor site) in patients with breast cancer and melanoma (152). If radiocolloid is introduced into into the interstitial fluid, it drains into the lymphatic vessels and then into regional lymph nodes. Colloidal particles smaller than 0.1 μm show rapid clearance from the interstitial space into lymphatic vessels and significant retention in lymph nodes. Normal lymph nodes appear as hot spots, but cancerous nodes do not sequester colloids, which results in false-negative identification. Because of their small particle size, ^{99m}Tc-antimony sulfide colloid (0.002 to 0.015 μm) and ^{99m}Tc-human serum albumin, or nanocolloid (0.01 to 0.02 μm), are ideal for lymphoscintigraphy studies. Because these agents are not available in United States, a filtered (with a 0.2-μm filter) preparation of ^{99m}Tc-sulfur colloid is being used for sentinel node detection (152).

Bone-seeking Radiopharmaceuticals

Bone scanning with ^{99m}Tc-labeled phosphonates (MDP, HDP) is extensively used in nuclear medicine to evaluate bone involvement or metastatic spread to bone in patients with a wide variety of cancers. These bone-seeking agents accumulate in hydroxyapatite crystal matrix as new bone is formed in response to tumor destruction of bone mineral matrix. The principal mechanism of uptake of the radiotracer is simply "physicochemical adsorption" in hydroxyapatite. Primary bone tumors like osteogenic sarcoma avidly accumulate bone agents because of the production of bone matrix in extraosseous tissue. Metastatic deposits that produce a vigorous osteoblastic response appear as hot spots in a bone scan, whereas the lesions that generate osteolytic reactions may not accumulate the bone agent (153).

The localization of bone-seeking radiotracers in increased amounts at the tumor–bone interface is the basis for the use of radionuclides in the treatment of bone pain. Several radiopharmaceuticals (Table 3.2) are indicated for relief (palliation) of pain in patients with confirmed osteoblastic bone lesions (154). However, their exact mechanism of action in relieving the pain of bone metastases is not known.

RADIOPHARMACEUTICALS TO IMAGE GENE EXPRESSION

The discovery of molecular mechanisms of carcinogenesis and significant advances in "gene therapy" and "antisense chemotherapy" have created new and exciting opportunities for the development of radiopharmaceuticals to image specific genes and gene expression in tumors. During the next 5 years, a new generation of radiotracers emitting positrons and single photons will be under intense clinical evaluation for "gene imaging" and "antisense imaging" in nuclear medicine. Several interesting mechanisms are involved in targeting these radiopharmaceuticals to localize in genetically altered tumor cells.

Two distinct classes of normal regulatory genes are involved in carcinogenesis. Oncogenes, or cancer-causing genes (such as *ras*, *erb*-B, N-*ras*, c-*myc*), are derived from protooncogenes, cellular genes that promote normal growth and differentiation. Oncogenes encode oncoproteins (growth factors, growth factor receptors, nuclear regulatory proteins), which stimulate cell division. In contrast, tumor-suppressor genes (*Rb*, *p53*, *WT-1*) counter the action of oncogenes and regulate cell growth. The loss, inactivation, or mutation of these genes may be a key event in triggering carcinogenesis.

Antisense Imaging

Oncogenes encode specific oncoproteins through the process of transcription and translation. Messenger RNA (mRNA) is a key component of this process and is present in large amounts in the cytoplasm of cells. Antisense oligonucleotides are synthetic single-strand DNA (or RNA) molecules designed to bind with high affinity to the complementary sequences of mRNA (155). Several antisense oligodeoxynucleotide pharmaceuticals have been developed as therapeutic agents that act to block protein synthesis by inactivating mRNA. To develop radiopharmaceuticals for imaging studies, oligodeoxynucleotides can be labeled efficiently with one of several radionuclides (155), such as ^{123}I, ^{99m}Tc, or ^{111}In. In 1994, Dewanjee et al. (156) developed an ^{111}In-labeled antisense oligonucleotide (15 bases long) to image c-*myc* oncogene mRNA expression. The radiolabeled oligonucleotide demonstrated specific binding to isolated mRNA *in vitro*. In addition, it was possible to image the oncogene or mRNA expression in the tumor tissue of nude mice bearing mammary adenocarcinoma. The potential of antisense imaging to quantify mRNA expression and the advantages and disadvantages of using radiolabeled oligonucleotides as probes have been the subject of recent reviews (155,157).

Gene Imaging

Gene therapy protocols in oncology are designed to manipulate the expression of genes so as to inhibit tumor growth. For example, the so-called drug sensitivity or "suicide gene therapy" protocols involve retroviral transfer of *HSV1-tk* gene to tumor cells (158). Subsequently, the gene encodes the enzyme HSV1-tk (thymidine kinase), which can selectively convert a normally nontoxic prodrug, such as ganciclovir, into a toxic compound that results in cell death (158). Based on this mechanism, several groups have recently proposed a "gene-imaging" technique to monitor and quantify gene expression, identify the optimal time to initiate treatment with the prodrug, and assess response to therapy (159,160). To image and quantify the *HSV1-tk* (marker or reporter) gene, a number of radiolabeled substrates (marker substrate or reporter probe) have been developed. Tjuvajev et al. (159) demonstrated that 5-iodo-2′-fluoro-2′-deoxy-1-β-D-arabinofuranosyluracil (FIAU) tagged with ^{131}I is potentially useful as a reporter probe for SPECT imaging of the expression of transfected *HSV1-tk* gene. Subsequently, they also developed [124]I-FIAU as a tracer for PET imaging studies (159). Compared with FIAU, acycloguanisine analogues, acyclovir, and ganciclovir (antiviral drugs) show very high specificity to the viral HSV1-tk enzyme (160). Among several labeled ganciclovir analogues, [8-^{18}F]fluoroganciclovir (FGCV) and 9-[3-^{18}F]fluoro-1-hydroxy-2-propoxymethylguanine (FHPG) have been reported recently to image gene expression *in vivo* with PET (160,161).

REFERENCES

1. Vaupel P. Oxygen supply to malignant tumors. In: Peterson HI, ed. *Tumor blood circulation: angiogenesis, vascuar morphology and blood flow of experimental and human tumors.* Boca Raton, FL: CRC Press, 1979:143–168.
2. Cleton FJ. Chemotherapy: general aspects. In: Peckham M, Pinedo HM, Veronesi U, eds. *Oxford textbook of oncology.* Oxford: Oxford University Press, 1998:445–468.
3. Britton KE, Granowska M. Tumor identification using radiopharmaceuticals. *Clin Radiol* 1997;52:731–738.
4. Wieland DM, Swanson DP, Brown LE, et al. Imaging the adrenal medulla with an I-131-labeled anti-adrenergic agent. *J Nucl Med* 1979;20:155–158.
5. Basmadjian GP, Hetzel KR, Ice RD, et al. Purity of adrenal scanning agents 19-iodocholesterol and 6-iodomethylnorcholesterol. *J Nucl Med* 1977;18:494–498.
6. Virgolini I, Raderer M, Kurtaran A, et al. Vasoactive intestinal peptide receptor imaging for the localization of intestinal adenocarcinomas and endocrine tumors. *N Engl J Med* 1994;331:1116–1121.
7. Kaminski MS, Zasadny KR, Francis IR, et al. Radioimmunotherapy of B-cell lymphoma with [^{131}I]anti-B1 (anti-CD20) antibody. *N Engl J Med* 1993;329:459–465.
8. Zalutsky MR, Narula AS. Radioiodination of a monoclonal antibodies using an *N*-succinimidyl 3-(tri-*n*-butylstannyl)benzoate intermediate. *Cancer Res* 1988;48:1446–1450.
9. Hansen HJ, Jones AL, Sharky RM, et al. Preclinical evaluation of an "instant" ^{99m}Tc-labeling kit for antibody imaging. *Cancer Res* 1990;50[Suppl]:794s–798s.
10. Bakker WH, Albert R, Bruns C, et al. [^{111}In-DTPA-D-Phe[1]]-octreotide, a potential radiopharmaceutical for imaging of somatostatin receptor-positive tumors: synthesis, radiolabeling and *in vitro* validation. *Life Sci* 1991;49:1583–1591.
11. Rodwell JD, Alvarez VL, Lee C, et al. Site-specific covalent modification of monoclonal antibodies: *in vitro* and *in vivo* evaluations. *Proc Natl Acad Sci U S A* 1986;83:2632–2636.
12. Burgers JK, Hinkle GH, Haseman MK. Monoclonal antibody imaging of recurrent and metastatic prostate cancer. *Semin Urol* 1995;13:102–112.
13. Meares CF, Moi MK, Diril H, et al. Macrocyclic chelates of radiometals for diagnosis and therapy. *Br J Cancer Suppl* 1990;10:21–26.
14. Hamachaer K, Coenen HH, Stocklin G. Efficient stereospecific synthesis of no carrier added 2-[^{18}F]fluoro-2-deoxy-D-glucose using aminopolyether-supported nucleophilic substitution. *J Nucl Med* 1986;27:235–238.
15. Crouzel C, Langstrom B, Pike VW, et al. Recommendations for a practical production of [^{11}C]methyl iodide. *Int J Appl Radiat Isot* 1987;38:601–604.
16. Langstrom B, Halldin C, Antoni G, et al. Synthesis of L- and D-methyl-^{11}C-methionine. *J Nucl Med* 1987;28:1037–1040.
17. Vaalburg W, Coenen HH, Crouzel C, et al. Amino acids for the measurement of protein synthesis *in vivo* by PET. *Nucl Med Biol* 1992;19:227–237.
18. Pauwels EKJ, McCready VR, Stoot JHMB, et al. The mechanism of accumulation of tumor-localizing radiopharmaceuticals. *Eur J Nucl Med* 1998;25:277–305.
19. Lebowitz E, Greene MW, Greene R, et al. [201]Tl for myocardial use. 1. *J Nucl Med* 1975;16:151–155.
20. Tonami N, Hisada K. Clinical experience of tumor imaging with ^{201}Tl-chloride. *Clin Nucl Med* 1977;2:75–81.
21. Elgazzar AH, Fernandez-Ulloa M, Silberstein EB. [201]Tl as a tumor-localizing agent. Current status and future considerations. *Nucl Med Commun* 1993;14:96–103.
22. Ando A, Ando I, Katayama M, et al. Biodistribution of Tl-201 in tumor-bearing animals and inflammatory lesions-induced animals. *Eur J Nucl Med* 1987;12:567–572.
23. Gehring PJ, Hammond PB. The uptake of thallium by rabbit erythrocytes. *J Pharmacol Exp Ther* 1964;145:215–221.
24. Britton J, Blank M. Thallium activation of the (Na+-K+)-activated ATPase of rabbit kidney. *Biochim Biophys Acta* 1968;159:160–166.
25. Sessler M, Maul FD, Geck P, et al. Kinetics and mechanism of thallium uptake in malignant tumors *in vivo* and *in vitro*. In: Raynaud C, ed. *Proceedings of the 3rd World Congress of Nuclear Medicine and Biology*, Paris, August 29–September 2, 1982:2281–2284.
26. Sessler MJ, Geck P, Maul FD, et al. New aspects of cellular Tl-201 uptake: T+NA+-2CL-cotransport is the central mechanism of ion uptake. *Nucl Med* 1986;25:24–27.
27. Muller S, Guth-Tougelidis B, Creutzig H. Imaging of malignant tumors with Tc-99m-MIBI SPECT. *J Nucl Med* 1987;28:562(abst).
28. Delmon-Moingeon LI, Piwinca-Wormas D, Van den Abbeele AD, et al. Uptake of the cation hexakis (2-methoxyisobutylisonitrile)-technetium-99m by human carcinoma cell lines *in vitro*. *Cancer Res* 1990;50:2198–2202.
29. Crane P, Laliberte R, Heminway S, et al. Effect of mitochondrial viability and metabolism on technetium-99m-sestamibi myocardial retention. *Eur J Nucl Med* 1993;20:20–25.
30. Piwnica-Worms D, Kronauge JF, Chiu ML. Uptake and retention of hexakis (2-methoxyisobutyl isonitrile) technetium (I) in cultured chick myocardial cells. Mitochondrial and plasma membrane potential dependence. *Circulation* 1990;82:1826–1838.
31. De Jong M, Bernard BF, Breeman WAP, et al. Comparison of uptake of ^{99m}Tc-MIBI, ^{99m}Tc-tetrofosmin and ^{99m}Tc-Q12 into human breast cancer cell lines. *Eur J Nucl Med* 1996;23:1361–1366.
32. Arbab AS, Koizumi K, Toyama K, et al. Uptake of technetium-99m-tetrofosmin, technetium-99m-MIBI and thallium-201 in tumor cell lines. *J Nucl Med* 1996;37:1551–1556.
33. Maublant JC, Moins N, Gachon P, et al. Uptake of technetium-99m-teboroxime in cultured myocardial cells: comparison with thallium-201 and technetium-99m-sestamibi. *J Nucl Med* 1993;34:255–259.

34. Piwnica-Worms D, Chiu ML, Budding M, et al. Functional imaging of multidrug-resistant P-glycoprotein with an organotechnetium complex. *Cancer Res* 1993;53:977–984.

35. Gottesman MM, Pastan I. Biochemistry of multidrug resistance mediated by the multidrug transporter. *Ann Rev Biochem* 1993;6: 385–427.

36. Piwnica-Worms D, Chiu ML, Croop JM, et al. Enhancement of Tc-99m sestamibi accumulation in multidrug resistant (MDR) cells by cytotoxic drugs and MDR reversing agents. *J Nucl Med* 1993;34:140P(abst).

37. Ballinger JR, Bannerman J, Boxen I, et al. Technetium-99m-tetrofosmin as a substrate for P-glycoprotein: *in vitro* studies in multidrug-resistant breast tumor cells. *J Nucl Med* 1996;37: 1578–1582.

38. Crankshaw CL, Marmion M, Luker GD, et al. Novel technetium (III)-Q complexes for functional imaging of multidrug resistance (MDR-1) P-glycoprotein. *J Nucl Med* 1998;39: 77–86.

39. Bernard BF, Krenning EP, Breeman WAP, et al. ^{99m}Tc-MIBI, ^{99m}Tc-tetrofosmin and ^{99m}Tc-q12 *in vitro* and *in vivo*. *Nucl Med Biol* 1998;25:233–240.

40. Hendrikse NH, Franssen EJ, van der Graaf WT, et al. ^{99m}Tc-sestamibi is a substrate for P-glycoprotein and the multi-drug resistance-associated protein. *Br J Cancer* 1998;77:353–358.

41. Dudley HC, Maddox GE, La Rue HC. Studies of the metabolism of gallium. *J Pharmacol Exp Ther* 1949;96:135–138.

42. Edwards CL, Hayes RL. Tumor scanning with ^{67}Ga citrate. *J Nucl Med* 1969;10:103–105.

43. Anghileri LJ, Heidbreder M. On the mechanism of accumulation of ^{67}Ga by tumors. *Oncology* 1977;34:74–77.

44. Larson SM. Mechanism of localization of gallium-67 in tumors. *Semin Nucl Med* 1978;8:193–204.

45. Hoffer P. Gallium: mechanisms. *J Nucl Med* 1980;21:282–285.

46. Tsan MF, Scheffel U. Mechanism of gallium-67 accumulation in tumors. *J Nucl Med* 1986;27:1215–1219.

47. Weiner RE. The mechanism of ^{67}Ga localization in malignant disease. *Nucl Med Biol* 1996;23:745–751.

48. Vallabhajosula SR, Harwig JF, Siemsen JK, et al. Radiogallium localization in tumors: blood binding and transport and the role of transferrin. *J Nucl Med* 1980;21:650–656.

49. Sephton RG. Relationships between the metabolism of ^{67}Ga and iron. *Int J Nucl Med Biol* 1981;8:323–331.

50. Logan KJ, Ng PK, Turner CJ, et al. Comparative pharmacokinetics of ^{67}Ga and ^{59}Fe in humans. *Int J Nucl Med Biol* 1981;8: 271–276.

51. Tzen KY, Oster ZH, Wagner HN Jr, et al. Role of iron-binding proteins and enhanced capillary permeability in the accumulation of gallium-67. *J Nucl Med* 1980;21:31–35.

52. Guillino PM, Clark SH, Grantham FH. The interstitial fluid of solid tumors. *Cancer Res* 1964;24:780–793.

53. Larson SM, Rasey JS, Allen DR, et al. Common pathway for tumor cell uptake of gallium-67 and iron-59 via a transferrin receptor. *J Natl Cancer Inst* 1980;64:41–53.

54. Sohn MH, Jones BJ, Whiting JH Jr, et al. Distribution of gallium-67 in normal and hypotransferrinemic tumor-bearing mice. *J Nucl Med* 1993;34:2135–2143.

55. Richardson DR, Ponka P. The molecular mechanisms of the metabolism and transport of iron in normal and neoplastic cells. *Biochim Biophys Acta* 1997;1331:1–40.

56. Hayes RL, Rafter JJ, Byrd BL, et al. Studies of the *in vivo* entry of Ga-67 into normal and malignant tissue. *J Nucl Med* 1981;22: 325–332.

57. Vallabhajosula SR, Harwig JF, Wolf W. Effect of pH on tumor cell uptake of radiogallium *in vitro* and *in vivo*. *Eur J Nucl Med* 1982;7:462–468.

58. Vallabhajosula S, Goldsmith SJ, Lipszyc H, et al. ^{67}Ga-transferrin and ^{67}Ga-lactoferrin binding to tumor cells: specific vs. nonspecific glycoprotein-cell interaction. *Eur J Nucl Med* 1983;8: 354–357.

59. Harris WR. Thermodynamics of gallium complexation by human lactoferrin. *Biochemistry* 1986;25:803–808.

60. Luttropp CA, Jackson JA, Jones BJ, et al. Uptake of gallium-67 in transfected cells and tumors absent or enriched in the transferrin receptor. *J Nucl Med* 1998;39:1405–1411.

61. Luttropp CA, Vu C, Morton KA. Photodegraded nifedipine promotes transferrin-independent gallium uptake by cultured tumor cells. *J Nucl Med* 1999;40:159–165.

62. Warburg O. On the origin of cancer cells. *Science* 1956;123: 309–314.

63. Hatanaka M. Transport of sugars in tumor cell membranes. *Biochim Biophys Acta* 1974;355:77–104.

64. Mueckler M. Facilitative glucose transporters. *Eur J Biochem* 1994;219:713–725.

65. Hiraki Y, Rosen OM, Birnbum MJ. Growth factors rapidly induce expression of the glucose transporter gene. *J Biol Chem* 1988;27:13655–13662.

66. Arora KK, Fancuilli M, Pedersen PL. Glucose phosphorylation in tumor cells. Cloning, sequencing, overexpression in active form of a full-length cDNA encoding a mitochondrial bindable form of hexokinase. *J Biol Chem* 1990;265:6381–6488.

67. Solos A, Crane RK. Substrate specificity of brain hexokinase. *J Biol Chem* 1954;210:581–595.

68. Coe EL. Inhibition of glycolysis in ascites tumor cells preincubated with 2-deoxy-2-fluoro-D-glucose. *Biochim Biophys Acta* 1972;264:319–327.

69. Ido T, Wan C-N, Fowler JS, et al. Fluorination with F_2. A convenient synthesis of 2-deoxy-2-fluoro-D-glucose. *J Org Chem* 1977; 42:2341–2342.

70. Som P, Atkins HL, Bandoypadhyay D, et al. A fluorinated glucose analog, 1-fluoro-2-deoxy-D-glucose (F-18): nontoxic tracer for rapid tumor detection. *J Nucl Med* 1980;21:670–675.

71. Gallagher BM, Fowler JS, Gutterson NI, et al. Metabolic trapping as a principle of radiopharmaceutical design: some factors responsible for the biodistribution of [^{18}F]2-deoxy-2-fluoro-D-glucose. *J Nucl Med* 1978;19:1154–1161.

72. Kubota R, Yamada S, Kubota K, et al. Intratumoral distribution of fluorine-18-fluorodeoxyglucose *in vivo*: high accumulation in macrophages and granulation tissues studied by microautoradiographic comparison with FDG. *J Nucl Med* 1992;33: 1872–1980.

73. Majno G, Joris I. Apoptosis, oncosis, and necrosis. An overview of the cell death. *Am J Pathol* 1995;146:3–15.

74. Folkman J, D'Amore PA. Blood vessel formation: what is the molecular basis? *Cell* 1996;87:1153–1155.

75. Livingston RB, Ambus U, George SL, et al. *In vitro* determination of thymidine-[^{3}H] labeling index in human solid tumors. *Cancer Res* 1974;34:1376–1380.

76. Goethals P, Lameire N, van Eijkeren M, et al. Methyl-carbon-11 thymidine for *in vivo* measurement of cell proliferation. *J Nucl Med* 1996;37:1048–1052.

77. Kassis AI, Adelstein SJ. Preclinical animal studies with radioiododeoxyuridine. *J Nucl Med* 1996;37[Suppl]:10s–12s.

78. O'Donoghue JA. Strategies for selective targeting of Auger electron emitters to tumor cells. *J Nucl Med* 1996;37[Suppl]:3s–6s.

79. Vaalburg W, Coenen HH, Crouzel C, et al. Amino acids for the measurement of protein synthesis *in vivo* by PET. *Nucl Med Biol* 1992;19:227–237.

80. Wester HJ, Herz M, Weber W, et al. Synthesis and radiopharmacology of O-[2-^{18}F]fluoroethyltyrosine for tumor imaging. *J Nucl Med* 1999;40:205–212.

81. Nuutinen J, Leskinen S, Lindholm P, et al. Use of carbon-11 methionine positron emission tomography to assess malignancy

grade and predict survival in patients with lymphomas. *Eur J Nucl Med* 1998;25:729–735.

82. Ishiwata K, Kubota K, Murakami M, et al. A comparative study on protein incorporation of L-[methyl-³H]methionine, L-[1-¹⁴C]leucine and L-[2-¹⁸F]fluorotyrosine in tumor-bearing mice. *Nucl Med Biol* 1993;20:895–899.

83. Willemsen ATM, van Waarde A, Paans AMJ, et al. *In vivo* protein synthesis rate determination in primary recurrent brain tumor L-[1-¹¹C]tyrosine and PET. *J Nucl Med* 1995;36: 411–419.

84. Kole AC, Boudewijn EC, Plaat EC, et al. FDG and L-[1-¹¹C]-tyrosine imaging of soft tissue tumors before and after therapy. *J Nucl Med* 1999;40:381–386.

85. Inoue T, Shibasaki T, Oriuchi N, et al. ¹⁸F-α-methyl-tyrosine PET studies in patients with brain tumors. *J Nucl Med* 1999;40: 399–405.

86. Shoup TM, Olson J, Hoffman JM, et al. Synthesis and evaluation of [¹⁸F]1-amino-3-fluorocyclobutane-1-carboxylic acid to image brain tumors. *J Nucl Med* 1999;40:331–338.

87. Beierwalters WH, LiebermanLM, Ansari AN, et al. Visualization of human adrenal glands *in vivo* by scintillation scanning. JAMA 1971;216:275–277.

88. Basmadjian GP, Hetzel KR, Ice RD, et al. Purity of adrenal scanning agents 19-iodocholesterol and 6-iodomethylnorcholesterol. *J Nucl Med* 1977;18:494–498.

89. Sudell CJ, Blake GM, Gosgages AAR, et al. Adrenal scintigraphy with ⁷⁵Se-selenonorcholesterol: a review. *Nucl Med Commun* 1985;6:519–527.

90. Beierwalters WH, Weiland DM, YU T, et al. Adrenal imaging agents. Rationale, synthesis, formulation and metabolism. *Semin Nucl Med* 1978;8:5–21.

91. Langley JN. On the contraction of muscle, chiefly in relation to the presence of "receptive" substances, part 1. *J Physiol* 1907;36: 347.

92. Goldsmith SJ. Receptor imaging: competitive or complementary to antibody imaging? *Semin Nucl Med* 1997;27:85–93.

93. Reubi JC, Laissue J, Krenning EP, et al. Somatostatin receptors in human cancer: incidence, characteristics, functional correlates and clinical implication. *J Steroid Biochem Mol Biol* 1992;43: 27–35.

94. Reubi JC. *In vitro* identification of vasoactive intestinal peptide receptors in human tumors: implications for tumor imaging. *J Nucl Med* 1995;36:1846–1853.

95. Patel YC, Greenwood MT, Panetta R, et al. Minireview: the somatostatin receptor family. *Life Sci* 1995;57:1249–1265.

96. Sreedharan SP, Kodama KT, Peterson KE, et al. Distinct subtypes of somatostatin receptors on cultured human lymphocytes. *J Biol Chem* 1989;264:949–953.

97. Krenning EP, Kwekkeboom DJ, Bakker WH, et al. Somatostatin receptor scintigraphy with [¹¹¹In-DTPA-D-Phe¹]- and [¹²³I-Tyr³]-octreotide: the Rotterdam experience with more than 1000 patients. *Eur J Nucl Med* 1993;20:716–731.

98. Virgolini I, Pangerl T, Bischof C, et al. Somatostatin receptor subtype expression in human tissues: a prediction for diagnosis and treatment of cancer? *Eur J Clin Invest* 1997;27:645–647.

99. Gomez-Pan A, Rodriguez-Arnao MD. Somatostatin and growth hormone-releasing factor: synthesis, location, metabolism and function. *Clin Endocrinol Metab* 1983;12:469–507.

100. Parmar H, Bogden A, Mollard M, et al. Somatostatin and somatostatin analogues in oncology. *Cancer Treat Rev* 1989;16: 95–115.

101. Bakker WH, Krenning EP, Breeman WA, et al. *In vivo* use of a radioiodinated somatostatin analogue: dynamics, metabolism, and binding to somatostatin receptor-positive tumors in man. *J Nucl Med* 1991;32:1184–1189.

102. Vallabhajosula S, Moyer BR, Lister-James J, et al. Technetium-99m-labeled somatostatin receptor-binding peptides for tumor imaging: preclinical evaluation of ⁹⁹ᵐTc-P587 and ⁹⁹ᵐTc-P829. *J Nucl Med* 1996;37:1016–1022.

103. Virgolini I, Leimer M, Handmaker H, et al. Somatostatin receptor subtype specificity and *in vivo* binding of a novel tumor tracer, ⁹⁹ᵐTc-P829. *Cancer Res* 1998;58:1850–1859.

104. Blum JE, Handmaker H, Rinne NA, et al. The utility of a somatostatin-type receptor binding peptide radiopharmaceutical (P829) in the evaluation of solitary pulmonary nodules. *Chest* 1999;115:224–232.

105. Breeman WAP, Hofland LJ, Bakker WH. Radioiodinated somatostatin analogue RC-160: preparation, biological activity, *in vivo* application in rats and comparison with [¹²³I-Tyr³] octreotide. *Eur J Nucl Med* 1993;20:1089–1094.

106. Breeman WAP, van Hagen PM, Kwekkeboom DJ. Somatostatin receptor scintigraphy using [¹¹¹In-DTPA⁰]RC-160 in humans: a comparison with [¹¹¹In-DTPA⁰]octreotide. *Eur J Nucl Med* 1998;25:182–186.

107. Thakur ML, Kolan H, Li J, et al. Radiolabeled somatostatin analogs in prostate cancer. *Nucl Med Biol* 1997;24:105–113.

108. Anderson CJ, Pajeau TS, Edwards WB, et al. *In vitro* and *in vivo* evaluation of copper-64 octreotide conjugates. *J Nucl Med* 1995;36:2315–2325.

109. Smith-Jones PM, Stolz B, Bruns C, et al. Gallium-67/gallium-68-[DFO]-octreotide: a potential radiopharmaceutical for PET imaging of somatostatin receptor-positive tumors: synthesis and radiolabeling, *in vitro* and preliminary *in vivo* studies. *J Nucl Med* 1994;35:317–325.

110. Wester HJ, Brockmann J, Rosch F, et al. PET-pharmacokinetics of ¹⁸F-octreotide: a comparison with ⁶⁷Ga-DFO and ⁸⁶Y-DTPA-octreotide. *Nucl Med Biol* 1997;24:275–286.

111. Krenning EP, de Jong M, Kooij PPM, et al. Radiolabeled somatostatin analogue(s) for peptide receptor scintigraphy and radionuclide therapy. *Ann Oncol* 1999;10[Suppl 2]: s23–s29.

112. Kozak RW, Raubitschek A, Mirzadeh S, et al. Nature of the bifunctional chelating agent used for radioimmunotherapy with yttrium-90 monoclonal antibodies: critical factors in determining *in vivo* survival and organ toxicity. *Cancer Res* 1989;49: 2639–2644.

113. Albert R, Smith-Jones PM, Stolz B, et al. Direct synthesis of [DOTA-D-Phe¹]-octreotide and [DOTA-D-Phe¹-Tyr³]-octreotide (SMT487): two conjugates for systemic delivery of radiotherapeutical nuclides to somatostatin receptor-positive tumors in man. *Bioorg Med Chem Lett* 1998;8:1207–1210.

114. de Jong M, Bakker WH, Krenning EP, et al. ⁹⁰Y and ¹¹¹In labeling, receptor binding and biodistribution of [DOTA⁰, D-Phe¹, Tyr³]octreotide, a promising somatostatin analog for radionuclide therapy. *Eur J Nucl Med* 1997;24:368–371.

115. Stolz B, Weckbecker G, Smith-Jones PM, et al. The somatostatin receptor-targeted radiotherapeutic [⁹⁰Y-DOTA-D-Phe¹-Tyr³]-octreotide (SMT487) eradicates experimental rat pancreatic CA 20948 tumors. *Eur J Nucl Med* 1998;25:668–674.

116. Virgolini I, Szilvasi I, Kurtaran A, et al. Indium-111-DOTA-lanreotide: biodistribution, safety and tumor dose in patients evaluated for somatostatin receptor-mediated radiotherapy. *J Nucl Med* 1998;39:1928–1936.

117. Smith-Jones PM, Bischof C, Leimer M, et al. DOTA-lanreotide: a novel somatostatin analog for tumor diagnosis and therapy. *Endocrinology* 1999;140:5136–5148.

118. Pincus DW, DiCicco-Bloom EM, Black IB. Vasoactive intestinal polypeptide regulates mitosis, differentiation, and survival of cultured sympathetic neuroblasts. *Nature* 1990;343:564–567.

119. Virgolini I, Yang Q, Li S, et al. Cross-competition between

vasoactive intestinal peptide and somatostatin for binding to tumor cell membrane receptors. *Cancer Res* 1994;54: 690–700.

120. Pallela VR, Thakur ML, Chakder S, et al. ^{99m}Tc-labeled vasoactive intestinal peptide receptor agonist: functional studies. *J Nucl Med* 1999;40:352–360.

121. Katzenellenbogen JA. Designing steroid receptor-based radiotracers to image breast and prostate tumors. *J Nucl Med* 1995; 36[Suppl]:8s–13s.

122. Dehdashti F, Mortimer JE, Siegel BA, et al. Positron tomographic assessment of estrogen receptors in breast cancer: comparison with FDG-PET and *in vitro* receptor studies. *J Nucl Med* 1995;36:1766–1774.

123. Rijks LJM, Boer GJ, Endert E, et al. The stereoisomers of 17α-[^{123}I]iodovinyloestradiol and its 11β-methoxy derivative evaluated for their estrogen receptor binding in human MCF-7 cells and rat uterus, and their distribution in immature rats. *Eur J Nucl Med* 1996;23:295–307.

124. Rijks LJM, Bakker PJM, Van Tienhoven G, et al. Imaging of estrogen receptors in primary and metastatic breast cancer patients with iodine-123-labeled Z-MIVE. *J Clin Oncol* 1997; 15:2536–2545.

125. Wieland DM, Swanson DP, Brown LE, et al. Imaging the adrenal medulla with an I-131-labeled anti-adrenergic agent. *J Nucl Med* 1979;20:155–158.

126. Wieland DM, Brown LE, Tobes MC, et al. Imaging the primate adrenal medulla with [^{123}I] and [^{131}I] meta-iodobenzylguanidine. *J Nucl Med* 1981;22:358–364.

127. Wafelman AR, Hoefnagel CA, Maes RA, et al. Radioiodinated metaiodobenzylguanidine: a review of its biodistribution and pharmacokinetics, drug interactions, cytotoxicity and dosimetry. *Eur J Nucl Med* 1994;21:545–559.

128. Beirwalters WH. Endocrine imaging: parathyroid, adrenal cortex and medulla, and other endocrine tumors. Part II. *J Nucl Med* 1991;32:1627–1639.

129. Jaques S Jr, Tobes MC, Sisson JC, et al. Comparison of sodium dependency of uptake of metaiodobenzylguanidine and norepinephrine into cultured bovine adrenomedullary cells. *Mol Pharmacol* 1984;26:539–546.

130. Glowniak JV, Kilty JE, Amara SH, et al. Evaluation of metaiodobenzylguanidine uptake by the norepinephrine, dopamine, and serotonin transporters. *J Nucl Med* 1993;34: 1140–1146.

131. de Herder WW, Reijs AE, Kwekkeboom DJ, et al. *In vivo* imaging of pituitary tumors using a radiolabeled dopamine D_2 receptor radioligand. *Clin Endocrinol* 1996;45:755–767.

132. de Herder WW, Reijs AE, de Swart J, et al. Comparison of iodine-123 epidepride and iodine-123 IBZM for dopamine D_2 receptor imaging in clinically non-functioning pituitary macroadenomas and macroprolactinomas. *Eur J Nucl Med* 1999;26: 46–50.

133. Maffioli L, Mascheroni L, Mongioj V, et al. Scintigraphic detection of melanoma metastases with a radiolabeled benzamide, [iodine-123]-(S)-IBZM. *J Nucl Med* 1994;35: 1741–1747.

134. Larisch R, Schulte K-W, Vosberg H, et al. Differential accumulation of iodine-123-iodobenzamide in melanotic and amelanotic melanoma metastases *in vivo*. *J Nucl Med* 1998;39: 996–1001.

135. Turner M. Antibodies and their receptors. In: Roitt I, Brostoff J, Male D, eds. *Immunology*. St. Louis: Mosby International, 1998:71–82.

136. Stoldt HS, Aftab F, Chinol M, et al. Pretargeting strategies for radioimmunoguided tumor localization and therapy. *Eur J Cancer* 1997;33:186–192.

137. Zuckier LS, DeNardo GL. Trials and tribulations: oncological antibody imaging comes to the fore. *Semin Nucl Med* 1997;27: 10–29.

138. Knox S, Goris M, Trisler K, et al. Yttrium-90-labeled anti-CD20 monoclonal antibody therapy of recurrent B-cell lymphoma. *Clin Cancer Res* 1996;2:457–470.

139. Chilkoti A, Stayton PS. Molecular origins of the slow dissociation kinetics of the streptavidin-biotin complex. *J Am Chem Soc* 1995;117:10622–10628.

140. Hnatowich DJ, Virzi F, Rusckowski M. Investigations of avidin and biotin for imaging applications. *J Nucl Med* 1987;28: 1294–1302.

141. Paganelli G, Magnani P, Zito F, et al. Three-step monoclonal antibody tumor targeting in carcinoembryonic antigen-positive patients. *Cancer Res* 1991;51:5960–5966.

142. Casalini P, Luison E, Menard S, et al. Tumor pretargeting: role of avidin/streptavidin on monoclonal antibody internalization. *J Nucl Med* 1997;38:1378–1381.

143. Hockel M, Schlenger K, Aral B, et al. Association between tumor hypoxia and malignant progression in advanced cancer of the uterine cervix. *Cancer Res* 1996;56:4509–4515.

144. Nunn A, Linder K, Strauss HW. Nitroimidazoles and imaging hypoxia. *Eur J Nucl Med* 1995;22:265–280.

145. Chapman JD, Franko AJ, Sharplin J. A marker for hypoxia cells in tumors with potential clinical applicability. *Br J Cancer* 1981; 43:546–550.

146. Rasey JS, Koh WJ, Evans ML, et al. Quantifying regional hypoxia in tumors with positron emission tomography of [^{18}F]fluoromisonidazole: a pretherapy study of 37 patients. *Int J Radiat Oncol Biol Phys* 1996;36:417–428.

147. Dearling JLJ, Lewis JS, Mullen GED, et al. Design of hypoxia-targeting radiopharmaceuticals: selective uptake of copper-64 complexes in hypoxic cells *in vitro*. *Eur J Nucl Med* 1998;25: 788–792.

148. Lewis JS, McCarthy DW, McCarthy TJ, et al. Evaluation of ^{64}Cu-ATSM *in vitro* and *in vivo* in a hypoxic tumor model. *J Nucl Med* 1999;40:177–183.

149. Parliament MB, Chapman JD, Urtasunn RC, et al. Noninvasive assessment of human tumor hypoxia with ^{123}I-iodoazomycin arabinoside: preliminary report of a clinical study. *Br J Cancer* 1992; 65:90–95.

150. Ballinger JR, Kee JWM, Rauth AM. *In vitro* and *in vivo* evaluation of a technetium-99m-labeled 2-nitroimidazole (BMS181321) as a marker of tumor hypoxia. *J Nucl Med* 1996; 37:1023–1031.

151. Cook GJR, Houston S, Barrington SF, et al. Technetium-99m-labeled HL91 to identify tumor hypoxia: correlation with fluorine-18-FDG. *J Nucl Med* 1998;39:99–103.

152. Alazraki NP, Eshima D, Eshima LA, et al. Lymphoscintigraphy, the sentinel node concept, and the intraoperative gamma probe in melanoma, breast cancer, and other potential cancers. *Semin Nucl Med* 1997;27:55–67.

153. Krasnow AZ, Hellman RS, Timins ME, et al. Diagnostic bone scanning in oncology. *Semin Nucl Med* 1997;27: 107–141.

154. McEwan AJB. Unsealed source therapy of painful bone metastases: an update. *Semin Nucl Med* 1997;27:165–182.

155. Hnatowich DJ. Antisense and nuclear medicine. *J Nucl Med* 1999;40:93–103.

156. Dewanjee MK, Ghafouripour AK, Kapadvanjwala M, et al. Noninvasive imaging of c-*myc* oncogene messenger RNA with indium-111-antisense probes in a mammary tumor-bearing mouse model. *J Nucl Med* 1994;35:1054–1063.

157. Urbain JL. Oncogenes, cancer and imaging. *J Nucl Med* 1999;40: 498–504.

158. Larson SM, Tjuvajev JG, Blasberg R, et al. Triumph over mischance: a role for nuclear medicine in gene therapy. *J Nucl Med* 1997;38:1230–1233.

159. Tjuvajev JG, Finn R, Watanabe K, et al. Noninvasive imaging of herpes virus thymidine kinase gene transfer and expression: a potential method for monitoring clinical gene therapy. *Cancer Res* 1996;56:4087–4095.

160. Gambhir SS, Barrio JR, Wu L, et al. Imaging of adenoviral-directed herpes simplex virus type 1 thymidine kinase reporter gene expression in mice with radiolabeled ganciclovir. *J Nucl Med* 1998;39:2003–2011.

161. De Vries EFJ, Hospers GAP, Doze P, et al. PET imaging of HSV thymidine kinase activity with 9-[3-^{18}F]fluoro-1-hydroxy-2-propoxymethylguanine ([^{18}F]FHPG) in a two-sided tumor-bearing rat model. *J Label Comm Radiopharm* 1999;42[Suppl 1]:s7–s9.

4

MULTIDRUG RESISTANCE

PART A: BREAST CANCER

DAVID PIWNICA-WORMS
KATHRYN E. LUKER
AULA M. FRACASSO

In the United States, breast cancer is the most common malignancy in women. It is estimated that breast cancer will be diagnosed in 182,800 women and that 40,800 will die of this disease in 2000 (1). Although adjuvant chemotherapy improves survival of early-stage breast cancer, approximately 50% of all patients eventually relapse (2). In addition, although most women with advanced disease initially respond to chemotherapy, most women die of recurrent and refractory disease.

The emergence of multidrug resistance (MDR) in breast cancer mediated by the *MDR1* P-glycoprotein (Pgp) has been associated with a poor response to treatment and a shorter overall survival. Pgp, a 170-kd membrane glycoprotein, acts as an adenosine triphosphate (ATP)-dependent efflux transporter to reduce the intracellular accumulation of many chemotherapeutic drugs. The MDR-associated protein (MRP1), a homologue of Pgp, may also play a role in the therapeutic response in breast cancer, but this is less well defined. Recently, several novel MDR inhibitors highly selective for Pgp have been commercially developed. Thus, functional identification of Pgp, and perhaps MRP1, might provide important information to direct the choice of chemotherapeutic agents for patients with breast cancer. Diagnostic radiopharmaceuticals that are recognized as transport substrates by the human *MDR1* Pgp and MRP1 may enable functional identification of transporter-mediated resistance *in vivo* by breast scintigraphy.

D. Piwnica-Worms and K. E. Luker: Mallinckrodt Institute of Radiology, Washington University School of Medicine; Department of Medical Oncology, Barnes-Jewish Hospital, St. Louis, Missouri 63110.

P. M. Fracasso: Department of Internal Medicine, Washington University School of Medicine; Department of Medical Oncology, Barnes-Jewish Hospital, St. Louis, Missouri 63110.

BIOCHEMISTRY OF MULTIDRUG RESISTANCE: *MDR1* P-GLYCOPROTEIN AND MULTIDRUG RESISTANCE-ASSOCIATED PROTEIN

The development of resistance to antineoplastic drugs is thought to be responsible for treatment failure in many cancers. This problem is compounded by the emergence of cross-resistance to multiple chemotherapeutic agents unrelated in structure and function to the original selective agent. The phenomenon of MDR is caused by several different mechanisms. The most extensively characterized mechanism is that associated with the *MDR1* gene and its protein product, Pgp (3–7). Pgp, a 170-kd membrane glycoprotein, acts as an ATP-dependent efflux pump to reduce the intracellular accumulation of anthracyclines, vinca alkaloids, taxanes, epipodophyllotoxins, dactinomycin, and other natural products (4). Normally expressed in many tissues, such as liver, kidney, and adrenal in addition to brain capillaries and choroid plexus epithelium, *MDR1* Pgp may have a physiologic role in the excretion of xenobiotics or intracellular trafficking of sterols (8).

Another recently identified gene, known as *MRP1*, also confers MDR *in vitro* (9). Also a transporter, *MRP1* and its protein product, MRP1, have subsequently been shown to be overexpressed in many cell lines that display the MDR phenotype (10,11, and references therein). Pgp and MRP1 transport an overlapping, but distinct, array of structurally and functionally unrelated toxic xenobiotics, natural product chemotherapeutic drugs, phospholipids, and hydrophobic charged compounds (12). Whereas substrates transported by Pgp generally are hydrophobic and cationic, compounds recognized by MRP1 generally are hydrophobic and anionic, such as glutathione conjugates. However, some compounds appear to be co-transported with, but not conjugated to, glutathione (13). MRP1 is widely expressed in various normal tissues, including heart, skeletal muscle, lung, kidney, testes, and epithelia (14). Indeed, *mrp1(-/-)* gene-disrupted mice show elevated levels of glutathione in lung, heart, kidney, muscle, and colon, but no change in organs known to express little if any *mrp1*, such as liver and small intestine (13).

MDR1 is overexpressed in many human cancers (6), including breast cancer (15), in which it has been associated with a shorter overall survival (16). Many other tumor types, such as sarcomas, lymphomas, neuroblastomas, acute lymphocytic leukemia, and chronic myelogenous leukemia, also have shown high levels of Pgp expression (6). Expression of *MDR1* Pgp and MRP1 is an independent prognostic indicator of a poor outcome in patients with selected cancers, and increased levels of *MDR1* Pgp and MRP1 are often detected in tumor biopsy specimens from relapsing cancer patients (17–21).

Whether Pgp is indeed responsible for treatment failure by outwardly transporting and thereby reducing the intracellular accumulation of certain chemotherapeutic agents or whether its overexpression is a simply a marker for a more malignant phenotype has been under investigation. For example, many anticancer agents, irrespective of their intracellular target, may exert their biologic effect in target cells by triggering a common final death pathway, known as *apoptosis* (22,23). Thus, mounting evidence exists that many anticancer treatments kill through apoptosis by activating intracellular death machinery in the target cell rather than by simply crippling various components of cellular metabolism (22,23). Of interest, recent data show that overexpression of *MDR1* Pgp delays progression of the apoptotic cascade (24,25). These data support the model that Pgp may also be viewed as a marker of a more malignant phenotype, resistant to execution of the apoptotic cascade. Thus, it has been suggested that Pgp has a prognostic significance independent of its involvement in drug transport (26).

BREAST CANCER MULTIDRUG RESISTANCE MEDIATED BY P-GLYCOPROTEIN

In untreated breast carcinoma, reported levels of *MDR1* expression have ranged broadly, depending on the quality, sensitivities, and specificities of the various detection techniques (15,27–33). Careful examination of these studies suggests that at least a third of untreated breast cancers overexpress *MDR1* (34). Furthermore, the percentage of breast carcinomas that overexpress *MDR1* has been shown to increase after chemotherapy (28,31,33). Importantly, the expression of *MDR1* has been associated with a poor prognosis in breast carcinoma (16), as has previously been described in acute myeloid leukemia, sarcoma, and neuroblastoma (19,35,36).

Several individual studies have been able to demonstrate the presence of Pgp in a significant proportion of breast tumors and to make a compelling case for Pgp expression as an independent prognostic indicator. In a study correlating Pgp detection by immunohistochemical assays with other prognostic indicators, 53% (113 of 213) of untreated breast cancers with a wide variety of histologic features were immunohistochemically positive for Pgp (37). Pgp expression was observed to be independent of various histochemical prognostic indicators, tumor size, histologic type, grade, Nottingham prognostic index, and nodal status. In another report, 35% (7 of 20) of untreated advanced breast cancers were strongly positive for Pgp by immunohistochemistry, and all seven of these failed to respond to chemotherapy (30). Similarly, Pgp expression was inversely correlated with pathologic response to a regimen of doxorubicin, cyclophosphamide, vincristine, and prednisone in breast tumors examined at mastectomy; 100% (3 of 3) of tumors that progressed and 83% (5 of 6) of tumors that exhibited a minor response expressed immunodetectable Pgp, whereas only 38% (12 of 31) of tumors with a complete or partial response to treatment were Pgp expressors (38). Because doxorubicin and vincristine are transported by Pgp, one may speculate that these treatment failures occurred in part because these drugs were transported out of the tumor cells that expressed Pgp.

A recent metaanalysis of 31 published studies examining *MDR1* Pgp expression in breast cancer attempted to evaluate the proportion of breast tumors that express *MDR1* Pgp and to correlate that expression with response to therapy (39). The overall findings of this analysis were as follows: (a) Pgp was expressed in 41.2% of breast tumors according to the various detection methods used in the studies; (b) chemotherapy and hormone treatment were associated with an increase in the proportion of tumors that expressed Pgp; and (c) patients with tumors expressing Pgp were *three times* more likely to fail chemotherapy than those with tumors that were Pgp-negative. Furthermore, Pgp was found to be an independent prognostic indicator of poor outcome.

BREAST CANCER MULTIDRUG RESISTANCE MEDIATED BY MULTIDRUG RESISTANCE-ASSOCIATED PROTEIN

Flens and colleagues (14) reported that 46 of 119 untreated tumors from various organs showed MRP1 staining. Although the majority of colon and lung cancers showed MRP1 staining, only 1 of 7 breast tumors showed strong staining for MRP1. Similarly, in a quantitative RNase protection assay, MRP1 was found to be expressed in a wide variety of tumors, but MRP1 mRNA levels in breast tumors generally were found only at low levels (40). In one study of breast cancer patients, a clear association between breast cancer progression and MRP1 was not found except by subgroup analysis. In patients with small tumors and negative nodes, and in patients with positive nodes who received adjuvant chemotherapy, MRP1 expression was associated with an increased risk for failure (41). In this study, MRP1 overexpression was not associated with reduced relapse-free survival or overall survival. Furthermore, this study did not address the functional assessment of MRP1 transport activity in breast cancer. Thus, although MRP1 has been identified in many tumors, the clinical significance of MRP1 expression, particularly in breast cancer, remains to be defined.

MODULATORS OF MULTIDRUG RESISTANCE

Because many studies have shown *MDR1* Pgp expression in tumors to be clinically relevant, the reversal of MDR by non-toxic agents that block the transport activity of *MDR1* Pgp has been an important target for pharmaceutical development (42). When co-administered with a cytotoxic agent, these nontoxic compounds, known as *MDR modulators* or *reversal agents*, enhance the net accumulation of cytotoxic drugs within the tumor cells. Many compounds known to have other pharmacologic sites of action initially were used to reverse MDR in cancer cells grown in culture (42). These compounds included verapamil, cyclosporin A, quinidine, and trifluperazine and derivatives thereof (42). However, the clinical utility of these agents is limited because of unacceptable toxicities at the serum levels of drug needed to modulate *MDR1* Pgp. New, second-generation modulators [dexverapamil, Knoll Pharmaceutical; valspodar (PSC 833), Novartis Pharmaceuticals] and third-generation modulators [GG918 (GF120918), Glaxo Wellcome; LY335979, Eli Lilly; VX-710, Vertex Pharmaceuticals] have been subsequently developed, and phase I/II clinical trials are currently in progress with these new, more potent compounds (43–47). Most specifically target *MDR1* Pgp, but data indicate that VX-710 also has cross-reactive inhibitory activity on MRP1 (46). Thus, the MDR phenotype may be modulated more effectively with these more potent and selective reversal agents designed to improve the efficacy of chemotherapy.

FUNCTIONAL DETECTION OF MULTIDRUG RESISTANCE

Increasingly, the choice of systemic therapy for breast cancer is based on tumor markers such as estrogen/progesterone receptor status and, more recently, *Her-2/neu*. If improvement in the therapeutic index is shown with MDR modulators currently in clinical trials, then measurement of MDR will be another important marker in planning systemic therapy. However, a general dilemma in the MDR field has been that correlation of *MDR1* Pgp expression with failure of chemotherapy has been difficult to demonstrate unequivocally in each patient. Differences in detection methods and reagents between laboratories have made comparisons of results of various studies difficult, although the recommendations of a consensus panel were published in the hope of unifying future studies (48). Furthermore, there has been lack of agreement on the optimal methodology for characterizing Pgp expression. For example, insufficient sensitivity of immunologic reagents appears to be a significant problem with low levels of Pgp expression, and analysis of extracted RNA has been hampered by the inclusion of tissue stroma containing capillaries and lymphocytes that may express high levels of endogenous Pgp (49). Thus, major efforts are under way to demonstrate the function of Pgp-mediated transport in tumors. Assays of Pgp-mediated transport activity provide the advantage of directly quantifying the potential to transport substrates out of cancer cells (50) and do not rely on an inference between the amount of protein or RNA and transport activity (49). Functional assays directly quantify the accumulation of fluorescent (*in vitro*) or radioactive substrates in tumor cells as markers of Pgp function. Imaging with a radiopharmaceutical that is transported by *MDR1* Pgp promises to identify those tumors in which the transporter is not only expressed but also functional. In addition, determination *in vivo* of the effect of MDR modulators in tumors and in nontarget tissues may direct the selection of chemotherapeutic agents and predict unanticipated toxicities, respectively. These applications potentially may improve the efficacy of chemotherapy in patients with cancer.

Noninvasive detection of Pgp utilizes gamma-emitting compounds characterized as substrates for *MDR1* Pgp. We and others have synthesized, developed, or validated several radiopharmaceuticals targeting Pgp (51–55) (Fig. 4A.1). Of the ^{99m}Tc-labeled compounds, ^{99m}Tc-sestamibi [*hexakis*(2-methoxyisobutylisonitrile)technetium-99m] and ^{99m}Tc-tetrofosmin [({1,2-*bis*[*bis*(2-ethoxyethyl)phosphino]-ethane}$_2$O$_2$)technetium-99m] are lipophilic cationic radiotracers that are commercially available (56–58). Each compound is a nonmetabolizable radiopharmaceutical with a monocationic charge, like most chemotherapeutic agents in the MDR phenotype (57–61). Additionally, substrates of *MDR1* Pgp suitable for positron emission tomography (PET) are under development for possible applications in oncologic imaging (55,62–65).

The mechanisms of uptake and retention of ^{99m}Tc-sestamibi and analogous ^{99m}Tc-based agents have been extensively studied in a variety of cellular and subcellular preparations *in vitro*. Net cell content of these ^{99m}Tc-based agents generally is a function of both passive, potential-dependent influx and *MDR1* Pgp-mediated extrusion. For example, biophysical analysis has shown that ^{99m}Tc-sestamibi is a high-fidelity probe of transmembrane potential (66,67); passive inward movement of this lipophilic cation is driven (in the absence of *MDR1* Pgp) by the transmembrane potentials generated in living cells (66,68). The complex is reversibly sequestered within mitochondria by the serial

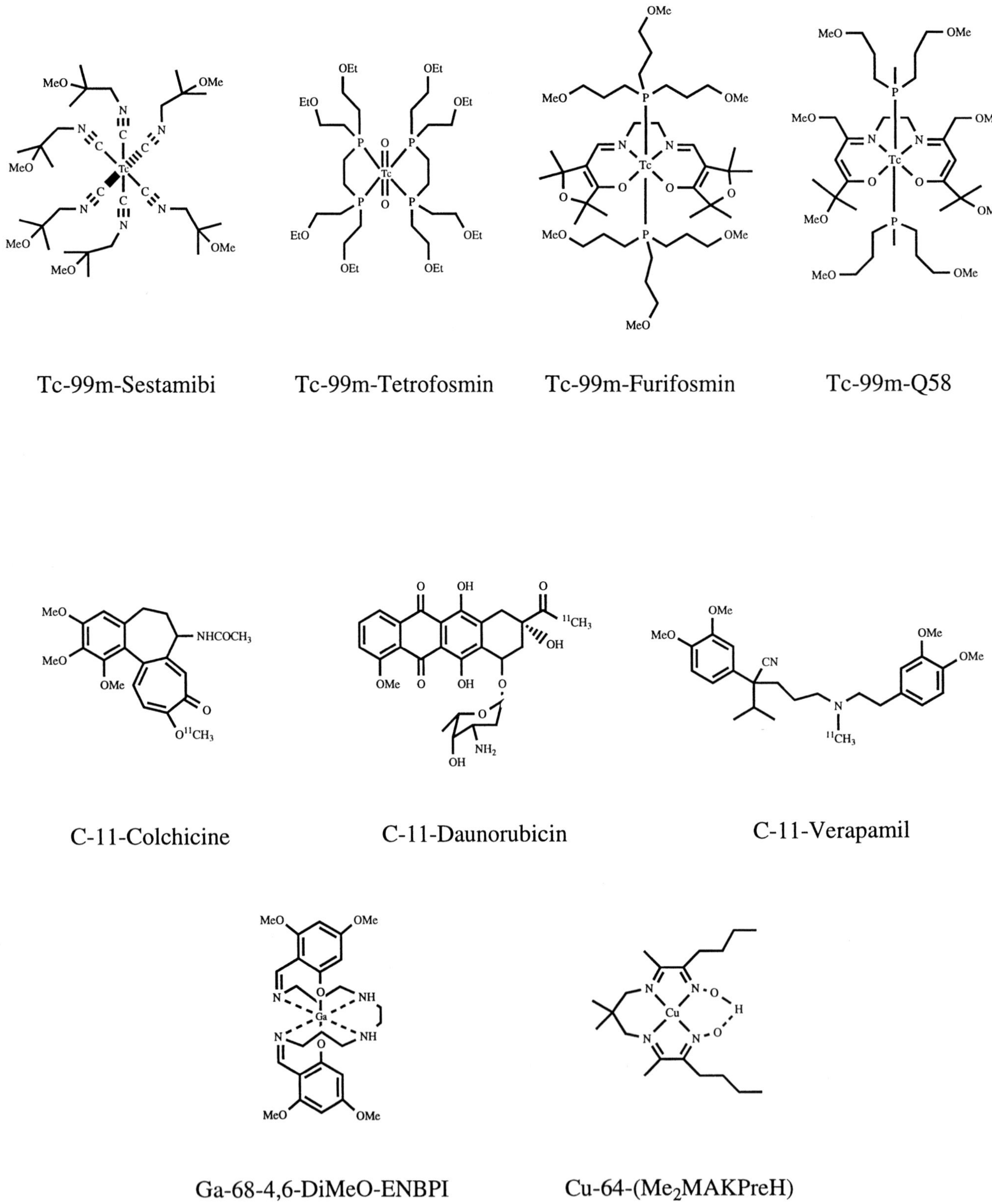

Tc-99m-Sestamibi   Tc-99m-Tetrofosmin   Tc-99m-Furifosmin   Tc-99m-Q58

C-11-Colchicine   C-11-Daunorubicin   C-11-Verapamil

Ga-68-4,6-DiMeO-ENBPI   Cu-64-(Me₂MAKPreH)

FIGURE 4A.1. Structures of single-photon emission computed tomography (*SPECT*) (*top row*) and positron emission tomography (*PET*) radiopharmaceuticals (*middle and bottom rows*) recognized as transport substrates by *MDR1* P-glycoprotein.

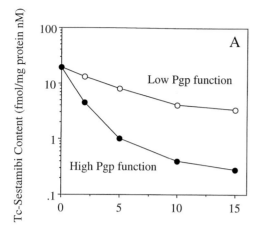

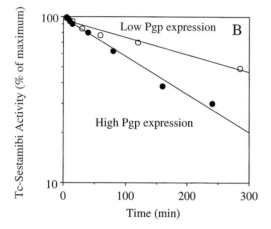

FIGURE 4A.2. Functional detection of transport activity mediated by P-glycoprotein (*Pgp*) *in vitro* and *in vivo* with a radiopharmaceutical. **A:** Pgp-mediated efflux of ^{99m}Tc-sestamibi from cells *in vitro*. Pgp-expressing V79 cells were equilibrated (15 minutes) in loading buffer containing ^{99m}Tc-sestamibi, then transferred to isotope-free solution in the absence (●) or presence (○) of the multidrug resistance (*MDR*) inhibitor verapamil (10 μM) for the times indicated. Cell-associated activity during washout is plotted. Each point is the mean of three to four determinations; standard error of the mean did not exceed 15% of mean values. Note semilogarithmic scale. (Data are replotted from Piwnica-Worms D, Chiu ML, Budding M, et al. Functional imaging of multidrug-resistant P-glycoprotein with an organotechnetium complex. *Cancer Res* 1993;53:977–984, with permission.) **B:** Pgp-mediated efflux of ^{99m}Tc-sestamibi from breast tumors *in vivo*. Tumor clearance of ^{99m}Tc-sestamibi was assessed by region-of-interest analysis of sequential images of two representative breast tumors expressing high (●) or low (○) levels of Pgp. Tumor-associated activity during washout is plotted as a percentage of maximum tumor accumulation. Note semilogarithmic scale. (Data are replotted from Del Vecchio S, Ciarmiello A, Potena MI, et al. *In vivo* detection of multidrug resistance (MDR1) phenotype by technetium-99m-sestamibi scan in untreated breast cancer patients. *Eur J Nucl Med* 1997;24:150–159, with permission.)

thermodynamic driving forces of the negative plasma membrane and mitochondrial inner membrane potentials (69).

Opposing passive influx is the action of *MDR1* Pgp (51, 70,71). For example, baculoviral expression of recombinant human *MDR1* in insect cells confers decreased accumulation of ^{99m}Tc-sestamibi (70), and furthermore, MDR cells expressing Pgp accumulate ^{99m}Tc-sestamibi at rates decreased in inverse proportion to the amount of immunodetectable transporter (51,72). Reduced cell efflux of ^{99m}Tc-sestamibi is observed on administration of inhibitors of MDR such as verapamil (Fig. 4A.2A). ^{99m}Tc-Tetrofosmin and ^{99m}Tc-furifosmin, another ^{99m}Tc-based cationic agent, also have been validated as transport substrates for Pgp in a variety of MDR human and rodent cells (53,54, 73–75). Net cellular accumulation of these tracers is decreased in proportion to the level of Pgp expression, and enhancement of radiotracer net content is observed on administration of inhibitors of MDR such as verapamil, cyclosporin A, or the new high-potency agents such as GG918 or valspodar (76,77). Addition of an MDR modulator that selectively blocks the function of Pgp and thus enables the tracer to accumulate within the cell forms the basis for a functional approach to the assessment of *MDR1* Pgp in patients.

Recent data indicate that ^{99m}Tc-sestamibi, in addition to being transported by Pgp, is also recognized as a substrate by MRP1 in cells in culture, putatively as a co-transported substrate with glutathione (78–80). For example, Morretti et al. (79) have shown that the net accumulation of ^{99m}Tc-sestamibi in human tumor cell lines expressing MRP1 is less than that in their matched, non–MRP1-expressing control cells and furthermore that it is enhanced by depletion of cellular glutathione with buthionine sulfoximine. However, the differences in ^{99m}Tc-sestamibi net uptake associated with MRP1 expression are significantly *less* than the differences associated with Pgp expression under similar conditions (78). Thus, although net accumulation (and putatively efflux) of ^{99m}Tc-sestamibi in tumors are potentially functionally affected by expression of MRP1, the effect may further depend on intrinsic levels of glutathione within a given tumor. Importantly, the functional impact of MRP1 expression on ^{99m}Tc-sestamibi kinetics has never been tested in patients.

FUNCTIONAL IMAGING OF MULTIDRUG RESISTANCE IN BREAST CANCER

Rates of efflux of ^{99m}Tc-sestamibi were determined by Del Vecchio et al. (81) in 30 patients with untreated breast cancer. Dynamic imaging of tumors was performed for 15 minutes, followed by static planar imaging at 0.5, 1, 2, and 4 hours after injection of 20 mCi of ^{99m}Tc-sestamibi. Tumor specimens were obtained 24 hours after scintigraphy, and Pgp levels were measured in each tumor by quantitative autoradiography for correlation with the calculated rate of efflux. Half-times ($t_{1/2}$) for rates of efflux ranged from 41 to 574 minutes. Rates of efflux of ^{99m}Tc-sestamibi were 2.7-fold greater in tumors expressing increased *MDR1* Pgp than in tumors expressing Pgp at a level comparable to that in benign breast lesions (Fig. 3A.2B). Estimates of sensitivity and specificity for *in vivo* detection of *MDR1* Pgp with ^{99m}Tc-sestamibi were 80% and 95%, respectively. These data suggest that efflux rate constants of ^{99m}Tc-sestamibi may be useful for noninvasive identification of *MDR1* Pgp.

Fractional retention values of ^{99m}Tc-sestamibi in breast cancers has also been compared with *MDR1* Pgp expression. In one study, 27 patients with histologically proven breast carcinoma were injected with ^{99m}Tc-sestamibi and static planar images of the breast were obtained at 10, 60, and 240 minutes (82). Fractional retention of ^{99m}Tc-sestamibi in the tumors was calculated from ratios of regions-of-interest drawn over the tumor images between 60 and 10 minutes (R60/10) and between 240 and 10 minutes (R240/10). Subsequently, Pgp expression in excised tumors was determined by quantitative autoradiography performed with radiolabeled MRK16, an *MDR1* Pgp-targeted monoclonal antibody, and correlated with tracer retention. Fractional retention, in particular the R240/10 values, was significantly higher in the group with low levels of Pgp expression than in the group with high levels of Pgp expression ($r = -.74$). Sensitivity for the detection of high levels of Pgp expression by analysis of fractional retention was 78% to 100% (depending on the cutoff value chosen), with an associated specificity of 95% to 83%. The investigators concluded that this practical protocol has the potential to identify noninvasively tumors with a high probability of expressing *MDR1* Pgp.

Similar data also were reported by Kostakoglu et al. (83) in a prospective study of 48 patients with either breast (30 patients) or lung (18 patients) cancer at the time of presentation (37 patients) or after therapy (11 patients). Scintigraphy was performed with whole-body planar imaging and single-photon emission computed tomography (SPECT) beginning 30 minutes after injection of 20 mCi of ^{99m}Tc-sestamibi. Tumor-to-background ratios of radioactivity from regions-of-interest were correlated with immunohistochemistry of specimens obtained 3 to 5 days after imaging. Overall, tumor-to-background ratios of ^{99m}Tc-sestamibi correlated inversely with expression of *MDR1* Pgp, although exceptions were noted. The authors also showed that strong but focal expression of *MDR1* Pgp in a specimen does not alter uptake ratios of ^{99m}Tc-sestamibi. In a retrospective analysis of breast tumor planar scintigraphy, a less robust correlation between 30-minute uptake of ^{99m}Tc-sestamibi and Pgp expression was reported (84).

The prospective value of high tumor *clearance rates* of ^{99m}Tc-sestamibi to predict poor therapeutic outcomes was recently reported for locally advanced breast cancer. In this study by Ciarmiello and colleagues (85), 39 patients with stage III disease were enrolled in a prospective clinical trial to receive pretreatment mammoscintigraphy with ^{99m}Tc-sestamibi before administration of neoadjuvant chemotherapy. Breast tumor clearance of ^{99m}Tc-sestamibi was determined out to 4 hours after injection, and half-times were calculated from the image sets by means of monoexponential curve fitting. Patients were subsequently treated with standard chemotherapy (epirubicin) for 6 weeks and then underwent surgery within 3 weeks of completion of chemotherapy. Tumor burden was assessed by pathologic examination of the mastectomy specimens. Of the 39 patients, 17 showed a tumor clearance half-time of less than 204 minutes, a value previously shown by this group to correspond to the mean tracer clearance rate minus 1 standard deviation in tumors with a high Pgp content. Of these 17 patients with rapidly effluxing tumors, 15 showed a highly cellular residual tumor, indicating a lack of response to neoadjuvant chemotherapy. Conversely, 22 patients showed prolonged tumor clearance ($t_{1/2} > 204$ minutes), and of these, only eight showed highly cellular residual tumor at the time of surgery. As pointed out by the investigators, the fact that slow clearance rates are not highly predictive of a good response is consistent with the existence of mechanisms of drug resistance other than Pgp in breast cancer patients. Interestingly, no patient with a half-time of less than 164 minutes (which was approximately 2 standard deviations faster than the mean half-time of breast tumors with high levels of Pgp expression) showed evidence of a pathologic response to neoadjuvant chemotherapy (81). Thus, results of pretreatment scintigraphy of advanced breast tumor were highly predictive of subsequent response to neoadjuvant chemotherapy. Especially noteworthy was the ability of dynamic mammoscintigraphy to identify a subset of patients with very rapid clearance rates, all of whom failed chemotherapy.

These scintigraphic approaches recently have been extended to SPECT to investigate the influence of heterogeneity of Pgp expression on the magnitude of ^{99m}Tc-sestamibi accumulation in breast tumors (86). The investigative team examined a total of 30 patients with breast cancer, 20 patients at initial presentation and 10 patients after completion of chemotherapy consisting of drugs included in the MDR phenotype. SPECT was performed starting 45 minutes after injection of a standard dose of ^{99m}Tc-sestamibi, and tumor-to-background uptake ratios were obtained by region-of-interest analysis of tumors and contralateral tissue. The SPECT images were correlated with immunohistochemical analysis of multiple sections of the tumor stained with JSB-1, a well-characterized Pgp-specific monoclonal antibody. The scintigraphic tumor-to-background ratios were lower for the strong Pgp expression group than for those with a heterogeneous pattern of strong-to-weak expression or those with weak-to-no expression. A statistically significant difference was observed between all groups, and no overlapping values were noted between the strong expression group and the weak-to-no expression group. The tumor-to-background values for the heterogeneous expression group, although they tended to cluster within the middle of the range, overlapped both the strong and weak expression groups. The investigators concluded that because of the heterogeneity of Pgp expression in some tumors, caution is warranted in assuming that immunohistochemistry is the "gold standard" if only a single tumor section is analyzed. When ^{99m}Tc-sestamibi scintigraphy yields apparently confounding results, tumor heterogeneity for expression of Pgp must also be considered.

Further analysis of the breast tumor-to-background data indicates some interesting trends (86). All six of the strong Pgp expression tumors had ^{99m}Tc-sestamibi SPECT tumor-to-background values of less than 2.0. In addition, 7 of 13 heterogeneous strong-to-weak tumors, but only 2 of 13 weak-to-negative tumors, had tumor-to-background values of less than 2.0. Thus, if one were to assume that strong plus strong-to-weak expression of Pgp would correlate with clinical MDR, then a ^{99m}Tc-sestamibi SPECT tumor-to-background cutoff value of less than 2.0 would have a sensitivity of 76% for detection of clinical MDR and a specificity of 85% for excluding MDR in breast cancer. If only strong expression of Pgp is assumed to be relevant, then a cutoff value of tumor-to-background ratio of less than 2.0 results in 100% sensitivity for detection of Pgp in breast cancer and a specificity of 63%. However, if the cutoff is more stringent, at a tumor-to-background ratio of 1.6 or less, then 100% sensitivity for detection of strong MDR is retained, and overall specificity improves to 80%. Interestingly, at this stringent level, all weak-to-negative tumors are excluded. Of course, these are only preliminary estimates and further validation is required with larger patient populations, but these estimates are in general agreement with those reported by Del Vecchio and colleagues (81) for scintigraphic detection of Pgp-mediated MDR in breast cancer.

All these studies showed a correlation of Pgp expression with ^{99m}Tc-sestamibi pharmacokinetics in tumors *in vivo*. However, the role of MRP1 expression on the efflux rate constants and the effects of potent MDR modulators need to be examined in the future.

FUNCTIONAL IMAGING OF MULTIDRUG RESISTANCE IN BREAST CANCER VERSUS CONVENTIONAL MAMMOSCINTIGRAPHY

Scintigraphy with ^{99m}Tc-sestamibi and ^{99m}Tc-tetrofosmin has been widely investigated for breast tumor imaging, and the radiopharmaceuticals have shown some utility to diagnose and distinguish malignant from benign breast tumors (87–90). Conventional mammoscintigraphy has been found to be useful for imaging breast tumors larger than 1 cm in selected patient populations (90), with high false-negative rates for smaller tumors. Identifying MDR in

advanced breast cancer by ^{99m}Tc-sestamibi functional imaging is quite different from conventional mammoscintigraphy with ^{99m}Tc-sestamibi. Conventional applications are based on early static imaging of the breast and do not evaluate washout kinetics. Furthermore, as pilot data indicate, an additional reason for false-negative results with conventional mammoscintigraphy (which reduces overall sensitivity for malignancy) may be strong expression of *MDR1* Pgp. In such cases, Pgp may lead to a low net uptake of ^{99m}Tc-sestamibi in a tumor, and the conventional practitioner may falsely conclude the presence of a benign lesion rather than the correct diagnosis of a malignant tumor with an aggressive MDR phenotype. The exact frequency of these false-negative results needs to be rigorously determined in cancer patient populations with dynamic ^{99m}Tc-sestamibi breast scanning *in vivo*.

CONCLUSIONS

Chemotherapy plays an important role in the management of all stages of breast cancer. For localized disease, adjuvant chemotherapy is credited with a decline in the death rate from breast cancer. In the neoadjuvant setting, operability of initially inoperable disease has been enhanced with combination chemotherapy. However, because populations of chemotherapy-resistant cells typically exist within advanced-stage tumors (either primary or acquired resistance), metastatic breast cancer is incurable and treatment is only palliative. Pgp (and possibly MRP1) appear to be important mechanisms of drug resistance in all stages. If drug resistance in metastatic disease can be overcome by using modulators of Pgp, MRP1, or both, patient survival may be prolonged. Functional *dynamic* imaging of tracer pharmacokinetics may assist in the evaluation of MDR and guide therapeutic and modulation regimens in advanced breast cancer. As results are validated in advanced disease, the potential exists for functional imaging of MDR to be applied to early-stage breast cancer.

ACKNOWLEDGMENTS

The authors thank all our colleagues and collaborators (both past and present) for their contributions, which have led to the successful execution of this review. Financial assistance for work from the Laboratory of Molecular Radiopharmacology was provided by the U.S. Department of Energy (DE-FG02-94ER61885) and the National Institutes of Health (RO1 CA65735; P20 CA86251).

REFERENCES

1. Greenlee RT, Murray T, Bolden S, et al. Cancer statistics, 2000. *CA Cancer J Clin* 2000;50:7–33.

2. Harris JR, Lippman ME, Veronesi U, et al. Breast cancer. *N Engl J Med* 1992;327:473–480.

3. Ling V. Charles F. Kettering Prize. P-glycoprotein and resistance to anticancer drugs. *Cancer* 1992;69:2603–2609.

4. Gottesman MM, Pastan I. Biochemistry of multidrug resistance mediated by the multidrug transporter. *Annu Rev Biochem* 1993;62:385–427.

5. Gottesman MM, Hrycyna CA, Schoenlein PV, et al. Genetic analysis of the multidrug transporter. *Annu Rev Genet* 1995;29:607–649.

6. Bosch I, Croop J. P-glycoprotein multidrug resistance and cancer. *Biochim Biophys Acta* 1996;1288:F37–F54.

7. Bradshaw DM, Arceci RJ. Clinical relevance of transmembrane drug efflux as a mechanism of multidrug resistance. *J Clin Oncol* 1998;16:3674–3690.

8. Rao V, Dahlheimer J, Bardgett M, et al. Choroid plexus epithelial expression of MDR1 P-glycoprotein and multidrug resistance-associated protein contribute to the blood–cerebrospinal fluid drug-permeability barrier. *Proc Natl Acad Sci U S A* 1999;96:3900–3905.

9. Cole SPC, Bhardwaj G, Gerlach JH, et al. Overexpression of a transporter gene in a multidrug-resistant human lung cancer cell line. *Science* 1992;258:1650–1654.

10. Zaman GJR, Versantvoort CHM, Smit JJM, et al. Analysis of the expression of *MRP1*, the gene for a new putative transmembrane drug transporter, in human multidrug-resistant lung cancer cell lines. *Cancer Res* 1993;53:1747–1750.

11. Breuninger LM, Paul S, Gaughan K, et al. Expression of multidrug resistance-associated protein in NIH/3T3 cells confers multidrug resistance associated with increased drug efflux and altered intracellular drug distribution. *Cancer Res* 1995;55:5342–5347.

12. Lautier D, Canitrot Y, Deeley R, et al. Multidrug resistance mediated by the multidrug resistance protein (*MRP1*) gene. *Biochem Pharmacol* 1996;52:967–977.

13. Lorico A, Rappa G, Finch R, et al. Disruption of the murine *MRP1* (multidrug resistance protein) gene leads to increased sensitivity to etoposide (VP-16) and increased levels of glutathione. *Cancer Res* 1997;57:5238–5242.

14. Flens MJ, Zaman GJR, van der Valk P, et al. Tissue distribution of multidrug resistance protein. *Am J Pathol* 1996;148:1237–1247.

15. Merkel D, Fuqua S, Tandon A, et al. Electrophoretic analysis of 248 clinical breast cancer specimens for P-glycoprotein overexpression or gene amplification. *J Clin Oncol* 1989;7:1129–1136.

16. Goldstein LJ, Pastan I, Gottesman MM. Multidrug resistance in human cancer. *Crit Rev Oncol/Hematol* 1992;12:243–253.

17. Yoshimura A, Shudo N, Ikeda SI, et al. Novel screening method for agents that overcome classical multidrug resistance in a human cell line. *Cancer Lett* 1990;50:45–51.

18. Goldstein LJ, Fojo AT, Ueda K, et al. Expression of the multidrug resistance, MDR1, gene in neuroblastomas. *J Clin Oncol* 1990;8:128–136.

19. Chan HSL, Haddad G, Thorner PS, et al. P-glycoprotein expression as a predictor of the outcome of therapy for neuroblastoma. *N Engl J Med* 1991;325:1608–1614.

20. Baldini N, Scotlandi K, Barbanti-Brodano G, et al. Expression of P-glycoprotein in high-grade osteosarcomas in relation to clinical outcome. *N Engl J Med* 1995;333:1380–1385.

21. Norris M, Bordow S, Marshall G, et al. Expression of the gene for multidrug-resistance-associated protein and outcome in patients with neuroblastoma. *N Engl J Med* 1996;334:231–238.

22. Fulda S, Sieverts H, Friesen C, et al. The CD95 (APO-1/Fas) system mediates drug-induced apoptosis in neuroblastoma cells. *Cancer Res* 1997;57:3823–3829.

23. Fisher DE. Apoptosis in cancer therapy: crossing the threshold. *Cell* 1994;78:539–542.

24. Robinson L, Roberts W, Ling T, et al. Human MDR1 protein overexpression delays the apoptotic cascade in Chinese hamster ovary fibroblasts. *Biochemistry* 1997;36:11169–11178.

25. Smyth MJ, Krasovskis E, Sutton VR, et al. The drug efflux protein P-glycoprotein additionally protects drug-resistant tumor cells from multiple forms of caspase-dependent apoptosis. *Proc Natl Acad Sci U S A* 1998;95:7024–7029.

26. Pinedo H, Giaccone G. P-glycoprotein—marker of cancer-cell behavior. *New Engl J Med* 1995;333:1417–1419.

27. Schneider J, Bak M, Efferth T, et al. P-glycoprotein expression in treated and untreated human breast cancer. *Br J Cancer* 1989;60:815–818.

28. Wishart GC, Plumb JA, Going JJ, et al. P-glycoprotein expression in primary breast cancer detected by immunocytochemistry with two monoclonal antibodies. *Br J Cancer* 1990;62:758–761.

29. Wallner J, Depisch D, Hopfner M, et al. MDR1 gene expression and prognostic factors in primary breast carcinomas. *Eur J Cancer* 1991;27:1352–1355.

30. Verrelle P, Meissonnier F, Fonck Y, et al. Clinical relevance of immunohistochemical detection of multidrug resistance P-glycoprotein in breast carcinoma. *J Natl Cancer Inst* 1991;83:111–116.

31. Noonan KE, Beck C, Holzmayer TA, et al. Quantitative analysis of MDR1 gene expression in human tumors by polymerase chain reaction. *Proc Natl Acad Sci U S A* 1990;87:7160–7164.

32. Sanfilippo O, Ronchi E, De Marco C, et al. Expression of P-glycoprotein in breast cancer tissues and *in vitro* resistance to doxorubicin and vincristine. *Eur J Cancer* 1991;27:155–158.

33. Lehnert M. Reversal of multidrug resistance in breast cancer: many more open questions than answers. *Ann Oncol* 1993;4:11–13.

34. Linn S, Giaccone G, van Diest P, et al. Prognostic relevance of P-glycoprotein expression in breast cancer. *Ann Oncol* 1995;6:679–685.

35. Campos L, Guyotat D, Archimbaud E, et al. Clinical significance of multidrug resistance P-glycoprotein expression on acute nonlymphoblastic leukemia cells at diagnosis. *Blood* 1992;79:473–476.

36. Chan H, Thorner P, Haddad G, et al. Immunohistochemical detection of P-glycoprotein: prognostic correlation in soft tissue sarcoma of childhood. *J Clin Oncol* 1990;8:689–704.

37. Charpin C, Vielth P, Duffaud B, et al. Quantitative immunocytochemical assays of P-glycoprotein in breast carcinomas: corelation to messenger RNA expression and to immunohistochemical prognostic indicators. *J Natl Cancer Inst* 1994;86:1539–1545.

38. Ro J, Sahin A, Ro JY, et al. Immunohistochemical analysis of P-glycoprotein expression correlated with chemotherapy resistance in locally advanced breast cancer. *Hum Pathol* 1990;21:787–791.

39. Trock B, Leonessa F, Clarke R. Multidrug resistance in breast cancer: a meta-analysis of MDR1/gp170 expression and its possible functional significance. *J Natl Cancer Inst* 1997;89:917–931.

40. Nooter K, Westerman A, Flens M, et al. Expression of the multidrug resistance-associated protein (*MRP1*) gene in human cancers. *Clin Cancer Res* 1995;1:1301–1310.

41. Nooter K, Brutel de la Riviere G, Look M, et al. The prognostic significance of expression of the multidrug resistance-associated protein (MRP1) in primary breast cancer. *Br J Cancer* 1997;76:486–493.

42. Ford JM, Hait WN. Pharmacology of drugs that alter multidrug resistance in cancer. *Pharmacol Rev* 1990;42:155–199.

43. Gaveriaux C, Boesch D, Jachez B. PSC 833, a non-immunosuppressive cyclosporin analog, is a very potent multidrug-resistance modifier. *J Cell Pharmacol* 1991;2:225–234.

44. Hyafil F, Vergely C, Du Vignaud P, et al. *In vitro* and *in vivo* reversal of multidrug resistance by GF120918, an acridonecarboxamide derivative. *Cancer Res* 1993;53:4595–4602.

45. Dantzig A, Shepard R, Cao J, et al. Reversal of P-glycoprotein-mediated multidrug resistance by a potent cyclopropyldibenzosuberane modulator, LY335979. *Cancer Res* 1996;56:4171–4179.

46. Germann U, Ford P, Schlakhter D, et al. Chemosensitization and drug accumulation effects of VX-710, verapamil, cyclosporin A, MS-209, and GF120918 in multidrug-resistant HL60/ADR cells expressing the multidrug resistance-associated protein MRP1. *Anticancer Drugs* 1997;8:141–155.

47. Toppmeyer D, Overmoyer B, Seidman A, et al. A phase II study of VX-710 (Incel) in combination with paclitaxel in women with advanced breast cancer refractory to paclitaxel. *Proceedings of the 21st Annual Breast Cancer Symposium*, San Antonio, Texas, 1998: 320.

48. Beck W, Grogan T, Willman C, et al. Methods to detect P-glycoprotein-associated multidrug resistance in patients' tumors: consensus recommendations. *Cancer Res* 1996;56:3010–3020.

49. Bosch I, Crankshaw C, Piwnica-Worms D, et al. Characterization of functional assays of P-glycoprotein transport activity. *Leukemia* 1997;11:1131–1137.

50. Homolya L, Hollo Z, Germann UA, et al. Fluorescent cellular indicators are extruded by the multidrug resistance protein. *J Biol Chem* 1993;268:21493–21496.

51. Piwnica-Worms D, Chiu ML, Budding M, et al. Functional imaging of multidrug-resistant P-glycoprotein with an organotechnetium complex. *Cancer Res* 1993;53:977–984.

52. Herman LW, Sharma V, Kronauge JF, et al. Novel *hexakis* (areneisonitrile)technetium(I) complexes as radioligands targeted to the multidrug resistance P-glycoprotein. *J Med Chem* 1995;38: 2955–2963.

53. Ballinger JR, Bannerman J, Boxen I, et al. Technetium-99m-tetrofosmin as a substrate for P-glycoprotein: *in vitro* studies in multidrug-resistant breast tumor cells. *J Nucl Med* 1996;37: 1578–1582.

54. Crankshaw C, Marmion M, Luker G, et al. Novel Tc(III)-Q-complexes for functional imaging of the multidrug resistance (*MDR1*) P-glycoprotein. *J Nucl Med* 1998;39:77–86.

55. Hendrikse N, Franssen E, van der Graaf W, et al. Visualization of multidrug resistance *in vivo*. *Eur J Nucl Med* 1999;26: 283–293.

56. Wackers FJ, Berman D, Maddahi J, et al. Tc-99m-*hexakis*-2-methoxy isobutylisonitrile: human biodistribution, dosimetry, safety and preliminary comparison to thallium-201 for myocardial perfusion imaging. *J Nucl Med* 1989;30:301–309.

57. Higley B, Smith FW, Smith T, et al. Technetium-99m-1,2-*bis*[*bis*(2-ethoxyethyl)phosphino]ethane: human biodistribution, dosimetry and safety of a new myocardial perfusion imaging agent. *J Nucl Med* 1993;34:30–38.

58. Rossetti C, Vanoli G, Paganelli G, et al. Human biodistribution, dosimetry and clinical use of technetium(III)-99m-Q12. *J Nucl Med* 1994;35:1571–1580.

59. Abrams MA, Davison A, Jones AG, et al. Synthesis and characterization of *hexakis*(alkyl isocyanide) and *hexakis*(arylisocyanide) complexes of technetium(I). *Inorganic Chem* 1983;22:2798–2800.

60. Kronauge JF, Kawamura M, Lepisto E, et al. Metabolic studies of the myocardial perfusion agent Tc-(MIBI). In: Nicolini M, Bandoli G, Mazzi U, eds. *Technetium and rhenium in chemistry and nuclear medicine*. Verona, Italy: Cortina International, 1990: 677–682.

61. Platts E, North T, Pickett R, et al. Mechanism of uptake of Tc-tetrofosmin I: uptake into isolated rat venticular myocytes and subcellular localization. *J Nucl Cardiol* 1995;2:317–326.

62. Mehta B, Rosa E, Biedler J, et al. *In vivo* uptake of carbon-14-colchicine for identification of tumor multidrug resistance. *J Nucl Med* 1994;35:1179–1184.

63. Sharma V, Wey SP, Bass L, et al. Monocationic N4O2 Schiff-base phenolate complexes of gallium(III): novel PET imaging agents of the human multidrug resistance (*MDR1*) P-glycoprotein. *J Nucl Med* 1996;37:51P.

64. Elsinga PH, Franssen JF, Hendrikse NH, et al. Carbon-11-labeled daunorubicin and verapamil for probing P-glycoprotein in tumors with PET. *J Nucl Med* 1996;37:1571–1575.

65. Packard A, Barbarics E, Kronauge J, et al. Copper(II)diiminedioxime complexes for imaging multidrug resistance. *Proceedings of the 215th American Chemical Society Meeting*, Dallas, Texas, 1998.

66. Piwnica-Worms D, Kronauge JF, Chiu ML. Uptake and retention of *hexakis* (2-methoxy isobutyl isonitrile) technetium(I) in cultured chick myocardial cells: mitochondrial and plasma membrane potential dependence. *Circulation* 1990;82:1826–1838.

67. Chernoff DM, Strichartz GR, Piwnica-Worms D. Membrane potential determination in large unilamellar vesicles with *hexakis*(2-methoxyisobutyl isonitrile) technetium(I). *Biochim Biophys Acta* 1993;1147:262–266.

68. Delmon-Moingeon LI, Piwnica-Worms D, Van den Abbeele AD, et al. Uptake of the cation *hexakis* (2-methoxy isobutylisonitrile) technetium-99m by human carcinoma cell lines *in vitro*. *Cancer Res* 1990;50:2198–2202.

69. Backus M, Piwnica-Worms D, Hockett D, et al. Microprobe analysis of Tc-MIBI in heart cells: calculation of mitochondrial potential. *Am J Physiol (Cell)* 1993;265:C178–C187.

70. Rao VV, Chiu ML, Kronauge JF, et al. Expression of recombinant human multidrug resistance P-glycoprotein in insect cells confers decreased accumulation of technetium-99m-SESTAMIBI. *J Nucl Med* 1994;35:510–515.

71. Ballinger JR, Sheldon KM, Boxen I, et al. Differences between accumulation of Tc-99m-MIBI and Tl-201-thallous chloride in tumor cells: role of P-glycoprotein. *Q J Nucl Med* 1995;39: 122–128.

72. Piwnica-Worms D, Rao V, Kronauge J, et al. Characterization of multidrug-resistance P-glycoprotein transport function with an organotechnetium cation. *Biochemistry* 1995;34:12210–12220.

73. Ballinger J, Hua H, Berry B, et al. ^{99m}Tc-Sestamibi as an agent for imaging P-glycoprotein-mediated multi-drug resistance: *in vitro* and *in vivo* studies in a rat breast tumour cell line and its doxorubicin-resistant variant. *Nucl Med Commun* 1995;16:253–257.

74. Crankshaw CL, Marmion M, Burleigh BD, et al. Non-reducible mixed ligand Tc(III) cations (Q complexes) are recognized as transport substrates by the human multidrug-resistance (MDR) P-glycoprotein. *J Nucl Med* 1995;36:130P.

75. Cordobes M, Starzec A, Delmon-Moingeon L, et al. Technetium-99m-sestamibi uptake by human benign and malignant breast tumor cells: correlation with mdr gene expression. *J Nucl Med* 1996;37:286–289.

76. Luker G, Rao V, Crankshaw C, et al. Characterization of phosphine complexes of technetium (III) as transport substrates of the multidrug resistance (MDR1) P-glycoprotein and functional markers of P-glycoprotein at the blood–brain barrier. *Biochemistry* 1997;36:14218–14227.

77. Barbarics E, Kronauge J, Cohen D, et al. Characterization of P-glycoprotein transport and inhibition *in vivo*. *Cancer Res* 1998; 58:276–282.

78. Crankshaw C, Piwnica-Worms D. Tc-99m-Sestamibi may be a transport substrate of the human multidrug resistance-associated protein (MRP1). *J Nucl Med* 1996;37:247P.

79. Moretti J-L, Cordobes M, Starzec A, et al. Involvement of glutathione in loss of technetium-99m-MIBI accumulation related to membrane MDR protein expression in tumor cells. *J Nucl Med* 1998;39:1214–1218.

80. Hendrikse N, Franssen E, van der Graaf W, et al. ^{99m}Tc-sestamibi is a substrate for P-glycoprotein and the multidrug resistance-associated protein. *Br J Cancer* 1998;77:353–358.

81. Del Vecchio S, Ciarmiello A, Potena MI, et al. *In vivo* detection of multidrug resistance (MDR1) phenotype by technetium-99m-sestamibi scan in untreated breast cancer patients. *Eur J Nucl Med* 1997;24:150–159.

82. Del Vecchio S, Ciarmiello A, Pace L, et al. Fractional retention

of technetium-99m-sestamibi as an index of P-glycoprotein expression in untreated breast cancer patients. *J Nucl Med* 1997; 38:1348–1351.

83. Kostakoglu L, Elahi N, Kirarli P, et al. Clinical validation of the influence of P-glycoprotein on technetium-99m-sestamibi uptake in malignant tumors. *J Nucl Med* 1994;38:1003–1008.

84. Moretti J, Azaloux H, Boisseron D, et al. Primary breast cancer imaging with technetium-99m sestamibi and its relation with P-glycoprotein overexpression. *Eur J Nucl Med* 1996;23: 980–986.

85. Ciarmiello A, Del Vecchio S, Silvestro P, et al. Tumor clearance of technetium-99m-sestamibi as a predictor of response to neoadjuvant chemotherapy for locally advanced breast cancer. *J Clin Oncol* 1998;16:1677–1683.

86. Kostakoglu L, Ruacan S, Ergun E, et al. Influence of the hetero-geneity of P-glycoprotein expression in technetium-99m-MIBI uptake in breast cancer. *J Nucl Med* 1998:1021–1026.

87. Khalkhali I, Mena I, Diggles L. Review of imaging techniques for the diagnosis of breast cancer: a new role of prone scintimammography using technetium-99m sestamibi. *Eur J Nucl Med* 1994;21: 357–362.

88. Khalkhali I, Mena I, Jouanne E. Prone scintimammography in patients with suspicion of carcinoma of the breast. *J Am Coll Surg* 1994;178:491–497.

89. Khalkhali I, Cutrone J, Mena I, et al. Scintimammography: the complementary role of Tc-99m sestamibi prone breast imaging for the diagnosis of breast carcinoma. *Radiology* 1995;196: 421–426.

90. Maublant J. Scintigraphic imaging of breast tumors. *Eur J Radiol* 1997;24:2–10.

4

MULTIDRUG RESISTANCE

PART B: OTHER TUMORS

LALE KOSTAKOGLU

Intrinsic or acquired resistance of cancer cells to chemotherapeutic agents plays a crucial role in clinical resistance to certain anticancer agents. Multidrug resistance (MDR) is a phenomenon in which malignant cells demonstrate resistance to multiple chemotherapeutic agents, even without exposure to a particular drug. This is usually a manifestation of activation of an intracellular mechanism that results in exclusion of the drug from the cell. MDR-associated antineoplastic agents have in common the following properties: They are lipophilic, their molecular weights range from 300 to 900 d, and they enter cells by passive diffusion. The accumulation and retention of these drugs is lower in MDR cells than in drug-sensitive cells, which results in attenuation of the cytotoxic signal.

Historically, MDR was considered to be caused exclusively by expression of *MDR1* P-glycoprotein (Pgp). More recent developments have demonstrated that MDR is a multifactorial phenomenon that may include overexpression of other drug resistance proteins, such as MDR-associated protein (MRP1) and lung resistance protein (LRP) (1,2), which are also associated with reduced intracellular drug accumulation and retention (3,4).

The recognition that ^{99m}Tc-sestamibi and other lipophilic cations act as transport substrates for Pgp and MRP1 has provided a tool for the clinical assessment of transmembrane efflux pumps in patients with malignant neoplasms.

GENERAL ASPECTS OF MULTIDRUG RESISTANCE

MDR1 P-glycoprotein

The best-defined type of MDR in cancer occurs as a result of the amplification of the *MDR1* gene, which encodes a transmembrane glycoprotein, Pgp (5–7). This form of

MDR is defined as the ability of cells exposed to a single drug to develop resistance to a broad range of structurally unrelated drugs as a result of enhancement of outward transport of these drugs by Pgp, a 170-kd transmembrane glycoprotein that acts as an adenosine triphosphate (ATP)-dependent efflux pump.

Some agents, so-called *modulators*, can regulate *MDR1*. The modulators also bind to Pgp and interfere with drug transport, thereby allowing more chemotherapeutic agent to reach its intracellular cytotoxic targets. As a result, some modulators, such as cyclosporin A, verapamil, dexverapamil, and SDZ PSC 833, have been successfully used to overcome this obstacle to treatment (8,9). Several studies have shown that *MDR1* regulation is possible at the transcriptional and post-transcriptional levels and also by the cell cycle checkpoint protein p53 (10–22).

The *p53* Gene and Its Association with Multidrug Resistance in Cancer

Inactivation of p53, a nuclear phosphoprotein and tumor suppressor, is strongly correlated with human cancers. Chemotherapy-induced apoptosis (programmed cell death) occurs to a lesser extent in tumor cells that lack *p53* gene (16,17). As functional inactivation of p53 would prevent DNA damage-induced apoptosis and contribute to the progression to higher levels of drug resistance, changes within *p53* gene are very common in neoplasms with MDR phenotype (18). Previous data have reported a correlation between mutations in *p53* gene and resistance to chemotherapeutic agents such as etoposide, Adriamycin, and fluorouracil (16). *MDR1* gene expression is regulated by mutant *p53*, which specifically stimulates the *MDR1* promoter (19,20). In malignant tumors, expression of Pgp is activated by mutant *p53*. The correlation of these two genes would be useful to identify a more aggressive and resistant phenotype (20,21). Importantly, concurrent Pgp and p53

L. **Kostakoglu:** Department of Radiology, Division of Nuclear Medicine, New York Presbyterian Hospital–Weill Medical College of Cornell University, New York, New York 10021.

positivity can be overcome in part by moderately high-dose chemotherapy or by transfection of wild-type *p53* (20,22).

Multidrug Resistance-associated Protein

Transfection experiments have shown that *MRP1* gene confers resistance to a similar, but not identical, spectrum of drugs as Pgp (23). *MRP1* gene encodes a 180- to 195-kd, ATP-binding transport protein, MRP1, that resides in the plasma membrane with homology to *MDR1* Pgp (3,24). It is expressed in the cell membrane and also in the cytoplasm, in the endoplasmic reticulum or Golgi apparatus (25–27). MRP1 has been found to be remarkably similar to Pgp in that it acts as an efflux pump, extruding hydrophobic compounds against a concentration gradient (23). Its mechanism of action differs somewhat from that of Pgp. MRP1 acts as a glutathione *S*-conjugate efflux pump (GS-X) by transporting drugs that are conjugated or co-transported with glutathione (28–30). The exact role of glutathione in MRP1-mediated transport is uncertain, although it is theorized that glutathione may function as a co-transporter to pump cationic drugs via MRP1 out of the cell. When cellular glutathione was depleted by administration of buthionine sulfoximine as an inhibitor of τ-glutamylcysteine synthetase, resistance to vincristine, doxorubicin, and daunorubicine was observed to be reversed (31,32). There are differences between MRP1 and *MDR1* Pgp (Table 4B.1). Transfection of *MRP1* cDNA does not result in the acquisition of resistance to cisplatin and paclitaxel (23). In the same context, cyclosporin A, an effective reversal agent for *MDR1* Pgp, does not inhibit MRP1 function (23). By contrast, the isoflavinoid genistein, a drug that does not inhibit *MDR1* Pgp-mediated drug transport, reduces the action of MRP1 (30).

Lung Resistance Protein

The complexity of MDR has gained a new dimension with the identification of so-called *lung resistance protein* (LRP) (33). *LRP* gene encodes a 110-kd protein that has been shown to be a major human vault protein (34). Vaults are newly described cellular organelles that play a prominent role in mediating intracellular transport of a wide variety of substrates. LRP expression is cytoplasmic, in contrast to the plasma membrane location of Pgp and MRP1. The distribution of LRP in normal tissues is remarkably similar to that of other drug resistance-related proteins. High levels of LRP were detected in bronchial and digestive tract epithelial cells, keratinocytes, macrophages, and adrenal cortex (35). A high frequency of LRP expression has been found in breast cancer (3), but more interestingly, the fact that LRP expression was frequently found in Pgp-positive patients after treatment with chemosensitizers has raised the possibility that elimination of Pgp with modulators might select for LRP resistance (36).

Other Forms of Multidrug Resistance

Altered levels of the enzyme DNA topoisomerase II (topo II) may also result in MDR. The DNA topoisomerases relieve the tortional stress on DNA during replication, transcription, and cell division through religation of the broken DNA. "Classic" anthracyclines (e.g., doxorubicin, daunorubicin), the epipodophyllotoxins (etoposide, teniposide), and aminoacridines (e.g., amsacrine) all block strand religation and stabilize DNA–protein complexes. Resistance to most of these topo II inhibitors manifests itself in two forms: a decrease in the amount of enzyme and a decrease in topo II activity by mutations.

The tripeptide glutathione has an important function. It reduces the cellular toxicity of several drugs, such as the anthracyclines, by facilitating their metabolism to less active compounds. Furthermore, glutathione plays a role in the detoxification of drug-induced free radicals (37). Currently, scintigraphic methods for evaluating these two resistance mechanisms, topo II and glutathione, are not available.

The overlapping of MDR phenotypes may result in a complex clinical situation. Accordingly, co-expression of two or three MDR-related proteins has been observed in 64% of the cell lines (35). Combining resistance modifiers that reverse Pgp, MRP1, and LRP may be necessary to achieve a durable response in certain diseases.

CLINICAL RELEVANCE OF MULTIDRUG RESISTANCE IN VARIOUS MALIGNANCIES

Lung Cancer

Although the best-defined type of MDR in lung cancer occurs as a result of the amplification of *MDR1* Pgp, resistance in most lung tumor cell lines is frequently multifactorial. Other mechanisms may be more important than Pgp. Lung tumors, especially small cell lung cancers, are the least amenable to evaluation for MDR protein or *MDR* gene distribution because most specimens are obtained through bronchoscopic biopsy and so might not represent all the tumor characteristics. The contamination of tumor samples with normal cells is also a big drawback in interpreting such

TABLE 4B.1. RESISTANCE SPECTRUM OF MULTIDRUG RESISTANCE PROTEINS

Drug	MDR1/Pgp	MRP1	LRP
Doxorubicin	+	+	+
Daunorubicin	+	+	+
Cisplatin	+	–	+
Vincristine	+	+	+
Etoposide (VP-16)	+	+	+
Paclitaxel	+	–	?

MDR, multidrug resistance; Pgp, P-glycoprotein; MRP1, multidrug resistance protein; LRP, lung resistance protein.

measurements in biopsy specimens. Furthermore, the limited amounts of tissue available, particularly in small cell lunger cancer, usually make it impossible to measure and compare multiple parameters, such as levels of MDR proteins and their mRNA and transport function, in a single sample.

Although small cell lung cancer is associated with progressive unresponsiveness to chemotherapy, the prevalence of *MDR1* Pgp in lung cancer is consistent. Different detection methods may be a contributing factor to these discrepancies. Although some investigators found a correlation between response to therapy and *MDR1* Pgp expression when they used a polymerase chain reaction assay in a rather limited group of patients with small cell lung cancer (38), expression of the *MDR1* gene responsible for Pgp is extremely low. It is generally undetectable in most human lung cancers. An extensive study by Lai et al. (39) revealed only low levels of *MDR1* mRNA expression in patients with small cell lung cancer. No obvious relationship was observed between the response to therapy and *MDR1* Pgp (40). This finding was supported by another study in which the *MDR1* gene was not associated with small cell lung cancer and tumor progression or drug resistance (41). Additionally, no significant differences have been observed in *MDR1* Pgp levels in pretherapy and post-therapy specimens of small cell lung cancer, which suggests that resistance to chemotherapy is unlikely to be caused by overexpression of Pgp. Also, up to 20% of non-small cell lung cancers, which are generally unresponsive to chemotherapy, are negative for *MDR1* Pgp (42).

There are strong indications that non–Pgp-mediated MDR and other mechanisms may be responsible for drug resistance in lung cancers (39,43–47). Pgp belongs to a superfamily of ATP-binding cassette transporters. Recently, a new member of this family, MRP1, has been cloned from human lung cancer cell lines. Expression of the *MRP1* gene may be a significant factor determining the response of lung cancer to therapy. Direct evidence for the function of MRP1 as an ATP-driven pump is lacking, but it has shown to be a primary export pump for lipophilic compounds with glutathione and other anionic residues (28,48). MRP1 was found to be expressed in 87% of all histologic subtypes of non-small cell lung cancer, especially in adenocarcinomas (55%) and squamous cell carcinomas (28%) (49,50). Both the level and frequency of MRP1 expression in untreated small cell lung cancer was significantly lower (56%). MRP1 immunoreactivity was also detected in reactive type 2 pneumocytes in hyperplastic alveoli. Furthermore, a significant correlation between MRP1 expression and resistance to daunorubicin, doxorubicin, and etoposide has been detected (51). Patients with high or moderate levels of MRP1 expression had a significantly worse prognosis than those with weak or absent expression of MRP1, which suggests that MRP1 is a factor in the prognosis of non-small cell lung cancer (52). Verapamil, rifamycins, genistein, and quinoline derivatives have been effective in modulating the function of the *MRP1* gene product (44,47,53).

Expression of LRP is another factor in the development of MDR phenotype, both acquired and intrinsic, in cancer patients (35,54). LRP was found to be a superior predictor for *in vitro* resistance to MDR-related drugs in comparison with Pgp and MRP1 (35). Intrinsically resistant non-small cell lung cancer cells were reported to exhibit a complex pattern of MDR proteins, with co-expression of LRP and MRP1, and carcinomas in heavy smokers were more frequently LRP-positive than those in nonsmokers (55–57). The correlation between the level of *LRP* mRNA expression and cisplatin sensitivity was significant in lung cancer (58). Although LRP expression at diagnosis has been described as an independent predictor of a poor response to chemotherapy and reduced overall survival in acute myeloid leukemia and ovarian carcinoma in a preliminary analysis, LRP expression was not predictive of response to therapy in lung cancer (59). Further investigation of cytoplasmic vault function is warranted to provide effective strategies to circumvent drug resistance and its clinical impact.

Hematologic Malignancies

Multidrug resistance phenotype has been suspected as a major cause of treatment failure in hematologic malignancies. By far the greatest number of analyses of *MDR1* Pgp expression in hematologic malignancies have been performed in acute nonlymphoblastic leukemia. Most of the studies have shown approximately 50% of patients to be positive for MDR phenotype at the time of diagnosis; also, the number of positive cases seems to be slightly higher after treatment (60). Furthermore, better remission rates were reported for *MDR1* Pgp-negative patients following induction therapy, and *MDR1* Pgp expression was an independent prognostic factor in regard to disease-free and overall survival (61).

In acute lymphocytic leukemia, MDR positivity is not as common as in acute nonlymphoblastic leukemia. The average number of MDR-positive cases is 22% at diagnosis, versus 58% at relapse or a refractory stage of disease. Again, better remission rates for MDR-negative patients and a correlation between the MDR phenotype and disease-free and overall survival were reported (62). In chronic myelogenous leukemia, it seems that *MDR1* Pgp expression is intrinsic, not treatment-related. *MDR1* gene is expressed in a majority of B-cell chronic lymphocytic leukemias, regardless of the stage or duration of disease or disease progression (63–65)

In multiple myeloma, evidence of an association of the MDR phenotype with disease progression is accumulating, and increased Pgp expression has been detected in cases with preceding anthracycline/vinca alkaloid treatment (66). For this reason, patients with multiple myeloma seem to be especially suitable for the testing of MDR modulator substances.

Because of the difficulties involved in obtaining sufficient material, lymphomas have been studied less extensively. The threshold for *MDR1* gene positivity between studies vary between 1% and 30%, thus it is virtually impossible to come to a conclusive result concerning the relevance of *MDR1* gene expression in lymphoma. Nevertheless, tendency toward a higher level of expression in treated patients has been noted, and successful modulation of the MDR phenotype has been shown for refractory lymphoma.

Soft-tissue Sarcomas

On multivariate analysis, Pgp expression was found to be an independent prognostic indicator, along with Ki-67 and nondiploid DNA content, that correlated with a poor outcome in soft-tissue sarcomas (67). On the other hand, *MDR1* mRNA expression was not predictive of survival. In another study, of Pgp, MRP1, and LRP, Pgp was the most commonly expressed marker, and its expression was correlated with survival (68). The co-expression of MRP1 and *MDR1* Pgp was recognized in 38% of soft-tissue sarcomas (69). Although the outcome of osteosarcoma has improved considerably since the addition of chemotherapy to surgery, systemic relapses still occur in 40% to 50% of cases (70). A group of investigators found that high levels of Pgp, determined by immunohistochemistry in tumor cells, were prognostic in osteosarcoma (70).

Other Malignant Neoplasms

The expression of *MDR1* Pgp in the capillary endothelial cells of the central nervous system has been demonstrated. Moreover, *MDR1* Pgp was found to be expressed in the newly formed capillaries of brain tumors (71). In light of this finding, MDR in brain tumors may result not only from the expression of resistance markers in neoplastic cells but also from the expression of *MDR1* Pgp in endothelial cells of tumor capillaries.

Drugs associated with MDR can induce overexpression of *MDR1* gene and result in the appearance of the MDR phenomenon in other malignancies, such as ovarian carcinoma, neuroblastoma, and renal cell carcinoma. In the same context, MRP1 and LRP have been found to play a role in the MDR phenotype of ovarian carcinoma and renal cell carcinoma (35,72).

MDR1 Gene Therapy in the Treatment of Cancer

Myelosuppression is a major dose-limiting factor in cancer chemotherapy. Little or no expression of Pgp occurs in normal bone marrow cells; therefore, they are particularly susceptible to killing by MDR-associated drugs such as vinca alkaloids, anthracyclines, and paclitaxel and its congeners. The introduction of drug resistance genes into bone marrow cells of cancer patients has been proposed to overcome this limitation. Recently, clinical trials of *MDR1* gene ther-

apy have been started for breast cancer patients undergoing high-dose chemotherapy with autologous hematopoietic stem cell transplantation; the intent is to prevent myelosuppression by protecting cells against the toxic effects of chemotherapy (73,74). Phase I studies have indicated the feasibility and safety of bone marrow gene therapy with the *MDR1* gene (74).

CONTROVERSIES IN THE DETECTION OF MULTIDRUG RESISTANCE PROTEINS

Discordant results may emerge when various techniques are compared because the sensitivity and specificity of a certain technique are always limited by unpredictable parameters; these include the diversity of tumor tissues, simultaneous presence of other resistance mechanisms, and heterogeneous expression of the proteins, particularly Pgp, all of which can make the results of efforts to detect MDR equivocal (75–78).

Shortcomings of Detection Techniques at the Protein Level

Immunohistochemical techniques provide specific information on the distribution of Pgp in different tumor sections, along with a definition of morphology and localization of the Pgp-expressing tumor and stromal cells (79). However, immunocytochemistry is subjective in interpretation, so that the use of a consistent scoring system by an experienced pathologist is necessary to provide better comparisons between different studies. Moreover, antigenic heterogeneity influences the interpretation of immunohistochemistry studies (76,77). A metaanalysis of studies of Pgp expression revealed that significant heterogeneity was present in the malignant breast tumors expressing Pgp. This finding could be attributed to the use of different immunohistochemical techniques, application of immunologic reagents with variable Pgp specificity, and differences in methods of analysis (80), in addition to other factors, such as co-expression of multiple resistance mechanisms and varying functional capacity of the Pgp efflux pump (5,6,81). Because Pgp might be expressed in the tissue but might not be functional, functional studies such as rhodamine 123 efflux studies should be carried out.

Shortcomings of Detection Techniques at the DNA and RNA Level

In a recent study, concordance between values for *MDR1* expression determined at the RNA level with reverse transcriptase polymerase chain reaction (RT-PCR) and dot blot and values determined at the protein level with immunohistochemistry was found in only 47% of the comparable specimens (69,82). It has been reported that most of these disparities originate from low levels and heterogeneous expression of Pgp (76,83). With immunohistochemistry, interpretation of *MDR1* Pgp measurements is complicated by heterogeneity among tumor cells and by a possible contribution from nontumor cells, which are usually associated with abundant stromal cells. The same levels of Pgp expression could result from homogeneous expression in all cells or from strong expression in a small population of tumor or stromal cells and no expression in others. This discrepancy between mRNA and protein expression may also be related to one of the post-transcriptional control mechanisms, such as negative translational control (84).

Furthermore, the characterization of MDR proteins by current techniques requires that serial tissue specimens be obtained; therefore, the usefulness of these approaches has been limited by sampling errors, the high degree of sensitivity required of RNA and antibody probes, and the labor intensiveness and invasiveness of the procedures.

FUNCTIONAL IMAGING OF MULTIDRUG RESISTANCE PHENOTYPE

In light of the discordant results and shortcomings of the currently available MRP1 and gene detection techniques, an imaging method that could be used as a noninvasive probe of tissue expression of MRPs should be the ultimate modality in the detection of MDR. The potential advantage of an imaging modality would be its ability to diagnose the MDR phenotype noninvasively *in vivo*. The information derived from images might prove quite useful in patient management and the design of effective therapy protocols.

^{99m}Tc-Sestamibi

Scintigraphy with ^{99m}Tc-sestamibi [*hexakis*(2-methoxy-isobutylisonitrile) technetium(I)] (MIBI) has proved valuable in tumor diagnosis. Although the accumulation rates are driven by negative transmembrane potentials (85), the accumulation and retention of MIBI are reduced in cells expressing MDR phenotype owing to the energy-dependent Pgp efflux pump that expels its substrates from the cell and causes a concomitant decrease in levels (86–95).

Current Clinical Data in Imaging P-glycoprotein

Prior studies have shown an inverse relationship between levels of Pgp and the magnitude of MIBI uptake and washout in tumor cells (86–95). In studies of lung and breast cancer, a statistically significant difference was noted in tumor-to-background ratios between the group with strong Pgp expression and the group with weak or no expression (86–88). However, contrasting points were also raised in the published data, such as the finding of high levels of Pgp expression associated with unexpectedly high tumor-to-background ratios

or vice versa. These discrepancies could be attributed to the presence of subsets of cells simultaneously expressing varying and multiple resistance mechanisms, or poor penetration of MIBI because of reduced blood flow in tumors undergoing necrosis (86,87,90).

Kao et al. (96), using ^{99m}Tc-sestamibi uptake in small cell lung cancer, studied the relationship between chemotherapy response and survival time. In a group of 15 patients, ^{99m}Tc-sestamibi predicted the chemotherapy response, with a high correlation between positive images and a good response and between negative images and a poor response. Also, the uptake ratios correlated well with survival time. In advanced non-small cell lung cancer, increased tumor clearance of ^{99m}Tc-sestamibi was significantly correlated with resistance to chemotherapy and the presence of distant metastases (97), which suggests a role for this agent in the prediction of response to cytotoxic therapy and in identifying tumors with aggressive behavior. In a recent study of a group of 27 patients with small cell lung cancer, the ^{99m}Tc-sestamibi uptake ratios in therapy responders were higher than those in nonresponders. In the same study, the authors reported the modulating ability of dipyridamole, a known Pgp modulator, which induced increased ^{99m}Tc-sestamibi uptake in all patients showing no response to therapy (98).

^{99m}Tc-Sestamibi was reported to identify MDR phenotype noninvasively in patients with acute myeloid leukemia or acute lymphocytic leukemia (89). An inverse correlation was noted between levels of Pgp and ^{99m}Tc-sestamibi uptake when flow cytometry and RT-PCR were used as detection methods for Pgp overexpression. Nevertheless, the results of RT-PCR, flow cytometry, and imaging were discordant; therefore, the authors concluded that a combination of current techniques, ideally one at the molecular level and one at the imaging level, would be ideal to avoid false-negative or false-positive results. In another study, functional imaging with ^{99m}Tc-sestamibi was performed in 21 patients with multiple myeloma to determine its value in detecting MDR phenotype (99). Although the presence of MDR was not confirmed at the tissue level, the authors found that ^{99m}Tc-sestamibi uptake was negative in drug-resistant cases with high total cumulative doses of doxorubicin.

The correlation of ^{99m}Tc-sestamibi accumulation in tumor with response to therapy was studied in children with lymphoma before and after therapy. The patients who had positive scans had a complete response to chemotherapy, whereas those with no uptake failed therapy irrespective of the lymphoma type (100). Although in this study the absence of determination of MDR-related protein expression in tissue was a shortcoming, the results suggest that ^{99m}Tc-sestamibi might predict response to therapy.

By contrast, in brain tumors, ^{99m}Tc-sestamibi levels were markedly high in patients with a higher grade of tumor and clinical deterioration, whereas no uptake was seen in patients who showed no sign of recurrence. The reason for this is that Pgp expression is inversely correlated with grade of malignancy in gliomas. Hence, the main cause of chemoresistance in gliomas is probably not an increased drug efflux associated with Pgp; ^{99m}Tc-sestamibi is useful for detecting active lesions but may not be useful for predicting the response to chemotherapy (101).

In a phase I trial of the Pgp reversal agent PSC 833, its effects were demonstrated in patients with renal cell carcinoma. Tumor visualization and ^{99m}Tc-sestamibi tumor uptake were observed to be enhanced by the administration of PSC 833 (102).

Current Clinical Data in Imaging Multiresistance Protein

Recently, MRP1 was found to play an important role in extruding MIBI from resistant cell lines (103). Accordingly, MIBI imaging characteristics should not be strictly related to Pgp expression. They should also provide a useful imaging tool for assessing functional resistance mediated by MRP1. The influence of the MRP1 pump mechanism on MIBI accumulation has been investigated in human cell lines; however, its significance has yet to be validated in clinical studies. Because MRP1 has been found to be remarkably similar to the drug-transporting Pgp in its mode of action as an efflux pump, breast cancers overexpressing MRP1 should be investigated with respect to MIBI accumulation and retention to establish the possible clinical implications of MIBI. To date, no data have been published correlating *in vivo* LRP overexpression with MIBI accumulation and retention.

^{99m}Tc-Tetrofosmin

^{99m}Tc-Tetrofosmin [*trans*-di-oxo-*bis* (diphosphine) technetium(V) cation] is a lipophilic phosphine cation, like ^{99m}Tc-sestamibi. It was developed for myocardial perfusion imaging and has recently been shown to accumulate in some tumors (104,105). When ^{99m}Tc-tetrofosmin was compared with ^{99m}Tc-sestamibi, the two tracers were found to behave similarly in sensitive and resistant MCF-7 breast cancer cell lines. On the other hand, the modulator PSC 833 was effective in reversing the resistance and enhancing the accumulation of both tracers, but higher concentrations of the modulator were required for ^{99m}Tc-tetrofosmin than for ^{99m}Tc-sestamibi, which suggests that ^{99m}Tc-sestamibi is a more specific tracer for Pgp.

In a clinical study of 18 patients with non-small cell lung cancer, the authors reported a statistically significant difference in uptake indices between Pgp-positive and Pgp-negative tumors. Furthermore, they noted an inverse relationship between the ^{99m}Tc-tetrofosmin uptake index and the level of Pgp expression according to immunohistochemistry data (106).

^{99m}Tc-Teboroxime, a neutral lipophilic myocardial agent, was found not to be a substrate for Pgp (107).

^{99m}Tc(III)-Q Complexes

^{99m}Tc-Q complexes are a class of nonreducible ^{99m}Tc(III) cations. These agents retain the desired modest lipophilicity and delocalized cationic charge of many other Pgp substrates and modulators while enabling selective exploration of single or paired modified functionalities. Various ^{99m}Tc-Q complexes have been developed to optimize these complexes as transport substrates of Pgp. ^{99m}Tc-Q63, ^{99m}Tc-Q58, and ^{99m}Tc-Q57 were found to have accumulation ratios of the sensitive to the resistant cell line equal to or higher than those for ^{99m}Tc-sestamibi and ^{99m}Tc-tetrofomin (108). ^{99m}Tc-Furifosmin (Q12) has also been validated as a transport substrate for *MDR1* Pgp *in vivo* (109).

IMAGING WITH POSITRON EMISSION TOMOGRAPHY

The pharmacokinetics of an MDR-associated cytotoxic agent, colchicine, may be favorable for positron emission tomography (PET) studies. Mehta et al. (110) studied the distribution and metabolism of ^{14}C-colchicine and found the accumulation of this agent in sensitive tumors of tumor-bearing mice to be twice as great as that in resistant tumors. These findings have been confirmed by quantitative autoradiography (111). The studies suggest the feasibility of imaging Pgp function in tumors with ^{11}C-colchicine PET. However, biodistribution studies have revealed high colchicine uptake in the liver and intestines, which may obviate its use for monitoring Pgp function in abdominal tumors.

Additionally, the cytotoxic agent daunorubicin and the modulator verapamil have been studied in cell lines to probe Pgp activity with the PET radiotracer ^{11}C. The accumulation ratio of ^{11}C-daunorubicin in drug-sensitive/drug-resistant cell lines was as high as 16. Addition of verapamil resulted in an increased uptake of ^{11}C-daunorubicin in the resistant cell lines. These results suggest that PET tracers have potential for *in vivo* probing of Pgp function (112).

Leukotrienes, the mediators of hypersensitivity reactions, shock, and inflammation, are specific substrates for MRP1. However, no *in vitro* or *in vivo* study has been performed to evaluate their role in PET imaging of MRP1 in resistant tumors.

CONCLUSION: IMPACT OF FUNCTIONAL IMAGING IN THE DETECTION OF MULTIDRUG RESISTANCE PROTEINS

Although the results of studies are controversial, MDR is widely accepted as a major hindrance in chemotherapy. The addition of neoadjuvant chemotherapy to protocols has led to a substantial improvement in patient survival, with 35% to 50% of patients surviving beyond 5 years (18). Despite these therapeutic advances, the development of MDR phenotype is still the most significant obstacle to cancer therapy. The observed association between Pgp expression and a worse prognosis, in addition to the possibility of modulating MRP1-mediated resistance by agents capable of reversing MDR, have stimulated the development of various methods to increase the sensitivity and accuracy of detection techniques (113). However, current methods are invasive, laborious, and vulnerable to sampling errors. Because an *in vivo* screen would facilitate the detection of MRPs and the evaluation of response to therapy, we believe that the potential advantage of imaging agents lies in their ability to detect the presence of MRPs noninvasively, especially Pgp overexpression *in vivo*. In this context, the information derived from images, either to detect MRPs before therapy or evaluate response to therapy, might prove useful in the selection of effective drug combinations and might guide the development of new programs using MDR modifiers.

REFERENCES

1. Morrow CS, Chiu J, Cowan KH. Posttranscriptional control of glutathione S-transferase pi gene expression in human breast cancer cells. *J Biol Chem* 1992;267:10544–10550.
2. Tuccari G, Rizzo A, Giuffre G, et al. Immunohistochemical detection of DNA topoisomerase type II in primary breast carcinomas: correlation with clinico-pathological features. *Virchows Arch Pathol Anat Histopathol* 1993;423:51–55.
3. Linn SC, Pinedo HM, van Ark Otte J, et al. Expression of drug resistance proteins in breast cancer, in relation to chemotherapy. *Int J Cancer* 1997;71:787–795.
4. Schneider E, Horton JK, Yang CH, et al. Multidrug resistance-associated protein gene overexpression and reduced drug sensitivity of topoisomerase II in a human breast carcinoma MCF7 cell line selected for etoposide resistance. *Cancer Res* 1994;54: 152–158.
5. Juliano Rl, Ling V. A surface glycoprotein modulating drug permeability in Chinese hamster ovary cell mutants. *Biochim Biophys Acta* 1976;455:152–162.
6. Shen DW, Fojjo A, Chin JE, et al. Human multidrug-resistant cell lines: increased MDR1 expression can precede amplification. *Science* 1986;232:643–645.
7. Verelle P, Missonnier F, Fonck F, et al. Clinical relevance of immunohistochemical detection of multidrug resistance of Pgp in breast carcinoma. *J Natl Cancer Inst* 1991;83:111–116.
8. Luker GD, Fracasso PM, Dobkin J, et al. Modulation of the multidrug resistance P-glycoprotein: detection with technetium-99m-sestamibi *in vivo*. *J Nucl Med* 1997;38:369–372.
9. Wilson B, Bates S, Fojo A, et al. Controlled trial of dexverapamil, a modulator of multidrug resistance, in lymphomas refractory to EPOCH chemotherapy. *J Clin Oncol* 1995;13:1995–2004.
10. Hartwell LH, Kastan MB. Cell cycle control and cancer. *Science* 1994;266:1821–1828.
11. Fearnhead HO, McCurrach ME, O'Neill J, et al. Oncogene-dependent apoptosis in extracts from drug-resistant cells. *Genes Dev* 1997;11:1266–1276.
12. Chomcyznski P, Sacchi N. Single-step method for RNA isolation by acid guanidium thiocyanate-phenol chloroform extraction. *Ann Biochem* 1979;162:156–159,.
13. Ryan JJ, Prochownik E, Gottlieb CA, et al. *c-myc* and *bcl-2* mod-

14. Minn AJ, Rudin CM, Boise LH, et al. Expression of Bcl-X$_L$ can confer a multidrug resistance phenotype. *Blood* 1995;86: 1903–1910.
15. O'Connor PM, Kohn KW. A fundamental role for cell cycle regulation in the chemosensitivity of cancer cell. *Semin Cancer Biol* 1992;3:409–416.
16. Lowe SW, Ruley HE, Jacks T, et al. P53-dependent apoptosis modulates the cytotoxicity of anticancer agents. *Cell* 1993;74: 957–967.
17. Thottassery JV, Zambetti GP, Arimori K, et al. P53-dependent regulation of MDR1 gene expression causes selective resistance to chemotherapeutic agents. *Proc Natl Acad Sci U S A* 1997;4: 11037–11042.
18. Beck WT, Dalton WS. Mechanisms of drug resistance. In: DeVita VT, Hellman S, Rosenberg SA, eds. *Principles and practice of oncology*. Philadelphia: JB Lippincott Co, 1997:498–512.
19. Kaye SB. Multidrug resistance in breast cancer—is the jury in yet? *J Natl Cancer Inst* 1997;89:902–903.
20. Linn SC, Honkoop AH, Hoekman K, et al. P53 and P-glycoprotein are often co-expressed and are associated with poor prognosis in breast cancer. *Br J Cancer* 1996;74:63–68.
21. Bodey B, Bodey B Jr, Groger AM, et al. Immunocytochemical detection of the p170 multidrug resistance (MDR) and the p53 tumor suppressor gene proteins in human breast cancer cells: clinical and therapeutical significance. *Anticancer Res* 1997;17: 1311–1318.
22. Fujiwara T, Grimm EA, Mukhopadhyay T, et al. Induction of chemosensitivity in human lung cancer cells *in vivo* by adenovirus-mediated transfer of wild-type p53 gene. *Cancer Res* 1994; 54:2287–2291.
23. Zaman GJR, Flens MJ, van Leusden MR, et al. The human multidrug resistance-associated protein MRP1 is a plasma membrane drug-efflux pump. *Proc Natl Acad Sci U S A* 1994;91:8822–8826.
24. Cole SPC, Bhardwaj G, Gerlach JH, et al. Overexpression of a transporter gene in a multidrug-resistant human cancer cell line. *Science* 1992;258:1650–1656.
25. Almquist KC, Loe DW, Hipfner DR, et al. Characterization of the M 190 000 multidrug resistance protein (MRP1) in drug-selected and transfected human tumor cells. *Cancer Res* 1995;55: 102–110.
26. Flens MJ, Izquierdo MA, Schaffer GL, et al. Immunohistochemical detection of the multidrug resistance-associated protein MRP1 in human multidrug-resistant tumour cells by monoclonal antibodies. *Cancer Res* 1994;54:4556–4563.
27. Van Luyn MJA, Muller M, Renes J, et al. Transport of glutathione conjugates into secretory vesicles is mediated by the multidrug-resistance protein 1. *Int J Cancer* 1998;76:55–62.
28. Leier I, Jedlitschky G, Bucholz U, et al. The MRP1 gene encodes an ATP-dependent export pump for leukotriene C and structurally related conjugates. *J Biochem Chem* 1994:269: 27807–27810.
29. Muller M, Meijer C, Zaman GJ, et al. Overexpression of the gene encoding the multidrug resistance-associated protein results in increased ATP-dependent glutathione S-conjugate transport. *Proc Natl Acad Sci U S A* 1994;91:13033–13037.
30. Versantvoort CHM, Broxterman HJ, Bagrij T, et al. Regulation by glutathione of drug transport in multidrug-resistant human lung cancer cell lines overexpressing multidrug resistance-associated protein. *Br J Cancer* 1995;72:82–89.
31. Hendrikse NH, Franssen EJF, van der Graaf WTA, et al. Tc-99m-sestamibi is a substrate for P-glycoprotein and the multidrug resistance-associated protein. *Br J Cancer* 1998;77: 353–358.
32. Hendrikse NH, Franssen EJF, van der Graaf WTA, et al. Visual-

ization of multidrug resistance *in vivo. Eur J Nucl Med* 1999;26: 283–293.

33. Raviv Y, Pollard HB, Bruggeman EP, et al. Photosensitized labeling of a functional multidrug transporter in living drug-resistant tumor cells. *J Biol Chem* 1990;265:3975–3980.

34. Scheffer GL, Wijngaard PLJ, Flens MJ, et al. The drug resistance-related protein LRP is the human major vault protein. *Nat Med* 1995;1:578–582.

35. Izquierdo MA, Scheffer GL, Flens MJ, et al. Relationship of LRP-human major vault protein to *in vitro* and clinical resistance to anticancer drugs. *Cytotechnology* 1996;19:191–197.

36. List AF, Spier CS, Grogan TM, et al. Overexpression of the major vault transporter protein lung-resistance protein predicts treatment outcome in acute myeloid leukemia. *Blood* 1996;87: 2464–2469.

37. Meijer C, Mulder NH, de Vries EGE. The role of detoxifying systems in resistance of tumor cells to cisplatin and Adriamycin. *Cancer Treat Rev* 1990;17:389–407.

38. Savaraj , Wu CJ, Xu R, et al. Multidrug-resistant gene expression in small-cell lung cancer. *Am J Clin Oncol* 1997;20:398–403.

39. Lai SL, Goldstein LJ, Gottesman MM, et al. MDR1 gene expression in lung cancer. *J Natl Cancer Inst* 1989;81:1144–1150.

40. Canitrot Y, Bichat F, Cole SP, et al. Multidrug resistance genes (MRP1) and MDR1 expression in small cell lung cancer xenografts: relationship with response to chemotherapy. *Cancer Lett* 1998;130:133–141.

41. Oka M, Fukuda M, Sakamato A, et al. The clinical role of MDR1 gene expression in human lung cancer. *Anticancer Res* 1997;17: 721–724.

42. Holzmayer TA, Hilsenbeck S, Von Doff DD, et al. Clinical correlates of MDR1 (P-glycoprotein) gene expression in ovarian and small cell lung carcinomas. *J Natl Cancer Inst* 1992;84: 1486–1491.

43. Giaccone G, van Ark-Otte J, Rubin GJ, et al. MRP1 is frequently expressed in human lung-cancer cell lines, in non-small-cell lung cancer and in normal lungs. *Int J Cancer* 1996;66: 760–767.

44. Binaschi M, Supino R, Gambetta RA, et al. MRP1 gene overexpression in a human doxorubicin-resistant SCLC cell line: alterations in cellular pharmacokinetics and in pattern of cross-resistance. *Int J Cancer* 1995;62:84–89.

45. Goldstein LJ, Gaski H, Fojo A, et al. Expression of a multidrug resistance gene in human cancers. *J Natl Cancer Inst* 1989;81: 116–124.

46. Eijdems EW, de Haas M, Coco-Martin JM, et al. Mechanisms of MRP1 over-expression in four human lung-cancer cell lines and analysis of the MRP1 amplicon. *Int J Cancer* 1995;60:676–684.

47. Narasaki F, Oka M, Fukuda M, et al. Multidrug resistance-associated protein gene expression and drug sensitivity in lung cancer cell. *Anticancer Res* 1997;17:3493–3497.

48. Nooter K, Westerman A, Flens MJ, et al. Expression of the multidrug resistance-associated protein (MRP1) gene in human cancers *Clin Cancer Res* 1995;1:1301–1310.

49. Berger W, Elbling L, Hauptmann E, et al. Expression of the multidrug resistance-associated protein (MRP1) and chemoresistance of human non-small-cell lung cancer. *Int J Cancer* 1997;73:84–93.

50. Wright SR, Boag AH, Valdimarsson G, et al. Immunohistochemical detection of multidrug resistance protein in human lung cancer and normal lung. *Clin Cancer Res* 1998;4: 2279–2289.

51. Gonzales Manzano R, Versanvoort C, Wright K, et al. Rapid recovery of a functional MDR phenotype caused by MRP1 after a transient exposure to MDR drugs in a revertant human lung cancer cell line. *Eur J Cancer* 1996;32:2136–2141.

52. Ota E, Abe Y, Oshika Y, et al. Expression of the multidrug resis-

tance-associated protein (MRP1) gene in non-small-cell lung cancer. *Br J Cancer* 1995;71:550–554.

53. Courtois A, Payen L, Vernhet L, et al. Inhibition of multidrug resistance-associated protein (MRP1) activity by rifampicin in human multidrug-resistant tumor cells. *Cancer Lett* 1999;139: 97–104.

54. Beck J, Bohnet B, Brugger D, et al. Multiple gene expression analysis reveals distinct differences between G2 and G3 stage breast cancers and correlations of PKC with MDR1, MRP1 and LRP gene expression. *Br J Cancer* 1998;77:87–91.

55. Laurencot CM, Scheffer GL, Scheper RJ, et al. Increased LRP mRNA expression is associated with the MDR phenotype in intrinsically resistant human cancer cell lines. *Int J Cancer* 1997; 72:1021–1026.

56. Trussardi A, Poitevin G, Gorisse MC, et al. Sequential overexpression of LRP and MRP1 but not p-gp 170 in VP-16-selected A549 adenocarcinoma cells. *Int J Oncol* 1998;13:543–548.

57. Volm M, Mattern J, Koomagi R. Expression of lung resistance-related protein (LRP) in non-small cell lung carcinomas of smokers and non-smokers and its predictive value for doxorubicin resistance. *Anticancer Drugs* 1997;8:931–936.

58. Ikeda K, Oka M, Narasaki F, et al. Lung resistance-related protein gene expression and drug sensitivity in human gastric and lung cancer cells. *Anticancer Res* 1998;18:3077–3080.

59. Dingemans AM, van Ark-Otte J, van der Valk, et al. Expression of the human major vault protein LRP in human lung cancer samples and normal lung tissues. *Ann Oncol* 1996;7:625–630.

60. Ball ED, Lawrence D, Malnar M, et al. Correlation of CD34 and multi-drug resistance P170 with FAB and cytogenetics but not prognosis in acute myeloid leukemia (AML). *Blood* 1990;76:252(abst).

61. Campos L, Guyotat D, Archimbaud E, et al. Clinical significance of multidrug resistance P-glycoprotein expression on acute nonlymphoblastic leukemia cells at diagnosis. *Blood* 1992;79: 473–476.

62. Goasguen JE, Dossot JM, Fardel O, et al. Expression of multidrug resistance-associated P-glycoprotein (P-170) in 59 cases of *de novo* acute lymphoblastic leukemia: prognostic implications. *Blood* 1993;81:2394–2398.

63. El Rouby S, Thomas A, Costin D, et al. P53 gene mutation in B-cell chronic lymphocytic leukemia is associated with drug resistance and is independent of MDR1/MDR3 gene expression. *Blood* 1993;82:3452–3459.

64. Ludescher C, Hilbe W, Eisterer W, et al. Activity of p-glycoprotein in B-cell chronic lymphocytic leukemia determined by a flow cytometric assay. *J Natl Cancer Inst* 1993;85:11751–11758.

65. Sparrow LR, Hall FJ, Siregar H, et al. Common expression of the multidrug resistance marker P-glycoprotein in B-cell chronic lymphocytic leukemia and correlation with *in vitro* drug resistance. *Leuk Res* 1993;17:941–947.

66. Grogan TM, Spier CM, Salmon SE, et al. P-glycoprotein expression in human plasma cell myeloma: correlation with prior chemotherapy. *Blood* 1993;81:490–495.

67. Levine EA, Holzmayer T, Bacus S, et al. Evaluation of newer prognostic markers for adult soft tissue sarcomas. *J Clin Oncol* 1997;15:3249–3257.

68. Coley HM. Drug resistance studies using fresh human ovarian carcinoma and soft tissue sarcoma samples. *Keio J Med* 1997;46: 142–147.

69. Oda Y, Schneider-Stock R, Rys J, et al. Reverse transcriptase-polymerase chain reaction amplification of MDR1 gene expression in adult soft tissue sarcomas. *Diagn Mol Pathol* 1996;5: 98–106.

70. Baldini N, Scotlandi K, Barbanti-Brodano G, et al. Expression of P-glycoprotein in high-grade osteosarcomas in relation to clinical outcome. *N Engl J Med* 1995;333:1380–1385.

71. Toth K, Vaughan MM, Slocum HK, et al. New immunohisto-chemical sandwich staining method for mdr1 P-glycoprotein detection with JSB-1 monoclonal antibody in formalin-fixed paraffin-embedded human tissues. *Am J Pathol* 1994;144:227–236.

72. Gamelin E, Mertins SD, Regis JT, et al. Intrinsic drug resistance in primary and metastatic renal cell carcinoma. *J Urol* 1999;162:217–224.

73. Moscow JA, Huang H, Carter C, et al. Engraftment of MDR1 and NeoR gene-transduced hematopoietic cells after breast cancer chemotherapy. *Blood* 1999;94:52–61.

74. Hersdorffer C, Ayello J, Ward M, et al. Phase-1 trial of retroviral-mediated transfer of the human MDR1 gene as marrow chemoprotection in patients undergoing high-dose chemotherapy and autologous stem-cell transplantation. *J Clin Oncol* 1998;16:165–172.

75. Kessel D, Beck WT, Kukuruga D, et al. Characterization of multidrug resistance by fluorescent dyes. *Cancer Res* 1991;51:4665–4670.

76. Charpin C, Vielh P, Duffaud F, et al. Quantitative immunocytochemical assays of Pgp in breast carcinomas: correlation to messenger RNA expression and to immunohistochemical prognostic indicators. *J Natl Cancer Inst* 1994;86:1539–1545.

77. van der Heyden S, Gheuens E, DeBruijn E, et al. P-glycoprotein: clinical significance and methods of analysis. *Crit Rev Clin Lab Sci* 1995;32:221–264.

78. Rabkin-D, Chieng-DC, Miller-MB, et al. Pgp expression in the squamous cell carcinoma of the tongue base. *Laryngoscope* 1995;105:1294–1299.

79. Decker DA, Morris LW, Levine AJ, et al. Immunohistochemical analysis of P-glycoprotein expression in breast cancer: clinical correlations. *Ann Clin Lab Sci* 1995;25:52–59.

80. Trock BJ, Leonessa F, Clarke R. Multidrug resistance in breast cancer: a meta-analysis of MDR1/gp170 expression and its possible functional significance. *J Natl Cancer Inst* 1997;89:917–931.

81. Ambudkar SV, Lelong JH, Zhang J, et al. Partial purification and reconstitution of the human multidrug resistance pump: characterization of the drug-stimulatable ATO hydrolysis. *Proc Natl Acad Sci U S A* 1992;89:8472–8476.

82. Chan H, Thorner P, Haddad G, et al. Immunohistochemical detection of P-glycoprotein: prognostic correlation in soft tissue sarcoma of childhood. *J Clin Oncol* 1990;8:689–704.

83. Cardon Cardo C, O'Brien JB, Boccia J, et al. Expression of multidrug resistance gene product (Pgp) in human normal and tumor tissues. *J Histochem Cytochem* 1990;38:1277–1287.

84. Melefors O, Hentze MW. Translational regulation by mRNA/protein interactions in eucaryotic cells: ferritin and beyond. *Bioassays* 1993;15:85–90.

85. Piwnica-Worms D, Krounage JF, Chiu ML. Uptake and retention of hexakis (2-methoxyisobutyl isonitrile) technetium(I) in cultured chick myocardial cells. Mitochondrial and plasma membrane potential dependence. *Circulation* 1990;82:1826–1838.

86. Kostakoglu L, Elahi N, Kiratli P, et al. Clinical validation of influence of Pgp on the uptake of Tc-99m-sestamibi in patients with malignant tumors. *J Nucl Med* 1997;38:1003–1008.

87. Kostakoglu L, Kiratli P, Ruacan S, et al. Association of tumor wash-out rates and accumulation of Tc-99m-MIBI with the expression of Pgp in lung cancer. *J Nucl Med* 1998;39:228–234.

88. Kostakoglu L, Ruacan S, Ergun EL, et al. Influence of the heterogeneity of P-glycoprotein expression on technetium-99m-MIBI uptake in breast cancer. *J Nucl Med* 1998;39:1021–1026.

89. Kostakoglu L, Guc D, Canpinar H, et al. Determination of P-glycoprotein using Tc-99m-MIBI in patients with hematologic malignancy: comparison of the results with flow cytometric analyses. *J Nucl Med* 1998;39:1191–1196.

90. Del Vecchio S, Ciarmiello A, Potena MI, et al. *In vivo* detection of multi-drug resistant (MDR1) phenotype by technetium-99m sestamibi scan in untreated breast cancer patients. *Eur J Nucl Med* 1997;24:150–159.

91. Duran Cordobes M, Starzes A, Delmon-Moingeon L, et al. Technetium-99m uptake by human benign and malignant breast tumor cells: correlation with mdr gene expression. *J Nucl Med* 1996;37:286–289.

92. Piwnica-Worms D, Chiu ML, Budding M, et al. Functional imaging of multidrug-resistant Pgp with an organotechnetium complex. *Cancer Res* 1993;53:977–984.

93. Rao VV, Chiu ML, Kronauge JF, et al. Expression of recombinant human multidrug resistance Pgp in insect cells confers decreased accumulation of technetium-99m-sestamibi. *J Nucl Med* 1994;35:510–515.

94. Andrews DW, Das R, Kim S, et al. Technetium MIBI as a glioma imaging agent for the assessment of multidrug resistance. *Neurosurgery* 1997;40:1323–1332.

95. Piwnica-Worms D, Rao VV, Kronauge JF, et al. Characterization of multidrug resistance P-glycoprotein function with an organotechnetium complex. *Biochemistry* 1995;34:12210–12220.

96. Kao CH, Chang Lai SP, Chieng PU, et al. Technetium-99m methoxyisobutylisonitrile chest imaging of small cell lung carcinoma: relation to patient prognosis and chemotherapy response—a preliminary report. *Cancer* 1998;83:64–68.

97. Koukourakis MI, Koukoraki S, Giatromanolaki A, et al. Non-small cell lung cancer functional imaging: increased hexakis-2-methoxy-isobutyl-isonitrile tumor clearance correlates with resistance to cytotoxic treatment. *Clin Cancer Res* 1997;3:749–754.

98. Bom HS, Kim YC, Song HC, et al. Technetium-99m-MIBI uptake in small cell lung cancer. *J Nucl Med* 1998;39:91–94.

99. Tirovola EB, Biassoni C, Britton KE, et al. The use of 99m Tc-MIBI scanning in multiple myeloma. *Br J Cancer* 1996;74:1815–1820.

100. Kapucu LO, Akyuz C, Vural G, et al. Evaluation of therapy response in children with untreated malignant lymphomas using technetium-99m-sestamibi. *J Nucl Med* 1997;38:243–247.

101. Yokogami K, Kawano H, Moriyama T, et al. Application of SPET using technetium-99m-sestamibi in brain tumors and comparison with expression of the MDR1 gene: is it possible to predict the response to chemotherapy in patients with gliomas by means of ^{99m}Tc-sestamibi SPET? *Eur J Nucl Med* 1998;25:401–409.

102. Chen G, Jaffrezou JP, Fleming WH, et al. Prevalence of multidrug resistance related to activation of the mdr1 gene in human sarcoma mutants derived by single-step doxorubicin selection. *Cancer Res* 1994;54:4980–4987.

103. Duran Cordobes M, Moretti JL, de Veco B, et al. Sestamibi Tc 99m (MIBI) uptake in human cell lines exhibiting multidrug resistance related to MDR or MRP1 genes. *J Nucl Med* 1997;38:253P(abst).

104. Mansi l, Rambaldi PF, La Provitera A, et al. Technetium-99m-tetrofosmin uptake in breast tumors. *J Nucl Med* 1995;36:83P(abst).

105. Klain N, Maurea S, Lastoria S, et al. Technetium-99m-tetrofosmin imaging of differentiated mixed thyroid cancer. *J Nucl Med* 1995;36:2248–2251.

106. Tabuenca MJ, Vargas JA, Varela A, et al. Inverse correlation between Tc-99m-tetrofosmin uptake and P-glycoprotein in non-small cell lung cancer. *J Nucl Med* 1999;40;1224–1225.

107. Gros P, Talbot F, Tang-Wai D, et al. Lipophilic cations: a group of model substrates for multidrug-resistance transporter. *Biochemistry* 1992;31:1992–1998.

108. Crankshaw CL, Marmion M, Luker GD, et al. Novel technetium (III)-Q complexes for functional imaging of multidrug resistance (MDR1) P-glycoprotein. *J Nucl Med* 1998;39:77–86.

109. Ballinger JR, Bannerman J, Boxen I, et al. Technetium-99m-

tetrofosmin as a substrate for P-glycoprotein: *in vitro* studies in multidrug-resistant breast tumor cells. *J Nucl Med* 1996;37: 1578–1582.

110. Mehta BM, Rosa E, Biedler JL, et al. *In vivo* uptake of [C-14]-colchicine for identification of tumor multidrug resistance. *J Nucl Med* 1994;35:1179–1184.

111. Mehta BM, Levchenko A, Rosa E, et al. Evaluation of [C-14]-colchicine biodistribution with whole body quantitative autora-diography in colchicine-sensitive and -resistant xenografts. *J Nucl Med* 1996;37:312–314.

112. Elsinga PH, Franssen EJF, Hendrikse NH, et al. [C-11]-labeled daunorubicin and verapamil for probing P-glycoprotein in tumours with PET. *J Nucl Med* 1996;37:1571–1575.

113. Beck WT, Grogan TM, Willman CL, et al. Methods to detect Pgp-associated multidrug resistance in patients' tumors: consensus recommendations. *Cancer Res* 1996;56:3010–3020.

5

RADIOLABELED MONOCLONAL ANTIBODIES

PART A: IMAGING

LIONEL S. ZUCKIER
RENEE M. MOADEL-SERNICK

Within the last several years, four commercially produced radiolabeled antibodies have achieved regulatory approval in the United States (1) (Table 5A.1). The successful appearance of these agents marks the initial realization of the long-standing dream of harnessing the diversity and specificity of the immune system to create effective, safe, and convenient radioimmunoimaging agents. These radiopharmaceuticals represent only the first generation of what is likely to become a series of ever-more sophisticated imaging agents. Ongoing discoveries in the laboratory are actively being incorporated into second- and third-generation radioimmunologic agents. For example, techniques in molecular immunology are being used to design immunologic moieties with variable regions optimized for superior tumor binding. Constant regions are also being engineered to reduce immunogenicity and improve pharmacokinetics and biodistribution. Advances in tumor biology have identified new and promising antigens for targeting, such as those related to angiogenesis or ability to metastasize.

This chapter reviews the fundamental background concepts and nomenclature relevant to present and future radioimmunoimaging agents. Formerly theoretical questions regarding the optimization of targeting, such as the issue of optimal affinity or the impact of polymerization, take on relevance and practicality when these attributes can be altered by antibody engineering.

IMMUNOGLOBULIN

Structure

The composition of the antibody molecule, and the structure–function relationships that govern its behavior, are basic to understanding radioimmunoscintigraphy (2–6). The term *immunoglobulin*, although historically defined from the perspective of electrophoresis, can be used synonymously with *antibody*. An antibody is a member of a family of structurally related glycoproteins, secreted by B cells or their progeny, that have the potential to bind to an antigen. An antigen is a foreign or endogenous macromolecule to which an antibody binds. The specific region of the antigen molecule to which an antibody binds is termed an *epitope*.

To date, the majority of immunoglobulins employed in clinical studies have been murine IgG molecules. The typical IgG antibody (Fig. 5A.1) is a heterodimer composed of two identical heavy and two identical light polypeptide chains, covalently linked by disulfide bonds to form a *Y*-shaped structure with paired antigen-binding arms. Mice, like humans, have five classes of antibodies (IgM, IgD, IgG, IgE, and IgA) and four subclasses of IgG. Each class or subclass of immunoglobulin shares a similarity of functional and structural properties encoded by a specific and unique heavy-chain immunoglobulin gene.

Heavy and light chains of immunoglobulins are divided into relatively compact globular regions approximately 110 amino acids, termed *domains*. Those located at the terminus of the antigen-binding arms are considerably more variable in composition than those situated elsewhere in the molecule and have been termed the *variable-heavy* (V_H) and *variable-light* (V_L) domains. It has been noted that three specific sites within both V_H and V_L are especially varied ("hypervariable") and are interspersed between more-constant ("framework") residues. It is now understood that these framework residues serve to fold and inter-

---

L. S. Zuckier: Departments of Nuclear Medicine and Radiology, Albert Einstein College of Medicine; Department of Nuclear Medicine, Jacobi Hospital, New York, New York 10461.

R. M. Moadel-Sernick: Department of Nuclear Medicine, Albert Einstein College of Medicine and Montefiore Medical Center, New York, New York 10461.

TABLE 5A.1. FDA-APPROVED RADIOIMMUNOIMAGING AGENTS

	OncoScint CR/OV	CEA-Scan	Verluma	ProstaScint
Tradename				
Pharmacopeia name	Satumomab pendetide	Arcitumomab	Nofetumomab merpentan	Capromab pendetide
Aliases	CYT-103	NP-4	OncoTrac	CYT-356
Antibody (amount)	B72.3 (1.0 mg)	IMMU-4 (1.0 mg)	NR-LU-10 (5–10 mg)	7E11-C5.3 (0.5 mg)
Label (activity)	^{111}In (5 mCi)	^{99m}Tc (20–25 mCi)	^{99m}Tc (15–30 mCi)	^{111}In (5 mCi)
Description	Murine IgG1, whole mAb	Murine IgG1, Fab'	Murine IgG2b, Fab	Murine IgG1, whole mAb
Epitope	TAG-72	200-kd CEA	40-kd cell surface glycoprotein	100-kd glycoprotein, LNCaP cells
FDA indications	Colorectal carcinoma, ovarian carcinoma	Colorectal carcinoma	Small cell lung carcinoma	Prostate carcinoma
Date of approval	December 1992	June 1996	August 1996	October 1996
Sponsor	Cytogen	Immunomedics	Boehringer Ingelheim, NeoRx	Cytogen

mAb, monoclonal antibody; CEA, carcinoembryonic antigen.

act so as to assemble the six hypervariable regions into a contiguous antigen-binding groove. It is therefore the properties of these hypervariable regions that dictate the epitope to which the antibody will bind, and they have therefore also been termed *complementarity-defining regions* (CDRs).

In addition to V_H, the IgG heavy chain is composed of three constant-region domains (C_H1, C_H2, and C_H3) and a hinge that provides segmental flexibility between C_H1 and C_H2 (Fig. 5A.1). A carbohydrate moiety is present in the C_H2 region. The light chain is composed of only a single constant-region domain (C_L) in addition to V_L. Composition of the heavy-chain constant domains determines the class and subclass of an immunoglobulin and confers specific effector functions (4–6), such as binding to Fc receptors or phagocytic cells, activation of the complement cascade, and regulation of the catabolic rate of the immunoglobulin molecule (7,8). Both IgD and IgA resemble IgG in that they

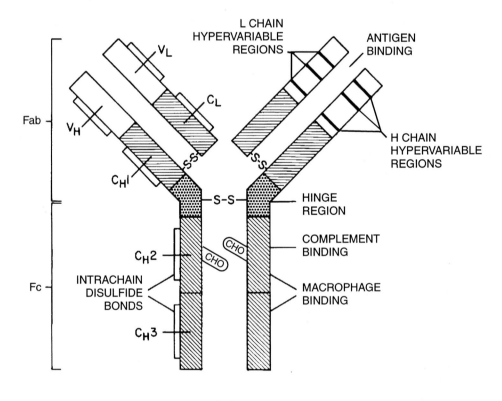

FIGURE 5A.1. Schematic structure of IgG molecule. Interchain and intrachain disulfide bonds (-*S-S*-) and the C_H2 region carbohydrates (*CHO*) are indicated schematically on the molecule. (Modified from Zuckier LS, Rodriguez LD, Scharff MD. Immunologic and pharmacologic concepts of monoclonal antibodies. *Semin Nucl Med* 1989;19:166–186, with permission.)

have three constant and one variable domain within their heavy chain, whereas IgE and IgM have an additional, fourth heavy domain (C_H4) that contributes to a higher molecular weight. IgE is monomeric, like IgG; however, IgA is assembled into bimeric or trimeric forms, and IgM forms pentamers, based on secretion of IgA and IgM from the B cell with an attached "joining" or J chain. With multimeric antibodies and adequate antigen density, *avidity* of binding, referring to the sum total of interactions between the immunoglobulin and antigen, is markedly increased. In contrast, the *affinity* of binding, which refers to the interaction between a single binding site and antigen, is by definition unaffected by multivalence. The increased avidity of binding afforded by multivalence is of crucial importance in the course of a normal immune response. IgM molecules initially formed in response to infection or antigenic challenge are of low affinity, yet they are able to bind effectively because of their multimeric nature.

IgG molecules have been digested by the enzymes papain and pepsin to form well-described subunits. When digested by papain, the heavy chains are cleaved above the disulfide bonds between them, and the resultant "Fab" fragment consists of the V_H, V_L, C_L, and C_H1 domains. The residual duplicated C_H2 and C_H3 domains, the "Fc" (crystallizable) fragment, do not bind antigen. Pepsin cleaves the heavy chains below their interchain disulfide bonds to produce a bivalent "F(ab')$_2$" fragment and small polypeptide fragments derived from the Fc region. F(ab')$_2$ may be reduced to two Fab' fragments, each slightly larger than the Fab fragment described above.

Monoclonal Antibody Technology

It is now understood that the immune response begins with a moderate number of B cells, each expressing products of the "germline" variable region genes on their surface. When exposed to antigen, the clones of cells that bind best to the antigen are stimulated to proliferate, and in doing so, they undergo random mutations in the DNA coding for their binding sites. The progeny that bind to the antigen most effectively are then further stimulated to divide and mutate and are thereby selected. This phenomenon of "affinity maturation" consists of successive rounds of mutation and selection that ultimate result in the emergence of new antibodies of higher affinity. In a second phenomenon that is also relevant to the immune response, termed *class and subclass switching*, a given variable region may successively associate with a series of different heavy-chain constant regions, based on rearrangement of the constant-region genes. It is interesting to note that through the concurrent processes of affinity maturation and class switching that take place as the antibody response evolves from pentameric IgM to monomeric IgG molecules, increases in antibody affinity compensate for the effect of a decrease in valence and thereby ensure adequate binding. Additionally, affinity maturation and subclass switching serve to explain the diversity

of binding and multiplicity of class and subclass within the immune system (9), which is quite astonishing in light of the finite number of germline immunoglobulin genes.

Despite the ability of the immune system to produce a diverse array of antibodies with high affinity and great specificity, the task of harnessing this potential for targeted delivery of radionuclides has been daunting. The concept of tissue targeting with antibodies can be traced back five decades to the work of Pressman and Keighly (10,11), who in 1948 targeted rat renal tissue with radiolabeled polyclonal antibodies derived from rabbit immune sera. Successful realization of this concept awaited numerous subsequent developments in immunology, cell biology, and molecular biology that revolutionized our understanding of the immune response and antibody structure–function relationships. For example, the response of an organism to immunization remains highly unpredictable and results in an assorted mixture of antibodies of different classes, subclasses, and affinities. It is therefore often very difficult to generate large amounts of high-affinity antibody to a given antigen, and it is virtually impossible to replicate a similar response when additional supplies are needed. This problem of consistency and availability of substrate, necessary requisites of a well-manufactured product, was solved only after Kohler and Milstein developed the hybridoma technique in 1975 (12), which allowed immunologic targeting to begin to mature as a commercially viable technique. In this method, antibody-forming B cells from an immunized subject (usually a mouse) are fused to a tissue culture-adapted malignant plasma cell to make hybrids that retain the properties of both the immunized antibody-forming cell and the immortal myeloma fusion partner (Fig. 5A.2). Single-cell clones are then cultured into homogeneous antibody-producing cell lines that can be individually typed and characterized. Antibodies produced from these cell lines are termed *monoclonal*, in contrast to the *polyclonal* antibodies obtained from immunized serum, which derive from multiple B cells within the immunized host. Monoclonal antibodies (mAbs) have universally replaced the use of pooled sera as the vehicle for targeting radionuclides to tumors. Unlimited amounts of homogeneous reagent can be produced from the cell line, so that mAb production is economically feasible (13). A second feature of mAb technology is the ability to select a reagent individually based on its attributes, including the class and subclass of the antibody (which determine half-life and bioavailability), the epitope to which the antibody binds, and the affinity of interaction between the antibody and the antigen. Finally, mAbs, in contrast to polyclonal sera, are amenable to antibody engineering (14–18), so that novel constructs can be created, as described below.

Human Anti-mouse Antibody and Humanization

A limitation of many of the antibodies presently in clinical trials is that they are murine in origin and can stimulate an

Immunization

10^8 Spleen Cells

2×10^7 Myeloma Cells

Fusion

Screen for Antibody

Selection (HAT)

Clone Positive Hybrids

Screen for Antibody

Grow up Clones

Produce Ascites

Freeze Cells

Ig gene

H chain vector

Neo

DNA

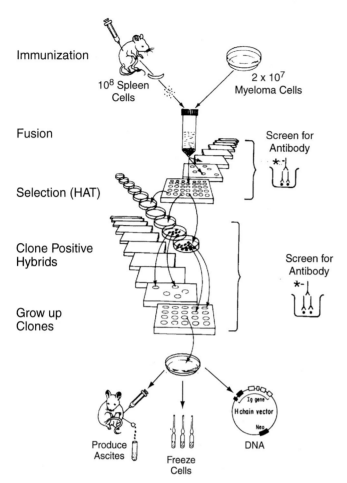

FIGURE 5A.2. Production of mouse monoclonal antibodies. The labor-intensive steps of immunization, fusion, selection of fused cells by heterophil antibody titer media, and screening are illustrated. Once a specific clone of cells has been characterized and selected, it is grown in culture and secretes antibody into the media, which can be obtained and purified. Cells can also be injected into animals to produce ascitic fluid containing high titers of antibody; this is frozen for future use or used as a source of DNA for recombinant antibody engineering. (Modified from Zuckier LS, Rodriguez LD, Scharff MD. Immunologic and pharmacologic concepts of monoclonal antibodies. *Semin Nucl Med* 1989;19:166–186, with permission.)

immune response in the human recipient. This so-called HAMA (human anti-mouse antibody) response does not result in acute injury, but it does limit the future use of identical or even antigenically related reagents because the presence of HAMA will result in rapid clearance of the infused antibody from the blood and its nonspecific accumulation in the reticuloendothelial system.

The obvious solution of replacing murine immunoglobulins with human antibodies has been limited by ethical problems in obtaining immunized human lymphocytes and by intrinsic technical difficulties in the human hybridoma process (19,20). As an alternative, researchers have developed methods for combining murine-derived binding specificity

with the constant-region structure of human immunoglobulins. Initially, murine DNA coding for the variable region was spliced onto human DNA coding for the constant region and expressed in previously nonsecreting lymphocytes to produce "chimeric" antibodies (21,22). Although functionally similar to human antibodies (23), the murine-derived variable regions may still elicit an immune response (24). To minimize this problem, "humanized" or "CDR-grafted" antibodies have been constructed in which both the constant regions and framework portion of the variable regions are derived from human immunoglobulins, with only the hypervariable regions cloned from the immunized mouse (15,25,26). The antigen binding of these antibodies is often diminished because of altered interactions between the native framework regions and the grafted murine hypervariable regions (27,28). To compensate, modeling (28,29) and labor-intensive substitution of flanking amino acids (28,30) has been used to restore affinity.

Progress in human hybridoma technology has led to greater ease in directly generating human monoclonal antibodies by Epstein-Barr virus transformation (31–33) or by human–mouse or human–human fusions (34,35), and these methods were in fact used to generate hu-mAb 88BV59, an antibody that has been in clinical trials for colorectal, ovarian, and breast carcinoma (1). Transgenic mice carrying human immunoglobulin genes have also been developed as a means of generating human antibodies from an animal species (36–38). These animals, endowed genetically with a functional human humoral immune system, may be immunized with a given antigen and their B cells used for subsequent hybridoma production.

An additional method of producing small antigen-binding proteins utilizes immunoglobulin genes expressed in bacteria, so that the need for immunization of live subjects is circumvented. In this method, termed the *phage-display library* (39–42), hundreds of thousands of variable region-derived amino acid sequences are expressed or "displayed" on the surface of filamentous phage, which are then screened for binding to the antigen of interest. By using multiple rounds of "panning" with the phage-display library, sequences that bind are retained and enriched, so that it is ultimately possible to isolate peptides with desired specificity.

Modification of Size

Many of the currently used radioimmunoimaging agents are antibody fragments enzymatically generated by digestion of the whole antibody with pepsin or papain (43–45) (Fig. 5A.3). The resultant (Fab')$_2$, Fab', or Fab fragments retain antigen binding (although avidity of Fab and Fab' fragments may be reduced because of loss of bivalence), but by virtue of their smaller size, they have an accelerated intravascular half-life (7), decreased immunogenicity, and superior penetration into the tumor interstitium (46). Recombinant DNA techniques, including the phage-display library, may be used to produce Fab fragments (41,47) or even smaller immunologically active reagents (48), such as single-chain variable regions (49,50), also known as single-chain Fvs (51), single-chain antigen-binding proteins (SCAs) (52), and single-chain molecules (SCMs) (3). These are composed of the heavy- and light-chain variable regions, attached by linker peptides (Fig. 5A.3). To increase valence, various dimeric constructs have been created as variants of the single-chain Fc. These include diabodies [(scFv')₂] and minibodies (Fig. 5A.3).

Even smaller molecules, such as single heavy-chain variable regions (40), termed *single-* or *variable-domain antibodies* (dAbs), and single hypervariable regions or CDRs (53,54), termed *molecular recognition units* (MRUs), have been described. Small peptides such as single-chain Fvs have been shown to exhibit more rapid and homogeneous penetration of tumor in comparison with larger immunoglobulin forms, with tumor-to-normal tissue ratios equal or superior to those of larger fragments (50,55). Increased kidney uptake, seen with ^{125}I-Fab and ^{125}I-F(ab')₂, is not noted (50). One of the major advantage of small peptides such as MRUs is that they may be chemically synthesized *de novo* without the complexity and regulatory difficulties of utilizing biologic cell lines for their production.

Disadvantages of MRUs are that binding is limited to a single hypervariable region, whereas in a native immunoglobulin molecule, the six hypervariable regions within each Fab contribute jointly to binding with the epitope. Taking the hypervariable regions out of their normal context may also alter them conformationally. It is therefore unlikely that a typical MRU will exhibit strong binding to the antigen. In certain cases, low affinity can

be overcome by tandem repeats of the MRU-binding sequence, which increases avidity (56,57), or by conformationally constraining the peptides to resemble the native conformation (56).

In contrast to this trend of miniaturizing binding agents, the generation of larger multimeric antibodies to increase the avidity of binding is also being studied. For example, an IgG1 constant-region mutation, leading to formation of covalently linked oligomers, has been shown to demonstrate increased antigen binding (58). With the use of methods of antibody engineering, recombinant polymeric immunoglobulins have been constructed from IgG (59,60).

Recombinant and Chemically Modified Proteins

In addition to modifications of size and immunogenicity, described above, numerous other changes to the antibody have been described, including those made to add to or alter the functionality of the immunoglobulin molecule. For example, mutations in critical amino acid residues, to improve binding, may be created based on specific details of antibody and antigen structure (61). The function of an additional biologic agent can be chemically or genetically engineered into the antibody molecule, such as a cytokine (62), hormone (63), or ligand (64). The isoelectric point of an antibody has been altered to modify its pharmacokinetics and improve tumor targeting (65). By somatic cell or chemical means, it is possible to construct antibodies with dual binding specificity (i.e., one of the Fab fragments binds a given antigen while the second binds another) (66–72), or to add functional groups to the constant region, such as avidin or biotin (73–76), discussed below. Bifunc-

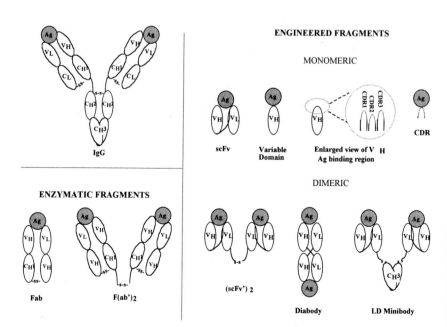

FIGURE 5A.3. Structure of various antibody-based molecules. Intact IgG molecules (*upper left panel*) can be enzymatically digested to yield Fab and F(ab')₂ fragments (*lower left panel*). By using antibody engineering techniques, a variety of monomeric and dimeric molecules have been described (*right panel*). (Reprinted from Adams GP. Improving the tumor specificity and retention of antibody-based molecules. *In Vivo* 1998;12:11–22, with permission.)

tional antibodies that bind two distinct antigens that coexist only in a given tumor tissue may be a potential means of increasing the specificity of tumor targeting.

Biologic response modifiers may play a role as adjuvants in mAb-based procedures (77). These biologically active proteins also may be directly attached to the antibody by chemical (78) or genetic (62) means. The modifiers may be used to increase capillary permeability, which results in greater tumor accretion of antibody (77), or to increase antigen expression on the tumor, which leads to increased antibody binding (79,80). Because the blood–brain barrier is generally impervious to systemically administered antibodies, ligands that are actively transported through it, such as transferrin, may be attached to an immunoglobulin molecule to ferry the antibody across the blood–brain barrier (64).

Recently, major advances have been made in the understanding of structural factors that govern antibody catabolism (81,82). A three-fold variation in serum half-life is found within the four subclasses of human IgG, ranging from approximately 3 weeks for IgG1, IgG2, and IgG4 to 1 week for IgG3 (7,8). The half-lives of the non-IgG antibody classes are considerably shorter. Hybridomas may be switched in culture by somatic mutation to specific antibody classes, or may be altered by recombinant DNA techniques to produce antibodies of any selected class or subclass. By selection of novel heavy-chain domain sequences, not normally found in nature, it may be possible to create immunoglobulins with prolonged (83) or shortened (84) serum half-lives.

RADIOLABEL

Early antibody imaging studies utilized iodinated mAbs, chiefly with ^{131}I (85). This reflected the familiarity and ease of use of ^{131}I as a diagnostic label. Shortcomings of ^{131}I include a relatively long physical half-life and poor imaging qualities of the 364-keV gamma photons on newer-generation gamma cameras (86). Additionally, despite the covalent attachment of iodine to amino acid residues on the antibody molecule, significant dehalogenation tends to occur *in vivo* (87). ^{123}I possesses a more readily imaged 159-keV photon. Because it is cyclotron-produced, it is expensive. It has a somewhat short 13-hour physical half-life and does not overcome the biologic limitations of iodine-labeled proteins. At the present time, commercially available antibodies use either ^{111}In or ^{99m}Tc as the diagnostic label (Table 5.1).

The energy and half-life characteristics of ^{111}In are very suitable for imaging; the 2.8-day physical half-life is well matched with the biologic clearance and behavior of intact immunoglobulins. The chemistry by which this metal is attached to proteins has been developed with the use of chelators such as DTPA (diethylenetriamine pentaacetic acid) and DOTA (tetraazacyclododecane-N,N',N'',N'''-tetraacetic acid) (87). In the two commer-

cially available ^{111}In-labeled antibodies, capromab pendetide and satumomab pendetide (Table 5.1), ^{111}In is attached by a linker chelator to the carbohydrate within the C_H2 region to minimize stearic interference with the distally located binding sites. A limitation of ^{111}In is that free radionuclide tends to accumulate in the reticuloendothelial system. To decrease this phenomenon, improved metal-binding chelators (88), such as isothiocyanatobenzylmethyl DTPA (89), have been developed. As an alternate approach, peptide chelators designed to be metabolized by hepatic enzymes have been used to decrease nonspecific liver accretion (90).

The more rapid localization and clearance of antibody fragments made it feasible to utilize shorter-lived radionuclides, and various techniques for the use of a ^{99m}Tc label have therefore been developed (87,91). ^{99m}Tc has the advantages of a high rate of monoenergetic photon flux, absence of particulate radiation, and a low radiation burden to the patient (91). In "direct" methods of labeling, ^{99m}Tc is believed to be attached to reduced sulfhydryl groups directly on the antibody molecule, whereas in "indirect" methods of labeling, an exogenous chelating group is covalently linked to the antibody. Two of the agents presently approved by the Food and Drug Administration, arcitumomab and nofetumomab merpentan (Table 5A.1), are directly labeled with ^{99m}Tc.

An additional area of development for the diagnostic use of antibodies is with positron-emitting tracers, such as ^{64}Cu, ^{68}Ga, and ^{124}I, which have been incorporated into antibodies for imaging on positron emission tomography (PET) systems (92,93). One of the major advantages of PET is that is makes possible true quantification of the radiopharmaceutical distribution.

TARGETING PROTOCOLS

During a decade of experience, strategies for immunologic targeting have been refined. In general, requirements for imaging are less stringent in certain ways than those for radioimmunotherapy, in that lesions must be identified but every cell in the tumor mass need not be targeted.

One of the key issues addressed has been the ideal amount or mass of antibody needed for optimal imaging (7). Because of nonspecific uptake of antibody by various sites within the recipient's body, increasing the mass of antibody is generally a means of optimizing the ratio of tumor-to-nontumor uptake, although greater mass increases cost and immunogenicity. The optimal amount of antibody to be administered is one of the issues addressed in initial trials of a new agent, in which antibody dose is escalated to study safety and targeting efficacy.

Issues that are difficult to analyze, such as the optimal antibody affinity, are still not resolved, although they have been addressed both experimentally (94–97) and in theoretical models (96,98). For example, it has been postulated that in one circumstance, a high-affinity antibody may be less desirable than one of low affinity because of complexation with circulating antigens (99,100), whereas in another case, high affinity may be needed to effect greater tumor binding and retention (97). It is clear that each antibody has its own optimal mode of administration that depends on tumor type and possibly even patient-specific factors. Specialized routes of administration, such as intracavitary (101) or intradermal (for lymphatic drainage) routes, have generally fallen out of favor.

The creation of biotinylated or bifunctional antibodies has been described. These reagents have been used in strategies for pretargeting of tumors; an unlabeled immunoglobulin molecule is targeted to the antigen site, followed subsequently by a radiolabeled moiety that attaches and binds with high specificity to the initially targeted immunologic agent (102). For example, streptavidinylated mAbs may be administered and allowed sufficient time to bind to the tumor. Several days later, radiolabeled biotin is administered, some of which binds strongly to the pretargeted avidin while the remainder is promptly excreted, thereby reducing background. In the same manner, bifunctional antibodies may be used as the initial reagent, with binding specificity to both the tumor and a second small, radiolabeled moiety. Strategies for pretargeting of tumors are entering clinical trials at the present time (103). These techniques have been successful in improving tumor-to-background ratios, although issues relating to antigenicity remain.

TECHNICAL FACTORS

In addition to the optimization of biologic factors to improve binding, new developments in nuclear medicine technology and more sophisticated application of this technology have also benefited antibody imaging. For example, the development and refinement of single-photon emission tomography (SPECT) has clearly improved modern antibody imaging; it allows foci of activity deep within the body to be differentiated from overlying regions of nonspecific uptake. With methods of simultaneously imaging a ^{99m}Tc-labeled blood pool marker, such as red blood cells, in conjunction with ^{111}In-labeled mAbs, areas of apparent ^{111}In uptake can be differentiated from the blood pool, so that specificity is increased. Other groups have developed methods of "fusion" imaging, in which the antibody images are overlaid onto images obtained from a cross-sectional anatomic modality, such as computed tomography (CT) or magnetic resonance imaging (MRI). Imaging may be performed with a fiduciary marker to enable precise co-registration of images (104), or even with a dual-purpose imaging device (106). In this manner, functional attributes of radioimmunoscintigraphy have been combined with the superior anatomic resolution of CT or MRI.

CURRENT STATUS AND FUTURE TRENDS

Despite all the technical advances and excitement generated in the laboratory, progress in the clinical application of mAbs has been slow. To understand this, it is worthwhile to contemplate the regulatory process, which has a controlling influence on the clinical development of these reagents (1). The process of obtaining Food and Drug Administration approval is long, arduous, and expensive. The several-year delay in the approval process leads to a long lag between the current development of radioimmunologic pharmaceuticals and their ultimate incorporation and approval as products for routine clinical use. Furthermore, the regulatory burden necessary to obtain pharmaceutical approval plays a major role in limiting the number of agents under clinical development by discouraging industry from pursuing promising agents that have only a limited potential revenue or that may be replaced after a short cycle with more innovative molecules.

Nonetheless, radioimmunoimaging has a unique ability to specifically target cancer-related antigens and allow a degree of characterization at the molecular and cellular levels (105). This is most advantageous in situations in which normal tissue architecture may be disrupted, such as following radiation, surgery, or chemotherapy. In these cases, conventional anatomic criteria of interpretation, used with CT, MRI, and ultrasonography, are not necessarily predictive of viable tumor. In addition to improving specificity, radioimmunoimaging may also affect sensitivity; when antibodies target sites of antigen excess in tissues that appear structurally normal, earlier detection of an abnormality becomes possible. These factors have been shown to affect clinical management positively by leading to an improved ability to localize and potentially treat malignant tissue (1).

The field of radioimmunoimaging is poised to experience a growth spurt based on progress in the fields of immunology and molecular biology. Although the regulatory and financial hurdles of introducing new biologically based imaging agents are great, the potential to image tissues at the molecular and cellular levels is a unique advantage of this method.

REFERENCES

1. Zuckier LS, DeNardo GL. Trials and tribulations: oncological antibody imaging comes to the fore. *Semin Nucl Med* 1997;27:10–29.
2. Pirofski L, Casadevall A, Rodriguez L, et al. Current state of the hybridoma technology. *J Clin Immunol* 1990;10:5s–14s.
3. Pirofski L-A, Casadevall A, Scharff MD. Current state of hybridoma technology. *ASM News* 1992;58:613–617.
4. Winkelhake JL. Immunoglobulin structure and effector functions. *Immunochemistry* 1978;15:695–714.
5. Burton DR. Immunoglobulin G: functional sites. *Mol Immunol* 1985;22:161–206.
6. Ward ES, Ghetie V. The effector functions of immunoglobulins: implications for therapy. *Ther Immunol* 1995;2:77–94.

7. Zuckier LS, Rodriguez LD, Scharff MD. Immunologic and pharmacologic concepts of monoclonal antibodies. *Semin Nucl Med* 1989;19:166–186.

8. Waldmann TA, Strober W. Metabolism of immunoglobulins. *Progr Allergy* 1969;13:1–110.

9. Wabl M, Steinberg C. Affinity maturation and class switching. *Curr Opin Immunol* 1996;8:89–92.

10. DeLand FH. A perspective of monoclonal antibodies: past, present, and future. *Semin Nucl Med* 1989;19:158–165.

11. Pressman D, Keighley G. The zone of activity of antibodies as determined by the use of radioactive tracers; the zone of activity of nephrotoxic antikidney serum. *J Immunol* 1948;59:141–146.

12. Kohler G, Milstein C. Continuous cultures of fused cells secreting antibodies of predefined specificity. *Nature* 1975;256:295–297.

13. Bogard WC Jr, Dean RT, Deo Y, et al. Practical consideration in the production, purification, and formulation of monoclonal antibodies for immunoscintigraphy and immunotherapy. *Semin Nucl Med* 1989;19:202–220.

14. Neuberger MS, Williams GT, Fox RO. Recombinant antibodies possessing novel effector functions. *Nature* 1984;312:604–608.

15. Winter G, Milstein C. Man-made antibodies. *Nature* 1991;349:293–299.

16. Morrison SL. *In vitro* antibodies: strategies for production and application. *Annu Rev Immunol* 1992;10:239–265.

17. Wright A, Shin S-U, Morrison SL. Genetically engineered antibodies: progress and prospects. *Crit Rev Immunol* 1992;12:125–168.

18. Hand PH, Kashmiri SVS, Schlom J. Potential for recombinant immunoglobulin constructs in the management of carcinoma. *Cancer* 1994;73[Suppl]:1105–1113.

19. James K, Bell GT. Human monoclonal antibody production: current status and future prospects. *J Immunol Methods* 1987;100:5–40.

20. James K. Human monoclonal antibodies and engineered antibodies in the management of cancer. *Semin Cancer Biol* 1990;1:243–253.

21. Morrison SL, Johnson MJ, Herzenberg LA, et al. Chimeric human antibody molecules: mouse antigen-binding domains with human constant region domains. *Proc Natl Acad Sci U S A* 1984;81:6851–6855.

22. Morrison SL. Generations of human monoclonal antibodies reactive with cellular antigens. *Science* 1985;229:1202–1207.

23. Bruggemann M, Williams GT, Bindon CI, et al. Comparison of the effector functions of human immunoglobulins using a matched set of chimeric antibodies. *J Exp Med* 1987;166:1351–1361.

24. Bruggemann M, Winter G, Waldmann H, et al. The immunogenicity of chimeric antibodies. *J Exp Med* 1989;170:2153–2157.

25. Jones PT, Dear PH, Foote J, et al. Replacing the complementarity-determining regions in a human antibody with those from a mouse. *Nature* 1986;321:522–525.

26. Reichmann L, Clark M, Waldmann H, et al. Reshaping human antibodies for therapy. *Nature* 1988;332:323–327.

27. Verhoeyen M, Milstein C, Winter G. Reshaping human antibodies: grafting an antilysozyme activity. *Science* 1988;239:1534–1536.

28. Queen C, Schneider WP, Selick HE, et al. A humanized antibody that binds to the interleukin 2 receptor. *Proc Natl Acad Sci U S A* 1989;86:10029–10033.

29. Roberts S, Cheetham JC, Rees AR. Generation of an antibody with enhanced affinity and specificity for its antigen by protein engineering. *Nature* 1987;328:731–734.

30. Co MS, Queen C. Humanized antibodies for therapy. *Nature* 1991;351:501–502.

31. Steinitz M, Klein G, Koskimies S, et al. EB virus-induced B lymphocytic cell lines producing specific antibody. *Nature* 1977;269:420–422.

32. Nakamura M, Burastero SE, Ueki Y, et al. Probing the normal and autoimmune B cell repertoire with Epstein-Barr virus. Frequency of B cells producing monoreactive high affinity autoantibodies in patients with Hashimoto's disease and systemic lupus erythematosus. *J Immunol* 1988;141:4165–4172.

33. Kozbor D, Lagarde AE, Roder JC. Human hybridomas constructed with antigen-specific Epstein-Barr virus-transformed cell lines. *Proc Natl Acad Sci U S A* 1982;79:6651–6655.

34. Ostberg L, Pursch E. Human X (mouse X human) hybridomas stably producing human antibodies. *Hybridoma* 1983;2:361–367.

35. Cote RJ, Morrissey DM, Houghton AN, et al. Specificity analysis of human monoclonal antibodies reactive with cell surface and intracellular antigens. *Proc Natl Acad Sci U S A* 1986;83:2959–2963.

36. Mosier DE, Gulizia RJ, Baird SM, et al. Transfer of a functional human immune system to mice with severe combined immunodeficiency. *Nature* 1988;335:256–259.

37. McCune JM, Namikawa R, Kaneshima H, et al. The SCID-hu mouse: murine model for the analysis of human hematolymphoid differentiation and function. *Science* 1988;241:1632–1639.

38. Bruggemann M, Neuberger MS. Strategies for expressing human antibody repertoires in transgenic mice. *Immunol Today* 1996;17:391–397.

39. Sastry L, Alting-Mees M, Huse WD, et al. Cloning of the immunological repertoire in *Escherichia coli* for generation of monoclonal catalytic antibodies: construction of a heavy chain variable region-specific cDNA library. *Proc Natl Acad Sci U S A* 1989;86:5728–5732.

40. Ward ES, Gussow D, Griffiths AD, et al. Binding activities of a repertoire of single immunoglobulin variable domains secreted from *Escherichia coli*. *Nature* 1989;341:544–546.

41. Huse WD, Sastry L, Iverson SA, et al. Generation of a large combinatorial library of the immunoglobulin repertoire in phage lambda. *Science* 1989;246:1275–1281.

42. Wells JA, Lowman HB. Rapid evolution of peptide and protein binding properties *in vitro*. *Curr Opin Biotechnol* 1992;3:355–362.

43. Larson SM, Carrasquillo JA, Krohn KA, et al. Localization of ^{131}I-labeled p97-specific Fab fragments in human melanoma as a basis for radiotherapy. *J Clin Invest* 1983;72:2101–2114.

44. Parham P. On the fragmentation of monoclonal IgG1, IgG2a, and IgG2b from BALB/c mice. *J Immunol* 1983;131:2895–2902.

45. Wahl RL, Parker CW, Philpott GW. Improved radioimaging and tumor localization with monoclonal F(ab')2. *J Nucl Med* 1983;24:316–325.

46. Sutherland R, Bucheggar F, Schreyer M, et al. Penetration and binding of radiolabeled anti-carcinoembryonic antigen monoclonal antibodies and their antigen-binding fragments in human colon multicellular tumor spheroids. *Cancer Res* 1987;47:1627–1633.

47. Kang AS, Barbas CF, Janda KD, et al. Linkage of recognition and replication functions by assembling combinatorial antibody Fab libraries along phage surfaces. *Proc Natl Acad Sci U S A* 1991;88:4363–4366.

48. Adams GP. Improving the tumor specificity and retention of antibody-based molecules. *In Vivo* 1998;12:11–22.

49. Bird RE, Hardman KD, Jacobson JW, et al. Single-chain antigen-binding proteins. *Science* 1988;242:423–426.

50. Milenic DE, Yokota T, Filpula DR, et al. Construction, binding properties, metabolism, and tumor targeting of a single-chain Fv

derived from the pancarcinoma monoclonal antibody CC49. *Cancer Res* 1991;51:6363–6371.

51. Huston JS, Levinson D, Mudgett-Hunter M, et al. Protein engineering of antibody binding sites: recovery of specific activity in an anti-digoxin single-chain Fv analogue produced in *Escherichia coli*. *Proc Natl Acad Sci U S A* 1988;85: 5879–5883.

52. Schlom J. New approaches to improved antibody targeting. *Antibody Immunoconjug Radiopharm* 1991;4:819–828.

53. Williams WV, Moss DA, Kieber-Emmons T, et al. Development of biologically active peptides based on antibody structure. *Proc Natl Acad Sci U S A* 1989;5537–5541.

54. Taub R, Gould RJ, Garsky VM, et al. A monoclonal antibody against the platelet fibrinogen receptor contains a sequence that mimics a receptor recognition domain in fibrinogen. *J Biol Chem* 1989;264:259–265.

55. Yokota T, Milenic DE, Whitlow M, et al. Rapid tumor penetration of a single-chain Fv and comparison with other immunoglobulin forms. *Cancer Res* 1992;52:3402–3408.

56. Williams WV, Kieber-Emmons T, VonFeldt J, et al. Design of bioactive peptides based on antibody hypervariable region structures: development of conformationally constrained and dimeric peptides with enhanced affinity. *J Biol Chem* 1991;266: 5182–5190.

57. Knight LC, Radcliffe R, Maurer AH, et al. Thrombus imaging with technetium-99m synthetic peptides based upon the binding domain of a monoclonal antibody to activated platelets. *J Nucl Med* 1994;35:282–288.

58. Pollock RR, French DL, Gefter ML, et al. Identification of mutant monoclonal antibodies with increased antigen binding. *Proc Natl Acad Sci U S A* 1988;85:2298–2302.

59. Smith RIF, Morrison SL. Recombinant polymeric IgG: an approach to engineering more potent antibodies. *Biotechnology* 1994;12:683–688.

60. Poon PH, Morrison SL, Schumaker VN. Structure and function of several anti-dansyl chimeric antibodies formed by domain interchanges between human IgM and mouse IgG2b. *J Biol Chem* 1995;270:8571–8577.

61. Riechmann L, Weill M, Cavanagh J. Improving the antigen affinity of an antibody Fv-fragment by protein design. *J Mol Biol* 1992;224:913–918.

62. Fell HP, Gayle MA, Grosmaire L, et al. Genetic construction and characterization of a fusion protein consisting of a chimeric F(ab′) with specificity for carcinomas and human IL-2. *J Immunol* 1991; 146:2446–2452.

63. Shin S-U, Morrison SL. Expression and characterization of an antibody binding specificity joined to insulin-like growth factor 1: potential applications for cellular targeting. *Proc Natl Acad Sci U S A* 1990;87:5322–5326.

64. Shin S-U, Friden P, Moran M, et al. Transferrin-antibody fusion proteins are effective in brain targeting. *Proc Natl Acad Sci U S A* 1995;92:2820–2824.

65. Sharifi J, Khawli LA, Hornick JL, et al. Improving monoclonal antibody pharmacokinetics via chemical modification. *Q J Nucl Med* 1998;42:242–249.

66. Suresh MR, Cuello AC, Milstein C. Bispecific monoclonal antibodies from hybrid hybridomas. *Methods Enzymol* 1986;121: 210–228.

67. Clark M, Gilliland L, Waldmann H. Hybrid antibodies for therapy. *Progr Allergy* 1988;45:31–49.

68. Phelps JL, Beidler DE, Jue RA, et al. Expression and characterization of a chimeric bifunctional antibody with therapeutic applications. *J Immunol* 1990;145:1200–1204.

69. Moran TM, Usuba O, Shapiro E, et al. A novel technique for the production of hybrid antibodies. *J Immunol Methods* 1990;129: 199–205.

70. Stickney DR, Anderson LD, Slater JB, et al. Bifunctional antibody: a binary radiopharmaceutical delivery system for imaging colorectal carcinoma. *Cancer Res* 1991;51:6650–6655.

71. LeDoussal J-M, Chetanneau A, Gruaz-Guyon A, et al. Bispecific monoclonal antibody-mediated targeting of an indium-111-labeled DTPA dimer to primary colorectal tumors: pharmacokinetics, biodistribution, scintigraphy and immune response. *J Nucl Med* 1993;34:16662–11671.

72. Peltier P, Curtet C, Chatal J-F, et al. Radioimmunodetection of medullary thyroid cancer using a bispecific anti-CEA/anti-indium-DTPA antibody and an indium-111-labeled DTPA dimer. *J Nucl Med* 1993;34:1267–1273.

73. Paganelli G, Magnani P, Siccardi AG, et al. Clinical application of the avidin-biotin system for tumor targeting. In: Goldenberg DM, ed. *Cancer therapy with radiolabeled antibodies*. Boca Raton, FL: CRC Press, 1995:239–254.

74. Paganelli G, Malcovati M, Fazio F. Monoclonal antibody pretargeting techniques for tumour localization: the avidin-biotin system. *Nucl Med Commun* 1991;12:211–234.

75. Kalofonos HP, Rusckowski M, Siebecker DA, et al. Imaging of tumor in patients with indium-111-labeled biotin and streptavidin-conjugated antibodies: preliminary communication. *J Nucl Med* 1990;31:1791–1796.

76. Hnatowich DJ, Virzi F, Rusckowski M. Investigations of avidin and biotin for imaging applications. *J Nucl Med* 1987;28: 1294–1302.

77. Guadagni F, Roselli M, Nieroda C, et al. Biological response modifiers as adjuvants in monoclonal antibody-based treatment *in vivo*. 1993;7:591–599.

78. LeBerthon B, Khawli LA, Alauddin M, et al. Enhanced tumor uptake of macromolecules induced by a novel vasoactive interleukin 2 immunoconjugate. *Cancer Res* 1991;51:2694–2698.

79. Greiner JW, Guadagni F, Noguchi P, et al. Recombinant interferon enhances monoclonal antibody-targeting of carcinoma lesions *in vivo*. *Science* 1987;235:895–898.

80. Greiner JW, Ullmann CD, Nieroda C, et al. Improved radioimmunotherapeutic efficacy of an anticarcinoma monoclonal antibody (^{131}I-CC49) when given in combination with gamma-interferon. *Cancer Res* 1993;53:600–608.

81. Junghans RP. Finally: the Brambell receptor (FcRB). Mediator of transmission of immunity and protection from catabolism for IgG. *Immunol Res* 1997;16:29–57.

82. Kim JK, Tsen MF, Ghetie V, et al. Localization of the site of the murine IgG1 molecule that is involved in binding to the murine intestinal Fc receptor. *Eur J Immunol* 1994;24:2429–2434.

83. Zuckier LS, Chang CJ, Scharff MD, et al. Chimeric human-mouse IgG antibodies with shuffled constant region exons demonstrate that multiple domains contribute to *in vivo* half-life. *Cancer Res* 1998;58:3905–3908.

84. Pollock RR, French DL, Metlay JP, et al. Intravascular metabolism of normal and mutant mouse immunoglobulin molecules. *Eur J Immunol* 1990;20:2021–2027.

85. Eckelman WC, Paik CH, Reba RC. Radiolabeling of antibodies. *Cancer Res* 1980;40:3036–3042.

86. Zuckier LS, Axelrod MS, Wexler JP, et al. The implications of decreased performance of new generation gamma-cameras on the interpretation of ^{131}I-hippuran renal images. *Nucl Med Commun* 1987;8:49–61.

87. Hnatowich DJ. Recent developments in the radiolabeling of antibodies with iodine, indium, and technetium. *Semin Nucl Med* 1990;20:80–91.

88. Fritzberg AR, Wilbur DS. Radiolabeling of antibodies for targeted diagnostics. In: Torchilin VP, ed. *Handbook of targeted delivery of imaging agents*. Boca Raton, FL: CRC Press, 1995: 83–101.

89. Brechbiel MW, Gansow OA, Atcher RW, et al. Synthesis of 1-(*p*-

isothiocyanatobenzyl) derivatives of DTPA and EDTA. Antibody labeling and tumor-imaging studies. *Inorganic Chem* 1986;25: 2772–2781.

90. DeNardo SJ, Zhong G-R, Salako Q, et al. Pharmacokinetics of chimeric L6 conjugated to indium-111- and yttrium-90-DOTA-peptide in tumor-bearing mice. *J Nucl Med* 1995;36: 829–836.

91. Hnatowich DJ. Is technetium-99m the radioisotope of choice for radioimmunoscintigraphy? *J Nucl Biol Med* 1994;38[Suppl]: 22–32.

92. Kairemo KJA. Positron emission tomography of monoclonal antibodies. *Acta Oncol* 1993;32:825–830.

93. Philpott GW, Schwarz SW, Anderson CJ, et al. Radioimmuno-PET: detection of colorectal carcinoma with positron-emitting copper-64-labeled monoclonal antibody. *J Nucl Med* 1995;36: 1818–1824.

94. Sakahara H, Endo K, Koizumi M, et al. Relationship between *in vitro* binding activity and *in vivo* tumor accumulation of radiolabeled monoclonal antibodies. *J Nucl Med* 1988;29: 235–240.

95. Andrew SM, Johnstone RW, Russell SM, et al. Comparison of *in vitro* cell binding characteristics of four monoclonal antibodies and their individual tumor localization properties in mice. *Cancer Res* 1990;50:4423–4428.

96. Sung C, Shockley TR, Morrison PF, et al. Predicted and observed effects of antibody affinity and antigen density on monoclonal antibody uptake in solid tumors. *Cancer Res* 1992; 527:377–384.

97. Schlom J, Eggensperger D, Colcher D, et al. Therapeutic advan-tage of high-affinity anticarcinoma radioimmunoconjugates. *Cancer Res* 1992;52:1067–1072.

98. Fujimori K, Covell DG, Fletcher JE, et al. A modeling analysis of monoclonal antibody percolation through tumors: a bind-ing-site barrier. *J Nucl Med* 1990;31:1191–1198.

99. Sharkey RM, Goldenberg DM, Goldenberg H, et al. Murine monoclonal antibodies against carcinoembryonic antigen: immunological, pharmacokinetic, and targeting properties in humans. *Cancer Res* 1990;50:2823–2831.

100. Goldenberg DM, Larson SM. Radioimmunodetection in can-cer identification. *J Nucl Med* 1992;33:803–814.

101. Wahl RL, Barrett J, Geatti O, et al. The intraperitoneal delivery of radiolabeled monoclonal antibodies: studies on the regional delivery advantage. *Cancer Immunol Immunother* 1988;26: 187–201.

102. Stoldt HS, Aftab F, Chinol M, et al. Pretargeting strategies for radio-immunoguided tumour localisation and therapy. *Eur J Cancer* 1997;33:186–192.

103. Goodwin DA. Tumor pretargeting: almost the bottom line. *J Nucl Med* 1995;36:876–879.

104. Kramer EL, Noz ME. CT-SPECT fusion for analysis of radio-labeled antibodies: applications in gastrointestinal and lung car-cinoma. *Nucl Med Biol* 1991;18:27–42.

105. DeNardo GL. Role of imaging in radioimmunotherapy. In: Haseman MK, ed. The American College of Nuclear Physicians, 1991:69–93.

106. Bocher M, Balan A, Krausz Y, et al. Gamma camera-mounted anatomical x-ray tomography: technology, system characteristics and first images. *Eur J Nucl Med* 2000;27:619–627.

RADIOLABELED MONOCLONAL ANTIBODIES

PART B: THERAPY

CHAITANYA R. DIVGI

Radioimmunotherapy involves the use of radionuclide-conjugated antibodies in the treatment of disease. The premise underlying this treatment modality in cancer is that preferential accumulation in tumor of a radionuclide-conjugated antibody will permit selective delivery of cytotoxic radioactivity and thus cause tumor regression.

Preferential accumulation of radiolabeled antibody in tumor is also the premise behind radioimmunodetection. However, several important features distinguish radioimmunotherapy from radioimmunodetection:

1. Relative versus absolute accumulation of radiolabeled antibody. The relative (tumor-to-nontumor) accumulation in tumor is important in both radioimmunotherapy and radioimmunodetection because it is the contrast between target and background that permits detection of a lesion, and it is the distribution of activity in the tumor and surrounding tissue that determines the target-to-nontarget ratio of radiation absorbed dose. In radioimmunotherapy, however, absolute tumor uptake (usually defined as percentage of the injected dose per gram of tumor) is equally important; the greater the number of radionuclide-carrying molecules that accumulate in tumor, the greater the therapeutic potential.

2. Uptake in nontarget tissues. Radioimmunotherapy involves the use of cytotoxic radionuclides; therefore, lack of uptake in nontumor tissue is important in the preferential delivery of cytotoxic radioactivity to tumor. Skeletal uptake of nuclides, for example, is of relatively little importance in radioimmunodetection when parenchymal disease is being evaluated, but such uptake in radioimmunotherapy would increase the radiation absorbed dose to bone marrow and decrease the therapeutic target-to-nontarget ratio.

3. Clearance characteristics. The optimal detection of tumor with radionuclides depends on rapid detection and a low radiation burden. Both of these features are enhanced by rapid serum clearance of the radioconjugate. The residence time of the antibody on the tumor is not of critical importance. Preferential tumor accumulation during the interval required for imaging is the only important feature. Whereas rapid serum clearance is equally important in radioimmunotherapy (a decrease in serum activity reduces marrow radiation absorbed dose and consequent hematologic toxicity), a long tumor residence time is of far greater importance in radioimmunotherapy than in radioimmunodetection. The longer the radioconjugate stays on tumor cells, the greater the likelihood of a cytotoxic effect.

4. Immunobiologic characteristics. The antigen that is recognized by the antibody will influence the choice of radioconjugate in both radioimmunodetection and radioimmunotherapy, albeit with differences. Antibodies that recognize shed antigens [e.g., carcinoembryonic antigen (CEA) or tumor-associated glycoprotein 72 (TAG-72)] may be useful in radioimmunodetection. The binding of cytotoxic radioconjugate to circulating antigen, however, may increase marrow toxicity in radioimmunotherapy.

The specificity of expression of antigen in tumor versus normal tissue is another important variable. Generally, the more ubiquitous the antigen expression, the greater the mass amount of antibody required for suitable targeting. On the other hand, the number of antigen sites per tumor cell is also important. The mass amount of antibodies is based on antigen expression in tumor and must be minimized when antigen expression per tumor cell is relatively low.

The fate of the radioimmunoconjugate subsequent to interaction with antigen (i.e., the fate of the radiolabeled antibody after attachment to tumor) is of similar relevance. Antibodies that internalize into lysosomes following interaction with antigen must be conjugated with radiometals for favorable targeting. Dehalogenases, abundant in lysosomes, preclude the effective use of halogens, such as iodine. It would appear, therefore, that nonhalogens are preferred radionuclides for both radioimmunodetection and radioimmunotherapy. The radiochemical characteristics of such conjugates, however, determine their utility for these applications.

C. R. Divgi: Department of Radiology, Weill Medical College of Cornell University; Department of Radiology and Medicine, Memorial Sloan-Kettering Cancer Center, New York, New York 10021.

5. Radioimmunoconjugate characteristics. Radiometals labeled to antibodies are of varying stability *in vivo*. This results in transchelation and increased hepatic and osseous uptake, which is obviously far more important in tumor cytotoxic therapy than in the detection of extrahepatic, extraosseous disease.

Similarly, current direct labeling methods for transitional element conjugation to antibodies result in radioimmunoconjugates that are of varying stability *in vivo*. This is not critical in radioimmunodetection so long as the conjugate is stable during the period of imaging. It is of far greater importance in radioimmunotherapy because an unstable radioconjugate may decrease tumor cytotoxicity and also increase normal tissue toxicity, which results in a decreased therapeutic ratio.

RADIOIMMUNOTHERAPY WITH RADIOIODINE

Antibodies labeled with iodine 131 have been studied most extensively, and the features of this nuclide warrant mention.

Iodine 131 has been used extensively in the treatment of differentiated thyroid cancer (1). Its biodistribution is well understood. The accumulation of free radioiodine in the body can be easily and successfully prevented by the administration of stable iodide, and also by the use of agents such as potassium perchlorate.

The iodination of proteins is relatively simple (2) and results in a compound that is stable *in vivo*. Radioiodinated antibody with a relatively high specific activity (up to 800 MBq of ^{131}I per milligram) and intact immunobiologic function can be produced and has been shown to be stable, under appropriate conditions, for long periods of time (3). This has made possible the centralized production of large amounts of ^{131}I-labeled antibody, which can then be shipped to remote centers, so that multicenter trials can be carried out with the same batch of radioiodinated antibody (4).

In addition to its potentially cytotoxic beta minus emission, ^{131}I emits high-energy gamma radiation that can be detected externally (5). This allows single-photon imaging to demonstrate the targeting of radioimmunoconjugate to tumor (Fig. 5B.1). It also permits the quantification of radioactivity in the body and in serum, so that dosimetric estimates can be made. Several trials are now under way that utilize this feature of ^{131}I. These trials are based on the radiation absorbed dose to critical normal organs, such as bone marrow (6) (and, in the case of myeloablative studies, to a second organ [7]).

The high-energy gamma emission is not without drawbacks. Exposure of staff and other personnel to radiation, which can be quite high, mandates patient isolation following high-dose therapy (8). Radiation absorbed dose to marrow (and other normal organs) is considerably increased, so that the amount of radioactivity that can be administered is limited.

Iodine is also a suboptimal nuclide for conjugation with antibodies that internalize following interaction with antigen (9). In most cases, the antigen–antibody complex resides in lysosomes after internalization, which are rich in enzymes, including dehalogenases. The resulting dehalogenation of the complex results in release of radioiodine from the cell, with a consequent decrease in cytotoxic potential.

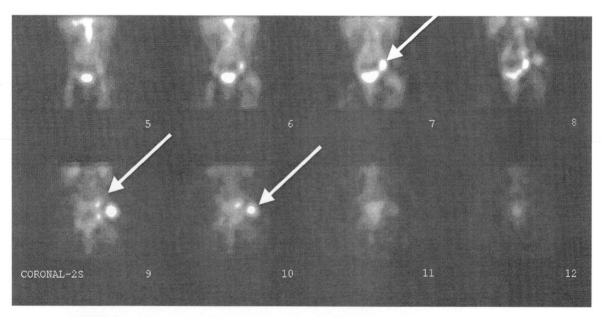

FIGURE 5B.1. Coronal SPECT (single-photon emission tomogram) slices (anterior to posterior, upper left to lower right) in a patient with transformed low-grade B-cell lymphoma treated with ^{131}I-labeled anti-CD20 antibody. Targeting to lymph node disease (*arrows*) is evident.

Important exceptions to the above are antigen–antibody systems that internalize into compartments (such as macropinosomes) that do not contain dehalogenases (10). In such cases, not only is ^{131}I a suitable radionuclide, but ^{125}I, with its high-energy Auger electron emission, may also have potential (11).

OTHER RADIONUCLIDES WITH THERAPEUTIC POTENTIAL

The limitations of ^{131}I have spurred the development of other radioimmunoconjugates. Radionuclides (including radioiodine) with potential in radioimmunotherapy are listed in Table 5B.1; their salient emissions and half-lives are included, and those radionuclides that have already been studied in clinical trials are marked with an asterisk.

Note that Table 5B.1 contains three major types of cytotoxic agents: pure beta emitters (either electron or positron), such as ^{67}Cu and ^{90}Y; alpha emitters (^{213}Bi, ^{211}At); and beta emitters that emit gamma radiation (^{131}I, ^{177}Lu, ^{186}Re). The list may also be divided into three large groups of radiochemicals: halogens (iodine, ^{211}At); metals (^{90}Y, ^{67}Cu, bismuth); and transitional elements (rhenium).

After ^{131}I, the most extensively studied radionuclide in radioimmunotherapy is ^{90}Y. It has a high-energy beta emission (5) with cytotoxic potential for large solid tumors and has shown promise in B-cell lymphoma (12). Moreover, radiometal-labeled antibodies are not as susceptible to intracellular degradation and may therefore be used in internalizing systems. Current chelation technology appears to be comparable for ^{111}In and ^{90}Y, so that the for-

mer can be used as a surrogate in the evaluation of biodistribution of the latter (13). Finally, with the positron emitter ^{86}Y, a true surrogate, external detection by means of positron emission tomography (PET) is possible (14).

The bone-seeking properties of yttrium have limited its utility as a therapeutic agent; bone marrow toxicity has occurred with relatively low doses of radionuclide (13). Radiometals such as ^{177}Lu (15,16) and ^{67}Cu (17) do not concentrate in bone and have therefore been studied. However, transchelation *in vivo* can be significant and result in considerable hepatic (and bone marrow) uptake of radiometals. This has spurred the development of more stable immunoconjugates, which are currently being investigated.

The radioisotopes of rhenium, a transitional element, are increasingly being explored for their potential as cytotoxic agents. Antibodies have been labeled with both ^{186}Re and ^{188}Re, usually through a suitable linker. ^{186}Re has been more extensively studied (18). As with the radiometals, stable conjugation of rhenium to antibodies is not yet optimal. The gamma emissions of both isotopes are eminently suitable for imaging with standard gamma cameras. ^{188}Re has a shorter half-life and a more energetic beta minus emission (5). The ability to produce rhenium 188 with a tungsten 188 generator system (19) offers the potential of easy availability, but its relatively short (17-hour) half-life will probably limit its use to locoregional applications or studies in which it is conjugated to antibody fragments or smaller molecules.

Recent developments in radiochemistry have also made possible the clinical study of antibodies labeled with alpha emitters. Astatine 211 is a halide ($t_{1/2}$, 7 hours) that has been stably conjugated to antibodies by means of a linker (unlike iodine, this halide cannot be directly labeled). Antibodies labeled with ^{211}At are being studied in trials of locoregional radioimmunotherapy in patients with malignant intracranial neoplasms (20). An alpha emitter with a much shorter (45-minute) half-life is being studied in myelogenous leukemia; this radiometal may be conjugated to antibodies with use of a methodology established for other radiometals, including ^{90}Y and ^{111}In (21).

Alpha-based radioimmunotherapy may be limited to locoregional therapy and therapy of hematologic neoplasms, in which the binding of radioimmunoconjugate to tumor is relatively rapid. Its extremely high energy deposition (linear energy transfer, or LET) may preclude its use in systemic therapy (except perhaps in the adjuvant situation), in which irradiation of normal tissue may preclude delivery of adequate cytotoxic radiation to tumor. High LET nuclides also include those that emit Auger electrons on decay. ^{125}I is the prototypical nuclide, although its long half-life makes it less than optimal for successful therapy. However, Auger electron emission is cytotoxic only when the decay occurs in or near the nucleus because the high energy deposition occurs over a very short distance (less than the diameter of a cell). This limits the use of Auger emitters to internalizing antibodies, although the extremely

TABLE 5B.1. RADIONUCLIDES (INCLUDING RADIOIODINE) WITH POTENTIAL IN RADIOIMMUNOTHERAPY

Radionuclide	Decay mode (energy, MeV)	Half-life
Iodine 131*	Beta minus (0.182), gamma (0.364)	8.0 d
Iodine 125*	EC	60.2 d
Iodine 124	EC, beta plus (0.188)	4.2 d
Rhenium 188*	Beta minus (0.8), gamma (0.16)	17 h
Rhenium 186*	EC, beta minus (0.323), gamma (0.14)	3.8 d
Copper 64	EC, beta plus (0.656)	12.8 h
Copper 67*	Beta minus (0.142)	62 h
Gallium 67	EC, gamma	3.3 d
Yttrium 90*	Beta minus (0.934)	64 h
Lutetium 177*	Beta minus (0.149), gamma (0.208)	6.7 d
Bismuth 212	Alpha (2.17), beta minus (0.492)	1 h
Bismuth 213*	Alpha, beta (multiple), gamma (0.44)	45 min
Actinium 225	Alpha (multiple)	10 d
Astatine 211*	Alpha (2.447)	7.2 h

*Have been studied in clinical radioimmunotherapy trials.

low passive irradiation of normal tissues makes possible the administration of large amounts of radioactivity.

APPROACHES TO CLINICAL RADIOIMMUNOTHERAPY

Systemic Therapy

The dose-limiting toxicity in radioimmunotherapy is myelosuppression, caused by the passive irradiation of bone marrow. Most radioimmunotherapy studies have been carried out at the maximum tolerated dose (MTD) for bone marrow (6,12,15,16,22–24). A few studies have explored the utility of myeloablative doses of radioimmunoconjugate; second-organ dose-limiting toxicity has usually been to the lung (7), although at least one study has demonstrated that failure of engraftment (of transplanted marrow) may be an important determinant of dose-limiting toxicity (25). Myeloablative radioimmunotherapy in B-cell lymphoma has resulted in response rates comparable with those achieved with nonmyeloablative radioimmunotherapy; it has been suggested that progression-free survival may be greater with myeloablative therapy (26). Because of the relative radioresistance of solid tumors, nonmyeloablative therapy may not result in significant response rates. Mye-

loablative radioimmunotherapy has shown promise in the therapy of neuroblastoma, a relatively radiosensitive tumor. It is not clear whether such therapy will be efficacious in other solid tumor systems.

Systemic radioimmunotherapy has been shown to be of considerable promise in B-cell lymphoma; pivotal phase III trials are being carried out with radiolabeled anti-CD20 antibodies in these lymphomas, and early results are indeed promising (27). Myeloablative radioimmunotherapy with ^{131}I-labeled anti-CD20 antibodies in B-cell lymphoma has resulted in significant overall response rates and in increased progression-free and overall survival; however, the prohibitive cost and specialized nature of this therapy make its wider application unlikely (26). The relative lack of an anti-antibody response in B-cell lymphoma makes it possible to repeat therapy, except perhaps in the adjuvant situation.

Similarly, radioimmunotherapy has shown considerable promise in the therapy of leukemia (28–30). Studies with anti-CD33 antibody labeled with a variety of cytotoxic nuclides (^{131}I, ^{90}Y, [213]Bi) have shown significant remission rates (Fig. 5B.2). However, in patients with leukemia (unlike those with B-cell lymphoma), anti-antibody responses have necessitated the development of nonimmunogenic forms of antibody. The relatively low expression of CD33 on myelogenous leukemia cells has limited the

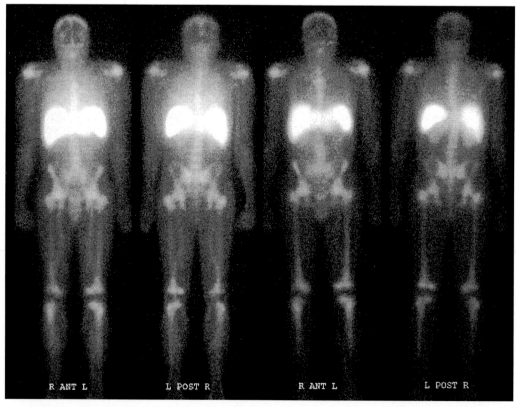

FIGURE 5B.2. Anterior and posterior whole-body images obtained 3 hours (*left pair*) and 3 days (*right pair*) after 5 mCi of ^{111}In-labeled anti-CD33 humanized antibody (as a surrogate to determine ^{90}Y biodistribution). Targeting to disease in marrow is immediate, with little clearance over time.

mass amount that may be optimally administered (28), although the consequent constraints on specific activity have not precluded therapy.

Progress in the treatment of solid tumors with radioimmunotherapy has been minimal (31) (Fig. 5B.3). The invariable development of an immune response requires the development of nonimmunogenic antibody. The relative inaccessibility of solid tumors to systemically administered macromolecules, combined with their innate radioresistance, has limited the delivery of adequate radiation to tumor at nonmyeloablative doses of radioimmunoconjugate. As in chemotherapy, progress in systemic radioimmunotherapy is probably going to be greater for hematologic than for solid neoplasms.

Locoregional Therapy

Locoregional radioimmunotherapy allows the relatively rapid access of radiolabeled antibody to tumor. Such therapy has been carried out, with considerable success, largely in intracranial neoplasms; direct intratumoral injection of

radioimmunoconjugate has resulted in improved progression-free survival, especially after surgical debulking (20,32). Intraperitoneal radioimmunotherapy has been successful (16,33), again in the adjuvant situation, in ovarian cancer, and results of limited studies with intrathecal radioimmunotherapy have been promising. In summary, this modality offers the potential to deliver high amounts of radiation to tumor cells while sparing normal tissue, such as bone marrow. Nonimmunogenic constructs are probably going to be necessary for repeated administration; the issue of whether the success of intratumoral radioimmunotherapy depends on the specificity of the antibody will probably never be resolved.

FUTURE DIRECTIONS IN RADIOIMMUNOTHERAPY

Dosimetry-based Radioimmunotherapy

Seminal studies (34) carried out in human melanoma demonstrated the concept of administering an initial dose of

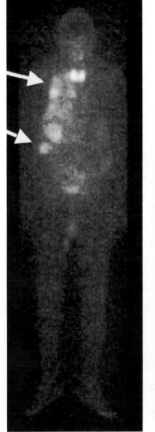
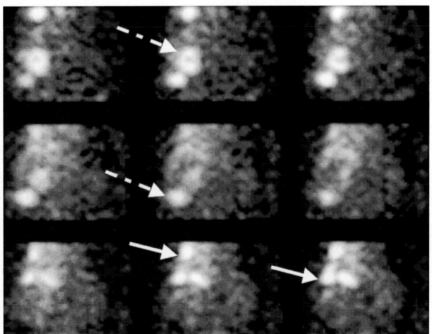

FIGURE 5B.3. Anterior whole-body (*left*) and thorax/upper abdomen coronal (*right*) SPECT (single-photon emission tomogram) obtained 1 week after 75 mCi of ^{131}I-murine A33 per square meter. A *solid arrow* indicates the pleura-based posterior lung lesions; the hepatic lesions (the larger with its photopenic center) are indicated by a *broken arrow*. This patient had a sustained partial response.

radioactivity with a tracer to predict organ-specific dose-limiting toxicity, for subsequent calculation of the maximum tolerated dose. Radioimmunotherapy studies in B-cell lymphoma were carried out based on radiation absorbed dose to critical organs [marrow for nonmyeloablative therapy (6, 27), lungs for myeloablative therapy (7,26)]. These studies, and retrospective evaluation of data from solid tumor radioimmunotherapy trials (35), demonstrated that the radiation absorbed dose to critical normal organs is the most important predictor of toxicity. Most trials of solid tumors have used a design in which escalation of the radioactivity dose was based on weight or body surface area, either because the immunogenicity of the murine protein precluded the administration of multiple doses or because the radionuclide was a pure beta emitter, so that external quantification was obviated.

The development of relatively nonimmunogenic antibodies has led to the increasing use of an initial dose of radioimmunoconjugate to study clearance and determine the radiation absorbed dose to critical organs, which in turn determines the amount of radioactivity administered in subsequent radioimmunotherapy. These treatment schemata are similar to those used to determine the maximum safe dose of ^{131}I for thyroid carcinoma, and those currently used in ^{131}I-labeled anti-CD20 radioimmunotherapy trials.

Measurement of the radiation absorbed dose necessitates the use of a nuclide that can be detected externally, and for measurement of the dose to organs other than the red marrow, imaging also is necessary. This is feasible for most nuclides with therapeutic potential, including ^{131}I, ^{186}Re, ^{188}Re, and ^{177}Lu. For nuclides like ^{90}Y and ^{67}Cu, which cannot be measured in this manner, suitable surrogates need to be identified. Developments in radiochemistry have permitted the use of ^{111}In as a surrogate in most cases. Moreover, developments in cyclotron chemistry have allowed the use of the positron emitters, ^{124}I (35), ^{86}Y (14), and ^{64}Cu (36), as "true" surrogates; positron emission tomography of positron-labeled antibodies permits quantification *in vivo*. It seems likely, therefore, that future radioimmunotherapy trials will increasingly employ estimates of radiation absorbed dose to determine toxicity, so that optimal therapy can be delivered with minimal and predictable toxicity.

Radioimmunotherapy with a Single Large Dose and Fractionated Radioimmunotherapy

The conventional wisdom that low-dose radiation, such as that delivered by radioimmunotherapy, is best administered as a single large dose may have important caveats (37). The twin limitations of antigen density and specific activity may necessitate multiple treatments, as with anti-CD33 antibodies.

Xenograft studies have suggested that fractionation may improve the efficacy of radioimmunotherapy (38,39). This may be a consequence of changes over time in tumor interstitial pressure and vascular flow, among other poorly understood factors. Like external beam radiotherapy, fractionated radioimmunotherapy may permit recovery of radiation-injured normal cells. Theoretical models have indicated that although the tumor cell survival fraction is less following single-large-dose radioimmunotherapy, cell repopulation following fractionated radioimmunotherapy may occur at a slower rate (37). Our group is comparing single-large-dose and fractionated radioimmunotherapy (Fig. 5B.4) in metastatic renal cell cancer. These studies should shed light on the relative merits of each schedule.

Constructs

Initially, antibodies were of murine origin, and this resulted (except in B-cell lymphoma) in the invariable development of an anti-antibody response, manifested in serum by the presence of human anti-mouse antibody (HAMA) and *in vivo* by rapid clearance and lack of specific targeting to tumor of subsequently administered antibody (22,25). The development of genetic engineering made possible the development of antibodies that incorporate portions of human immunoglobulin. It is now possible to determine the gene sequence for murine monoclonal antibodies and isolate the gene(s) responsible for the antigen-binding or complementarity-determing region (CDR) in addition to the variable region (Fv) of the murine immunoglobulin. Transfection of a suitable mammalian immunoglobulin-producing cell with the gene sequence for the Fv along with that for human immunoglobulin constant (Fc) regions results in the production of *chimeric* antibody (40). Generally, chimeric antibodies are less immunogenic than their murine counterparts. However, their immunogenicity (resulting in the development of human antichimeric antibody, or HACA) and their serum clearance have been extremely variable (41). Attention is thus now focused on *humanized* monoclonal antibodies, with murine CDRs on a human IgG backbone (42). The development of human anti-humanized antibody, or HAHA, has been reported, although it is rare. Carlos Barbas and his colleagues at the Scripps Clinic are addressing this problem by replacing murine sequences in the CDR with human sequences, without loss of immunobiologic characteristics, and these constructs should enter clinical trials shortly. Clinical radioimmunotherapy trials with chimeric and humanized antibodies are well under way. It is noteworthy that an unlabeled antibody approved by the Food and Drug Administration for the treatment of B-cell lymphomas is chimeric, and a humanized antibody has been approved for the treatment of refractory breast cancer. An advantage of these constructs is that the immune effector function of the molecule can enhance the cytotoxicity of the radioimmunoconjugate; potential disadvantages include slow clearance and human Fc receptor binding.

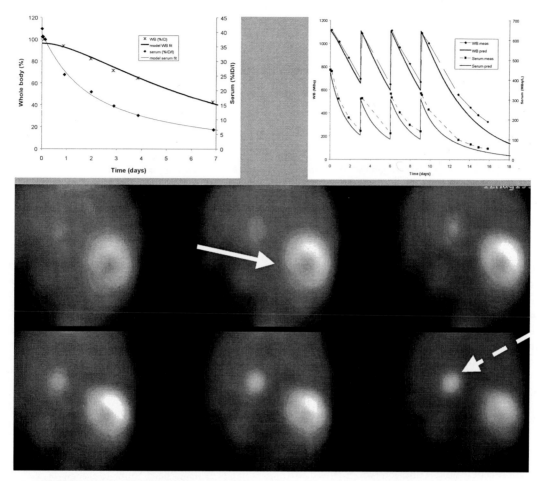

FIGURE 5B.4. Fractionated radioimmunotherapy with ¹³¹I-cG250. Upper left figure demonstrates two-compartmental model fitted on whole-body and serum radioactivity clearance data obtained during 1 week. Upper right figure demonstrates actual (*broken curves*) and predicted (*solid curves*) clearances in the same patient. The images represent coronal slices (posterior to anterior, upper left to lower right) obtained 3 days after 1,110 MBq of ¹³¹I-cG250 per 5 mg in a patient with renal cell carcinoma (with its photopenic center, *solid arrow*) and liver (*broken arrow*) metastases.

Availability of the gene sequence for the antigen-binding protein and its transfection into suitable mammalian or bacterial cells makes it theoretically possible to produce a host of antigen-binding proteins, ranging from intact immunoglobulin to CDR constructs. None has been studied in clinical trials to date. *Single-chain antigen-binding proteins* (sFv) are constructs of CDRs, produced by transfection of *Escherichia coli* with the CDR-encoding gene along with suitable linker genes (43). These sFvs have been shown to clear the blood rapidly and specifically localize in xenograft models, and, unlike Fab´ fragments, they are not retained in renal parenchyma. In addition, penetration into tumor appears greater with these smaller molecules. We carried out a phase I trial with ¹²³I-sFv CC49 in presurgical patients with colon cancer (45). The radiolabeled sFv was stable *in vivo*, with no evidence of dimerization or dehalogenation. Although tumor uptake was lower than that of

intact IgG, the rapid clearance allowed early imaging and use of ¹²³I, a short-lived nuclide. Other constructs, again soon to enter clinical trials, include diabodies (46), which consist of two sFv molecules bridged by disulfide bonds or other linkers, and minibodies (47), which consist of two sFvs linked to an appropriate protein, either a component of the constant region (typically the CH₃ fragment) or another immunobiologic agent. An excellent review by Winter (44) details the potential of genetic engineering in the creation of immunobiologic proteins with tailored characteristics for (radio)immunotargeting.

Pretargeting

The relatively low absolute uptake of antibodies in tumor led to the exploration of novel multistep targeting systems. The considerable advantages of PET have intensified efforts

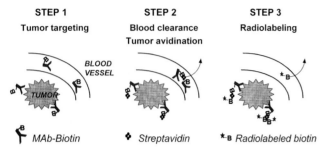

FIGURE 5B.5. Schema for three-step radioimmunotargeting.

to develop antibody-mediated tumor imaging methods appropriate for use with short-lived positron emitters. Goodwin et al. (48) pioneered the development of this technique; seminal studies by Paganelli et al. (49) and Barbet et al. (50) in Europe and the NeoRx group (51) in the United States have demonstrated the feasibility of the method. In essence, the tumor is pretargeted by an antibody that has a tumor-recognition domain and another that recognizes a fast-clearing ligand that can be suitably radiolabeled. After a period of time sufficient to allow for tumor targeting and systemic clearance of unbound antibody, sometimes accelerated by the use of a "clearing agent" (Fig. 5B.5), the radiolabeled ligand is administered. The rapid targeting of the radioligand to the antibody and its rapid systemic clearance result in images of high contrast. These pretargeting approaches hold considerable potential for scintigraphy with single-photon or positron emitters.

CONCLUSIONS

The specificity and low toxicity of monoclonal antibodies make them attractive, when suitably radiolabeled, for the therapy of cancer. Murine antibodies have been studied extensively and have permitted us to acquire an understanding of constraints and opportunities. The next generation of radioimmunotargeting agents is being explored in clinical trials; these studies involve tailored nonimmunogenic molecules with optimal clearance that have been conjugated with nuclides with suitable characteristics. Also being studied are multistep targeting methods that result in higher rates of selective tumor uptake of radioactivity than are currently attainable. PET with positron-labeled antigen-binding molecules is also in its infancy; pretargeting methodology, and the development of genetically engineered antigen-binding constructs, is likely to increase significantly the utility of antibody PET. Genetically engineered constructs will also permit the delivery of novel forms of cytotoxic radiation, such as alpha emission, which can deliver highly selective radiation while sparing normal tissue. The future utility of radioimmunotargeting appears promising indeed.

REFERENCES

1. Maxon HR, Thomas SR, Hertzberg VS, et al. Relation between effective radiation dose and outcome of radioiodine therapy for thyroid carcinoma. *N Engl J Med* 1983;309:937.
2. Eary J, Krohn KA, Kishore R, Welp WB. Radiochemistry of halogenated antibodies. In: Zalutsky MR, ed. *Antibodies in radiodiagnosis and therapy.* Boca Raton, FL: CRC Press, l989:240.
3. Ferns JM, Krohn K , Beaumier PL, et al. High-level iodination of monoclonal antibody fragments for radiotherapy. *J Nucl Med* 1984;75:367–370.
4. Colcher D. Centralized radiolabeling of antibodies for radioimmunotherapy. *J Nucl Med* 1998;39:11S–13S.
5. *http://nucleardata.nuclear.lu.se/Database/nudat/.*
6. Kaminski MS, Zasadny KR, Francis IR, et al. Radioimmunotherapy of B-cell lymphoma with [131I]anti-B1 (anti-CD20) antibody. *N Engl J Med* 1993;329:459–465.
7. Press OW, Eary JF, Appelbaum FR, et al. Radiolabeled-antibody therapy of B-cell lymphoma with autologous bone marrow support. *N Engl J Med* 1993;329:1219–1224.
8. Zanzonico PB. Internal radionuclide radiation dosimetry: a review of basic concepts and recent developments. *J Nucl Med* 2000;41:297–308.
9. Carrasquillo JA, Mulshine JL, Bunn PA, et al. Tumor uptake of 111In-T101 monoclonal antibody is superior to 131I-T101 in cutaneous T-cell lymphoma. *J Nucl Med* 1987;28:281–287.
10. Daghighian F, Barendswaard E, Welt S, et al. Enhancement of radiation dose to the nucleus by vesicular internalization of iodine-125-labeled A33 monoclonal antibody. *J Nucl Med* 1996;37:1052–1057.
11. Welt S, Scott AM, Divgi CR, et al. Phase I/II study of iodine 125-labeled monoclonal antibody A33 in patients with advanced colon cancer. *J Clin Oncol* 1996;14:1787–1797.
12. Knox SJ, Goris ML, Trisler K, et al. Yttrium-90-labeled anti-CD20 monoclonal antibody therapy of recurrent B-cell lymphoma. *Clin Cancer Res* 1996;2:457–470.
13. Carrasquillo JA, Bunn PA Jr, Keenan AM, et al. Radioimmunodetection of cutaneous T-cell lymphoma with 111In-labeled T101 monoclonal antibody. *N Engl J Med* 1986;315:673–680.
14. Herzog H, Rosch F, Stocklin G, et al. Measurement of pharmacokinetics of yttrium-86 radiopharmaceuticals with PET and radiation dose calculation of analogous yttrium-90 radiotherapeutics. *J Nucl Med* 1993;34:2222–2226.
15. Mulligan T, Carrasquillo JA, Chung Y, et al. Phase I study of intravenous 177Lu-labeled CC49 murine monoclonal antibody in patients with advanced adenocarcinoma. *Clin Cancer Res* 1995;1:1447–1454.
16. Alvarez RD, Partridge EE, Khazaeli MB, et al. Intraperitoneal radioimmunotherapy of ovarian cancer with 177Lu-CC49: a phase I/II study. *Gynecol Oncol* 1997;65:94–101
17. DeNardo GL, Kukis DL, Shen S, et al. 67Cu- versus 131I-labeled Lym-1 antibody: comparative pharmacokinetics and dosimetry in patients with non-Hodgkin's lymphoma. *Clin Cancer Res* 1999;5:533–541.
18. Breitz HB, Fisher DR, Wessels BW. Marrow toxicity and radiation absorbed dose estimates from rhenium-186-labeled monoclonal antibody. *J Nucl Med* 1998;39:1746–1751.
19. Seitz U, Neumaier B, Glatting G, et al. Preparation and evaluation of the rhenium-188-labelled anti-NCA antigen monoclonal antibody BW 250/183 for radioimmunotherapy of leukaemia. *Eur J Nucl Med* 1999;26:1265–1273.
20. Zalutsky MR, Bigner DD. Radioimmunotherapy with alpha-particle-emitting radioimmunoconjugates. *Acta Oncol* 1996;35:373–379.
21. Nikula TK, McDevitt MR, Finn RD, et al. Alpha-emitting bis-

muth cyclohexylbenzyl DTPA constructs of recombinant humanized anti-CD33 antibodies: pharmacokinetics, bioactivity, toxicity and chemistry. *J Nucl Med* 1999;40:166–176.

22. Welt S, Divgi CR, Kemeny N, et al. Phase I/II study of iodine 131-labeled monoclonal antibody A33 in patients with advanced colon cancer. *J Clin Oncol* 1994;12:1561–1571.

23. Divgi CR, Scott AM, Dantis L, et al. Phase I radioimmunotherapy trial with I-131 CC49 in metastatic colon carcinoma. *J Nucl Med* 1995;36:586–592.

24. Divgi CR, Bander NH, Scott AM, et al. Phase I/II radioimmunotherapy trial with iodine-131-labeled monoclonal antibody (Mab) G250 in metastatic renal cell carcinoma. *Clin Cancer Res* 1998;4:2729–2739.

25. Tempero M, Leichner P, Dalrymple G, et al. High-dose therapy with iodine-131-labeled monoclonal antibody CC49 in patients with gastrointestinal cancers: a phase I trial. *J Clin Oncol* 1997;:1518–1528.

26. Liu SY, Eary JF, Petersdorf SH, et al. Follow-up of relapsed B-cell lymphoma patients treated with iodine-131-labeled anti-CD20 antibody and autologous stem-cell rescue. *J Clin Oncol* 1998;16:3270–3278.

27. Wahl RL, Zasadny KR, MacFarlane D, et al. Iodine-131 anti-B1 antibody for B-cell lymphoma: an update on the Michigan phase I experience. *J Nucl Med* 1998;39:21S–27S.

28. Scheinberg DA, Lovett D, Divgi CR, et al. A phase I trial of monoclonal antibody M195 in acute myelogenous leukemia: specific bone marrow targeting and internalization of radionuclide. *J Clin Oncol* 1991;9:478–490.

29. Jurcic JG, Caron PC, Miller WH Jr, et al. Sequential targeted therapy for relapsed acute promyelocytic leukemia with all-trans retinoic acid and anti-CD33 monoclonal antibody M195. *Leukemia* 1995;9:244–248.

30. Caron PC, Jurcic JG, Scott AM, et al. A phase 1B trial of humanized monoclonal antibody M195 (anti-CD33) in myeloid leukemia: specific targeting without immunogenicity. *Blood* 1994;83:1760–1768.

31. Larson SM, Sgouros G, Cheung N-K V. Radioisotope conjugates. In: DeVita VT Jr, Hellman S, Rosenberg SA, eds. *Biologic therapy of cancer: principles and practice*, 2nd ed. Philadelphia: JB Lippincott Co, 1995:534–552.

32. Riva P, Franceschi G, Frattarelli M, et al. ^{131}I-radioconjugated antibodies for the locoregional radioimmunotherapy of high-grade malignant glioma—phase I and II study. *Acta Oncol* 1999;38:351–359.

33. Hird V, Maraveyas A, Snook D, et al. Adjuvant therapy of ovarian cancer with radioactive monoclonal antibody. *Br J Cancer* 1993;68:403–406.

34. O'Donoghue JA. Dosimetric aspects of radioimmunotherapy. *Tumor Targeting* 1998;3:105–111.

35. Larson SM, Raubitschek A, Reynolds JC, et al. Comparison of bone marrow dosimetry and toxic effect of high-dose ^{131}I-labeled monoclonal antibodies administered to man. *Int J Radiat Appl Instr B* 1989;16:153–158.

36. Larson SM, Pentlow KS, Volkow ND, et al. PET scanning of iodine-124-3F8 as an approach to tumor dosimetry during treatment planning for radioimmunotherapy in a child with neuroblastoma. *J Nucl Med* 1992;33:2020–2023.

37. Shen S, DeNardo GL, DeNardo SJ, et al. Dosimetric evaluation of copper-64 in copper-67-2IT-BAT-Lym-1 for radioimmunotherapy. *J Nucl Med* 1996;37:146–150.

38. O'Donoghue JA. The implications of non-uniform tumor doses for radioimmunotherapy. *J Nucl Med* 1999;40:1337–1341.

39. Schlom J, Molinolo A, Simpson JF, et al. Advantage of dose fractionation in monoclonal antibody-targeted radioimmunotherapy. *J Natl Cancer Inst* 1990;82:763–771.

40. Sun LQ, Vogel CA, Mirimanoff RO, et al. Timing effects of combined radioimmunotherapy and radiotherapy on a human solid tumor in nude mice. *Cancer Res* 1997;57:1312–1319.

41. Shaw DR, Khazaeli MB, LoBuglio AF. Mouse/human chimeric antibodies to a tumor-associated antigen: biologic activity of the four human IgG subclasses. *J Natl Cancer Inst* 1988;80:1553–1559.

42. LoBuglio AF, Wheeler RH, Trang J, et al. Mouse/human chimeric monoclonal antibody in man: kinetics and immune response. *Proc Natl Acad Sci U S A* 1989;86:4220–4224.

43. Caron PC, Co MS, Bull MK, et al. Biological and immunological features of humanized M195 (anti-CD33) monoclonal antibodies. *Cancer Res* 1992;52:6761–6767.

44. Winter G. Making antibody and peptide ligands by repertoire selection technologies. *J Mol Recognit* 1998;11:126–127.

45. Larson SM, El-Shirbiny AM, Divgi CR, et al. Single chain antigen binding protein (sFv CC49): first human studies in colorectal carcinoma metastatic to liver. *Cancer* 1997;80:2458–2468.

46. Reiter Y, Pastan I. Antibody engineering of recombinant Fv immunotoxins for improved targeting of cancer: disulfide-stabilized Fv immunotoxins. *Clin Cancer Res* 1996;2:245–252.

47. Hu S, Shively L, Raubitschek A, et al. Minibody: a novel engineered anti-carcinoembryonic antigen antibody fragment (single-chain Fv-CH3) which exhibits rapid, high-level targeting of xenografts. *Cancer Res* 1996;56:3055–3061.

48. Goodwin DA, Meares CF, Watanabe N, et al. Pharmacokinetics of pretargeted monoclonal antibody 2D12.5 and [88]Y-*janus*-2-(*p*-nitrobenzyl)-1,4,7,10-tetraazacyclododecanetetraacetic acid (DOTA) in BALB/c mice with KHJJ mouse adenocarcinoma: a model for ^{90}Y radioimmunotherapy. *Cancer Res* 1994;54:5937–5946.

49. Grana C, Chinol M, Magnani P, et al. *In vivo* tumor targeting based on the avidin-biotin system. *Tumor Targeting* 1996;2:230–239.

50. Le Doussal J-M, Chetanneau A, Gruaz-Guyon A, et al. Bispecific monoclonal antibody-mediated targeting of an indium-111-labeled DTPA dimer to primary colorectal tumors: pharmacokinetics, biodistribution, scintigraphy and immune response. *J Nucl Med* 1993;34:1662–1671.

51. Fritzberg AR. Antibody pretargeted radiotherapy: a new approach and a second chance. *J Nucl Med* 1998;39:20N–22N.

6

RADIOPHARMACEUTICAL THERAPY OF OSSEOUS METASTATIC DISEASE

EDWARD B. SILBERSTEIN

Our diagnostic methods detect with great difficulty tumor masses containing a million cells and having a volume of only 1 mm^3. Although oncologic science continues to make great strides in the cure of many cancers, palliation of cancers remains a significant function for physicians providing care to these patients. Significant cytocidal effects are obtained with chemotherapy and radiation. In addition, symptomatic relief is central to maintaining the patient's quality of life. This chapter addresses radiotherapy for the amelioration of pain caused by metastatic disease. The emphasis is on "unsealed sources" of beta particles or electrons emitted from radiopharmaceuticals that can be administered by injection or ingestion to reduce or eliminate bone pain and decrease the mass of neoplastic cells in bone metastases.

SCOPE OF THE PROBLEM

Bone metastases are seen in up to 85% of patients dying of highly prevalent cancers (e.g., breast, lung, and prostate carcinoma) (1). More than 125,000 cases of osseous metastases are diagnosed in the United States annually. Half to three fourths of patients with cancer metastatic to bone experience significant pain. The effects of this bone pain can be devastating: narcotic use with all its side effects, depression, withdrawal from the family, decreased mobility with resultant generalized weakness and increased risk for thromboembolism and pneumonia, hypercalcemia, and pathologic fracture.

BIOLOGY OF PAINFUL BONE METASTASES

Bone metastases generally develop late in the course of a malignancy, requiring multiple mutations to be able to sur-

vive separately from the primary cancer in the vascular compartment and to break down the endothelial and sinusoidal barriers that permit these cells to enter the bone. Direct extension of tumor to bone occurs less often. Evidence has been found for a variety of chemical stimuli that can cause tumor migration to, and growth within, bone (2). It is possible that tumors directly stimulate bone resorption because they are frequently seen adjacent to resorbed bone margins. Some tumors can stimulate mineral release and matrix resorption *in vitro* (2). Often, bone destruction is preceded by osteoblastic activation by a variety of tumor-derived factors (Table 6.1). Some of these cytokines have direct bone-resorbing capabilities.

Several of the mechanisms of bone pain caused by the presence of osseous metastases are obvious. Mechanical stretching of periosteum is clearly painful. Similarly, it is obvious that a pathologic fracture is always painful. It is not uncommon for pain to resolve within 1 to 3 days after the commencement of teletherapy or, less frequently, the injection of radiopharmaceuticals. So soon after treatment the tumor mass is still present, and there has not been sufficient time for shrinkage. If the pain has improved impressively in such a short time, then other mechanisms must be invoked. Often, cells of the immune system are present in the tumor microenvironment, among them lymphocytes,

TABLE 6.1. TUMOR-DERIVED FACTORS ALTERING OSTEOCLAST AND OSTEOBLAST FUNCTION

Eicosanoids
Granulocyte-macrophage colony-stimulating factor
Interleukin-1
Interleukin-6
Parathyroid hormone-related protein
Transforming growth factor-alpha
Transforming growth factor-beta
Tumor necrosis factor-alpha
Tumor necrosis factor-beta

From Garrett IR. Bone destruction in cancer. *Semin Oncol* 1993;20: 4–9, with permission.

E. B. Silberstein: Departments of Radiology and Medicine, University of Cincinnati Medical Center, Department of Nuclear Medicine, University Hospital, Cincinnati, Ohio 45219.

in which apoptosis is triggered at low radiation doses. These are sources of several cytokines and interferons that modulate pain, so it seems reasonable to hypothesize that when the source of pain modulation stops functioning, the pain may abate.

MANAGEMENT OF CANCER PAIN

A vast medical literature on the management of pain resulting from cancer is available, which is well summarized in a document from the Agency for Health Care Policy and Research of the U.S. Department of Health and Human Services (3). A stepwise approach to pain management is urged; multiple options are available before the use of narcotics, with their adverse effects of constipation and lethargy. Newer techniques of administration make these side effects somewhat more tolerable for most patients, but no patient must be allowed to suffer.

Hormone therapy reduces pain in at least half of patients with responsive tumors (i.e., prostate and breast cancer). The responses may be rapid and last for months. Successful chemotherapy may also reduce bone pain. Unfortunately, when osseous metastases occur later in the course of cancer, few drug regimens are effective.

A recent addition to the clinical analgesic armamentarium is the bisphosphonate group of drugs. These are characterized by a covalent carbon-to-phosphorus bond that no human enzyme can cleave. By chemisorption to calcium in surface hydroxyapatite, and also through a direct toxic effect on osteoclasts, bone resorption is inhibited. These agents reduce the fracture rate, decrease bone pain, prolong the time until repeated radiotherapy is required, and control hypercalcemia. Oral etidronate appears to decrease the development of metastases in high-risk breast cancer (4), as does intravenous pamidronate.

RADIOTHERAPY OF PAINFUL BONE METASTASES

External beam radiation (teletherapy) was utilized to treat tumor in bone within a year of Roentgen's description of x-rays. In patients with multiple involved sites, wide-field radiation therapy (usually hemibody) has been used for at least four decades (5). Strontium 89 was injected into patients to treat bone pain as early as 1942 (6). The use of wide-field radiotherapy has diminished at this time, and the roles of teletherapy and internal radiation emitters have become clearer.

Teletherapy has been used to reduce or eliminate bone pain throughout the 20th century, but unanimity regarding the number of fractions required, the radiation dose per fraction, and the total amount of radiation needed has not been attained. Solitary and multiple metastases have been treated with fractionated doses of 3 to 5 Gy, with a total of 20 to 40 Gy given. With all these variables, the overall response rates are indistinguishable, ranging from 80% to 93% during the 12 to 20 weeks after treatment (7,8). A randomized trial of 8 Gy in one fraction versus 20 Gy in five fractions and 30 Gy in 10 fractions gave the same response rates, although complete responses may have been higher at the higher doses (7). Recent reviews of teletherapy have demonstrated a rate of palliation of pain of more than 90%; in 40% to 65% of patients, however, complete pain relief is not achieved (7,8).

Hemibody radiation has been used for the palliation of pain from multiple osseous metastases. A Radiation Therapy Oncology Group report found an overall response rate of 73%, with complete relief in 20% of patients (9). Nearly 50% of the patients responded in 48 hours, and 80% in a week. The most effective safe doses were found to be 600 rads to the upper body, and 800 rads for the lower or middle hemibody. Although no fatalities occurred, 9% of patients with middle or lower hemibody and 16% of patients with upper hemibody irradiation experienced severe or life-threatening nausea and vomiting. In 10% of the middle or lower hemibody group and 32% of the upper hemibody patients, hematologic toxicity was severe or life-threatening (10).

The first publication on the use of radiotracers to palliate bone cancer appeared in 1942; many years later, clinical trials are still being developed to optimize the utilization of this modality. Table 6.2 summarizes the physical properties of the radionuclides in the radiopharmaceuticals currently in use or clinical trial. The various radiopharmaceuticals differ remarkably in several ways; the physical half-life ranges from 0.7 days for ^{188}Re to 50.0 days for ^{89}Sr, a variation by a factor of 72. The mean beta electron energies range from 0.94 MeV for ^{90}Y to 0.13 for ^{117m}Sn, a variation by a factor of 7.2. As a result, the mean range of these particles in tissue is between 0.2 and 3.0 mm. Some are gamma emitters and others emit only minor, insignificant *bremsstrahlung*. With these differences, one would expect a wide variation in efficacy of the radiopharmaceuticals, but the prevalence of pain reduction is not greatly different. Their effectiveness is probably related to cytocidal effects of the emitted particle. All the agents have a beta emission except ^{117m}Sn, which decays by isomeric transition, emitting abundant conversion electrons. One can assume that if ^{117m}Sn and ^{32}P, the latter with a path length 10 times greater than that of the former, are equally effective, the target cells must lie, on average, within 200 to 300 μ of the trabecular bone, where these radiopharmaceuticals are largely deposited. *If* they are all equally effective, then the differences in dose rate also do not have an effect.

It is difficult, also, to compare total radiation dose. Complete pain relief has been seen with 1 to 3 days of fractionated teletherapy, which suggests that doses of 200 to 600 rads may be adequate if delivered at a high dose rate. The dosimetry of radiopharmaceuticals deposited in metastatic bone tumor is

TABLE 6.2. BETA OR ELECTRON-EMITTING RADIOPHARMACEUTICALS FOR PAINFUL METASTASES

Radiopharmaceutical	Half-life (d)	Maximum E_B (MeV)	Mean E_B (MeV)	Mean range (mm)	Gamma MeV (% abundance)
^{188}Re (Sn)-HEDP	0.7	2.12	0.73	2.7	0.155 (10%)
			0.79	3.1	
^{153}Sm-EDTMP	1.9	0.81	0.22	0.6	0.103 (28%)
					0.041 (49%)
^{90}Y citrate	2.7	2.27	0.94	2.5	—
^{186}Re(Sn)-HEDP	3.8	1.07	0.33	1.1	0.137 (9%)
^{131}I-BDP	8.1	0.81	0.19	0.8	0.374 (82%)
^{117m}Sn-DTPA	13.6	—	0.15	0.3	0.159 (86%)
			0.13	0.2	
^{32}P-phosphate	14.3	1.71	0.70	3.0	—
^{89}Sr chloride	50.5	1.46	0.58	2.4	0.909 (0.01%)

EDTMP, ethylenediaminetetramethylphosphonate; DTPA, diethylenetriaminepentaacetic acid.

quite complex. Osteoblastic lesions with a high bone mineral content must be distinguished from osteolytic lesions with a high soft-tissue content, even if the percentage of uptake and biologic half-life of the radiopharmaceutical are identical. One commonly employed dosimetry model assumes homogeneous lesion morphology, uniform radionuclide dispersion, and complete energy deposition within the lesion by the emitted particles. These erroneous simplifications yield only very approximate doses. The uniform deposition model can underestimate a radiation dose to blastic lesions by as much as 80% (range, 7% to 84%) and to mixed blastic/lytic lesions by as much as almost 40% (range, 19% to 39%) (11). A review of ^{32}P dosimetry showed a fourfold range in estimates of rads/mCi injected based on variations in lesion uptake, another important dosimetric variable, among other assumptions required in these calculations (12).

Total-body retention of these radiotracers parallels that of the common ^{99m}Tc bisphosphonate scintigraphic agents, ranging from 40% to 100%. This results in considerable variation in total-body dosimetry. Individual-lesion dosimetry may be required to determine if sufficient radiopharmaceutical can be deposited to deliver a therapeutic dose. A single 800-rad dose from teletherapy has been found to be adequate to relieve bone pain from metastatic disease, so the required effective radiation dose from the beta electron emitters may have to exceed this level by at least a factor of 2 if the dose-reduction factor of 2 to 10 suggested by the National Council on Radiation Protection for the biologic effects of low-dose-rate ionizing radiation proves to be applicable to this model.

The administered dose or activity for each radiopharmaceutical is generally specified per kilogram of body weight. The radiation dose in rads or grays is much more difficult to determine.

In evaluating the efficacy data for each radiopharmaceutical, determination of the response is also problematic. Sub-jective pain, by its very nature, is difficult to measure. The perception of pain is probably best quantified by a simple graphic representation that has been shown to be reproducible and is widely accepted. This measurement tool is known as the Visual Analogue Scale. It is represented as a 10-cm horizontal line, with the left edge representing the absence of pain and the right edge representing pain as severe as the patient can conceive (13). The patient places a mark on the line to indicate the degree of pain. If the patient has less pain after a radiopharmaceutical treatment, it is crucial to learn whether an analgesic dose has been increased. When different opiate drugs are substituted, a dose equivalent chart for opiate analgesics should be used (3).

If the treated patient becomes bedridden, pain may be reduced but activities of daily living (ADL) have declined. This concept of ADL is best measured by a scale developed by the Eastern Cooperative Oncology Group in which a grade of zero means fully active and able to perform activities without restriction. Grade 4 indicates a patient who is completely disabled, cannot carry out any self-care, and is totally confined to bed (14). The three measures, pain, drug use, and ADL, have been graphically combined in a scale that is recommended to determine whether a therapeutic response to a radiopharmaceutical has occurred (15).

Any radiopharmaceutical used to relieve bone pain resulting from metastatic disease must have a very high affinity for bone and a still higher affinity for and longer biologic half-life in metastatic disease. Abnormal bone-to-normal bone ratios of uptake and retention of 3:1 to 5:1 (or higher) do, in fact, occur commonly. ^{89}Sr, ^{186}Re etidronate, and ^{117m}Sn pentetate have all been demonstrated to be retained significantly longer in the "woven" bone around metastases than in normal bone.

Although the physical half-life should ideally be equal to, or longer than, the biologic half-life to maximize the dose to tumor, it is not clear that this is extremely important because radionuclides with a short half-life (e.g., [153]Sm) seem to be associated with response rates similar to those of longer half-lived radioisotopes (e.g., ^{89}Sr).

In the United States, many of these radiopharmaceuticals cost in the range of $2,000, whereas oral ^{32}P, without requirements for sterility or absence of pyrogenicity, is available at less than half of this figure.

These radiopharmaceuticals should be used only if a diagnostic bone scan with ^{99m}Tc-MDP (methylene diphosphonate) or ^{99m}Tc-HMDP (hydroxymethylene disphosphonate) shows uptake in the painful regions. The distribution and degree of uptake have been shown to be identical to those of the conventional diagnostic bone-scanning agents.

Phosphorus 32

Phosphorus 32 is a pure beta emitter that is incorporated into hydroxyapatite as the phosphate moiety. This radiopharmaceutical, given as sodium phosphate either intravenously or orally, was the first radioactive material to be widely employed to alleviate the pain of osseous metastatic disease (16,17). The range of response to oral and intravenous ^{32}P has been reported as 50% to 100%. Few studies with ^{32}P had excellent pain measurements until 1992, when a small but carefully conceived study showed a response (pain reduction of at least 50%) in 14 of 15 patients given 12 mCi orally. A dose–response relationship (increasing response to pain with increasing activity administered) has not been shown (12). Many of the earlier investigations attempted to stimulate bone uptake of ^{32}P with androgens or parathyroid hormone, but the response was no greater than without these stimuli. A 1999 study comparing ^{89}Sr and ^{32}P showed a response rate of 93% for oral ^{32}P given without any of these osteoblast-stimulating adjuvants (18).

Strontium 89

Strontium 89 was given to patients in 1942, the same year that ^{32}P therapy was initiated (6). [89]Sr, injected as strontium chloride, is incorporated into hydroxyapatite, like calcium. Both elements circulate as divalent cations. It was demonstrated that the [85]Sr isotope detects all lesions identified by ^{99m}Tc-MDP, and a remarkably long biologic half-life has been found in reactive bone around tumor (19).

A double-blinded placebo study (20) confirmed the efficacy of ^{89}Sr that had been reported earlier (21–23). Two of these reports involved dose-escalation studies. No improvement in the response rate was noted with an increase in administered activity (21,23), as was observed with the analysis of [32]P. The reported response rates for ^{89}Sr have been between 50% and 80%.

The Trans-Canada study, unusual for using ^{89}Sr as an adjuvant to teletherapy, demonstrated that with 10.8 mCi, which is 2.7 times greater than the maximum activity employed in the United States, significant improvement in pain control was achieved in comparison with a placebo. In

this study, ^{89}Sr was shown to delay the onset of new painful metastases and to prolong the time until teletherapy to initially painful lesions was again required. Reduced analgesic requirements and improved quality of life were found in the ^{89}Sr group (24). Quilty et al. (25) compared 5.4 mCi of intravenous ^{89}Sr with either wide-field radiation therapy or local teletherapy and found no significant difference. As in the Trans-Canada study, significant delays before additional radiotherapy was required were observed in the ^{89}Sr group, which suggests an important effect of the long physical and biologic half-life of ^{89}Sr in bone. Most clinical trials have been reported in prostate cancer, but equal efficacy, about 80%, has been shown for breast cancer (26). McEwan and co-workers, reviewing the Trans-Canada study data, also found a clear cost benefit for the group of prostate cancer patients receiving ^{89}Sr of more than $5,000 per patient (27).

How to predict responders to these radiopharmaceuticals remains uncertain. Higher Karnofsky performance scores predicted responses to ^{89}Sr in one study (28), but not in another (21). It would be unfortunate if these conflicting data were used to argue that sicker cancer patients should be denied this form of nonopiate analgesia.

In the only comparative study of any two of the radiopharmaceuticals listed in Table 6.2, no difference in degree or duration of pain relief was found between ^{32}P given orally (12 mCi), with 14 of 15 patients experiencing at least a 50% reduction in pain, and ^{89}Sr, with a similar response in 14 of 16 patients (18). The onset of therapeutic response, time to maximal pain relief, and degree and duration of relief were not significantly different. [32]P was associated with a slight increase in grade 2 thrombocytopenia (platelet count, 50,000 to 75,000/μL), a level that does not cause spontaneous bleeding or require transfusion. No difference in leukopenia was found between patients receiving ^{32}P and [89]7Sr (15).

Strontium has been combined with chemotherapeutic agents such as cisplatin, carboplatin, and doxorubicin. A group treated with carboplatin at 7 and 21 days after ^{89}Sr was said to have a clearly superior pain response in comparison with those patients treated with strontium only. Nevertheless, no survival advantage was noted (29), nor was a survival advantage seen in the Trans-Canada study (24). Cisplatin has also been used with [89]Sr (30), but no controlled study has been published. Studies combining ^{89}Sr with mitoxantrone and hydrocortisone, doxorubicin, and estramustine plus vinblastine are in progress.

[153]Sm-Lexidronam

Samarium 153, produced by neutron irradiation of [152]Sm, was found to be optimally chelated for bone localization by ethylenediamine tetramethylphosphonate (EDTMP) (31), now called *lexidronam*. Clearance from blood and urine is complete by 6 hours. The mechanisms of retention include some chemisorption of the tetraphosphonate by hydroxyapatite, and also the formation of samarium oxide involving an oxygen of hydroxyapatite. Like ^{89}Sr, [153]Sm-lexidronam has been approved by the U.S. Food and Drug Administration for the treatment of bone pain. The short half-life of [153]Sm-lexidronam results in a significantly greater dose rate than that of ^{89}Sr, but the response rates do not seem to differ. Because of this shorter half-life, however, [153]Sm-lexidronam does not provide significant cytocidal radiation to bone metastases for weeks after its administration, in contrast to [89]Sr. It has not been determined whether these characteristics provide any advantage.

An early controlled trial with [153]Sm-lexidronam compared dosages of 0.5 mCi/kg and 1.0 mCi/kg and found no significant difference at 4 weeks in patient-reported pain relief, although the difference in improved sleep and relief of "daytime discomfort" was said to be statistically significant in favor of the higher dosage (32). Another study, comparing 0.75 mCi/kg with 1.5 mCi/kg, found no clear dose–response relationship (33). A double-blinded comparison of a single dose of either 0.5 or 1.0 mCi of [153]Sm-lexidronam per kilogram and a placebo indicated a better response for both groups receiving the active drug, with responses favoring the higher dose until the fourth week after injection, at which time they were identical (34). The response with [153]Sm-lexidronam was observed in 61% to 80% of the patients.

Rhenium Re 186 Etidronate

Rhenium is a group VIIA element, as is technetium. Reduced rhenium reoxidizes to some extent after chemisorption to hydroxyapatite, and perrhenate may therefore be found in the urine for several days after administration of [186]Re etidronate. As with any agent with an affinity for hydroxyapatite, skeletal uptake may approach 100% for diffuse metastatic disease. Elegant Monte Carlo dosimetry has been performed for [186]Re (11), but the use of individual-lesion dosimetry is quite difficult. A double-blinded, crossover study has been reported showing the superiority of [186]Re etidronate to placebo (35). Evidence has been found of increasing response with increasing dose (36). However, these investigators reported response rates as low as 55%, far less than the 75% to 80% initially reported with [186]Re etidronate.

When greater amounts of tumor evoke an osteoblastic response, greater amounts of radiopharmaceutical will be retained, and hence higher levels of marrow irradiation will result in cytopenia. The Utrecht group has correlated toxicity, primarily thrombocytopenia, with the measurement of the extent of skeletal involvement to predict the maximal safe dosage of [186]Re etidronate in individual patients (26).

Tin-117m-Diethylenetriamine Pentaacetic Acid

[117m]Sn-DTPA differs from the other bone-seeking radionuclides in that decay occurs by isomeric transition. The particulate radiation emitted is a conversion electron of low energy and very short range, about 0.2 to 0.3 mm. The chelated tin forms an oxide on the surface of hydroxyapatite. The short path of the conversion electron has been perceived as an advantage because myelotoxicity may well be less as a result of a particulate range that is only about 10% that of [32]P. Accordingly, less marrow is irradiated per decay (37).

Because [117m]Sn-DTPA is one of the newer radiopharmaceuticals evaluated for the reduction of pain from bone metastases, fewer clinical trials have been reported (37,38). No clear correlation between dose and response has been noted (38). An overall response rate of 75% has been observed in 40 patients, with complete pain relief achieved in 12 (30%). Toxicity is not marked; only two grade 2 cases (white blood cell count, 2,000 to 2,900/μL) and one grade 3 case (white blood cell count, 1,000 to 1,900/μL) of leukopenia have been observed, and no thrombocytopenia. These authors concluded that [117m]Sn-DTPA causes less myelotoxicity than the other radiopharmaceuticals. This may be the result of the high ratio of bone surface to red marrow absorbed dose because of the limited range of the electron emitted.

RADIOPHARMACEUTICAL EFFICACY

It is clear that these beta electron emitters reduce the pain of osseous metastases in most patients treated, roughly 55% to 80%. A minority of the responders may have complete resolution of pain. It is not possible to predict which patients will respond to treatment, although it is clear that if the bone scan results at a painful site are negative, there will be no selective uptake and no response. All the radiopharmaceuticals discussed are effective, and no good, clear evidence has been found that any one is more efficacious or takes effect more rapidly than another. In 1999, a double-blinded study was initiated to determine whether [117m]Sn-DTPA is less myelotoxic than [89]Sr. Data are not available at this time.

The time to response averages 1 to 3 weeks, although responses have occurred within 3 days after therapy or as late as 30 days. Successful retreatment has been reported in responders, usually at 12-week intervals, for up to seven repeated injections, with response rates of 50% to 60%.

Although the evidence for a cytocidal effect of the injected radiation is good (e.g., a falling level of prostate-specific antigen and healing of radiographic and scintigraphic abnormalities), no data are available to suggest any prolongation of survival (24), probably because the bone metastases are only a fraction of the tumor burden, which proves lethal.

ADVERSE REACTIONS

Some degree of myelosuppression is regularly observed, although in patients with normal leukocyte and platelet counts before therapy, clinical sequalae are rare. Treating patients with leukocyte counts below 3,000/μL or platelet counts under 60,000 to 100,000/μL can lead to infection and bleeding, respectively. The platelet count is usually affected to a greater degree than the leukocyte count, but both may fall to 40% to 70% of pretreatment values by 4 to 6 weeks; they usually recover by 8 to 10 weeks.

Other causes of pancytopenia must be excluded. Disseminated intravascular coagulation accompanies some malignancies and leads to thrombocytopenia, with the possibility of a very rapid drop in platelet counts if megakaryocytic proliferation is slowed by radiation. Measurement of fibrin split products or an analogous screening test should be performed before therapy with unsealed sources that have an affinity for bone. Prior radiotherapy or chemotherapy may have depleted marrow stem cells, which makes severe cytopenia more likely. Concurrent chemotherapy or teletherapy should be avoided for this reason. Marrow replacement by metastases is another cause of cytopenia.

A consent form spelling out these dangers is suggested, as deaths related to thrombocytopenia have been reported for all these radiopharmaceuticals except ^{117m}Sn-DTPA, of which far fewer doses have thus far been administered. The second side effect of all these radiopharmaceuticals is a "flare" response, which is increased pain at one or more of the sites being treated, usually within 2 to 3 days of injection and rarely as late as 10 days, that lasts 1 to 3 days.

RADIATION SAFETY

The U.S. Nuclear Regulatory Commission allows all these therapeutic agents to be administered on an outpatient basis. Patients receiving beta plus gamma-emitting radiopharmaceuticals must have a count rate below a specified maximum before discharge, or have the appropriate calculations performed to indicate that household members will receive less than 500 mrad and children and pregnant women less than 100 mrad. Written instructions should be given to the patient concerning radiation safety and personal hygiene. All these radiopharmaceuticals are excreted in the urine. Accordingly, a few basic precautions are suggested, including handling soiled undergarments with gloves and washing them separately, flushing the toilet twice for 1 week after injection, and washing hands thoroughly after urination or defecation. Patients should be reassured that they are not a radiation hazard to family members.

TECHNIQUE OF ADMINISTRATION

Beta electron emitters produce *bremsstrahlung*, which increases with higher atomic number shielding. For pure beta emitters, plastic syringe shields are suggested.

Injection should be administered through a running intravenous line, both to avoid infiltration of a form of radiation that can cause local subcutaneous necrosis and to reduce

TABLE 6.3. CLINICAL PREPARATION FOR TREATING A PATIENT WITH BONE PAIN FOR METASTASES

Obtain informed consent.
Recent bone scan must demonstrate uptake at painful sites.
Obtain leukocyte and platelet count and fibrin split product assays.
Perform pregnancy test in women of childbearing age.
Start intravenous line.
Use syringe shield.
Inject slowly.

exposure to the hand of the therapist, which might result from excess handling of the syringe during venipuncture.

A bolus injection should be avoided. ^{89}Sr may cause flushing or cardiotoxicity if given rapidly because its physiologic sequelae are similar to those of calcium. Chelates can lower plasma ionized calcium and magnesium levels acutely if given too rapidly. A 1- to 3-minute period of injection is suggested. Table 6.3 summarizes the preparations for treatment.

OTHER TREATMENT CONSIDERATIONS

In addition to avoiding treatment in the presence of severe pancytopenia or disseminated intravenous coagulation, during active chemotherapy, or when the bone scan shows no increased uptake on a painful site, one must ascertain that no pathologic fracture is present at the site of pain because pain resulting from fracture will not respond to beta electron therapy. Epidural metastases pressing on the spinal cord and soft-tissue masses causing nerve pressure elsewhere must also be excluded.

Teletherapy is more appropriate for a single painful site because the remainder of the marrow will receive little radiation. Teletherapy is the treatment of choice for preventing or treating pathologic fracture, cord compression, or pain from soft-tissue tumor extending to bone. Patients with an Eastern Cooperative Oncology Group scale score of more than 2 (Karnofsky performance score < 50)—that is, those who are more debilitated—should not be denied the opportunity to receive these pain-reducing radiopharmaceuticals. Patients with as little as 1 month to live can still obtain pain relief from this form of treatment. The literature is divided about response frequency in advanced disease (20,27).

FUTURE TRENDS

The combination of a beta electron emitter with either a bisphosphonate or one or more forms of chemotherapy still needs to be assessed. The bisphosphonates may reduce uptake of these radiotracers. Large, comparative studies could indicate any advantage of one of the agents over another, but such studies are expensive to perform. Careful dose-escalation studies are also needed to determine whether the increased myelotoxicity associated with higher administered doses is offset by truly higher response rates.

REFERENCES

1. Lote K, Walloe A, Bjersand A. Bone metastases: prognosis, diagnosis and treatment. *Acta Radiol Oncol* 1986;25:227–232.
2. Garrett IR. Bone destruction in cancer. *Semin Oncol* 1993;20:4–9.
3. Jacox A, Carr DB, Payne R, eds. *Management of cancer pain.* US Department of Health and Human Services, Agency for Health Care Policy and Research, publication No. 94-0592, 1994:257.
4. Diel U, Solomayer EF, Goerner R, et al. Reduction of new metastases in breast cancer by clodronate. *N Engl J Med* 1997;339:657–663.
5. Saenger EL, Silberstein EB, Aron B, et al. Whole and partial body radiotherapy of advanced cancer. *Am J Roentgenol* 1973;117:670–685.
6. Pecher C. Biological investigations with radioactive Ca and Sr: preliminary report on the use of radioactive Sr in treatment of bone cancer. *U Calif Pub Pharmacol* 1942;11:117–139.
7. Bates T. A review of local radiotherapy in the treatment of bone metastases and cord compression. *Int J Radiat Oncol Biol Phys* 1992;23:217–227.
8. Janjan NA. Radiation for bone metastases: conventional techniques and the role of systemic radiopharmaceuticals. *Cancer* 1997;80[Suppl]:1628–1640.
9. Blitzer PH. Reanalysis of the RTOG study of the palliation of symptomatic osseous metastases. *Cancer* 1985;55:1468–1475.
10. Salazar OM, Rubin P, Hendrickson FR, et al. Single-dose half-body irradiation for palliation of multiple bone metastases from solid tumors. *Cancer* 1986;58:29–36.
11. Samaratunga RC, Thomas SR, Hinnefield JD, et al. A Monte Carlo simulation model for radiation dose to metastatic skeletal tumor from rhenium-186(Sn)-HEDP. *J Nucl Med* 1995;36:336–350.
12. Silberstein EB, Elgazzar AH, Kapilivsky A. Phosphorus-32 radiopharmaceuticals for the treatment of painful osseous metastases. *Semin Nucl Med* 1992;22:17–27.
13. Scott J, Huskisson EC. Graphic representation of pain. *Pain* 1976;2:175–184.
14. Zibrod CG, Schneiderman M, Frei E, et al. Appraisal of methods for the study of chemotherapy of cancer in man: comparative therapeutic trial of nitrogen mustard and trimethylene thiophosphoramide. *J Chronic Dis* 1960;11:7–32.
15. Quirijnen JMSP, Shiuw HH, Zonnenberg BA, et al. Efficacy of rhenium-186-etidronate in prostate cancer patients with metastatic bone pain. *J Nucl Med* 1996;37:1511–1515.
16. Friedell HL, Storaasli JP. The use of radioactive phosphorus in the treatment of carcinoma of the breast with widespread metastases to bone. *Am J Roentgenol* 1950;64:557–559.
17. Maxfield JR, Maxfield JGS, Maxfield WS. The use of radioactive phosphorus and testosterone in metastatic bone lesions from breast and prostate. *Southern Med J* 1958;51:320–328.
18. Nair N. Relative efficacy of ^{32}P and ^{89}Sr in palliation of skeletal metastases. *J Nucl Med* 1999;40:256–261.
19. Blake GM, Zivanovic MA, Blaquiere RM, et al. Strontium-89 therapy: measurement of absorbed dose to skeletal metastases. *J Nucl Med* 1988;29:549–555.
20. Lewington VJ, McEwan AJ, Ackery DM, et al. A prospective, randomized double-blind crossover study to examine the efficacy of strontium-89 in pain palliation in patients with advanced prostatic cancer metastatic to bone. *Eur J Cancer* 1991;27:961–965.
21. Silberstein EB, Williams C. Strontium-89 therapy for the pain of osseous metastases. *J Nucl Med* 1985;26:345–349.
22. Laing AH, Ackery DM, Bayly RJ, et al. Strontium-89 chloride for pain palliation in prostatic skeletal malignancy. *Br J Radiol* 1991;64:816–824.
23. Robinson RG, Preston DF, Schiefelbein M, et al. Strontium-89 therapy for the palliation of pain due to osseous metastases. *JAMA* 1995;274:420–425.
24. Porter AT, McEwan AJB, Power JE, et al. Results of a randomized phase III trial to evaluate the efficacy of strontium-89 adjuvant to local field external beam irradiation in the management of endocrine-resistant metastatic prostatic cancer. *Int J Radiat Oncol Biol Phys* 1993;25:805–816.
25. Quilty PM, Kirk D, Bolger JJ, et al. A comparison of the palliative effects of strontium-89 and external beam radiotherapy in metastatic prostatic cancer. *Radiother Oncol* 1994;31:33–41.
26. Baziotis N, Yakoumakis E, Zissimopoulos A, et al. Strontium-89 chloride in the treatment of bone metastases from breast cancer. *Oncology* 1998;55:377–384.
27. McEwan AJB, Amyotte GA, McGowan DG, et al. A retrospective analysis of the cost-effectiveness of treatment with Metastron (^{89}Sr-chloride) in patients with prostate cancer metastatic to bone. *Nucl Med Commun* 1994;15:499–507.
28. Schmeler K, Bastin K. Strontium-89 for symptomatic metastatic prostate cancer to bone: recommendations for hospice patients. *Hosp J* 1996;11:1–4.
29. Sciuto R, Mami CL, Tofani A, et al. Radiosensitization with low-dose carboplatin enhances pain palliation in radioisotope therapy with strontium-89. *Nucl Med Commun* 1996;17:699–804.
30. Mertens WC, Porter AT, Reid RH, et al. Strontium-89 and low-dose infusion cisplatin for patients with hormone-refractory prostate carcinoma metastatic to bone: a preliminary report. *J Nucl Med* 1992;33:1437–1443.
31. Goeckler WF, Edwards B, Volkert WA, et al. Skeletal localization of samarium-153 chelates: potential therapeutic agents. *J Nucl Med* 1987;28:495–503.
32. Resche I, Chatal J-F, Pecking P, et al. A dose-controlled study of ^{153}Sm-ethylenediaminetetramethylphosphonate (EDTMP) in the treatment of patients with painful bone metastases. *Eur J Cancer* 1997;33:1583–1591.
33. Alberts AS, Smit BJ, Louw WKA, et al. Dose-response relationship and multiple dose efficacy and toxicity of samarium-153-EDTMP in metastatic cancer to bone. *Radiother Oncol* 1997;43:175–179.
34. Serafini AN, Houston SJ, Resche I, et al. Palliation of pain associated with metastatic bone cancer using samarium-153 lexidronam: a double-blind placebo-controlled clinical trial. *J Clin Oncol* 1998;16:1574–1582.
35. Maxon HR, Schroder LE, Hertzberg VS, et al. Rhenium-186(Sn) HEDP for treatment of painful osseous metastases: results of a double-blind crossover and comparison with placebo. *J Nucl Med* 1991;27:954–960.
36. DeKlerk JMH, Zonnenberg BA, van het Schip AD, et al. Dose escalation study of rhenium-186-etidronate in prostate cancer patients with metastatic bone pain. *J Nucl Med* 1996;37:1511–1521.
37. Atkins HL, Mausner L, Srivastava SC, et al. Biodistribution of Sn-117m(4+) DTPA for palliative therapy of painful osseous metastases. *Radiology* 1993;186:279–287.
38. Srivastava SC, Atkins HL, Krishnemurthy GT, et al. Treatment of metastatic bone pain with tin-117m stannic diethylenetriaminepentaacetic acid: a phase I/II clinical study. *Clin Cancer Res* 1998;4:61–68.

7

PEDIATRIC NUCLEAR ONCOLOGY

LEONARD P. CONNOLLY
LAURA A. DRUBACH
S. TED TREVES

Cancer is rare during childhood. Pediatric cancers, which are generally defined as cancers occurring before the age of 15 years, account for only about 2% of all cancers. Nevertheless, cancer is the most common cause of death from disease during childhood. Approximately 10% of deaths during childhood are attributable to cancer (1).

The incidence of cancer is estimated to be 133.3 per million children (2). Table 7.1 provides the estimated incidence rates of the more commonly encountered cancers in American children. This table makes it quite apparent that childhood cancers often differ from those encountered in adults. The incidence of some pediatric cancers varies markedly with age. Some tumors occur predominantly in children younger than 5 years of age. Examples include neuroblastoma and Wilms' tumor. Other malignancies, such as Hodgkin's lymphoma and osteosarcoma, predominantly affect children older than 10 years of age.

The pediatric cancers for which nuclear medicine has proved most valuable in diagnosis, staging, and long-term surveillance are emphasized in this chapter. Before the discussion of clinical applications, a brief review of nuclear medicine studies in children is offered.

IMAGING THE PEDIATRIC PATIENT

Patient Preparation, Immobilization, and Sedation

Patient cooperation is a prerequisite to optimal performance of nuclear medicine examinations. To gain this cooperation, any fears a child has concerning an examination must be allayed. This requires patience and understanding on the part of all personnel with whom the child has contact. The nuclear medicine facility must have a "child-friendly" environment. Because parental attitudes and anxieties are readily conveyed to children, it is essential that parents be well informed and that any parental concerns be addressed. Parents should be

encouraged to accompany their children during the course of a study and provide needed emotional support.

Once a child's trust has been gained, continued cooperation is usually ensured by relatively simple methods. Sheets wrapped around the body, sandbags, or special holding devices are often sufficient for immobilization. Entertainment in the form of television, videotapes, music, or reading and the proximity of favorite toys or blankets is helpful in calming and distracting older children.

Sedation is indicated when, on the basis of careful consideration, it is anticipated that the methods described above will prove inadequate or when they unexpectedly prove unsuccessful. Sedation may also be employed when a young cancer victim is finding it difficult to cope with the extensive testing involved in diagnosis or follow-up. For imaging procedures, the usual goal of sedation is a minimally depressed level of consciousness in which the patient

TABLE 7.1. CANCER INCIDENCE RATES PER MILLION CHILDREN YOUNGER THAN 15 YEARS OF AGE IN THE UNITED STATES AS DERIVED FROM THE SURVEILLANCE, EPIDEMIOLOGY, AND END RESULTS (SEER) PROGRAM

Cancer	Rate	Peak rate	Age (y) at peak
All cancers	133.3	218.4	<1
Acute lymphoid leukemia	30.9	76.6	2
Central nervous system tumors	27.6	34.9	4
Neuroblastoma	9.7	55.2	<1
Non-Hodgkin's lymphoma	8.4	12.0	14
Wilms' tumor	8.1	21.7	<1
Hodgkin's lymphoma	6.6	23.1	14
Acute myeloid leukemia	5.6	10.6	<1
Rhabdomyosarcoma	4.5	7.8	5
Retinoblastoma	3.9	24.7	<1
Osteosarcoma	3.4	10.6	14
Ewing's sarcoma	2.8	6.8	13
All others	21.8	—	—

From Gurney JG, Serverson RK, Darris S, et al. Incidence of cancer in children in the United States. *Cancer* 1995;75:2186–2195, with permission.

L. P. Connolly, L. A. Drubach, and S. T. Treves: Department of Radiology, Harvard Medical School; Division of Nuclear Medicine, Children's Hospital, Boston, Massachusetts 02115.

remains responsive to physical stimulation and verbal commands and a patent airway and protective reflexes are independently maintained (3). This level of sedation is referred to as *conscious sedation*. Only extremely rare cases require deeper levels of sedation.

Sedation protocols, particularly regarding the recommended medications and their dosages, vary from institution to institution. These protocols are continually being reevaluated and are frequently customized to the needs of an individual patient. Chloral hydrate is commonly used in infants. Parenteral sedation is used in older children. Commonly used parenteral sedatives include barbiturates, such as pentobarbital sodium, and opiates, such as fentanyl. An institutional sedation program should be a collaborative effort between imaging specialists, clinical practitioners, anesthesiologists, and nursing personnel. Guidelines, such as those advanced by the Society of Nuclear Medicine (4), are useful.

Personnel trained in pediatric advanced life support, monitoring, and resuscitative equipment and an active quality assurance program are essential components of a sedation program.

Administered Dose

In determining the radiopharmaceutical dose to be administered for pediatric studies, the goal is to keep the absorbed radiation dose at a minimum while retaining the ability to obtain a study of diagnostic quality. Administered doses are generally calculated by adjusting recommended adult radiopharmaceutical doses according to body weight or body surface area. Special consideration must be given to neonates and infants, in whom the concept of *minimal total dose* is applied. This is the radiopharmaceutical dose below which a study will be inadequate regardless of the body weight or surface area. The minimal total dose is determined by the type of examination, the time over which the examination is to be performed, and the specifications of the equipment with which the examination is to be performed. Table 7.2 provides the dosage schedule used at Children's Hospital in Boston for radiopharmaceuticals of principal importance in pediatric nuclear oncology (5,6).

CLINICAL APPLICATIONS

Neuroblastoma

Clinical Considerations

Neuroblastoma is the most common extracranial solid malignancy of children. The tumor is predominantly encountered in the very young. The mean age of patients at presentation is 20 to 30 months (7). It is the most commonly diagnosed neoplasm in the first year of life, during which it accounts for approximately 25% of all malignancies. The incidence decreases thereafter. The age of children at presentation with neuroblastoma is rarely more than 5 years (2).

Neuroblastoma originates from the embryonal neural crest anywhere along the sympathetic ganglion chain or within the adrenal medulla. Approximately 70% of tumors are located in the abdomen or pelvis. The most common primary site is adrenal, where 40% to 50% of primary neuroblastomas are found. Other abdominal sites of origin include the paravertebral and presacral sympathetic chain and the

TABLE 7.2. RADIOPHARMACEUTICALS OF PRINCIPAL IMPORTANCE IN PEDIATRIC NUCLEAR ONCOLOGY

Procedure	Radiopharmaceutical	Route of administration	Dose/kg		Minimum administered dose		Maximum administered dose	
			mCi	MBq	mCi	MBq	mCi	MBq
Skeletal scintigraphy	^{99m}Tc-MDP	Intravenous	0.2	7.4	1.0	37.0	20.0	740.0
Neuroblastoma detection or viability assessment	^{123}I-MIBG	Intravenous	0.2	7.4	1.0	37.0	10.0	370.0
Neuroblastoma detection or viability assessment	^{131}I-MIBG	Intravenous	0.014	0.52	0.1	3.7	1.0	37.0
Neuroblastoma detection or viability assessment	^{111}In-pentetreotide	Intravenous	0.04	1.5	0.5	18.5	3.0	111.0
Tumor detection or viability assessment	^{201}Tl chloride	Intravenous	0.03	1.11	0.5	18.5	2.0	74.0
Tumor detection or viability assessment	^{99m}Tc-MIBI	Intravenous	0.4	14.8	2.0	74	20.0	740.0
Tumor detection or viability assessment	^{67}Ga citrate	Intravenous	0.04	1.48	0.25	9.25	6.0	222.0
Tumor detection or viability assessment	^{18}F-FDG	Intravenous	0.15	5.55	0.5	18.5	10.0	370.0

MDP, methylene diphosphonate; MIBG, metaiodobenzylguanidine; MIBI, methoxyisobutylisonitrile; FDG, fluorodeoxyglucose.

organ of Zuckerkandl. Thoracic tumors, which are usually located in the posterior mediastinal sympathetic ganglia, and cervical tumors, which arise from sympathetic plexuses in the lower neck, account for 15% and 5% of tumors, respectively. A primary tumor may not be detected in as many as 10% of children who present with disseminated neuroblastoma (8).

Neuroblastoma is characterized by small round cells that contain neurofilaments and form tumor rosettes in bone marrow and blood. Gross or microscopic calcification is often present in the tumor. Neuroblastomas are typically solid masses. The size varies. Abdominal tumors tend to be larger than those in the thorax or neck. Areas of hemorrhage or necrosis are frequently present in larger tumors (7,8).

Two related neural crest tumors, ganglioneuroma and ganglioneuroblastoma, have been described. Ganglioneuroma contains mature ganglion cells. Some neuroblastomas spontaneously regress or mature into this benign tumor. The peculiar capacity of neuroblastoma to mature into a histologically benign tumor or occasionally regress completely is a unique aspect of this malignancy. The unpredictability and infrequency of these occurrences and the consequences of delaying therapy require that treatment be instituted at diagnosis, however. Ganglioneuroblastoma is a malignant tumor that contains both undifferentiated neuroblasts and mature ganglion cells. Its histologic differentiation from neuroblastoma is somewhat arbitrary and subject to sampling variations (7,8).

The clinical manifestations of neuroblastoma are protean in scope. The tumor may produce a palpable mass, or symptoms may be caused by invasion or compression of adjacent structures. Many children present with nonspecific signs and symptoms, including fever, weight loss, irritability, an elevated sedimentation rate, and anemia. Signs and symptoms may result from distant metastases. Bone pain or refusal to move an extremity because of skeletal metastases may be the presenting complaint. Paraneoplastic syndromes also occur. A syndrome of diarrhea, hypokalemia, and achlorhydria resulting from secretion of vasoactive intestinal peptide occurs in about 7% of cases. A syndrome that potentially includes opsoclonus, myoclonus, and cerebellar ataxia occurs in about 2% of patients with neuroblastoma. Cross-reaction between tumor antigens and cerebellar tissue is believed to account for the association between this syndrome, which is referred to as *infantile myoclonic encephelopathy*, and neuroblastoma. As many as 50% of patients with infantile myoclonic encephalopathy have neuroblastoma (8).

Disseminated disease is present in up to 70% of cases at diagnosis. The distribution of metastases varies with the age of the child. Through 1 year of age, metastatic involvement is frequently confined to the bone marrow, liver, and skin. In this group, the bone marrow is often sparsely involved and hepatic metastases tend to be diffusely infiltrative. Despite dissemination, infants with this pattern of disease have a favorable prognosis and often require only excision of the primary tumor for treatment. In children who are older at diagnosis, metastases usually involve cortical bone, bone marrow, liver, and lymph nodes. The marrow is often extensively infiltrated, and liver metastases are commonly well defined in these older children (7). This pattern of metastatic disease carries a poor prognosis.

Three different systems are used in staging neuroblastoma. The Evans, International, and Pediatric Oncology Group staging systems are summarized in Table 7.3 (7–10).

TABLE 7.3. STAGING SYSTEMS FOR NEUROBLASTOMA

Stage	Description
Evans staging system for neuroblastoma	
I	Tumor confined to organ of origin (totally excised).
II	Tumor extension beyond organ of origin. Tumor does not cross midline. Regional lymph nodes may be involved.
III	Tumor extension across midline with encroachment on contralateral tissues.
IV	Distant metastases (skeletal, other organs, soft tissues, distant lymph nodes).
IV-S	Localized primary tumor not crossing midline. Remote disease confined to liver, subcutaneous tissues, and bone marrow. Cortical bone not involved.
International neuroblastoma staging system	
1	Localized tumor, complete gross resection with or without microscopic residual disease. Nonadherent lymph nodes microscopically negative for tumor.
2A	Localized tumor, incomplete gross resection. Nonadherent lymph nodes microscopically negative for tumor.
2B	Localized tumor, complete or incomplete gross resection. Nonadherent lymph nodes microscopically positive, contralateral lymph nodes microscopically negative for tumor.
3	Unresectable unilateral tumor infiltrating across midline with or without regional nodal involvement. OR Localized unilateral tumor with contralateral nodal involvement. OR Midline tumor with bilateral infiltration or nodal involvement.
4	Any tumor with dissemination to distant lymph nodes, bone, bone marrow, liver, skin, and/or other organs (except as defined for stage 4S).
4S	Localized primary tumor with dissemination limited to skin, liver, and/or marrow with marrow involvement < 10% by biopsy or aspirate. MIBG should be negative in the marrow. Limited to infants < 1 year of age.
Pediatric Oncology Group staging system for neuroblastoma	
A	Localized primary tumor, completely resected.
B	Incomplete research of primary tumor. Lymph nodes and liver uninvolved.
C	Complete or incomplete resection of primary tumor. Lymph nodal involvement, liver uninvolved.
D	Disseminated metastatic tumor.

MIBG, metaiodobenzylguanidine.

In addition to stage, age at diagnosis and location of disease are important prognostic determinants. Patients younger than 1 year of age have a better prognosis than older patients. Thoracic tumors are associated with longer survival than abdominal tumors. Other prognostic factors include cellular differentiation, mitotic activity, and DNA analysis. A karyotype analysis of a neuroblastoma revealing deletion of the short arm of chromosome 1 or amplification of the N-*myc* oncogene indicates a poor prognosis (7,11–13).

Surgical excision is the preferred treatment of localized neuroblastoma. Complete gross excision is not always possible, and some tumor may have to be left *in situ*. When local disease is extensive, intensive preoperative chemotherapy may be utilized. Surgical removal is not likely to improve survival for children with Evans stage IV or International stage 4 disease. The prognosis in these cases is poor, but high-dose chemotherapy, total-body irradiation, and bone marrow reinfusion are beneficial for some children with this presentation.

Metaiodobenzylguanidine

Metaiodobenzylguanidine (MIBG) is structurally similar to the neurotransmitter norepinephrine and the adrenergic neuron blocker guanethidine. At doses used for imaging, a neuronal sodium- and energy-dependent transport mechanism is responsible for uptake of MIBG into the cytosol of neuroblastoma cells. At higher doses, passive diffusion may prevail. MIBG that has been transported into neuroblastoma cells largely remains free within the cytoplasm (14). Retention of MIBG in neuroblastomas is a consequence of rapid reuptake of tracer that escapes from the cell (15).

A number of medications interfere with MIBG uptake into tumors (16). These include sympathomimetics, antihypertensives, tricyclic antidepressants, calcium channel blockers, a few long-acting beta blockers, and cocaine (16,17). Although few children with neuroblastoma are taking these medications, some are receiving nonprescription medications used in the treatment of upper respiratory or ear infections that contain ephedrine, phenylephrine, phenylpropanolamine, or other potentially interfering agents. Specific recommendations regarding the time between discontinuation of various medications and MIBG administration have been published (16).

Radioiodine labels of MIBG that have been described include ^{131}I, ^{125}I, [124]I, and [123]I. Of these, ^{131}I and ^{123}I have been most widely used clinically. To study children with neuroblastoma, ^{123}I is preferable to [131]I. Even in higher administered doses, radiation dosimetry is more favorable with ^{123}I because of its shorter physical half-life and paucity of particulate emission. Additionally, the 159-keV gamma photon of ^{123}I is more optimal for imaging than the 364-keV gamma photon of [131]I. High-quality single-photon emission computed tomography (SPECT) is readily performed in a reasonable acquisition time with ^{123}I-MIBG but not with ^{131}I-MIBG. Although ^{123}I-MIBG is the preferable radiopharmaceutical, commercially available ^{131}I-MIBG is also an excellent agent that is reasonable and appropriate to use if ^{123}I-MIBG is not available. In the United States, ^{123}I-MIBG is currently available only at institutions where it has been granted Investigational New Drug status from the Food and Drug Administration.

Metaiodobenzylguanidine is administered slowly because it is possible to precipitate a hypertensive crisis by competitive displacement of norepinephrine from storage sites. Pretreatment and post-treatment with supersaturated potassium iodide decreases thyroidal uptake of unbound radioiodine.

Imaging should encompass the entire body because of the propensity of neuroblastoma to disseminate widely. Imaging is performed the day after administration of ^{123}I-MIBG. SPECT can increase the number of lesions detected in a patient with metastatic disease (18) or, at least, increase the certainty of interpretation (19). We perform SPECT of the chest and abdomen and planar imaging of the head and extremities. Supplementing images obtained on the first day following ^{123}I-MIBG administration with additional planar imaging on the second day does not appear to increase the sensitivity of the examination (18), but it may enable better delineation of some lesions (20) and can assist in differentiating tracer within bowel from sites of disease. SPECT on the first day following ^{123}I-MIBG administration usually obviates the need for this second set of images. When ^{131}I-MIBG is used, planar imaging is performed 1, 2, and occasionally 3 or 4 days after administration. Anatomic definition is poorer at the later times, but some lesions become more conspicuous (15).

The normal distribution of MIBG includes salivary glands, lacrimal glands, nasopharynx, myocardium, liver, spleen, adrenals, kidneys, bladder, bowel, and muscle. The thyroid may be faintly demonstrated (21). In some children, MIBG localizes in the lungs, either diffusely or in the lower zones. MIBG uptake is often prominent in muscles of the neck, shoulders, and upper thorax of infants and small children (20). Myocardial uptake is frequently depressed or absent in patients with high levels of circulating catecholamines (22). Cerebellar localization of MIBG has been described (23) but is highly unusual (15).

Although this chapter reviews only the imaging aspects of MIBG, it is worth noting that advanced MIBG-avid disease has been treated with ^{131}I-MIBG (24–27) and ^{125}I-MIBG (28).

Imaging of Neuroblastoma

The diagnostic imaging of children with neuroblastoma varies with the mode of presentation. Often, a mass is first detected on abdominal or chest radiographs obtained to evaluate symptoms resulting from local effects of the tumor. Calcification is demonstrated radiographically in approximately 15% of thoracic and 66% of abdominal tumors (7).

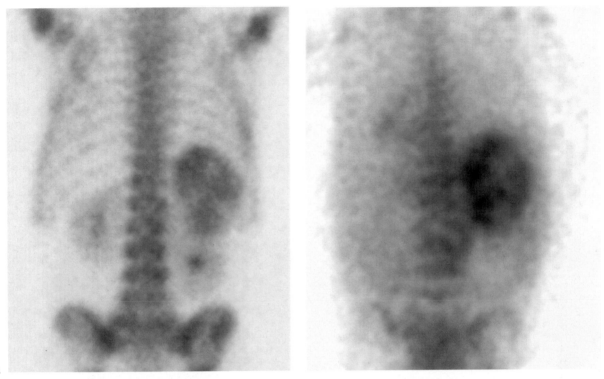

FIGURE 7.1. Metastatic neuroblastoma. Posterior planar images show accumulation of ⁹⁹ᵐTc-methylene diphosphonate (*MDP*) (**A**) and ¹²³I-metaiodobenzylguanidine (*MIBG*) (**B**) in a neuroblastoma of the right adrenal of a 4-year-old girl. Both studies also show evidence of vertebral and pelvic metastases.

Because ultrasonography is widely utilized in children with abdominal masses, it is often the first study to suggest the diagnosis. Bone radiographs or skeletal scintigraphy (29) may be the first study to suggest the diagnosis in patients who present with symptoms attributable to skeletal involvement. Although the radiographic and scintigraphic manifestations of skeletal metastases are fairly characteristic, identification of calcification or skeletal tracer uptake in the primary tumor increases the level of diagnostic certainty. Skeletal uptake of tracer is present in 40% to 85% of primary tumors (30–34) (Figs. 7.1–7.3). It is postulated to reflect active calcium metabolism by viable tumor (33). The likelihood of skeletal tracer localization in the primary site increases with tumor size but does not independently carry

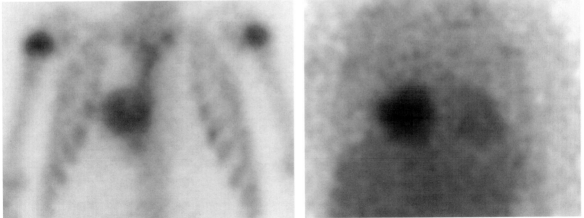

FIGURE 7.2. Neuroblastoma. Skeletal scintigraphy (**A**) shows localization of ⁹⁹ᵐTc-methylene diphosphonate (*MDP*), and ¹²³I-metaiodobenzylguanidine (MIBG) imaging (**B**) shows ¹²³I-MIBG uptake in a right posterior mediastinal neuroblastoma of a 12-month-old boy.

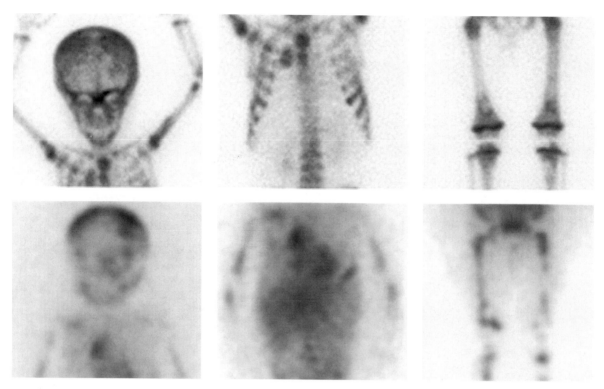

FIGURE 7.3. Metastatic neuroblastoma. Selected anterior planar images from ^{99m}Tc-methylene diphosphonate (*MDP*) skeletal scintigraphy (*upper row*) and ^{123}I-metaiodobenzylguanidine (*MIBG*) scintigraphy (*lower row*) show abnormal accumulation of both tracers in a right paraspinal neuroblastoma in a 25-month-old boy. Metastatic involvement of the calvarium, facial bones, ribs, spine, and extremities is shown by both studies.

prognostic significance (33) or correlate with the demonstration of calcification by radiography or CT (32).

In cases that present with disseminated disease or with a paraneoplastic syndrome, identification of the primary site is sometimes challenging. Scintigraphy with MIBG can facilitate this process. The sensitivity of MIBG imaging for demonstrating a primary site of neuroblastoma has been reported to approach or exceed 90% (15,24,35–41) (Figs. 7.1, 7.3, 7.4). Absence of the mechanism by which MIBG is transported into neuroblastoma cells and small tumor size account for the absence of demonstrable MIBG uptake in some neuroblastomas (42). MIBG scintigraphy can also be of value in planning surgery for patients with suspected neuroblastoma and a known mass. In the appropriate clinical setting, uptake of MIBG into a mass virtually establishes a diagnosis of neuroblastoma. The possibility of an MIBG-avid pheochromocytoma being mistaken for a neuroblastoma should not pose a significant problem because pheochromocytomas are extremely rare in childhood (particularly in the age group affected by neuroblastoma) and are typically manifested by characteristic clinical symptoms. Reports of MIBG uptake into non-neural crest tumors in children are rare (43). Importantly, although localization of MIBG has been reported in Wilms' tumor (44), which may be difficult to differentiate from neuroblastoma by CT,

magnetic resonance imaging (MRI), or ultrasonography, none of 14 Wilms' tumors included in one series accumulated MIBG (43).

The staging of neuroblastoma involves determining the extent of local disease and identifying metastatic disease. Anatomic delineation of the extent of local disease is achieved with MRI or CT. Scintigraphy has proved essential for the detection of skeletal metastases. For this purpose, skeletal scintigraphy has been traditionally used, but MIBG scintigraphy has gained favor in recent years.

Metastases to cortical bone usually appear lytic radiographically, but some appear partially or completely sclerotic. Cortical bone metastases are typically multiple and most commonly involve the long bones, spine, pelvis, ribs, calvarium, and periorbital facial bones. Involvement of the long bones is characteristically metaphyseal and occasionally diaphyseal. The distribution of metastases in the long bones is usually asymmetric, but symmetric lesions are frequently encountered. Vertebral involvement may result in vertebral body collapse. Calvarial metastases radiographically appear as permeative osteolysis, often associated with areas of sclerosis or cortical thickening. Vertical osseous striations may extend from the outer table ("hair-on-end" appearance). Sutural diastasis suggests increased intracranial pressure secondary to a dura-based metastasis. Local tumor

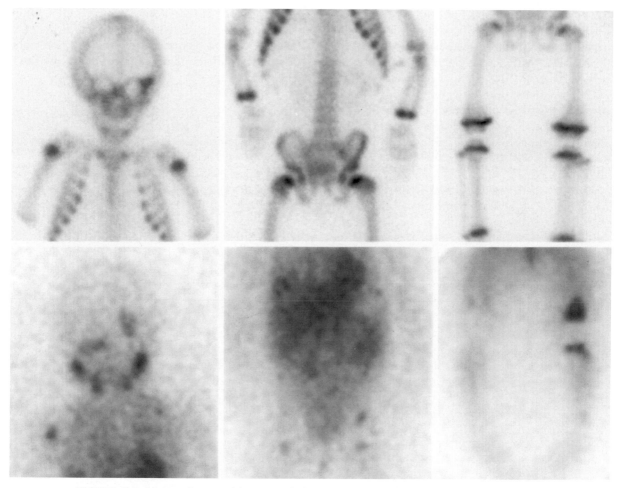

FIGURE 7.4. Metastatic neuroblastoma. Skeletal scintigraphy *(upper row)* shows increased uptake centered on the left superolateral orbital wall. Uptake is asymmetrically higher in the right maxilla, in the region above the left acetabulum, and at the left distal femoral and proximal tibial physes. These findings are relatively subtle. Planar scintigraphy with ^{123}I-metaiodobenzylguanidine *(MIBG)* shows abnormal uptake in the left superolateral orbital wall, right maxilla, right proximal humerus, left shoulder, lower ribs bilaterally, left supraacetabular region, both proximal and distal femoral metaphyses, left proximal tibial metaphysis, and left proximal fibular metaphysis. Localization of ^{99m}Tc-methylene diphosphonate *(MDP)* and MIBG in the left adrenal neuroblastoma of this 14-month-old girl were better shown on posterior images.

extension can produce enlargement of an intervertebral foramen, widening of an interpedicular or intercostal space, and erosive changes (7,8,45,46).

Cortical metastases are detected earlier with skeletal scintigraphy than with radiography. For the detection of cortical metastases, skeletal scintigraphy has been shown to be superior to radiography, in regard to both the number of cases of metastatic disease detected and the number of lesions demonstrated (8,32,34,47). Proper positioning of the child, high-resolution imaging, and familiarity with the normal distribution of skeletal tracer in the growing skeleton are essential. Cortical bone metastases typically appear as areas of high uptake on skeletal scintigraphy (Figs. 7.1, 7.3, 7.4). Decreased uptake is demonstrated in areas of highly aggressive bone destruction or ischemia. Metastases occasionally produce relatively little alteration in skeletal

tracer uptake (Fig. 7.4). This can be problematic with symmetric metaphyseal lesions. Although because of this limitation some lesions escape detection by skeletal scintigraphy, it is highly unusual for skeletal scintigraphic images to be interpreted as normal in a child with radiographic evidence of cortical bone metastases (32,34,48).

Because uptake of MIBG is not identified in normal bone or bone marrow, MIBG scintigraphy readily demonstrates skeletal metastases (Figs. 7.1, 7.3, 7.4). Definitive differentiation between cortical and marrow metastases is not possible with MIBG scintigraphy, however. Cortical and marrow metastases both appear as areas of abnormal MIBG localization within the skeleton.

On a per patient basis, the overall sensitivities of skeletal scintigraphy and MIBG scintigraphy for detecting skeletal metastatic disease probably do not differ significantly (49).

Either study may reveal metastases of neuroblastoma when the other does not. This reflects the different mechanisms by which these agents localize at metastatic sites. In patients whose skeletal and MIBG scintigrams both demonstrate metastases, however, MIBG scintigraphy frequently provides a better assessment of the extent of disease by revealing more sites of skeletal involvement (50) (Fig. 7.4). A study indicating that the extent of disease shown by MIBG scintigraphy is a strong prognostic indicator for children older than 1 year of age (51) suggests that this feature is of practical importance.

The choice of whether to perform skeletal scintigraphy, MIBG scintigraphy, or both is often based on the impact that results may have on staging with the system used at a given institution, the requirements of the chemotherapy protocol to be used in treatment, and individual preferences. In general, MIBG scintigraphy offers some distinct advantages over skeletal scintigraphy in addition to the ability to indicate extent of disease more accurately. First, MIBG does not localize at sites of bone repair associated with healing metastases, bone marrow biopsy and harvest sites, or other trauma (50,52,53). Skeletal tracers do. This eliminates a potential source of uncertainty in some cases and renders MIBG scintigraphy more useful than skeletal scintigraphy for evaluating therapeutic response. Second, accurate detection of skeletal metastases seems to be less dependent on interpretative experience with MIBG scintigraphy than with skeletal scintigraphy (32). Third, MIBG scintigraphy is also useful to show nonskeletal metastases, with the exception of hepatic metastases (54). Uptake of skeletal tracers in nonskeletal metastases of neuroblastoma is not common (55, 56). The main disadvantage of MIBG is its high cost. Although an inability to distinguish cortical from marrow metastases with MIBG is often cited as a limitation, the prognostic implication may be the same for marrow infiltration that is sufficiently extensive to be detected with MIBG scintigraphy as it is for cortical metastases (10).

Following therapy, serial evaluation with laboratory measurements and imaging studies is required for early identification of children whose treatment has failed or whose remission is not sustained. MIBG scintigraphy is an effective means of whole-body surveillance. Identification of an abnormal site of MIBG uptake is strong evidence of viable neuroblastoma, although some ganglioneuromas accumulate MIBG (15,57). The meaning of a negative study result is less certain. In one study, some thoracic and abdominal lesions that were identified by CT and subsequently shown to represent viable deposits of neuroblastoma were not revealed by ^{131}I-MIBG scintigraphy. These lesions were predominantly 2.0 to 4.0 cm in diameter (53). ^{123}I-MIBG scintigraphy with SPECT improves the detectability of uptake in lesions of this size but is unlikely to completely eliminate this potential pitfall.

Although experience is limited, radioguided surgery with use of a gamma probe to detect emissions from radiolabeled MIBG localized at sites of disease appears to be helpful in defining tumor limits and identifying nodes for resection (58,59). Whether better macroscopic resection improves survival in children with disseminated disease remains to be determined.

Imaging of Neuroblastoma with Other Tracers

Other radiotracers have also been used or are being studied in patients with neuroblastoma.

More than 80% of neuroblastomas have been reported to accumulate pentetreotide labeled with indium 111 (^{111}In) (60). This reflects the presence of somatostatin type 2 receptors on some neuroblastoma cells (61). Experience is more limited with this radiopharmaceutical than with MIBG. Because ^{111}In-pentetreotide localizes in a number of non-neuroendocrine and neuroendocrine tumors and at sites of inflammation, it is less specific than MIBG for neuroblastoma. Reports suggest that ^{111}In-pentetreotide scintigraphy is also less sensitive than ^{131}I-MIBG for detecting neuroblastoma (62–65). Nevertheless, some tumors that accumulate ^{111}In-pentetreotide do not accumulate MIBG. Scintigraphy with ^{111}In-pentetreotide may therefore be most useful in assessing patients whose neuroblastomas are not MIBG-avid. Based on a small number of cases, it has been suggested that ^{111}In-pentetreotide uptake is greater in well-differentiated and aneuploid tumors (62), so that this tracer might be of some value in prognostic stratification (60,62,66). By identifying neuroblastomas with high-affinity somatostatin receptors, ^{111}In-pentetreotide scintigraphy might indicate tumors that would benefit from targeted therapy with synthetic somatostatin analogues.

Gallium 67 (^{67}Ga) citrate localizes in a high percentage of primary neuroblastomas, but its nonspecificity and reportedly poor sensitivity for skeletal metastases limit its use (67). Although an early report indicated bone marrow scintigraphy with technetium (99mTc) sulfur colloid to be an effective means of identifying marrow disease (68), this technique has failed to gain widespread favor. Thallium 201 (69) and [99m]Tc-*hexakis*-2-methoxyisobutylisonitrile (MIBI) (70) localize poorly or not at all in neuroblastomas. Radiolabeled monoclonal antibodies are being studied as imaging and radioimmunotherapy agents (71–75).

Because neuroblastomas are usually metabolically active tumors that avidly concentrate fluorodeoxyglucose (FDG) tagged with fluorine 18, FDG positron emission tomography (PET) has been evaluated as a potential alternative to MIBG scintigraphy in detecting neuroblastoma (57). Although the ability to complete FDG-PET within 1 to 2 hours after tracer administration is a definite advantage over MIBG scintigraphy, one study indicates that MIBG scintigraphy is superior in terms of lesion visibility and the ability to provide whole-body evaluation (57). The utility of FDG-PET may be greatest for patients whose primary tumor does not concentrate MIBG. An important consideration regarding the potential application of FDG-PET in neuroblastoma is the accumulation of FDG by normal bone marrow constituents. The limitation that this places on FDG-PET for assessing skeletal disease is accentuated following chemotherapy. A high rate of uptake of FDG by bone marrow following chemotherapy, which is especially common when colony-stimulating factors have been used as an adjunct (76,77), may be mistakenly interpreted as indicating the presence of disseminated metastatic disease.

Osteosarcoma

Clinical Considerations

Osteosarcoma is the most common primary bone malignancy of childhood. This tumor usually originates within the medullary space. Histologically, the diagnosis of osteosarcoma requires the demonstration of neoplastic osteoid and osseous tissue (78). Chondroid or fibrous tissue is frequently present. Osteosarcoma is classified as osteoblastic, chondroblastic, or fibroblastic, or as of mixed cellularity, based on the relative distribution of tissue types; when large cystic spaces are present that contain blood, scant osteoid, and massive cellular necrosis, it is classified as telangiectatic.

The etiology of osteosarcoma is unknown. In a minority of cases, osteosarcoma develops as a late complication of radiation therapy or chemotherapy (Fig. 7.5). A predisposition to osteosarcoma is present in children with the hereditary type of retinoblastoma. Very rarely, osteosarcoma develops in benign lesions, including fibrous dysplasia, infarction, chronic osteomyelitis, osteoblastoma, and aneurysmal bone cyst (79–81).

The incidence of osteosarcoma is highest between the ages of 12 and 25 years. The tumor rarely affects children younger than 6 years of age (2). Patients typically present with localized pain or swelling, or both. Pathologic fracture, which occurs in approximately 5% of patients, disturbs normal barriers to tumor spread and worsens the prognosis (45,82).

Osteosarcoma is predominantly a lesion of the long bones, where it is typically metaphyseal in location. The distal femur (Fig. 7.6), proximal tibia, and proximal humerus (Fig. 7.7) are most commonly affected (83,84). Because osteosarcoma is related to the production of bone, it is not surprising that it primarily occurs in these, the regions of fastest skeletal growth. Flat bones, particularly the ilium and mandible, are involved in 10% of cases (45).

The most common location of osteosarcoma metastases are lung and bone. Pulmonary metastases usually precede skeletal metastases. Skeletal metastases involve sites remote from the primary tumor or the same bone in which the primary tumor is located. The latter are often referred to as "skip" metastases. In a small percentage of patients, multiple skeletal lesions are detected at the time of diagnosis. This presentation is referred to as *osteosarcomatosis* (Fig. 7.8). The lesions most commonly involve the metaphyses of the long bones, pelvis, vertebrae, and ribs and are associated with a single radiographically dominant lesion in more than 90% of cases. Although some believe that osteosarcomatosis represents multiple primary lesions, it is more likely that osteosarcomatosis represents the skeletal metastases of a single primary lesion (85).

The treatment of choice for osteosarcoma is wide resection and limb-sparing surgery. Limb-sparing procedures entail the resection of tumor with a cuff of surrounding normal tissue at all margins, skeletal reconstruction, and muscle and soft-tissue transfers. Skeletal reconstruction is accomplished with a cadaveric allograft, bone prosthesis, or both (82). When current chemotherapeutic regimens are

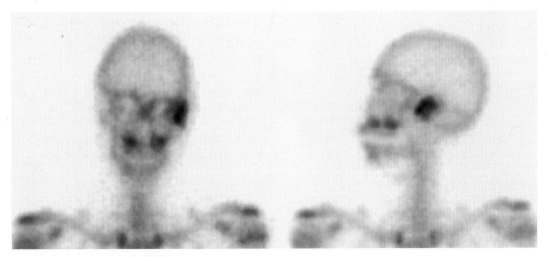

FIGURE 7.5. Osteosarcoma. Skeletal scintigraphy shows markedly increased uptake in a left temporal osteosarcoma. The 15-year-old boy whose images are depicted had been treated with chemotherapy and radiation therapy for choroid plexus carcinoma at 2 years of age.

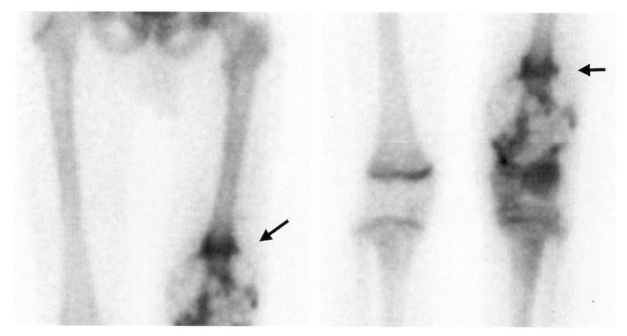

FIGURE 7.6. Osteosarcoma. Skeletal scintigraphy of a 14-year-old boy shows areas of high and low uptake in a left distal femoral osteosarcoma. Uptake abnormalities extend into the soft tissues, where a large mass is present. The linear diaphyseal area of increased uptake extending across the diaphysis (*arrow*) represents pathologic fracture. Uptake throughout the left femur and in the left tibia and fibula is higher than uptake contralaterally. In this patient, the extended pattern was attributable to hyperemia.

used preoperatively and postoperatively and imaging is performed preoperatively to define tumor extent and tumor viability, limb-sparing procedures can be appropriately carried out in 80% of patients with osteosarcoma (86).

The 10-year survival rate of osteosarcoma patients treated with current methods exceeds 70% (87). Death is frequently caused by pulmonary metastases. Survival rates are highest in patients without metastatic disease at presentation whose tumor is more than 90% to 95% necrotic before resection (87–89).

Imaging of Osteosarcoma

Osteosarcoma is usually revealed with radiographs (45,46, 84). Findings include bone destruction, sclerosis, periosteal reaction, and in some cases a contiguous soft-tissue mass that may contain areas of neoplastic bone. Further imaging is required at diagnosis to define the extent of the primary tumor. Following treatment, imaging is employed to evaluate the response to preoperative chemotherapy and to detect the development of local recurrence or complications of therapy. At diagnosis and during follow-up, imaging plays a central role in detecting metastatic disease. Scintigraphic techniques are useful in variable degrees for each of these purposes.

Osteosarcomas typically demonstrate marked tracer uptake on skeletal scintigraphy. Regions of decreased tracer

uptake within viable nonossified tumor and necrotic tumor are also frequently present (Fig. 7.6). Skeletal tracers often localize in the soft-tissue component of the tumor. Increased tracer uptake often extends beyond the pathologic confines of the tumor (90–92) (Fig. 7.6). The intensity varies from faint to marked. This extended pattern of high uptake typically involves bone in immediate continuity with, or immediately across the joint adjacent to, the tumor. Less often, it affects the entire ipsilateral extremity. Marrow hyperemia, medullary reactive bone, and periosteal new bone have been demonstrated in some cases exhibiting

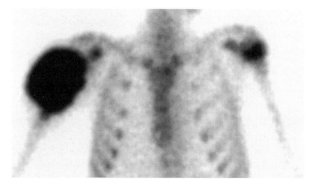

FIGURE 7.7. Osteosarcoma. Markedly increased uptake is shown in a right proximal humeral osteosarcoma of a 10-year-old girl.

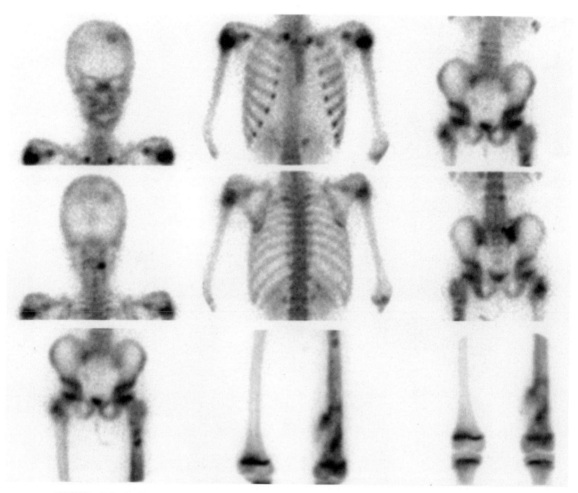

FIGURE 7.8. Osteosarcomatosis. Skeletal scintigraphy of a 7-year-old with a left femoral osteosarcoma demonstrates the primary tumor and metastatic sites in the left proximal tibial metaphysis, right intertrochanteric femur, right distal femoral and proximal tibial metaphyses, left ischium, sacrum, L-4, C-2, left third rib posteriorly, and calvarium. Shown are anterior and posterior projections of the head, chest, abdomen, and pelvis and anterior projections of the lower extremities. (Reprinted from Connolly LP, Treves ST. *Pediatric skeletal scintigraphy with multimodality imaging correlation.* New York: Springer-Verlag, 1998, p. 221, with permission.)

this pattern (90). The occurrence of an extended pattern of high uptake limits the ability of skeletal scintigraphy to define the margins of an osteosarcoma. Margin definition is better achieved with MRI, although MRI can overestimate tumoral extent because signal abnormalities result from peritumoral edema (93,94).

An important role of nuclear medicine in osteosarcoma is detection of osseous metastases at diagnosis and during follow-up (Figs. 7.8, 7.9). Skeletal metastases typically appear as areas of increased tracer uptake. They are often radiographically occult and/or asymptomatic at the time of scintigraphic detection (95,96).

Pulmonary metastases are best detected with CT, but because of osteoid production by the metastatic deposits, they are occasionally demonstrated with skeletal scintigraphy (96–99). Other extraosseous metastases, including nodal, renal, adrenal, hepatic, and cerebral, have been iden-

tified with skeletal scintigraphy but are also better detected with other modalities (Fig. 7.9).

Because the degree of histologic necrosis following chemotherapy is a strong predictor of long-term survival for patients with nonmetastatic osteosarcoma (87,89), much attention has been directed toward development of a noninvasive method to assess the histologic response to chemotherapy. Prolonged ineffective chemotherapy and a resultant delay in surgical treatment can be avoided by identification of treatment failures. Identification of a favorable response facilitates the performance of limb salvage surgery. Skeletal scintigraphy has not proved to be an effective method of predicting the histologic response (100,101). Imaging with ^{67}Ga citrate is slightly more reliable than skeletal scintigraphy, but results are frequently inaccurate (100–102). Structural imaging modalities have also not been highly successful in this regard. Although increased tumor volume (103,104) and increased

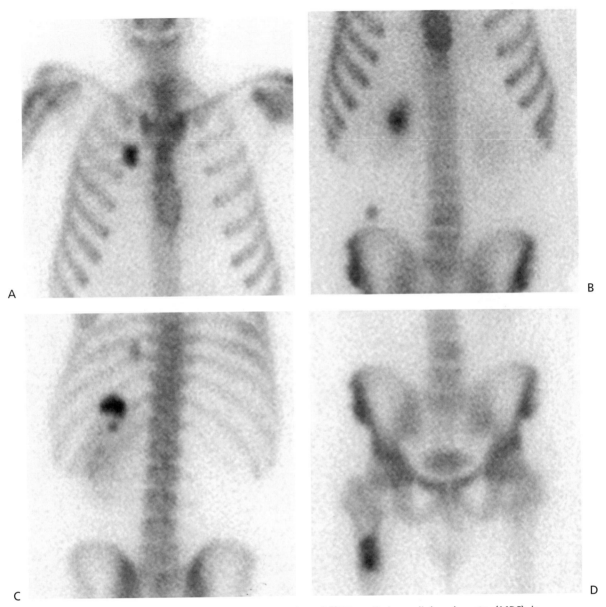

FIGURE 7.9. Metastatic osteosarcoma. Uptake of ^{99m}Tc-methylene diphosphonate (*MDP*) is shown in a right pulmonary nodule 7 years after resection of a right humeral osteosarcoma with allograft reconstruction (**A**, anterior projection). Uptake along the allograft represents known allograft fracture. Ten months after resection of the pulmonary nodule, ^{99m}Tc-MDP is shown localizing in right renal and right lower quadrant omental metastases (**B**, anterior projection). Nine months after resection of the omental metastasis and right nephrectomy, ^{99m}Tc-MDP localizes in left pulmonary, left adrenal, left renal, and right femoral metastases (**C**, posterior projection; **D**, anterior projection).

or unchanged peritumoral edema (103) shown by MRI independently indicate a poor response, MRI is not highly reliable for confirming successful treatment. This partly reflects the nonspecific appearance of viable tumor on MRI (100, 103,104). Enhancement following gadolinium is a sensitive but nonspecific indicator of residual viable tumor because granulation tissue and edema may also be enhanced.

The uptake of certain radiopharmaceuticals reflects tumor viability, and these have been utilized in predicting the therapeutic response of osteosarcoma. The ability to provide semiquantitative analysis with nuclear medicine techniques is particularly appealing in this regard. Osteosarcomas usually show intense uptake of ^{201}Tl before treatment (Figs. 7.10, 7.11). Tumor cell death resulting from chemotherapy leads to a decrease in tumoral ^{201}Tl uptake. This phenomenon has been assessed visually with use of a subjective grading system: 0, no tumor uptake; 1, tumor uptake equivocally higher than uptake in background; 2,

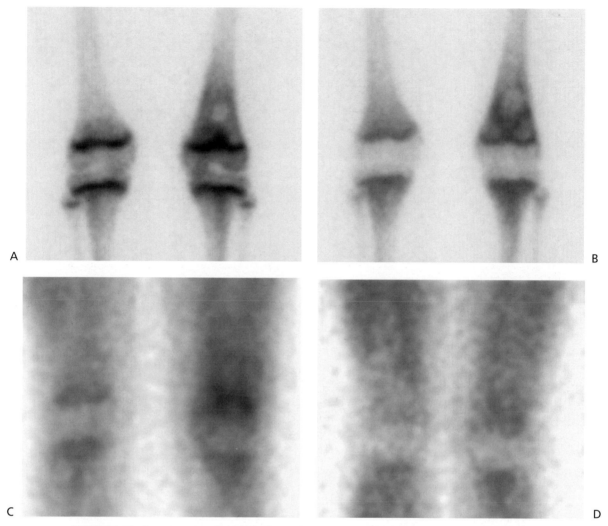

FIGURE 7.10. Osteosarcoma: favorable chemotherapeutic response. Skeletal scintigraphy at diagnosis (**A**) shows abnormal increased uptake with an associated ovoid area of lower uptake affecting the left distal femoral metadiaphysis of a 14-year-old boy. Following chemotherapy, the uptake abnormality persists (**B**), and a zone of high uptake is present along the inferior aspect of the ovoid area of lower uptake. Tumor ^{201}Tl uptake at diagnosis was high (**C**). Following chemotherapy, tumor ^{201}Tl uptake was only slightly above background levels (**D**). Histopathologic analysis showed more than 90% necrosis.

tumor uptake definitely higher than uptake in background but lower than cardiac uptake; 2, tumor uptake equal to cardiac uptake; 3, tumor uptake greater than cardiac uptake (101). Methods of semiquantitative analysis comparing tumor with background (usually contralateral) uptake, ratio of tumor-to-background uptake before and after therapy, and percentage change in the ratio have been described (105–110). Although these methods have tended to be somewhat institution-specific, taken as a whole they show value for ^{201}Tl imaging. Osteosarcomas in which ^{201}Tl uptake decreases to background levels following chemotherapy typically demonstrate more than 90% tumor necrosis and often 100% tumor necrosis on histologic examination (Fig. 7.10). Conversely, tumors in which ^{201}Tl uptake fol-

lowing chemotherapy is equal to or greater than that shown before chemotherapy typically exhibit little or no histologic evidence of response (Fig. 7.11). Histologic evaluation of tumors in which the degree of ^{201}Tl uptake decreases but remains higher than background generally reveals a partial response, with some areas of viable tumor remaining.

In addition to ^{201}Tl, other nonspecific tumor-depicting tracers may also be applicable in assessing therapeutic response in osteosarcoma. ^{99m}Tc-MIBI localizes in osteosarcoma (109,110). One series has shown a correlation between percentage reduction in tumor ^{99m}Tc-MIBI uptake following chemotherapy and histologic evidence of necrosis (111). ^{99m}Tc-MIBI studies of tumors must be interpreted in light of the multidrug resistance phenomenon that develops

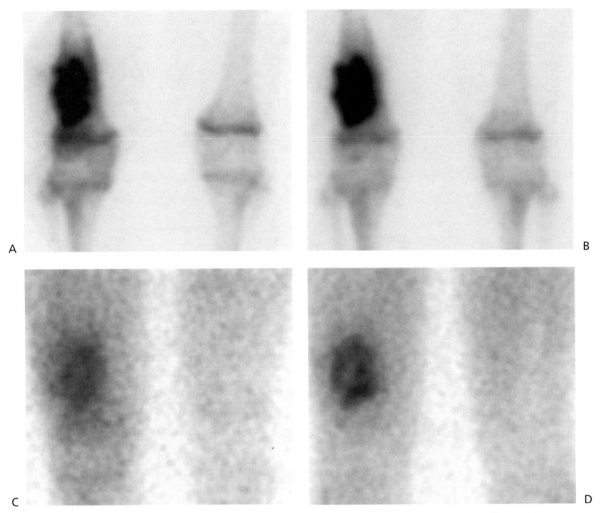

FIGURE 7.11. Osteosarcoma: poor chemotherapeutic response. Skeletal scintigrams at diagnosis (**A**) and following chemotherapy (**B**) show intense uptake in a distal right femoral osteosarcoma of a 15-year-old boy. Scintigraphy with ^{201}Tl shows that the high ^{201}Tl uptake in the tumor at diagnosis (**C**) persisted following chemotherapy (**D**). Histopathologic analysis showed less than 50% necrosis.

after the use of certain chemotherapeutic agents. One mechanism by which this resistance develops is through P-glycoprotein (Pgp). This membrane glycoprotein transports lipophilic compounds, including ^{99m}Tc-MIBI and various chemotherapeutic agents, out of cells (112,113). It has yet to be established whether ^{99m}Tc-MIBI is either a suitable substitute for ^{201}Tl in assessing tumor response or a reliable means of assessing the functional status of the Pgp transport system. A role for FDG-PET in osteosarcoma also has not been established, but it has been suggested that FDG-PET will eventually be important in the assessment of therapeutic response (114).

Because skeletal scintigraphy is employed for the detection of skeletal metastases during follow-up of children with osteosarcoma, imaging specialists must be aware of the normal scintigraphic appearance of allografts and amputation stumps, scintigraphic abnormalities not related to metasta-

tic disease, and the occurrence of the "flare phenomenon" in osseous metastatic deposits.

Transplantation of a cadaveric bone allograft is frequently performed as part of a limb-sparing procedure. Osteoarticular allografts include the epiphysis and articulating surfaces (Fig. 7.12). Intercalary allografts are used to reestablish a segment of the diaphysis of a long bone exclusive of the epiphysis and articulating surfaces (Fig. 7.13). Allografts are incorporated into the skeleton by a process referred to as *creeping substitution*. Host capillaries initially invade the allograft. Host osteocytes then deposit new bone on the allograft matrix and resorb the allogeneic bone. Remodeling takes place in response to mechanical strains (115,116). A study on retrieved cadaveric bone allografts shows that this process is limited to the allograft ends and superficial layers and involves no more than 20% of the allogeneic bone by 5 years (117).

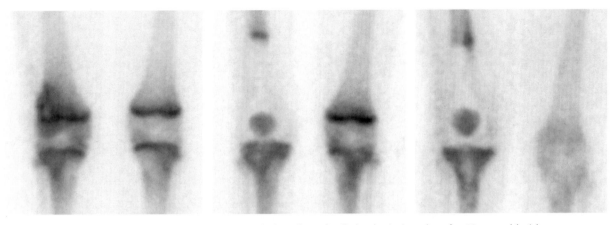

A,B   C

FIGURE 7.12. Osteosarcoma, osteoarticular allograft. Skeletal scintigraphy of a 12-year-old girl shows increased uptake in a right distal femoral osteosarcoma (**A**). Eight months following resection and osteoarticular allograft, increased uptake is present in the native femur at the osteotomy site, in the native patella, and in the tibial surfaces articulating with the allograft. The allograft itself shows only minimal uptake along its periphery (**B**). Three years later, the distribution of uptake at the osteotomy site, in the native patella, and in the tibia have changed, reflecting mechanical stresses. The allograft continues to show only minimal uptake along its periphery (**C**).

Allografts have a characteristic scintigraphic appearance that reflects this incorporation process (118,119) (Figs. 7.12, 7.13). Increased tracer uptake is typically seen at the junction between host and allograft bone, where host bone unites with the allograft by callus formation, and at sites of plate and screw fixation. The allograft itself is visualized as an area of decreased tracer uptake, with its periphery outlined by a rim of tracer uptake that is slightly greater than that in adjacent soft tissues. The rim likely corresponds to a thin seam of new bone that develops on allograft surfaces (117) and has been described as imparting a "tramline" appearance on anterior or posterior planar projections (119). With long-term follow-up, more diffuse uptake may be observed (120). Increased tracer uptake is noted in joint surfaces articulating with osteoarticular allografts. This results from stress-induced changes in host joints secondary to degeneration of allograft cartilage (117).

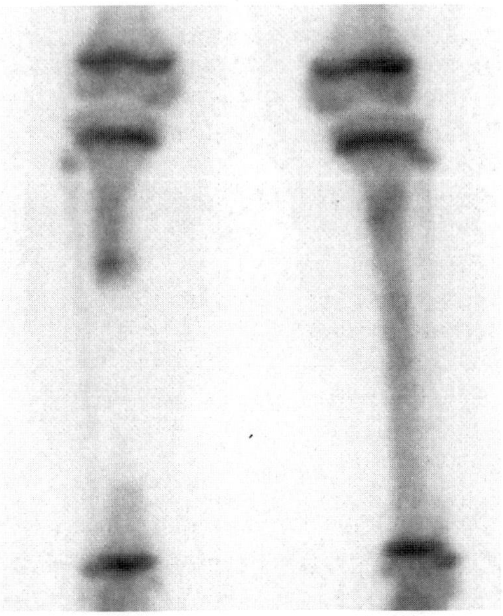

Deviation from the typical scintigraphic pattern associated with allografts suggests complication (Figs. 7.9, 7.14). The most common complication is allograft fracture (120). Most allograft fractures occur 2 or more years postoperatively and are caused by mechanical stresses. Fracture may also result from rejection, in which case it typically occurs within 18 months of surgery and is associated with allograft dissolution (121). Most allograft infections occur in the first months postoperatively, but some develop later (122,123). Local recurrence usually develops in host bone or adjacent soft tissue but may extend to involve the allograft (119).

Following amputation and the fitting of a prosthesis, increased tracer uptake is usually seen at the tip of the bone that has been amputated (124).

Skeletal scintigraphy typically reveals evidence of bone stress after allograft reconstruction or amputation of a lower extremity (Fig. 7.15). Typical locations of skeletal stress are the lower extremity contralateral to an allograft or amputation, the lower extremity ipsilateral to an allograft, and the pelvis. Stress-related abnormalities also occur in the upper extremities of patients ambulating with the assistance of crutches. On a single study, the distinction between skeletal stress and metastatic disease can be difficult. In general, stress changes tend to appear as more diffuse areas of abnormal uptake than do metastases. When focal, stress abnormalities

FIGURE 7.13. Intercalary allograft. Increased uptake is present in the native tibia at the site of fixation hardware just proximal to the junction between allograft and native right tibia. The allograft appears as an area of low to absent uptake extending to its junction with the native distal tibial diaphysis.

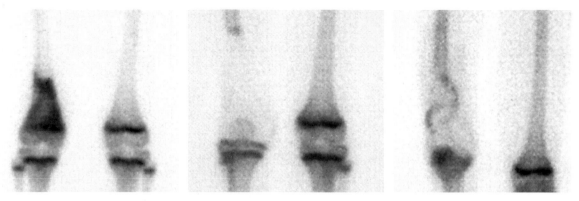

FIGURE 7.14. Osteosarcoma: allograft and fracture. Skeletal scintigraphy of a 10-year-old girl shows markedly increased uptake in a right distal femoral osteosarcoma (**A**). Twenty-one months following resection and osteoarticular allograft, increased uptake is present along the tibial articulating surfaces and at the junction between the allograft and native femur (**B**). The allograft shows only minimal uptake along the periphery of the femoral condyles. The rounded area projecting over the allograft distally is the native patella. Skeletal scintigraphy performed 5 months later shows curvilinear areas of increased uptake related to the allograft (**C**). The leg is held in a foreshortened position because of a fracture that had been detected radiographically. The fractured allograft was surgically removed and replaced with a prosthesis.

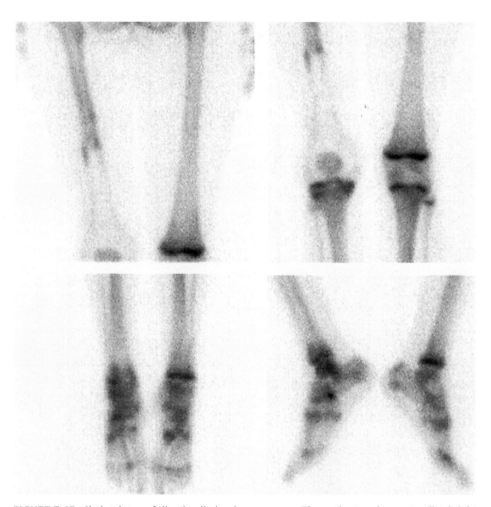

FIGURE 7.15. Skeletal stress following limb salvage surgery. The patient underwent a distal right femoral osteoarticular allograft for osteosarcoma. The allograft appears as a photon-deficient area outlined by a faint rim of tracer localization. Immediately related to the allograft, increased uptake is seen corresponding to callus at the allograft–host junction, along the right femur related to fixation hardware, in the right patella, and in the right tibial articulating surfaces. Increased uptake in the right medial and lateral malleoli, right talus and cuboid, right second metatarsal, and first tarsometatarsal joints bilaterally suggests skeletal stress. (Reprinted from Connolly LP, Treves ST. *Pediatric skeletal scintigraphy with multimodality imaging correlation.* New York: Springer-Verlag, 1998, p. 239, with permission.)

tend to show less intense uptake than do metastases. Focal abnormalities in the skull or spine are likely to be of metastatic origin (124). A high level of suspicion for metastatic disease must be maintained, and further imaging with radiography, CT, or MRI is frequently required. Some uncertainties are resolved only with clinical and imaging follow-up. Skeletal stress changes often show variability on sequential studies, reflecting changes in weight-bearing patterns and levels of physical activity.

Chemotherapeutic regimens for osteosarcoma frequently include methotrexate. Use of this folic acid analogue, which impedes purine synthesis and DNA biosynthesis, is associated with skeletal abnormalities in some children. The typical radiographic findings of methotrexate osteopathy resemble those seen in scurvy: severe osteopenia, dense zones of provisional calcification, transverse metaphyseal bands, and metaphyseal fractures. The mechanism of skeletal injury is postulated to result from osteoblast suppression and osteoclast recruitment (125). Initially described in children receiving low-dose, long-term, oral maintenance methotrexate for acute leukemia (122,126–128), this complication also develops in some children with osteosarcoma who undergo high-dose, short-term, intravenous methotrexate therapy (129). Methotrexate osteopathy should be considered as a possible cause of metaphyseal abnormalities seen on skeletal scintigrams of children receiving, or who have recently received, this agent. Correlation with radiographs permits the diagnosis to be reached and methotrexate to be discontinued. This is important, as rapid improvement is seen after discontinuation of the drug (122,126). Non-union and angulation may occur at fracture sites despite adequate immobilization when methotrexate therapy is continued (122). Compression fractures of the spine and a sacral insufficiency fracture have also been noted secondary to methotrexate osteopathy (129).

Osteosarcoma metastases may demonstrate the scintigraphic flare phenomenon during therapy (123). This pattern is characterized by increasing intensity of tracer uptake at sites of known metastases or the appearance of new foci of increased tracer uptake on a study obtained within months of a therapeutic intervention, despite a patient's apparent clinical improvement (130). It is likely a consequence of bone repair. The flare phenomenon should be considered when the appropriate findings are observed, especially within 2 months of the onset of therapy, in patients who appear to be responding well clinically. Excluding disease progression remains the primary concern, particularly when new abnormalities are detected. Close correlation with clinical and other imaging parameters is, therefore, essential. Unfortunately, a patient's subsequent clinical course and imaging findings are the only reliable arbiters in some cases. Skeletal scintigraphy typically shows regression of a flare phenomenon during 4 to 6 months (130).

Ewing's Sarcoma

Clinical Considerations

Ewing's sarcoma is the second most common primary bone malignancy of childhood. Ewing's sarcoma has several different genotypes that share a common neuroectodermal origin and, with primitive neuroectodermal tumor, constitute what is considered to be the Ewing's sarcoma family of tumors (131).

Ewing's sarcoma is composed of small round cells. The absence of lobular rosettes, neuron-specific enolase, and neurosecretory granules helps differentiate Ewing's sarcoma from primitive neuroectodermal tumor (132). In some cases, it can be difficult to distinguish the histologic features of Ewing's sarcoma from those of other small round cell tumors of childhood, such as neuroblastoma, leukemia, and lymphoma (133,134).

The incidence of Ewing's sarcoma is highest in the second decade of life. Almost all cases occur between the ages of 5 and 30 years. Whites are predominantly affected (45, 46,79,83,84).

Pain and swelling are the most common symptoms at presentation. A palpable mass is often present. The patient may be febrile. Hematologic analysis reveals elevation of the erythrocyte sedimentation rate, leukocytosis, and anemia in some cases. The constellation of clinical and hematologic findings occasionally suggests a diagnosis of osteomyelitis.

Through the age of 20 years, Ewing's sarcoma most often affects the appendicular skeleton, particularly the femur, tibia, and humerus. Ewing's sarcoma of the long bones is centered in the metaphysis slightly more often than in the diaphysis (Fig. 7.16). Metaphyseal lesions are typically eccentrically positioned and tend to extend into the diaphysis. Pelvic, rib, and vertebral lesions predominate in patients older than 20 years of age but also occur at younger ages (45,135). A soft-tissue mass is frequently present with Ewing's sarcoma. The mass is often large. In some cases, the tumor is predominantly within the soft tissues. Skeletal metastases usually precede pulmonary metastases and are present in 10% to 20% of patients at diagnosis (46).

The reported 5-year survival rate of patients with Ewing's sarcoma ranges from 54% to 74% and is less than 30% in patients with metastatic disease (133,136). Therapy for Ewing's sarcoma entails the use of chemotherapy with multiple agents to eradicate microscopic or overt metastatic disease and the use of irradiation, surgery, or both for control of the primary lesion. Because late recurrence is not uncommon, resection of the primary tumor is gaining favor for local disease control (136). The limb-sparing surgeries described for osteosarcoma are also used in managing Ewing's sarcoma of the long bones.

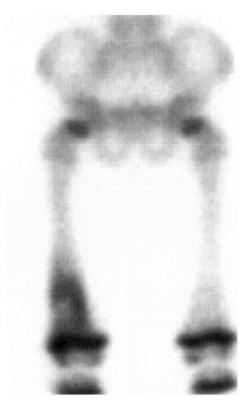

FIGURE 7.16. Ewing's sarcoma. Increased uptake with an associated area of lower uptake is present in a right distal femoral metadiaphyseal Ewing's sarcoma of a 3-year-old girl.

Imaging of Ewing's Sarcoma

Ewing's sarcoma is usually revealed with radiographs. The radiographic manifestations are variable. Permeative osteolysis and a laminated or spiculated periosteal reaction are relatively common findings. A large soft-tissue mass may be identified (45,46,84).

When a tumor escapes radiographic detection because of referral of pain or the presence of only subtle radiographic manifestations, the lesion may be first detected by skeletal scintigraphy (Fig. 7.17). Marked skeletal tracer uptake is typically present in the affected bone, but aggressive lesions may appear as areas of predominantly or entirely decreased uptake (137). An extended pattern occurs in some cases (84). Skeletal tracer uptake in the soft-tissue component of a Ewing's sarcoma is unusual but is occasionally observed (Fig. 7.18).

In patients with Ewing's sarcoma, skeletal scintigraphy is most valuable for identifying skeletal metastases, which typically appear as focal areas of increased uptake (Fig. 7.19). CT is used for detection of pulmonary metastases.

In tumors treated with radiation therapy, marked diminution in skeletal tracer uptake is often seen within 4

months (138) (Fig. 7.17). Persistent or new areas of increased uptake elicit concern for recurrence, fracture, or infection but are nonspecific. A flare response may occur in skeletal metastases during chemotherapy. Skeletal tracer localization in the soft-tissue component of Ewing's sarcoma has been reported as a manifestation of the flare phenomenon (139) but can also be seen with recurrent or residual disease. The postoperative appearance of allografts is the same as has been described for osteosarcoma.

As with osteosarcoma, neither skeletal scintigraphy nor ^{67}Ga citrate imaging has proved consistently accurate in defining tumor extent or therapeutic response in Ewing's sarcoma (101,102,140). The published experience on ^{201}Tl imaging of Ewing's sarcoma is too limited to allow strong conclusions to be drawn concerning its value in assessing therapeutic response. Small series have shown a correlation between tumor regression and reduced ^{201}Tl uptake on serial studies (101,141). Ewing's sarcoma tends to show less avidity for ^{201}Tl than does osteosarcoma. The uptake of ^{99m}Tc-MIBI in Ewing's sarcoma is too variable (142,143) for ^{99m}Tc-MIBI scintigraphy to be useful in assessing therapeutic response in this malignancy. ^{99m}Tc-MIBI imaging may be useful in cases in which a high uptake is shown at diagnosis, however. ^{201}Tl and ^{99m}Tc-MIBI imaging of Ewing's sarcoma involving the pelvis or spine is better accomplished with SPECT than with planar techniques because of the physiologic localization of these agents in genitourinary and gastrointestinal structures. A role for FDG-PET in evaluating therapeutic response in Ewing's sarcoma has been suggested but not established (114,144).

Central Nervous System Tumors

Clinical Considerations

Taken as a group, tumors of the central nervous system (CNS) are the most common solid tumors of childhood. Tumors of the CNS are categorized as being of neuroepithelial or non-neuroepethelial origin. The majority of pediatric brain tumors arise from neuroepithelial tissue. CNS tumors are further classified histopathologically by cell type and graded for degree of malignancy according to criteria that include mitotic activity, infiltration, and anaplasia (145,146).

From a clinical and imaging perspective, pediatric brain tumors are grouped according to the major anatomic compartment involved. In the posterior fossa, medulloblastoma, cerebellar astrocytoma, ependymoma, and brain stem gliomas are most common. Tumors about the third ventricle include those that arise in the suprasellar area, pineal region, or ventricle. The most common neoplasms about the third ventricle are optic glioma, hypothalamic glioma,

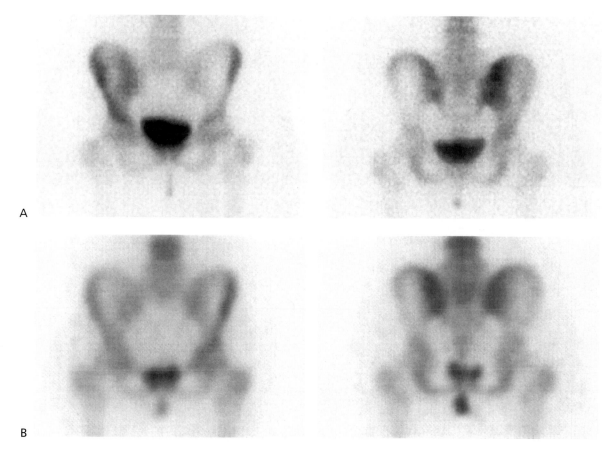

FIGURE 7.17. Ewing's sarcoma. Skeletal scintigraphy (anterior and posterior projections) of a 14-year-old girl experiencing right leg pain shows diffusely increased uptake affecting the right ilium, highest along the sacroiliac (*SI*) joint **(A)**. Following additional imaging and biopsy, Ewing's sarcoma was diagnosed. Skeletal scintigraphy 6 months following chemotherapy and local radiation therapy shows uptake to be asymmetrically lower in the right ilium and along the right SI joint **(B)**. Note also low uptake in L-5, which was within the radiation port.

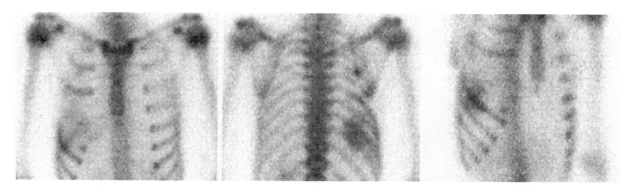

FIGURE 7.18. Ewing's sarcoma. Skeletal scintigraphy of a 14-year-old girl with an 11 x 10 x 14-cm right chest wall mass and rib destruction seen radiographically demonstrates ^{99m}Tc-methylene diphosphonate (*MDP*) localizing within the mass, absence of uptake within portions of the right fourth through sixth ribs, and increased uptake in the right second, third, fifth, and seventh ribs (anterior, posterior, and right anterior oblique projections).

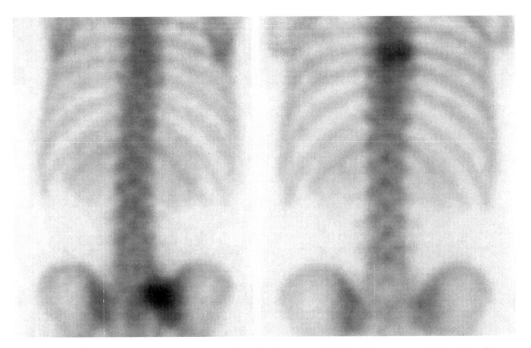

FIGURE 7.19. Ewing's sarcoma. Increased uptake is present in the right sacrum at the site of a Ewing's sarcoma in a 12-year-old boy (**A**, posterior projection). No evidence of metastatic disease was present at this time. The patient received local radiation therapy and chemotherapy. Three years later, skeletal scintigraphy performed as part of an evaluation for back pain shows increased uptake in T-8 (**B**, posterior projection). Biopsy confirmed metastatic involvement.

craniopharyngioma, and germ cell tumor. Supratentorial tumors are most often astrocytomas. Many are considered to be low-grade tumors, but it is often difficult to make this determination (146).

The incidence of pediatric CNS tumors is increased in children with neurofibromatosis and tuberous sclerosis. Children who have received cranial irradiation as part of the treatment for leukemia or other disorders are also at increased risk.

Imaging of Pediatric Brain Tumors

The principle imaging modalities used in staging and following children with CNS tumors are CT and MRI. Their main limitation is an inability to distinguish viable recurrent or residual tumor from abnormalities resulting from surgery or radiation. Enhancement following intravenous administration of contrast reflects disruption of the blood–brain barrier and not necessarily viable tumor. Because ^{201}Tl, ^{99m}Tc-MIBI, and FDG uptake in brain tumors reflects active cellular metabolism in addition to disruption of the blood–brain barrier, imaging with these agents can complement MRI and CT.

Two studies have reported that between 75% and 80% of histologically diverse pediatric brain tumors demonstrate ^{201}Tl uptake (147,148). Residual ^{201}Tl uptake following therapy indicates the presence of viable tumor (Fig.

7.20). The absence of ^{201}Tl uptake following therapy, however, even in tumors that localized ^{201}Tl at diagnosis, is not an absolute indicator of the absence of viable tumor cells. This has led some to conclude that SPECT with ^{201}Tl adds little to the information available with MRI (149). That conclusion ignores the potential importance of early, noninvasive confirmation of residual or recurrent tumor. ^{201}Tl-SPECT is a powerful tool to obtain this confirmation and adds specificity to the findings of MRI or CT. Three-dimensional registration and alignment algorithms enable the fusion of SPECT with MRI or CT (150). SPECT results similar to those obtained with ^{201}Tl have been obtained with ^{99m}Tc-MIBI (148). We prefer ^{201}Tl because of the absence of normal choroid plexus uptake with ^{99m}Tc-MIBI. One caveat in evaluating pediatric brain tumors with ^{201}Tl-SPECT regards the use of semiquantitative techniques. Because of a pediatric preponderance of low-grade tumors, which typically accumulate ^{201}Tl less avidly than do high-grade tumors (151), values to differentiate treatment changes from viable tumor that are derived from an adult population (152) may not be applicable in children.

The use of FDG-PET in brain tumors has been widely reported in series including predominantly adult patients. FDG-PET has proved valuable in distinguishing viable tumor from post-therapeutic changes (153–156). Increased FDG uptake relative to adjacent brain indicates residual or

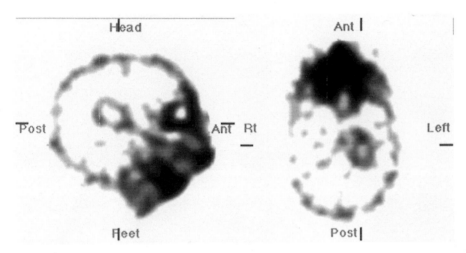

FIGURE 7.20. Thalamic astrocytoma. Single-photon emission computed tomography (*SPECT*) with ^{201}Tl in a 7-year-old girl who had undergone radiation therapy following resection of a left thalamic astrocytoma shows a rim of abnormal ^{201}Tl localization in the left thalamic region. Results of magnetic resonance imaging were indeterminate for viable tumor versus effects of radiation.

recurrent tumor, whereas decreased FDG uptake is observed in areas of necrosis. This distinction is most readily made in high-grade tumors with a high rate of FDG uptake at diagnosis. However, even with high-grade tumors, the presence of microscopic tumor foci is not excluded by an FDG-PET study that does not show an increased uptake. This is particularly true after intensive radiation therapy, when FDG-PET results may not accurately correlate with tumor progression (157).

One study has indicated that collimated (noncoincidence) FDG-SPECT is less sensitive than ^{201}Tl-SPECT to show viable tumor following therapy of pediatric brain tumors (158). Additional studies comparing FDG imaging by coincidence and noncoincidence detection gamma camera techniques, FDG imaging performed with a dedicated PET system, and ^{201}Tl-SPECT are needed to establish the relative sensitivities of these methods.

Both ^{201}Tl-SPECT and FDG-PET have been used for tumor grading and prognostic stratification in adults. High-grade aggressive tumors typically exhibit higher rates of [201]Tl (151) or FDG uptake (159) than do low-grade tumors. In some low-grade tumors, ^{201}Tl or FDG uptake is insufficient for them to be identified. With FDG-PET, some low-grade tumors appear hypometabolic relative to adjacent brain. The development of hypermetabolism, evidenced by increased [201]Tl (160) or FDG (161) uptake in a low-grade tumor, indicates degeneration to a higher grade. The biologic behavior of high-grade tumors may be reflected in their appearance on ^{201}Tl-SPECT or FDG-PET. Shorter survival times have been reported for patients whose tumors show the highest degree of [201]Tl (160) or FDG uptake (162). Some data, although limited, suggest that FDG-PET findings also correlate well with pathology and clinical outcome in children (163–165); for example, an excellent correlation has been reported between FDG-PET findings and clinical outcome in children affected by neurofibromatosis who

have low-grade astrocytomas (153). In that series, a high rate of tumor glucose metabolism shown by FDG-PET was a more accurate predictor of tumor behavior than was histologic analysis.

[11]C-Methionine has also been used to study brain tumors. Uptake of this positron-emitting amino acid reflects transmethylation pathways present in some tumors. ^{11}C-Methionine localizes to only a minimal degree in normal brain, which offers the potential advantage of higher tumor-to-background ratios than can be obtained with FDG. Nevertheless, as with FDG, some low-grade gliomas may escape detection (166,167). PET with ^{11}C-methionine has been reported to be useful in differentiating viable tumor from treatment-induced changes (166,167) and in assessing glioma grade (168).

Other Radionuclide Techniques

The patency of cerebrospinal fluid (CSF) shunts can be assessed by instillation of ^{99m}Tc-pertechnetate into the shunt reservoir. In cases in which CSF loculation or CSF leakage is a postoperative concern, radionuclide cisternography with [99m]Tc- or ^{111}In-diethylenetriamine pentaacetic acid (DTPA) is effective. Radionuclide cisternography is also applicable in difficult cases in which results of MRI to determine whether leptomeningeal metastases have blocked CSF flow are equivocal (169). Radionuclide ventriculography, performed following instillation of tracer into an Ommaya reservoir, has also been used for this purpose (170,171) (Fig. 7.21). Because incomplete distribution of intrathecally administered chemotherapeutic agents is a potential cause of treatment failure and may increase the risk for neurotoxicity, radionuclide ventriculography can provide important information in cases in which CSF dynamics are uncertain following MRI. Radionuclide ventriculography is an alternative to contrast myelography or CT myelography when the question of CSF block arises in any patient with an Ommaya reservoir.

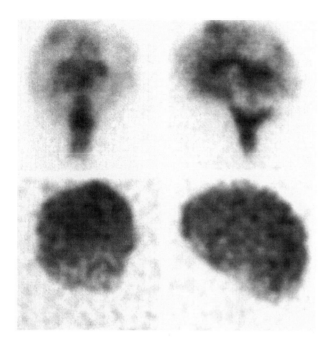

FIGURE 7.21. Block to cerebrospinal fluid (*CSF*) flow secondary to leptomeningeal metastases in a 7-year-old girl with a malignant mixed neuroepithelial parietal neoplasm. Radionuclide ventriculography was performed to assess CSF block after magnetic resonance imaging revealed cord compression at the C-3 to C-7 level. Posterior and lateral images obtained 4 hours following administration of ^{99m}Tc-diethylenetriamine pentaacetic acid (*DTPA*) via an Ommaya reservoir (*upper row*) show that tracer has not descended below the midcervical level. Normally in children, tracer reaches the lumbar level within 90 minutes of intraventricular administration. Posterior and lateral images obtained at 24 hours (*lower row*) show tracer in the cerebral fissures and over the convexities. Imaging over the thoracic and lumbar spine showed no tracer at those levels. On the basis of this study, it was decided to administer additional radiation treatments rather than to proceed with planned intrathecal chemotherapy. (Reprinted from Connolly LP, Dinh L, Treves ST. The detection of CSF block with Tc-99m DTPA cerebral ventriculography. *Clin Nucl Med* 1996; 21:71–72, with permission.)

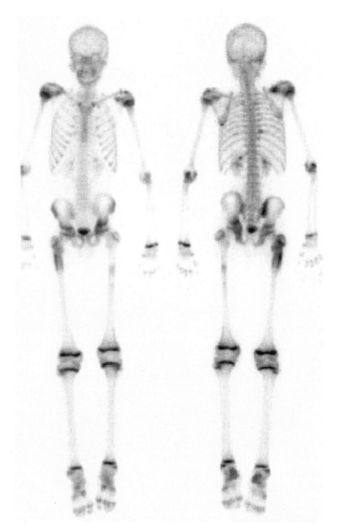

FIGURE 7.22. Metastatic medulloblastoma. Whole-body images of a 16-year-old boy obtained 18 months following posterior fossa medulloblastoma resection show sites of increased uptake in the right scapula, right and left ninth posterior ribs, left 12th rib, right sacrum and ilium along the sacroiliac joint, left acetabulum, and proximal femora. The patient complained only of mild hip pain.

Skeletal scintigraphy plays an important role in evaluating and following children with medulloblastoma, which is the childhood CNS tumor with the greatest likelihood of spreading outside the CNS (7) (Fig. 7.22).

Lymphoma

Clinical Considerations

Hodgkin's and non-Hodgkin's lymphomas account for between 10% and 15% of pediatric malignancies. Non-Hodgkin's lymphoma occurs throughout childhood. Lymphoblastic and small cell tumors, including Burkitt's lymphoma, are the most common histologic types. The disease is usually widespread at diagnosis. Mediastinal and hilar involvement is common with lymphoblastic lymphoma. Burkitt's lymphoma most often occurs in the abdomen.

Hodgkin's lymphoma has a peak incidence during adolescence. It is extremely rare in children less than 5 years of age. Nodular sclerosing and mixed cellularity are the most common histologic types. Unlike lymphomas, the disease is rarely widespread at diagnosis. In the vast majority of cases, however, intrathoracic nodes are involved (2,7).

Imaging of Lymphoma

A multimodality imaging approach is applied in children with lymphoma. Pediatric imaging strategies more often include radionuclide imaging with ^{67}Ga citrate in Hodgkin's lymphoma than in non-Hodgkin's lymphoma. The roles of radionuclide imaging in staging and monitoring

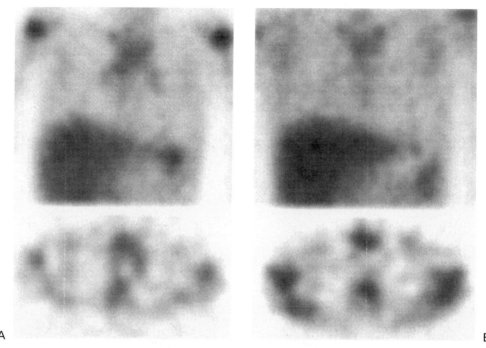

A   B

FIGURE 7.23. Thymic uptake of ^{67}Ga citrate. Planar imaging and single-photon emission computed tomography (*SPECT*) of a 5-year-old boy with Hodgkin's lymphoma show ^{67}Ga-avid tissue in the anterior mediastinum (**A**). The child had no mediastinal disease at diagnosis, had completed chemotherapy 3 weeks previously, and had what was believed to be thymic enlargement on CT. When the child returned 7 months later without having received further treatment, the gallium-avid tissue was no longer present (**B**).

therapeutic response are the same in children as in adults. An important point, however, is that ^{67}Ga citrate often localizes in the thymus of children who have undergone chemotherapy despite an absence of thymic involvement (172–177) (Fig. 7.23). This is generally attributed to "rebound" thymic hyperplasia. It can present a problem when associated thymic enlargement is inconclusively distinguished from residual mediastinal disease by CT, MRI, or plain film radiography. Other radionuclides have been used to assist with this differentiation. Uptake of either ^{201}Tl or ^{99m}Tc-MIBI suggests lymphomatous involvement but does not exclude benign enlargement (102,178–181). Because FDG localizes in the thymus of children, FDG-PET is not helpful in the differential diagnosis (182,183). In rare instances, localization of ^{67}Ga citrate has also been observed in the thymus of ill or recently ill children who have not received chemotherapy (174,184).

Leukemia

Leukemia is the most common malignancy of childhood. Approximately 75% of all cases are acute lymphoid leukemia.

Radionuclide techniques are not routinely used to evaluate or follow children with leukemia. It is not unusual, however, for a child with leukemia to come to clinical attention because of skeletal symptoms (Figs. 7.24, 7.25).

In such cases, skeletal scintigraphy may be the first study to yield abnormal results. As many as 80% of children with leukemia have abnormalities on skeletal scintigraphy at the time of diagnosis. Abnormalities of cortical bone are detected radiographically in more than 40% of cases and are symptomatic in approximately 20% of cases at diagnosis. Radiographic manifestations include osteopenia, transverse metaphyseal bands, periosteal reaction, and focal lytic lesions (185). Scintigraphic abnormalities are most often sites of increased uptake affecting metaphyses or diaphyses of the long bones, the spine, and the flat bones. Regional decreased uptake may occur with an aggressive lesion or may indicate ischemia resulting from packing of leukemic cells in the bone marrow (186) (Fig. 7.25). Although common, osseous disease does not affect treatment or prognosis.

Scintigraphic studies may be used to assess potential complications of treatment. Suspected corticosteroid-induced avascular necrosis of bone is evaluated well by skeletal scintigraphy. Abnormalities related to methotrexate osteopathy (127) may also be identified with skeletal scintigraphy. Brain SPECT and PET have shown abnormalities in regional cerebral blood flow (187,188) and glucose utilization (189,190) following treatment of leukemia with high-dose methotrexate, intrathecal methotrexate, and cerebral irradiation. A pattern of abnormalities predicting

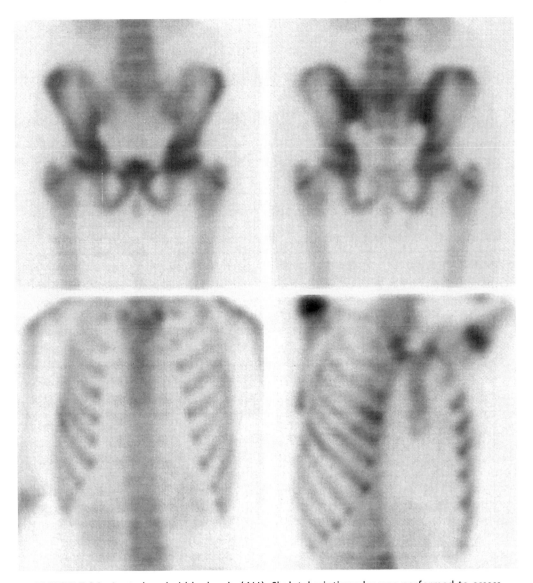

FIGURE 7.24. Acute lymphoid leukemia (*ALL*). Skeletal scintigraphy was performed to assess right buttock pain associated with an elevated erythrocyte sedimentation rate in the 11-year-old girl whose images are depicted here. The white blood cell count was normal. Sites of increased uptake were shown in the right ilium and the right sixth and seventh anterolateral ribs. Subsequent pelvic magnetic resonance imaging showed a focal signal abnormality in the right ilium and diffuse signal abnormality within all bones of the pelvis, the lower lumbar vertebral bodies, and the femoral diaphyses. Bone marrow aspiration and biopsy resulted in a diagnosis of ALL.

which children are at increased risk for long-term clinical manifestations of treatment-related neurotoxicity has not been identified, however.

Wilms' Tumor

Wilms' tumor is the most common renal malignancy of childhood. It is predominantly seen in infants and young children and is uncommonly encountered after the age of 5 years. Bilateral renal involvement occurs in about 5% of all cases and can be identified synchronously or metachronously. Histologically, Wilms' tumor contains blastemic, stromal, and epithelial cells (7).

Scintigraphy has not played an important role in imaging Wilms' tumor. Radiographs, ultrasonography, CT, and MRI are utilized in anatomic staging and detection of metastases, which predominantly involve lung, occasionally liver, and only rarely other sites. Clear cell sarcoma and rhabdoid tumor, which some consider variants of Wilms' tumor, have a tendency to metastasize to bone (7).

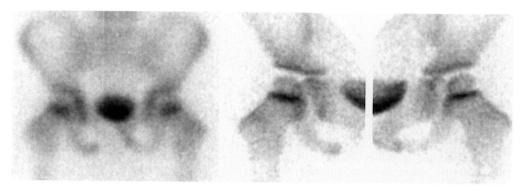

FIGURE 7.25. Acute lymphoid leukemia (*ALL*). These images are of a 4-year-old boy who presented with refusal to walk and right hip pain. Skeletal scintigraphy demonstrates absent tracer localization in the right inferior pubic ramus and slightly increased tracer localization in the right acetabulum. Subsequent pelvic magnetic resonance imaging showed signal abnormality within the right iliac wing, acetabulum, and ischium, particularly in the region of the right ischial tuberosity. Bone marrow aspiration and biopsy resulted in a diagnosis of ALL. (Reprinted from Connolly LP, Treves ST. *Pediatric skeletal scintigraphy with multimodality imaging correlation.* New York: Springer-Verlag, 1998, p. 264, with permission.)

Skeletal scintigraphy is used in staging and following these entities. The principal limitation of structural cross-sectional imaging has been assessment of the tumor bed for residual or recurrent disease. Although uptake of FDG has been observed in Wilms' tumor (191), a role for FDG-PET in this determination has not been established.

Rhabdomyosarcoma

Rhabdomyosarcoma is the most common soft-tissue malignancy of childhood. The peak incidence is between 3 and 6 years of age. Rhabdomyosarcomas can develop in any organ or tissue. Contrary to what its name might imply, this tumor does not usually arise in muscle. The most common anatomic locations are the head, particularly the orbit and paranasal sinuses, the neck, and the genitourinary tract. Imaging with CT or MRI is important to assess the extent of local disease. Radiographs and CT are used to detect pulmonary metastases. Skeletal scintigraphy is used to identify osseous metastases (Fig. 7.26). Rhabdomyosarcomas show variable degrees of accumulation of ^{67}Ga citrate, ^{201}Tl, and FDG (69,144). Clinical applications for these agents in patients with rhabdomyosarcoma have been suggested but not established.

Retinoblastoma

Retinoblastoma is the only primary intraocular malignancy with an appreciable incidence during childhood. Histologically, the tumor is composed of small round cells. More than 80% of cases occur before the age of 3 years. Retinoblastoma is familial in about 10% of cases. Many other cases are hereditary and are caused by a spontaneous mutation involving chromosome 13. Children with hereditary retinoblastoma are at increased risk for the development of a second malignancy. Radiation-induced cancers, particularly osteosarcoma, are most common. Between 20% and 30% of retinoblastomas are bilateral. All bilateral tumors are considered hereditary. Treatment is individualized. Options include enucleation, cryotherapy, photocoagulation, radiation therapy, and chemotherapy (7,192, 193).

A yellowish white appearance of the pupil (leukokoria) is the typical manifestation of this tumor. Although the differential diagnosis of leukokoria includes many entities, a diagnosis of retinoblastoma can be reached clinically with confidence in the majority of cases. CT and MRI are used to evaluate local extent of disease and assess for the possibility of ectopic pineal disease (192). Reports from one institution of ^{123}I-MIBG uptake by retinoblastoma, which is histologically similar to neuroblastoma, suggested that MIBG scintigraphy might prove useful in confirming the diagnosis in difficult cases (194,195). This has not been substantiated by subsequent data, which, although sparse, indicate that retinoblastomas do not typically accumulate MIBG (37,43). In this regard, it must be emphasized that negative examination results are not useful; the likelihood of survival is high if disease is confined to the globe. The likelihood of survival is low if tumor spreads beyond the eye (192). False-positive results caused by metastasis of neuroblastoma to the orbit are also a concern.

Because bone is one of the more common sites of metastases, skeletal scintigraphy may be performed to evaluate and observe children with retinoblastoma. Skeletal scintigraphy is most strongly indicated when clinical or pathologic evidence of extraocular disease is found at diagnosis (196). During follow-up, imaging specialists must remain aware of the possibility of a second malignancy.

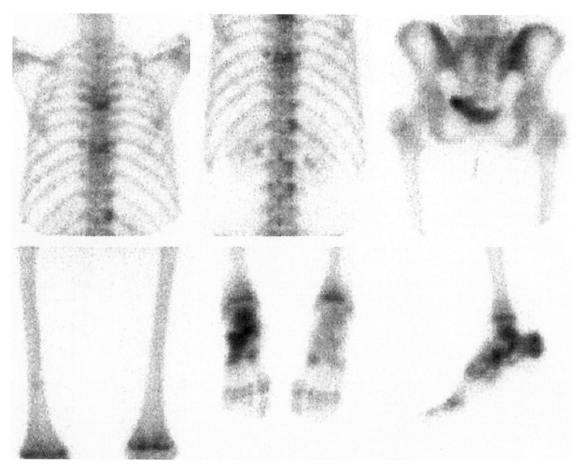

FIGURE 7.26. Metastatic rhabdomyosarcoma. These images were obtained following emergency T-8 laminectomy and evacuation of an epidural mass necessitated by lower extremity weakness and sensory loss. Selected images show multiple sites of increased uptake at metastases in the thoracic and lumbar spine, right ilium along the sacroiliac joint, right distal femoral diaphysis, right talus, right calcaneus, and right cuboid.

SUMMARY

This chapter has emphasized the applications of nuclear medicine that have proved valuable in the diagnosis and management of malignancies in children. The increasing importance of nuclear medicine in pediatric oncology is indicated by the references made to newer applications. The expansion of PET capability in children's hospitals is enabling practitioners of pediatric nuclear medicine to define the role of PET in pediatric oncology and harness the great potential of PET to improve the care of children with cancer. The continued development of radiotracers with a high specificity for malignancies, the emerging field of nuclear genetics, new compact imaging devices that facilitate radiotracer-guided surgery, and advances in fusing PET or SPECT images with CT or MR images should greatly enhance the value of nuclear medicine in pediatric nuclear oncology. Practitioners of nuclear medicine must continue to refine imaging techniques, dosimetry, and image interpretation to bring the full benefits of the evolving field of nuclear oncology to children.

REFERENCES

1. Robison LL. General principles of the epidemiology of childhood cancer. In: Pizzo PA, Poplack DG, eds. *Principles and practice of pediatric oncology.* Philadelphia: Lippincott–Raven Publishers, 1997:1–10.
2. Gurney JG, Severson RK, Davis S, et al. Incidence of cancer in children in the United States. *Cancer* 1995;75:2186–2195.
3. Committee on Drugs, Section on Anesthesiology. Guidelines for the elective use of conscious sedation, deep sedation and general anesthesia in pediatric patients. *Pediatrics* 1985;76:317–321.
4. Mandell GA, Cooper JA, Majd M, et al. Procedure guideline for pediatric sedation in nuclear medicine. *J Nucl Med* 1997;38: 1640–1643.
5. Treves ST. Introduction. In: Treves ST, ed. *Pediatric nuclear medicine,* 2nd ed. New York: Springer-Verlag, 1995:1–11.
6. Connolly LP, Treves ST. *Pediatric skeletal scintigraphy with multimodality imaging correlation.* New York: Springer-Verlag, 1998.

7. Cohen MD. *Imaging of children with cancer.* St. Louis: Mosby–Year Book, 1992.

8. Bousvaros A, Kirks DR, Grossman H. Imaging of neuroblastoma: an overview. *Pediatr Radiol* 1986;16:89–106.

9. Brodeur GM, Seeger RC, Barrett A, et al. International criteria for diagnosis, staging, and response to treatment in patients with neuroblastoma. *J Clin Oncol* 1988;6:1874–1881.

10. Brodeur GM, Pritchard J, Berthold F, et al. Revisions of international criteria for neuroblastoma diagnosis, staging, and response to treatment. *J Clin Oncol* 1993;11:1466–1477.

11. Barnewolt CE, Paltiel HJ, Lebowitz RL, et al. Genitourinary tract. In: Kirks DR, ed. *Practical pediatric imaging. Diagnostic radiology of infants and children*, 3rd ed. Philadelphia: Lippincott–Raven Publishers, 1997:1009–1170.

12. Woods WG, Lemieux B, Tuchman M. Neuroblastoma represents distinct clinical-biologic entities: a review and perspective from the Quebec neuroblastoma screening project. *Pediatrics* 1992;89:114–118.

13. Shimada H, Chatten J, Newton WA, et al. Histopathologic prognostic factors in neuroblastic tumors: definition of subtypes of ganglioneuroblastoma and an age-linked classification of neuroblastomas. *J Natl Cancer Inst* 1984;73:405–416.

14. Smets LA, Loesberg C, Janssen M, et al. Active uptake and extravesicular storage of *m*-iodobenzylguanidine in human neuroblastoma SK-N-SH cells. *Cancer Res* 1989;49:2941–2944.

15. Shulkin BL, Shapiro B. Current concepts on the diagnostic use of MIBG in children. *J Nucl Med* 1998;39:679–688.

16. Solanki KK, Bomanji J, Moyes J, et al. A pharmacological guide to medicines which interfere with the biodistribution of radiolabelled meta-iodobenzylguanidine (MIBG). *Nucl Med Commun* 1992;13:513–521.

17. Gelfand MJ, Harris RE. Meta-iodobenzylguanidine in children. *Semin Nucl Med* 1986;23:231–242.

18. Rufini V, Fisher GL, Shulkin BL, et al. Iodine-123-MIBG imaging of neuroblastoma: utility of SPECT and delayed imaging. *J Nucl Med* 1996;37:1464–1468.

19. Gelfand MJ, Elgazzar AH, Kriss VM, et al. Iodine-123-MIBG SPECT versus planar imaging in children with neural crest tumors. *J Nucl Med* 1994;35:1753–1757.

20. Paltiel HJ, Gelfand MJ, Elgazzar AH, et al. Neural crest tumors: ^{123}I-MIBG imaging in children. *Radiology* 1994;190:117–121.

21. Nakajo M, Shapiro B, Copp J, et al. The normal and abnormal distribution of the adrenal medullary imaging agent *m*-[I-131] iodobenzylguanidine (I-131-MIBG) in man: evaluation by scintigraphy. *J Nucl Med* 1983;24:672–682.

22. Nakajo M, Shapiro B, Glowniak J, et al. Inverse relationship between cardiac accumulation of meta-[131I]iodobenzylguanidine (^{131}I-MIBG) and circulating catecholamines in suspected pheochromocytoma. *J Nucl Med* 1985;24:1127–1134.

23. Hattner RS, Pounds TR, Matthay KK. Normal cerebellar MIBG localization. Implications in the interpretation of delayed scans. *Clin Nucl Med* 1994;19:985–988.

24. Hoefnagel CA, Voute PA, de Kraker J, et al. Radionuclide diagnosis and therapy of neural crest tumors using iodine-131 metaiodobenzylguanidine. *J Nucl Med* 1987;28:308–314.

25. Voute PA, Hoefnagel CA, de Kraker J. ^{131}I-meta-iodobenzylguanidine in diagnosis and treatment of neuroblastoma. *Bull Cancer* 1988;75:107–111.

26. Klingebiel T, Bader P, Bares R, et al. Treatment of neuroblastoma stage 4 with ^{131}I-meta-iodo-benzylguanidine, high-dose chemotherapy and immunotherapy. A pilot study. *Eur J Cancer* 1998; 34:1398–1402.

27. van Hasselt EJ, Heij HA, de Kraker J, et al. Pretreatment with [131I]metaiodobenzylguanidine and surgical resection of advanced neuroblastoma. *Eur J Pediatr Surg* 1996;6:155–158.

28. Sisson JC, Shapiro B, Hutchinson RJ, et al. Survival of patients with neuroblastoma treated with ^{125}I-MIBG. *Am J Clin Oncol* 1996;19:144–148.

29. Applegate KA, Connolly LP, Treves ST. Neuroblastoma presenting clinically as hip osteomyelitis: a signature diagnosis on skeletal scintigraphy. *Pediatr Radiol* 1995;25:S93–S97.

30. Smith FW, Gilday DL, Ash JM, et al. Primary neuroblastoma uptake of ^{99m}Tc-methylene diphosphonate. *Radiology* 1980;137: 501–504.

31. Young G, L'Hereux P. Extraosseous tumor uptake of ^{99m}Tc phosphate compounds in children with abdominal neuroblastoma. *Pediatr Radiol* 1978;7:159–163.

32. Podrasky AE, Stark DD, Hattner RS, et al. Radionuclide bone scanning in neuroblastoma: skeletal metastases and primary tumor localization of ^{99m}Tc-MDP. *Am J Roentgenol* 1983;141: 469–472.

33. Martin-Simmerman P, Cohen MD, Siddiqui A, et al. Calcification and uptake of Tc-99m diphosphonates in neuroblastomas: concise communication. *J Nucl Med* 1984;25:656–660.

34. Howman-Giles RB, Gilday DL, Ash JM. Radionuclide skeletal survey in neuroblastoma. *Radiology* 1979;131:497–502.

35. Geatti O, Shapiro B, Sisson JC. ^{131}I-metaiodobenzylguanidine (^{131}I-MIBG) scintigraphy for the localization of neuroblastoma: preliminary experience in 10 cases. *J Nucl Med* 1985;34: 1140–1146.

36. Hoefnagel CA, Voute PA, de Kraker J, et al. Total body scintigraphy with ^{131}I-metaiodobenzylguanidine for detection of neuroblastoma. *Diagn Imaging Clin Med* 1985;54:21–27.

37. Jacobs A, Delree M, Desprechins B, et al. Consolidating the role of *I-MIBG-scintigraphy in childhood neuroblastoma: five years of clinical experience. *Pediatr Radiol* 1990;20:157–159.

38. Neunschwander S, Ollivier L, Tobeau M, et al. Local evaluation of abdominal neuroblastoma stage III and IV: use of US, CT, and ^{123}I-metaiodobenzylguanidine (MIBG) scintigraphy. *Ann Radiol* 1987;30:491–496.

39. Lumbroso JD, Guermazi F, Hartmann O, et al. Meta-iodobenzylguanidine (MIBG) scans in neuroblastoma: sensitivity and specificity: a review of 115 scans. *Prog Clin Biol Res* 1988;271: 689–705.

40. Edeling CJ, Frederiksen PB, Kamper J, et al. Diagnosis and treatment of neuroblastoma using metaiodobenzylguanidine. *Clin Nucl Med* 1987;12:632–637.

41. Troncone L, Rufini V, Danza FM, et al. Radioiodinated metaiodobenzylguanidine (*I-MIBG) scintigraphy in neuroblastoma: a review of 160 studies. *J Nucl Med Allied Sci* 1990;34: 279–288.

42. Shapiro B, Gross MD. Radiochemistry, biochemistry, and kinetics of ^{131}I-metaiodobenzylguanidine (MIBG) and ^{123}I-MIBG. Clinical applications of the use of ^{123}I-MIBG. *Med Pediatr Oncol* 1987;15:170–177.

43. Leung A, Shapiro B, Hattner R, et al. The specificity of radioiodinated MIBG for neural crest tumors in childhood. *J Nucl Med* 1997;38:1352–1357.

44. Schmiegelow K, Simes MA, Agertoft L, et al. Radio-iodobenzylguanidine scintigraphy of neuroblastoma: conflicting results, when compared with standard investigations. *Med Pediatr Oncol* 1989;17:127–130.

45. Laor T, Jaramillo D, Oestrich A. Skeletal system. In: Kirks DR, ed. *Practical pediatric imaging. Diagnostic radiology of infants and children*, 3rd ed. Philadelphia: Lippincott–Raven Publishers, 1997:327–510.

46. Sty JR, Wells RG, Starshak RJ, et al. The musculoskeletal system. In: Sty JR, Wells RG, Starshak RJ, et al., eds. *Diagnostic imaging of infants and children*. Gaithersburg: Aspen Publishers, 1992: 233–405 (vol 3).

47. Baker M, Siddiqui AR, Provisor A, et al. Radiographic and scintigraphic skeletal imaging in patients with neuroblastoma: concise communication. *J Nucl Med* 1983;24:467–469.

48. Heisel MA, Miller JH, Reid BS, et al. Radionuclide bone scan in neuroblastoma. *Pediatrics* 1983;71:206–209.

49. Gordon I, Peters AM, Gutman A, et al. Tc-99m bone scans are more sensitive than I-123 MIBG scans for bone imaging in neuroblastoma. *J Nucl Med* 1990;31:129–134.

50. Shulkin BL, Shapiro B, Hutchinson RJ. Iodine-131-metaiodobenzylguanidine and bone scintigraphy for the detection of neuroblastoma. *J Nucl Med* 1992;33:1735–1740.

51. Suc A, Lumbroso J, Rubie H, et al. Metastatic neuroblastoma in children older than one year: prognostic significance of the initial metaiodobenzylguanidine scan and proposal for a scoring system. *Cancer* 1996;77:805–811.

52. Ortiz SS, Miller JH, Villablanca JG, et al. Bone abnormalities detected with skeletal scintigraphy after bone marrow harvest in patients with childhood neuroblastoma. *Radiology* 1994;192:755–758.

53. Englaro EE, Gelfand MJ, Harris RE, et al. I-131 MIBG imaging after bone marrow transplantation for neuroblastoma. *Radiology* 1992;182:515–520.

54. Dessner DA, DiPietro MA, Shulkin BL. MIBG detection of hepatic neuroblastoma: correlation with CT, US and surgical findings. *Pediatr Radiol* 1993;23:276–280.

55. Connolly LP, Bloom DA, Kozakewich H, et al. Localization of Tc-99m MDP in neuroblastoma metastases to liver and lung. *Clin Nucl Med* 1996;21:629–633.

56. Mandell GA, Heyman S. Extraosseous uptake of technetium-99m MDP in secondary deposits of neuroblastoma. *Clin Nucl Med* 1986;11:337–341.

57. Shulkin BL, Hutchinson RJ, Castle VP, et al. Neuroblastoma: positron emission tomography with 2-[fluorine-18]-fluoro-2-deoxy-D-glucose compared with metaiodobenzylguanidine scintigraphy. *Radiology* 1996;199:743–750.

58. Heij HA, Rutgers EJ, de Kraker J, et al. Intraoperative search for neuroblastoma by MIBG and radioguided surgery with the gamma detector. *Med Pediatr Oncol* 1997;28:171–174.

59. Martelli H, Ricard M, Larroquet M, et al. Intraoperative localization of neuroblastoma in children with [123]I- or ^{125}I-radiolabeled metaiodobenzylguanidine. *Surgery* 1998;123:51–57.

60. Krenning EP, Kwekkeboom DJ, Bakker WH, et al. Somatostatin receptor scintigraphy with [In-111-DTPA-D-Phe[1]] and [^{123}I-Tyr[3]]-octreotide: the Rotterdam experience with more than 1000 patients. *Eur J Nucl Med* 1993;20:716–731.

61. Briganti V, Sestini R, Orlando C, et al. Imaging of somatostatin receptors by indium-111-pentetreotide correlates with quantitative determination of somatostatin receptor type 2 gene expression in neuroblastoma tumor. *Clin Cancer Res* 1997;3:2385–2391.

62. Manil L, Edeline V, Lumbroso J, et al. Indium-111-pentetreotide scintigraphy in children with neuroblast-derived tumors. *J Nucl Med* 1996;37:893–896.

63. Limouris GS, Giannakopoulos V, Stavraka A, et al. Comparison of In-111 pentetreotide, Tc-99m (V)DMSA and I-123 MIBG scintimaging in neural crest tumors. *Anticancer Res* 1997;17:1589–1592.

64. Kropp J, Hofmann M, Bihl H. Comparison of MIBG and pentetreotide scintigraphy in children with neuroblastoma. Is the expression of somatostatin receptors a prognostic factor? *Anticancer Res* 1997;17:1583–1588.

65. Shalaby-Rana E, Majd M, Andrich MP, et al. In-111 pentetreotide scintigraphy in patients with neuroblastoma. Comparison with I-131 MIBG, N-*myc* oncogene amplification, and patient outcome. *Clin Nucl Med* 1997;22:315–319.

66. Dorr U, Sautter-Bihl ML, Schilling FH, et al. Somatostatin receptor scintigraphy: a new diagnostic tool in neuroblastoma? *Prog Clin Biol Res* 1994;385:355–361.

67. Garty I, Friedman A, Sandler MP, et al. Neuroblastoma: imaging evaluation by sequential Tc-99m MDP, I-131 MIBG, and Ga-67 citrate studies. *Clin Nucl Med* 1989;14:515–522.

68. Siddiqui AR, Oseas RS, Wellman HN, et al. Evaluation of bone-marrow scanning with technetium-99m sulfur colloid in pediatric oncology. *J Nucl Med* 1979;20:379–386.

69. Howman-Giles R, Uren RF, Shaw PJ. Thallium-201 scintigraphy in pediatric soft-tissue tumors. *J Nucl Med* 1995;36:1372–1376.

70. De Moerloose B, Van de Wiele C, Dhooge C, et al. Technetium-99m sestamibi imaging in paediatric neuroblastoma and ganglioneuroma and its relation to P-glycoprotein. *Eur J Nucl Med* 1999;26:396–403.

71. Berthold F, Waters W, Sieverts H, et al. Immunoscintigraphic imaging of mIBG-negative metastases in neuroblastoma. *Am J Pediatr Hematol Oncol* 1990;12:61–62.

72. Reuland P, Handgretinger R, Smykowsky H, et al. Application of the murine anti-Gd-2 antibody 14.Gd-2a for diagnosis and therapy of neuroblastoma. *Int J Radiat Appl Instr B* 1991;18:121–125.

73. Yeh SD, Larson SM, Burch L, et al. Radioimmunodetection of neuroblastoma with iodine-131-3F8: correlation with biopsy, iodine-131-metaiodobenzylguanidine and standard diagnostic modalities. *J Nucl Med* 1991;32:769–776.

74. Larson SM, Pentlow KS, Volkow ND, et al. PET scanning of iodine-124-3F9 as an approach to tumor dosimetry during treatment planning for radioimmunotherapy in a child with neuroblastoma. *J Nucl Med* 1992;33:2020–2023.

75. Seregni E, Chiti A, Bombardieri E. Radionuclide imaging of neuroendocrine tumours: biological basis and diagnostic results. *Eur J Nucl Med* 1998;25:639–658.

76. Hollinger EF, Alibazoglu H, Ali A, et al. Hematopoietic cytokine-mediated FDG uptake simulates the appearance of diffuse metastatic disease on whole-body PET imaging. *Clin Nucl Med* 1998;23:93–98.

77. Sugawara Y, Fisher SJ, Zasadny KR, et al. Preclinical and clinical studies of bone marrow uptake of fluorine-18-fluorodeoxyglucose with or without granulocyte colony-stimulating factor during chemotherapy. *J Clin Oncol* 1998;16:173–180.

78. Mirra JM. *Bone tumors*. Philadelphia: Lea & Febiger, 1989.

79. Resnick D, Kyriakos K, Greenway GD. Tumors and tumor-like lesions of bone: imaging and pathology of specific tumors. In: Resnick D, ed. *Diagnosis of bone and joint disorders*, 3rd ed. Philadelphia: WB Saunders, 1995:3662–3697 (vol 6).

80. Meadows AT, Baum E, Fassati-Bellani F, et al. Second malignant neoplasms in children: an update from the Late Effects Study Group. *J Clin Oncol* 1985;3:532–538.

81. Link MP, Eilber F. Osteosarcoma. In: Pizzo PA, Poplack DG, eds. *Pediatric oncology*, 2nd ed. Philadelphia: Lippincott–Raven Publishers, 1997:889–920.

82. Aboulafia AJ, Malawer MM. Surgical management of pelvic and extremity osteosarcoma. *Cancer* 1993;71[Suppl]:3358–3366.

83. Resnick D. Tumors and tumor-like lesions of bone: radiographic principles. In: Resnick D, ed. *Diagnosis of bone and joint disorders*, 3rd ed. Philadelphia: WB Saunders, 1995:3613–3627 (vol 6).

84. Hudson TM. *Radiologic-pathologic correlation of musculoskeletal lesions*. Baltimore: Williams & Wilkins, 1987.

85. Hopper KD, Moser RP, Haseman DB, et al. Osteosarcomatosis. *Radiology* 1990;175:233–239.

86. McDonald DJ. Limb salvage surgery for sarcomas of the extremities. *AJR Am J Roentgenol* 1994;163:509–513.

87. Glasser DB, Lane JM, Huvos AG, et al. Survival, prognosis, and therapeutic response in osteogenic sarcoma: the Memorial Hospital experience. *Cancer* 1992;69:698–708.

88. Bacci G, Picci P, Ruggieri P, et al. Primary chemotherapy and

delayed surgery (neoadjuvant chemotherapy) for osteosarcoma of the extremities. *Cancer* 1990;65:2539–2553.

89. Meyers PA, Heller G, Healey J, et al. Chemotherapy for non-metastatic osteogenic sarcoma: the Memorial Sloan-Kettering experience. *J Clin Oncol* 1992;10:5–15.

90. Chew FS, Hudson TM. Radionuclide bone scanning of osteosarcoma: falsely extended uptake patterns. *Am J Roentgenol* 1982; 139:49–54.

91. Goldman B, Braunstein P. Augmented radioactivity on bone scans of limbs bearing osteosarcomas. *J Nucl Med* 1978;16: 423–424.

92. Thrall JH, Geslein GE, Corcoran RJ, et al. Abnormal radionuclide deposition patterns adjacent to focal skeletal lesions. *Radiology* 1975;115:659–663.

93. Beltran J, Simon DC, Katz W, et al. Increased MR signal intensity in skeletal muscle adjacent to malignant tumors: pathologic correlation and clinical relevance. *Radiology* 1987;162:251–255.

94. Jaramillo D, Laor T, Gebhardt M. Pediatric musculoskeletal neoplasms. Evaluation with MR imaging. *Magn Reson Imaging Clin N Am* 1996;4:1–22.

95. McKillop JH, Etcubanus E, Goris ML. The indications for and limitations of bone scintigraphy in osteogenic sarcoma: a review of 55 patients. *Cancer* 1981;48:1133–1138.

96. Rees CR, Siddiqui AR, duCret R. The role of bone scintigraphy in osteogenic sarcoma. *Skeletal Radiol* 1986;15:365–367.

97. Vanel D, Henry-Amar M, Lumbrosus J, et al. Pulmonary evaluation of patients with osteosarcoma: roles of standard radiography, tomography, CT, scintigraphy, and tomoscintigraphy. *Am J Roentgenol* 1984;143:519–523.

98. Kirks DR, Cook TA, Merten DF, et al. The value of radionuclide bone imaging in selected patients with osteosarcoma metastatic to lung. *Pediatr Radiol* 1980;9:139–143.

99. Hoefnagel CA, Bruning PF, Cohen P, et al. Detection of lung metastases from osteosarcoma by scintigraphy using ^{99m}Tc-methylene diphosphonate. *Diagn Imaging* 1981;50:277–284.

100. Erlemann R, Sciuk J, Bosse A, et al. Response of osteosarcoma and Ewing sarcoma to preoperative chemotherapy: assessment with dynamic and static MR imaging and skeletal scintigraphy. *Radiology* 1990;175:791–796.

101. Ramanna L, Waxman A, Binney G, et al. Thallium-201 scintigraphy in bone sarcoma: comparison with gallium-67 and technetium-99m MDP in the evaluation of chemotherapeutic response. *J Nucl Med* 1990;31:567–572.

102. Nadel HR, Rossleigh MA. Tumor imaging. In: Treves ST, ed. *Pediatric nuclear medicine*, 2nd ed. New York: Springer-Verlag, 1995:496–527.

103. Holscher HC, Bloem JL, Vanel D, et al. Osteosarcoma: chemotherapy-induced changes at MR imaging. *Radiology* 1992;182: 839–844.

104. Lawrence JA, Babyn PS, Chan HS, et al. Extremity osteosarcoma in childhood: prognostic value of radiologic imaging. *Radiology* 1993;189:43–47.

105. Kostakoglu L, Panicek DM, Divgi CR, et al. Correlation of the findings of thallium-201 chloride scans with those of other imaging modalities and histology following therapy in patients with bone and soft tissue sarcomas. *Eur J Nucl Med* 1995;22: 1232–1237.

106. Sato O, Kawai A, Ozaki T, et al. Value of thallium-201 scintigraphy in bone and soft tissue tumors. *J Orthop Sci* 1998;3: 297–303.

107. Ohtomo K, Terui S, Yokoyama R, et al. Thallium-201 scintigraphy to assess effect of chemotherapy to osteosarcoma. *J Nucl Med* 1996;37:1444–1448.

108. Lin J, Leung WT. Quantitative evaluation of thallium-201 uptake in predicting chemotherapeutic response of osteosarcoma. *Eur J Nucl Med* 1995;22:553–555.

109. Imbriaco M, Yeh SD, Yeung H, et al. Thallium-201 scintigraphy for the evaluation of tumor response to preoperative chemotherapy in patients with osteosarcoma. *Cancer* 1997;80:1507–1512.

110. Connolly LP, Laor T, Jaramillo D, et al. Prediction of chemotherapeutic response of osteosarcoma with quantitative thallium-201 scintigraphy and magnetic resonance imaging. *Radiology* 1996; 201(P):349(abst).

111. Soderlund V, Larsson SA, Bauer SCF, et al. Use of ^{99m}Tc-MIBI scintigraphy in the evaluation of response of osteosarcoma to chemotherapy. *Eur J Nucl Med* 1997;24:511–515.

112. Kartner N, Riordan JR, Ling V. Cell surface P-glycoprotein associated with multidrug resistance in mammalian cell lines. *Science* 1983;221:1285–1288.

113. Piwnica-Worms D, Chiu ML, Budding M, et al. Functional imaging of multidrug-resistant P-glycoprotein with an organotechnetium complex. Cancer Res 1993;53:977–984.

114. Abdel-Dayem HM. The role of nuclear medicine in primary bone and soft tissue tumors. *Semin Nucl Med* 1997;27: 355–363.

115. Friedlaender GE. Bone grafts. Current concepts [Review]. *J Bone Joint Surg Am* 1987;69:786–790.

116. Mankin HJ, Springfield DS, Gebhardt MC, et al. Current status of allografting for bone tumors. *Orthopedics* 1992;15:1147–1152.

117. Enneking WF, Mindell ER. Observations on massive retrieved human allografts. *J Bone Joint Surg Am* 1991;73:1123–1142.

118. Bar-Sever Z, Connolly LP, Treves ST. Scintigraphy of lower extremity cadaveric bone allografts in osteosarcoma patients. *Clin Nucl Med* 1995;22:532–535.

119. Roebuck DJ, Griffith J, Kumta SM, et al. Imaging following allograft reconstruction in children with malignant bone tumors. *Pediatr Radiol* 1999;29:785–793.

120. Alman BA, De Bari A, Krajbich JI. Massive allografts in the treatment of osteosarcoma and Ewing sarcoma in children and adolescents. *J Bone Joint Surg Am* 1995;77:54–64.

121. Berrey BH Jr, Lord CF, Gebhardt MC, et al. Fractures of allografts. Frequency, treatment, and end-results. *J Bone Joint Surg Am* 1990;72:825–833.

122. Stanisavljevic S, Babcock AL. Fractures in children treated with methotrexate for leukemia. *Clin Orthop* 1977;125:139–144.

123. Herrlin K, Willen H, Wiebe T. Flare phenomenon in osteosarcoma after complete remission. *J Nucl Med* 1995;36:1429–1431.

124. Ben Ami T, Treves ST, Tumeh S, et al. Stress fractures after surgery for osteosarcoma: scintigraphic assessment. *Radiology* 1987;163: 157–162.

125. May KP, West SG, McDermott MT, et al. The effect of low-dose methotrexate on bone metabolism and histomorphometry in rats. *Arthritis Rheum* 1994;37:201–206.

126. Nesbit M, Krivit W, Heyn R, et al. Acute and chronic effects of methotrexate on hepatic, pulmonary, and skeletal systems. *Cancer* 1976;37:1048–1054.

127. Ragab AH, Frech RS, Vietti TJ. Osteoporotic fractures secondary to methotrexate therapy of acute leukemia in remission. *Cancer* 1970;25:580–585.

128. Schwartz AM, Leonidas JC. Methotrexate osteopathy. *Skeletal Radiol* 1984;11:13–16.

129. Ecklund K, Laor T, Goorin AM, et al. Methotrexate osteopathy in patients with osteosarcoma. *Radiology* 1995;202:543–547.

130. Podoloff DA. Malignant bone disease. In: Henkin RE, Boles MA, Dillehay GL, et al., eds. *Nuclear medicine*, 2nd ed. Philadelphia: Mosby–Year Book, 1996:1208–1222.

131. Triche TJ. Pathology and molecular diagnosis of pediatric malignancies. In: Pizzo PA, Poplack DG, eds. *Principles and practice of pediatric oncology*, 3rd ed. Philadelphia: Lippincott–Raven Publishers, 1997:141–186.

132. Marina NM, Etcubanas E, Parham DM, et al. Peripheral primitive neuroectodermal tumor (peripheral neuroepithelioma) in

children. A review of the St. Jude experience and controversies in diagnosis and management. *Cancer* 1989;64:1952–1960.

133. Horowitz ME, Malawer MM, Woo SY, et al. Ewing's sarcoma family of tumors: Ewing's sarcoma of bone and soft tissue and the peripheral primitive neuroectodermal tumors. In: Pizzo PA, Poplack DG, eds. *Pediatric oncology*, 3rd ed. Philadelphia: Lippincott–Raven Publishers, 1997:831–864.

134. Crist WM, Kun LE. Common solid tumors of childhood. *N Engl J Med* 1991;324:461–471.

135. Parker BR, Castellino RA. *Pediatric oncologic radiology*. St. Louis: Mosby, 1977.

136. O'Connor MI, Pritchard DJ. Ewing's sarcoma. Prognostic factors, disease control, and the reemerging role of surgical treatment. *Clin Orthop* 1991;262:78–87.

137. Bushnell D, Shirazzi P, Khedkar N. Ewing's sarcoma seen as "cold" lesions on bone scan. *Clin Nucl Med* 1983;8:173–174.

138. McNeil BJ, Cassidy JR, Geiser CF, et al. Fluorine-18 bone scintigraphy in children with osteosarcoma or Ewing's sarcoma. *Radiology* 1973;109:627–631.

139. Meyer JR, Shulkin BL. Flare response in Ewing's sarcoma. *Clin Nucl Med* 1991;16:807–809.

140. Simon MA, Kirchner PT. Scintigraphic evaluation of primary bone tumors: comparison of technetium-99m phosphonate and gallium citrate imaging. *J Bone Joint Surg Am* 1980;62:758–764.

141. Menendez LR, Fideler BM, Mirra J. Thallium-201 scanning for the evaluation of osteosarcoma and soft tissue sarcoma. *J Bone Joint Surg Am* 1993;75:526–531.

142. Bar-Sever Z, Connolly L, Treves ST, et al. Technetium-99m MIBI in the evaluation of children with Ewing sarcoma. *J Nucl Med* 1997;38:13P–14P(abst).

143. Caner B, Kitapci M, Unlu M, et al. Technetium-99m MIBI uptake in benign and malignant bone tumors: a comparative study with technetium-99m MDP. *J Nucl Med* 1992;33:319–324.

144. Shulkin BL, Mitchell DS, Ungar DR, et al. Neoplasms in a pediatric population: 2-[F-18]-fluoro-2-deoxy-D-glucose PET studies. *Radiology* 1995;194:495–500.

145. Kleihues P, Burger PC, Scheithauer BW. The new WHO classification of brain tumours. *Brain Pathol* 1993;3:255–268.

146. Robertson RL, Ball WS Jr, Barnes PD. Skull and brain. In: Kirks DR, ed. *Practical pediatric imaging. Diagnostic radiology of infants and children*, 3rd ed. Philadelphia: Lippincott–Raven Publishers, 1997:65–200.

147. Maria BL, Drane WB, Quisling RJ, et al. Correlation between gadolinium-diethylenetriaminepentaacetic acid contrast enhancement and thallium-201 chloride uptake in pediatric brainstem glioma. *J Child Neurol* 1997;12:341–348.

148. O'Tuama LA, Janicek MJ, Barnes PD, et al. [201]Tl/^{99m}Tc-HMPAO SPECT of treated childhood brain tumors. *Pediatr Neurol* 1991;11:249–257.

149. Rollins NK, Lowry PA, Shapiro KN. Comparison of gadolinium-enhanced MR and thallium-201 single-photon emission computed tomography in pediatric brain tumors. *Pediatr Neurosurg* 1995;22:8–14.

150. Habboush IH, Mitchell KD, Mulkern RV, et al. Registration and alignment of three-dimensional images: an interactive visual approach. *Radiology* 1996;199:573–578.

151. Black KL, Hawkins RA, Kim KT, et al. Use of thallium-201 SPECT to quantitate malignancy grade of gliomas. *J Neurosurg* 1989;71:342–346.

152. Kosuda S, Aoki S, Suzuki K, et al. Re-evaluation of quantitative thallium-201 brain SPECT for brain tumor. *J Nucl Med* 1992;33:844(abst).

153. Molloy PT, Defeo R, Hunter J, et al. Excellent correlation of FDG-PET imaging with clinical outcome in patients with neu-

rofibromatosis type I and low-grade astrocytomas. *J Nucl Med* 1999;40:129P(abst).

154. Valk PE, Budinger TF, Levin VA, et al. PET of malignant cerebral tumors after interstitial brachytherapy. Demonstration of metabolic activity and correlation with clinical outcome. *J Neurosurg* 1988;69:830–838.

155. Di Chiro G, Oldfield E, Wright DC, et al. Cerebral necrosis after radiotherapy and/or intraarterial chemotherapy for brain tumors: PET and neuropathologic studies. *Am J Roentgenol* 1988;150:189–197.

156. Glantz MJ, Hoffman JM, Coleman RE, et al. Identification of early recurrence of primary central nervous system tumors by [18F]fluorodeoxyglucose positron emission tomography. *Ann Neurol* 1991;29:347–355.

157. Janus T, Kim E, Tilbury R, et al. Use of [18F]fluorodeoxyglucose positron emission tomography in patients with primary malignant brain tumors. *Ann Neurol* 1993;33:540–548.

158. Maria BL, Drane WE, Mastin ST, et al. Comparative value of thallium and glucose SPECT imaging in childhood brain tumors. *Pediatr Neurol* 1998;19:351–357.

159. Schifter T, Hoffman JM, Hanson MW, et al. Serial FDG-PET studies in the prediction of survival in patients with primary brain tumors. *J Comput Assist Tomogr* 1993;17:509–561.

160. Oriuchi N, Tamaru M, Shibazaki T, et al. Clinical evaluation of thallium-201 SPECT in supratentorial gliomas: relationship to histologic grade, prognosis, and proliferative activities. *J Nucl Med* 1993;34:2085–2089.

161. Francavilla TL, Miletich RS, Di Chiro G, et al. Positron emission tomography in the detection of malignant degeneration of low-grade gliomas. *Neurosurgery* 1989;24:1–5.

162. Patronas NJ, Di Chiro G, Kufta C, et al. Prediction of survival in glioma patients by means of positron emission tomography. *J Neurosurg* 1985;62:816–822.

163. Molloy PT, Belasco J, Ngo K, et al. The role of FDG-PET imaging in the clinical management of pediatric brain tumors. *J Nucl Med* 1999;40:129P(abst).

164. Holthof VA, Herholz K, Berthold F, et al. *In vivo* metabolism of childhood posterior fossa tumors and primitive neuroectodermal tumors before and after treatment. *Cancer* 1993;72:1394–1403.

165. Hoffman JM, Hanson MW, Friedman HS, et al. FDG-PET in pediatric posterior fossa brain tumors. *J Comput Assist Tomogr* 1992;16:62–68.

166. O'Tuama LA, Phillips PC, Strauss LC, et al. Two-phase [11C]L-methionine PET in childhood brain tumors. *Pediatr Neurol* 1990;6:163–170.

167. Mosskin M, von Holst H, Bergstrom M, et al. Positron emission tomography with 11C-methionine and computed tomography of intracranial tumours compared with histopathologic examination of multiple biopsies. *Acta Radiol* 1987;28:673–681.

168. Ericson K, Lilja A, Bergstrom M, et al. Positron emission tomography with ([11C]methyl)-L-methionine, [11C]D-glucose, and [68Ga]EDTA in supratentorial tumor. *J Comput Assist Tomogr* 1985;9:683–689.

169. Treves ST, O'Tuama LA, Kuruc A. Cerebrospinal fluid. In: Treves ST, ed. *Pediatric nuclear medicine*, 2nd ed. New York: Springer-Verlag, 1995:109–120.

170. Connolly LP, Dinh L, Treves ST. The detection of CSF block with Tc-99m DTPA cerebral ventriculography. *Clin Nucl Med* 1996;21:71–72.

171. Chamberlain MC. Pediatric leptomeningeal metastasis: ^{111}In-DTPA cerebrospinal fluid flow studies. *J Child Neurol* 1994;9:150–154.

172. Donahue DM, Leonard JC, Basmadjian GP, et al. Thymic gallium-67 localization in pediatric patients on chemotherapy: concise communication. *J Nucl Med* 1981;22:1043–1048.

173. Drossman SR, Schiff RG, Kronfeld GD, et al. Lymphoma of

the mediastinum and neck: evaluation with Ga-67 imaging and CT correlation. *Radiology* 1990;174:171–175.

174. Handmaker H, O'Mara RE. Gallium imaging in pediatrics. *J Nucl Med* 1977;18:1057–1063.

175. Hibi S, Todo S, Imashuku S. Thymic localization of gallium-67 in pediatric patients with lymphoid and nonlymphoid tumors. *J Nucl Med* 1987;28:293–297.

176. Peylan-Ramu N, Haddy TB, Jones E, et al. High frequency of benign mediastinal uptake of gallium-67 after completion of chemotherapy in children with high-grade non-Hodgkin's lymphoma. *J Clin Oncol* 1989;7:1800–1806.

177. Rossleigh MA, Murray IP, Mackey DW, et al. Pediatric solid tumors: evaluation by gallium-67 SPECT studies. *J Nucl Med* 1990;31:168–172.

178. Nadel H. Thallium-201 for oncological imaging in children. *Semin Nucl Med* 1993;23:243–254.

179. Roebuck DJ, Nicholls WD, Bernard EJ, et al. Misleading leads. Thallium-201 uptake in rebound thymic hyperplasia. *Med Pediatr Oncol* 1998;30:297–300.

180. Campeau RJ, Ey EH, Varma DG. Thallium-201 uptake in a benign thymoma. *Clin Nucl Med* 1986;11:524.

181. Fukuda T, Itami M, Sawa H, et al. A case of thymoma arising from undescended thymus. High uptake of thallium-201 chloride. *Eur J Nucl Med* 1980;5:465–468.

182. Weinblatt ME, Zanzi I, Belakhlef A, et al. False-positive FDG-PET imaging of the thymus of a child with Hodgkin's disease. *J Nucl Med* 1997;38:888–890.

183. Patel PM, Alibazoglu H, Ali A, et al. Normal thymic uptake of FDG on PET imaging. *Clin Nucl Med* 1996;21:772–775.

184. Johnson PM, Berdon WE, Baker DH, et al. Thymic uptake of gallium-67 citrate in a healthy 4-year-old boy. *Pediatr Radiol* 1978;7:243–244.

185. Rogalsky RJ, Black B, Reed MH. Orthopedic manifestations of leukemia in children. *J Bone Joint Surg Am* 1986;68:494–501.

186. Clausen N, Gotze H, Pedersen A, et al. Skeletal scintigraphy and radiography at onset of acute lymphocytic leukemia in children. *Med Pediatr Oncol* 1983;11:291–296.

187. Osterlundh G, Bjure J, Lannering B, et al. Studies of cerebral blood flow in children with acute lymphoblastic leukemia: case reports of six children treated with methotrexate examined by single-photon emission computed tomography. *J Pediatr Oncol* 1997;19:28–34.

188. Harila-Saari AH, Ahonen AK, Vainionpaa LK, et al. Brain perfusion after treatment of childhood acute lymphoblastic leukemia. *J Nucl Med* 1997;38:82–88.

189. Komatsu K, Takada G, Uemura K, et al. Decrease in cerebral metabolic rate of glucose after high-dose methotrexate in childhood acute lymphocytic leukemia. *Pediatr Neurol* 1990; 303–306.

190. Phillips PC, Moeller JR, Sidtis JJ, et al. Abnormal cerebral glucose metabolism in long-term survivors of childhood acute lymphocytic leukemia. *Ann Neurol* 1991;29:263–271.

191. Shulkin BL, Chang E, Strouse PJ, et al. PET FDG studies of Wilms' tumors. *J Pediatr Hematol Oncol* 1997;19:334–338.

192. Donaldson SS, Eghert PR, Newsham I, et al. Retinoblastoma. In: Pizzo PA, Poplack DG, eds. *Principles and practice of pediatric oncology*, 3rd ed. Philadelphia: Lippincott–Raven Publishers, 1997:699–716.

193. Robson CD, Kim FM, Barnes PD. Head and neck. In: Kirks DR, ed. *Practical pediatric imaging. Diagnostic radiology of infants and children*, 3rd ed. Philadelphia: Lippincott–Raven Publishers, 1997:201–325.

194. Bomanji J, Kingston JE, Hungerford JL, et al. ^{123}I-metaiodobenzylguanidine scintigraphy of ectopic intracranial retinoblastoma. *Med Pediatr Oncol* 1989;17:66–68.

195. Bomanji J, Hungerford JL, Kingston JE, et al. ^{123}I-metaiodobenzylguanidine (MIBG) scintigraphy of retinoblastoma: preliminary experience. *Br J Ophthalmol* 1989;73:146–150.

196. Pratt CB, Crom DB, Magill L, et al. Skeletal scintigraphy in patients with bilateral retinoblastoma. *Cancer* 1990;65:26–28.

8

CARDIOTOXICITY IN CANCER THERAPY

JEAN C. MAUBLANT
FRANCESCO GIAMMARILE
MARC FERRIERE

Cardiotoxicity ranks among the leading side effects of cancer therapy, and it must be considered against the oncologic risk because it can produce greater morbidity than the cancer itself. Myocardial toxicity is primarily related to chemotherapy with anthracyclines or anthracycline-like drugs, but it also can occur following external radiation therapy of the cardiac region. Scintigraphy plays an important role in the early detection of cardiotoxicity, influencing proper treatment.

CARDIOTOXICITY OF ANTHRACYCLINES

Anthracyclines are chemotherapeutic agents with well-documented efficacy in adults and children against a wide range of solid neoplasms and hematologic malignancies. The most responsive are breast and esophageal carcinomas, sarcomas, and lymphomas, but digestive and endometrial carcinomas are also good indications for its use. The leading compound with the widest tumoricidal effect in this class of drugs is doxorubicin, with a response rate of 40% in patients who have not undergone prior chemotherapy (1). However, the efficacy of anthracyclines is limited by two major factors: (a) development of resistance that generally extends to other agents (multidrug resistance), and (b) development of a frequently fatal dose-dependent cardiac toxicity.

The cardiotoxic effects of doxorubicin have been known since the first clinical trials (2). Unlike the other complications of this treatment, which include stomatitis, nausea, vomiting, and alopecia, cardiac toxicity is generally irreversible. Although studies involving several hundreds and even thousands of patients have been performed, the exact incidence remains imprecise because of the lack of standardized long-term follow-up studies and a lack of homogeneity in regard to methodology, patient inclusion criteria, methods

J. C. Maublant: Division of Nuclear Medicine, Anticancer Centre Jean Perrin; Department of Biophysics, Auvergne University, 63011 Clermont-Ferrand, France.

F. Giammarile: Division of Nuclear Medicine, Centre Leon Berard, 69373 Lyon, France.

M. Ferriere: Division of Cardiology, University Hospital Arnaud de Villeneuve, 34295 Montpellier, France.

of evaluating cardiac function, and duration of follow-up. Moreover, the development of cardiotoxicity is characterized by marked individual variations, particularly in children (3).

Cardiac complications of doxorubicin can appear at any stage during the course of therapy and can be divided into acute, subacute, and chronic effects. Acute and subacute effects are dose-independent. Acute effects are very rare but severe. They occur around the time of infusion and involve mainly supraventricular arrythmias (rarely significant) and myopericarditis. Symptoms are usually delayed and appear progressively. Subacute effects are also uncommon and are represented by transient episodes of left ventricular dysfunction or episodes of pericarditis/myocarditis. The mean incidence of these various cardiac complications is 16% (4) to 23% (5).

The most frequent and clinically significant complications are chronic, mainly a dose-dependent, generally irreversible cardiomyopathy that is followed by congestive heart failure associated with elevated diastolic and pulmonary capillary pressures and a decreased cardiac output. The median time interval between anthracycline infusion and the first signs of cardiac insufficiency is between 2 and 3 months (6), but complications can be delayed for up to 20 years (7). In a retrospective study of 6,493 children, 90% of the cardiac complications, which involved 1.6% of the overall population, occurred within 1 year after completion of the anthracycline treatment (8). In adults, an incidence of 23% has been reported during a 20-year follow-up (7).

The cumulative dose plays a major role in the occurrence of cardiac toxicity; the threshold dose is 550 mg/m^2 of body surface area, although histologic damage and cardiac insufficiency have been described for lower doses (9). In a single study, the risk for development of congestive heart failure was about 3% with a dose in the range of 450 to 550 mg/m^2, but it rose to 18% with a cumulative dose of 551 to 600 mg/m^2 and to 36% for higher doses (10). With doses higher than 500 mg/m^2 (in a follow-up lasting more than 10-years), abnormal cardiac findings were detected in 63% of 201 patients (7). Alterations of myocardial histology are always present at cumulative doses higher than 200 or 250 mg/m^2. These alterations occur two to three times faster for doses of more than 400 mg/m², although wide individual variations are observed.

MECHANISMS OF ANTHRACYCLINE CARDIOTOXICITY

Doxorubicin-induced cell injury is recognized at histology as loss of myofibrils and vacuolization of cytoplasm. Although the exact mechanism by which the cardiac toxicity of the iron-chelating doxorubicin is induced is still not fully understood (11), production of oxygen free radicals appears to play a predominant role. Indeed, in addition to causing DNA damage, such as binding, alkylation, or cross-linking leading to inhibition of topoisomerase II, doxorubicin also generates free radicals, such as superoxide and hydrogen peroxide, which are believed to be responsible for its antitumor activity as well as its cumulative dose-related cardiotoxicity. In the same way, cardiac production of endogenous antioxidants such as glutathione peroxidase is impaired, so that the development of an oxidative stress is favored, to which the myocardium is particularly responsive. Possibly through the same biochemical effects, lipid metabolism is also linked to doxorubicin efficacy and cardiotoxicity; for instance, increased levels of myocardial and plasma lipids have been reported with doxorubicin therapy. Conversely, a protective cardiac effect has been observed with dexrazoxane (12) and with the antioxidant and lipid-lowering agent probucol in animals (13). This opens interesting perspectives to adjunctive therapy.

MANAGEMENT OF ANTHRACYCLINE CARDIOTOXICITY

During and after doxorubicin treatment, clinical and electrocardiographic signs of doxorubicin-induced cardiomyopathy and congestive heart failure (e.g., gallop rhythms, jugular vein distention, T-wave flattening, prolongation of the QT interval, loss of R-wave voltage) are not specific, but their sudden occurrence should suggest the diagnosis. Morphologic evaluation of endomyocardial biopsy specimens is the most sensitive, specific, and unquestioned method of determining the extent of cardiotoxicity; however, this method is invasive, expensive, and not available everywhere. Cardiac systolic dysfunction can be detected through measurement of the left ventricular ejection fraction (LVEF), which is considered to be the most useful functional parameter. A robust, precise, and reproducible method is therefore necessary.

Prevention is based first on a proper knowledge of anthracycline cardiotoxicity. It is also based on the detection of patients at higher risk for the development of congestive heart failure than the general population. Risk factors include age above 70 years, history of hypertension, prior mediastinal radiotherapy, or cardiotoxic chemotherapy. The presence of a documented cardiomyopathy is not an absolute contraindication to therapy so long as the LVEF is not lower than 50%, assuming that the normal value is in the range of 60% to 65%. In the absence of any of these factors, other abnormalities can be detected through "complementary tests," such as cardiac hypertrophy on chest roentgenography, rhythm or conduction abnormalities on electrocardiography, or impaired systolic function of the left ventricle, encountered in 5% to 10% of asymptomatic patients.

In practice, after initial staging, some patients should fall into one of three groups. (a) The first group comprises patients with an absolute *contraindication* to doxorubicin treatment: cardiac insufficiency documented by an LVEF below 45% or related to previous anthracycline therapy. (b) The second group includes patients at *high risk*. It is recommended that the frequency of LVEF measurement be increased once the dose limit of 300 mg/m² has been reached. This procedure must be repeated at each treatment if the LVEF has decreased or if the cumulative dose has reached 400 mg/m². From the start of treatment, the cardiologist can administer a continuous intravenous infusion over 6 hours rather than a bolus injection. This significantly decreases the risk for cardiotoxicity. The most efficient criteria on which to base a decision to interrupt chemotherapy appear to be a decline of more than 10% in LVEF between two treatments plus a residual value of less than 50% (4), or 45% for some authors (5). The presence of only one of these two abnormalities requires evaluation before each successive treatment. (c) The third group comprises patients for whom *long-term, high-dose chemotherapy* is planned. An intravenous continuous infusion is indicated, but it is also necessary to assess cardiac function at each successive treatment once the dose of 450 mg/m² has been reached. A second LVEF measurement must be performed at the end of treatment. If the LVEF is normal, it is not necessary to follow these patients further because clinical cardiac insufficiency will subsequently develop in very few of them. If the LVEF is altered, it must be measured again 1 year later because a further decrease will occur in about 30% of patients, possibly with the appearance of clinical signs. In children, a repeated evaluation is mandatory at 6 months or 1 year. If the LVEF is normal, it should be checked every 3 to 5 years.

Once cardiomyopathy and congestive heart failure become clinically apparent, medical treatment with digitalis, beta blockers, diuretics, and angiotensin-converting enzyme inhibitors produces only transient effects and is overall not effective. Fatal congestive heart failure eventually develops in about one third of these patients within a short time after onset of symptoms. Previous mediastinal irradiation increases the risk for death related to congestive heart failure and decreases the median survival time (14). The combination of doxorubicin with taxane has been reported to enhance the risk for congestive heart failure by increasing plasma retention of doxorubicin by approximately 30% (15).

Continuous infusion has been shown to be less cardiotoxic than the usual bolus injection (16). Doxorubicin derivatives such as epirubicin, with a lower cardiotoxicity, have also been tested. In 285 patients, congestive heart failure occurred less often (4.4%) than in doxorubicin-treated patients (13.4%) (17). The cumulative risk was 4% at 900 mg/m^2 and increased exponentially to 15% at 1,000 mg/m^2 (18). In an effort to lower the administered dose, doxorubicin has also been administered concurrently with other cytotoxic drugs, such as cyclophosphamide and 5-fluorouracil.

If not detected in time, cardiac complications can eventually cause more morbidity than the treated tumor. If cardiac involvement is detected early, in particular through LVEF evaluation, doxorubicin can be discontinued and the cardiac impairment stabilized (4,19). For example, in the study of Schwartz et al. (4), the incidence of congestive heart failure was significantly lower in patients managed properly than in patients in whom these criteria were not applied (2.9% vs. 20.8%, respectively; *p* < .001). Prevention and early detection of cardiac toxicity in patients for whom anthracycline therapy is being planned is therefore of major importance. Because this complication can also occur in patients without risk factors who are treated with doses smaller than 500 mg/m^2, continuous cardiac monitoring and follow-up are important for all patients.

NONINVASIVE EVALUATION OF LEFT VENTRICULAR FUNCTION

Cardiac gated blood pool scintigraphy (GBPS) at equilibrium with the use of ^{99m}Tc-labeled red blood cells has long been recognized as a precise and reproducible method to measure LVEF; echocardiography is an alternative approach. GBPS is a standard scintigraphic procedure that will not be described here. High-quality acquisition and a validated computer program are central to obtaining a reliable and reproducible LVEF measurement. Careful selection of the best septal left anterior oblique projection is important. Angulation parameters must be noted in the patient's file so that the same acquisition can be reproduced during follow-up. A database of normal LVEF values helps define the threshold of abnormality in each center. The LVEF can also be measured with the nuclear stethoscope, a nonimaging, ambulatory device (20).

The choice of method is guided by several criteria: availability of the technique, patient echogenicity, reproducibility of the measurement, and experience of the technical staff. In any case, a baseline study is necessary. Echocardiography is generally preferred in children and for frequent evaluations. It is easier to perform, although more time-consuming for the physician, and is less expensive than GBPS. Scintigraphy is not hampered by poor echogenicity and has a higher rate of reproducibility. It is important to utilize the same technique throughout follow-up. It has been proposed that echocardiography be used in children whose dose is below 300 mg/m^2 and during the first year of follow-up, and that GBPS be used for patients who have received higher doses and for follow-up after 1 year (3).

With either echocardiography or GBPS, LVEF is the most important parameter; a value of 65 ± 5% is considered normal, and signs of heart failure with a fall below 45% or a decrease of more than 10% between two consecutive measurements are considered to represent cardiotoxicity. Parameters of diastolic function are sensitive indicators of early cardiac toxicity. With echocardiography, several parameters of diastolic function have been found to deteriorate before parameters of systolic function (21). With GBPS, the peak filling rate appeared to be more sensitive than LVEF in several studies (22,23). Other parameters, such as the one-third peak filling rate and one-third filling fraction, have been found to be significantly decreased in patients treated with anthracyclines whose LVEF was not altered, suggesting silent myocardial damage (24). This is at variance with a report in which the development of diastolic dysfunction before systolic dysfunction was uncommon (25); others have observed a simultaneous impairment of diastolic and systolic left ventricular function between baseline measurement and 1- or 12-month follow-up (26, 27). There is no consensus regarding which parameter is most useful in the evaluation of diastolic function. Several methods of normalizing the parameters have been proposed (e.g., by heart rate, end-diastolic volume, LVEF, or peak ejection rate). Overall, the assessment of diastolic function requires further confirmatory studies before the LVEF measurement can be replaced.

Apparent improvement in echographic parameters of left ventricular contractility during the 6-month period following discontinuation of anthracycline has been reported in children (28), but this seems to be only a temporary rebound effect.

Other imaging tests, such as scintigraphy with ^{111}In-antimyosin antibodies or ^{123}I-metaiodobenzylguanidine, have been reported to be useful in cases of anthracycline cardiotoxicity. Uptake of antimyosin antibodies is related to the extent and severity of damage and precedes LVEF abnormalities (29), but such relatively complex procedures cannot be used as routine screening tests.

MYOCARDIAL DAMAGE AFTER EXTERNAL RADIATION THERAPY

Myocardial damage is a possible complication in patients who have received therapeutic doses of mediastinal irradiation for lymphoma, or adjuvant radiotherapy to the internal mammary chain after mastectomy for left-sided breast cancer. It is probably secondary to ischemia resulting from microvascular damage at the capillary level, which can sometimes lead to fibrosis and progressive cardiac dysfunction (30). Conflicting data have been reported in the literature on the incidence of this complication, probably because its onset is much less dramatic than that of radiotherapy-induced pericarditis (31). It may not develop for several years after irradiation has been completed. Associated factors, such as clinical or subclinical thyroid or pulmonary disease, can also contribute to the appearance of cardiopathy. Even while cardiac function remains generally normal (32), perfusion scintigraphy with ^{201}Tl or with ^{99m}Tc-labeled agents to image blood flow can detect radiation-induced abnormalities, particularly during exercise and predominantly on the anterior wall (30,33). The possible role of myocardial irradiation in the development of coronary artery disease remains unknown. In practice, many believe that a cardiac risk does exist and try to optimize the irradiation technique by utilizing computed tomography to define the target. Long-term follow-up and a reduction of associated risk factors is encouraged for these patients.

It is important that specialists in nuclear medicine be aware of the central role that scintigraphy plays in the management of cardiotoxicity induced by anthracycline treatment, a major form of chemotherapy. High-quality and reproducible procedures to measure LVEF will ensure the best compromise between tumoricidal effect and cardiotoxicity.

REFERENCES

1. Weiss RB. The anthracyclines: will we ever find a better doxorubicin? *Semin Oncol* 1992;19:670–686.
2. Tan C, Tasaka H, Yu KP, et al. Daunomycin, an antitumor antibiotic, in the treatment of neoplastic disease. *Cancer* 1967;20: 333–353.
3. Steinherz LJ, Graham T, Hurwitz R, et al. Guidelines for cardiac monitoring of children during and after anthracycline therapy: report of the Cardiology Committee of the Children's Cancer Study Group. *Pediatrics* 1992;89:942–949.
4. Schwartz RG, McKenzie WB, Alexander J, et al. Congestive heart failure and left ventricular dysfunction complicating doxorubicin therapy. Seven-year experience using serial radionuclide angiocardiography. *Am J Med* 1987;82:1109–1118.
5. Venturini M, Michelotti A, Del Mastro L, et al. Multicenter randomized controlled clinical trial to evaluate cardioprotection of dexrazoxane versus no cardioprotection in women receiving epirubicin chemotherapy for advanced breast cancer. *J Clin Oncol* 1996; 14:3112–3120.
6. Ferriere M, Donadio D, Ramirez R. Cardiotoxicity of anthracyclines. *Arch Mal Coeur* 1993;86:53–58.
7. Steinherz LJ, Steinherz PG, Tan CT, et al. Cardiac toxicity 4 to 20 years after completing anthracycline therapy. *JAMA* 1991;266: 1672–1677.
8. Krischer JP, Epstein S, Cuthbertson DD, et al. Clinical cardiotoxicity following anthracycline treatment for childhood cancer: the Pediatric Oncology Group experience. *J Clin Oncol* 1997;15: 1544–1552.
9. Billingham ME, Mason JW, Bristow MR, et al. Anthracycline cardiomyopathy monitored by morphologic changes. *Cancer Treat Rep* 1978;62:865–872.
10. Lefrak EA, Pitha J, Rosenheim S, et al. A clinicopathologic analysis of Adriamycin cardiotoxicity. *Cancer* 1973;32:302–314.
11. Gewirtz DA. A critical evaluation of the mechanisms of action proposed for the antitumor effects of the anthracyclines antibiotics Adriamycin and daunorubicin. *Biochem Pharmacol* 1999; 57:727–741.
12. Wiseman LR, Spencer CM. Dexrazoxane: a review of its use as a cardioprotective agent in patients receiving anthracycline-based chemotherapy. *Drugs* 1998;56:385–403.
13. Iliskovic N, Li T, Khaper N, et al. Modulation of Adriamycin-induced changes in serum free fatty acids, albumin and cardiac oxidative stress. *Mol Cell Biochem* 1998;188:161–166.
14. Shapiro CL, Hardenbergh PH, Gelman R, et al. Cardiac effects of adjuvant doxorubicin and radiation therapy in breast cancer patients. *J Clin Oncol* 1998;16:3493–3501.
15. Martin M, Lluch A, Ojeda B, et al. Paclitaxel plus doxorubicin in metastatic breast cancer: preliminary analysis of cardiotoxicity. *Semin Oncol* 1997;24:S17-26–S17-30.
16. Shapira J, Gotfried M, Lishner M, et al. Reduced cardiotoxicity of doxorubicin by a 6-hour infusion regimen: a prospective randomized evaluation. *Cancer* 1990;65:870–873.
17. Mouridsen HT, Alfthan C, Bastholt L, et al. Current status of epirubicin (Farmorubicin) in the treatment of solid tumours. *Acta Oncol* 1990;29:257–285.
18. Ryberg M, Nielsen D, Skovsgaard T, et al. Epirubicin cardiotoxicity: an analysis of 469 patients with metastatic breast cancer. *J Clin Oncol* 1998;16:3502–3508.
19. Alexander J, Dainiak N, Berger HJ, et al. Serial assessment of doxorubicin cardiotoxicity with quantitative radionuclide angiocardiography. *N Engl J Med* 1979;8:278–283.
20. Wagner HN Jr, Rigo P, Baxter RH, et al. Monitoring ventricular function at rest and during exercise with a nonimaging nuclear detector. *Am J Cardiol* 1979;43:975–979.
21. Schmitt K, Tulzer G, Merl M, et al. Early detection of doxorubicin and daunorubicin cardiotoxicity by echocardiography: diastolic versus systolic parameters. *Eur J Pediatr* 1995;154:201–204.
22. Ganz WI, Sridhar KS, Forness TJ. Detection of early anthracycline cardiotoxicity by monitoring the peak filling rate. *Am J Clin Oncol* 1993;16:109–112.
23. Cottin Y, Touzery C, Dalloz F, et al. Comparison of epirubicin and doxorubicin cardiotoxicity induced by low doses: evolution of the diastolic and systolic parameters studied by radionuclide angiography. *Clin Cardiol* 1998;21:665–670.
24. Suzuki J, Yanagisawa A, Shigeyama T, et al. Early detection of anthracycline-induced cardiotoxicity by radionuclide angiocardiography. *Angiology* 1999;50:37–45.
25. Parmentier S, Melin JA, Piret L, et al. Assessment of left ventricular diastolic function in patients receiving anthracycline therapy. *Eur J Nucl Med* 1988;13:563–567.
26. Cottin Y, Touzery C, Coudert B, et al. Impairment of diastolic function during short-term anthracycline chemotherapy. *Br Heart J* 1995;73:61–64.
27. Cottin Y, Touzery C, Coudert B, et al. Diastolic or systolic left and right ventricular impairment at moderate doses of anthracycline? A 1-year follow-up study of women. *Eur J Nucl Med* 1996; 23:511–516.
28. Lewis AB, Crouse VL, Evans W, et al. Recovery of left ventricular function following discontinuation of anthracycline chemotherapy in children. *Pediatrics* 1981;68:67–72.
29. Estorch M, Carrio I, Berna L, et al. Indium-111-antimyosin scintigraphy after doxorubicin therapy in patients with advanced breast cancer. *J Nucl Med* 1990;31:1965–1969.
30. Cowen D, Gonzague-Casabianca L, Brenot-Rossi I, et al. Thallium-201 perfusion scintigraphy in the evaluation of late myocar-

dial damage in left-side breast cancer treated with adjuvant radiotherapy. *Int J Radiat Oncol Biol Phys* 1998;41:809–815.

31. Gyenes G, Fornander T, Carlens P, et al. Morbidity of ischemic heart disease in early breast cancer 15 to 20 years after adjuvant radiotherapy. *Int J Radiat Oncol Biol Phys* 1994;28:1235–1241.

32. Gustavsson A, Bendahl PO, Cwikiel M, et al. No serious late effects after adjuvant radiotherapy following mastectomy in premenopausal women with early breast cancer. *Int J Radiat Oncol Biol Phys* 1999;43:745–754.

33. Gyenes G, Fornander T, Carlens P, Glas U, Rutqvist LE. Detection of radiation-induced myocardial damage by technetium-99m sestamibi scintigraphy. Eur J Nucl Med 1997;24:286–292.

9

NEPHROTOXICITY IN CANCER THERAPY

GARY F. GATES

Cancer has been a challenge for physicians since the dawn of medicine. Initially, surgery was the only hope for cure. Roentgen's discovery of x-rays in 1895 and the Curies' discovery of radium in 1898 led to the eventual use of radiation as a treatment for malignancy. A stroke of fortune occurred during a systemic analysis of nitrogen mustards in 1942 when a tumor-bearing mouse responded to mustard, showing the potential beneficial effects of this agent. The first patient treated had Hodgkin's disease, which responded, albeit temporarily. Thus, the era of chemotherapy had begun.

Undesirable side effects of radiation and chemotherapy were soon evident and presented complex challenges. The toxicity of cancer chemotherapy agents exceeds that of any other pharmacologic group and limits the use of these drugs. Radiation can also produce adverse results, but these are usually confined to the region being treated, unlike the effects of chemotherapy, which are systemic and widespread. Kidney function can be reduced by radiation or chemotherapy, and changes may range from minor and subclinical to devastating and life-threatening. Radiation and chemotherapy have different nephropathic effects, but a compounding effect may occur when both are used in the same patient.

RADIATION THERAPY

Radiation effects are categorized as acute, subacute, or late, depending on the time elapsing from irradiation to the presentation of symptoms. Acute changes occur within hours to days following radiation and involve tissues with a rapid cell turnover, such as gastrointestinal mucosa, bone marrow, skin, and testis (germinal cells). Subacute changes occur several months after exposure and are caused by failure of a critical cell line having a longer turnover time than the cells involved in acute responses. These changes occur during the remodeling phase in irradiated tissue and include conditions such as subacute radiation pneumonitis, which occurs 2 to 3 months after the start of lung radiation. Late effects develop months to years following irradiation and are caused by progressive damage secondary to depletion of slowly proliferating crucial cell lines; affected tissues include the endothelium of the blood vessels and renal tubules. Any tissue can exhibit both acute and late changes, depending on the affected cell type, and acute injury can result in chronic fibrosis, atrophy, and ulceration.

Radiation nephropathy is generally a late consequence of fractionated therapy; it affects the glomeruli and tubules, producing fibrosis and vascular lesions that result in renal atrophy. Fibrosis is one of the most common delayed consequences of irradiation and can result in urinary strictures. Vascular lesions are found more often in capillaries or sinusoids than in larger vessels because of the sensitivity of endothelial cells, which are the most important part of the walls of these small vessels. The radiosensitivity of arteries is less than that of capillaries, and veins are affected least. Glomerular tufts show increased density, altered nuclei, and reduced capillary lumina. Eventually, atrophy and fibrosis affect glomeruli and tubules.

Radiation-induced renal changes initially occur in the arteriolar–glomerular area and are caused by endothelial vascular cell injury, which precedes tubular damage (1). A progressive, dose-related glomerulosclerosis is marked by thickening of afferent arterioles (2). Medullary tubules are less involved than cortical ones. This initial effect is associated with a reduction of total capillary blood flow, measured by rubidium 86 (3). Larger arteries are not affected even though glomeruli are being lost, which likely reflects the relative radiosensitivity of these vascular structures; however, arterial damage can eventually occur as a consequence of hypertension. Thus, the functional changes of radiation nephropathy are the result of vascular injury of glomerular capillaries and afferent arterioles, which occurs before tubular depletion (4). This process is the reverse of the usual nephrotoxic effects of chemotherapy, which are mainly tubular, and underscores the potential toxic effects

G. F. Gates: Department of Diagnostic Radiology, Oregon Health Science University School of Medicine, Portland, Oregon 97201; Department of Nuclear Medicine, Providence St. Vincent Medical Center, Portland, Oregon 97225.

of combined therapy with drugs such as cisplatin. The sequence of chemotherapy and radiation therapy is important, as was demonstrated in a rat model, which showed more nephrotoxic effects when cisplatin was given before radiation than after (5). Several drugs may promote radiation nephropathy, such as dactinomycin, vincristine, cyclophosphamide, and doxorubicin, used in the treatment of Wilms' tumor (4), or combination therapies of actinomycin D and vincristine or vinblastine and bleomycin (6).

The radiation tolerance of tissue depends on target cell radiosensitivity and also on the number of target cells in the functional units being irradiated. The nephron is the functional unit for the kidney, and its tubule cannot regenerate if it is completely deepithelialized. Thus, tolerance to renal radiation is determined by the number of tubule cells per nephron. Histologic evidence for renal tubular cell depletion may be lacking for many months after irradiation, after which a long time (months to more than a year) elapses before the onset of repopulation. Tissue tolerance to radiation is expressed as $TD_{5/5}$ or $TD_{50/5}$, which are guidelines for determining the consequences of a specific radiation dose in terms of the 5% ($TD_{5/5}$) or 50% ($TD_{50/5}$) incidence of an adverse effect at 5 years (7). Renal $TD_{5/5}$ tolerance is 20 Gy (2,000 rads) when both kidneys are irradiated according to Cassady (8), who also published renal dose–response curves indicating the initial threshold for radiation injury to be 15 Gy, with a nearly linear increase thereafter to a plateau at 30 Gy, at which point the incidence of radiation injury is 100%. Philips (9) reported a 5% risk of radiation nephropathy after 20 Gy; this increased to 50% after 25 Gy, which is close to the 2,300 rad (23 Gy) reported by Schilsky (6) as the level above which radiation nephritis occurs.

Various clinical syndromes appear following radiation therapy (10). Acute changes (before 6 months) are usually not symptomatic; at first, the glomerular filtration rate (GFR) and renal plasma flow (usually expressed as effective renal plasma flow, or ERPF) are increased because of glomerular vasodilation and permeability, which occur as an initial radiation response; later, both decrease following tuft scarring (11). Subacute changes (6 to 12 months) result in increased fluid retention, dyspnea on exertion, hypertension, anemia, elevated serum creatinine, albuminuria, and abnormal findings on urinalysis, which shows microscopic hematuria and granular or hyaline casts. Chronic or late changes (usually 18 months following therapy) may present as hypertension, the severity depending on the degree of renal dysfunction. The mildest and most delayed form of chronic radiation nephropathy (up to 10 years or more after irradiation) is "hyperreninemic hypertension," which develops secondary to a Goldbatt kidney. Exceptions to this outline of clinical syndromes occur when acute nephritis results in renal failure or infection complicates chronic radiation nephritis.

CHEMOTHERAPY

Toxic responses to chemotherapy can be life-threatening and may limit drug use. Some adverse effects are organ-specific (e.g., nephrotoxic), whereas others are less specific (e.g., hypersensitivity reactions, vascular toxicity). This section initially addresses the direct nephrotoxic and metabolic effects of chemotherapy drugs, after which hypersensitivity reactions and the vascular toxicity of nephrotoxic drugs are discussed.

Direct Nephrotoxic and Metabolic Effects

Nephrotoxicity results in reduced renal function with metabolic and electrolyte complications. Renal tubular injuries are more common than glomerular damage and result in renal failure and decreasing creatinine clearance rather than in hypertension and proteinuria (4). Proximal tubular dysfunction can result in aminoaciduria, phosphaturia, increased urate excretion, acidosis, glucosuria, hypokalemia, hypomagnesemia with hypocalcemia, and renal sodium wasting. Distal tubular dysfunction results in polyuria and renal tubular acidosis. Some patients may have symptomatic hyponatremia caused by to the syndrome of inappropriate secretion of antidiuretic hormone (SIADH) (12–14).

In patients with either a large tumor mass or rapidly proliferating lesions (e.g., Burkitt's lymphoma, diffuse histiocytic lymphoma, acute leukemia), rapid cell lysis may follow chemotherapy and result in elevated serum levels of uric acid, which is cleared by the kidneys. Hyperuricemic nephropathy develops when conditions of a low urine pH and preexisting renal dysfunction result in the precipitation of uric acid crystals in the distal renal tubules and collecting ducts to produce intrarenal obstruction (6,13). This complication can be reduced by intravenous hydration to maintain a high rate of urine flow, alkalinization of the urine (pH $\geq$ 7.0), and the use of allopurinol to inhibit uric acid formation. Allopurinol is not risk-free and can lead to the precipitation of oxypurinol or xanthine crystals with stone formation or occasionally cause acute interstitial nephritis.

"Rapid tumor lysis syndrome," the consequence of a massive release of intracellular ions following tumor cell lysis, results in electrolyte and metabolic disturbances (6,13). Severe hyperkalemia, hyperphosphatemia, and hypocalcemia may occur within 24 hours after initiation of chemotherapy and can be rapidly fatal. The presence of hyperuricemic nephropathy, azotemia, bulky tumors, or ureteral obstruction increases the likelihood of this syndrome, which ordinarily lasts only 5 to 7 days after the start of chemotherapy, as the period of rapid cytolysis is finite.

The features of some of the many nephrotoxic chemotherapeutic drugs (6,12–15) are summarized below:

- Nitrosoureas. Streptozotocin, lomustine (CCNU), and carmustine (BCNU) are nitrosoureas. Streptozotocin damages the proximal tubules to produce tubulointerstitial nephritis and renal atrophy. Hypokalemia, proximal renal tubular acidosis, Fanconi's syndrome (aminoaciduria, phosphaturia, glycosuria), and diminished renal function occur. Nephrotoxicity is a dose-limiting effect of this agent. CCNU and BCNU may produce similar injuries of chronic interstitial nephritis and renal failure.

- Cisplatin (CDDP). Nephrotoxicity is a dose-limiting side effect of CDDP. The presentation can be acute or chronic. Proximal and distal tubular necrosis can be extensive, with relatively less glomerular damage. Acute injury tends to occur in inadequately hydrated patients. Electrolyte abnormalities also develop, including hypomagnesemia, hypocalcemia, and renal sodium wasting. Preexisting renal disease or the simultaneous administration of other nephrotoxic drugs may result in an increased risk for renal failure. Cisplatin nephrotoxicity can be reduced by amifostine (16,17), a sulfhydryl compound that does not protect tumors from the cytotoxic effects of cisplatin. Sodium thiosulfate (17) is used with intraperitoneal cisplatin therapy to protect the patient from the nephrotoxic effects of absorbed cisplatin. Mesna is a second-generation agent used to protect against the toxic monohydroxy monochloro species of cisplatin without reducing its therapeutic benefit (17). CDDP has also been associated with thrombotic microangiopathic syndrome, a vascular toxicity.
- Carboplatin is a cisplatin analogue associated with less nephrotoxicity and hypomagnesemia. Thrombotic microangiopathic syndrome occurs
- Methotrexate does not directly damage the kidneys, but more than 90% is eliminated by renal excretion, and it can precipitate in renal tubules and collecting ducts to result in reduced renal function. This effect is diminished by diuresis and urine alkalinization during administration.
- Mitomycin C may cause renal failure in up to 40% of patients by damaging the proximal and distal tubules or inducing the thrombotic microangiopathic syndrome.
- Cyclophosphamide. Impaired water excretion and secondary dilutional hyponatremia may be caused either by a direct toxic effect on the distal renal tubules and collecting ducts or by SIADH. The effect is symptomatic hyponatremia resulting from water intoxication. Nephrogenic diabetes insipidus has also been reported. A further complication is hemorrhagic cystitis.
- Ifosfamide. This alkylating agent is an analogue of cyclophosphamide and commonly produces proximal tubular injury that results in renal tubular acidosis, hypokalemia, and Fanconi's syndrome of glycosuria, aminoaciduria, and phosphaturia. Ifosfamide can also cause hypophosphatemic rickets in children. Distal renal tubular damage and nephrogenic diabetes insipidus have been reported, in addition to SIADH. Mild reductions in the GFR occur commonly; acute renal failure is seen less often. Sometimes, chronic renal failure develops, requiring dialysis. Ifosfamide is also urotoxic and causes hemorrhagic cystitis; mesna is used to protect against this but does not prevent nephrotoxicity.
- Vincristine may be associated with severe hyponatremia and sodium wasting or SIADH.
- Bleomycin does not have any significant direct nephrotoxic effects but is associated with fevers following administration and thrombotic microangiopathic syndrome.
- L-Asparaginase. Azotemia can occur, but its cause is unclear. This agent is associated with the highest incidence of hypersensitivity reactions.
- Mithramycin. Azotemia develops in up to 40% of patients as a result of necrosis of the proximal and distal tubules.
- Interleukin 2 (IL-2). Severe, but not necessarily permanent, nephrotoxicity occurs as a consequence of reduced renal perfusion and direct tubular injury. Electrolyte abnormalities include hypokalemia, hypomagnesemia, hypophosphatemia, and hypocalcemia.

Hypersensitivy Reactions

Hypersensitivity reactions may follow the administration of chemotherapeutic drugs and have been classified into four types (18) (Table 9.1). Some reactions are immunologic in origin and others are not; often, the mechanism of the reaction is unknown. All four types of hypersensitivity reactions

TABLE 9.1. CLASSIFICATION OF HYPERSENSITIVE REACTIONS

	Clinical signs and symptoms	Mechanism
Type 1	Urticaria, angioedema, rash, bronchospasm, abdominal cramping, hypotension	Degranulation of mast cells and basophils releasing histamine; complement activation producing anaphylatoxins; neurogenic release of vasoactive substances
Type 2	Hemolytic anemia	Antibody reacts with cell-bound antigen and activates complement
Type 3	Tissue injury resulting from deposition of immune complexes	Tissue deposition of antigen-antibody complexes that form intravascularly
Type 4	Contact dermatitis, homograft rejection, formation of granuloma	Lymphokine release from sensitized T lymphocytes following antigenic reaction

From Gell PGH, Coombs RRA. *Clinical aspects of immunology.* Oxford: Blackwell Science, 1975, with permission (18).

can occur with chemotherapeutic agents (19,20) except the nitrosoureas, altretamine, and dactinomycin. Type 1 reactions are the most common; some are IgE-mediated, whereas others are caused by the release of vasoactive substances from mast cells and basophils. L-Asparaginase and mitomycin (when instilled into the bladder) are associated with the highest frequency of hypersensitivity reactions. The incidence and type of reaction vary, as summarized below (in decreasing frequency) for some commonly used nephrotoxic drugs.

- L-Asparaginase is the agent associated with the highest risk for hypersensitivity reactions, with a dose-related incidence of type 1 reactions of up to 43%.
- Cisplatin and analogues have a dose-related incidence of type 1 and type 2 reactions of 6% to 14%.
- Methotrexate and analogues produce occasional type 1 and type 3 hypersensitivity reactions.
- Cyclophosphamide causes occasional type 1 reactions.
- Ifosfamide and mesna. Ifosfamide causes a chemical cystitis, and mesna is administered at the same time to minimize this toxicity, but both agents can produce type 1 reactions.
- Mitomycin. No type 1 reactions have been reported when mitomycin is given intravenously, but type 4 hypersensitivity reactions in the form of contact dermatitis occur in up to 10% of patients following postvoiding skin contamination when this agent is used to treat bladder cancer by topical administration.
- Bleomycin. Fevers (with rare constitutional symptoms of hypotension, delirium, and death) commonly occur after administration and have been described as "anaphylactic" reactions, but these by definition are related to IgE-mediated release of vasoactive substances after an interval of sensitization. Bleomycin-induced symptoms are not caused by any of the four types of hypersensitivity reactions, nor are they immunologically mediated; they are the result of a direct release of pyrogens and in some instances may be associated angioedema and erythematous rash.

Vascular Toxicity

Chemotherapy can be associated with vascular toxicity syndromes (21), some of which affect specific organs (e.g., venoocclusive disease of the lungs and liver); others, like hypotension or hypertension, are less specific. Several mechanisms have been proposed to account for vascular toxicity, including (a) direct damage to endothelial cells secondary to chemotherapeutic drugs or their metabolites; (b) drug-induced changes of the clotting system or platelet activation; (c) hypomagnesemia as a causative factor in the development of vasospasm; and (d) autonomic neuropathy and dysfunction enhancing arterial vasospasm. Several of these possibilities may be in effect simultaneously, or,

on the other hand, the syndromes may be caused by the underlying malignancy and not the chemotherapeutic drugs at all. Two of these syndromes directly affect the kidneys:

- Thrombotic microangiopathic syndrome comprises the clinical triad of microangiopathic hemolytic anemia, thrombocytopenia, and renal insufficiency and is usually fatal within a few months after diagnosis as a result of renal failure. Abnormalities in the renal vasculature are the principal histopathologic findings; these include fibrin deposition and endothelial proliferation in glomerular capillaries and afferent arterioles along with thickening of glomerular basement membranes and glomerular infarcts with necrosis. Ninety percent of these patients have adenocarcinomas; tumors of the stomach, breast, and colorectum are the most frequent types, although lymphomas and acute leukemia have also been reported. Mitomycin is the agent most commonly associated with this condition. Clinical onset is usually within 4 to 9 weeks after the last administered dose but can occur as late as 4 to 15 months after treatment. The histopathologic features of mitomycin-induced thrombotic microangiopathic syndrome are similar to those of the hemolytic uremic syndrome and thrombotic thrombocytopenic purpura. Mitomycin appears to produce renal insufficiency, either with or without microangiopathic hemolytic anemia. This vascular syndrome also can occur with cisplatin and bleomycin regimens, carboplatin, or various combination therapies.
- Hypertension. Sustained hypertension can occur following cisplatin, vinblastine, or bleomycin therapy, with an incidence of up to 17% incidence in testicular cancer patients treated with all three agents. The hypertension is associated with narrowing of interlobular renal arteries and fibrin thrombosis of afferent arterioles, features similar to the histologic findings in thrombotic microangiopathic syndrome following mitomycin or cisplatin therapy.

ROLE OF NUCLEAR MEDICINE IN NEPHROTOXICITY

Radionuclide studies are useful in patients whose kidney function has been compromised by radiation therapy and/or chemotherapy, providing the following information: (a) qualitative assessment of renal perfusion; (b) morphologic evaluation of the kidneys; (c) assessment of urine drainage; and (d) quantification of kidney function. Quantification of renal function is probably the most unique contribution of nuclear medicine in the setting of nephrotoxicity, although the evaluation of renal perfusion and urine drainage is also important. It is possible to determine accurately both total and individual kidney GFR or ERPF, expressed as milliliters per minute. It is beyond the scope of this communication to describe the various techniques used for measuring renal function except to mention that two general methods exist—blood sampling and gamma camera techniques. In both, a single intravenous injection of a tracer is administered to estimate either GFR [with ^{99m}Tc-DTPA (diethylenetriamine pentaacetic acid) or sometimes ^{125}I-iothalamate] or ERPF (with ^{131}I- or ^{123}I-hippurate or sometimes ^{99m}Tc-MAG-3). However, determining the function of each kidney requires imaging with a gamma camera, which is a limitation to the use of ^{125}I-iothalamate.

The glomerular filtration rate is regarded as the single most important parameter of renal function by nephrologists and is regularly mentioned in the literature as a benchmark for determining the adverse effects of either radiation or chemotherapy. Furthermore, the GFR is used in determining the dose of some chemotherapeutic agents that can be safely given to patients (6,13), as shown in Table 9.2. The serum creatinine level is a function of the GFR but is relatively insensitive for detecting early renal insufficiency because it has a logarithmic relationship to the GFR. This means that significant decreases in the GFR can be accompanied by only small numeric changes in the serum creatinine. This limitation is offset in clinical practice by either measuring the creatinine clearance (a function of the GFR) or estimating it from the serum creatinine with the use of published formulas (22). These approaches have limitations for the following reasons: (a) rapid decreases in the GFR are not reflected by equally prompt increases in the serum creatinine; (b) determination of the creatinine clearance usually requires a 24-hour urine collection and may not accurately estimate a low GFR because some tubular secretion of creatinine can occur in these circumstances; and (c) individual kidney function (or dysfunction, as the case may be)

cannot be determined. These limitations are avoided by using DTPA to measure the GFR; when used in combination with a gamma camera, determination of individual kidney GRF is also possible. The advantage of imaging combined with measurement of function is illustrated in Fig. 9.1, in which multiple renal infarcts were uncovered in the setting of increasing serum creatinine and normal renal ultrasonographic findings, and in Fig. 9.2, in which a renogram was performed to evaluate a patient with ovarian carcinoma who was thought to have a partially obstructed kidney, only to have the examination show a striking reduction of function on the affected side.

Proximal tubular function is determined in most clinical situations by urinary dipstick to detect glucose and protein or by measuring pH. More sensitive tests of proximal tubular function measure urinary amino acids, phosphates, and uric acid. Distal tubular dysfunction presents with renal tubular acidosis and polyuria.

Ideally, nuclear medicine techniques would be used to establish baseline values of renal function before treatment with radiation fields that include the kidneys or with nephrotoxic chemotherapy drugs, and then to follow renal function with serial studies over time. The excellent reproducibility of the results of nuclear medicine studies allow for accurate comparison of follow-up studies through many years. In many circumstances, however, a pretreatment renogram is not performed, and a patient's first study is performed when nephrotoxic effects are suspected. Useful information is still available and can be augmented by comparing the radionuclide GFR with pretreatment measured or estimated creatinine clearance. Radionuclide renography does not replace computed tomography or ultrasonography to assess renal anatomy but does provide unique physiologic information regarding the function of each kidney that cannot be obtained easily by any other means.

TABLE 9.2. SUGGESTED PERCENTAGES OF DOSES OF SOME CHEMOTHERAPEUTIC DRUGS BASED ON GLOMERULAR FILTRATION RATE

GFR	>60 mL/min	30–60 mL/min			10–30 mL/min		<10 mL/min	
Dose (%)	100%	75%	50%	Omit	75%	Omit	50%	Omit
	BLEO CDDP CTX MTX MITH MITO NUREAS	BLEO MITH MITO	CDDP MTX	NUREAS	BLEO MITH MITO	CDDP MTX NUREAS	BLEO CTX MITH MITO	CDDP MTX NUREAS

BLEO, bleomycin; CDDP, cisplatin; CTX, cyclophosphamide; MTX, methotrexate; MITH, mithramycin; MITO, mitomycin C; NUREAS, nitrosoureas.
From Patterson WP, Reams GP. Renal toxicities of chemotherapy. *Semin Oncol* 1992;19:521, with permission (13).

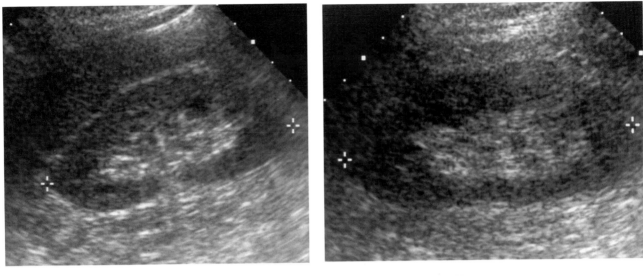

A   B

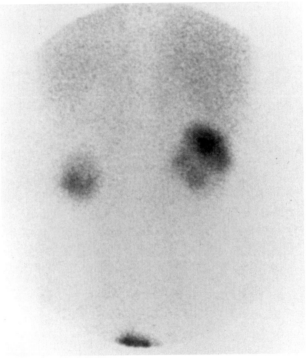

C

FIGURE 9.1. A 53-year-old woman with renal insufficiency had normal findings on renal ultra-sonography in both the right (**A**) and left (**B**) kidneys. Radionuclide renography the next day determined the glomerular filtration rate (by gamma camera technique and diethylenetriamine pentaacetic acid) to be 24 mL/min, which was nearly the same as the creatinine clearance of 21 mL/min estimated by using that day's serum creatinine level of 3.1 mg/dL (22). The right kidney accounted for 76% of function (18 mL/min) and the left kidney for 24% (6 mL/min). **C:** Scintigraphy (MAG-3 injected after measurement of the glomerular filtration rate) showed distorted kidneys with cortical defects caused by multiple infarcts. Camera imaging made possible a full diagnosis, which was not determined by ultrasonography or measurements of the glomerular filtration rate alone.

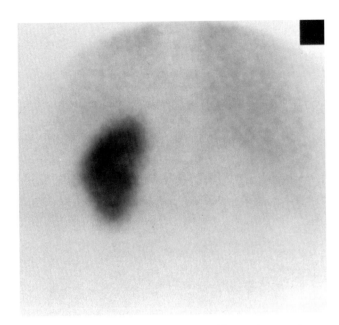

FIGURE 9.2. A 63-year-old woman with ovarian carcinoma underwent computed tomography, which showed a partially obstructed right kidney caused by midureteral narrowing. Six months later, diuretic renography showed that the right kidney accounted for only 8% of the glomerular filtration rate (total was 46 mL/min). Determination of the glomerular filtration rate alone could not identify unilateral renal dysfunction, but it was clearly evident when quantification was combined with gamma camera imaging.

REFERENCES

1. Maier JG, Casarett GW. *Pathophysiologic aspects of radiation nephritis in dogs.* University of Rochester, Atomic Energy Commission Report UR-626, 1963.
2. Gladstein E, Fajardo LF, Brown JM. Radiation injury in the mouse kidney. I. Sequential light microscopic studies. *Int J Radiat Oncol Biol Phys* 1977;2:933.
3. Gladstein E, Brown RC, Zanelli GD, et al. The uptake of rubidium-86 in kidneys irradiated with fractionated doses of x-rays. *Radiat Res* 1975;61:417.
4. Rubin P, Constine LS, Williams JP. Late effects of cancer treatment: radiation and drug toxicity. In: Perez CA, Brady LW, eds. *Principles and practice of radiation oncology*, 3rd ed. Philadelphia: Lippincott–Raven Publishers, 1998:155–211.
5. Moulder JE, Fish BL. Influence of nephrotoxic drugs on the late renal toxicity associated with bone marrow transplant conditioning regimens. *Int J Radiat Oncol Biol Phys* 1991;20:333.
6. Schilsky RL. Renal and metabolic toxicities of cancer chemotherapy. *Semin Oncol* 1982;9:75–83.
7. Rubin P. Basic concepts of radiation pathology: radiation tolerance doses and tolerance volumes of specific tissues and organs. In: Busch DB, ed. Radiation and chemotherapy injury: pathophysiology, diagnosis, and treatment. *Crit Rev Oncol Hematol* 1993;15:52.
8. Cassady JR. Clinical radiation nephropathy. *Int J Radiat Oncol Biol Phys* 1995;31:1249.
9. Phillips TL. Urinary radiation and chemotherapy pathology. In: Busch DB, ed. Radiation and chemotherapy injury: pathophysiology, diagnosis, and treatment. *Crit Rev Oncol Hematol* 1993;15:72.
10. Rubin P, Casarett GW. Urinary tract: the kidney. In: *Clinical radiation pathology*. Philadelphia: WB Saunders, 1968:293–333 (vol 1).
11. Avioli LV, Lazor MZ, Cotlove E, et al. Early effects of radiation on renal function in man. *Am J Med* 1963;34:329.
12. Rich PS. *Cis*-dichlorodiammineplatinum II-induced syndrome of inappropriate secretion of antidiuretic hormone. *Cancer* 1988;61:448–450.
13. Patterson WP, Reams GP. Renal toxicities of chemotherapy. *Semin Oncol* 1992;19:521–528.
14. Berns JS, Ford PA. Renal toxicities of antineoplastic drugs and bone marrow transplantation. *Semin Nephrol* 1997;17:54–66.
15. Lestingi TM, Thompson JA. Management of interleukin 2. In: Vogelzang NJ, Scardino PT, Shipley WU, et al., eds. *Comprehensive textbook of genitourinary oncology*. Baltimore: Lippincott Williams & Wilkins, 1999:255–261.
16. Markman M. Amifostine in reducing cisplatin toxicity. *Semin Oncol* 1998;15:522–524.
17. Hausheer FH, Kanter P, Cao S, et al. Modulation of platinum-induced toxicities and therapeutic index: mechanistic insights and first- and second-generation protecting agents. *Semin Oncol* 1998;25:584–599.
18. Gell PGH, Coombs RRA. *Clinical aspects of immunology*. Oxford: Blackwell Science, 1975.
19. Weiss RB. Hypersensitivity reactions to cancer chemotherapy. *Semin Oncol* 1982;9:5–13.
20. Weiss RB. Hypersensitivity reactions. *Semin Oncol* 1992;19:458–477.
21. Doll DC, Yarbro JW. Vascular toxicity associated with antineoplastic agents. *Semin Oncol* 1992;19:580–596.
22. Gates GF. Creatinine clearance estimation from serum creatinine values: an analysis of three mathematical models of glomerular function. *Am J Kidney Dis* 1985;3:199–205.

APPLICATIONS

10

POSITRON EMISSION TOMOGRAPHY IMAGING

PETER S. CONTI

The ability to identify structural alterations in diseased tissues, such as those seen in brain cancer, has increased dramatically in the last two decades with the development of noninvasive cross-sectional imaging techniques, including computed tomography (CT) and magnetic resonance imaging (MRI). Although significant advances have been made in anatomic imaging, until recently, less attention has been given to the development of *in vivo* methods of quantifying metabolism in normal and diseased tissues (1). Positron emission tomography (PET) is one example of a technique that has the potential to yield the information necessary not only to diagnose cancers based on altered tissue metabolism, but also to serve as a tool to monitor the effects of therapy (2–5). Correlative metabolic–anatomic imaging makes it possible to study biochemical processes in the morphologic loci in which they occur, and perhaps detect changes indicative of tumor response to therapy before structural alterations occur.

Currently, the best imaging methods available for the diagnosis and monitoring of brain neoplasms are MRI and CT; both procedures are based on tissue morphology and rely heavily on contrast enhancement for differential diagnosis. Although MRI and CT can provide precise anatomic delineation of such lesions, frequently in ways that exceed views at surgery, and also determine changes in tumor volume in response to therapeutic manipulation, they fall short in their ability to assess response to therapy rapidly, when changes in treatment planning could be most effective—that is, before changes in tumor volume occur (1). In addition, little or no information is provided that can be used to predict response to therapy other than referral to the natural history of similar lesions once the diagnosis has been made.

Because the early detection of either a primary or metastatic neoplasm and rapid administration of effective therapeutic intervention are major clinical goals, new techniques are needed that could be used to diagnose expeditiously, provide prognostic information, and assess response to therapy (1). Two new technologies are beginning to provide such information: magnetic resonance spectroscopy (MRS) and PET. Although MRS is capable of providing useful biochemical information with the use of ^{1}H, ^{31}P, ^{19}F, and ^{13}C, its clinical utility has thus far been limited. This is likely to change with further advances in technology. Imaging tumor metabolism with these technologies will provide complementary information to the morphologic assessment of human cancers. In clinical practice, the combination of anatomic and metabolic imaging techniques will be used to assess the effectiveness of surgery, radiation therapy, and chemotherapy, and will provide earlier documentation of the extent of disease in addition to progression or regression as a result of treatment. Such data should permit the treatment plan to be modified sooner than can be done based on clinical response or changes in lesion morphology alone.

These newer metabolic imaging techniques will extend the diagnosis and monitoring of cancers on the basis of physiologic and biochemical characteristics and changes therein. PET provides information about *in vivo* regional chemistry with a sensitivity and specificity comparable with that of radioimmunoassay in studies of body fluids, and can often detect abnormalities before structural changes have occurred. As gross changes in anatomy are no longer adequate endpoints for therapy protocols, treatment need no longer be based solely on clinical response, lesion morphology, and histopathologic findings in biopsy specimens. *In vivo* biochemical characterization of tumors with labeled tracers is becoming a new method for classifying tumors and planning and monitoring their treatment (1,6–8). *In vivo* assessment of the metabolic activity of tumors, specifically measurement of DNA synthesis, protein synthesis, and glucose utilization by means of PET, is proving useful for both diagnosing and monitoring the effects of therapy on tumors. PET makes it possible to measure the rate of utilization of substrates such as sugars and amino acids, which supply energy to tumors, and nucleotides, which reflect DNA metabolism, and to obtain pharmacokinetic and pharmacodynamic data concerning radiolabeled cancer chemotherapeutic agents.

P. S. Conti: Department of Radiology and PET Imaging Science Center, University of Southern California, Los Angeles, California 90033.

It is also important to recognize that malignancy can be manifested by multiple histologic patterns, variable cell types with variable degrees of differentiation, and differences in antigenicity, immunogenicity, biochemical properties, growth behavior, and cellular susceptibility to chemotherapeutic drugs (9,10). Although tumors of the same histologic type often follow a relatively predictable and reproducible pattern of clinical progression in most hosts (9), the biologic behavior of one cancer cannot always be inferred from that of another because of the presence of heterogeneous cell populations that may dominate as the tumor grows and so change its behavior (10). Heterogeneity occurs at all levels of neoplastic organization. It is seen not only in similar tumors from different patients, but also within the same tumor from a single patient (11). Likewise, in animal tumors of diverse histologic origin, significant variation has been noted in the metastatic capabilities of subpopulations of cells isolated from the same tumor (9). Neither MRS nor PET techniques are able to evaluate tumors at the level of the individual cell, although advances in technology have significantly improved resolution capabilities. Currently, the issues of tumor heterogeneity can be addressed only on a macroscopic level from an imaging viewpoint—that is, in regions of tumor tissue determined by the resolution of the imaging device.

Malignant cells generally also have an enhanced requirement for metabolic substrates, such as certain amino acids, sugars, and nucleosides, because of cell membrane-related changes, an enhanced growth rate, and changes in biochemical functions. A potential strategy for evaluating malignancy may involve identifying perturbations in normal tissue metabolic processes with the use of *in vivo* radiotracers (7,8). Likewise, if the specific metabolic behavior of a tumor measured *in vivo* can be correlated with anatomy, histochemical findings, and clinical outcome, it may be possible not only to identify tumor types *in vivo*, but also to monitor and perhaps predict response or lack of response to therapeutic intervention. PET radiotracers, such as ^{18}F-fluorodeoxyglucose (^{18}F-FDG), have proved helpful in determining diagnosis, prognosis, and response of tumor tissue to therapy, and have been used to determine tumor grade and histology and distinguish viable tumor from necrosis. In the field of oncology, ^{18}F-FDG, a positron-emitting glucose analogue, has been the most widely used radiotracer for the study of intracranial tumors.

CLINICAL APPLICATIONS IN DIAGNOSIS AND LESION CHARACTERIZATION

Fluorodeoxyglucose in the Detection of Primary Brain Tumors

Glucose is the primary metabolic substrate of the adult brain under most circumstances. Cerebral glucose utilization is a measure of cerebral energy metabolism and an index of functional activity. In the autoradiographic deoxyglucose technique of Sokoloff et al. (12), local cerebral glucose utilization is measured with [^{14}C]2-deoxy-D-glucose (DG) as a radiotracer for glucose metabolism. It has been used in animals to demonstrate a close relationship between glucose consumption and local cerebral function in a variety of experimental and pathologic states. The regional cerebral metabolic rate of glucose (rCMRglu) can be measured in humans by PET after injection of the short-lived radiotracer ^{18}F-fluorine-2-deoxyglucose, an analogue of DG (12–15). This method allows simultaneous measurement of glucose utilization in multiple regions of the brain. The accumulation of DG in tissues reflects the degree of glucose uptake and phosphorylation to the 6-phosphate product. The phosphorylated derivative of DG, which is not metabolized further, is trapped in the tissue and released at a very slow rate. The degree of tissue trapping and release may be correlated with the relative concentration of phosphorylating tissue enzymes (16). Metabolic trapping of DG permits determination of regional glucose metabolism, which would be difficult to accomplish if metabolism were able to proceed.

Imaging with FDG-PET has been used clinically for about 20 years to assess glucose metabolism in a number of clinical settings, such as dementia of Alzheimer's type, epilepsy, brain tumors, somatic cancers, and heart disease. In the field of oncology, because many tumor tissues exhibit accelerated glycolysis, DG labeled with ^{11}C or ^{18}F is being used successfully for the detection of neoplasms *in vivo* based on the fact that it is avidly accumulated in most tumor tissues (1,2,4,5,17–24).

By 1982, data were emerging that showed a correlation between the rate of glucose utilization and the histologic grade of malignant brain tumors. FDG was also shown to be useful to distinguish recurrent tumor from radiation changes (25–27). Figure 10.1 demonstrates a case of known tumor recurrence, seen as focal hypermetabolism on FDG-PET, associated with an enhancing lesion on MRI. Although some investigators have reported variability in the rates of glucose utilization within tumors of similar pathologic grade (28), new data continue to support many of the basic applications for tumor imaging with FDG and PET. Goldman et al. (29), for example, analyzed histologic features and corresponding metabolic rates in 161 biopsy samples from 20 procedures guided by FDG-PET in patients with brain tumors. When glucose metabolic rates, identified from stereotactic coordinates, were normalized to the cortex or white matter, a highly significant difference between anaplastic and non-anaplastic tumor samples was demonstrated ($p < .0001$); approximately 75% of samples metabolically graded 3 or 4 demonstrated anaplasia histologically, compared with 10% of samples graded 0 or 1.

A grading system for cerebral gliomas based on FDG-PET was proposed nearly a decade ago (30). More recently, cutoff levels have been proposed as a means of differentiating low-grade from high-grade brain tumors with the use of FDG (31). In this latter study, 32 high-grade tumors (including

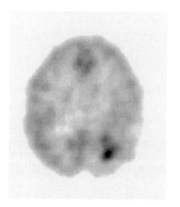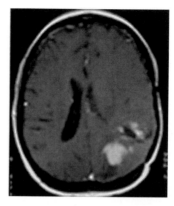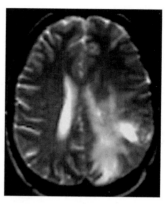

FIGURE 10.1. Contrast enhancing mass on magnetic resonance imaging and recurrent high-grade glioma seen on fluorodeoxyglucose positron emission tomography.

primary gliomas, lymphoma, atypical meningiomas, choroid plexus carcinomas, and metastases outside the central nervous system), and 26 low-grade lesions (including gliomas, schwannomas, craniopharyngiomas, germinomas, and epidermoid cysts) were studied. The investigators determined the best cutoff levels to be 1.5 for tumor-to-white matter ratios and 0.6 for tumor-to-normal cortex ratios. These cutoff values were appropriate for the subgroup of gliomas and also for all the tumors taken together. The sensitivity was 94% and the specificity 77% for high-grade tumors when the tumor-to-white matter ratio was greater than 1.5.

Juvenile pilocytic astrocytomas appear to display a markedly increased uptake of FDG, similar to that seen in anaplastic astrocytoma, yet these tumors generally have a better prognosis than low-grade astrocytomas. In one study, the five patients evaluated showed no signs of progressive disease despite the PET findings (32). These investigators suggested that even though juvenile pilocytic astrocytomas may undergo malignant degeneration, the uptake may be related more to increased glucose transporter expression in the vasculature supporting these tumors than to aggressive behavior of the tumor cells themselves.

Several other types of less common primary intracranial tumors also have been studied with PET. Pleomorphic xanthoastrocytoma has been shown to have a rate of FDG uptake lower than that of contralateral gray matter but still consistent with an intermediate- or high-grade primary brain tumor (33). Minuera et al. (34) observed that the rCMRglu is generally low in neurocytomas in comparison with that in contralateral gray matter, although lesions can on occasion demonstrate more pronounced uptake. In one such case, follow-up studies demonstrated an increase in size after partial resection, whereas in the other patients with low uptake, no tumor regrowth was observed. In ganglioglioma, FDG-PET and ²⁰¹Tl appear to be equally useful in predicting the histologic grade of lesions (35). Finally, gliomatosis cerebri has been seen on FDG-PET as an extensive region of hypometabolism of the superficial and deep gray matter (36). Although this is a lesion principally

involving the white matter, no white matter disease was detected by FDG-PET. These findings are likely consistent with the slowly growing, infiltrative nature of the disease.

Glucose consumption measured by quantitative analysis of FDG uptake also has been used to categorize recurrent gliomas. In astrocytoma, cell density rather than nuclear polymorphism appears to correlate with glucose consumption measured with FDG (37). In one study of 18 recurrences, a high rate of glucose consumption generally correlated with a "hot spot" that was higher than or similar to contralateral cortex, along with histologic evidence of malignancy (38). However, half of the known recurrences demonstrated low consumption, and two thirds of this latter group were high-grade recurrences at histologic analysis. Although the data did not reach significance, patients displaying lower rates of tumor glucose consumption had a longer survival. The authors cautioned that because viable tumor cells can exist in the presence of low levels of glucose consumption, small recurrences can be missed because of poor spatial resolution.

Based on these findings, FDG has become the principal radiotracer used to grade primary brain tumors and determine prognosis (28,39–43). Imaging with FDG, however, is not without problems regarding the differential diagnosis of intracranial masses. Hypometabolism can be observed with a number of entities, such as infarct, interictal epilepsy, and radiation changes in addition to low-grade brain tumors. Boon et al. (44), for example, noted that although FDG-PET has a role in identifying interictal disease in epilepsy in cases with low-grade or benign lesions, it can demonstrate hypometabolism in structural lesions leading to the disorder. Hence, more specific markers of disease are needed, as described in a subsequent section.

Fluorodeoxyglucose in the Detection of Metastatic Disease to the Brain

The sensitivity of FDG-PET in detecting brain metastases from non-central nervous system (CNS) primary tumors is

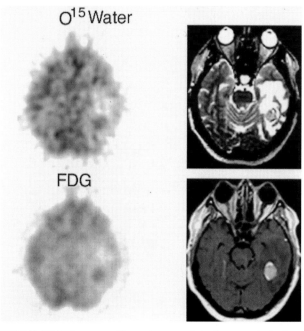

FIGURE 10.2. Large, solitary, hypermetabolic metastasis from lung cancer with surrounding edema. Note the elevated accumulation of ^{15}O-water on the perfusion study, compatible with the highly vascular nature of the lesion.

lower than its sensitivity in identifying high-grade glial tumors. In one study, a detection rate of 68% was reported in a spectrum of disease (45). Although small size accounted for several of the missed lesions, several larger lesions displayed low rates of FDG uptake. Given the limited sensitivity described, the generally small size of many of these lesions, and their usual close proximity to the gray matter, these investigators felt that further study is necessary to determine the utility of this imaging approach in screening for brain metastases. In fact, screening for cerebral metastases in patients with suspected malignancy has been performed. In a large study of 273 such patients evaluated with whole-body PET, a total of four patients (1.5%) had cerebral metastases, only two of which were unsuspected (46). These investigators suggested that the yield of this type of screening is low and may not be clinically useful.

The uptake in CNS metastases also may be variable. In one study, PET measurements of rCMRglu, regional cerebral blood flow (rCBF), or regional cerebral blood volume (rCBV) in patients with lung metastases to brain varied widely among 12 tumor sites in six patients, but they were higher than the corresponding values in white matter and higher than or similar to those of gray matter (47). Figure 10.2 demonstrates a case of solitary metastasis from lung cancer. As in primary brain tumors, however, PET appears superior to CT and MRI in the differentiation between recurrence of irradiated brain metastases and radiation necrosis (48). An example of the latter application is shown in Fig. 10.3 in a patient with recurrent esthesioneuroblastoma of the ethmoid sinus.

In addition, PET may have a role in staging disease in patients with suspected or proven extracranial malignancies who present with intracranial lesions. Gupta et al. (49) used FDG to evaluate 31 patients with solitary intracranial lesions; 22 of them had histologic or clinical evidence of metastatic disease, and nine had documented benign disease. PET was able to document focal hypermetabolism in 19 of the 22 proven metastases and hypometabolism in all nine of the lesions determined to be benign. The extracranial primary tumor sites were identified in 82% of the 22 patients with proven disease, of which 55% were found only on PET and not on conventional imaging studies. The primary tumors identified included cancers of the lung, cancers of the head and neck, lymphomas, renal cell cancers, melanomas, and colon cancers. In addition, in nine of the 22 patients, additional somatic lesions were demonstrated and confirmed by clinical or radiographic follow-up, whereas six of the nine had had negative results on initial conventional imaging studies of those sites.

Imaging of Brain Stem and Spinal Cord Tumors with Fluorodeoxyglucose

The utility of PET has been demonstrated in imaging primary spinal cord malignancies. Marked elevation in glucose metabolic rates can be observed in high-grade lesions, and reduction in low-grade gliomas and other non-neoplastic lesions in the brain stem and spinal cord (40,50). Observed

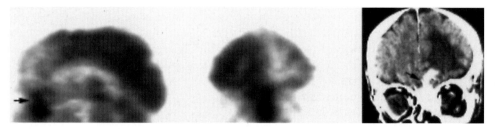

FIGURE 10.3. Suspected recurrent metastatic cancer to the inferior left frontal lobe versus radiation necrosis. Hypermetabolism in the inferior frontal lobe (*arrow*) is seen along with locally recurrent disease below the cribriform plate.

absolute levels are different from the corresponding levels in cerebral lesions of equivalent grade, but these can be appropriately evaluated by taking into consideration the relative differences in baseline activity of normal cord versus normal cerebral gray or white matter (50). Ratios of activity in regions of interest (ROIs) in cerebral gray and white matter, as well as cord tissue in attenuation-corrected scans agree well with ratios calculated by using literature values for absolute metabolic rates; that is, cerebral gray matter is approximately twice as active as white matter, which in turn is approximately twice as active as average cord tissue (22). Likewise, clinical studies can be performed without calculations of absolute glucose metabolic rate in cord lesions by using a similar methodology for tumor grading. Importantly, Bruggers et al. (51) have found that FDG-PET is helpful in confirming tumor progression in brain stem gliomas when MRI results demonstrate stable disease in a patient who is deteriorating clinically.

Cranial and spinal schwannomas, including acoustic neuromas associated with neurofibromatosis type 2, can be visualized with ^{18}F-FDG (52). The extracerebral lesions are seen well because surrounding normal structures generally demonstrate a low accumulation of tracer. Preliminary studies also suggest that the lesions can be graded in regard to aggressiveness and potential for recurrence (52).

Finally, visualization of metastatic disease to spinal cord with PET has been reported. Intense uptake of FDG has been demonstrated by Bakheet et al. (53) in a primary pineoblastoma of the brain, along with accumulation in metastatic disease to the spinal cord. Spinal metastases from high-grade astrocytoma have been clearly visualized with the use of FDG (54).

Comparative Studies with Fluorodeoxyglucose and ^{11}C-Methionine

Several investigators have found ^{11}C-methionine to be superior to FDG in delineating tumor margins, acquiring information to be used in planning and performing brain surgery, and differentiating tumor recurrence from radiation necrosis (55–61). High rates of accumulation of ^{11}C-methionine have been observed in patients with high-grade glioma and also low-grade tumor. In one study, although the difference in uptake of tracer between the two groups of patients was significant ($p < .001$), the investigators found it difficult to discriminate between tumor types on the basis of accumulation of tracer alone in individual cases (62). The distribution of the tracer identified tumor boundaries more clearly than CT did, which led to the conclusion that PET with ^{11}C-methionine is more useful in defining extent of disease than tumor grade.

Derlon et al. (63) evaluated the differences between low-grade astrocytomas and oligodendrogliomas based on uptake patterns of ^{11}C-methionine and FDG. Their study demonstrated that although accumulation of ^{11}C-methionine varies in astrocytoma, uptake in oligodendroglioma is generally substantially higher. In both tumor lines, accumulation of FDG was generally similar, albeit lower than that of ^{11}C-methionine, with only a slightly higher accumulation seen in astrocytomas. This study demonstrated that the two lines of tumors display different patterns of metabolism and hence biologic characteristics. Holzer (64) also found that ^{11}C-methionine uptake is significantly higher in oligodendrogliomas than in astrocytomas. Although further study is required, such differences could correlate with variations in treatment response and help in determining prognosis.

A comparative evaluation of ^{11}C-methionine and FDG in a preoperative patient population demonstrated that ^{11}C-methionine is superior in delineating low-grade lesions (65). However, although ^{11}C-methionine uptake was high in glioblastoma, imaging could not be used to discriminate low-grade lesions from anaplastic astrocytomas. In this study, low-grade oligodendrogliomas demonstrated a high rate of uptake of both FDG and ^{11}C-methionine. A good correlation was found between histologic grade and FDG uptake. Both tracers were useful to predict patient survival, and the combination of tracers better predicted histologic grade and survival than either tracer alone. ^{11}C-Methionine has also been shown to be useful in detecting recurrence of oligodendroglioma (66).

The superiority of lesion delineation with ^{11}C-methionine has been demonstrated in a study of crossed cerebellar diaschisis in patients with brain tumors. Otte et al. (67) utilized ^{11}C-methionine studies to discriminate tumor from surrounding edema, and then correlated the ROIs thus determined with matched FDG scans in subsequent analysis. Evaluation of the FDG data showed frontal lobe tumors to be associated with the highest rates of crossed cerebellar diaschisis. In addition, diaschisis increased with increasing lesion size and was more frequent in malignant lesions than in low-grade tumors.

Some investigators utilize imaging studies of blood flow with ^{11}C-methionine because the incorporation of ^{11}C-methionine into glioma, but not brain tissue, appears to depend on blood flow (68). In some cases of low-grade tumor and heterogeneous higher-grade lesions, uptake of ^{11}C-methionine is the same in tumor lesions as in areas of normal brain with diminished blood flow, so that tumor grade might be underestimated without a correction for blood flow. A study by Roelke et al. (69) demonstrated an association between uptake of ^{82}Rb and ^{11}C-methionine in primary brain tumors, including gliomas and meningiomas. Both active as well as passive uptake of ^{11}C-methionine appears to account for the accumulation of tracer in brain tumor, potentially limiting the use of ^{11}C-methionine in differentiating recurrent tumor from radiation necrosis; the blood–brain barrier would be disrupted in both circumstances.

Goldman et al. (70) evaluated the use of ^{11}C-methionine and FDG-PET to guide stereotactic biopsy of brain tumors.

Anaplasia and heterogeneity influence the uptake of both ^{11}C-methionine and FDG. Uptake of both tracers is elevated in regions of anaplasia. ^{11}C-Methionine appeared to be superior in discriminating tumor from gray matter, detecting regions of infiltrating neoplastic cells, and distinguishing non-neoplastic cellular components in regions of necrosis from tumor. These observations are supported by autoradiographic data demonstrating that ^{14}C-methionine uptake is proportional to the number of viable tumor cells and is low in macrophages and other non-neoplastic cellular components, whereas FDG uptake is significant in tumor-associated macrophages and pre-necrotic neoplastic cells (71). Although uptake of FDG is independent of blood–brain barrier disruption, the latter could influence methionine uptake, as noted above. Nonetheless, the investigators stressed the complementary nature of these tracers and the overall role of PET as a guide for stereotactic biopsy.

Methionine labeled with ^{11}C and FDG-PET imaging have been used to visualize spinal cord tumors (72), although no direct comparisons have been performed. A cervical cord ependymoma in a patient with progressive weakness of the left extremity was imaged with conventional techniques, including myelography and CT, which demonstrated an intramedullary mass with cystic cavities extending from C-2 to T-1. ^{11}C-Methionine accumulated in the solid components of the tumor and in other nearby normal structures, including the submandibular glands and saliva collecting in the piriform recesses (72).

Rationale for a Multitracer Approach to Tumor Imaging and Characterization

Whereas individual radiotracers may be useful for diagnosis and evaluation of response to therapy, a combination of metabolic probes may be required to describe the metabolic profile of a tumor more accurately. By providing several parameters with which to evaluate tissue heterogeneity, multiple tracers provide a more reliable assessment of tumor activity before and after treatment (7,8). Differential diagnosis is difficult in certain circumstances when one relies on single-agent imaging, a situation that can occur, for example, when FDG is used to assess the presence of tumor versus inflammation or infection, both of which may be associated with elevated glucose utilization. Not infrequently, it is difficult to distinguish tumor from surrounding normal tissue on FDG-PET because of uptake of the radiolabeled agent by normal tissue, such as cerebral cortex.

Techniques of multiparametric analysis of experimental and human brain tumors have used radiolabeled markers of perfusion and metabolism such as ^{15}O-water (perfusion), ^{11}C-methionine (amino acid uptake), and ^{18}F-FDG (glucose utilization) (6–8,58,73–77). In such studies, data representing the accumulation of these tracers in tumors are generally presented as ratios of uptake between tumor and normal surrounding tissue, or as quantitative metabolic rates deter-

mined with the use of mathematical modeling. The accumulation of ^{11}C-methionine or FDG into intracranial lesions can be used to evaluate patients for recurrent tumor versus radiation necrosis. FDG should be used initially to determine the presence of hypermetabolism in the lesion. If a lesion is hypermetabolic in comparison with normal brain, radiation necrosis can be ruled out. However, if a lesion is hypometabolic on FDG-PET, it may be a low-grade tumor, infarct, or necrosis. A follow-up study with ^{11}C-methionine is required to evaluate the presence of viable tissue—that is, tumor.

The use of radiolabeled thymidine (TdR), or another radiolabeled DNA precursor analogue, is appropriate in a multiparametric analysis of glioma metabolism because such a tracer provides the most direct assessment of cellular division, which is the primary focus of therapeutic intervention in tumor treatment. Multiparametric *in vivo* imaging of gliomas with ^{18}F-FDG, ^{11}C-TdR, and ^{11}C-methionine has been evaluated in clinical trials (78,79).

A number of other primary CNS lesions, several of which are not malignant, have been studied. For example, accumulation of ^{11}C-methionine is significantly greater than accumulation of FDG in intracranial hemangiopericytoma, which is an aggressive lesion with an 80% recurrence rate following treatment and a propensity for metastasizing to distant sites (23% of cases) (80). These lesions are highly vascular and can be seen as sites of hyperperfusion with ^{15}O-water, as in this case. Minuera et al. (34) observed that rCRF and rCBV are elevated in neurocytomas, corresponding to angiographic findings in these lesions. Although rCMRgl was generally lower in tumors than in contralateral gray matter, ^{11}C-methionine was able to demonstrate a clear outline of the mass, with a tumor-to-contralateral gray matter ratio of 1.51.

Blood flow and oxygen metabolism have also been evaluated in cavernous angiomas and arteriovenous malformations (81). In cavernous angiomas, no significant changes in blood flow were observed, although oxygen consumption was decreased in the cortex supplied by the arterial branches of the angiomas. In arteriovenous malformations, blood flow was elevated in the territories feeding the lesions, and oxygen extraction rates were increased in vascular areas remote from the supply area of the larger lesions, which suggests chronic ischemia. Unlike cavernous angiomas, large arteriovenous malformations may be associated with a chronic vascular steal phenomenon. Cavernous angiomas and arteriovenous malformations demonstrate little if any accumulation of FDG. Another highly vascular lesion, meningioma, also demonstrates elevated perfusion on ^{15}O-water studies and has long been known to display elevated FDG uptake, according to the aggressiveness of the tumor (25). Finally, as would be expected, aneurysms demonstrate marked hyperperfusion, but no significant metabolic activity, on FDG studies (Fig. 10.4).

By choosing the appropriate combination of radiotracers, it may be possible to reduce substantially the differential diagnosis of an unknown lesion. Entities that frequently

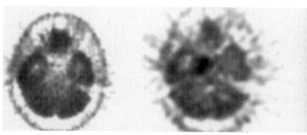
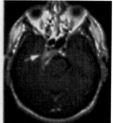

FIGURE 10.4. Low rate of metabolic activity and hyperperfusion in a patient with a known aneurysm (*arrow*).

confuse the anatomic picture can be separated on the basis of differences in metabolic profiles. In addition, such combinations may provide information on (a) similarities of uptake of individual tracers between tumor and normal tissues, (b) whether tumor can be distinguished from surrounding normal tissue and which agent or agents are most successful in doing so, (c) the presence of significant changes in uptake of individual tracers versus global or total uptake of all tracers following therapy, and (d) whether uptake by normal tissues is changed by the presence of tumor, therapy, or both. Both increases and decreases in accumulation of radiolabeled biomolecules have been observed in animal tumor models following chemotherapy. Similar findings have been demonstrated clinically. Such information may provide a more accurate assessment of tumor biology and response to therapy, and perhaps lead to better patient management.

Emerging Radiotracers for Positron Emission Tomography

In many malignant tumors, the rates of glycolysis and glucose transport into cells are accelerated in comparison with the rates in most surrounding normal tissues (6,82–84). Thus, the accumulation of FDG, a glucose analogue, can be used to measure regional glucose utilization. Amino acid transport across tumor cell membranes also has been found to differentiate many malignant from nonmalignant tumors (85–88). Not only membrane transport but also protein synthesis can be examined if suitable mathematical modeling is used in data analysis. Another important characteristic of neoplastic tissue is its increased rate of cell division. In general, accumulation of TdR into neoplasms is increased when DNA synthesis is increased (79,89–99). Analogues of these basic biomolecules, and many others, have potential utility for cancer evaluation with PET.

To develop other suitable tracers to image malignant tumors, metabolic processes must be identified that occur to a greater or lesser extent in neoplasms relative to the surrounding tissues or organs (3,6–8). To map the metabolic status of a tumor, biologically observable radiotracers are required that localize in neoplasms in concentrations sufficient to detect changes in uptake within the primary tumor

or metastases. Positron-emitting isotopes have been incorporated into a variety of biologically active compounds to probe tumor metabolism *in vivo* with PET (4).

In addition to ^{11}C-methionine, other amino acids may be found useful in the evaluation of tumor metabolism as data from experimental studies continue to demonstrate altered amino acid transport and protein synthesis in malignant cells (85–88). Derivatives of natural and synthetic amino acids are being studied in patients with brain tumors, including fluorotyrosine (100), glutamate (101), fluorophenylalanine (102,103), and a number of noncatabolized derivatives (104–107). Although the measurement of protein synthesis in tumors with radiolabeled natural amino acids, such as ^{11}C-methionine, provides specific biologic information regarding tumor behavior, data now available suggest that rates of amino acid transport rather than of protein synthesis are strongly correlated to tumor grade (60). If this is the case, further studies with transport-specific nonmetabolized amino acids may be warranted (103,107).

Tyrosine labeled with ^{11}C has been used to image primary brain tumors in a small number of patients ($n = 22$) with a sensitivity of 92%, specificity of 67%, and accuracy of 89%, although the number of patients studied without tumor was small (108). Background activity in normal brain was found to be relatively low. Although establishment of any relationship between protein synthesis rates and uptake of this tracer requires further investigation, its potential ability to quantify amino acid turnover may provide distinct advantages over other labeled amino acids, such as ^{11}C-methionine, uptake of which may be more reflective of transport and utilization and confounded by the presence of significant transmethylation.

The uptake of ^{18}F-fluorophenylalanine is elevated in brain tumor independently of grade, and the molecule appears to be transported by a carrier-mediated process into tumor tissue (103). This agent seems to be more useful for detection of tumor than for grading of malignancy. Another amino acid, L-(3-^{18}F)-α-methyltyrosine, has been studied in patients with a variety of intracranial tumors, and in general it has demonstrated tumor-to-normal cortex and tumor-to-white matter ratios superior to those of FDG (109). Although all lesions were clearly identified and uptake in normal brain was low, the tracer was unable to discriminate between high- and low-grade tumors. Like other amino acids, however, this agent has a potential role in the delineation of tumor extent, which is valuable in the planning of radiation treatment or resection.

The synthetic amino acid ^{11}C-ACBC (aminocyclobutane carboxylic acid) has been used to image a variety of neoplasms. In a study comparing uptake of FDG with uptake of ^{11}C-ACBC in a series of brain tumors of varying grades, Hubner (106) demonstrated a sensitivity, specificity, and accuracy of 93%, 71%, and 90%, respectively, for ^{11}C-ACBC, in comparison with 76%, 50%, and 68% for FDG. More recently, an ^{18}F-labeled analogue of ACBC was compared with FDG, and both agents displayed avid accumulation in the patient studied (110). ^{18}F-FACBC showed an initially low rate of accumulation in normal brain, but this increased during the 60-minute period of study. At 20 minutes, the ratio of tumor to normal brain tissue was approximately 6, which suggests that its ability to distinguish brain tumors from normal brain structures is superior to that of FDG. In human and animal studies, this agent is not metabolized. Like other synthetic analogues that have been proposed as PET agents, it could be used to assess amino acid transport in malignancy.

Choline labeled with ^{11}C has been used to visualize primary brain tumors against a background of relatively low uptake in normal brain parenchyma (111). In this group of patients, about half of whom had received prior radiation or chemotherapy, no correlation could be established with blood flow measured with PET and ^{15}O-water. Interestingly, because choline is also incorporated into the endothelium of cerebral blood vessels, the investigators speculated that the net uptake in brain lesions might represent a combination of tumor cells and endothelial cells within the tumor vasculature. This observation may have important implications in the design of radiopharmaceuticals to image the process of angiogenesis.

In addition to uptake in primary brain tumors, metastases, and pituitary adenoma, it has been noted that accumulation of tracer can be observed in tuberculous meningitis (112). Uptake was not seen in brain infarct or hemorrhage. The investigators also noted that in their experience, ^{11}C-choline provided better images of brain tumors than ^{11}C-methionine did. ^{11}C-Choline also appears to offer distinct advantages over FDG in that it provides clearer images of tumors and lesion borders and allows faster acquisition of data because of its more rapid clearance from blood. Additionally, tissue uptake stabilizes within the first 5 minutes after injection.

Nucleoside derivatives will play an important role in imaging cancer, especially brain tumors, because in most cases accumulation of exogenous nucleoside is minimal in normal brain tissue. ^{11}C-TdR has been considered as an *in vivo* radiotracer of nucleotide metabolism and DNA synthesis. The accumulation of radiolabeled TdR into tumor tissue and organs with high proliferative rates reflects the relative degree of DNA synthesis and serves as an index of metabolic activity. In human trials, tritiated TdR was administered to patients with solid tumors, and its incorporation into cell nuclei, measured by serial biopsies with autoradiography, reflected incorporation into DNA tumor cells during mitosis (94). In addition, alterations in tumor growth rates, such as occur during effective therapeutic manipulation, may be followed by measuring variations in uptake of radiolabeled TdR (94).

Unlike other currently available radiotracers used in PET, ^{11}C-TdR potentially can provide the most direct *in vivo* measurement of cellular proliferation. Accumulation of ^{11}C-TdR, labeled either in the 5-methyl position or in the 2 position of the base ring, has been demonstrated in newly diagnosed, treated, and recurrent primary brain neoplasms (4,78,79,113,114). However, in one study, uptake was not found to reflect tumor grade (113); FDG was compared with TdR and appeared more effective in discriminating low- from high-grade lesions.

According to De Reuck et al. (114), ^{11}C-TdR labeled in the methyl position appears to act as a tracer of blood flow in early dynamic images; afterward, uptake depends on radiolabeled metabolites crossing the blood–brain barrier. Although complicated by the presence of radiolabeled catabolic by-products, which vary depending on the labeling position of the parent molecule, analysis of ^{11}C-TdR data obtained from PET studies in which mathematical modeling techniques are used may provide a means for quantifying DNA synthesis and cellular replication rates *in vivo* (115). It is most likely that development of a partially catabolized or noncatabolized analogue will be necessary to avoid the complications of circulating radiolabeled metabolites in plasma and tissues (116,117).

Other nucleosides, such as ^{18}F-FUdR (fluorodeoxyuridine), have been proposed to investigate the metabolism of nucleic acids in brain tumors (118). Kameyama et al. (119) demonstrated elevated uptake of this tracer in high- versus low-grade primary brain tumors and generally low rates of background uptake in normal brain parenchyma. These investigators had previously demonstrated similar accumulation of ^{18}F-FUdR and ^{14}C-TdR in experimental rat brain tumor (120). In a case of multicentric anaplastic astrocytoma, uptake of ^{11}C-methionine was elevated in both left- and right-sided lesions, more so on the right, whereas accumulation of ^{18}F-FUdR was seen only on the right (121). In this case, pathologic assessment showed that the density of undifferentiated tumor cells was higher in the right-sided lesion.

Agents that can potentially bind to receptor sites in primary and metastatic brain tumors are being developed (122). Dopamine receptors, for example, are often increased in pituitary adenomas, and appropriately labeled receptor ligands can be used to image these sites in tumor cells (123). A positive correlation between peripheral benzodiazepine receptor density, measured *in vitro* with ^{3}H-PK-11195 and *in vivo* with FDG, has been observed in untreated cerebral tumors of various grades (124,125). This correlation is not present in tumors after either radiation therapy or chemotherapy. An additional correlation was observed between elevated uptake of FDG and PK-11195 and degree of malignancy, which suggests that ^{11}C-PK-11195 or similar agents may have a clinical role in the future for lesion characterization.

Putrescine labeled with ^{11}C is being developed as a tracer of polyamine synthesis (125–127). Activity in this synthetic pathway is known to be elevated in many tumor types and coupled to cellular replication. Limited clinical trials have demonstrated a correlation between uptake and tumor malignancy (126,127). Likewise, a number of agents designed to evaluate other physiologic and biochemical changes associated with malignancy and therapy are under development. These include [82]Rb to monitor transport across blood–brain and blood–tumor barriers and provide insight into the mechanisms of edema and the effects of glucocorticoid treatment or radiation therapy (128).

Calcium influx is essential in both cell death and leukocyte infiltration. [55]Co chloride has been studied in a small number of patients as a marker of calcium influx in decaying brain tumor tissue (129). In this study, the tracer did not appear to accumulate in viable cells or in regions of necrosis. The investigators suggested that uptake of this agent may be independent of the integrity of the blood–brain barrier.

Unraveling the uncertainties of the regulation of brain tumor pH, or evaluating hypoxia with agents such as ^{11}C-DMO (dimethyloxazolindinedione) (130,131) and ^{18}F-labeled imidazole derivatives (132–134), are possible subjects of future study. In addition, chemotherapeutic agents are being labeled with positron-emitting isotopes, several of which already have been evaluated in brain tumors (135, 136). Such labeled derivatives may prove helpful in acquiring an understanding the delivery and metabolism of the parent therapeutics used to treat brain malignancies and should be investigated further. The clinical and investiga-

TABLE 10.1. TRACERS USED FOR POSITRON EMISSION TOMOGRAPHY IN THE EVALUATION OF BRAIN TUMORS

Applied in clinical setting
  ^{18}F-Fluorodeoxyglucose
  ^{11}C-Methionine
Investigational
  ^{18}F-Fluorodeoxyuridine
  ^{18}F-Fluorophenylalanine
  ^{18}F-FACPC
  ^{11}C-Thymidine
  ^{11}C-ACPC
  ^{11}C-Tyrosine
  ^{11}C-α-methyltyrosine
  ^{11}C-Choline

ACPC, aminocyclopentane carboxylic acid.

tional PET radiotracers used for brain tumor imaging are summarized in Table 10.1.

Positron Emission Tomography versus Single-photon Emission Computed Tomography for Lesion Detection

A few studies have appeared recently comparing the use of ^{201}Tl and single-photon emission computed tomography (SPECT) with FDG-PET. For example, Black et al. (137) observed that ^{201}Tl and FDG demonstrate similar ability to predict histologic grade in cerebral gliomas, although in 35 paired studies, ^{201}Tl had a slight advantage in distinguishing tumor recurrence (sensitivity, 100%; positive predictive value, 97.1%) in comparison with FDG-PET (sensitivity, 90.9%; positive predictive value, 93.7%). Tamura et al. (138) found that in tumors with labeling indices of 5 or higher, measured with BRdU, ^{201}Tl-SPECT was slightly more sensitive than FDG-PET, whereas in tumors with labeling indices of 1 or less, FDG was better for lesion identification. However, they also observed that accumulation of ^{201}Tl in some low-grade tumors could yield false-positive results. In another study, of 23 patients with newly diagnosed astrocytomas, ^{201}Tl was found to be better than methionine or FDG in differentiating high- from low-grade tumors (139). Methionine was very useful for detecting lesions, differentiating benign from malignant lesions, and evaluating extent of disease, whereas FDG was not helpful in differentiating benign from malignant lesions or in grading tumors. The latter finding appears to contradict those of most other studies regarding the use of FDG in lesion grading, discussed above.

Kahn et al. (140) were unable to detect a statistically significant difference in sensitivity or specificity between ^{201}Tl and FDG in patients with evidence of tumor recurrence on CT or MRI. A total of 21 studies were performed in 19 patients, with recurrence based on biopsy findings or clinical follow-up. Follow-up revealed 16 cases of tumor and five cases of radiation necrosis, with 14 cases confirmed by clinical criteria. The tumors included five grade 1/2 lesions, 11 grade 3/4 lesions, one renal cell metastasis, and one locally invading esthesioblastoma. The sensitivity for tumor detection was 69% for ^{201}Tl and 81% for PET; both had the same specificity. In this study, scintigraphic results did not correlate with patient survival.

[11]C-Methionine appears to be superior to ^{201}Tl-SPECT in differentiating radiation necrosis from recurrent tumor, and in delineating the extent of the lesion. In a study of 10 patients, with two patients studied twice, both ^{201}Tl and ^{11}C-methionine identified all five known recurrences (141). In the remaining seven cases of radiation necrosis, elevated ^{201}Tl uptake was observed in four, whereas elevated uptake was observed in only one with ^{11}C-methionine.

Radiolabeled amino acids prepared for SPECT imaging are useful agents for brain tumor detection. In a study comparing the utility of FDG-PET and SPECT imaging with ^{123}I-IMT (α-methyl-L-tyrosine), Weber et al. (142) found IMT to be superior to FDG for tumor delineation and lesion detection, despite the inferior resolution and sensitivity of SPECT instrumentation. Interobserver variability was significantly lower when IMT was used to define the extent of lesions. Other investigators have found no significant differences in the ability of FDG and ^{123}I-IMT to discriminate between high- and low-grade primary brain tumors, and they suggest that the less expensive SPECT technology may have advantages over PET (143). In a comparison between IMT and ^{11}C-methionine, Langen et al. (144) determined that imaging of tumor extent was similar with both agents, which suggests that the results of SPECT could potentially rival those of PET.

Although perfusion imaging appears to have a limited diagnostic role in patients with brain tumors, data from the SPECT and PET literature suggest that measurement of tumor perfusion and oxygenation status may influence treatment outcome in cancer patients. Blood flow measured with PET techniques is usually variable in brain tumors, whereas oxygen extraction is generally decreased in and around these lesions in comparison with that normal brain tissue (145). Only limited data are available from comparative studies of blood flow and oxygen metabolism to date. However, given the need to understand further the complex pathophysiology of brain tumors and the potential confounds introduced with therapeutic intervention in the clinical setting, further studies exploring tumor oxygen metabolism and the relationship between tumor perfusion and metabolism are required. SPECT perfusion agents such as ^{99m}Tc-HMPAO (hexamethylpropylenamine oxime) and tumor hypoxia agents such as ^{123}I-IAZA (iodoazomycin arabinoside), are being used in patient studies (146). Although an association (*p* < .05) was observed between perfusion deficit and hypoxia in most tumors studied, including brain metastases and somatic lesions, it was not seen in glioblastoma multiforme, which suggests that malignant glial cells might be more sensitive to ischemic death and that only a small number of viable hypoxic cells exist within such tumors.

Multimodality Imaging Trials

The complementary use of MRS, SPECT, and PET in the imaging of brain tumors has been reviewed (147). Multimodal and multitracer approaches have been recommended in this patient population to improve lesion characterization (1,6–8,148,149). Recently, Go et al. (150) compared localized proton spectroscopy and spectroscopic imaging with PET and FDG or ^{11}C-tyrosine in the evaluation of cerebral gliomas. The ratio of lactate to creatinine was elevated in two of three patients with increased FDG uptake in tumor, and was normal in the third. A fourth patient displayed low FDG uptake and no lactate in the spectrum.

Although lactate is the end product of glycolysis, the elevated signal could be related to a number of factors, such as anaerobic glycolysis, ischemic or hypoxic conditions, or predominance of glycolysis over oxidative phosphorylation. Previous studies by Alger et al. (151) showed a lack of correlation between glucose utilization, measured by FDG-PET, and lactate signal on ^{1}H-MRS. This observation is relevant, given that PET studies have generally shown that FDG uptake is related to enhancement of glycolysis, with upregulation of hexokinase activity (6,152–154). Alger et al. observed that FDG was elevated on the periphery of the tumor masses, whereas lactate was elevated more centrally, which suggests that ischemic factors are involved in the latter situation. When Go et al. (150) studied ^{11}C-tyrosine, they found uptake to be elevated peripherally, corresponding to the choline signal on MRS, and suggested that both processes are related to cellular proliferation.

In a comparison of enhanced MRI with PET, Davis et al. (155) rated FDG uptake and gadolinium enhancement independently in 36 intracranial lesions and found a 93% concordance between enhancement and elevated FDG uptake. However, they noted that FDG uptake may be elevated in benign lesions, such as meningioma and radiation necrosis, although in the latter cases, concomitant tumor may be present despite negative results on histologic sampling. The authors also noted that although elevated FDG uptake and enhancement are usually associated with high-grade lesions, certain lesions, such as anaplastic astrocytomas, may not enhance and can be hypometabolic. In another study, metastatic and primary brain cancers were detected with FDG-PET in 11 of 20 patients thought to have intracranial malignancy, whereas only 9 of the 11 were seen with conventional CT or MRI (156). The false-negative rate with FDG-PET was 15.4%, and it was 30.7% with conventional imaging. No false-positives occurred with PET or conventional workups.

Finally, distinguishing neoplastic from non-neoplastic hematomas may be difficult with CT or MRI, but the diagnosis can be improved with the use of ^{11}C-methionine (157). Although ^{11}C-methionine appears to accumulate in the contrast-enhancing borders of both types of lesions, uptake beyond the contrast-enhancing boundaries observed with anatomic imaging and the higher degree of accumulation of tracer seen in the neoplastic lesions appear to be important features in making this distinction.

PATIENT MANAGEMENT

Clinical Decision Making

The role of FDG-PET in clinical decision making has been reviewed by Deshmukh et al. (158). They found its primary use (87% of 75 cases) to be in the differentiation between radiation necrosis and recurrent tumor. This study was conducted retrospectively through inspection of patient records.

TABLE 10.2. CLINICAL INDICATIONS FOR FLUORODEOXYGLUCOSE IN BRAIN TUMORS

Discrimination of high-grade from low-grade primary brain tumors
Evaluation of metastatic disease to the brain
Evaluation of primary and metastatic disease to the spinal cord
Exclusion of recurrent malignancy from post-therapy necrosis
Evaluation of treatment response
Aid in treatment planning

In 25% of cases, the results of PET were the sole basis for a clinical decision, whereas the majority of cases relied on both the clinical course and results of imaging with several modalities. PET had little impact on the number or type of other imaging studies performed to determine patient management, and no records were found that indicated that PET had influenced the decision to obtain or postpone other studies. Although PET was applied in post-therapeutic assessment, patients were always evaluated with either CT or MRI in addition to PET. The second most frequent indication for PET was as a substitute for biopsy in the assessment of malignancy (11%). Other indications included mapping before treatment or biopsy (4%), postsurgical evaluation for residual tumor (2%), and pretreatment baseline studies (1%). This experience is likely reflective of the scenarios in most centers employing PET technology in the management of patients with brain tumors. The clinical indications for FDG-PET in brain tumros are summarized in Table 10.2.

Determination of Prognosis and Survival from Baseline Examinations

In addition to identifying a correlation between histologic grade and aggressiveness of lesions and accumulation of ^{18}F-FDG, early studies also showed a relationship between tracer uptake and the prognosis or survival of patients with primary brain neoplasms (41,152,159). Thus, in addition to clinical parameters, such as performance status and histologic grade, FDG uptake is a significant factor for predicting survival.

Minuera et al. (160) demonstrated the median survival time of patients with a median rCMRglu value of 4.4 mg/100 mL per minute or higher to be 9 months, whereas patients with lower values had survivals of 113 months or longer. In addition, these investigators observed longer survival times in patients with elevated blood flow and oxygen metabolism in gray matter. In a prospective cohort study of 15 patients undergoing surgery followed by radiation therapy and chemotherapy under a standardized protocol, the prognostic value for patient survival and tumor recurrence was correlated with the metabolic index, measured by the ratio of maximum residual tumor metabolism to contralateral normal brain metabolism (161). On follow-up studies beyond the first postoperative PET assessment, contralat-

eral brain metabolism began to correlate with prognosis, as opposed to tumor metabolism alone.

Serial studies of FDG metabolism in patients with primary brain tumors generally also show that higher uptake in tumor than in gray matter is associated with shorter survival. In a study of 20 patients with untreated and previously treated tumors, Schifter et al. (162) evaluated initial FDG scans versus serial examinations and demonstrated that the relationship between high uptake and shorter survival is significant only when the persistent elevation observed on serial studies is considered. As in other studies, these investigators noted the high frequency of heterogeneous tumor uptake of tracer. They also suggested that studies designed to evaluate the relationship between prognosis and tumor metabolism based on absolute quantification could underestimate malignancy because of partial volume averaging in the ROI, and that visual inspection might be more accurate in determining tumor metabolism.

Low-grade gliomas may demonstrate areas of increased uptake of FDG, possibly a signal of the advent of malignant degeneration. De Witte et al. (163) studied 28 patients with low-grade glioma and demonstrated that elevated FDG uptake in such lesions usually antedates a deleterious outcome. Although FDG uptake has been reported to be increased in the malignant transformation of low-grade tumors (43), no relationship has been established between the level of FDG uptake in pathologically demonstrated low-grade gliomas and the risk for malignant transformation. In another study, two patients with slowly progressive gliomas were evaluated serially with PET to determine changes in rCBF, rCBV, oxygen extraction and oxygen metabolism, and glucose utilization over time (164). These studies demonstrated a good correlation between oxygen metabolism and regional blood flow, which indicates that oxygen extraction is a reasonable indicator of oxygen metabolism. Oxygen extraction was low initially and remained low throughout the serial evaluations, which suggests that this parameter might be useful in detecting the early stage of glioma development. FDG uptake remained similar to or increased above uptake in ipsilateral and contralateral gray matter in these two patients during the course of the serial examinations.

Although several studies have been published regarding the utility of FDG for predicting tumor grade and survival, less is known about its role in determining the prognosis of patients in whom tumor recurrence is suspected. A few studies have reported trends toward longer survival in patients with low rates of glucose uptake at the time of suspected recurrences, but no statistically significant differences in survival have been demonstrated (38,140,165). In a study by Barker et al. (166), the prognostic value of FDG-PET was determined in 55 patients with a diagnosis of brain tumor recurrence versus radiation necrosis based on MRI or CT findings. In this study, FDG-PET scans were graded visually on a scale of 4 (0, no visible activity; 1, activity visible but less than adjacent cortical activity; 2, activity greater than adjacent cortical activity but less than contralateral cortical activity; 3, activity greater than contralateral cortical activity). The FDG-PET score was a significant predictor of survival time after scanning ($p = .005$); median survival was 10 months for scores of 2 or 3, and 20 months for score of 0 or 1. The score was also a significant predictor of survival ($p = .019$) in a multivariate proportional hazards analysis when patient age, recurrence number, and score were considered in the model. No differences were observed for grade 3 or 4 tumors, first or subsequent recurrence, standard fractionation or hyperfractionation photon irradiation, or stereotactic irradiation before the PET study.

Finally, the effectiveness of different radiotracers and techniques in determining prognosis or survival has been studied. Kahn et al. (140) evaluated the uptake of ^{201}Tl and FDG in patients with evidence of tumor recurrence on CT or MR images. In this study, although both tracers were reasonably sensitive for tumor detection, scintigraphic results did not appear to correlate with patient survival. However, another study evaluated ^{11}C-methionine and FDG in a preoperative patient population (65). In this case, both tracers were useful in predicting patient survival, and the combination of tracers predicted the histologic grade and survival better than either tracer alone.

Treatment Planning

Eloquent areas have been mapped with ^{15}O-water and PET in patients with structural brain lesions requiring surgical resection. In a study by Vinas et al. (167), PET obtained during performance of motor, visual, and language tasks was compared with intraoperative cortical stimulation in 11 patients and visual evoked potentials in another, and results were found to be concordant. During resection, however, intraoperative stimulation was helpful in identifying additional sites not observed with PET. The authors concluded that although ^{15}O-water-PET can be used for the preoperative identification of functional cortex and neurosurgical planning, intraoperative mapping remains the best means to prevent neurologic damage and guide the surgical procedure. This is particularly relevant, given the limited utility of the ^{15}O-water technique for mapping subcortical regions in comparison with the cerebral cortex and basal ganglia.

In a study by Nyberg et al. (168) of 11 patients undergoing surgical resection of tumor or vascular lesions, analysis of results of PET showed that in most patients, the important relationship between the lesion and the sensorimotor cortex could be determined. The authors point out the need for noninvasive techniques to identify eloquent areas, given the increasing use of stereotactically focused irradiation in the treatment of arteriovenous malformations and tumors. Sequential resting and motor activation FDG scans also have been used for brain mapping (169). Subtractive techniques following FDG examination may be useful in the case of low-grade lesions, in which FDG uptake is low. However, the presence of high-grade lesions, which accumulate FDG at a high rate, will likely complicate the application of this approach.

Fusion of PET and MRI or CT data will likely aid in surgical navigation and determination of tumor volume (170). Likewise, the co-registration of high-resolution FDG-PET and MRI may be very useful in identifying small lesions near the cortex and in situations in which FDG uptake is altered by treatment or is heterogeneous because of the coexistence of tumor and necrosis. The accuracy of current registration techniques has been estimated to be 1 to 2 mm (171).

The effect of FDG-PET on delineation of the target volume in planning three-dimensional radiation treatment of primary brain tumors has been studied (172). The volume of abnormal FDG uptake appeared larger than the area of contrast enhancement on MRI in only 1 of 18 patients. In this study, FDG provided additional information in a minority of patients, with a key limitation being high rates of uptake in surrounding normal brain tissue. The investigators noted that FDG-PET may be of use in delineating regions of brain tumor requiring a boost in radiation dose.

Pardo et al. (173) explored the use of functional imaging data, including cerebral blood volume obtained with MRI and FDG uptake determined with PET, in planning three-dimensional radiation therapy. Imaging data were obtained before therapy and at 3-month intervals during the course of radiation therapy in eight patients. In this pilot study, the investigators found that in two of the eight patients studied, the addition of functional imaging data to information obtained with conventional anatomic imaging resulted in a modification of the treatment plan. Although they observed a correlation between a high rate of FDG uptake and an elevated CBV determined by functional MRI in most of the cases studied, they cautioned that further studies are required to investigate the prognostic role of CBV measurement in patient care.

Methods for obtaining patient-specific target-to-surrounding normal tissue ratios of absorbed dose are being developed for use in antibody treatment planning (174). These efforts utilize anatomic imaging modalities, in addition to PET or SPECT, to determine the volume of a source of radioactivity after administration of a diagnostic level of a substance such as ^{124}I-labeled antibody; this information is used to calculate a spatially varying absorbed dose, which can be superimposed on the patient's anatomic imaging data. Such approaches will likely prove beneficial in planning treatment with a variety of ligands bearing therapeutic isotopes.

Positron emission tomography imaging agents for use in planning boron neutron capture therapy are being developed. An ^{18}F-labeled derivative of *p*-boronophenylalanine (FBPA) has been prepared for use in neutron capture therapy of malignant melanoma (175). The agent has been designed for use with PET in the detection and three-dimensional imaging of melanoma during the planning of noninvasive treatment. These investigators were able to demonstrate accumulation of the agent in both intracranial and somatic lesions of melanoma. ^{18}F-FBPA also was evaluated in patients with gliomas of various grades (176). Quantitative analysis based on Gjedde-Patlack plots revealed that K1 (amino acid transport) is the primary factor determining accumulation of the agent and that uptake correlates with degree of malignancy. Metabolism, measured as K3 in a three-compartment model, did not appear to correlate with degree of malignancy. The ability to direct boron neutron capture therapy effectively will be applied clinically as the technology evolves.

Finally, integration of FDG-PET studies into the planning of stereotactic biopsy of brain lesions has been evaluated (177–182). The application of PET in such situations can increase the diagnostic yield of the biopsy procedure and reduce the number of passes required to achieve adequate material in comparison with traditional approaches using CT alone. In 10 of 38 patients, consecutive acquisitions with ^{11}C-methionine and FDG were performed before biopsy, and results demonstrated a good correlation between glucose and amino acid uptake (182). In one case, in which uptake of FDG was low in a low-grade tumor, ^{11}C-methionine proved useful in guiding the biopsy procedure. Goldman et al. (70) also evaluated the use of ^{11}C-methionine and FDG-PET to guide stereotactic biopsy of brain tumors and demonstrated the complementary nature of these tracers in addition to the overall role of PET to guide stereotactic biopsy.

Assessment of Treatment Response

The use of radiotracers and multimodality imaging to assess tumor response to therapy has emerged as an integral component of the management of cancer patients. In addition, the choice of therapeutic regimens has been expanded. As a consequence, the role of PET now extends beyond aiding in the differential diagnosis of necrosis versus tumor recurrence after traditional approaches to radiation therapy. PET and other technologies, such as MRS, have been applied to distinguish radiation injury from tumor regrowth following radiosurgery of primary and metastatic tumors (183,184). Yoshino et al. (184), for example, used ^{18}F-FBPA to identify changes in the metabolism of metastatic brain tumors on PET and MRS. Uptake of ^{18}F-FBPA decreased at 15 days following therapy and continued to decrease progressively at 43 days and 15 months. Serial MRS studies displayed decreasing levels of choline.

In a series of patients with intracranial metastases (breast, lung, melanoma) treated with gamma knife, FDG made it possible to discriminate between radiation necrosis and tumor necrosis based on visual inspection, and was superior to CT and MRI (185). Six patients with elevated uptake died within 54 weeks, whereas four of five without elevated uptake were alive 1.7 years after the scan; the fifth patient died of peptic ulcer disease at 56 weeks. However, a rim of hypermetabolism has been observed following gamma knife treatment of primary brain tumors that may lead to an erroneous interpretation of PET results (186). Figure 10.5 illustrates a patient who underwent gamma knife surgery for a brain lesion and subsequently had an enhancing lesion on MRI. PET revealed a rim of mild tracer uptake, later shown to be related to inflammatory changes rather than tumor. Nodularity associated with such a rim of activity, on the other hand, suggests malignancy in patients who have undergone gamma knife treatment (186).

Early studies presented evidence that PET is useful in assessing the response of brain tumors to chemotherapy or radiochemotherapy (187–190). More recent work has demonstrated clinical improvement and reduction or stabilization of FDG uptake in 4 of 11 patients treated with high-dose tamoxifen; the remaining subjects had clinical and radiologic evidence, including evidence on PET, of disease progression (191,192). All patients entered into the study had failed previous radiation, chemotherapy, or

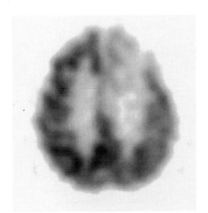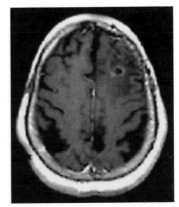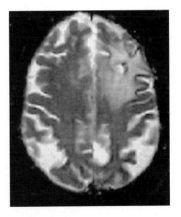

FIGURE 10.5. Ring enhancing mass on magnetic resonance imaging, with extensive radiation-related necrosis and a ring of minimal hypermetabolism on fluorodeoxyglucose positron emission tomography, representing inflammatory changes resulting from prior gamma knife therapy.

both and had clinically and radiographically documented progression or recurrence of disease. One such case is shown in Fig. 10.6.

De Witte et al. (193) have suggested that a hypermetabolic reaction, assessed according to the ratio of FDG metabolism before and after treatment of glioblastoma with carmustine (BCNU), may predict longer survival. In this study, 10 patients were evaluated before and 24 hours after administration of chemotherapy during 2 days. No significant changes in cortical or white matter metabolism were observed, although a spectrum of changes was observed in the tumors of the various subjects. The investigators reported a significant positive correlation ($p <$ .002) between post-therapy and prechemotherapy ratios of glucose metabolism and survival length.

Rozental et al. (194) determined that the percentage of change in glucose uptake ratio (tumor to normal contralateral white matter) between the baseline scan and the 24-hour scan after administration of the first cycle of adjuvant treatment with BCNU are of prognostic significance; the patients with the largest percentage of change in FDG accumulation had the shortest survival. In this protocol, the investigators found that neither the baseline ratio nor the tumor grade based on visual inspection accurately predicted survival. Whereas Rozental et al. (194) studied patients 2 to 4 weeks after brain irradiation, De Witte et al. (193) delayed their study until a minimum of 20 weeks after irradiation to lessen the likelihood of irradiation having an effect on tumor and brain glucose metabolism.

The case of a patient with multifocal malignant astrocytoma who received recombinant human tumor necrosis factor (rH-TNF) as part of a therapy protocol and underwent serial PET with FDG, ^{15}O-water, and ^{15}O-carbon monoxide to assess glucose metabolism, blood flow, and blood volume, respectively, has been published (195). In this study, the patient was studied before treatment, at 24 hours, and again at 2 weeks after the final intracarotid administration of rH-TNF. Although the MRI results did not change during the study, metabolism and flow decreased in one of the two lesions and later rose above pretreatment levels on the last scan. The second lesion remained unchanged throughout the study. The administration of the drug had no effect on

ipsilateral or contralateral normal brain tissue, except for a transient decrease in blood volume in the ipsilateral cortex. In this case, although a rising metabolism is suggestive of progressive disease (196,197), the patient remained symptom-free for 4 months following the therapy and showed no evidence of tumor regrowth. These results demonstrate that significant physiologic alterations following therapy can be observed in brain tumors early after treatment with PET, despite the lack of changes observed on MRI.

Intracavitary treatment of brain tumors presents an interesting issue with regard to FDG uptake. FDG activity outlining a tumor bed following intracavitary administration of ^{131}I-antibody may not necessarily represent the presence of malignant disease (198). These hypermetabolic rims were observed 1 to 3 months after therapy and persisted for 2 to 26 months during follow-up. Although the number of patients studied was small (10), the development of a metabolic rim appeared to be dose-dependent. Pathologic assessment revealed the presence of macrophage infiltrates in this rim area. As noted above, nodularity associated with such a rim of activity following gamma knife treatment suggests the presence of malignancy (186)

In a study by Ericson et al. (48) of metastatic disease to brain, the survival time of patients with an increased accumulation of FDG in irradiated lesions was significantly shorter than the survival of those without evidence of elevated tracer uptake, although the optimal timing of the PET examinations requires further investigation. However, others could not demonstrate a correlation between survival and metabolic or hemodynamic parameters with the use of PET measurements of rCMRglu, rCBF, or rCBV in patients with lung metastases to brain (47). In this case, the investigators were also unable to identify a significant change in any of the parameters measured in tumor tissue following radiotherapy.

The use of radiation in the treatment of low-grade primary brain tumors in the early postoperative period remains a subject of controversy. Although PET has a role in identifying malignant degeneration of low-grade primary brain tumors, little is known regarding its role in assessing the response to treatment of such lesions before degeneration. In a study by Roelcke et al. (199), malignant progression

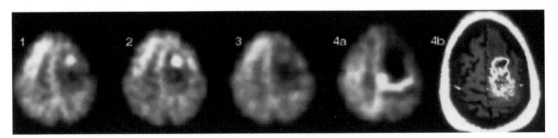

FIGURE 10.6. Serial positron emission tomographic (*PET*) scans in a patient receiving chemotherapy for brain tumor show initial response and subsequent disease progression. Enhanced magnetic resonance imaging scan corresponds to final PET scan.

occurred at the same rate in a group of 30 patients regardless of whether they received radiation treatment; 17 of them did not receive radiotherapy. The tumor-to-contralateral brain ratios were generally higher in the malignant recurrences than in the nonmalignant recurrences in both groups, irrespective of radiotherapy, when they were evaluated with either ^{11}C-methionine or FDG. Thus, although the results show a relative lack of effect of radiotherapy on course of disease or tracer uptake at the time of recurrence, both tracers appeared useful for detecting malignant progression.

Few data are available at this time to demonstrate the utility of amino acids such as ^{11}C-methionine in the evaluation of treatment response. Wurker et al. (200) have shown that ^{11}C-methionine is more suitable than FDG for monitoring the therapeutic effects of brachytherapy in low-grade tumor; a significant dose-dependent decrease in uptake was shown for methionine, whereas FDG uptake remained nearly unchanged through 1 year following treatment. Long-term follow-up during a 2-year period in a patient who received radiochemotherapy for a primary brain tumor revealed a continued reduction of amino acid metabolism, measured with ^{11}C-methionine and serial PET (201).

Effects of Therapy on Central Nervous System Metabolism

The effect of therapy on surrounding brain tissue, as opposed to the tumor itself, remains an important although thus far poorly studied parameter. It has long been observed that one of the manifestations of radiation therapy on surrounding and remote brain tissue is depression of FDG uptake on brain scans (189,190,202–206). Although a number of processes may contribute to the overall picture of cortical hypometabolism, such as edema and frank necrosis, such decreased accumulation of FDG can be observed in their absence following treatment. In fact, alterations in tumor metabolism following treatment, rather than physical changes in tumor tissues (e.g., changes in volume), may influence the metabolism of nontumoral brain tissue (207).

FDG-PET has been used to evaluate the effects of surgery on cerebral metabolism (208). In a study of 15 patients who underwent resection of cavernous angiomas and had PET preoperatively and 1 year after resection, results indicated no significant change in global cerebral glucose metabolism, but persistent decreases in the ipsilateral hemisphere and perilesional regions of the brain. Thus, the metabolic changes in brain associated with the lesion are maintained long after surgical treatment, perhaps as a result of replacement of the lesion by a surgical cavity. Surgery *per se* therefore does not appear to produce metabolic variations, at least in the time course studied here. The authors also suggest that the decreases in the ipsilateral cortex are related to deafferentation, whereas those surrounding the lesion are related to chronic bleeding in this patient population.

It is well known that a variety of drugs, both therapeutics and substances of abuse, can alter brain metabolism as measured by PET. Although PET data regarding the effects of chemotherapeutic agents on brain tumor metabolism are accumulating, as noted above, little is known about the effects of these agents on normal brain tissue, if any. On the other hand, drugs such as barbiturates, used in many of these patients as part of disease management, affect normal brain tissue but have little influence on glioma metabolism (209). The latter observation is of clinical relevance because barbiturates or similar agents could enhance tumor uptake relative to background activity in normal brain and potentially influence image interpretation, especially if ratios of tumor to cortical activity are used in the assessment process.

The effect of glucose levels on brain tumor uptake of FDG has been discussed in the literature. Although only limited information has been published to date regarding this subject, one study of three patients with glioblastoma compared uptake of FDG in the glucose-loaded versus the fasting state (210). In this study, imaging at a minimum of 2 hours revealed a clearer delineation of tumors in the glucose-loaded state, with a mean increase in tumor-to-normal cortex ratios of 27% in comparison with the fasting state. The basis for this, at least in part, could be the decreases observed in uptake of deoxyglucose in normal brain when serum glucose levels are elevated (211,212). In another study by the same group, eight patients with glioma and one with metastasis were studied in the glucose-loaded versus the fasting state (213). All patients demonstrated a decrease in uptake in both normal brain and tumor, although the tumor-to-cortex ratio increased by 26% because the depression in tumor uptake was relatively less. These investigators noted that any observed alterations in tumor uptake might reflect a more complicated process than competitive transport.

Glucose levels are also relevant when steroids are administered as part of the management of patients with high-grade lesions. Early studies suggested that uptake of FDG by anaplastic gliomas and primary CNS lymphomas does not appear to be affected by steroids (19,214). However, more recent data suggest that FDG uptake is altered by dexamethasone, as opposed to FDG metabolism, perhaps as a result of elevated serum glucose (215). In Cushingoid patients with brain tumor, glucose metabolic rates are reduced in uninvolved areas of brain in comparison with rates in normal individuals (216). This effect appears to be independent of radiotherapy, concurrent anticonvulsant medication, and trans-hemispheric diaschisis. Evidence has also been found of a specific reduction in hippocampal metabolism as measured with FDG in normal elderly patients after the administration of pharmacologic doses of cortisol (217). In this group of subjects, serum glucose levels were also elevated above control patient levels. The effect, however, was not observed in Alzheimer's patients, possibly because of alterations in the glucocorticoid-mediated regulation of glucose transport in these patients. Thus, understanding the relationship between the effects of glucose levels, or agents influencing them, on tumor tissue and their effects on normal brain may be relevant in image interpretation.

Patients with previously resected low-grade gliomas have been shown to have a global reduction of cerebral glucose metabolism in comparison with control patients (218). Metabolism is reduced regardless of whether the patient has received follow-up radiation therapy. Interestingly, however, despite the use of localized external beam therapy, an additional 17% reduction in uptake was observed in remote brain in radiated patients when they were compared with nonirradiated patients. Metabolic suppression of remote brain was therefore observed in response both to the presence of tumor and to radiation therapy. Although this study did not attempt to correlate neuropsychological impairment with imaging results, other data have demonstrated a relationship between irradiation and performance (219–223). In addition, evidence has been found of a relationship between results of neuropsychological testing or degree of subjective complaints and reduction in cerebral metabolism as measured by FDG. Such evidence has been reported in patients with Alzheimer's disease (224,225), brain injury (226,227), somatic cancers (228), and multiple sclerosis (229), and also in elderly healthy subjects (230). To establish such relationships and understand the effect of the interaction of co-existing pathologic and normal processes on brain metabolism, however, more extensive study is required to determine the clinical relevance of imaging results.

Finally, altered metabolic patterns in normal brain tissues in patients receiving therapy for their primary brain tumor have been observed with other tracers, such as ^{11}C-methionine. An example is found in the report of a patient who received radiochemotherapy for a primary brain tumor (201). This study revealed a reduction of tracer uptake in both tumor and normal brain tissue. Uptake continued to decrease long after the cessation of therapy, which demonstrates the protracted effects of such therapy on tissue metabolism.

Differential Diagnosis of Infection versus Malignancy

The need to differentiate infection or other benign entities from malignancy with accuracy poses a challenge to many of today's imaging modalities. Although advances in morphologic imaging have aided clinicians, many cases of uncertain diagnosis remain. This is particularly true, for example, in patients afflicted with AIDS. In this population, intracranial mass lesions can be seen in associated with primary lymphoma, toxoplasmosis, candidal abscess, tuberculosis, cryptococcosis, herpes, Kaposi's sarcoma, and bacterial abscess, in addition to noninfectious disorders, such as inflammatory cerebritis, infarction, and hematoma (231).

The differential diagnosis would also include other primary brain tumors and metastatic disease from other cancers. The CT or MRI finding of a ring enhancing lesion, for example, could occur in primary or metastatic brain tumor, cerebritis, resolving hematoma, abscess, granuloma, or cerebral infarction (232,233).

One of the more frequent problems in the workup of intracranial mass lesions in AIDS patients is the distinction between primary lymphoma and toxoplasmosis. Although symptomatic toxoplasmosis occurs more commonly in Hodgkin's disease than in any other malignant condition (234), it is frequently observed in AIDS patients. Toxoplasmosis affects 10% of all AIDS patients (235–238). The incidence of chronic positive serologic titers for toxoplasmosis in the normal population is as high as 70%, which limits the diagnostic use of a single serologic value in predicting or excluding *Toxoplasma gondii* CNS abscess (239). On the other hand, the incidence of primary malignant lymphoma is rare, between 0.2% and 2%, and the 3- to 5-month survival may be altered by early radiotherapy (240,241). Remission is sometimes achievable with radiotherapy, although death usually occurs within 2 months (240,241). Primary lymphoma is observed in approximately 6% of AIDS patients and therefore is less common than toxoplasmosis (242).

The most common CT presentation for toxoplasmosis is multiple ring enhancing lesions with surrounding edema. Homogeneous enhancement or lack of enhancement is uncommon. Pathologically, the abscesses are usually multiple, with thin capsules and necrotic centers. Toxoplasmosis findings on MRI include a low T_1 signal, a medium to high T_2 signal with a high signal from surrounding edema, and either ring or homogeneous enhancement (243). CT of primary lymphoma demonstrates a focus of homogeneous enhancement in half of patients (240,241,244,245). Before administration of contrast, a focus of increased or isodense attenuation in comparison with surrounding tissue is noted. The remainder of the patients demonstrate peripheral enhancement relative to the central portion. Fifty percent of patients demonstrate multiple lesions, typically in peripheral supratentorial white matter. On MRI, primary lymphoma demonstrates a low signal on T_1 and a medium to high signal on T_2, with either ring or homogeneous enhancement.

Although it has been possible to localize intracerebral brain lesions by CT or MRI, and to use stereotactic techniques to reduce morbidity and mortality during biopsy, histology may not provide the correct diagnosis (239,246,247). In AIDS patients with CNS mass lesions who are being evaluated for primary lymphoma versus toxoplasmosis, protocols frequently include treatment with antibiotics before biopsy because toxoplasmosis is more common (231). During a 2-week period, one should observe a rapid response if the lesion represents toxoplasmosis. If no response occurs or the patient has atypical clinical findings, a biopsy might then be recommended. Otherwise, radiation therapy can be administered if no response to antibiotics is noted.

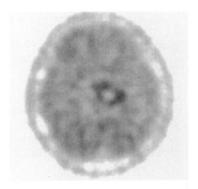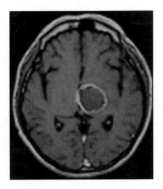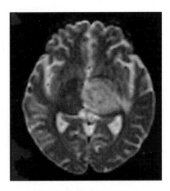

FIGURE 10.7. Fluorodeoxyglucose positron emission tomography in pathologically proven AIDS-related lymphoma of the central nervous system.

Clearly, additional *in vivo* diagnostic information, such as the metabolic information provided by PET, would be helpful in these situations. However, elevated or decreased FDG accumulation is seen in conditions that frequently are included in the differential diagnosis of intracranial mass lesions or that may simultaneously occur with tumor, such as infection, inflammation, seizure activity, radiation necrosis, edema, and infarct (6–8,77,78,248). Minuera et al. (77), for example, have noted an increased accumulation of FDG in both tumor and other entities, such as cerebral sarcoidosis and abscess, and suggest that other tracers, such as $^{15}O_2$, be used for further metabolic analysis designed to differentiate such lesions.

AIDS patients who demonstrate an enhancing CNS mass lesion could harbor one of several types of pathology. Recent PET studies regarding the differential diagnosis of infection versus tumor have detailed methods to distinguish intracranial toxoplasmosis from primary lymphoma (249,250). Although the accumulation of FDG can be seen in both malignant and infected tissue, these researchers have successfully applied PET-FDG techniques to this area. An absence of uptake of FDG in an enhancing lesion is more consistent with toxoplasmosis than primary lymphoma when the two entities are being considered. Figure 10.7 demonstrates a case of known primary CNS lymphoma in a patient with AIDS. These successes represent important preliminary steps in the application of PET in the differential diagnosis of infectious disease and malignancy. However, more specific radiotracers will be required in the future to distinguish between and characterize these various disease processes (116,117,251–254).

SUMMARY

The need for the prompt and detailed evaluation and treatment of malignant tumors requires increasingly sophisticated methodologies for *in vivo* assessment. The morphologic detail provided by CT and MRI has made possible significant advances in diagnostic medicine. Despite such advances, the means of improving the quality and duration of life in many cancer patients, particularly those with brain tumors, remain elusive. Although neither morphologic imaging *in vivo* with CT or MRI nor physiologic imaging with PET or MRS can provide the resolution necessary for assessment at the microscopic or cellular level, all can provide macroscopic or regional data. With PET, exploration of the kinetics of chemical processes occurring at the cellular level provides a "biologic resolution" not heretofore achieved with *in vivo* imaging. Application of this complementary morphologic and biochemical diagnostic information may lead to significant advances in the management of patients with brain tumors in the immediate future.

Numerous investigators at multiple institutions have evaluated PET-FDG in patients with brain tumors. This technique is effective in distinguishing high-grade from low-grade lesions and radiation necrosis from residual or recurrent tumor. It can detect malignant degeneration in tumors originally of a low grade and can provide metabolic information regarding tumor biochemistry and response to therapy that cannot be acquired with morphologic imaging techniques. It is likely, however, that multiple PET radiotracers along with multimodality imaging will be used for diagnosis and monitoring of the effects of therapeutic intervention in the future. The rationale for this is based partly on the heterogeneous nature of malignant tumors and partly on the need to evaluate multiple biochemical parameters so as to be able to classify lesions and assess their response to treatment accurately.

REFERENCES

1. Wagner HN Jr, Conti PS. Advances in medical imaging for cancer diagnosis and treatment. *Cancer* 1991;67:1121–1128.
2. Brownell GL, Kariento AL, Swartz M, et al. PET in oncology: the Massachusetts General Hospital experience. *Semin Nucl Med* 1985;15:201–209.
3. Conti PS, Bading JR, Wong DF, et al. Positron-emitting radio-

tracers: potential aids in the diagnosis and management of neoplasms. *Tumor Diagn Therapy* 1988;9:175–176.

4. Strauss LG, Conti PS. The applications of PET in clinical oncology. *J Nucl Med* 1991;32:623–648.

5. Conti PS, Lilien DL, Grafton ST, et al. PET and [18F]-FDG: a clinical update. *Nucl Med Biol* 1996;23:717–735.

6. Schmall B, Conti PS, Kleinert E, et al. Metabolic characterization of rat prostatic carcinoma *in vivo* with radiolabeled alpha-aminoisobutyric acid (AIB), aminocyclopentane carboxylic acid (ACPC), 2-deoxy-D-glucose (2-DG), and thymidine (TdR). *Biochemistry* 1983;22:36A.

7. Zanzonico PB, Bigler RE, Leonard RW, et al. The enzymatic basis of the biodistribution of FDG: implications for tumor imaging. *J Nucl Med* 1985;26:P64.

8. Schmall B, Conti PS, Kleinert EL, et al. Tumor and organ biochemical profiles determined *in vivo* following uptake of a combination of radiolabeled substrates: potential applications for PET. *Am J Physiol Imaging* 1992;7:2–11.

9. Schmall B, Conti PS, Schaeffer DJ, et al. Radiotracer-derived biochemical profiles via a mathematical model: implications for therapeutic intervention [Letter]. *Nucl Med Biol* 1998;25:799–801.

10. Poste G, Greig R. On the genesis and regulation of cellular heterogeneity in malignant tumors. *Invasion Metastasis* 1982;2:137–176.

11. Henson DE. Heterogeneity in tumors. *Arch Pathol Lab Med* 1982;106:597–598.

12. Sokoloff L, Reivich M, Kennedy M, et al. The (14C) deoxyglucose method for the measurement of local cerebral glucose utilization: theory, procedure and normal values in the conscious and anesthetized albino rat. *J Neurochem* 1977;28:897–916.

13. Phelps ME, Huang SC, Hoffman EJ, et al. Tomographic measurement of local cerebral glucose metabolic rate in humans with (F-18) 2 fluoro-2-deoxy-D-glucose: validation of method. *Ann Neurol* 1979;5:371–388.

14. Reivich M, Kuhl D, Wolf A, et al. The (18F) fluorodeoxyglucose method for the measurement of the local cerebral glucose utilization in man. *Circ Res* 1979;44:127–137.

15. Reivich M, Alavi A, Wolf A, et al. Use of 2-deoxy-D-(1-11C) glucose for the determination of local cerebral glucose metabolism in humans: variation within and between subjects. *J Cereb Blood Flow Metab* 1982;2:307–309.

16. Mazziotta JC, Phelps ME, Kuhl DE. Tomographic mapping of human cerebral metabolism: normal unstimulated state. *Neurology* 1981;31:503–516.

17. Conti PS, Grafton ST. Functional brain imaging using positron emission tomography: applications in oncology and neurology. In: Kelley RE, ed. *Functional neuroimaging.* Armonk, NY: Futura Publishing, 1994:19–50.

18. Coleman RE, Hoffman JM, Hanson MW, et al. Clinical application of PET for the evaluation of brain tumors. *J Nucl Med* 1991;326:616–622.

19. Glantz MJ, Hoffman JM, Coleman RE, et al. Identification of early recurrence of primary central nervous system tumors by [18F]fluorodeoxyglucose positron emission tomography. *Ann Neurol* 1991;29:347–355.

20. Schwaiger M, Hicks R. The clinical role of metabolic imaging of the heart by positron emission tomography. *J Nucl Med* 1991;32:565–578.

21. Schelbert HR. Metabolic imaging to assess myocardial viability. *J Nucl Med* 1994;35:8S–14S.

22. Conti PS. Brain and spinal cord tumors. In: Wagner HN Jr, ed. *Principles of nuclear medicine,* 2nd ed. Philadelphia: WB Saunders, 1995:1041–1054.

23. Conti PS. Introduction to imaging brain tumor metabolism with positron emission tomography. *Cancer Invest* 1995;13:244–259.

24. Derlon JM. The *in vivo* metabolic investigation of brain gliomas with positron emission tomography. *Adv Tech Stand Neurosurg* 1998;24:41–76.

25. DiChiro G, Hatazawa J, Katz, DA, et al. Glucose utilization by intracranial meningiomas as an index of tumor aggressivity and probability of recurrence: a PET study. *Radiology* 1987;164:521–526.

26. Patronas NJ, DiChiro G, Brooks RA, et al. (18F)Fluorodeoxyglucose and positron emission tomography in evaluation of radiation necrosis of the brain. *Radiology* 1982;144:885–889.

27. Doyle WK, Budinger TF, Valk PE, et al. Differentiation of cerebral radiation necrosis from tumor recurrence by [18F] FDG and 82Rb positron emission tomography. *J Comput Assist Tomogr* 1987;11:563–570.

28. Tyler JL, Diksic M, Villemure J-G, et al. Metabolic and hemodynamic evaluation of gliomas using positron emission tomography. *J Nucl Med* 1987;28:1123–1133.

29. Goldman S, Levivier M, Pirotte B, et al. Regional glucose metabolism and histopathology of gliomas. A study based on positron emission tomography-guided stereotactic biopsy. *Cancer* 1996;78:1098–1106.

30. Kim CK, Alavi JB, Alavi A, et al. New grading system of cerebral gliomas using positron emission tomography with F-18 fluorodeoxyglucose. *J Neurooncol* 1991;10:85–91.

31. Delbeke D, Meyerowitz C, Lapidus RL, et al. Optimal cutoff levels of F-18 fluorodeoxyglucose uptake in the differentiation of low-grade from high-grade brain tumors with PET. *Radiology* 1995;195:47–52.

32. Fulham MJ, Melisi JW, Nishimiya J, et al. Neuroimaging of juvenile pilocytic astrocytomas: an enigma. *Radiology* 1993;189:221–225.

33. Bicik I, Raman R, Knightly JJ, et al. PET-FDG of pleomorphic xanthoastrocytoma. *J Nucl Med* 1995;36:97–99.

34. Mineura K, Sasajima T. Itoh Y, et al. Blood flow and metabolism of central neurocytoma: a positron emission tomography study. *Cancer* 1995;76:1224–1232.

35. Kincaid PK, El-Saden SM, Park SH, et al. Cerebral gangl, ogliomas: preoperative grading using FDG-PET and 201Tl-SPECT. *Am J Neuroradiol* 1998;19:801–806.

36. Dexter MA, Parker GD, Besser M, et al. MR and positron emission tomography with fluorodeoxyglucose F-18 in gliomatosis cerebri. *Am J Neuroradiol* 1995;16:1507–1510.

37. Herholz K, Pietrzyk U, Voges J, et al. Correlation of glucose consumption and tumor cell density in astrocytomas. A stereotactic PET study. *J Neurosurg* 1993;79:853–858.

38. Ishikawa M, Kikuchi H, Miyatake S, et al. Glucose consumption in recurrent gliomas. *Neurosurgery* 1993;33:28–33.

39. DiChiro G, DeLaPaz RL, Brooks RA, et al. Glucose utilization of cerebral gliomas measurement by (18F)fluorodeoxyglucose and positron emission tomography. *Neurology* 1982;32:1323–1329.

40. DiChiro G, Oldfield E, Bairamian D, et al. *In vivo* glucose utilization of tumors of the brain stem and spinal cord. In: Greitz T, Ingvar DH, Widen L, eds. *The metabolism of the human brain: studies with positron emission tomography.* New York: Raven Press, 1985:351–361.

41. DiChiro G. Positron emission tomography using [18F]fluorodeoxyglucose in brain tumors: a powerful diagnostic and prognostic tool. *Invest Radiol* 1986;22:360–371.

42. Alavi JB, Alavi A, Chawluk J, et al. Positron emission tomography in patients with glioma: a prediction of prognosis. *Cancer* 1988;62:1074–1078.

43. Francavilla TL, Miletich RS, Dichiro G, et al. Positron emission tomography in the detection of malignant degeneration of low-grade gliomas. *Neurosurgery* 1989;24:1–5.

44. Boon P, Calliauw L, De Reuck J, et al. Clinical and neurophysiological correlations in patients with refractory partial epilepsy

and intracranial structural lesions. *Acta Neurochir* 1994;128:68–83.

45. Griffeth LK, Rich KM, Dehdashti F, et al. Brain metastases from non-central nervous system tumors: evaluation with PET. *Radiology* 1993;186:37–44.

46. Larcos G, Maisey MN. FDG-PET screening for cerebral metastases in patients with suspected malignancy. *Nucl Med Commun* 1996;17:197–198.

47. Lassen U, Andersen P, Daugaard G, et al. Metabolic and hemodynamic evaluation of brain metastases from small cell lung cancer with positron emission tomography. *Clin Cancer Res* 1998;4:2591–2597.

48. Ericson K, Kihlstrom L, Mogard J, et al. Positron emission tomography using ^{18}F-fluorodeoxyglucose in patients with stereotactically irradiated brain metastases. *Stereotact Funct Neurosurg* 1996;66[Suppl 1]:214–224.

49. Gupta NC, Nicholson P, Bloomfield SM. FDG-PET in the staging workup of patients with suspected intracranial metastatic tumors. *Ann Surg* 1999;230:202–206.

50. DiChiro G, Oldfield E, Bairamian D, et al. Metabolic imaging of the brain stem and spinal cord: studies with positron emission tomography using F-18 2-deoxyglucose in normal and pathological cases. *J Comput Assist Tomogr* 1983;7:937–945.

51. Bruggers CS, Friedman HS, Fuller GN, et al. Comparison of serial PET and MRI scans in a pediatric patient with a brain-stem glioma. *Med Pediatr Oncol* 1993;21:301–306.

52. Borbely K, Fulham MJ, Brooks RA, et al. PET-fluorodeoxyglucose of cranial and spinal neuromas. *J Nucl Med* 1992;33:1931–1934.

53. Bakheet SM, Hassounah M, Al-Watban J, et al. F-18 FDG PET scan of a metastatic pineoblastoma. *Clin Nucl Med* 1999;24:198–199.

54. Woesler B, Kuwert T, Probst-Cousin S, et al. Spinal metastases of a high-grade astrocytoma visualized with FDG-PET. *Clin Nucl Med* 1997;22:863–864.

55. Bergstrom M, Ericson K, Hagenfeldt L, et al. PET study of methionine accumulation in glioma and normal brain tissue: completion with branched-chain amino acids. *J Comput Assist Tomogr* 1987;11:208–213.

56. Bergstrom M, Muhr C, Lundberg PO, et al. Amino acid distribution and metabolism in pituitary adenomas using positron emission tomography with D-[^{11}C]methionine and L-[^{11}C]methionine. *J Comput Assist Tomogr* 1987;11:384–389.

57. O'Tuama LA, Guilarte TR, Douglass KH, et al. Assessment of [^{11}C]-L-methionine transport into the human brain. *J Cereb Blood Flow Metab* 1988;8:341–345.

58. Ericson K, Lilja A, Bergstrom M, et al. Positron emission tomography with 11-C-methyl-L-methionine, 11-C-D-glucose, and 68-Ga-EDTA in supratentorial tumors. *J Comput Assist Tomogr* 1985;9:683–689.

59. Lilja A, Bergstrom K, Hartvig P, et al. Dynamic study of supratentorial gliomas with L-methyl ^{11}C-methionine and positron emission tomography. *Am J Neuroradiol* 1985;6:505–514.

60. Meyer GJ, Harre R, Orth F, et al. *In vivo* protein synthesis in human brain tumors measured with ^{11}C-L-methionine. *J Nucl Med* 1989;30:910–911.

61. Ogawa T, Kanno I, Shishido F, et al. Clinical value of PET with ^{18}F-fluorodeoxyglucose and 1-methyl-^{11}C-methionine for diagnosis of recurrent brain tumor and radiation injury. *Acta Radiol* 1991;32:197–202.

62. Ogawa T, Shishido F, Kanno I, et al. Cerebral glioma: evaluation with methionine PET. *Radiology* 1993;186:45–53.

63. Derlon JM, Petit-Taboue MC, Chapon F, et al. The *in vivo* metabolic pattern of low-grade brain gliomas: a positron emission tomographic study using ^{18}F-fluorodeoxyglucose and ^{11}C-L-methylmethionine. *Neurosurgery* 1997;40:276–287.

64. Holzer T. The *in vivo* metabolic pattern of low-grade brain gliomas: a positron emission tomographic study using F-18-fluorodeoxyglucose and C-11-L-methylmethionine. *Neurosurgery* 1998;42:1200–1201.

65. Kaschten B, Stevenaert A, Sadzot B, et al. Preoperative evaluation of 54 gliomas by PET with fluorine-18-fluorodeoxyglucose and/or carbon-11-methionine. *J Nucl Med* 1998;39:778–785.

66. Viader F, Derlon JM, Petit-Taboue MC, et al. Recurrent oligodendroglioma diagnosed with ^{11}C-L-methionine and PET: a case report. *Eur Neurol* 1993;33:248–251.

67. Otte A, Roelcke U, von Ammon K, et al. Crossed cerebellar diaschisis and brain tumor biochemistry studied with positron emission tomography, [^{18}F]fluorodeoxyglucose and [^{11}C]methionine. *J Neurol Sci* 1998;156:73–77.

68. Nariai T. Comparison of measurement between Xe/CT CBF and PET in cerebrovascular disease and brain tumor. *Acta Neurol Scand Suppl* 1996;166:10–12.

69. Roelcke U, Radu E, Ametamey S, et al. Association of rubidium-82 and C-11-methionine uptake in brain tumors measured by positron emission tomography. *J Neurooncol* 1996;27:163–171.

70. Goldman S, Levivier M, Pirotte B, et al. Regional methionine and glucose uptake in high-grade gliomas: a comparative study on PET-guided stereotactic biopsy. *J Nucl Med* 1997;38:1459–1462.

71. Kubota R, Kubota K, Yamada S, et al. Methionine uptake by tumor tissue: a microautoradiographic comparison with FDG. *J Nucl Med* 1995;36:484–492.

72. Higano S, Shishido F, Nagashima M, et al. PET evaluation of spinal cord tumor using C-11 methionine. *J Comput Assist Tomogr* 1990;14:297–299.

73. Mies G, Bodsch W, Paschen W, et al. Experimental application of triple-labeled quantitative autoradiography for measurement of cerebral blood flow, glucose metabolism and protein biosynthesis. In: Heiss WD, Phelps ME, eds. *Positron emission tomography of the brain*. Berlin: Springer-Verlag, 1983:19–28.

74. Kameyama M, Tsurumi Y, Shirane R, et al. Multiparametric analysis of brain tumor with PET. *J Cereb Blood Flow Metab* 1987;7:S466.

75. Abe Y, Matsuzawa T, Itoh M, et al. Regional coupling of blood flow and methionine uptake in an experimental tumor assessed with autoradiography. *Eur J Nucl Med* 1988;14:388.

76. Meyer GJ, Schober O, Gaab MR, et al. Multiparametric studies in brain tumors. In: Beckers C, Goffinet A, Bol A, eds. *Positron emission tomography in clinical research and clinical diagnosis*. Dordrecht: Kluwer Academy, 1989:229–248.

77. Mineura K, Sasajima T, Kowada M, et al. Indications for differential diagnosis of nontumor central nervous system diseases from tumors: a positron emission tomography study. *J Neuroimaging* 1997;7:8–15.

78. Conti PS, Camargo EE, Grossman SA, et al. Multiple radiotracers for evaluation of intracranial mass lesions using PET. *J Nucl Med* 1991;32:954.

79. Conti PS, Grossman SA, Wilson AA, et al. Brain tumor imaging with C-11 labeled thymidine and PET. *Radiology* 1990;177P:234.

80. Kracht LW, Bauer A, Herholz K, et al. Positron emission tomography in a case of intracranial hemangiopericytoma. *J Comput Assist Tomogr* 1999;23:365–368.

81. De Reuck J, De la Meilleure G, Boon P, et al. Comparison of cerebral haemodynamic and oxygen metabolic changes due to cavernous angiomas and arteriovenous malformations of the brain: a positron emission tomography study. *Acta Neurol Belg* 1994;94:239–244.

82. Flier J, Mueckler MM, Usher P, et al. Elevated levels of glucose transport and transporter messenger RNA are induced by *ras* or *src* oncogenes. *Science* 1987;235:1492–1495.

83. Persons DA, Schek N, Hall BL, et al. Increased expression of glycolysis-associated genes in oncogene-transformed and growth-accelerated states. *Mol Carcinog* 1989;2:88–94.

84. Warburg O. *The metabolism of tumors.* London: Arnold Constable, 1930:75–327.

85. Johnstone RM, Scholefield PG. Amino acid transport in tumor cells. *Adv Cancer Res* 1965;9:143–226.

86. Foster DO, Pardee AB. Transport of amino acids by confluent and nonconfluent 3T3 and polyoma virus-transformed 3T3 cells growing on glass cover slips. *J Biol Chem* 1969;244:2675–2681.

87. Isselbacher KJ. Sugar and amino acid transport by cells in culture: differences between normal and malignant cells. *New Engl J Med* 1972;286:929–933.

88. Parnes JR, Isselbacher KJ. Transport alterations in virus-transformed cells. *Prog Exp Tumor Res* 1978;22:79–122.

89. Taylor JH, Woods PS, Hughes WL. The organization and duplication of chromosomes as revealed by autoradiographic studies using tritium-labeled thymidine. *Proc Natl Acad Sci U S A* 1957;43:122–127.

90. Chang LO, Looney WB. A biochemical and autoradiographic study of the *in vivo* utilization of tritiated thymidine in regenerating rat liver. *Cancer Res* 1965;25:1817–1822.

91. Stewart PA, Quastler H, Skougaard MR, et al. Four-factor model analysis of thymidine incorporation into mouse DNA and the mechanism of radiation effects. *Radiat Res* 1965;24:521–537.

92. Lea MA, Morris HP, Weber G. Comparative biochemistry of hepatomas VI. Thymidine incorporation into DNA as a measure of hepatoma growth rate. *Cancer Res* 1966;26:465–469.

93. Cleaver JE. *Thymidine metabolism and cell kinetics.* Amsterdam: North Holland, 1967.

94. Frindel E, Malaise F, Tubiana M. Cell proliferation kinetics in five human solid tumors. *Cancer* 1968;22:611–620.

95. Shapiro WR. The effect of chemotherapeutic agents on the incorporation of DNA precursors by experimental brain tumors. *Cancer Res* 1972;32:2178–2185.

96. Tew KD, Taylor DM. The relationship of thymidine metabolites to the use of functional incorporation as measure of DNA synthesis and tissue proliferation. *Eur J Cancer* 1978;14:153–168.

97. Shields AF, Lim K, Grierson J, et al. Utilization of labeled thymidine in DNA synthesis: studies for PET. *J Nucl Med* 1990;31:337–342.

98. Conti PS, Hilton J, Wong DF, et al. High-performance liquid chromatography of methyl-C-11-thymidine and its major catabolites for clinical PET studies. *Nucl Med Biol* 1994;21:1045–1051.

99. Bizzi A, Wong DF, Mouton P, et al. Correlation of ^{11}C-thymidine PET and MRI with biopsy specimens of brain gliomas. *Radiology* 1996;198(P):280(abst).

100. Weinhard K, Herholz K, Coenen HH, et al. Increased amino acid transport into brain tumors measured by PET of L-(2-^{18}F) fluorotyrosine. *J Nucl Med* 1991;32:1338–1346.

101. Reiman RE, Benua RS, Gelbard AS, et al. Imaging of brain tumors after administration of L-(N-13) glutamate: concise communication. *J Nucl Med* 1982;23:682–687.

102. Katsuyoshi M, Kowada M, Shishido F. Brain tumor imaging with synthesized ^{18}F-fluorophenylalanine and positron emission tomography. *Surg Neurol* 1989;31:468–469.

103. Ogawa T, Miura S, Murakami M, et al. Quantitative evaluation of neutral amino acid transport in cerebral gliomas using positron emission tomography and fluorine-18 fluorophenylalanine. *Eur J Nucl Med* 1996;23:889–895.

104. Hayes RL, Washburn LC, Wieland BW, et al. Carboxy-labeled C-11 1-aminocyclopentane carboxylic acid, a potent agent for cancer detection. *J Nucl Med* 1976;17:748–751.

105. Hubner KF, Purvis JT, Mahaley SM Jr, et al. Brain tumor imaging by positron emission computed tomography using C-11 labeled amino acids. *J Comput Assist Tomogr* 1982;6:544–550.

106. Hubner KF. *Unnatural amino acids in PET oncology.* 5th Annual Meeting of the Institute for Clinical PET, McLean, Virginia, October 28–31, 1993.

107. Schmall B, Conti PS, Bigler RE, et al. Synthesis and quality assurance of C-11 alpha-aminoisobutyric acid (AIB), a potential radiotracer for imaging and amino acid transport studies in normal and malignant tissues. *Int J Nucl Med Biol* 1984;11:209–214.

108. Pruim J, Willemsen AT, Molenaar WM, et al. Brain tumors: L-[1-C-11]tyrosine PET for visualization and quantification of protein synthesis rate. *Radiology* 1995;197:221–226.

109. Inoue T, Shibasaki T, Oriuchi N, et al. ^{18}F alpha-methyl tyrosine PET studies in patients with brain tumors. *J Nucl Med* 1999;40:399–405.

110. Shoup TM, Olson J, Hoffman JM, et al. Synthesis and evaluation of [^{18}F]1-amino-3-fluorocyclobutane-1-carboxylic acid to image brain tumors. *J Nucl Med* 1999;40:331–338.

111. Shinoura N, Nishijima M, Hara T, et al. Brain tumors: detection with C-11 choline PET. *Radiology* 1997;202:497–503.

112. Hara T, Kosaka N, Shinoura N, et al. PET imaging of brain tumor with [methyl-^{11}C]choline. *J Nucl Med* 1997;38:842–847.

113. Vander Borght T, Pauwels S, Lambotte L, et al. Brain tumor imaging with PET and 2-[carbon-11]thymidine. *J Nucl Med* 1994;35:974–982.

114. De Reuck J, Santens P, Goethals P, et al. [Methyl-^{11}C]thymidine positron emission tomography in tumoral and non-tumoral cerebral lesions. *Acta Neurol Belg* 1999;99:118–125.

115. Shields AF, Graham MM, O'Sullivan F. Use of C-11 thymidine with PET and kinetic modeling to produce images of DNA synthesis. *J Nucl Med* 1992;33:1009–1010.

116. Conti PS, Alauddin MM, Fissekis J, et al. Synthesis of carbon-11 labeled 2'-fluoro-5-methyl-1-α-D-arabinofuranosyluracil (FMAU): a potential nucleoside analogue for *in vivo* study of cellular proliferation with PET. *Nucl Med Biol* 1995;22:783–789.

117. Conti PS, Alauddin MM, Fissekis JD, et al. Synthesis of F-18 2'-fluoro-5-methyl-1-β-D-arabinofuranosyluracil (F-18 FMAU). *J Nucl Med* 1999;40:83P.

118. Ishiwata K, Tsurumi Y, Kameyama M, et al. Brain tumor accumulation and plasma pharmacokinetic parameters of 2'-deoxy-5-^{18}F-fluorouridine. *Ann Nucl Med* 1993;7:199–205.

119. Kameyama M, Ishiwata K, Tsurumi Y, et al. Clinical application of ^{18}F-FUdR in glioma patients: PET study of nucleic acid metabolism. *J Neurooncol* 1995;23:53–61.

120. Tsurumi Y, Kameyama M, Ishiwata K, et al. ^{18}F-fluoro-2'-deoxyuridine as a tracer of nucleic acid metabolism in brain tumors. *J Neurosurg* 1990;72:110–113.

121. Sato K, Kameyama M, Ishiwata K, et al. Multicentric glioma studied with positron emission tomography: a case report. *Surg Neurol* 1994;42:14–18.

122. Thomas G, Szucs M, Mamone JY, et al. Sigma and opioid receptors in human brain tumors. *Life Sci* 1990;46:1279–1286.

123. Muhr C, Bergstrom M, Lundberg PO, et al. Dopamine receptors in pituitary adenomas: PET visualization. *J Comput Assist Tomogr* 1986;10:175–180.

124. Ferrarese C, Pierpaoli C, Linfante I, et al. Peripheral benzodiazepine receptors and glucose metabolism in human gliomas. *J Neurooncol* 1994;22:15–22.

125. Roelcke U. PET: brain tumor biochemistry. *J Neurooncol* 1994;22:275–279.

126. Volkow N, Goldman SS, Flam ES, et al. Labeled putrescine as a probe in brain tumors. *Science* 1983;221:673–675.

127. Hiesiger E, Follwer JS, Wolf AP, et al. Serial PET studies of human cerebral malignancy with [1-^{11}C]putrescine and [1-^{11}C]2-deoxy-D-glucose. *J Nucl Med* 1987;28:1251–1261.

128. Jarden JO. Pathophysiological aspects of malignant brain tumors studied with positron emission tomography. *Acta Neurol Scand Suppl* 1994;156:1–35.

129. Jansen HM, Dierckx RA, Hew JM, et al. Positron emission tomography in primary brain tumours using cobalt-55. *Nucl Med Commun* 1997;18:734–740.

130. Rottenberg DA, Ginoz KJ, Kearfott KJ, et al. *In vivo* measurement of brain tumor pH using ^{11}C-DMO and positron emission tomography. *Ann Neurol* 1985;17:70–79.

131. Kearfott KJ, Junck L, Rottenberg DA. ^{11}C-Dimethyloxazolindinedione (DMO): biodistribution, estimates of radiation absorbed dose and potential for positron emission tomographic (PET) measurement of regional brain tissue. *J Nucl Med* 1983; 8:805–811.

132. Valk PE, Mathis CA, Prados MD, et al. Hypoxia in human gliomas: demonstration by PET with fluorine-18-fluoromisonidazole. *J Nucl Med* 1992;33:2133–2137.

133. Graham MM, Peterson LM, Link JM, et al. Fluorine-18-fluoromisonidazole radiation dosimetry in imaging studies. *J Nucl Med* 1997;38:1631–1636.

134. Aboagye EO, Kelson AB, Tracy M, et al. Preclinical development and current status of the fluorinated 2-nitroimidazole hypoxia probe N-(2-hydroxy-3,3,3-trifluoropropyl)-2-(2-nitro-1-imidazolyl) acetamide (SR 4554, CRC 94/17): a non-invasive diagnostic probe for the measurement of tumor hypoxia by magnetic resonance spectroscopy and imaging, and by positron emission tomography. *Anticancer Drug Res* 1998;13:703–730.

135. Diksic M, Sako K, Feindel W, et al. Pharmacokinetics of positron-labeled 1,3-*bis* (2-chloroethyl) nitrosourea in human brain tumors using positron emission tomography. *Cancer Res* 1984;44:3120–3124.

136. Ginos JZ, Cooper AJL, Dhawan V, et al. [^{13}N]-Cisplatin PET to assess pharmacokinetics of intra-arterial versus intravenous chemotherapy for malignant brain tumors. *J Nucl Med* 1987;28:1844–1852.

137. Black KL, Emerick T, Hoh C, et al. Thallium-201 SPECT and positron emission tomography equal predictors of glioma grade and recurrence. *Neurol Res* 1994;16:93–96.

138. Tamura M, Shibasaki T, Zama A, et al. Assessment of malignancy of glioma by positron emission tomography with ^{18}F-fluorodeoxyglucose and single photon emission computed tomography with thallium-201 chloride. *Neuroradiology* 1998;40:210–215.

139. Sasaki M, Kuwabara Y, Yoshida T, et al. A comparative study of thallium-201 SPET, carbon-11 methionine PET and fluorine-18 fluorodeoxyglucose PET for the differentiation of astrocytic tumours. *Eur J Nucl Med* 1998;25:1261–1269.

140. Kahn D, Follett KA, Bushnell DL, et al. Diagnosis of recurrent brain tumor: value of ^{201}Tl SPECT vs ^{18}F-fluorodeoxyglucose PET. *AJR Am J Roentgenol* 1994;163:1459–1465.

141. Sonoda Y, Kumabe T, Takahashi T, et al. Clinical usefulness of ^{11}C-MET PET and ^{201}T1 SPECT for differentiation of recurrent glioma from radiation necrosis. *Neuromedicochir* 1998;38:342–347.

142. Weber W, Bartenstein P, Gross MW, et al. Fluorine-18-FDG PET and iodine-123-IMT SPECT in the evaluation of brain tumors. *J Nucl Med* 1997;38:802–808.

143. Woesler B, Kuwert T, Morgenroth C, et al. Non-invasive grading of primary brain tumours: results of a comparative study between SPET with ^{123}I-alpha-methyl tyrosine and PET with ^{18}F-deoxyglucose. *Eur J Nucl Med* 1997;24:428–434.

144. Langen KJ, Ziemons K, Kiwit JC, et al. 3-[^{123}I]Iodo-alpha-methyltyrosine and [methyl-^{11}C]-L-methionine uptake in cerebral gliomas: a comparative study using SPECT and PET. *J Nucl Med* 1997;38:517–522.

145. Leenders KL. PET: blood flow and oxygen consumption in brain tumors. *J Neurooncol* 1994;22:269–273.

146. Groshar D, McEwan AJ, Parliament MB, et al. Imaging tumor hypoxia and tumor perfusion. *J Nucl Med* 1993;34:885–888.

147. Slosman DO, Lazeyras F. Metabolic imaging in the diagnosis of brain tumors. *Curr Opin Neurol* 1996;9:429–435.

148. Alavi A, Alavi JB, Lenkinski RE. Complementary roles of PET and MR spectroscopy in the management of brain tumors. *Radiology* 1990;177:617–618.

149. Luyten PR, Marien Ad JH, Heindel W, et al. Metabolic imaging of patients with intracranial tumors: H-1 MR spectroscopic imaging and PET. *Radiology* 1990;176:791–799.

150. Go KG, Kamman RL, Mooyaart EL, et al. Localised proton spectroscopy and spectroscopic imaging in cerebral gliomas, with comparison to positron emission tomography. *Neuroradiology* 1995;37:198–206.

151. Alger JR, Frank JA, Bizzi A, et al. Metabolism of human gliomas: assessment with H-1 MR spectroscopy and F-18 fluorodeoxyglucose PET. *Radiology* 1990;177:633–641.

152. Patronas NJ, DiChiro G, Kufta C, et al. Prediction of survival in glioma patients by means of positron emission tomography. *J Neurosurg* 1985;62:816–822.

153. Graham JF, Cummins CJ, Smith BH, et al. Regulation of hexokinase in cultured gliomas. *Neurosurgery* 1985;17:537–542.

154. Kornblith PL, Cummins CJ, Smith BH, et al. Correlation of experimental and clinical studies of metabolism by PET scanning. *Prog Exp Tumor Res* 1984;27:170–178.

155. Davis WK, Boyko OB, Hoffman JM, et al. [^{18}F]2-fluoro-2-deoxyglucose-positron emission tomography correlation of gadolinium-enhanced MR imaging of central nervous system neoplasia. *Am J Neuroradiol* 1993;14:515–523.

156. Kim DG, Kim CY, Paek SH, et al. Whole-body [^{18}F]FDG PET in the management of metastatic brain tumours. *Acta Neurochir* 1998;140:665–673.

157. Ogawa T, Hatazawa J, Inugami A, et al. Carbon-11-methionine PET evaluation of intracerebral hematoma: distinguishing neoplastic from non-neoplastic hematoma. *J Nucl Med* 1995;36:2175–2179.

158. Deshmukh A, Scott JA, Palmer EL, et al. Impact of fluorodeoxyglucose positron emission tomography on the clinical management of patients with glioma. *Clin Nucl Med* 1996;21:720–725.

159. Valk PE, Budinger TF, Levin VA, et al. PET of malignant cerebral tumors after interstitial brachytherapy: demonstration of metabolic activity and correlation with clinical outcome. *J Neurosurg* 1988;69:830–838.

160. Mineura K, Sasajima T, Kowada M, et al. Perfusion and metabolism in predicting the survival of patients with cerebral gliomas. *Cancer* 1994;73:2386–2394.

161. Holzer T, Herholz K, Jeske J, et al. FDG-PET as a prognostic indicator in radiochemotherapy of glioblastoma. *J Comput Assist Tomogr* 1993;17:681–687.

162. Schifter T, Hoffman JM, Hanson MW, et al. Serial FDG-PET studies in the prediction of survival in patients with primary brain tumors. *J Comput Assist Tomogr* 1993;17:509–561.

163. De Witte O, Levivier M, Violon P, et al. Prognostic value of positron emission tomography with [^{18}F]fluoro-2-deoxy-D-glucose in the low-grade glioma. *Neurosurgery* 1996;39:470–476.

164. Mineura K, Sasajima T, Kowada M, et al. Long-term positron

emission tomography evaluation of slowly progressive gliomas. *Eur J Cancer* 1996;32:1257–1260.

165. Janus TJ, Kim EE, Tilbury R, et al. Use of [^{18}F]fluorodoxyglucose positron emission tomography in patients with primary malignant brain tumors. *Ann Neurol* 1993;33:540–548.

166. Barker FG, Chang SM, Valk PE, et al. 18-Fluorodeoxyglucose uptake and survival of patients with suspected recurrent malignant glioma. *Cancer* 1997;79:115–126.

167. Vinas FC, Zamorano L, Mueller RA, et al. [^{15}O]-water PET and intraoperative brain mapping: a comparison in the localization of eloquent cortex. *Neurol Res* 1997;19:601–608.

168. Nyberg G, Andersson J, Antoni G, et al. Activation PET scanning in pretreatment evaluation of patients with cerebral tumours or vascular lesions in or close to the sensorimotor cortex. *Acta Neurochir* 1996;138:684–694.

169. Schreckenberger M, Spetzger U, Sabri O, et al. Preoperative PET activation for assessment of motor cortex area in precentral chondroma. *Surg Neurol* 1999;52:24–29.

170. Kraus GE, Bernstein TW, Satter M, et al. A technique utilizing positron emission tomography and magnetic resonance/computed tomography image fusion to aid in surgical navigation and tumor volume determination. *J Image Guided Surg* 1995;1:300–307.

171. Nelson SJ, Day MR, Buffone PJ, et al. Alignment of volume MR images and high resolution [^{18}F]fluorodeoxyglucose PET images for the evaluation of patients with brain tumors. *J Comput Assist Tomogr* 1997;21:183–191.

172. Gross MW, Weber WA, Feldmann HJ, et al. The value of F-18-fluorodeoxyglucose PET for the 3-D radiation treatment planning of malignant gliomas. *Int J Radiat Oncol Biol Phys* 1998;41:989–995.

173. Pardo FS, Aronen HJ, Kennedy D, et al. Functional cerebral imaging in the evaluation and radiotherapeutic treatment planning of patients with malignant glioma. *Int J Radiat Oncol Biol Phys* 1994;30:663–669.

174. Sgouros G, Chiu S, Pentlow KS, et al. Three-dimensional dosimetry for radioimmunotherapy treatment planning. *J Nucl Med* 1993;34:1595–1601.

175. Mishima Y, Imahori Y, Honda C, et al. *In vivo* diagnosis of human malignant melanoma with positron emission tomography using specific melanoma-seeking ^{18}F-DOPA analogue. *J Neurooncol* 1997;33:163–169.

176. Imahori Y, Ueda S, Ohmori Y, et al. Fluorine-18-labeled fluoroboronophenylalanine PET in patients with glioma. *J Nucl Med* 1998;39:325–333.

177. Washington C, Tyler JL, Villemure JG. Sterotaxic biopsy and positron emission tomography correlation of cerebral gliomas. *Surg Neurol* 1987;27:87–92.

178. Hanson MW, Glantz MJ, Hoffman JM, et al. FDG-PET in selection of brain lesions for biopsy. *J Comput Assist Tomogr* 1991;15:796–801.

179. Levivier M, Goldman S, Bidaut LM, et al. Positron emission tomography-guided stereotactic brain biopsy. *Neurosurgery* 1992;31:792–797.

180. Levivier M, Goldman S, Pirotte B, et al. Diagnostic yield of stereotactic brain biopsy guided by positron emission tomography imaging-directed stereotactic neurosurgery. *J Neurosurg* 1995;82:445–452.

181. Pirotte B, Goldman S, Bidaut LM, et al. Use of positron emission tomography (PET) in stereotactic conditions for brain biopsy. *Acta Neurochir* 1995;134:79–82.

182. Pirotte B, Goldman S, David P, et al. Stereotactic brain biopsy guided by positron emission tomography (PET) with [F-18]fluorodeoxyglucose and [C-11]methionine. *Acta Neurochir Suppl* 1997;68:133–138.

183. Rozental JM, Levine Rl, Mehta MP, et al. Early changes in tumor metabolism after treatment: the effects of streotactic radiotherapy. *Int J Radiat Oncol Biol Phys* 1991;20:1053–1060.

184. Yoshino E, Ohmori Y, Imahori Y, et al. Irradiation effects on the metabolism of metastatic brain tumors: analysis by positron emission tomography and ^{1}H-magnetic resonance spectroscopy. *Stereotact Funct Neurosurg* 1996;66[Suppl 1]:240–259.

185. Mogard J, Kihlstrom L, Ericson K, et al. Recurrent tumor vs radiation effects after gamma knife radiosurgery of intracerebral metastases: diagnosis with PET-FDG. *J Comput Assist Tomogr* 1994;18:177–181.

186. Duma CM, Jacques DB, Rand RW, et al. *Poor concordance of PET and thallium imaging in differentiating tumor growth from radionecrosis after high-dose single fraction radiosurgery.* Gamma Knife Users' Meeting, Kyoto, Japan, May 5, 1994.

187. Di Chiro G, Oldfield E, Wright DC, et al. Cerebral necrosis after radiotherapy and for intraarterial chemotherapy for brain tumors: PET and neuropathologic studies. *Am J Neuroradiol* 1987;8:1083–1091.

188. Mineura K, Yasuda T, Kowada M, et al. Positron emission tomographic evaluations in the diagnosis and therapy of multifocal glioblastoma. *Pediatr Neurol* 1985;12:208–213.

189. Mineura K, Yasuada T, Kowada M, et al. Positron emission tomographic evaluation of radiochemotherapeutic effect on regional cerebral haemocirculation and metabolism in patients with gliomas. *J Neurooncol* 1987;5:277–285.

190. Mineura K, Suda Y, Yasuda T, et al. Early and late stage positron emission tomography (PET) studies on the haemocirculation and metabolism of seemingly normal brain tissue in patients with gliomas following radiochemotherapy. *Acta Neurochim* 1988;93:110–115.

191. Couldwell WT, Weiss MH, DeGiorgio CM, et al. Clinical and radiographic response in a minority of patients with recurrent malignant gliomas treated with high-dose tamoxifen. *Neurosurgery* 1993;32:485–489.

192. Conti PS, Wdowczyk J, Grafton ST, et al. Serial PET scans in patients receiving high-dose tamoxifen for primary brain malignancy. *J Nucl Med* 1995;36:225P.

193. De Witte O, Hildebrand J, Luxen A, et al. Acute effect of carmustine on glucose metabolism in brain and glioblastoma. *Cancer* 1994;74:2836–2842.

194. Rozental JM, Cohen JD, Mehta MP, et al. Acute changes in glucose uptake after treatment: the effects of carmustine (BCNU) on human glioblastoma multiforme. *J Neurooncol* 1993;15:57–66.

195. Sasajima T, Mineura K, Sasaki J, et al. Positron emission tomographic assessment of cerebral hemocirculation and glucose metabolism in malignant glioma following treatment with intra-arotid recombinant human tumor necrosis factor-alpha. *J Neurooncol* 1995;23:67–73.

196. Langen KJ, Roosen N, Kuwert T, et al. Early effects of intra-arterial chemotherapy in patients with brain tumors studied with PET: preliminary results. *Nucl Med Commun* 1989;10:779–790.

197. Rozental JM, Levine RL, Nickles RJ, et al. Glucose uptake by gliomas after treatment. *Arch Neurol* 1989;46:1302–1307.

198. Marriott CJ, Thorstad W, Akabani G, et al. Locally increased uptake of fluorine-18-fluorodeoxyglucose after intracavitary administration of iodine-131-labeled antibody for primary brain tumors. *J Nucl Med* 1998;39:1376–1380.

199. Roelcke U, von Ammon K, Hausmann O, et al. Operated low-grade astrocytomas: a long-term PET study on the effect of radiotherapy. *J Neurol Neurosurg Psychiatry* 1999;66:644–647.

200. Wurker M, Herholz K, Voges J, et al. Glucose consumption and methionine uptake in low-grade gliomas after iodine-125 brachytherapy. *Eur J Nucl Med* 1996;23:583–586.

201. Sato K, Kameyama M, Kayama T, et al. Serial positron emission tomography imaging of changes in amino acid metabolism in

low-grade astrocytoma after radio- and chemotherapy: case report. *Neuromedicochir* 1995;35:808–812.

202. De La Paz R, Patronas NJ, Brooks RA, et al. Positron emission tomographic study of the suppression of gray matter glucose utilization of brain tumors. *Am J Neuroradiol* 1983;4:826–829.

203. Patronas NJ, DiChiro G, Smith BH, et al. Depressed cerebellar glucose metabolism in supratentorial tumors. *Brain Res* 1984; 291:93–101.

204. Ito M, Patronas NJ, DiChiro G, et al. Effect of moderate level x-radiation to brain on cerebral glucose utilization. *J Comput Assist Tomogr* 1986;10:584–588.

205. Rozental JM, Levine RL, Nickles RJ, et al. Cerebral diaschisis in patients with malignant glioma. *J Neurooncol* 1990;8:153–161.

206. Valk PE, Dillon WP. Diagnostic imaging of central nervous system radiaton injury. In: Gutin PH, Leibel SA, Sheline GE, eds. *Radiation injury to the nervous system*. New York: Raven Press, 1991:211–237 (vol 12).

207. Wang G-J, Volkow ND, Lau YH, et al. Glucose metabolic changes in nontumoral brain tissue of patients with brain tumor following radiotherapy: a preliminary study. *J Comput Assist Tomogr* 1996;20:709–714.

208. Gogoleva SM, Ryvlin P, Sindou M, et al. Brain glucose metabolism with [^{18}F]-fluorodeoxyglucose and positron emission tomography before and after surgical resection of epileptogenic cavernous angiomas. *Stereotact Funct Neurosurg* 1997;69:225–228.

209. Blacklock JB, Oldfield EH, DiChiro G, et al. Effect of barbiturate coma on glucose utilization in normal brain versus gliomas. *J Neurosurg* 1987;67:71–75.

210. Ishizu K, Sadato N, Yonekura Y, et al. Enhanced detection of brain tumors by [^{18}F]fluorodeoxyglucose PET with glucose loading. *J Comput Assist Tomogr* 1994;18:12–15.

211. Brooks DJ, Beanye RP, Lammertsma AA, et al. Glucose transport across the blood–brain barrier in normal human subjects and patients with cerebral tumors studied using [^{11}C]-3-O-methyl-D-glucose and positron emission tomography. *J Cereb Blood Flow Metab* 1986;6:230–239.

212. Wahl RL, Henry CA, Ethier SP. Serum glucose: effects on tumor and normal tissue accumulation of 2-[^{18}F]-fluoro-2-deoxy-D-glucose in rodents with mammary carcinoma. *Radiology* 1992;183:643–647.

213. Ishizu K, Nishizawa S, Yonekura Y, et al. Effects of hyperglycemia on FDG uptake in human brain and glioma. *J Nucl Med* 1994;35:1104–1109.

214. Rosenfeld SS, Hoffman JM, Coleman RE, et al. Studies of primary central nervous system lymphoma with fluorine-18-fluorodeoxyglucose positron emission tomography. *J Nucl Med* 1992;33:532–536.

215. Roelcke U, Blasberg RG, von Ammon K, et al. Dexamethasone treatment and plasma glucose levels: relevance for fluorine-18-fluorodeoxyglucose uptake measurements in gliomas. *J Nucl Med* 1998;39:879–884.

216. Fulham MJ, Brunetti A, Aloj L, et al. Decreased cerebral glucose metabolism in patients with brain tumors: an effect of corticosteroids. *J Neurosurg* 1995;83:657–664.

217. De Leon MJ, McRae T, Rusinek H, et al. Cortisol reduces hippocampal glucose metabolism in normal elderly, but not in Alzheimer's disease. *J Clin Endocrinol Metab* 1997;82: 3251–3259.

218. Bruehlmeier M, Roelcke U, Amsler B, et al. Effect of radiotherapy on brain glucose metabolism in patients operated on for low-grade astrocytoma. *J Neurol Neurosurg Psychiatry* 1999;66: 648–653.

219. Armstrong C, Ruffer J, Corn B, et al. Biphasic patterns of memory deficits following moderate-dose partial-brain irradiation: neuropsychologic outcome and proposed mechanisms. *J Clin Oncol* 1995;13:2263–2271.

220. Roman DD, Sperduto PW. Neuropsychological effects of cranial radiation: current knowledge and future directions. *Int J Radiat Oncol Biol Phys* 1995;31:983–998.

221. Chadderton RD, West CG, Schuller S, et al. Radiotherapy in the treatment of low-grade astrocytomas: II. The physical and cognitive sequelae. *Childs Nerv Syst* 1995;11:443–448.

222. Crossen JR, Garwood D, Glatstein E, et al. Neurobehavioral sequela of cranial irradiation in adults: a review of radiation-induced encephalopathy. *J Clin Oncol* 1994;12:627–642.

223. Vigliani M-C, Sichez N, Poisson M, et al. A prospective study of cognitive functions following conventional radiotherapy for supratentorial gliomas in young adults: 4-year results. *Int J Radiat Oncol Biol Phys* 1996;35:527–533.

224. Nyback H, Nyman H, Blomqvist G, et al. Brain metabolism in Alzheimer's dementia: studies of ^{11}C-deoxyglucose accumulation, CSF monoamine metabolites and neuropsychological test performance in patients and healthy subjects. *J Neurol Neurosurg Psychiatry* 1991;54:672–678.

225. Sultzer DL, Mahler ME, Mandelkern MA, et al. The relationship between psychiatric symptoms and regional cortical metabolism in Alzheimer's disease. *J Neuropsychiatry Clin Neurosci* 1995;7:476–484.

226. Humayun MS, Presty SK, LaFrance ND, et al. Local cerebral glucose abnormalities in mild closed head injury patients with cognitive impairments. *Nucl Med Commun* 1989;10:335–344.

227. Bergsneider M, Hovda DA, Shalmon E, et al. Cerebral hyperglycolysis following severe traumatic brain injury in humans: a positron emission tomography study. *J Neurosurg* 1997;86: 241–251.

228. Tashiro M, Kubota K, Itoh M, et al. Hypometabolism in the limbic system of cancer patients observed by positron emission tomography. *Psychooncology* 1999;8:283–286.

229. Brooks DJ, Leenders KL, Head G, et al. Studies on regional cerebral oxygen utilization and cognitive function in multiple sclerosis. *J Neurol Neurosurg Psychiatry* 1984;47:1182–1191.

230. Small GW, Okonek A, Mandelkern MA, et al. Age-associated memory loss: initial neuropsychological and cerebral metabolic findings of a longitudinal study. *Int Psychogeriatr* 1994;6:23–44.

231. Federle MP. A radiologist looks at AIDS: imaging evaluation based on symptoms complexes. *Radiology* 1988;166:553–562.

232. Dobkin JF, Healton EB, Dickinson PCT, et al. Nonspecificity of ring enhancement in "medically cured" brain abscess. *Neurology* 1984;34:139–144.

233. Post MJ, Kursunoglu SJ, Hensley GT, et al. Cranial CT in acquired immunodeficiency syndrome: spectrum of diseases and optimal contrast enhancement technique. *Am J Roentgenol* 1985;145:929–940.

234. Summerfield GP. Demonstration of lesions of cerebral toxoplasmosis by computerized tomography. *Postgrad Med J* 1980;56: 112–114.

235. Moskowitz LB, Hensley GI, Chan JC, et al. The neuropathology of acquired immune deficiency syndrome. *Arch Pathol Lab Med* 1984;108:867–872.

236. Levy RM, Bredesan EE, Rosenblum ML. Neurological manifestations of the acquired immunodeficiency syndrome (AIDS): experience at UCSF and review of the literature. *J Neurosurg* 1985;62:475–495.

237. Navia BA, Jordan BD, Price RW. The AIDS dementia complex: I. Clinical features. *Ann Neurol* 1986;19:517–524.

238. Navia BA, Petito CK, Gold JWM, et al. Cerebral toxoplasmosis complicating the acquired immune deficiency syndrome: clinical and neuropathological findings in 27 patients. *Ann Neurol* 1986; 19:224–238.

239. Elkin CM, Leon E, Grenell SL, et al. Intracranial lesions in the acquired immunodeficiency syndrome: radiological (CT) features. *JAMA* 1985;253:393–396.

240. Tadmor R, Davis KR, Robertson GH, et al. Computed tomography in primary malignant lymphoma of the brain. *J Comput Assist Tomogr* 1978;2:135–140.

241. Kazner E, Wilske J, Steinhoff H, et al. Computer-assisted tomography in primary malignant lymphomas of the brain. *J Comput Assist Tomogr* 1978;2:125–134.

242. Petito CL, Cho ES, Lemann W, et al. Neuropathology of acquired immunodeficiency syndrome (AIDS): an autopsy review. *J Neuropathol Exp Neurol* 1986;45:635–646.

243. Zee CS, Segal HG, Rogers, et al. MR imaging of cerebral toxoplasmosis: correlation of computed tomography and pathology. *J Comput Assist Tomogr* 1985;9:797–799.

244. Lee YY, Bruner JM, Von Tassel P, et al. Primary central nervous system lymphoma: CT and pathologic correlation. *Am J Roentgenol* 1986;147:747–752.

245. Jack CR Jr, Reese DF, Scherthauer BW. Radiographic findings in 32 years of primary CNS lymphoma. *Am J Roentgenol* 1986;146:271–276.

246. Levy RM, Pons VG, Rosenblum ML. Central nervous system mass lesions in the acquired immunodeficiency syndrome (AIDS). *J Neurosurg* 1984;61:9–16.

247. Levy RM, Rosenbloom S, Perret LV. Neurologic findings in AIDS: a review of 200 cases. *Am J Roentgenol* 1986;147:977–983.

248. Grossman SA, Eller S, Dick J, et al. Thymidine, leucine, and 2-deoxyglucose incorporation in brain tumors and abscess: a quantitative autoradiographic (QAR) study with implications for PET scan. In: *Proceedings of the Annual Meeting of the American Association for Cancer Research* 1988;29:516.

249. Kuwabara Y, Ichiya Y, Otsuka M, et al. High [^{18}F] FDG uptake in primary cerebral lymphoma: a PET study. *J Comput Assist Tomogr* 1988;6:47–48.

250. Hoffman JM, Waskin HA, Schifter T, et al. FDG-PET in differentiating lymphoma from nonmalignant central nervous system lesions in patients with AIDS. *J Nucl Med* 1993;34:567–575.

251. Perlman MF, Conti PS, Schmall B, et al. Synthesis and purification of the antiviral agent 1-(2-deoxy-2-fluoro-beta-D-arabinofuranosyl)-5-iodocytosine (FIAC) labeled with iodine-125. *Int J Nucl Med Biol* 1984;11:215–218.

252. Wilson AA, Conti PS, Dannals RF, et al. Radiosynthesis of [^{11}C]-N-methylacyclovir. *J Lab Comp Radiopharm* 1991;29:765–768.

253. Alauddin MM, Conti PS, Mazza SM, et al. Synthesis of 9[(3-[^{18}F]-fluoro-1-propoxy)methyl]guanine ([^{18}F]-FHPG): a potential agent for *in vivo* imaging of viral infection and gene therapy using PET. *Nucl Med Biol* 1996;23:787–792.

254. Alauddin MM, Conti PS. Radiolabeled acyclic nucleosides for imaging viral infection and gene therapy: synthesis of 9-(4-[^{18}F]fluoro-3-hydroxy-methylbutyl)guanine ([^{18}F]-FHBG). *Nucl Med Biol* 1999;26:371–376.

11

CEREBROSPINAL FLUID AND SHUNT IMAGING

FRANKLIN C.L. WONG
DONALD A. PODOLOFF

In humans, the cerebrospinal fluid (CSF) is typically produced in the choroid plexus along the roof of the lateral ventricles and the fourth ventricle. It moves down the third ventricle to the fourth ventricle, then to the level of the cisterna magna, farther down the posterior portion of the spinal canal, up the anterior compartment of the spinal canal before joining at the basal cisterns, and then farther up to the cerebral convexity to return to the general circulation. In normal humans with no central nervous system (CNS) pathology, this pathway accounts for about 80% of the CSF drainage; the remaining 20% arises from transependymal flow and through the sleeves of the spinal nerve roots (1). In patients with primary CNS tumors (and leptomeningeal inflammation) or metastases, the CSF drainage pattern may vary greatly.

The dynamics of CSF are therefore of great interest to the clinical scientist. CSF flow varies greatly among animal species, although it remains relatively constant for each particular species (2). The CSF production rate in humans is about 700 mL/d, and the volume is about 150 mL (3). These values translate into a CSF turnover rate of approximately five times a day in normal humans. In CNS disease, the CSF turnover and excretion rates may change greatly, but the production rate largely remains constant except in patients with choroid plexus carcinoma.

Earlier methods of imaging human CSF included the pneumoencephalogram, contrast myelogram, and radionuclide cisternogram. Recent advances in magnetic resonance imaging (MRI) have made imaging possible without the administration of exogenous agents to evaluate CSF flow, but MRI techniques are expensive and may be limited to research. However, radionuclide imaging of the CSF provides a less expensive and more convenient means to evaluate CSF dynamics with the use of minute amounts (less

than a nanogram) of exogenous chemicals. This chapter addresses CSF radionuclide imaging, with particular attention given to the evaluation of ventriculoperitoneal (VP) shunts in patients with CNS tumors.

VENTRICULOPERITONEAL SHUNTS

The purpose of the VP shunt is to relieve the increased intracranial pressure that results from either structural or functional blockade of CSF excretion through its normal pathways. Exploration of various shunting routes, including ventriculoatrial, ventriculopleural, and VP shunts, has led to the conclusion that the VP shunt is preferred in terms of safety and ease of operation (4). Neurosurgeons have used various types of catheters, with or without valves, as shunts. Some of these valves are turned on or off manually by external maneuvers, whereas others respond to low, medium, or high pressure in the CSF. Various configurations in the proximal and distal openings have been designed, with or without a reservoir for intrathecal access (5).

When levels of protein and white blood cells in the CSF are increased (e.g., intracranial hemorrhage after neurosurgery, meningitis, chemotherapy, high tumor cell load), the shunt can become blocked by debris. This is a common condition that requires surgical intervention. The role of imaging studies is to confirm or exclude such blockade. It has been a common practice among pediatric neurosurgeons to introduce radioopaque contrast materials into the shunt, either directly into the tubing or into the valve/reservoir, and observe the flow by means of regular plain roentgenography or fluoroscopy. This practice is convenient, but the long-term effects of the intrathecal application of grams of iodine-containing contrast materials have not been studied. Arachnoiditis is a potential untoward effect that has been observed in adult patients after they have undergone myelography in which intrathecal iodine-

F. C. L. Wong and D. A. Podoloff: Department of Nuclear Medicine, University of Texas, M.D. Anderson Cancer Center, Houston, Texas 77030.

containing contrast materials were used. Radionuclide study of the VP shunt requires the introduction of only minimal amounts of foreign material. Because the tracers used have a high specific activity, only micrograms of the physical materials are injected, and no reaction is expected to such a small amount of material. As long as the radiation dose to the body and nervous tissues is low, radionuclide study of the VP shunt provides a distinct advantage because of its minimal toxicity. The obvious disadvantages are cost and the technical requirements involved.

TECHNIQUES OF RADIONUCLIDE STUDIES OF VENTRICULPERITONEAL SHUNTS

Few descriptions of the technical details are available in the literature. Some authors perform a quick dynamic study in which injection under the camera is immediately followed by serial imaging. The injection site is typically in the reservoir area, and a 0.5-mCi dose of ^{111}In-DTPA (diethylenetriamine pentaacetic acid) is usually used. ^{99m}Tc-DTPA is less expensive and allows a higher dose to be administered, with better photon flux and visualization. Because delayed images are not required for the purpose of verifying the patency of the shunt, its short half-life of 6 hours is not detrimental to the study. However, it is not approved or prepared for institutional use; ^{111}In-DTPA is the only intrathecal radiopharmaceutical approved by the Food and Drug Administration for clinical study. Historically, the pyrogenicity of the substances injected intrathecally, such as serum albumin tagged with radioactive iodine, were a concern. The availability of ^{111}In-DTPA has eliminated this problem.

The procedure involves acquiring sequential anterior or posterior planar projection images over the head, neck, and thorax at 1- to 2-minute intervals for a total of 30 to 60 minutes. Usually, the ventricles and the proximal portion of the shunt are identified by the presence of tracer progressing distally in the direction of the abdomen. Initial sequential imaging is followed by planar imaging of the distal sites, typically in the abdomen. If no tracer is identified in the distal abdominal site, the patient is instructed to get up and move about for a few minutes to allow decompression of the shunts. The entire study may require hours of imaging (Fig. 11.1). For patients with on-off valves in the reservoir, the evaluation of the patency of the shunt requires the valve to be in the *on* position. The sequential method allows affirmative visualization of the tracer descending the shunt; however, different disciplines are required for injection, positioning, timed acquisition, and interpretation of the images.

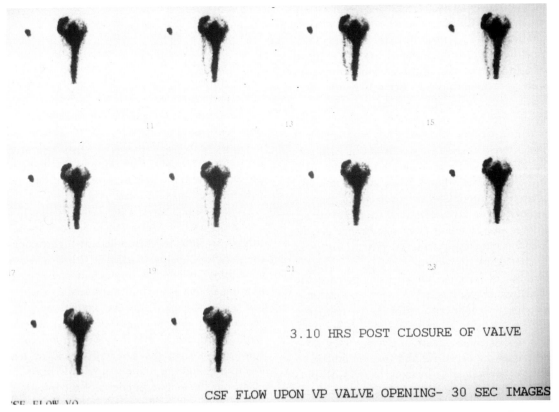

FIGURE 11.1. Serial 30-second anterior images of the head obtained after injection of 5 mCi of ^{99m}Tc-diethylenetriamine pentaacetic acid (*DTPA*) into the right-sided reservoir connected with a ventriculoperitoneal shunt.

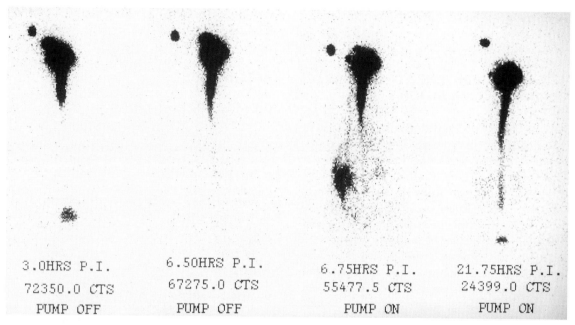

FIGURE 11.2. Twenty-minute whole-body images taken 3, 6.5, 6.75, and 21.75 hours after injection of 0.5 mCi of ^{111}In-diethylenetriamine pentaacetic acid (*DTPA*). The valve was turned on after the second image at 6.5 hours. No shunt was identified after it was turned on. The ventriculoperitoneal shunt is seen along with a collection of tracer in the abdomen. Tracer clears promptly from the abdomen, as can be seen in the 21.75-hour image.

In an alternative method, image acquisition is performed at delayed intervals after the initial intrathecal injection. An example is given in Fig. 11.2. After the injection of ^{111}In-DTPA via the reservoir of a VP shunt with a valve at a closed position, whole-body images are obtained at 3 hours and 6.5 hours later. The shunt is not visualized, as predicted. When the valve is turned to an open position, the subsequent whole-body images show prompt and distinct descent of tracer to the abdomen. Without sequential imaging, the duration of the initial delayed interval after injection is a concern because of the rapid dispersion of tracer in the peritoneal cavity. As seen in Fig. 11.3, the shunt is hardly visualized 3 hours after the injection of 5 mCi of ^{99m}Tc-DTPA into the reservoir. Nevertheless, our study of nine patients with this delayed method has shown that tracer is identified in the shunt up to 1 hour after injection of the tracer or opening of the valve. The presence of tracer activity in the peritoneal cavity is another indication of the patency of the shunt. Other advantages of delayed whole-body imaging include complete evaluation of CSF flow in the native CSF compartment and quantification of CSF dynamics with or without a patent VP shunt. The effective half-life of tracer in the CSF correlates with obstructive symptoms (6) and with the opening or closure of the valve (7). A delayed CSF clearance rate was observed in three patients with nonvisualization of initial peritoneal cavity tracer activity despite the valves being open. This pattern is consistent with subsequent confirmation of nonfunctioning shunts.

Delayed whole-body imaging involves less concerted efforts from various personnel and is therefore more practical. Furthermore, multiple, delayed whole-body imaging allows a more comprehensive evaluation of CSF flow in patients with a VP shunt. Certainly, the ideal study would be to perform sequential imaging followed by multiple whole-body imaging to obtain both dynamic and delayed CSF flow images. Such a comprehensive study would add

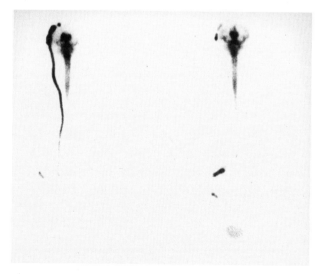

FIGURE 11.3. Three-hour delayed whole-body image of the patient in Fig. 11.1 after the injection of 5 mCi of ^{99m}Tc-diethylenetriamine pentaacetic acid (*DTPA*).

to the cost of the procedure and might not be practical, even in tertiary medical centers.

SIGNIFICANCE OF VENTRICULOPERITONEAL SHUNT RADIONUCLIDE STUDIES

Evaluation of a VP shunt is indicated to establish patency in patients who require CSF drainage to relieve increased intracranial pressure. More detailed inspection by means of whole-body delayed imaging provides information about the CSF flow in the native CSF pathways and the relative drainage of tracer by intracranial versus extracranial routes. Because ^{111}In-DTPA is a small, nondiffusible molecule and the CSF is predominantly driven by bulk flow, visualization of the tracer in the native pathway provides a glimpse of how small, nondiffusible molecules travel in the CSF. For instance, repeated intrathecal sampling has confirmed that the pharmacokinetics of methotrexate, a chemotherapeutic agent, closely parallel the pharmacokinetics of ^{111}In-DTPA in patients without a VP shunt (8). This relationship may also apply to patients with VP shunt because bulk flow remains the driving force behind CSF movement. The radionuclide VP shunt study with ^{111}In-DTPA may also make it possible to observe the pharmacokinetics of small, nondiffusible molecules within and outside the neuroaxis. Further investigation into the application of VP shunt studies to derive pharmacokinetic parameters may be useful therapeutically.

REFERENCES

1. Davson H, The return of the CSF to the blood: the drainage mechanism. In: Davson H, Segal MD, eds. *Physiology of the CSF and blood–brain barriers*. Boca Raton, FL: CRC Press, 1996:489–525.
2. Davson H. The secretion of the cerebrospinal fluid. In: Davson H, Segal MD, eds. *Physiology of the CSF and blood–brain barriers*. Boca Raton, FL: CRC Press, 1996:193–256.
3. Nilsson C, Stahlberg F, Thomesen C, et al. Circadian variation in human cerebrospinal fluid production measured by magnetic resonance imaging. *Am J Physiol* 1992;262:R20–R24.
4. Harbert JC. Radionuclide techniques in the evaluation of cerebrospinal fluid shunts. *Crit Rev in Diagn Imaging* 1977;9:207–228.
5. Drake JM, Sainte-Rose C, eds. *The shunt book*. Cambridge, UK: Blackwell Science, 1994.
6. Wong FCL, Jaeckle KA, Kim EE, et al. Whole-body ommayogram in the evaluation of CSF flow in patients with leptomeningeal carcinomatosis (LC). *Eur J Nucl Med* 1998;25:1075.
7. Wong FCL, Jaeckle KA, Kim EE, et al. Whole-body scintigraphic estimation of clearance of In-111 DTPA in the CSF of patients with VP shunt. *Neurology* 1999;52:A198.
8. Mason WP, Yeh SDJ, DeAngelis LM. In-111 DTPA cerebrospinal fluid flow studies predict distribution of intrathecally administered chemotherapy and outcome in patients with leptomeningeal metastases. *Neurology* 1998;50:438–444.

12

POSITRON EMISSION TOMOGRAPHY IMAGING

VAL J. LOWE
BRENDAN C. STACK

Head and neck cancer represents about 5% of all malignancies diagnosed annually. More than 90% of these tumors have a squamous cell pathology. Head and neck squamous cell carcinoma (HNSCC) is typically seen in men between the fifth and seventh decades of life.

Risk factors for HNSCC are classically reported as prolonged abuse of tobacco and ethanol. Each substance is an independent risk factor, but when combined, they act synergistically to raise a person's risk for the disease. Tobacco is a risk factor for HNSCC regardless of whether it is smoked or chewed. The risk for HNSCC of the oral cavity is increased more by masticatory tobacco than by its inhaled counterpart. Other purported risk factors, which are numerous, include marijuana use, chewing betel nuts, human papillomavirus infection, Epstein-Barr virus (EBV) infection, gastroesophageal reflux disease, long-term and excessive use of mouthwash (containing alcohol), and poor dental hygiene.

An increasing number of women and younger men have been presenting with HNSCC in recent years. This may represent, in part, an increase in smoking among women and teenagers, and an increased use of marijuana during the past three decades.

The geographic distribution of HNSCC is universal. However, some peculiar geographic patterns have been noted with respect to the subsites of head and neck involvement. The incidence of oral cavity tumors is particularly high on the Indian subcontinent and in adjacent regions, presumably because of dietary preferences (spicy foods) and the cultural acceptance of chewing betel nuts. The high incidence of nasopharyngeal carcinoma in southeast Asia is presumed to represent in part high rates of EBV exposure and infection.

V. J. Lowe: Department of Radiology, Mayo Medical School; Department of Radiology, Mayo Clinic, Rochester, Minnesota 55905.

B. C. Stack: Departments of Surgery and Head and Neck Oncology, Penn State Milton S. Hershey Medical Center, College of Medicine, Hershey, Pennsylvania 17033.

The prognosis for most subsites and stages of HNSCC has remained unchanged during the last 40 years. Organ-sparing approaches (chemotherapy and radiation) have gained an increased acceptance as therapeutic modalities but are still considered alternatives to the therapeutic gold standard, which is surgery with postoperative radiotherapy. Tumors of the larynx are an exception. An organ-sparing approach is first attempted at most cancer centers (1,2). Current work on new agents (taxane derivatives and novel compounds) may offer improvements in the organ-sparing approach to treatment. Other alternative treatments in the field that are being utilized include concomitant chemotherapy and radiation, intraarterial chemotherapy, repeated irradiation, implant irradiation (brachytherapy), stereotactic radiosurgery, and photodynamic therapy after administration of photosensitizers. Advanced reconstructive techniques (microvascular free-tissue reconstruction) have not affected the survival of patients with HNSCC but have improved the quality of life of patients after surgery.

POSITRON EMISSION TOMOGRAPHY IMAGING TECHNIQUES

The PET imaging of head and neck cancer depends on the increased metabolism and rapid cell proliferation of head and neck neoplasms. In the 1930s, it was shown that glucose metabolism is increased in malignant cells (3). The largest PET experience with head and neck neoplasms has been with ^{18}F-fluorodeoxyglucose (FDG), which capitalizes on the increased anaerobic metabolism of these malignancies. Other PET tracers, such as ^{11}C-methionine and ^{11}C-thymidine, have been used to evaluate head and neck neoplasms to a lesser extent. The rationale for the use of these tracers is the increased transport of amino acids and increased synthesis of proteins and nucleic acids in tumor cells.

Imaging with FDG is performed in the fasting state to minimize the competitive inhibition of ^{18}F-FDG uptake by glucose. The effect of diabetes on the uptake of FDG has

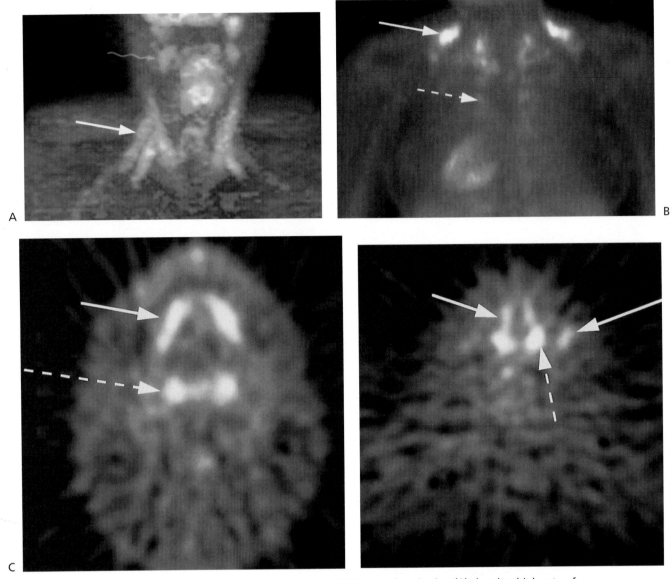

FIGURE 12.1. Positron emission tomography (*PET*) coronal projection (**A**) showing high rate of metabolism in neck muscles, probably scalene and sternocleidomastoid muscles (*arrow*). Pterygoid muscle uptake is also seen (*curved arrow*). PET coronal projection (**B**) showing high rate of metabolism at neck muscle insertions (*arrow*) and costovertebral articulations (*dashed arrow*). PET axial view (**C**) showing high rate of metabolism in muscles in floor of mouth, probably mylohyoid (*arrow*), and at palatine tonsils (*dashed arrow*). PET axial view (**D**) showing high rate of metabolism, probably in vocalis muscles (*short arrow*), cricoarytenoid posterior muscle (*dashed arrow*), and the inferior margin of a tumor-bearing lymph node (*long arrow*).

not been fully elucidated, but elevated serum glucose levels may result in decreased FDG accumulation in cancer cells. Serum glucose values should be checked before FDG imaging is performed; for patients with values above 150 dL/mg, testing should be postponed until their serum glucose is under better control.

Because tumor uptake of FDG continues to increase even up to 2.5 hours after injection, standardizing the delay from injection to imaging is advantageous. FDG emission scans should generally be performed approximately 50 min-

utes after the intravenous administration of FDG for head an neck cancer imaging (4). A dose of 10 mCi of FDG can be routinely administered, but higher doses are not uncommonly used. Emission images are generally acquired to contain 1 million counts per plane.

Images should be obtained to include regions at least from the maxillary sinuses to the aortic arch. The emission data should then be corrected with use of a measured attenuation map. The curvature around the mouth, nose, mandibles, and neck results in severe edge artifacts when

PET studies are performed without attenuation correction. Cervical lymph nodes may lie near the skin surface, and edge artifacts without attenuation correction can hamper identification. Anatomic relationships of the airways and osseous structures can also be more reliably assessed when an attenuation map is available for comparison. Semiquantitative analysis of the data with standardized uptake ratio (SUR) calculation may further aid in assessment and also requires attenuation correction. Imaging to include the liver is recommended to exclude distant metastatic disease in all but early-stage tumors (T1 or T2).

Imaging the head and neck presents unique challenges for PET. Substantial normal variations in uptake in the region can present dilemmas in the identification of pathology (Fig. 12.1). Uptake in adenoid, palatine, and lingual tonsil tissue is a normal variant that needs to be recognized. Uptake in the floor of the mouth and laryngeal musculature is also a common finding. Both these areas usually appear as symmetric regions of uptake in *v*-like patterns, which make them recognizable. On occasion, uptake in various other muscles, most commonly the sternocleidomastoid muscle in the neck, is seen. Scalene muscle uptake also occurs and is often seen in patients after neck dissection with removal of the sternocleidomastoid muscle. The lower neck may demonstrate uptake only at the insertion sites of the neck muscles in the clavicle. This can be easily confused with bilateral supraclavicular lymph node disease. However, the muscle uptake is usually symmetric, and palpation does not detect nodes large enough to cause the amount of uptake seen on the scan. On rarer occasions, temporalis, pterygoid, masseter, or other head and neck muscles accumulate tracer. Some have advocated the use of diazepam to induce muscle relaxation. Careful examination of all three orthogonal views enables the examiner to differentiate muscle uptake from disease based on the anatomic pattern of distribution.

STAGING

Clinical Considerations

The single most important factor in patient assessment, treatment planning, and prognosis is accurate staging of disease (5,6). The current staging guidelines for HNSCC are derived from the 1997 manual of the American Joint Committee on Cancer. Staging involves an accurate assessment of tumor at the primary site (T), regional lymphatic metastases (N), and distant metastases (M). Each primary tumor has a unique propensity for local and regional spread.

Evaluation of the patient begins at the first consultation with a physical examination. This includes direct visualization of the primary tumor, either through the mouth or nose or by endoscopy performed in the office. Next, the neck is palpated to determine the presence of cervical lymph node enlargement. Lymph nodes less than 1 cm in diameter are not reliable appreciated on physical examina-

tion. Features of the body habitus, such as obesity or a short neck, may make this assessment even more problematic. The next phase of the evaluation consists of a pathologic diagnosis (direct biopsy of the tumor or a needle biopsy of a neck mass) or anatomic imaging if the neoplastic process is not visualized, palpable, or accessible.

The most commonly used imaging modality for HNSCC is computed tomography (CT) with intravenous iodinated contrast. Lymph nodes larger than 1 cm in diameter (1.5 cm for jugulodigastric nodes) or with central necrosis are considered abnormal and suspect for metastasis. The obvious shortcoming to this approach is that the determination of metastasis is based on anatomic criteria alone and excludes the possibility of early (yet viable) nodal metastases that have failed to enlarge the lymph node.

Standard assessment for distant metastases in HNSCC, which are uncommon in patients presenting with a new tumor, can include chest roentgenography and liver function tests. CT of the chest or abdomen is most commonly used to evaluate abnormal results found on the preceding two studies.

Second primary disease (either synchronous or metachronous) is an occasional dilemma in HNSCC. These lesions are usually located in the head and neck, lung, or esophagus. Synchronous lesions are defined as second primaries discovered within 6 months of the diagnosis of the first. Metachronous primaries are discovered at an interval longer than 6 months. The standard approach to HNSCC to rule out a second primary has been operative endoscopy (laryngoscopy, bronchoscopy, esophagoscopy). Improvements in office endoscopy and CT (neck and chest) have resulted in a decrease in operative endoscopy. The precision of PET (head, neck, and whole body) may prove useful in the detection of synchronous second primaries detection and also surveillance for metachronous lesions.

The location of a head and neck primary tumor subsite is a strong predictor of cervical metastases. In many cases, failure to treat the regional lymphatics adequately results in subsequent recurrence and is the major cause of morbidity and mortality in these patients. An understanding of which primary tumors metastasize is imperative to avoid undertreating HNSCC. For example, tumors of the supraglottic larynx tend to spread to the cervical lymph nodes bilaterally, even though enlarged nodes are found only unilaterally by palpation or CT. Another example is the oral cavity. Thirty percent of lesions at this site have metastasized to regional lymph nodes at the time of presentation, although they escape detection by palpation or CT. Nasopharyngeal tumors have a propensity to metastasize bilaterally and to the posterior triangles of the neck. With laryngeal tumors, the incidence of nodal involvement is lower, even when they present at an advanced stage, presumably because of a paucity of lymphatics and other anatomic barriers to metastasis.

Once the patient has been adequately staged, a treatment plan is formulated. Usually, the primary tumor is surgically removed if an organ-sparing approach has not been selected. In conjunction with tumor removal, the primary site is reconstructed and the regional lymphatics are removed. If the neck has been staged as N0 or N1, neck dissection or radiation are considered equivalent treatment. Some clinicians opt to observe and treat regional failures expectantly in patients presenting with N0 disease. The advantage to surgical treatment for the N0 neck is that the presence or absence of nodal metastases can be confirmed by pathology; in the event of primary radiation to the neck, metastatic disease is not confirmed pathologically. For N2a disease (a single unilateral neck node > 3 cm), neck dissection with postoperative radiation is the standard of care.

The standard treatment for advanced (stages III and IV) head and neck cancer is surgery and postoperative radiation therapy (7). However, surgery and postoperative radiation cause long-term morbidity and disfigurement. In an effort to diminish morbidity, organ preservation has been achieved by a number of authors utilizing induction chemotherapy and radiation therapy, with surgical salvage. Despite this accomplishment, survival has remained constant (2). Therefore, considerable debate continues regarding which advanced-stage head and neck tumors should be treated with standard surgical resection and which with presurgical chemotherapy. For example, chemotherapy may be selected over more mor-

bid surgery, such as laryngectomy, whereas partial glossectomy may be preferred over chemotherapy. The impetus to treat with chemotherapy and avoid surgery may be greater when more extensive primary disease is identified by FDG-PET than by conventional imaging.

Staging with Positron Emission Tomography

The ability of PET to change disease stage by finding undetected malignancy affects treatment. Tumor staging is based on assessments of primary tumor, local nodal disease, and metastatic disease. Staging of the primary tumor (T) by PET has been described (8,9). The standard methods of CT and physical examination provide more anatomic information important in tumor staging than PET does. In approximately 5% of cases, however, the primary may not be identified by standard techniques in patients with other evidence of disease (the unknown primary). Some of these primary tumors become obvious over time. Others may spontaneously regress, and many are never diagnosed by conventional means. PET may identify the unknown primary in about 25% to 30% of such cases (10, 11) (Fig. 12.2).

The high accuracy of FDG-PET in local nodal staging of head and neck cancer has been described (8,9,12–16) (Fig.

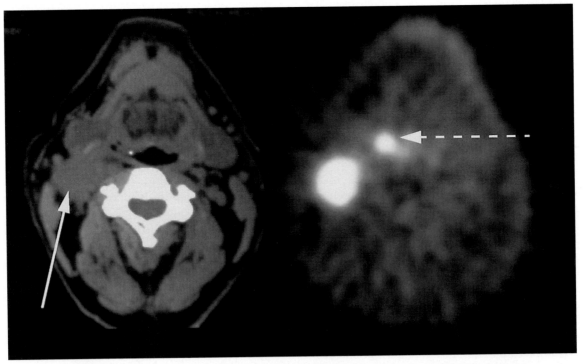

FIGURE 12.2. Computed tomographic (*CT*) and positron emission tomographic (*PET*) images of a patient with a mass in the right side of the neck showing squamous cell cancer on biopsy (*arrow*) and an unknown primary, even after review of the CT findings, physical examination, and negative panendoscopic biopsy results. Thereafter, PET demonstrated a primary in the right side of the base of tongue (*dashed arrow*).

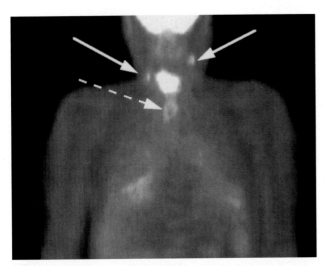

FIGURE 12.3. Improved staging by use of positron emission tomographic (*PET*) in a patient with laryngeal cancer. Computed tomography (*CT*) showed a laryngeal mass and adenopathy in the left side of the neck and below the carina. PET showed bilateral neck disease (*arrows*), the laryngeal primary, and no subcarinal disease. A tracheostomy site is also faintly seen secondary to inflammation (*dashed arrow*). Bilateral neck dissections confirmed bilateral neck disease, and a follow-up CT showed resolution of the subcarinal adenopathy.

12.3). All studies have shown PET to be equivalent or superior to anatomic methods of nodal staging (Table 12.1). In a study by Adams et al. (12), approximately 1,400 lymph nodes were sampled in 60 patients. The sensitivity of PET for detecting local nodal disease was 10% better than that of CT, magnetic resonance imaging (MRI), or ultrasonography. The specificity of PET was also 10% higher.

Metastatic disease to distant regions is less common with head and neck cancer than with other malignancies. This may relate to the earlier detection of head and neck cancer. Hence, FDG-PET is less likely to identify metastatic disease in initial staging. Nevertheless, body imaging with FDG-PET is still recommended at initial staging as a baseline evaluation for comparison with later imaging. For example, subtle uptake from inflammatory lung lesions can be documented so that it will not be confused with metastasis on future examinations. Such imaging also addresses the issue of second primary disease and possibly reduces the need for other testing. Additional imaging can usually be completed in approximately 15 minutes and entails no additional radiation exposure for the patient.

Therapy based on the more accurate staging provided by FDG-PET is more likely to be appropriate. Patients with locoregional disease that is more extensive than originally identified may undergo bilateral neck dissection rather than unilateral dissection. Patients with unknown primary disease of the head and neck may undergo radiation therapy with extensive radiation ports from the maxillary sinuses to the lower neck. Identification of an unknown primary

malignancy by FDG-PET can prevent extensive morbidity from such treatment. Patients with distant metastases that would otherwise go undetected may avoid unnecessary surgery of the head and neck or thorax.

EVALUATION OF THERAPY

Clinical Considerations

The potential role of PET in evaluating tumor response to nonoperative therapies is promising. Artifact resulting from chemotherapy or radiation therapy (fibrosis, erythema, edema) may confound the practitioner's ability to evaluate tumor response to therapy by physical examination or anatomic imaging. The ability of standard anatomic imaging with CT or MRI to evaluate the effect of radiation or chemotherapy on malignancy is limited. This is in part a consequence of the contrast enhancement or soft-tissue distortion that is apparent in previously treated regions on conventional imaging. Changes in tumor size may lag behind the metabolic effects of therapy. Because FDG-PET is a functional study of metabolism, it can be used to assess persistence of tumor in a setting of normal anatomy or absence of tumor in a setting of persistent anatomic abnormality.

Imaging with Positron Emission Tomography

Changes in tumor metabolism during therapeutic interventions can be identified with FDG-PET. Its utility in identifying therapeutic effects depends on the therapy used. Radiotherapy induces early, acute inflammatory hypermetabolism, which can be confused with tumor hypermetabolism (17).

Significantly increased FDG uptake is seen in normal soft-tissue regions that are irradiated. Most commonly, these are surface tissues that are more intensely exposed. Some normal deep structures may not show radiation-related changes in metabolism (18). The duration of increased uptake following radiation therapy is of interest for study interpretation. Increased FDG accumulation in regions of radiation therapy can be statistically significant even 12 to 16 months after treatment in some body regions (19). The SUR of radiation-related uptake is generally less than that of recurrent tumor. Nevertheless, FDG uptake resulting from radiation effects can be in a range that is worrisome for malignancy and needs to be recognized. Some investigators have concluded that an early decrease in tumor FDG uptake after radiation does not necessarily indicate a good prognosis.

Metabolic changes in tumor during chemotherapy may be somewhat more specific to tumor response. Some tumors demonstrate a significant reduction in metabolism that is associated with a good pathologic response. Gener-

TABLE 12.1. STUDIES COMPARING PET AND CT AND/OR MRI IN NODAL STAGING OF HEAD AND NECK CANCER

Author, y (ref)	Patients, No.	Study type	Nodal status: malignant/ benign (No. of)	Sensitivity PET (%)	Specificity PET (%)	Sensitivity compared test (%)	Specificity compared test (%)	Statistical significance PET vs. test
Benchaou, 1996 (13)	48	Blinded, prospective, single	54/414 (nodes)	72	99	67 (CT)	97 (CT)	p = .25
Braams, 1997 (11)	12	Blinding not noted, single institution	22/177 (nodes)	91	88	36 (MRI)	94 (MRI)	Not done
Laubenbacher, 1995 (8)	22	Blinding not noted, prospective, single	83/438 (nodes)	90	96	78 (MRI)	71 (MRI)	p < .05
McGuirt, 1995 (14)	49	Blinding not noted, prospective, single	23/22 (necks)	83	82	78 (CT)	86 (CT)	Not done
Myers, 1998 (15)	14 (no necks by palpation)	Blinding not noted, prospective, single institution	9/15 (necks)	78	100	57 (CT)	90 (CT)	p = .11
Rege, 1994 (16)	34	Blinding not noted, prospective, single	16/18 (stations)	88	89	81 (MRI)	89 (MRI)	Not done
Wong, 1997 (9)	16	Blinding not noted, prospective, single	NA	67	100	67 (CT/MRI)	25 (CT/MRI)	Not done
Adams, 1998 (12)	60	Blinded, prospective, single	117/1,284 (nodes)	90	94	82 (CT) 80 (MRI) 72 (US)	85 (CT) 79 (MRI)	p < .00001

PET, positron emission tomography; CT, computed tomography; MRI, magnetic resonance imaging; US, ultrasonography.

ally, a reduction of 80% in the SUR is predictive of a complete pathologic response. Hypermetabolism secondary to inflammation does not appear to be a significant problem after chemotherapy, as it is in radiation-treated tissue. Tumor metabolism can be at baseline soft-tissue levels as early as 1 week after therapy in responding patients (20). The sensitivity and specificity of FDG-PET in detecting residual disease after chemotherapy in this setting are 90%. In a blinded, prospective study of 27 patients at a single institution, FDG-PET was as sensitive as needle biopsy (90%) in detecting residual disease after therapy, and its specificity was 83% (20) (Fig. 12.4). Greven et al. (21), in a nonblinded, prospective study at a single institution, assessed 31 patients after radiation therapy and found an 80% sensitivity and 81% specificity for FDG-PET in the detection of residual or recurrent head and neck cancer.

Metabolic changes in tumor early in the course of chemotherapy are currently under investigation.

ASSESSMENT OF RECURRENCE

Clinical Considerations

All patients with HNSCC are at high risk for tumor recurrence in addition to second primary disease. This may be because of an underlying molecular or cellular abnormality of the cells lining the upper aerodigestive tract mucosal lin-ing, which have been similarly exposed to carcinogens. Risks for recurrence are related to initial stage, treatment, and ongoing exposure to risk factors. The more advanced the stage of the HNSCC at presentation, the greater the risk for recurrence. Pathologic findings such as nerve invasion, extracapsular spread to lymph nodes, and positive surgical margins are adverse risk factors. Continued smoking and alcohol consumption (a common clinical scenario) are also significant ongoing risk factors.

Most recurrences are in the first 24 months following therapy for HNSCC. Lesions appearing later are probably second primaries. Local recurrences can present many challenges, but when detected early, they can often be excised. Repeated excision will further compromise any preexisting dysfunction (speech, voice, swallowing, or airway) and will have a negative impact on the quality of life.

Regional recurrences (treatment failures) are associated with greater morbidity. They present in the operated neck, radiated neck, or a neck that has undergone both treatments. Carotid artery involvement is a significant issue in this population and can result in stroke or death from acute arterial hemorrhage. Treatment for these recurrences can include reoperation, repeated irradiation (external beam or implant), chemotherapy (with palliative intent), or comfort measures and support (hospice).

As a result, HNSCC patients require long-term surveillance for recurrence and are only deemed "cured" after 5

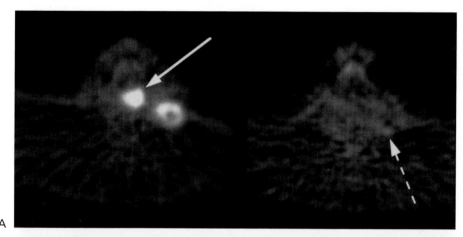

A

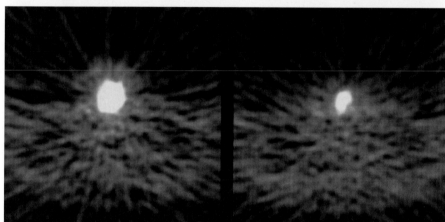

B

FIGURE 12.4. A: Positron emission tomographic (*PET*) images demonstrating hypermetabolism in a cancer of the base of the tongue (*arrow*) and a left jugulodigastric lymph node before therapy (*left*) and resolution of all abnormalities after neoadjuvant chemotherapy (*right*) except for minimal activity in the lymph node after therapy (*dashed arrow*). Neck dissection after chemotherapy documented residual disease in the lymph node. **B:** PET images demonstrating hypermetabolism in a larynx cancer before therapy (*left*) and reduced but persistent activity after neoadjuvant chemotherapy (*right*). Needle biopsy failed to document residual disease, but salvage laryngectomy confirmed residual disease.

disease-free years. The traditional approach includes serial physical examinations, annual chest roentgenography, and liver function tests. Other tests (CT or MRI) are ordered when physical examination findings or patient complaints arouse suspicion of a recurrent or second primary neoplasm. PET may serve as a post-treatment surveillance tool to detect new disease at a subclinical level earlier than by conventional means.

Detection of Recurrent Disease with Positron Emission Tomography

Standard anatomic methods of imaging can be especially difficult in evaluating recurrent disease because of contrast enhancement and soft-tissue distortion after surgery or other therapy. A recent evaluation of MRI and CT showed both to have a sensitivity of about 50%, with substantial

TABLE 12.2. STUDIES COMPARING PET AND CT AND/OR MRI IN DETECTING RECURRENT HEAD AND NECK CANCER

Author, y (ref)	Patients, No.	Sensitivity PET (%)	Specificity PET (%)	Sensitivity compared test (%)	Specificity compared test (%)	Statistical significance PET vs. test
Anzai, 1996 (23)	12	88	100	25 (CT/MRI)	75 (CT/MRI)	*p* = .03
Greven, 1997 (21)	31	80	81	58 (CT)	100 (CT)	Not done
Lapela, 1995 (24)	22	88	86	92 (CT)	50 (CT)	Not done
Rege, 1994 (16)	17	90	100	60 (MRI)	57 (MRI)	Not done
Wong, 1997 (9)	12	100 (accuracy)		54 (accuracy) (CT/MRI)		NA

PET, positron emission tomography; CT, computed tomography; MRI, magnetic resonance imaging.

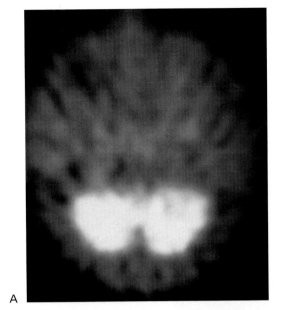
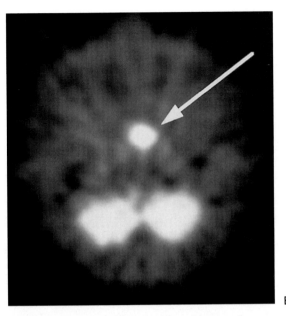

A   B

FIGURE 12.5. Positron emission tomographic (*PET*) images of a patient with a history of nasopharynx cancer showing no disease 2 months after completion of chemotherapy and radiation therapy (**A**) but high nasopharynx recurrence (*arrow*) at the 9-month post-therapy scan (**B**). Computed tomography (*CT*) showed stable post-therapy abnormalities at these times, not indicative of recurrence. Biopsy was difficult, given the location, and results were negative 2 months after the second PET. Disease was not confirmed pathologically until 1 year after the initially positive PET and had continued to enlarge on PET during this time.

interobserver variability (*k* = .563), for identifying recurrent nasopharyngeal cancer (22). Comparison of serial images is the most reliable method to detect recurrent disease.

The use of PET to detect recurrence of head and neck cancer is summarized in Table 12.2 (9,16,21,23,24). PET is more reliable than CT or MRI to detect recurrence because of the anatomic changes in the head and neck that result from surgery or radiation. However, Lapela et al. (24) showed a slightly higher sensitivity of CT (difference of 4%) for detecting recurrence in their series; PET had a 36% higher specificity. When FDG-PET is used in the surveillance of patients who have completed treatment for head

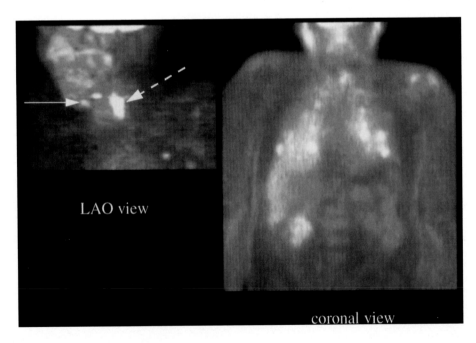

LAO view

coronal view

FIGURE 12.6. Positron emission tomographic (*PET*) images of a patient who had previously undergone laryngectomy and radiation treatment for larynx cancer. The patient presented with difficulty swallowing and a "suspicious" needle aspirate of a submental lymph node. Computed tomographic (*CT*) imaging showed only postoperative changes in the head and neck. The PET showed nodal disease (*arrow*), local laryngeal recurrence (*dashed arrow*), and lung metastasis.

and neck cancer, it identifies nearly twice as many cases of recurrent tumor as regular physical examination or routine CT (25). Most of these recurrences are small and require repeated biopsies for confirmation (Fig. 12.5). If an initial biopsy result is not positive when PET shows an abnormality, repeated biopsy or close follow-up should be undertaken. Surgical exploration should also be considered if the PET results are impressive, as they are rarely incorrect (Figs. 12.5 and 12.6).

CONCLUSIONS

Imaging with FDG-PET can make a significant contribution to the management of patients with head and neck cancer. Improved detection of unknown primaries and local nodal disease may alter initial therapeutic plans. The use of FDG-PET to assess therapy has just begun, but it has the potential to provide clearer information about the results of treatment. Detecting early recurrence more accurately with FDG-PET may provide a means of improving the currently dismal survival of patients with recurrent head and neck cancer. Further evaluation of tracers other than ^{18}F-FDG is necessary to determine their clinical value.

REFERENCES

1. Kraus DH, Pfister DG, Harrison LB, et al. Larynx preservation with combined chemotherapy and radiation therapy in advanced hypopharynx cancer. *Otolaryngol Head Neck Surg* 1994;111: 31–37.
2. Spaulding MB, Fischer SG, Wolf GT. Tumor response, toxicity, and survival after neoadjuvant organ-preserving chemotherapy for advanced laryngeal carcinoma. The Department of Veterans Affairs Cooperative Laryngeal Cancer Study Group. *J Clin Oncol* 1994;12:1592–1599.
3. Warburg O. *The metabolism of tumors.* London: Constable, 1930.
4. Lowe VJ, Delong DM, Hoffman JM, et al. Dynamic FDG-PET imaging of focal pulmonary abnormalities to identify optimum time for imaging. *J Nucl Med* 1995;36:883–887.
5. Bocca E, Calearo C, Marullo T, et al. Occult metastases in cancer of the larynx and their relationship to clinical and histological aspects of the primary tumor: a four-year multicentric research. *Laryngoscope* 1984;94:1086–1090.
6. Shuller DE, McGuirt WF, McCabe BF, et al. The prognostic significance of metastatic cervical lymph nodes. *Laryngoscope* 1980; 90:557–570.
7. Al-Sarraf M, Hussein M. Head and neck cancer: present status and future prospects of adjuvant chemotherapy. *Cancer Invest* 1995;13:41–53.
8. Laubenbacher C, Saumweber D, Wagner MC, et al. Comparison of fluorine-18-fluorodeoxyglucose PET, MRI and endoscopy for staging head and neck squamous-cell carcinomas. *J Nucl Med* 1995;36:1747–1757.
9. Wong WL, Chevretton EB, McGurk M, et al. A prospective study of PET-FDG imaging for the assessment of head and neck squamous cell carcinoma. *Clin Otolaryngol Appl Sci* 1997;22: 209–214.
10. Kole AC, Nieweg OE, Pruim J, et al. Detection of unknown occult primary tumors using positron emission tomography. *Cancer* 1998;82:1160–1166.
11. Braams JW, Pruim J, Kole AC, et al. Detection of unknown primary head and neck tumors by positron emission tomography. *Int J Oral Maxillofac Surg* 1997;26:112–115.
12. Adams S, Baum RP, Stuckensen T, et al. Prospective comparison of 18F-FDG PET with conventional imaging modalities (CT, MRI, US) in lymph node staging of head and neck cancer. *Eur J Nucl Med* 1998;25:1255–1260.
13. Benchaou M, Lehmann W, Slosman DO, et al. The role of FDG-PET in the preoperative assessment of N-staging in head and neck cancer. *Acta Otolaryngol* 1996;116:332–335.
14. McGuirt WF, Williams D3, Keyes JJ, et al. A comparative diagnostic study of head and neck nodal metastases using positron emission tomography. *Laryngoscope* 1995;105:373–375.
15. Myers LL, Wax MK, Nabi H, et al. Positron emission tomography in the evaluation of the N0 neck. *Laryngoscope* 1998;108: 232–236.
16. Rege S, Maass A, Chaiken L, et al. Use of positron emission tomography with fluorodeoxyglucose in patients with extracranial head and neck cancers. *Cancer* 1994;73:3047–3058.
17. Hautzel H, Muller GH. Early changes in fluorine-18-FDG uptake during radiotherapy. *J Nucl Med* 1997;38:1384–1386.
18. Rege SD, Chaiken L, Hoh CK, et al. Change induced by radiation therapy in FDG uptake in normal and malignant structures of the head and neck: quantitation with PET. *Radiology* 1993; 189:807–812.
19. Lowe VJ, Heber ME, Anscher MS, et al. Chest wall FDG accumulation in serial FDG-PET images in patients being treated for bronchogenic carcinoma with radiation. *Clin Positron Imaging* 1998;1:185–191.
20. Lowe V, Dunphy F, Varvares M, et al. Evaluation of chemotherapy response in patients with advanced head and neck cancer using FDG-PET. *Head Neck* 1997;19:666–674.
21. Greven KM, Williams D 3, Keyes JJ, et al. Can positron emission tomography distinguish tumor recurrence from irradiation sequelae in patients treated for larynx cancer? *Cancer J Sci Am* 1997;3:353–357.
22. Chong VFH, Fan Y-F. Detection of recurrent nasopharyngeal carcinoma: MR imaging versus CT. *Radiology* 1997;202: 463–470.
23. Anzai Y, Carroll WR, Quint DJ, et al. Recurrence of head and neck cancer after surgery or irradiation: prospective comparison of 2-deoxy-2-[F-18]fluoro-D-glucose PET and MR imaging diagnoses. *Radiology* 1996;200:135–141.
24. Lapela M, Grenman R, Kurki T, et al. Head and neck cancer: detection of recurrence with PET and 2-[F-18]fluoro-2-deoxy-D-glucose. *Radiology* 1995;197:205–211.
25. Lowe VJ, Dunphy F, Boyd J, et al. Surveillance for recurrent head and neck cancer using positron emission tomography. *J Clin Oncol* 2000;18:651–658.

13

THYROID CARCINOMA

STANLEY J. GOLDSMITH

The thyroid gland is a bilobed, butterfly-shaped organ composed predominantly of thyroid follicular cells that synthesize, store, and release the iodinated thyroid hormones triiodothyronine (T_3) and thyroxine (T_4). Other cells dispersed throughout the thyroid are not involved in thyroid hormone production: parafollicular "C" cells, which secrete calcitonin (a peptide hormone involved in bone mineral homeostasis), in addition to lymphocytes and stromal and other migratory cells. Any of these cells are capable of malignant transformation. The term *thyroid carcinoma*, however, refers to the diverse group of malignant tumors arising from the thyroid follicular cells and includes papillary thyroid carcinoma, follicular thyroid carcinoma, and poorly differentiated and anaplastic thyroid carcinoma. Depending on the degree of differentiation, these tumors (papillary and follicular carcinoma) have thyroid-stimulating hormone (TSH) receptors and intact iodine-trapping mechanisms, and they retain the capacity to synthesize thyroid hormones. Each subtype exhibits a characteristic histopathologic pattern; in addition, they vary in their clinical course, so that the clinical management differs for each subtype. The biology of medullary thyroid carcinoma, which arises from the parafollicular C cells, is entirely different and is addressed in a separate chapter.

Thyroid carcinoma is the most common malignant tumor of the endocrine glands; nearly 19,000 new cases were reported in the United States in 1999. This represents an increase from 11,300 new cases in 1989. Thyroid cancer-related mortality in the United States has also increased, from 1,000 deaths in 1989 to 1,500 deaths in 1999. Whether these changes reflect a true increase, better detection, or both is unclear.

Ninety percent of malignant thyroid nodules are well-differentiated thyroid cancers (papillary or follicular); approximately 7% are medullary carcinomas; anaplastic carcinoma, lymphoma, and other, less common tumors account for the remainder. Most differentiated thyroid carcinomas are of the papillary variety (70% to 80%), with a characteristic tissue and cellular histology. The remaining 20% to 30% of the differentiated tumors are follicular. These designations define different clinical patterns of disease expression; papillary carcinoma typically spreads via lymphatic drainage, with nodal and lung involvement, whereas hematogenous dissemination and metastasis to bone are more frequent in follicular carcinoma. Although these clinical generalizations are useful, exceptions are so frequent that physicians involved in the management of patients with differentiated thyroid carcinoma recognize that the natural history is unpredictable and variable despite the initial histopathologic classification. Papillary and follicular carcinoma may undergo variable degrees of de-differentiation, with loss of the capacity to concentrate radioactive iodine. This is usually associated with more aggressive clinical behavior.

Given the variations in the natural history of these tumors, in addition to individual variations between patients that appear to increase or decrease their risk for recurrence of the disease and death, no single therapeutic approach can be applied to all patients with thyroid cancer.

Medical opinions vary even among experienced physicians and organizations about the extent and details of the treatment of thyroid cancer. Practitioners with limited clinical experience may be confused by all the options. Some see the disease as a biologic curiosity, a malignancy that either progresses slowly and does not require aggressive treatment or is so aggressive that therapeutic intervention is not effective. The natural history of the patient with thyroid cancer is indeed quite variable. Those with papillary and follicular thyroid cancer who are not cured by surgical excision benefit from ^{131}I therapy. Used appropriately, ^{131}I extends disease-free survival and decreases mortality, even when all tumor cannot be surgically removed. Even patients with advanced metastatic disease have been "cured," or at least have been without evidence of disease, for many years.

A wide range of therapeutic options are available in the management of these patients. They should be classified according to the risk factors influencing disease-free survival or disease-related mortality, and an incremental effort should be applied to patients as is appropriate to their

S. J. Goldsmith: Departments of Radiology and Medicine, Weill Medical College of Cornell University; Department of Nuclear Medicine, New York Presbyterian Hospital—Weill Cornell Medical Center, New York, New York 10021.

degree of risk for recurrence and mortality. Therapeutic intervention itself should be based on analysis of patient-specific pathophysiology.

In 1895, iodine was demonstrated to be a component of thyroid tissue. Subsequently, Kendall isolated thyroxine, the physiologically active iodinated compound, from the thyroid gland in 1915. After the discovery of methods to produce radioactive versions of otherwise stable elements, Hertz and colleagues in 1938 (1) demonstrated thyroidal concentration of a radioactive isotope of iodine with a 25-minute half-life (^{128}I) after injection into 48 rabbits. In a brief article entitled "Radioactive Iodine as an Indicator in the Study of Thyroid Physiology," they concluded that "it is therefore logical to suppose that when strongly active materials are available, the concentrating power for radioactive iodine may be of clinical or therapeutic significance." This statement foresaw the eventual evolution of the central role of nuclear medicine in the management of patients with thyroid carcinoma. Because the follicular elements of the thyroid gland are primarily involved in the synthesis of the iodine-containing thyroid hormones, ^{131}I has been an essential part of the therapy of patients with differentiated thyroid carcinoma.

Numerous reviews, even complete texts, deal with thyroid carcinoma. This chapter provides a survey of the data and procedures as they affect the practice of nuclear medicine and formulates a contemporary approach to the management of patients with thyroid carcinoma. The approach is based on the natural history of the disease, advances in endocrinology (e.g., the recent availability of recombinant human TSH) and oncology (e.g., the use of serum thyroglobulin as a tumor marker), and the use of radiation dosimetry to determine appropriate therapeutic doses of ^{131}I.

DIAGNOSIS OF THYROID CANCER

Thyroid Nodule: Clinical

The presentation and course of thyroid cancer are extremely variable. It may be detected as a coincidental finding during pathologic examination of an otherwise benign nodule that has been surgically removed for a variety of reasons. Alternately, it may present as a nodule itself, either initially observed by the patient or found on physical examination by a physician, or be identified as a solitary "cold" nodule on thyroid scanning with ^{99m}Tc-pertechnetate or ^{123}I. On other occasions, a patient may present with metastases—an incidentally discovered pulmonary nodule or a pathologic fracture resulting from a lytic bone metastasis of an unidentified differentiated thyroid carcinoma.

The role of nuclear medicine in the evaluation of a thyroid nodule is primarily to determine if the nodule is "cold" or "warm." These terms describe the functional status of the nodule relative to the surrounding thyroid parenchyma. Cold nodules are more likely to be malignant than "warm"

or "hot" nodules that trap as much or more tracer than the surrounding tissue does. Solitary cold nodules are of particular concern because the incidence of malignancy in such nodules is as high as 20% to 35% (2–4), whereas the incidence of malignancy in warm or hot nodules is very low. Accordingly, solitary cold nodules merit further evaluation with direct sampling of tissue or outright surgical removal. Patients with a history of childhood neck irradiation are particularly at risk (5). Male sex and the extremes of age and youth likewise place the patient at greater risk. Even in a multinodular goiter, a nodule that increases in size is particularly suspect. In multinodular goiters, multiple nodules exhibit varying degrees of function. Cold nodules in a multinodular goiter have not been viewed with particular concern. A dominant cold nodule, however, even within the setting of a multinodular goiter, should be evaluated further. In a recent study (6), fine-needle aspiration of cold nodules was performed in 95 patients with multinodular goiter. In 16 of the 95, abnormal findings led to surgery. Differentiated thyroid cancer was found in 13 of the 16 patients (6 papillary carcinoma, 3 follicular carcinoma, 3 Hürthle cell carcinoma). Three of the 12 had a prior history of neck irradiation. Even when those patients with a history of neck irradiation were excluded (as this exposure may be an independent risk factor), the rate of malignant nodules in the group evaluated did not differ from the incidence in a contemporaneous group of patients with solitary cold nodules (8% to 10%).

Thyroid Nodule: Imaging Technique

Nuclear imaging to evaluate a palpable nodule or simply to evaluate the homogeneity of thyroid tissue function is best performed with a gamma camera having a pinhole collimator and ^{99m}Tc-pertechnetate (144 to 370 MBq; 4 to 10 mCi) or ^{123}I (7.2 to 144 MBq; 200 to 400 µCi). For many years, ^{131}I and a rectilinear scanner with a collimator suitable for the principal 364-keV γ photon were used for thyroid imaging. The gamma camera is more suitable to image low-energy photons, such as the 140-keV emission from ^{99m}Tc or the 159-keV photon from ^{123}I. Technetium 99m as the pertechnetate ion is sufficiently similar to the iodide ion in charge and ionic dimensions to be trapped by functioning thyroid tissue. Although pertechnetate does not subsequently bind to tyrosine (the first step in thyroid hormone synthesis), it provides high-quality images of functional thyroid tissue. The pinhole collimator is preferred over parallel-hole collimation because it provides magnification of the thyroid gland and better resolution in addition to oblique views that serve to assess nodules that may be at the margin of the thyroid lobes (Fig. 13.1). The greatest shortcoming of pinhole collimator imaging is its relative insensitivity in comparison with that of parallel hole collimation, which is caused by the distance of the object from the detector. Pinhole collimator imaging is also associated

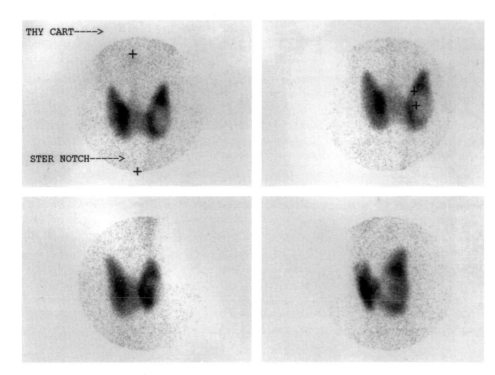

THY CART---->

STER NOTCH---->

FIGURE 13.1. Multiple views of the thyroid gland acquired with a pinhole collimator 20 minutes after administration of 130 MBq (4.0 mCi) of ^{99m}Tc-pertechnetate. Anterior (*upper panels*) and right and left anterior oblique (*lower panels*) projections demonstrate a solitary cold nodule in the left lobe of the thyroid. In this example, the nodule is well outlined on the anterior projection. The depth and extent of involvement can be more fully appreciated, however, on examination of the oblique projections.

with a variety of effects that distort the image to some degree. These include variation in size depending on the distance of the thyroid from the crystal, parallax distortion depending on displacement from the central axis, and pin cushion distortion resulting from a loss of counts related to the parallax effect. These effects, however, are minor. Provided a consistent technique is used, nuclear physicians with experience develop a capacity for mental calibration whereby the size of the thyroid image is used to estimate the clinical size. Alternately, a source of known dimensions can be imaged simultaneously. If the source is placed on a specific anatomic landmark, such as the sternal notch or clavicles, this technique provides additional useful information. Another imaging technique involves electronic magnification of an image acquired with parallel-hole collimation. This approach has the advantage of greater count sensitivity, but it does not provide oblique views. Tomographic techniques have been used infrequently for thyroid imaging, particularly in the assessment of thyroid nodules.

^{99m}Tc-Pertechnetate is more convenient to use than ^{123}I as a tracer for thyroid imaging. It is usually available in nuclear medicine facilities regardless of whether a ^{99}Mo/^{99m}Tc generator is used or daily supplies of ^{99m}Tc-pertechnetate are delivered. It is inexpensive and provides a greater photon flux than the usual diagnostic doses of ^{123}I. In the past, the biologic comparability of the two tracers was a topic of considerable discussion because pertechnetate, although readily trapped by differentiated thyroid tissue, does not undergo organification, unlike radioactive forms of iodine. Physicians were also concerned whether imaging with ^{123}I 2 to 4 hours after administration of the

agent allowed enough time to determine whether a nodule had an intact organification mechanism; in contrast, imaging is performed after 24 hours when ^{131}I is used. By 24 hours, iodine tracer trapped but not organified would "wash out" of a nodule, and the nodule would be imaged as cold. Imaging at 4 hours with ^{123}I or at 20 to 30 minutes with ^{99m}Tc-pertechnetate might not allow sufficient time for washout of the unorganified tracer. This concern is not a real issue. Kusic et al. (7) compared ^{99m}Tc-pertechnetate and ^{123}I imaging in 316 patients. They demonstrated that although in rare cases the ^{99m}Tc-pertechnetate scan differed from the ^{123}I scan, these instances rarely involved thyroid carcinoma as the underlying lesion. Accordingly, ^{99m}Tc-pertechnetate can be used as a surrogate tracer to image the thyroid gland and identify cold nodules.

In addition to classic radionuclide imaging of the thyroid, other techniques used to image a thyroid nodule include ultrasonography, computed tomography (CT) with or without contrast, and magnetic resonance imaging. Although all these techniques are useful to characterize the nodule, their role is less essential at this time because of the availability of thin-needle biopsy with or without ultrasonographic guidance, which allows direct assessment of tissue cytology (8). Despite the potential for sampling error, the technique has emerged as the method of choice for the assessment of palpable nodules in euthyroid patients. Accordingly, it is not unusual for a patient with a prominent palpable nodule to undergo needle biopsy without prior radionuclide imaging. Depending on clinical features and other risk factors, excision of the suspect nodule is a relatively benign procedure in the hands of a skilled thyroid surgeon and the use of contemporary anesthesia techniques. Removal of the nodule obviates concerns about sampling error during thin-needle biopsy. In many patients with a history of goiter or nodule who undergo multiple needle biopsies during a period of several years with benign results, thyroid carcinoma is ultimately diagnosed. Removal of a dominant cold nodule is therefore a reasonable clinical approach, even when histopathology confirms subsequently that the nodule was benign.

In summary, although differentiated thyroid carcinoma may present as a thyroid nodule, and although the likelihood of a cold nodule being malignant is 25% to 35%, many patients presenting to clinicians go on to needle biopsy or even excision with or without radionuclide imaging. The initial presentation to nuclear medicine for evaluation or consultation may be after thyroid carcinoma has been diagnosed.

MANAGEMENT AND THERAPY OF THYROID CARCINOMA

Risk Assessment

The patient with differentiated thyroid carcinoma may present with any one of a variety of clinical scenarios. In the most benign situation, a nest of malignant cells or a small tumor mass that is entirely encapsulated, without vascular invasion or abnormal lymph nodes, is discovered incidentally in a young woman with no history of childhood radiation exposure. As any of these features change, the risk increases that the patient will not be rendered free of disease with simple excision of the primary lesion or even total thyroidectomy. At the other end of the spectrum are the patients who have distal metastases at the time of presentation. Among all patients with the diagnosis of differentiated thyroid carcinoma, age at the time of initial diagnosis is the greatest determinant of outcome; the likelihood of recurrence or death increases significantly after age 45 (9). Other factors related to risk are sex (male sex is associated with a greater mortality risk in patients with papillary carcinoma), size of the primary lesion (risk increases with size), penetration of the thyroid capsule (invasion of surrounding tissue), invasion of blood vessels (in patients with either papillary or follicular carcinoma, although it is more common in the latter), lymph node metastases, and metastases to distal organs (10). These risk factors have been analyzed by several groups and correlate with the likelihood of recurrence and disease-related mortality.

Given the overall low incidence of thyroid carcinoma, the striking contrast between low-risk and high-risk patients with thyroid carcinoma is relatively unfamiliar to most physicians. It is thus easy to understand why a consensus regarding management and therapy is lacking. A review of the collected experience does, however, provide a basis for rational and consistent clinical management and the use of radioactive materials, principally ^{131}I, for diagnosis and treatment.

In Fig. 13.2, cumulative mortality data are plotted as a function of time during a 20-year period for patients with papillary thyroid carcinoma scored as being at low or high risk according to one of four different systems (11): the European Organization for Research on Thyroid Cancer (EORTC) (12); the Union Internationale Contre le Cancer (UICC), which uses the TNM (tumor–node–metastasis) staging system (13); the Mayo Clinic system (14). based on age, tumor grade, extent, and size (AGES); and the Lahey Clinic system (15), based on age, metastases, extent, and size (AMES). The data confirm the impression that in certain patients, classified as being at low risk, papillary carcinoma is indeed a benign disease with virtually no associated mortality following initial diagnosis and treatment. In other patients, scored adversely according to the criteria cited or

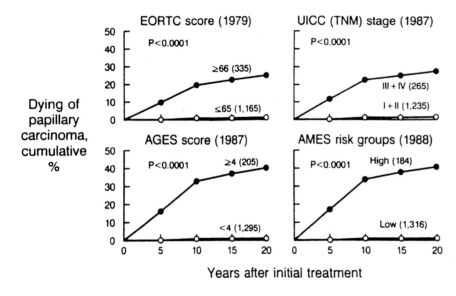

FIGURE 13.2. Cumulative mortality during a 20-year period in high- and low-risk patients with papillary carcinoma of the thyroid. Mortality risk is assessed by four different systems: the European Organization for Research on Thyroid Cancer (*EORTC*) system (12); the Union Internationale Contre le Cancer (*UICC*) system, based on the tumor–node–metastasis (*TNM*) staging system (13); the Mayo Clinic system (14), based on age, tumor grade, extent, and size (*AGES*); and the Lahey Clinic system (15), based on age, metastases, extent, and size (*AMES*). (From Hay D. Papillary thyroid carcinoma. *Endocrinol Metab Clin North Am* 1990;19:545–576, with permission.)

defined as being at high risk, a 20% to 30% cumulative mortality is noted within 10 years after diagnosis. The disease-associated mortality increases to a cumulative value of 40% by 20 years.

Similar risk stratification exists for patients with the somewhat more aggressive follicular thyroid carcinoma (16) (Fig. 13.3). Low-risk patients have perhaps a 5% mortality at 10 years. Mortality increases to 10% to 12% at 20 years. In contrast, patients with follicular carcinoma categorized as being at high risk (based on clinical and surgical findings) have a 70% mortality at 10 years and a greater than 90% mortality at 20 years after diagnosis.

Mazzaferri and Young (17) showed that ^{131}I therapy has a beneficial effect on survival in comparison with surgery alone or surgery augmented by thyroid hormone. More recently, Mazzaferri and Jhiang (18) developed a classification of risk factors and analyzed the effect of ^{131}I therapy among patients in their stages 2 and 3. In this analysis, they excluded patients at minimal risk for recurrence and death (stage 1, papillary or follicular thyroid carcinoma < 1.5 cm without distal metastases) and those in stage 4 (distant metastases) because these two groups represent extremes of risk. Among the patients who did not receive an ablative dose of ^{131}I, a marked increase in both recurrence (Fig. 13.4A) and mortality (Fig. 13.4B) is noted. At 10 years, the cumulative recurrence rate is 25% in the group without ^{131}I therapy and increases to 30% at 20 years, whereas in the group with ^{131}I ablative therapy, it is 6% at 10 years and 7% to 8% at 20 years. No disease-related deaths occurred during a 35-year follow-up period in stage 2 and 3 patients

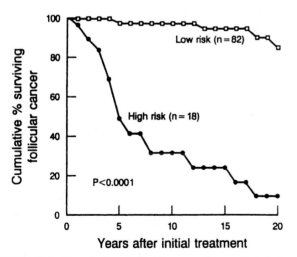

FIGURE 13.3. Cumulative survival (inverse of mortality) during a 20-year period in high- and low-risk patients with follicular carcinoma of the thyroid. Risk is assigned based on age, vascular invasion, and the presence of metastases at initial diagnosis. (From Brennan MD, Bergstrahl EJ, Van Heerden JA, et al. Follicular thyroid cancer treated at the Mayo Clinic, 1946 through 1970: initial manifestations, pathologic findings, therapy and outcome. *Mayo Clin Proc* 1991;66:11–22, with permission.)

who received ^{131}I ablative therapy (138 patients), whereas the cumulative death rate in the untreated group (802 patients) was 8%. Not all patients have been followed for 30 years, and many are lost to follow-up. Nevertheless, given the similarities in risk between those who received ^{131}I and those who did not, the difference in disease-associated mortality is striking. Whereas patients with minimal disease may be satisfactorily treated with even less than total thyroidectomy, patients in stages 2 and 3 (tumors > 1.5 cm, with or without cervical lymph node metastases and/or localized extension of tumor) should receive an appropriate dose of ^{131}I following total or near-total thyroidectomy.

In addition to effecting an overall improvement in disease-free survival, ablation of the thyroid remnant removes remnant thyroid tissue as a source of thyroglobulin during follow-up. In the absence of residual thyroid tissue, serum thyroglobulin is useful to monitor patients with thyroid carcinoma. Ablation of the remnant also eliminates competition for tracer or therapeutic doses of ^{131}I when these procedures are performed subsequently.

Ablative Dose

Once the patient to receive ablative ^{131}I therapy has been identified, the next issue is to determine the ^{131}I dose to be delivered to eradicate the thyroid tissue. For many years, 50 to 75 mCi of ^{131}I was recommended for this purpose (19).

As the number of patients receiving ^{131}I therapy increased, the cost of hospitalizing patients who were otherwise well for no other purpose than radiation isolation became an issue. The regulatory limit in the United States requires that patients be isolated until the emitted radiation flux is below 5 mR/h at 1 m, the rate equivalent to 30 mCi of [131]I. Ablative doses of 29.9 mCi of ^{131}I were suggested. This method is efficacious in 20% to 83% of the patients treated. Although in some patients ablation is successful with this "outpatient" dose, in may cases it is not (20–22). Hurley and Becker (22) have shown that 30 mCi results in a wide range of calculated radiation doses to the thyroid remnant in different patients. They demonstrated that 30 mCi delivers 50,000 to 250,000 cGy among various patients, which accounts for the variable clinical effects of a fixed dose of 30 mCi. In 1992, Maxon et al. (23) calculated the thyroid radiation absorbed dose in 85 patients and compared it with the success of ablation of residual thyroid tissue. They noted a regular relationship between radiation absorbed dose and subsequent ablation. The thyroid remnant was ablated in 79% to 83% of patients when a calculated dose of 30,000 cGy was delivered. The range of doses administered was from below 30 mCi to several hundred millicuries, as some patients were treated for more extensive disease at the same time. Absorbed doses were estimated for thyroid remnants and various areas of tumor involvement. Ablation was successful in some patients less than 30 mCi of ^{131}I, but only if the radiation absorbed dose to the thy-

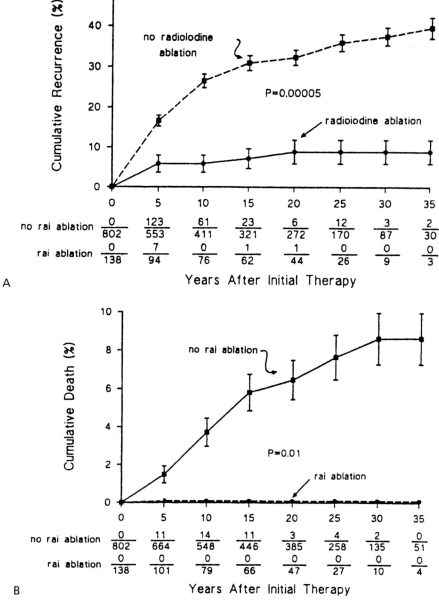

FIGURE 13.4. Effect of ^{131}I ablation on tumor recurrence (**A**) and mortality (**B**) in 940 patients with either papillary or follicular carcinoma larger than 1.5 cm without distant metastases at presentation. (From Mazzaferri EL, Jhiang SM. Long-term impact of initial surgical and medical therapy on papillary and follicular thyroid cancer. *Am J Med* 1994;97:418–428, with permission.)

roid remnant was in the range of 30,000 cGy. Cervical lymph node metastases were successfully ablated with 10,000 to 12,000 cGy to these foci. Cervical lymph node metastases and residual tumor may receive a sufficient ablative dose even if the fraction of the administered dose taken up by these deposits is less than the uptake of the thyroid remnant. Hence, radioactive iodine ablation of the supposedly normal thyroid remnant makes good sense because it frequently treats other disease in the local lymph node chains that was not identified on scans before therapy with

only 1 to 2 mCi of [131]I. The malignant tissue may be too small to be palpated at surgery. The small size favors a successful response, as radiation absorbed dose increases for a given amount of radioactivity delivered as the tumor mass decreases. The observations of Mazzaferri and Jhiang (18) of the improved survival associated with ^{131}I ablative therapy in patients with even minimal risk factors, combined with the data of Maxon et al. (23), provide the basis for the recommendation that patient-specific dosimetry be performed to determine the ablative dose of [131]I. The dose selected should deliver at least 300 Gy (30,000 rad) to the thyroid remnant when no other metastatic thyroid tissue is identified in the neck. To ablate tumor outside lymph nodes, considerably larger radiation absorbed doses may be necessary for a tumoricidal effect.

The regulatory limit in the United States recently has been revised so that patients can be released after receiving doses larger than 30 mCi of ^{131}I provided that it can be demonstrated that family members, caregivers, and members of the public are protected from exposure in excess of 5.0 mSv. A recent study observed that in fact the exposure of family members of patients with thyroid cancer treated with doses of ^{131}I ranging from 2.8 to 5.6 GBq is minimal (24). In many European countries, however, the regulatory limits are more restrictive than in the United States. In those circumstances, the arbitrary choice of 30 mCi (approximately 1,100 MBq) offers no cost advantage in the selection of an ablative dose.

In essence, patient-specific dosimetry incorporates the 29.9-mCi approach provided that the calculation demonstrates that a dose in this range will deliver approximately 30,000 rad to the tissue. Dosimetry permits administration of doses larger than 30 mCi when it is determined that larger doses are likely to be necessary to ablate the remnant tissue. Whereas 47% of the population studied by Maxon et al. (23) could be treated as outpatients, this simple estimate of radiation absorbed dose "allocates hospitalization and higher exposures to ^{131}I to those patients who require them." Likewise, it is inappropriate to hospitalize a patient to administer a larger dose of ^{131}I without demonstrating the necessity of doing so. Accordingly, nuclear medicine practitioners are encouraged to perform patient-specific dosimetry before selecting an ablative dose of [131]I. The additional effort involved is small, the overall results are better, and the insight gained in relating administered dose to radiation absorbed dose is valuable for other radionuclide therapy. In 1992, Maxon et al. (23) estimated the cost of thyroid remnant dosimetry to be $150 (23).

Dosimetry of Ablation

Although dosimetry, the calculation of a radiation absorbed dose, is a part of the training and competence of specialists in nuclear medicine, these concepts have been little utilized in practice. In the initial evaluation of diagnostic agents, these studies have been performed by a few investigators. Once the radiation absorbed doses have been determined, the calculated doses have been used by the rest of the nuclear medicine community without a repetition of the assessment of these values. The therapeutic use of radionuclides has been limited to thyroid disease until recently. Convenient dose regimens based on clinical experience have been developed for the treatment of both hyperthyroidism and thyroid carcinoma.

Several approaches are available: (a) treatment with a fixed dose for all patients; (b) modification of dose based on a number of factors, such as tissue mass and tracer uptake; and (c) patient-specific dosimetry. The latter method identifies a desirable radiation absorbed dose for the specific goal and determines the size of the dose to be administered based on patient-specific kinetics. Treatment with a specific radiation absorbed dose is inherently more logical than treatment with a uniform administered dose, as the former addresses patient-specific variables such as mass of the remnant, fractional uptake of the administered dose, and biologic turnover of the therapeutic radionuclide. To select a dose of ^{131}I to deliver a calculated radiation absorbed dose, it is necessary to perform a few simple measurements and calculations that are within the scope of all nuclear medicine facilities (Appendix A).

Basically, the radiation absorbed dose is the product of the amount of radiation to which a given amount of tissue is exposed and the duration of the exposure. Unlike external radiation, which is turned on and off, internally administered radionuclides deliver radiation to tissue while they decay to the degree that exposure of a specific tissue is maintained. The calculation of the radiation absorbed dose is based on a determination of the effective half-life in the region of interest, which is obtained by repeated measurement of the radioactivity in the tissue either after a test dose of the radioactive material or after the treatment dose is administered.

The unit of radiation absorbed dose, formerly called *rad*, is now assigned the unit *gray* and is defined as the product of the initial amount of radioactive material and the effective half-life divided by the mass of the tissue involved. For clinical purposes, the effective half-life is estimated by measuring the counts in the remnant at 24 and 48 hours, and preferably a third time for greater accuracy. If the results are not corrected for decay, the effective half-life is directly determined by plotting these values on semilogarithmic paper and determining the value for $t_{1/2}$. Alternately, of course, programmable calculators or computer programs can determine the $t_{1/2}$ with the measured uptakes used as input data. If the decay-corrrected 24-, 48-, and 72-hour uptakes are calculated and plotted, the biologic half-life is determined. This value is related to the effective half-life as follows:

$$t_{1/2 \text{ eff}} = \frac{t_{1/2 \text{ biologic}} \times t_{1/2 \text{ physical}}}{t_{1/2 \text{ biologic}} + t_{1/2 \text{ physical}}}$$

The radiation absorbed dose is equal to the product of the activity (MBq) in the tissue (which for purposes of this calculation is the product of the 24-hour uptake and the administered dose), the effective half-life, and a constant to adjust for the units used and the physical characteristics of the specific radionuclide (i.e., ^{131}I) divided by the mass of the tissue in which the radionuclide is distributed. This relationship is expressed by the following formula:

$$\text{Dose} = \frac{\text{Activity} \times \text{Average Half-life} \times K}{\text{Mass of Tissue}}$$

Because the dose is the radiation absorbed dose that we will select to be 30,000 cGy to the remnant, the administered dose (in microcuries) can be determined by rearranging terms (22) such that

$$\text{Admin Dose (\mu Ci)} = \frac{\text{Radiation Absorbed Dose} \times \text{Tissue Weight} \times 6.67}{t_{1/2\ eff}\ \text{(d)} \times \text{24-h uptake (\%)}}$$

The mass of tissue can be measured with either ultrasonography, CT, or MRI, or it can be estimated based on experience and the size of the functioning tissue seen on scanning. Often, it is advisable to define a best- and worst-case assumption. If a satisfactory dose can be delivered even given a worst-case assumption, it is reasonable to proceed with that dose. Basically, the recommendation of Maxon et al. (23) is to determine whether the 29.9 mCi (1,100 MBq) of ^{131}I is likely to deliver 300 Gy. If that is likely, it is reasonable to use 1,100 MBq (29.9 mCi) as an ablative dose; if it cannot be demonstrated that 1,100 MBq of ^{131}I is likely to deliver 300 Gy to the remnant, a larger dose, perhaps 2,200 to 3,300 MBq, is reasonably used. Given the many assumptions involved, no effort is made to select a specific number of microcuries or megabecquerels for the administered dose, which is based on a clinical assessment of the desired goal and the probability, based on the calculation, that the goal can be achieved with a dose larger or smaller than 1,100 MBq (30 mCi) of ^{131}I. Even enthusiasts for patient-specific ablative dosimetry are aware of the limitations and lack of precision of the method. In fact, in the publication of Maxon et al. (23), the value for $t_{1/2\ eff}$ was assigned because measurements were not available in many cases. Nevertheless, even this roughly estimated radiation absorbed dose achieves ablation more regularly than the arbitrary 30 mCi dose and makes it possible to avoid overtreating patients in whom it is demonstrated that ablation can be achieved with 30 mCi of ^{131}I.

LONG-TERM MONITORING

Clinical

The issue of appropriate long-term monitoring of patients with thyroid carcinoma is as complex as the scope of initial treatment. This is a consequence of the variety of clinical courses encountered, which vary from clinically benign disease that can be successfully managed at the time of initial presentation to disease that may recur at virtually any time after diagnosis and initial therapy, and even after follow-up therapy. The physician and the patient must recognize that no simple or standard protocol is applicable to all patients. At the same time, follow-up such as annual whole-body ^{131}I imaging is costly and inconvenient. Once again, the chal-lenge is to select the appropriate degree of monitoring for each patient's clinical situation. The question arises of what constitutes appropriate and cost-effective monitoring.

Withdrawal of Thyroid Hormone

The traditional approach to evaluating the patient with thyroid carcinoma has been to withdraw thyroid hormone replacement, allow a sufficient interval for the patient to become hypothyroid (4 to 5 weeks, confirmed by a serum TSH level above 30 μU/L), and perform neck and whole-body imaging. Because of the longer biologic effectiveness and slow turnover of T_4, most athyreotic patients are maintained on preparations of T_4. With thyroxine-binding globulin (TBG), a reservoir of T_4 that lasts for several weeks is maintained in the circulation. Following discontinuation of T_4 replacement, it takes 4 to 6 weeks before metabolism of the TBG-bound T_4 is sufficient for endogenous TSH to rise. The TSH level should be above 30 μU/L before an evaluation for functioning residual or metastatic thyroid carcinoma is performed, so that one can be confident that a negative scan result is an accurate assessment of functioning thyroid carcinoma metastases. The patient may be evaluated clinically to confirm the hypothyroid status as a basis to begin testing, but a serum TSH level should be obtained to confirm this impression *post hoc*. It is usually possible to proceed with the ^{131}I evaluation based on the clinical assessment without waiting for the TSH result. If a significant mass of functioning thyroid tissue is present, however, the patient may not become hypothyroid and adequate TSH elevation may not occur. In these instances, ^{131}I scanning and staging may proceed, as it will usually be possible to demonstrate many of the functioning thyroid metastases.

A kinder, gentler approach to patient preparation involves substituting replacement T_4 with T_3 at the time of (or several days after) T_4 is discontinued. This enables the patient to remain euthyroid and function more effectively in private, family, and vocational affairs while the T_4 is being consumed. Doses of 25 μg of T_3 (Cytomel) are prescribed, to be taken two or three times a day depending on body mass. After 3 to 4 weeks of this substitution, the T_3 is discontinued. The patient becomes hypothyroid more rapidly than after discontinuation of T_4 alone. In practice, this usually takes at least a full 2 weeks. Studies with ^{131}I are scheduled 2 weeks following discontinuation of the T_3. Both the patient and the nuclear medicine physician should be prepared to proceed to ^{131}I therapy if indicated approximately 7 days later. If for some reason the patient cannot be available for ^{131}I therapy during the week following diagnostic studies, T_3 replacement can be restarted and subsequently discontinued for 2 weeks to treat the patient with ^{131}I.

Until recently, ^{131}I imaging of the patient with thyroid carcinoma required discontinuation of thyroid hormone replacement to elevate endogenous TSH and stimulate ^{131}I uptake by malignant tissue for imaging or delivery of a therapeutic dose. Because this rendered the patient profoundly hypothyroid, it was a great inconvenience associated with temporary but significant morbidity. Other radioactive tracers have been evaluated to assess the possible or persistent presence of soft-tissue tumor without the need to discontinue thyroid hormone replacement; they can also be used in the patient at risk with a negative ^{131}I whole-body scan.

Recombinant Thyroid-stimulating Hormone

After many years of development and clinical assessment, human TSH has become available based on recombinant molecular biology synthesis. Several clinical studies have been performed to develop a satisfactory dosing scheme and evaluate the clinical reliability of whole-body ^{131}I imaging and/or serum thyroglobulin assay to detect thyroid carcinoma metastases. Meier at al. (25) compared findings following one or two doses of recombinant TSH (rTSH) with findings after withdrawal of thyroid hormone replacement therapy. Two injections given 24 hours apart produced higher serum TSH levels 24 hours after the second dose than were observed after a single injection. All the scans obtained following rTSH were compared with those obtained following discontinuation of thyroid hormone (T_3) replacement for 29 days. Blinded readings of unpaired scans rated the post-TSH scans equivalent in 17 of 19 instances (89%). When the scans were paired but the readers still blinded, an equivalent rating was obtained in 12 of 19 pairs; in four instances, the post-rTSH scans were rated better, whereas in three instances the thyroid hormone withdrawal scans were rated better than the post-rTSH scans.

Subsequently, a larger study comprising 152 patients, in which the now standardized 0.9-mg dose injected twice 24 hours apart and a 2- to 4-mCi dose of ^{131}I were used, demonstrated mean serum TSH levels of 132 mU/L 24 hours after the second injection, versus 101 mU/L 4 to 6 weeks following thyroid hormone withdrawal (26,27). Findings on scans after administration of human rTSH and scans after T_3/T_4 withdrawal were concordant in 66% of the patients with positive scans. Among the 34% scans rated to be discordant, the post-withdrawal scan was viewed as superior in 29% of the 152 studies; the post-human rTSH scan was rated superior in 5% of the studies. Although the serum thyroglobulin response was not evaluated for all patients in this study, when it was (35 patients), elevations in serum thyroglobulin were noted even when the scan was read as inadequate to identify metastatic disease. Accordingly, when rTSH is administered before whole-body imaging, serial thyroglobulin measurements should be performed, with the maximum response at 48 to 72 hours after the last injection of human rTSH. Unfortunately, the reproducibility of the serum thyroglobulin response at lower levels (< 10 ng/mL) is variable. The "threshold" incremental thyroglobulin value was 3 ng/mL. Sensitivity and specificity at this level were 72% and 95%,

respectively, after preparation with TSH and 71% and 100%, respectively, after thyroid hormone withdrawal. The combination of ^{131}I scanning and serum thyroglobulin assay appears to be as sensitive for the detection of thyroid carcinoma metastases as 30-day withdrawal of thyroid hormone replacement, and the discomfort and inconvenience of the latter can be avoided.

In summary, the following protocol is recommended: Before the first injection, baseline blood samples should be obtained specifically for thyroglobulin. The patient receives an intramuscular injection of 0.9 mg human rTSH freshly reconstituted with saline solution on days 1 and 2. On day 3, ^{131}I tracer is given; the patient is imaged on days 4 and 5. A second blood sample for serum thyroglobulin should be obtained on day 4. This represents the stimulated sample.

Human rTSH is not approved for use in preparing patients for ^{131}I therapy, but its use has been suggested, particularly in patients with sufficient thyroid hormone production by the tumor to preclude elevation of serum TSH following thyroid hormone withdrawal (28). Additionally, some patients cannot tolerate the delay involved in cessation of hormone therapy and spontaneous pituitary response. Finally, patients with hypothalamic or pituitary dysfunction are incapable of responding to thyroid hormone withdrawal.

In the initial clinical trials, the absolute fractional uptake of ^{131}I was observed to be less in patients after human rTSH than after T_3/T_4 withdrawal for 29 days (26,27). The whole-body retention of the ^{131}I diagnostic dose was also less. It seems likely that the somewhat improved detection of lesions in the hypothyroid subject in comparison with detection in the patient prepared with TSH injections may be a consequence of the increased background. This conclusion would suggest that when human rTSH is used, it may be worthwhile to administer a larger "tracer" dose of ^{131}I, perhaps 5 to 10 mCi. As yet, no comparative data are available to confirm the merit of this suggestion.

Thyroglobulin

The development of a radioimmunoassay to measure thyroglobulin has provided a serum marker for differentiated thyroid carcinoma that can be used for surveillance in a patient with no known tumor metastases and for monitoring response to therapy in a patient with known disease. The improved availability and quality of serum thyroglobulin determinations make it possible to assess patients for persistent or residual differentiated thyroid carcinoma at the same time that ^{131}I imaging is performed and also during intervals between imaging. In some patients, elevated thyroglobulin may be detected despite negative findings on ^{131}I scintigraphy. Serum thyroglobulin levels are very low (< 5 ng/mL) or undetectable in the normal or athyreotic patient but are elevated in patients with thyroiditis and thyroid carcinoma, probably because this tissue protein is able to gain access to the circulation.

Hence, it is appropriate to ablate residual thyroid tissue in patients with thyroid carcinoma who have undergone total or near-total thyroidectomy to improve the specificity of serum thyroglobulin as a tumor marker. In a patient who has been rendered athyreotic, elevation of thyroglobulin is evidence of residual thyroid carcinoma, even if ^{131}I-concentrating tissue is not detectable on whole-body imaging. Elevation of serum thyroglobulin values while the patient is euthyroid is indicative of recurrent tumor, but the absence of elevated levels does not exclude the presence of tumor. Accordingly, the assay is most sensitive for the detection of tumor and has the best negative predictive value when it is performed during adequate TSH stimulation. TSH stimulation is achieved either by discontinuing replacement thyroid hormone (T_4) for a period of 4 to 6 weeks or by injecting rTSH. The administration of two intramuscular injections of 0.9 mg of rTSH 24 hours apart is sufficient to stimulate thyroglobulin elevation in patients with differentiated thyroid carcinoma and to stimulate sufficient ^{131}I uptake that metastatic disease can be detected as well as with the traditional schema of discontinuation of thyroid hormone. Results comparing rTSH administration with thyroid hormone withdrawal indicate a high degree of correlation between the two techniques, sufficient to support Food and Drug Administration approval of the use of rTSH (Thyrogen) to identify patients with functioning metastases, either by measuring serum thyroglobulin as a marker or by performing whole-body ^{131}I imaging to detect functioning metastases from a differentiated thyroid carcinoma.

Elevation of thyroglobulin in the athyreotic euthyroid patient is certainly an indication of functioning thyroid metastases (26,27). Even in the patient with undetectable levels during suppression, periodic evaluation following cessation of replacement thyroid hormone is appropriate to determine if thyroid tissue is present that can be stimulated. Identification of residual activity in the thyroid bed on ^{131}I imaging is usually sufficient to explain the finding and justify ablation of the remnant, so that the serum thyroglobulin level will once again be valuable for the sensitive detection of functioning thyroid tissue, albeit not specific for malignant tissue. Thyroglobulin values above 30 ng/mL or a serial rise in thyroglobulin levels while the patient is on suppressive therapy should be investigated.

A management problem arises when elevated thyroglobulin is detected but no functioning thyroid tissue is identified. In the past, clinicians often restarted thyroid hormone replacement because "if the functioning tissue cannot be seen, it is too little to bother with" or "it is not possible to deliver sufficient ^{131}I for effective therapy."

Pineda et al. (29), Pacini et al. (30), and others have treated these patients with doses of 100 mCi of ^{131}I or more. In one third of the patients, functioning metastases are seen on post-therapy scans. In another third of the patients, the thyroglobulin levels are significantly lower after therapy.

Whole-body Imaging with [131]I

Whole-body imaging with ^{131}I is a *sine qua non* in assessing the extent of thyroid cancer in several clinical scenarios:

1. Following initial surgical treatment (total or near-total thyroidectomy)
2. During regular surveillance
3. In patients who present with metastases
4. In the reevaluation of patients after ^{131}I therapy of metastases

Patients are prepared either by discontinuing thyroid hormone replacement or by injecting rTSH, as described earlier. A diet low in iodine for at least 2 weeks before evaluation is recommended to augment ^{131}I uptake and retention (Table 13.1). If therapy is indicated, the low-iodine diet should be continued until after it is completed and the patient is restarted on thyroid hormone replacement.

Before the diagnostic dose is selected, it is worthwhile to perform a ^{99m}Tc-pertechnetate scan on initial visits to assess the volume of residual normal thyroid tissue (Fig. 13.5). If the patient is athyreotic, a vigorous evaluation with 185 MBq (5.0 mCi) of ^{131}I proceeds. If the patient has substantial residual thyroid and metastases are not evident or suspected, a relatively small dose (approximately 15 MBq) of ^{131}I is given to calculate the radiation absorbed dose to the remnant tissue, followed by an ablative dose of [131]I. A whole-body scan is performed several days after the ablative dose (10 to 20 GBq). If more extensive disease or distant metastases are demonstrated at that time, the patient is reevaluated in 6 to 12 months, with the intent of treating

TABLE 13.1. LOW IODINE DIET

No iodized salt (avoid salt in general; specifically, salted nuts, crackers, and pretzels)
No milk or dairy products (dietary iodine is excreted in milk)
No seafood (shellfish, fish, kelp, or seaweed)
No bakery products (commercial products with preservatives)
No red foods or medications (red food dye contains iodine, as does commercial canned tomato sauces)
No mineral supplements
No iodinated medication (radiographic contrast material)
Allowed foods
Red meat, pork, veal, chicken
Potatoes and vegetables (cooked without iodized salt)
Pasta and rice
Fresh vegetables, including tomatoes and sauces

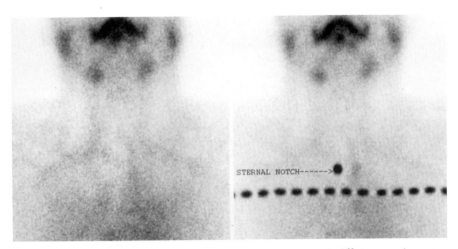

STERNAL NOTCH------>

FIGURE 13.5. Anterior neck and chest views obtained with 4.0 mCi of ^{99m}Tc-pertechnetate and a parallel-hole collimator in an athyreotic patient (previous total thyroidectomy). This image is obtained before selection of an ^{131}I dose to determine whether the patient will require ablation of a thyroid remnant (and hence appropriate measurement) or a larger dose to exclude metastatic disease.

with a maximum tolerated (recommended) dose at that time. Before the initial ^{99m}Tc-pertechnetate scan is performed, it is advisable to obtain a beta-human chorionic gonadotropin level to confirm the pregnancy status of young female patients. This result is available within a few hours before the administration of ^{131}I.

A range of doses of ^{131}I may be used for whole-body imaging, depending on which of the clinical situations is applicable. The standard dose was 1.0 mCi of ^{131}I. Because more limited disease with less uptake is identified with higher doses, doses as high as 10 mCi of ^{131}I have been recommended for diagnostic purposes. Doses in the range of 74 to 185 MBq (2 to 5 mCi) are commonly used because of concerns about possible "stunning" effects and the availability of thyroglobulin assays to detect disease even if the results of ^{131}I scintigraphy are negative.

Stunning is the phenomenon in which the initial diagnostic dose affects the iodine trapping or organification mechanism so that uptake of the subsequent therapeutic dose is impaired. Many reports have documented differences between uptake of the diagnostic and therapeutic dose (31,32). It is difficult, however, to demonstrate that a reduced uptake of the therapeutic dose is a consequence of the prior diagnostic dose rather than of the larger therapeutic dose.

The choice of the scanning dose of ^{131}I depends on patient-specific issues. It is appropriate to consider why the patient is being scanned. What previous information is available? What is planned for the patient? Has the patient received prior treatment for known disease? Has this scanning episode been planned to determine the efficacy of that therapy? Does the patient have demonstrable residual or metastatic disease? Does the patient presently have known tumor? Is the patient in a low-risk or relatively low-risk category and being scanned for completeness of evaluation with little expectation of disease being found?

In most circumstances, patients are scanned with 2 to 5 mCi of ^{131}I. This procedure is repeated annually for 3 to 5 years. If the results of imaging and thyroglobulin studies are negative, ^{131}I scanning at longer intervals (two or three times at 2-year intervals, then at 3-year intervals) can be scheduled. A patient who has been free of disease in several prior years might receive a larger dose of ^{131}I for evaluation before annual ^{131}I whole-body imaging is deferred. If a study result is negative with 5 to 10 mCi, the interval between observations can be extended with greater confidence. Conversely, in the patient suspected of having, or known to have, metastatic disease who is scheduled for ^{131}I therapy, there is no need to scan and document the extent of disease exhaustively with a "diagnostic" dose. Dosimetry (blood and whole-body counting) can be performed with 3.7 to 10 MBq (100 to 300 µCi) of ^{131}I. The extent of disease can be documented on the scan obtained approximately 7 days after ^{131}I therapy with a dose of 150 mCi or more.

Patients should be imaged at 24 to 72 hours after administration of ^{131}I. Organ mode (static) images of the neck and chest should be acquired, and also a whole-body image at 48 to 72 hours obtained with use of a high-energy collimator (Figs. 13.6–13.8). If daily imaging is inconvenient or impractical, the single best images are obtained in most patients at 72 hours after the diagnostic dose, particularly in hypothyroid patients who have been prepared for imaging by withdrawal of thyroid hormone replacement. Although experience is limited, patients prepared for surveillance imaging with rTSH have a faster body turnover of ^{131}I. In

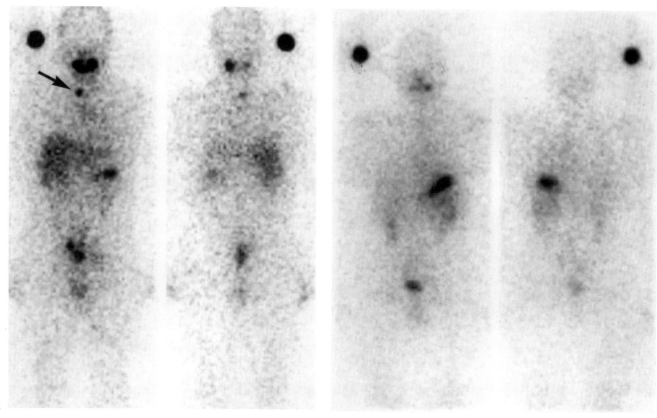

A

B

FIGURE 13.6. Whole-body ^{131}I scan performed with a gamma camera at 48 hours after administration of 5.0 mCi of [131]I. A standard source is positioned to the right of the patient's head. **A:** An *arrow* identifies a residual focus in the lower right side of the neck in a patient with a previous total thyroidectomy. Considerable activity in the liver indicates incorporation of ^{131}I into thyroid hormone, which is excreted by the liver. Activity in the left upper quadrant is interpreted as gastric secretion, but activity at the midline in the lower abdominal region may be nodal or osseous foci. Activity is often seen in the bladder (urine) and rectum (stool). The patient was treated with a large dose, approximately 250 mCi of [131]I. **B:** One year following ^{131}I therapy, the patient again underwent scanning with 5.0 mCi of [131]I. The cervical focus is no longer seen, nor is activity seen in the region of the liver. The activity in the left upper quadrant is clearly gastric. Given the absence of hepatic activity, the pelvic activity is interpreted as excreted radioiodine. The thyroglobulin level was unmeasurable.

these patients, optimal images in terms of lesion percentage dose and target-to-background ratio may be obtained at 48 hours.

In many instances, small foci in the neck or mediastinum may not be seen on initial 24- or 48-hour images but become distinctly visible after further background clearance. Finally, if the patient is treated with ^{131}I, imaging should be performed approximately 7 days later to document the extent of disease for future surveillance.

Regardless of the scanning dose selected, negative findings should be treated with caution. Given the propensity of the disease to recur after many years, it is worthwhile to maintain surveillance of the patient appropriate for the individual risk factors. The currently refined serum thyroglobulin assay provides a convenient means to follow even low-risk patients. Certainly any patient whose original

risk factors merited total or near-total thyroidectomy merits regular surveillance.

Whole-body Imaging with Alternate Agents

Metastatic thyroid carcinoma can be imaged with radiopharmaceuticals other than [131]I. This is relevant because lesions may be found inadvertently with these agents when they are being used for other indications. Alternate imaging techniques provide a method to determine tumor viability and biology without having to prepare the patient for ^{131}I imaging (T$_4$ withdrawal or rTSH stimulation). This technique also permits imaging of patients with thyroid carcinoma who have received contaminating doses of iodide either inadvertently or for medical reasons. CT and MRI

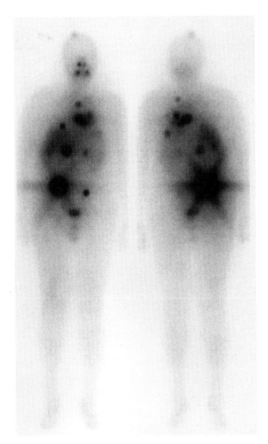

FIGURE 13.7. Whole-body ^{131}I scan in a 52-year-old man who had undergone a total thyroidectomy at another institution 7 years earlier after discovery of a 2.5-cm papillary carcinoma. Results of an immediate postoperative scan were negative, and the patient was discharged from follow-up on thyroid hormone. He began limping 6 weeks before presenting for roentgenography, which revealed a lytic lesion in the right iliac crest extending to the sacroiliac joint. This scan, performed 1 week after therapy with 400 mCi of ^{131}I, revealed extensive soft-tissue and osseous metastases. Many of the lesions have resolved, although several small osseous metastases concentrate iodine on follow-up imaging.

are useful to identify large tumors, but these techniques lack specificity and sensitivity for involved lymph nodes, as the detection limit is a lesion larger than 1 cm. In managing patients with thyroid carcinoma, one must be cautious about CT imaging to ensure that the patient does not receive iodinated contrast material that will interfere with ^{131}I uptake by functioning thyroid metastases. In this regard, MRI is a safer modality. Gadolinium contrast does not interfere with iodine trapping or the ability to treat the patient.

Bone Scintigraphy

Bone metastases may be visualized by ^{99m}Tc-methylene diphosphonate (MDP) bone scintigraphy. Even though bone metastases of thyroid carcinoma are predominantly osteolytic, a rim of osteoblastic activity is frequently present around lesions. In larger lesions, the photon-deficient focus is identifiable. Bone scintigraphy, however, is of limited utility in evaluating patients because it does not image soft-tissue metastases from thyroid carcinoma. Alam et al. (33) reported a 93.5% sensitivity with a combination of ^{99m}Tc-MDP bone scintigraphy and ^{201}Tl scintigraphy in 14 patients with thyroid carcinoma and negative findings on ^{131}I scans. In this group, the results of ^{201}Tl scintigraphy were positive in 10 of 14 cases, and the results of ^{99m}Tc-MDP bone scintigraphy were positive in all 14 patients.

Tumor Scintigraphy

Agents such as ^{201}Tl, ^{99m}Tc-MIBI (methoxyisobutylisonitrile), ^{18}F-FDG (fluorodeoxyglucose), and ^{111}In-octreotide have been used to image lymph node, soft-tissue, and osseous metastases without T_4 withdrawal. They are potentially useful to evaluate patients with tumors that have unusual histologic patterns, such as Hürthle cell and columnar or insular variants of papillary carcinoma because these tumors may be less iodine-avid than the more classic forms of papillary and follicular carcinoma. Another advantage of these agents is that they can be used to assess tumor extent while the patient is euthyroid (on replacement T_4 therapy). This is particularly useful to monitor patients after therapy during intervals between ^{131}I whole-body imaging.

Tumor Perfusion Agents

The results of regional or body imaging with ^{201}Tl have been variable (33–36). Positive results were reported in 10 of 14 patients with negative ^{131}I body images (33). Ugar et al. (36) reported 70% overall agreement between results of imaging with ^{201}Tl, ^{99m}Tc-MIBI, and [131]I. Both ^{201}Tl and ^{99m}Tc-MIBI, however, yielded false-negative results in patients in whom ^{131}I demonstrated functioning metastases. It has been reported that ^{99m}Tc-tetrofosmin performed better than either ^{201}Tl or ^{99m}Tc-MIBI (37). It is not clear why this should be the case based on a comparison of the imaging characteristics of the radionuclide and the extraction efficiency and mechanism of localization. In other studies, Tc-tetrofosmin performed as well as ^{201}Tl, but both were inconsistent in comparison with [131]I (38). Both ^{201}Tl and the ^{99m}Tc tumor perfusion agents may have some utility in patients with insular or Hürthle cell carcinoma, two variants that frequently have a diminished capacity to concentrate [131]I. These variant tumor types are sometimes detected with ^{131}I following optimal preparation with an iodine-deficient diet.

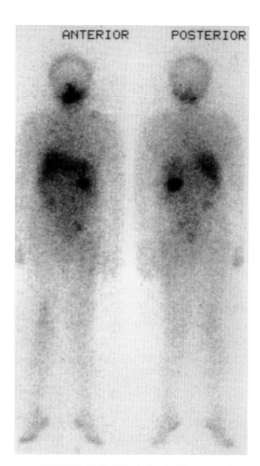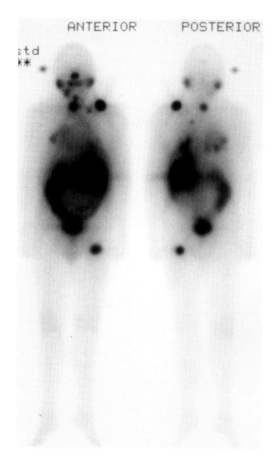

FIGURE 13.8. Whole-body ¹³¹I scans obtained 48 to 72 hours after administration of a 2-mCi scanning dose of ¹³¹I (*panels 1 and 2*) and 7 days after therapy (*panels 3 and 4*) with 10.7 GBq (350 mCi) of ¹³¹I in a patient with thyroid carcinoma evaluated as part of long-term surveillance. On the diagnostic procedure, a well-defined functioning metastasis is identified in a posterior left rib. This finding should not be confused with bowel excretion. The hepatic activity confirms the presence of functioning thyroid tissue and thyroid hormone synthesis because ¹³¹I as iodide ion is not excreted via the hepatobiliary pathway. On delayed post-therapy dose imaging, additional extensive sites of metastatic involvement are identified: the thyroid bed, left infraclavicular lymph node, left distal clavicle, multiple pulmonary nodules, and a focus in the left femoral shaft. In retrospect, some of the lesions can be identified on the diagnostic image, but the extent of disease is markedly underestimated on the low-dose scan.

In summary, imaging with either ²⁰¹Tl or ⁹⁹ᵐTc-MIBI is feasible and provides useful information in certain cases (Fig. 13.9). However, no clear recommendation can be made regarding the overall utility of these techniques except that they provide a convenient means to assess patients while they are on T₄ replacement and may detect thyroid carcinoma metastases in patients with negative findings on ¹³¹I scintigraphy. Positive results are useful, but the overall sensitivity and specificity of these techniques is not well defined.

Somatostatin Receptor Imaging

Few reports have described thyroid carcinoma imaging with ¹¹¹In-octreotide, an agent that localizes based on high-affinity binding to somatostatin receptors, particularly subtype

2. The uptake of ¹¹¹In-octreotide has been observed in both ¹³¹I-positive and ¹³¹I-negative thyroid tumors (Fig. 13.10). Baudin et al. (39) obtained positive ¹¹¹In-octreotide images in 12 of 16 patients with thyroid carcinoma that was negative on whole-body ¹³¹I scintigraphy. The results of ¹¹¹In-octreotide scintigraphy were positive in eight of nine patients with positive results on ¹³¹I scintigraphy. In another report, the results of ¹¹¹In-octreotideimaging of thyroid carcinoma were positive in five of eight patients (40). These observations are useful beyond simply providing another imaging technique. This information identifies a biologic feature of thyroid carcinoma in a subset of patients and suggests a potential alternative therapy with the pharmacologic agent octreotide or a long-acting octreotide analogue. Octreotide therapy may be useful to slow progression of more aggressive thyroid carcinoma that

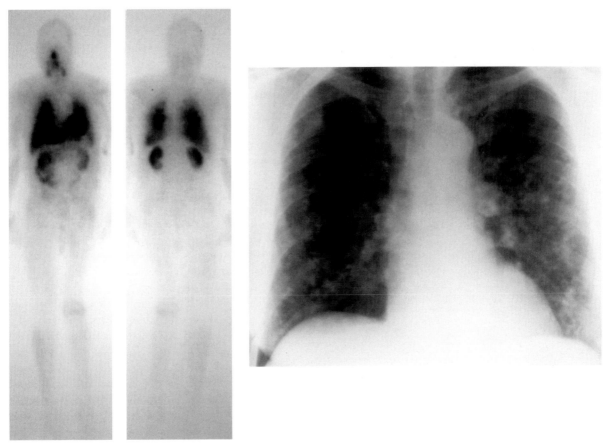

FIGURE 13.9. Whole-body scintigraphy with 20 mCi of Tc-MIBI (methoxyisobutylisonitrile) and chest roentgenography in a patient with a history of papillary thyroid carcinoma. Some suspect areas are seen on the chest roentgenogram, and the ^{99m}Tc-MIBI images reveal extensive pulmonary infiltration with tumor. Pulmonary metastases often respond well to ^{131}I therapy, but the therapeutic dose in the presence of diffuse lung involvement is limited to one that will result in not more than 80 mCi of ^{131}I being retained in the lungs at 48 hours. The dose limit is expressed in this manner because of difficulties with the assumptions involved in lung dosimetry (44–46).

is unresponsive to other therapies. Virgolini (41) has used repeated doses of ^{90}Y-labeled somatostatin receptor peptide ligands to treat patients with ^{131}I-negative, somatostatin receptor-positive thyroid carcinoma. In some instances, partial responses have been observed. This approach is still investigational and is not available in routine nuclear medicine practice.

Positron Emission Tomography with Fluorodeoxyglucose

Several large centers in Europe and the United States (42–44) have described the uptake of ^{18}F-FDG by thyroid carcinoma in a subset of patients. They observed both concordance and nonconcordance between ^{131}I and ^{18}F-FDG imaging. In some patients, positive results were obtained with both ^{18}F-FDG and ^{131}I, whereas some results were positive with ^{131}I only and others were positive with ^{18}F-FDG only. Tumors that are negative with both agents are

infrequent. These early findings merely provided another imaging option to identify disease not seen with ^{131}I imaging. More recently, however, additional observations suggest that ^{18}F-FDG uptake by thyroid carcinoma may provide significant prognostic information and therapeutic options. Wang et al. (44) correlated ^{18}F-FDG activity with tumor aggressiveness; their results were consistent with observations made in other tumors. The degree of ^{18}F-FDG uptake [whether quantified by standard uptake value (SUV) or semiquantitatively by image assessment] provides additional information about tumor biology and clinical prognosis. These patients present a therapeutic challenge for the nuclear medicine physician and oncologist. In a subset of patients with scans positive for tumor uptake of ^{18}F-FDG, scans were also positive for ^{111}In-octreotide uptake. Insufficient information is available at this time to determine whether treatment with either the pharmaceutical OctreoScan or radiolabeled somatostatin receptor ligands has a role in the management of these patients.

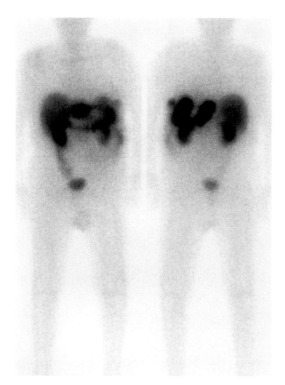

FIGURE 13.10. Anterior and posterior whole-body images at 24 hours after the administration of 6.0 mCi of ^{111}In-DTPA (diethylenetriamine pentaacetic acid) pentetreotide (OctreoScan) in a patient with known thyroid carcinoma metastatic to the thoracic spine. Prior ^{131}I scanning had demonstrated failure to take up iodine in this region, and biopsy confirmed unresectable papillary thyroid carcinoma. The OctreoScan images demonstrate physiologic distribution in the liver, spleen, and kidneys in addition to bowel excretion. A large mass positive for somatostatin receptors is best seen in the posterior projection in the midline, extending to the left. The finding is confirmed on the anterior image and corresponds to a mass seen on computed tomography. The thyroglobulin level was above 10,000 ng/mL.

THERAPY OF METASTATIC THYROID CARCINOMA

Based on the ability of functioning thyroid carcinoma to concentrate iodine, treatment with ^{131}I has been an essential component of management for more than 50 years. The early success of this modality, in fact, encouraged government and industry to make radionuclides available for medical applications, and served as a stimulus to physicians to develop and refine the clinical applications of these radioactive materials. As a result, nuclear medicine has evolved as a medical discipline. The initial therapy of thyroid carcinoma is usually surgical, with removal of the involved thyroid gland and identifiable lymph nodes if indicated, depending on the extent of disease. Metastatic disease involving cervical, mediastinal, or other lymph nodes, lungs, or bone may be present at the time of initial diagnosis, or it may become clinically apparent during subsequent surveillance, even after many years without evidence of disease. When feasible, isolated osseous metastases should be treated surgically

to "debulk" tumor and provide orthopedic management of bony structures at risk for fracture. Often, osseous metastases are amenable to external beam radiation therapy. Even when metastatic disease is treated by one of these alternate modalities, the patient should receive the benefit of ^{131}I scanning and therapy, as other disseminated disease is likely to be present that is not readily demonstrated by traditional imaging. More commonly, the disseminated nature of metastatic thyroid carcinoma makes ^{131}I therapy the treatment of choice in the management of this disease.

Dose Selection for [131]I Therapy

Once it has been determined that a patient has functioning residual, recurrent, or metastatic thyroid carcinoma, the treatment dose must be determined. Most of the nuclear medicine community uses the so-called "standard fixed dose" of 100 to 200 mCi of [131]I (3.7 to 7.4 GBq). Some have recommended adjusting the dose based on the site of involvement; thyroid bed tumor is treated with up to 150 mCi (5.5 GBq), lymph node metastases with 175 mCi, and metastases outside the neck with 200 mCi (7.4 GBq) (45). Harbert (46) endorses this approach and cites a report from the Atomic Energy Commission that failed to find evidence that doses greater than 200 mCi (7.4 GBq) are more effective. Harbert concludes that no evidence has been reported to prove that patient-specific dose determinations are more effective, and that use of the fixed-dose method reduces the cost of therapy and avoids time-consuming measurements (46).

Alternatively, the "maximum safe dose" method recognizes that bone marrow suppression at high levels of exposure is a problem, but that this complication is observed only when the bone marrow is exposed to more than 200 cGy (exposure determined by calculating the radiation absorbed dose to blood) (47–49). By measuring tracer doses in individual patients and estimating bone marrow exposure, it has been possible to treat many patients safely with doses of ^{131}I in excess of 200 mCi. Furthermore, this method identifies patients (15% to 20% of those studied) who would be at risk for adverse marrow effects if they received even a 200-mCi dose.

The method to estimate blood (marrow) dose was developed some time ago at the Memorial Sloan-Kettering Cancer Center in New York (47–49) (Appendix B). In the Benua-Leeper approach, in which the classic Marinelli-Quimby equations are used, the radiation absorbed dose to the blood in the marrow volume is estimated because of the difficulties encountered in models of marrow distribution and mass. The calculation notes the absence of direct uptake by the marrow elements. The marrow radiation absorbed dose is received from the β⁻ emission in the blood perfusing the marrow. An additional γ component is received from the total activity distributed throughout the body. To perform clinical dosimetry by this method, the blood radioactivity is measured over time by sampling blood at intervals and deriving the percentage administered dose per milliliter (Appendix B). This is the fraction of administered radioactivity perfusing and exposing the bone marrow mass. Bone marrow mass is obtained from standardized tables based on weight and height, with the assumption of no evidence of bone marrow uptake or involvement.

Some practitioners continue to use this approach even though the MIRD (medical internal radiation dose) formulation is now available. In general, either method will provide similar dosing guidelines and clinical results so long as appropriate assumptions are made. Doses of ^{131}I can be selected based on measuring whole-body activity and calculating a whole-body $t_{1/2\ eff}$ as an indicator of the radiation absorbed dose (50,51).

Regardless of whether the Benua-Leeper approach or the MIRD whole-body determination is used, calculation of at least some indices that reflect bone marrow exposure and absorbed dose provide an indication of whether the patient can tolerate administered doses in excess of 7.4 GBq (200 mCi) of ^{131}I or, for that matter, even a dose of 7.4 GBq. In about 80% of the patients evaluated by these techniques, doses of ^{131}I considerably in excess of 7.4 GBq have been determined to be safe. In fact, prolonged bone marrow suppression is not regularly seen until doses in excess of 300 cGy (calculated by the Benua-Leeper method) are received. The 200-cGy limit, however, provides sufficient flexibility to treat most patients. This technique of estimating marrow absorbed dose is not simply a method to give larger doses of [131]I. In 20% of the patients, the maximal recommended safe dose is less than 200 mCi.

It is important to remember that specific numeric values will change based on the assumptions made; the method used to calculate the blood, marrow, or whole-body radiation absorbed dose; and the number of data points used in the calculation. Despite the differences in the precise dose calculated depending on methodology, these calculations clarify the physiology influencing the calculated blood radiation absorbed dose. Values for the radiation absorbed dose per unit of radioactivity are high when the body turnover is prolonged by impaired renal excretion or incorporation of ^{131}I into T_4 by bulky metastatic tissue, with subsequent slow turnover as a result of binding to circulating TBG. Impaired excretion reflects renal failure to turn over the body iodine pool. In patients with impaired renal function, a larger calculated safe dose can be obtained after several days of enhancement of iodide pool turnover by diuretic therapy with sodium chloride replacement (52). No published series of randomized therapy doses are available to demonstrate the superiority of the maximal tolerated or recommended dose in terms of long-term outcome. However, the maximal tolerated dose provides a more rational approach to radionuclide therapy than a simple, fixed-dose method.

It is recommended that nuclear medicine physicians use a rational approach until it has been convincingly demonstrated that it provides no advantage. The additional effort involved is not great, and the arguments about reducing cost or the need to hasten ^{131}I therapy are not sound when one is dealing with the well-being of patients. Given the great variability in the clinical course of patients with thyroid carcinoma and the relatively low incidence of the disease, it is highly problematic that a randomized study will be performed in the near future. Nevertheless, several multicenter trials have been organized.

The dose of ^{131}I delivered to different sites and the tumor and body turnover of ^{131}I vary, and each tumor site will receive different a different radiation absorbed dose. Ablation of metastases with persistence of tumor at some sites is frequently observed, and new tumor sites may be found. In general, smaller metastases respond better than larger ones (53) (Figs. 13.6–13.8). Because individualized doses cannot be delivered to each tumor site, the "maximal tolerated dose" schema seeks to deliver the largest dose that avoids marrow and other adverse side effects. As indicated, this is possible in 80% of the patients evaluated. Authorities such as Hurley and Becker (54) use a modified approach; without performing dosimetry, they select a dose of ^{131}I between 1.1 and 7.4 GBq (30 to 200 mCi) for younger patients who have no known metastases, and they reserve the use of a maximal tolerated or recommended dose for patients identified as potentially requiring doses larger than 7.4 GBq or possibly having impaired renal function. The precise dose selected depends on other clinical features and risk factors.

[131]I Treatment of Patients with Negative Findings on [131]I Scintigraphy

The early method of dose selection based only on the site of metastatic disease did not provide a recommendation for treatment of patients with elevated serum thyroglobulin but no demonstrable functioning metastases when imaged with low doses of [131]I. It was the practice not to treat such patients with [131]I. Pineda et al. (29) and Pacini et al. (30) reported results following administration of 100 to 150 mCi ^{131}I in patients whose only evidence of disease was elevation of serum thyroglobulin. In this group, thyroglobulin levels fell in one third to one half of the patients, and functioning metastases were identified with scintillation scanning in approximately 50% of the patients when it was performed after administration of the therapy dose.

Even when functioning metastases have been identified on diagnostic scanning, more extensive involvement may be seen when the patients are imaged following the therapeutic dose (Fig. 13.8). Accordingly, the most appropriate treatment of a patient with metastatic thyroid carcinoma is to administer the largest possible safe dose of [131]I. The Benua-Leeper formulation or the MIRD calculation provide methodology to do this that is neither cumbersome nor inappropriately costly.

Efficacy of [131]I Therapy of Metastases

Mazzaferri and Jhiang (18) clearly demonstrated that early treatment with ^{131}I improves survival in patients with an increased risk for recurrence and mortality based on the risk factors reviewed earlier. Presumably, this is a consequence of treatment (ablation) of metastatic foci that may not have been identified on early imaging. The effectiveness of treating known metastases remains an issue, which is complicated by the many treatment schemes that have been employed, even at centers with large experience. Nevertheless, good results have been achieved, even in patients with distant metastases (48,53–56).

Survival is related to early detection (i.e., the smaller the extent of disease, the greater the likelihood of effective treatment). Favorable outcome is also determined by the vigor of ^{131}I uptake. The data on the relationship between uptake and outcome are complicated, however, by the various therapy dose schemes used; often, a smaller therapy dose is given than could be tolerated if a maximal recommended dose evaluation were performed.

Patients with lung metastases whose tumor is identified by scintigraphy alone have a better outcome than those whose disease is evident on roentgenography. Among those with abnormal roentgenogrphic findings, micronodular metastases are more likely than macronodular disease to be treated effectively with [131]I (53,54) (Table 13.2). Of patients in this category, the percentage surviving at 5 years increased from 8% to 72% with ^{131}I therapy. At 8 years, 50% of the patients with lung metastases treated with ^{131}I survived, whereas none without treatment survived (53).

Age is also a determinant of outcome; younger patients perform better than older patients. Whether this reflects a shorter duration of tumor proliferation or a more basic

dependency on factors related to youth is not clear. More than 95% of younger patients with limited disease and reasonable ^{131}I uptake responded to therapy, whereas 56% of patients over 40 years had effective uptake. Only 19% of this group responded to ^{131}I therapy.

Bone metastases are often associated with other metastatic involvement, so it is difficult to assess the response of bone metastases alone. In general, the presence of bone metastases denotes a worse overall prognosis than soft-tissue metastases alone. Furthermore, osseous metastases require surgical treatment, external radiation therapy, or both in addition to ^{131}I treatment because in isolated locations, a more effective radiation dose and dose rate can be delivered than with ^{131}I alone. [131]I should be used in addition to these modalities to treat any potential residual disease outside the radiation field, even if it is not demonstrated by routine techniques at the time of diagnosis and staging. Overall, the response to treatment is related to the degree of uptake and size of the therapy dose. Given the variation in dosing schemes and the complexity of the management of patients with soft-tissue and osseous involvement, the published results should be used as a call for more vigorous therapy rather than as an indication that little can be achieved (53,56). In this regard, Schlumberger et al. (53) observed an overall 30% increase in the survival of patients with distant metastases diagnosed after 1976 in comparison with the survival of patients with metastases discovered between 1960 and 1976, and a 140% increase in comparison with the survival of patients with metastases discovered before 1960.

Whereas the dose–response relationship for ^{131}I may not be linear over an entire range of possible therapy doses, the maximal tolerated dose evaluation that permits doses in excess of 7.4 GBq to be given may produce still better results in the future.

Finally, Fatourechi and Hay (57) suggest that failure to demonstrate ^{131}I uptake, even after treatment doses, may reflect a basic change in tumor biology that is more common among older patients, whereas failure to identify disease on diagnostic scanning in younger patients is more likely to be a consequence of geometric factors (small tumor foci) (53,57). The tumors of older patients that have lost iodide symporters and developed neuroendocrine characteristics may be amenable to treatment with innovative techniques, such as therapy with radiolabeled somatostatin receptor ligands (41,57).

Side Effects

Bone marrow toxicity is the primary concern in selecting and administering a dose of [131]I. Even though ^{131}I administered as sodium iodide does not concentrate or deposit in bone marrow, the bone is exposed to ^{131}I in the blood following absorption from the gastrointestinal tract. Even though the blood is cleared of ^{131}I relatively rapidly in most

TABLE 13.2. FACTORS ASSOCIATED WITH SURVIVAL IN PATIENTS WITH LUNG METASTASES

Factor	Number	Eight-year survival rate (%)
Micronodular metastases	14	77
Macronodular metastases	27	18
Mediastinal metastases	17	9
Bone and brain metastases	27	14
Cervical node metastases	30	40
Papillary carcinoma	27	51
Follicular carcinoma	30	11
Positive ^{131}I uptake	28	43
Negative ^{131}I uptake	23	26
All patients	58	28

From Massin JP, Savoie JC, Garnier H, et al. Pulmonary metastases in differentiated thyroid carcinoma. *Cancer* 1984;53:982–988, with permission.

patients, the exposure that the perfused active marrow receives during this interval accounts for most of the radiation absorbed dose, primarily as a result of β emissions from ^{131}I. The bone receives additional radiation exposure from τ emissions from iodine distributed throughout the body. The absolute value for bone marrow exposure varies with the methods and assumptions used. As stated previously, the Benua-Leeper method determines the "blood" dose, and usually a dose is selected that will not exceed 200 cGy to the blood. Although this methodology has not resulted in prolonged bone marrow suppression or aplastic marrow, a profound effect on hematologic indices is usually observed, including a mild anemia, leukopenia, and thrombocytopenia. These effects are transient, and a gradual return to pretreatment values is noted within 3 months. The absolute granulocyte count recovers, but prolonged suppression of lymphocytes usually results in an overall lowering of the white blood cell count. Despite the lower absolute lymphocyte count, immunodeficiency syndromes have not been reported in treated patients, even after many years of lymphocyte depletion.

Other side effects are observed following ^{131}I therapy, particularly when doses of 7.4 GBq (200 mCi) or more are used. These effects can be defined as acute, intermediate, and late in onset. Acute symptoms are observed during the first hours to days after therapy. The most common initial symptom is loss of appetite and nausea that may be accompanied by vomiting. Despite these symptoms, patients are usually able to maintain hydration following high-dose ^{131}I therapy. The possibility that these symptoms may occur should be discussed with the patient in advance to provide reassurance. A light diet is encouraged, and antiemetic medication should be made available, usually in the form of Compazine suppositories (25 mg every 4 to 6 hours as needed). Because vomiting does not occur for 6 to 8 hours after administration, absorption of ^{131}I is usually complete, and loss of the dose is generally not an issue. The vomitus may be contaminated, however, as iodide ion is secreted into the gastric acid. The gastrointestinal side effects clear within 1 to 3 days after therapy. Parotid swelling and discomfort are often seen on the second day. It is best avoided or reduced by discussing the urgency of adequate oral hydration with the patient in advance and advising the use of lemon-flavored candies and fruit juices to promote saliva flow. It is necessary to balance the need to maintain saliva flow with the potential for gastric distention followed by vomiting. Nevertheless, discussion of these issues with the patient with a view toward striking a balance between overhydration and underhydration is usually feasible. Analgesics should be made available for pain relief. Tylenol (650 mg every 4 to 6 hours) is usually sufficient.

In addition to the discomfort associated with parotid enlargement, patients experiencing significant parotitis are at greater risk for loss of taste and dry mouth. Both of these complications may clear in 4 to 6 weeks, but occasionally these symptoms persist. Despite the importance of treating distant metastases with adequate doses of ^{131}I, it is necessary to strike a balance between larger doses and these potential complications. In practice, permanent loss of taste and dry mouth are usually avoidable at doses below 450 to 500 mCi. Doses in excess of 500 mCi are usually not prescribed as a single administration, even when doses in this range are within a "maximal tolerated dose" level in terms of bone marrow exposure.

Other areas of concern include potential affects on fertility and possible second malignancies. Although not many studies of these potential complications have been performed, the available information is somewhat encouraging. Dottorini et al. (58) reported that women treated with 150 mCi of ^{131}I had subsequent fertility histories similar to those of women with thyroid carcinoma who were treated with surgery alone. The period of observation was 1 to 15 years. No data are available for higher doses of ^{131}I. A significant incidence of oligospermia has been observed in men who received ^{131}I therapy (59). This effect is related to Sertoli cell failure, probably as a result of the radiation received during the interval in which levels in the blood are high. Serum levels of follicle-stimulating hormone are elevated. The effect is dose-dependent. Accordingly, it is prudent to advise young men of this possibility and to consider sperm banking in advance of ^{131}I therapy. If this is opted, it should be performed while the patient is euthyroid.

The concern that large doses of ^{131}I are potentially carcinogenic has not been substantiated by experience (53,54,58). Second tumors are not more likely to develop in patients with thyroid carcinoma who have been treated with ^{131}I than in those not treated with ^{131}I. In particular, an increased incidence of chronic myelogenous leukemia, which is noted after marrow exposure to high radiation absorbed doses, has not been observed in patients treated with ^{131}I (53–58). In the report by Dottorini et al. (58), second tumors were not observed with a statistically significant increased frequency in women who received 150 mCi of ^{131}I.

CONCLUSIONS

The diagnosis and treatment of thyroid carcinoma evolving from the thyroid follicular cells are part of the foundation and evolution of nuclear medicine. ^{131}I continues to have a role in both the evaluation and therapy of patients with this disorder. This chapter has reviewed the elements of this disease as they relate to the practice of nuclear medicine. The perspective offered is that the disease represents a variable clinical picture for which no single protocol can be used, either by the surgeon, endocrinologist/oncologist, or nuclear medicine physician. The risk factors that predict a complex course have been defined. Some patients do indeed have minimal disease and can be effectively treated with minimally invasive procedures. Other patients require aggressive initial therapy and follow-up. It is the responsibility of nuclear medicine physicians to be aware of the array of procedures available and to supplement their technical knowledge with good judgment concerning the appropriate utilization of these procedures.

APPENDIX A. PROTOCOL FOR CALCULATION OF AN ABLATIVE DOSE OF ^{131}I BASED ON DOSIMETRY

1. Patient appears for evaluation.
2. Perform neck scan with ^{99m}Tc-pertechnetate; estimate weight of residual tissue (intact normal thyroid lobe weighs 10 g). Administer a 5- to 50-µCi tracer dose of ^{131}I.
3. Measure 24-hour uptake.
4. Measure 48-hour uptake.
5. Measure 72-hour uptake.
6. Plot uptake values on semilogarithmic paper; determine value for $t_{1/2\ eff}$.
7. Calculate dose to be administered with the following equation:

$$\text{Admin Dose (µCi)} = \frac{\text{Radiation Absorbed Dose} \times \text{Tissue Weight} \times 6.67}{t_{1/2\ eff}\ (d) \times 24\text{-h uptake (\%)}}$$

Example: A 53-year-old man recently underwent a near-total thyroidectomy to remove a 4.0-cm papillary carcinoma of the right lobe of the thyroid. The surgical specimen had "negative margins," and excised lymph nodes were negative for tumor. A ^{99m}Tc-pertechnetate scan demonstrated a virtually complete absence of thyroid tissue in the left side of the thyroid bed and a 2.0-cm focal area of tissue on the right side. Seven weeks after surgery, the patient is clinically hypothyroid, with a serum TSH level of 60 µIU/mL. The 24-hour "thyroid" uptake of the remnant is 8%. At 48 hours, the uptake is 7.2%, and at 96 hours, the uptake has decreased to 6%.

$$t_{1/2\ biologic} \approx 6\ d$$

$$t_{1/2\ eff} = (6 \times 8)/(6 + 8) = 48/14 = 3.4\ d$$

$$\text{Admin Dose (µCi)} = \frac{\text{Radiation Absorbed Dose} \times \text{Tissue Weight} \times 6.67}{t_{1/2\ eff}\ (d) \times 24\text{-h uptake (\%)}}$$

Desired Radiation Absorbed Dose = 3×10^4 cGy

Tissue Weight ≈ 3.14 g (assuming 1 g/cc; volume = πr^3)

$$t_{1/2\ eff} = 3.4\ d$$

24-h uptake = 8%

$$\text{Admin Dose (mCi)} = \frac{3 \times 10^4 \times 3.14 \times 6.67}{3.4 \times 8} = \frac{628.3}{27.2} = 23.1\ \text{mCi}\ ^{131}I$$

These calculations determine that 23.1 mCi of ^{131}I will deliver 300 Gy to the patient's thyroid remnant, which confirms that a dose of 1,100 MBq (30 mCi) of ^{131}I is likely to be effective to ablate the tissue. If the calculation determines that it is necessary to administer a larger dose, perhaps 2,000 MBq, the clinical decision is usually made to treat the patient with at least 2,800 MBq (75 mCi). It is no longer necessary to hospitalize patients for ^{131}I therapy in the United States, so the 1,100-MBq level has less significance because an economic component is no longer involved in the decision of whether to administer a dose larger or smaller than this amount. It is likely, however, that physicians will continue to segregate patients into a low-dose (1,100 MBq) and high-dose (2,800 MBq) categories. It is recommended that the selection of the actual administered dose be based on a calculation of the radiation absorbed dose delivered to the thyroid remnant.

APPENDIX B. PROTOCOL FOR CALCULATION OF A MAXIMAL THERAPY DOSE BASED ON LIMITING BONE MARROW RADIATION ABSORBED DOSE

An estimate of the radiation absorbed dose to the bone marrow can be calculated by either of two methods, the Quimby-Marinelli formulation used by Benua and Leeper at Memorial Sloan-Kettering Cancer Center or the MIRD Dose 3 formulation. The Benua-Leeper approach actually estimates the radiation absorbed dose to the blood based on the assumption that for ^{131}I therapy, the marrow exposure cannot exceed this value. This method continues to be used at a number of centers. The MIRD Dose 3 formulation provides many refinements, some of which are neither practical nor necessary to use in clinical practice. Centers using this approach "calculate" either the marrow or whole-body dose based on limited determinations of either the whole-body activity or whole-body activity and blood percentage administered dose per volume (i.e., % dose/L) and the turnover rate of each of these values.

Calculation with the Benua-Leeper method:

1. Patient appears for evaluation after withdrawal of thyroid hormone; clinical status confirmed; serum TSH, T_4, thyroglobulin, complete blood cell count determined.
2. A 1.0- to 5.0-mCi tracer dose of ^{131}I is administered.
3. At 2 to 4 hours, blood sample (heparinized) is drawn; whole-body count is performed.
4. At 24 hours, blood sample (heparinized) is drawn; whole-body count is performed.
5. At 48 hours, blood sample (heparinized) is drawn; whole-body count is performed.
6. At 72 to 120 hours, blood sample (heparinized) is drawn; whole-body count is performed.
7. Counts in 1 to 2 mL of blood are plotted versus time on semilogarithmic paper; blood $t_{1/2\ eff}$ is determined.
8. Whole-body counts are plotted versus time on semilogarithmic paper; whole-body $t_{1/2\ eff}$ is determined.
9. Radiation absorbed dose to blood per mCi (MBq) is calculated.

$$\text{Blood Radiation Absorbed Dose} = \text{Dose } \beta_{\text{ blood}} + \text{Dose } \gamma_{\text{ whole body}}$$

$$\text{Dose } \beta_{\text{ blood}} = 51.2 \text{ (constant)} \times E_\beta \text{ (average } \beta \text{ energy)} \times C(t) \text{ rad/d}$$

$$\text{Dose } \gamma_{\text{ whole body}} = 0.024 \text{ (constant)} \times \gamma\ t \times \rho \text{ (density} \approx 1) \times \Gamma \text{ (geometry factor) rad/d}$$

The dose for β and γ is the integral of the dose rate (described above) over time [average $t_{1/2} = 1.44 \times t_{1/2\ eff}$ (d)].

It is our practice to calculate the so-called "maximal recommended dose" with a programmed computer, although it is possible to perform the calculation "by hand." The calculation and approach use the so-called "blood dose" because it was not possible at the time to consider values for red marrow. Of course, methods presently exist either to determine marrow or to extrapolate from standardized tables, as the original biologic assumptions are still reasonably correct:

1. ^{131}I is not taken up directly by marrow elements.
2. Marrow exposure is derived from the nonpenetrating radiation (β) of the activity in the blood while it is perfusing marrow.
3. Marrow exposure from penetrating radiation (γ) is derived from the entire body distribution.

The radiation absorbed dose for the marrow is in fact a percentage of the dose calculated for the blood. The value varies between 30% and 60% of the calculated blood dose depending on the radiopharmaceutical. Of course, the experience garnered based on the clinical effects evolving from 200 rad to blood must be extrapolated down if estimates of bone marrow absorbed dose are to be used (i.e., for ^{131}I, 200 rad to blood might equate with 160 rad to red marrow).

The calculation can be made also with the MIRD formulation (MIRD Dose 3):

$$\text{Dose} = \text{Activity/Mass} \times \text{Average } t_{1/2\ eff} \times S$$

This calculation has been reviewed at length in the literature (46).

With the proper set of assumptions, the two formulations, Marinelli-Quimby and MIRD, will give similar results, although the MIRD is a more sophisticated formulation that allows many more variables to be considered. The Marinelli-Quimby formulation to calculate the "blood dose" continues to be used by many, as it provides continuity and consistency with the previous, albeit limited, published experience.

REFERENCES

1. Herz S, Roberts A, Evans RD. Radioactive iodine as an indicator in the study of thyroid physiology. *Proc Soc Exp Biol Med* 1938;38:510–514.
2. Christensen SB, Bondeson L, Ericsson UB, et al. Prediction of malignancy in the solitary thyroid nodule by physical examination, thyroid scan, fine-needle biopsy and serum thyroglobulin: a prospective study of 100 surgically treated patients. *Acta Chir Scand* 1984;150:433–440.
3. Belflore A, LaRosa GL, LaPorta GA, et al. Cancer risk in patients with cold thyroid nodules: relevance of iodine intake, sex, age, and multinodularity. *Am J Med* 1992;93:363–369.
4. Mazzaferri EL. Management of a solitary thyroid nodule. *N Engl J Med* 1993;328:553–558.
5. Schneider AB, Shore-Freedman E, Ryo UY, et al. Radiation-induced tumors of the head and neck following childhood irradiation: prospective studies. *Medicine* 1985;64:1–15.
6. Sachmechi I, Miller E, Varatharajah R, et al. Thyroid carcinoma in single cold nodules and in cold nodules of multinodular goiters. *Endocr Pract* 2000;6:5–7.
7. Kusic Z, Becker DV, Saenger EL, et al. Comparison of technetium-99m and iodine-123 imaging of thyroid nodules: correlation with pathologic findings, *J Nucl Med* 1990;31:393–399.
8. Ridgeway EC. Clinician evaluation of a solitary thyroid nodule. *J Clin Endocrinol Metab* 1992;8:215–224.
9. Bacourt F, Asselain B, Savoie JC, et al. Multifactorial study of prognostic factors in differentiated thyroid carcinoma and a re-evaluation of the importance of age. *Br J Surg* 1986;73:274–280.
10. Schelfhout LJ, Creutzberg CL, Hamming JF, et al. Multivariate analysis of survival in differentiated thyroid cancer: the prognostic significance of the age factor. *Eur J Cancer Clin Oncol* 1988;24:331–341.
11. Hay D. Papillary thyroid carcinoma. *Endocrinol Metab Clin North Am* 1990;19:545–576.
12. Byar DP, Green SB, Dor P, et al. A prognostic index for thyroid carcinoma: a study of the E.O.R.T.C. Thyroid Cancer Cooperative Group. *Eur J Cancer* 1979;15:1033–1041.
13. Fourquet A, Asselain B, Joly J. Cancer de la thyroïde: analyse multidimensionnelle des facteurs pronostiques. *Ann Endocrinol (Paris)* 1983;44:121–129.
14. McConahey WM, Hay ID, Woolner LB, et al. Papillary thyroid cancer treated at the Mayo Clinic, 1946 through 1970: initial manifestations, pathologic findings, therapy and outcome. *Mayo Clin Proc* 1986;61:978–988.
15. Cady B, Rossi R. An expanded view of risk-group definition in differentiated thyroid carcinoma. *Surgery* 1988;104:947–957.
16. Brennan MD, Bergstrahl EJ, Van Heerden JA, et al. Follicular thyroid cancer treated at the Mayo Clinic, 1946 through 1970:

initial manifestations, pathologic findings, therapy and outcome. *Mayo Clin Proc* 1991;66:11–22.

17. Mazzaferri EL, Young RL. Papillary thyroid carcinoma: a 10-year follow-up report of the impact of therapy in 576 patients. *Am J Med* 1981;70:511–518.

18. Mazzaferri EL, Jhiang SM. Long-term impact of initial surgical and medical therapy on papillary and follicular thyroid cancer. *Am J Med* 1994;97:418–428.

19. Beierwaltes VM, Rabbani R, Dmuchowski C, et al. An analysis of "ablation of thyroid remnants" with I-131 in 511 patients from 1947–1984: experience at University of Michigan. *J Nucl Med* 1984;25:1287–1293.

20. Sisson JC. Applying the radioactive eraser: I-131 to ablate normal thyroid tissue in patients from whom thyroid cancer has been resected. *J Nucl Med* 1983;24:743–745.

21. Goolden AW. The indications for ablating normal thyroid tissue with ^{131}I in differentiated thyroid cancer. *Clin Endocrinol* 1985;23:81–86.

22. Hurley JR, Becker DV. The use of radioiodine in the management of thyroid cancer. In: Freeman LM, Weissman HS, eds. *Nuclear medicine annual.* New York: Raven Press, 1983:329–384.

23. Maxon HR III, Englaro EE, Thomas SR, et al. Radioiodine-131 therapy for well-differentiated thyroid cancer—a quantitative radiation dosimetric approach: outcome and validation in 85 patients. *J Nucl Med* 1992;33:1132–1136.

24. Grigsby PW, Siegel BA, Baker S, et al. Radiation exposures from outpatient radioactive (^{131}I) therapy for thyroid carcinoma. *JAMA* 2000;283:2272–2274.

25. Meier CA, Braverman LE, Ebner SA, et al. Diagnostic use of recombinant human thyrotropin versus thyroid hormone withdrawal in patients with thyroid carcinoma (phase I/II study). *J Clin Endocrinol Metab* 1994;78:188–196.

26. Ladenson PW, Braverman LE, Mazzaferri EL, et al. Comparison of administration of recombinant human thyrotropin with withdrawal of thyroid hormone for radioactive iodine scanning in patients with thyroid carcinoma. *N Engl J Med* 1997;337:888–896.

27. Ladenson PW. Recombinant human thyrotropin symposium: strategies for thyrotropin use to monitor patients with treated thyroid carcinoma. *Thyroid* 1999;9:429–433.

28. Rudavsky AZ, Freeman LM. Treatment of I-131 scan-negative, thyroglobulin-positive metastaic thyroid carcinoma using radioactive I-131 and recombinant human thyroid-stimulating hormone. *J Clin Endocrinol Metab* 1997;82:11–14.

29. Pineda JD, Lee T, Ain K, et al. Iodine-131 therapy for thyroid cancer patients with elevated thyroglobulin and negative diagnostic scans. *J Clin Endocrinol Metab* 1995;80:1488–1492.

30. Pacini F, Lippi F, Formica N, et al. Therapeutic doses of iodine-131 reveal undiagnosed metastases in thyroid cancer patients with detectable serum thyroglobulin levels. *J Nucl Med* 1987;28:1888–1891.

31. Park H. Stunned thyroid after high-dose I-131 imaging. *Clin Nucl Med* 1992;17:501–502.

32. Jeevanram RK, Shah DH, Sharma SM, et al. Influence of initial large dose on subsequent uptake of therapeutic radioiodine in thyroid cancer patients. *Nucl Med Biol* 1986;13:277–279.

33. Alam MS, Takeuchi L, Kasagi K, et al. Value of combined technetium-99m hydroxymethylene diphosphate and thallium-201 imaging in detecting bone metastases from thyroid carcinoma. *Thyroid* 1997;7:705–712.

34. Tonami N, Hisada K. ^{201}Tl scintigraphy in post-operative detection of thyroid cancer. A comparative study with ^{131}I. *Radiology* 1980;136:461–465.

35. Balon HR, Fink-Bennett D, Stoffer SS. Technetium-99m sestamibi uptake by recurrent Hürthle cell carcinoma of the thyroid. *J Nucl Med* 1992;33:1393–1396.

36. Ugar O, Kostakoglu L, Caner B, et al. Comparison of 201-Tl, ^{99m}Tc-MIBI and 131-I imaging in the follow-up of patients with well-differentiated thyroid carcinoma. *Nucl Med Commun* 1996;17:373–377.

37. Lind P, Gallowitsch HJ, Landsteger W, et al. Technetium-99m tetrofosmin whole body scintigraphy in the follow-up of differentiated thyroid carcinoma. *J Nucl Med* 1997;38:348–352.

38. Unal S, Menda Y, Adalet I, et al. Thallium-201, technetium-99m-tetrofosmin and iodine-131 in detecting differentiated thyroid carcinoma metastases. *J Nucl Med* 1998;39:1897–1902.

39. Baudin E, Schlumberger M, Lumbroso J, et al. Octreotide scintigraphy in patients with differentiated thyroid carcinoma: contribution for patients with negative radioiodine scan. *J Clin Endocrinol Metab* 1996;81:2541–2544.

40. Krenning E, Kwekkeboom DJ, Bakker WH, et al. Somatostatin receptor scintigraphy with [^{111}In-DTPA-D-Phe]- and [^{123}I-Tyr^3]-octreotide: the Rotterdam experience with more than 1000 patients. *Eur J Nucl Med* 1993;20:716–731.

41. Virgolini I. *Personal communication.*

42. Feine V, Lietzenmayer R, Hanke JP, et al. Fluorine-18-FDG and iodine-131 uptake in thyroid cancer. *J Nucl Med* 1996;37:1468–1472.

43. Wang W, Macapinlac H, Finn R, et al. PET scanning with ^{18}F-fluorodeoxyglucose can localize residual differentiated thyroid carcinoma in patients with negative ^{131}I whole body scans. *J Clin Endocrinol Metab* 1999;84:2291–2302.

44. Wang W, Larson SM, Fazzari M, et al. Prognostic value of [^{18}F]fluorodeoxyglucose positron emission tomography scanning in patients with thyroid carcinoma. *J Clin Endocrinol Metab* 2000;85:1107–1113.

45. Beierwaltes WH. The treatment of thyroid carcinoma with radioactive iodine. *Semin Nucl Med* 1978;8:79–94.

46. Harbert JC. Radiiodine therapy of differentiated thyroid carcinoma. In: Harbert JC, Eckelman WC, Neumann RD, eds. *Nuclear medicine: diagnosis and therapy.* Stuttgart: Thieme Medical Publishers, 1996:975–1020.

47. Benua RS, Cicale NR, Sonenberg M, et al. The relation of radioiodine dosimetry to results and complications in the treatment of metastatic thyroid cancer. *Am J Roentgenol* 1962;87:171.

48. Leeper R. Controversies in the treatment of thyroid cancer. The New York Memorial Hospital approach. *Thyroid Today* 1982;5:1–4.

49. Leeper RD, Shimaoka K. Treatment of metastatic thyroid cancer. *Clin Endocrinol Metab* 1980;9:383–391.

50. Maxon MR, Smith HS. Radioiodine-131 in the diagnosis and treatment of metastatic well-differentiated thyroid cancer. *Endocrinol Metab Clin North Am* 1990;19:685–719.

51. Wahl RL, Kroll S, Zasadny KR. Patient-specific whole-body dosimetry: principles and a simplified method for clinical implementation. *J Nucl Med* 1998;39[Suppl]:14S–20S.

52. Hamburger JI. Diuretic augmentation of ^{131}I uptake in inoperable thyroid cancer. *N Engl J Med* 1969;280:1091–1094.

53. Schlumberger M, Challeton C, Vathaire FD, et al. Radioactive iodine treatment and external radiotherapy for lung and bone metastases from thyroid carcinoma. *J Nucl Med* 1996;37:598–605.

54. Hurley JR, Becker DV. Treatment of thyroid cancer with radioactive ^{131}I. In: Sandler MP, Coleman RE, Wackers FJ, et al., eds. *Diagnostic nuclear medicine,* 3rd ed. Baltimore: Williams & Wilkins, 1995:959–990.

55. Samaan NA, Schultz PN, Hickey RC, et al. The results of various modalities of treatment of well-differentiated thyroid carcinoma: a retrospective review of 1599 patients. *J Clin Endocrinol Metab* 1992;75:714–720.

56. Massin JP, Savoie JC, Gamier H, et al. Pulmonary metastases in differentiated thyroid carcinoma. *Cancer* 1984;53:982–992.

57. Fatourechi V, Hay ID. Treating the patient with differentiated thyroid cancer with thyroglobulin-positive iodine-131 diagnostic scan-negative metastases: including comments on the role of serum thyroglobulin monitoring in tumor surveillance. *Semin Nucl Med* 2000;30:107–114.

58. Dottorini ME, Lomuscio G, Mazzucchelli L, et al. Assessment of female fertility and carcinogenesis after iodine-131 therapy for differentiated thyroid carcinoma. *J Nucl Med* 1995; 36:21–27.

59. Pacini F, Gasperi M, Fugazzola L, et al. Testicular function in patients with thyroid carcinoma treated with radioiodine. *J Nucl Med* 1994;35:1418–1422.

14

PARATHYROID SCINTIGRAPHY

RAYMOND TAILLEFER

Primary hyperparathyroidism is a relatively common disorder that is most frequently detected as asymptomatic hypercalcemia. It is estimated that approximately 100,000 new cases of primary hyperparathyroidism are diagnosed each year in the United States, with an incidence that increases with age (1). Many advances have been made in recent years in the diagnosis, localization, and treatment of primary hyperparathyroidism. The clinical utilization of routine automated biochemical screenings to detect elevated serum calcium levels has contributed significantly to the early diagnosis of this disease, which has been supported by the availability of radioimmunoassay for parathyroid hormone. Surgical exploration and removal of the diseased glands is the treatment of choice, once the diagnosis of hyperparathyroidism has been established. The success of parathyroid surgery is based on many factors, such as knowledge of the pathologic conditions, accurate localization of normal and abnormal parathyroid glands, and the experience of the surgeon in performing a meticulous dissection during removal of the abnormal glands.

Although the methods for obtaining the initial diagnosis and the treatment of this condition are well defined and established in the medical literature, considerable controversy remains regarding the use of preoperative studies to localize abnormal parathyroid tissue before a primary neck exploration is undertaken (2). Because the rate of success in primary surgical exploration of the neck in patients presenting with primary hyperparathyroidism has been reported to exceed 90% in experienced hands, many authors have questioned the role of preoperative localization studies in these cases. Although the vast majority of them agree that localization studies should be used before a parathyroidectomy is contemplated in a patient who has undergone extensive thyroid surgery in the past or will undergo a second parathyroidectomy for recurrent or persistent hyperparathyroidism, most surgeons, according to Kaplan et al. (2), agree that localization studies are not needed when the patient has a "virgin neck." This argument is based on the fact that com-

mon localization procedures are reported to be about 75% to 80% accurate when performed by experienced specialists using modern imaging equipment.

Because an expert parathyroid surgeon is able to cure more than 90% of these patients, why should a preoperative localization study be performed? Although this question is legitimate, there are many indications for performing parathyroid localization before a primary neck exploration. Shaha et al. (3) recently elaborated these indications, which can be divided into three categories: diagnostic problems (hypercalcemic crisis for urgent diagnosis, mild asymptomatic hypercalcemia or associated malignancies); anticipated technical difficulties (patients with previous neck or thyroid surgery, obese persons with short necks, patients with cervical spine problems in whom extension may be difficult, and those with palpable thyroid lesions); and factors putting the patient at high risk (patients with cardiac problems in whom unilateral exploration is crucial or in whom surgery is to be performed under local anesthesia). It has been shown that a preoperative localization procedure may help to shorten operative and anesthesia time by directing the surgeon to the site of the lesions (4–7). Furthermore, because the primary reason for failure at the initial exploration is inability of the surgeon to identify a parathyroid lesion (multiple adenomas, diffuse parathyroid hyperplasia, adenomas in supernumerary glands, ectopic adenomas outside the accessible operative field), a preoperative localization study that helps the surgeon to find abnormal parathyroid tissue may also be useful in decreasing the number of reexplorations, especially in cases of ectopic glands (8). It has been reported that previously missed adenomas are found in up to 80% of patients undergoing reexploration of the neck, frequently in an ectopic location, which indicates that a safe, inexpensive, and precise localization procedure before surgery is valuable and necessary (9). Therefore, although the need for a noninvasive preoperative localization test in patients with primary hyperparathyroidism continues to be debated in the medical literature, definite clinical indications do exist for such investigation (Table 14.1).

Several techniques with varying degrees of accuracy have been evaluated for the preoperative localization of parathyroid adenoma in patients with biochemically proven hyper-

R. Taillefer: Department of Radiology, University of Montreal; Department of Nuclear Medicine, Hôtel-Dieu de Centre Hospitalier de Université de Montreal, Montreal, Quebec, H2W 1T8, Canada.

TABLE 14.1 INDICATIONS FOR PARATHYROID SCINTIGRAPHY IN PREOPERATIVE LOCALIZATION IN PATIENTS WITH HYPERPARATHYROIDISM

A. **Before a second neck exploration for recurrent or persistent hyperparathyroidism**
   - Ectopic adenoma
   - Supernumerary gland adenoma
   - Multiple adenomas
   - Diffuse parathyroid hyperplasia
B. **Before a first neck exploration**
   Diagnostic problems
   - Mild asymptomatic hypercalcemia
   - Hypercalcemic crisis, for urgent diagnosis
   - Associated malignancies
   Anticipated technical difficulties
   - Previous neck or thyroid surgery
   - Obese patients with short necks
   - Cervical spine problems with difficult extension
   - Palpable thyroid lesions
   High-risk factors
   - Cardiac problems
   - Central nervous system disease
   - Bleeding disorders
   - Other conditions in which local anesthesia is preferred

parathyroidism. These include intraoperative vital staining methods, cine-esophagography, thermography, mediastinography, computed axial tomography, arteriography, selective venography, ultrasonography, and, more recently, magnetic resonance imaging, digital subtraction arteriography, and needle aspiration combined with high-resolution ultrasonography (10–19). The introduction of nuclear medicine procedures was initially based on the concept of using metabolic markers directed to specific tissues, such as ^{57}Co-vitamin B_{12} (20), ^{75}Se-methionine (21), and ^{131}Ce chloride (22). In the late 1970s, ^{201}Tl-thallous chloride was introduced as an agent to visualize parathyroid glands (23). Concomitant ^{99m}Tc-pertechnetate imaging was introduced a few years later to provide computerized subtraction of ^{201}Tl uptake in the normal thyroid gland (24,25). Since then, several studies have demonstrated the clinical value of radionuclide imaging with dual radioisotopes, including ^{201}Tl, in the preoperative localization of abnormal parathyroid tissue before a first or second cervical exploration (26–28). Although parathyroid scintigraphy with dual radionuclides has yielded satisfactory results and good diagnostic accuracy, this procedure presents some disadvantages, mainly related to the physical characteristics of ^{201}Tl. ^{99m}Tc-Sestamibi was introduced in the early 1990s as a myocardial perfusion imaging radiopharmaceutical, with the potential of replacing ^{201}Tl. Besides its applications in cardiologic nuclear medicine, ^{99m}Tc-sestamibi has been investigated for radionuclide imaging in various oncologic disorders and thyroid diseases. More recently, ^{99m}Tc-tetrofosmin, another ^{99m}Tc-labeled myocardial perfusion imaging agent, has been used for parathyroid imaging. ^{99m}Tc-Furifosmin and radio-

pharmaceuticals used for positron emission tomography (PET) are also currently under investigation.

The purpose of this chapter is to review the concepts underlying the use of parathyroid scintigraphy with different radiotracers and imaging techniques, with emphasis on single- and dual-radionuclide ^{99m}Tc-sestamibi parathyroid imaging.

NORMAL PHYSIOLOGY OF THE PARATHYROID GLANDS

The inferior parathyroid glands are embryologically derived from the third branchial pouch and can be found anywhere along the entire course of migration of this pouch, so that the inferior parathyroid glands tend to be less constant in position than the superior glands, which are derived from the fourth pouch. The parathyroid glands generally measure 4 to 6 mm in length, 2 to 4 mm in width, and 1 to 2 mm in thickness. The mean glandular weight is 32 mg, with a maximum gland weight of 59 mg (29–31). Most normal adults, approximately 85%, have four parathyroid glands, whereas 13% of normal persons have more than four glands, and 3% have only three (32). Histologically, parathyroid chief cells comprise most of the glands, which have varying numbers of oncocytic cells and transitional oncocytic cells. Oncocytic cells are rich in oxidative enzymes and contain abundant mitochondria. Transitional cells are histologically intermediate between chief and oncocytic cells. Chief cells secrete parathyroid hormone, or parathormone (PTH); the function of the other cells remains uncertain. PTH is an 84-amino acid peptide that is synthesized within the cytoplasm of the chief cells and, to a lesser extent, within the oncocytes. PTH is one of the major hormones regulating calcium and phosphorus homeostasis. The major action of the hormone is on bone and results ultimately in the stimulation of bone resorption and the inhibition of bone formation. PTH secretion is regulated by the serum calcium level in a classic feedback loop (33).

PATHOPHYSIOLOGY OF THE PARATHYROID GLANDS

Pathologically, the anatomic disorders of the parathyroid glands are usually classified by their functional effects on the glands (i.e., hypoparathyroidism and hyperparathyroidism). The latter is further divided into primary, secondary, and tertiary hyperparathyroidism. Hyperparathyroidism is characterized by an excess secretion of PTH. The major biochemical features of primary hyperparathyroidism include elevated serum levels of PTH, hypercalcemia, hypophosphatemia, and excessive urinary excretion of calcium. Excess PTH originates in adenomatous, hyperplastic, or carcinomatous tissue. Hyperparathyroidism is a relatively common disease, occurring in approximately 1 of every 500 women over 40 years of age and approximately 1 of every 2,000 men. Hyperparathyroidism appears to be the most common cause of hypercalcemia in nonhospitalized patients. Secondary hyperparathyroidism is characterized by a compensatory hypersecretion of PTH induced by an end-organ resistance to PTH. The most important cause of secondary hyperparathyroidism is chronic renal insufficiency resulting in chronic hypocalcemia and hyperphosphatemia. Tertiary hyperparathyroidism refers to the development of autonomous parathyroid hyperfunction in patients with secondary hyperparathyroidism.

Most cases (80% to 85%) of primary hyperparathyroidism are the result of a single parathyroid adenoma; two adenomas occur in 2% to 3% of cases. Carcinomas are found in 2% to 3% of persons with parathyroid tumors, whereas about 10% to 15% of patients present with primary parathyroid hyperplasia. Parathyroid adenoma is a benign neoplasm composed of chief cells, oncocytic cells, transitional oncocytic cells, or mixtures of these cell types. Although adenomas may occur in either sex at any age, most become evident in the middle decades of life. Adenomas vary considerably in size and weight, with a usual range of 0.5 to 5.0 g. Occasionally, they are as large as 10 to 100 g. Although 80% to 85% of parathyroid adenomas are found adjacent to the thyroid gland in their normal locations (most often in the inferior parathyroid glands for unknown reasons), 15% to 20% are ectopic and can be found in such sites as the thymus and pericardium, or behind the esophagus. Uncommonly, an adenoma can be found high up in the neck, anterior to the carotid bifurcation, and in 3% to 5% of cases, parathyroid adenomas can be intrathyroidal.

^{201}TL/^{99m}Tc-PERTECHNETATE DUAL-RADIONUCLIDE SCINTIGRAPHY

Among the noninvasive imaging techniques used to detect abnormal parathyroid glands, dual-radionuclide parathyroid scintigraphy with ^{201}Tl/^{99m}Tc-pertechnetate was, until recently, certainly one of the most preferred (34). In the late 1970s, ^{201}Tl-thallous chloride was reported to visualize parathyroid glands. Increased perfusion, functional activity, and cellularity of parathyroid adenomas have been postulated as the main reasons for increased ^{201}Tl uptake in these lesions. Because ^{201}Tl is taken up by both the thyroid and enlarged parathyroid glands, a second image obtained with a radiopharmaceutical taken up only by the thyroid gland was needed. A few years later, ^{99m}Tc-pertechnetate imaging was added to provide an image of the thyroid tissue for comparison or for computerized subtraction of ^{201}Tl uptake by the normal thyroid gland. Since then, several studies of ^{201}Tl/^{99m}Tc-pertechnetate dual-radiotracer parathyroid scintigraphy have been reported. In an extensive review of 14 studies comprising a total of 317 patients

who had primary hyperparathyroidism and had undergone surgery, the accumulated sensitivity of parathyroid scintigraphy to detect parathyroid adenomas was 82% (35). The overall diagnostic accuracy rate was 78%, the positive predictive value 94%, and the false-positive rate 5%. The majority of false-positive results were in patients with coexisting thyroid diseases.

Although dual-radionuclide parathyroid scintigraphy with ^{201}Tl/^{99m}Tc-pertechnetate has provided satisfactory results and good diagnostic accuracy, results reported in the literature have been somewhat variable, and this technique may be highly operator-dependent. Many different protocols have been used for data acquisition and subtraction. Various technical aspects of the procedure are still either somewhat controversial or not completely resolved, including the choice of radiotracer (^{123}I vs. ^{99m}Tc-pertechnetate with ^{201}Tl), order of injection of tracers (^{201}Tl before or after ^{99m}Tc-pertechnetate), relative activities injected (related to the tracers and their order of injection), value of computer subtraction technique (with increased sensitivity and possibly decreased specificity), and computer alignment and display procedures (36–46). Furthermore, it is essential that the head and neck of the patient remain immobile during the entire process of image acquisition. For these reasons, investigators continued to seek another radionuclide for use in parathyroid scintigraphy.

^{99m}Tc-Sestamibi (^{99m}Tc-*hexakis*-2-methoxyisobutylisonitrile) is a ^{99m}Tc-labeled lipophilic cationic complex that was empirically designed for myocardial perfusion imaging (47–53). Because of the more favorable emission characteristics of ^{99m}Tc and its myocardial biodistribution proportional to the blood flow, ^{99m}Tc-sestamibi offered a good alternative to ^{201}Tl for this purpose. It soon became obvious that ^{99m}Tc-sestamibi would be an interesting radiopharmaceutical, not only for myocardial perfusion imaging but also for other uses of ^{201}Tl, especially the detection of various types of benign and malignant tumors (54–56). The step of replacing ^{201}Tl with ^{99m}Tc-sestamibi for parathyroid scintigraphy was also relatively easy given the physical characteristics of ^{99m}Tc-sestamibi, the inherent technical problems related to dual-radionuclide parathyroid scintigraphy with ^{201}Tl/^{99m}Tc-pertechnetate, and the results of some initial experimental physiologic and histologic studies of ^{99m}Tc-sestamibi pertinent to its use for parathyroid imaging.

^{99m}Tc-SESTAMIBI PARATHYROID SCINTIGRAPHY

Mechanism of Parathyroid Uptake of ^{99m}Tc-Sestamibi

The exact mechanisms of ^{99m}Tc-sestamibi uptake in parathyroid lesions are not precisely known at the present time. It is likely, however, that many nonspecific factors are simultaneously involved. These include the biochemical characteristics of ^{99m}Tc-sestamibi (its cationic charge and lipophilicity), the degree of local blood flow, transcapillary exchange, interstitial transport, and the negative intracellular charge of both mitochondria and cell membranes. It has been shown that ^{99m}Tc-sestamibi is sequestered within the cytoplasm and mitochondria of cultured mouse fibroblasts, and that its net cellular uptake and retention occur in response to electric potentials generated across the membrane bilayers of both cell and mitochondria (57). These results suggest that normal or abnormal tissues with a large number of mitochondria would take up ^{99m}Tc-sestamibi more avidly than a tissue containing fewer mitochondria. Myocytes, which contain a large number of mitochondria per cell, retain ^{99m}Tc-sestamibi longer than ^{201}Tl.

Piwnica-Worms et al. (58) found that the transport of ^{99m}Tc-sestamibi involves passive diffusion across plasma and mitochondrial membrane. At equilibrium, it is sequestered largely within mitochondria by the large transmembrane potentials (-150 mV). Crane et al. (59) confirmed that in guinea pigs hearts the mitochondrial fraction of myocardial homogenates contain close to 90% of the overall cellular ^{99m}Tc-sestamibi activity. Using quantitative electron probe x-ray, Backus et al. (60) showed that the concentration of ^{99m}Tc-sestamibi in the mitochondria is up to 1,000 times greater than that in the extracellular content. Sandrock et al. (61) reported a study comparing ultrastructural histology with the results of ^{201}Tl/^{99m}Tc-pertechnetate parathyroid subtraction scintigraphy. They found that true-positive lesions have a significantly higher number of oxyphil cells than false-negative or normal glands, and that the number of mitochondria per cell is higher in oxyphil cells in true-positive lesions than in chief or clear cells in false-negative or normal glands. These data indicate that the presence of mitochondria-rich oxyphil cells can be a significant factor influencing the detectability of abnormal parathyroid glands by ^{201}Tl/^{99m}Tc-pertechnetate scintigraphy.

The above-mentioned observations suggest that ^{99m}Tc-sestamibi would be taken up more avidly in adenomatous tissue than in surrounding thyroid parenchyma. Because ^{99m}Tc-sestamibi is retained longer than ^{201}Tl in tissue containing a large number of mitochondria per cell, such as cardiac tissue, ^{99m}Tc-sestamibi would be released more slowly from abnormal parathyroid cells following its initial uptake (62). This characteristic should allow the more selective visualization of abnormal parathyroid tissue. Carpentier et al. (63) performed a study to assess the relationship between parathyroid oxyphil cell content and early or delayed phases of ^{99m}Tc-sestamibi uptake. Various parathyroid lesions in patients with hyperparathyroidism were evaluated: 8 adenoma, 1 adenocarcinoma, and 2 hyperplasia. Seven of nine (78%) parathyroid lesions with an oxyphil cell content above 25% showed positive late ^{99m}Tc-sestamibi uptake, in comparison with two of six (33%) lesions

with an oxyphil cell content between 1% and 25% and none of three lesions with no oxyphil cells. These investigators showed that late-phase ^{99m}Tc-sestamibi uptake is more frequently positive in lesions with an oxyphil cell content above 50%. Early ^{99m}Tc-sestamibi uptake was associated with higher serum calcium levels and larger lesions. Therefore, it is not surprising, in some cases, to have a negative ^{99m}Tc-sestamibi delayed study in the presence of a parathyroid adenoma because a rapid ^{99m}Tc-sestamibi washout can be observed in an adenoma with few oxyphil cells.

^{99m}Tc-Sestamibi is a lipophilic isonitrile derivative of technetium that is positively charged. Thus, ^{99m}Tc-sestamibi shares some physical and chemical characteristics with the chemotherapeutic agents and various drugs and natural products transported by P-glycoprotein, a transmembrane protein that functions to protect cells from toxic substances. The overexpression of this protein through the activation of a mammalian *MDR1* gene (multidrug resistance) results in a cross-resistance of chemotherapeutic agents and other structurally related drugs. Mitchell et al. (64) recently reported the results of a study suggesting that expression of P-glycoprotein may be involved in the mechanism of parathyroid imaging. A decreased expression of P-glycoprotein in the membrane of abnormal parathyroid cells may be related to the visualization of parathyroid glands with ^{99m}Tc-sestamibi.

Before undertaking to use ^{99m}Tc-sestamibi for parathyroid scintigraphy, one must consider the normal uptake in surrounding tissues, especially the thyroid. The mechanism of ^{99m}Tc-sestamibi uptake in the thyroid is not yet clearly understood. Increased thyroid blood flow and capillary permeability, the characteristics of ^{99m}Tc-sestamibi, mitochondrial and plasma membrane potentials of the follicular cells, and mitochondrial content may all play a significant role in thyroid uptake. ^{99m}Tc-Sestamibi is rapidly taken up by the thyroid following intravenous injection; its retention half-life is approximately 60 minutes (64). This uptake is not affected by exogenous thyroxine therapy, perchlorate, iodine saturation, or thyroid-stimulating hormone control (65–69). Uptake of ^{99m}Tc-sestamibi has been detected in various thyroid lesions, such as medullary thyroid carcinoma (70), Hürthle cell carcinoma of the thyroid (71), differentiated thyroid carcinomas (72), primary thyroid lymphoma (73), and benign thyroid adenomas (74). Because these lesions may increase the uptake of ^{99m}Tc-sestamibi in the neck, they affect the specificity of parathyroid scintigraphy.

Protocols for Parathyroid Imaging with ^{99m}Tc-Sestamibi

Although the clinical use of ^{99m}Tc-sestamibi parathyroid scintigraphy is still relatively recent, various imaging protocols and modifications thereof have been described. Two distinct basic imaging strategies with ^{99m}Tc-sestamibi have been investigated for parathyroid scintigraphy (Fig. 14.1). The first reported [99mTc]-sestamibi imaging protocol for parathyroid scintigraphy entailed the use of this radiopharmaceutical as a substitute for [201Tl] in a dual-radionuclide approach with subtraction imaging. In the second approach, [99mTc]-sestamibi is used alone for early and delayed imaging to perform what is referred to as *double-phase study*. This imaging protocol is based on the differential washout of [99mTc]-sestamibi in the thyroid and in parathyroid lesions. Although the underlying principles of these protocols are different, their accuracy is similar in the detection of abnormal parathyroid glands. Each protocol has its clinical advantages and limitations.

Parathyroid Scintigraphy with Dual Radionuclides

Coakley et al. (74) in 1989 were the first to suggest the clinical use of [99mTc]-sestamibi for parathyroid imaging. Their preliminary study comparing [123I]/[99mTc]-sestamibi with

A) DUAL-RADIOTRACER TECHNIQUE

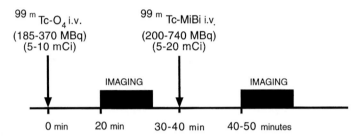

B) DUAL-PHASE TECHNIQUE

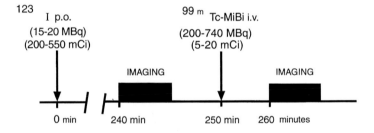

C) "COMBINED " TECHNIQUE

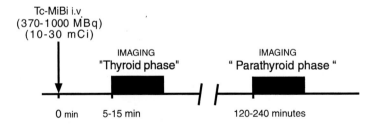

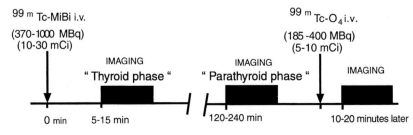

FIGURE 14.1. Schematic representation of different imaging protocols for parathyroid scintigraphy with [99mTc]-sestamibi (see text for explanations).

^{201}Tl/^{99m}Tc-pertechnetate parathyroid imaging included five patients. In three of four patients with parathyroid adenomas, the abnormal parathyroid gland was more obvious on the ^{99m}Tc-sestamibi study than on the ^{201}Tl study. Quantitative analysis showed a higher parathyroid-to-thyroid uptake ratio with ^{99m}Tc-sestamibi than with ^{201}Tl. Their limited data also showed that ^{201}Tl and ^{99m}Tc-sestamibi behave similarly in the thyroid gland, with peak uptake between about 3 and 5 minutes after injection and a subsequent rapid washout; peak activity in the parathyroid glands also occurs at the same time, but the washout of ^{99m}Tc-sestamibi is slower in the parathyroids than the washout of ^{201}Tl. The conclusion of this initial report was that ^{99m}Tc-sestamibi is a suitable alternative to ^{201}Tl in the preoperative localization of abnormal parathyroid glands. The authors hypothesized that the better visualization obtained in some cases with ^{99m}Tc-sestamibi might be related to the superior physical characteristics of ^{99m}Tc as a radiolabel and its slower washout from parathyroid glands in comparison with ^{201}Tl (Fig. 14.2).

Two years later, the same group of authors reported their clinical experience with a larger group of patients (75). They compared ^{99m}Tc-sestamibi with ^{201}Tl as a parathyroid imaging agent in 57 patients preoperatively. Thyroid localization was achieved with the use of oral ^{131}I-sodium iodide (0.5 mCi) administered 4 hours before parathyroid imaging with ^{201}Tl and ^{99m}Tc-sestamibi. All these imaging procedures were carried out on the same day. Forty patients had confirmed parathyroid adenomas. Thallium 201 detected 37 adenomas (sensitivity of 92.5%), whereas the ^{99m}Tc-sestamibi study was positive in 39 cases (sensitivity of 97.5%). The dynamic curves for ^{201}Tl and ^{99m}Tc-sestamibi uptake in the thyroid and parathyroid tissue showed that uptake reached a maximum at 4 to 6 minutes in both the thyroid gland and the parathyroid adenomas. The activity in the thyroid then decreased with both tracers. The ^{201}Tl activity in the parathyroid lesions steadily declined following the peak activity, whereas the ^{99m}Tc-sestamibi uptake remained relatively constant. Data obtained in a subgroup of 20 patients showed that the uptake of ^{99m}Tc-sestamibi per gram of parathyroid tissue was higher than the uptake per gram of thyroid tissue, whereas the difference in ^{201}Tl uptake was not statistically different in the two tissues. The authors stated that the use of ^{123}I is not essential for thyroid localization. This procedure was used in their study primarily to provide a constant thyroid background with which ^{201}Tl and ^{99m}Tc-sestamibi data could be compared.

Since the publication of that study, different investigators have used this approach to perform parathyroid scintigraphy (74–88). In summary, either ^{123}I or ^{99m}Tc-pertechnetate is administered before ^{99m}Tc-sestamibi is injected (89). Although different doses and different intervals of time after injection of the radiopharmaceuticals have been reported, Fig. 14.1 shows the most common and representative imaging protocols and doses used in dual-radionuclide ^{99m}Tc-sestamibi parathyroid imaging. In the protocol for ^{123}I, images are obtained 4 hours after the administration of an oral dose of ^{123}I. Then, ^{99m}Tc-sestamibi (5 to 25 mCi) is injected intravenously and images are obtained in either static or dynamic mode beginning 1 to 5 minutes after the injection and usually up to 20 to 30 minutes later. Anterior planar cervical and upper thoracic views (to include the mediastinum) are usually obtained first, and

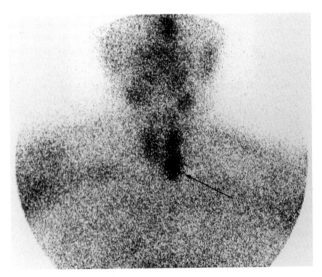
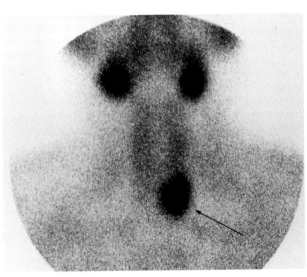

A   B

FIGURE 14.2. Comparison between ^{201}Tl (**A**) and ^{99m}Tc-sestamibi (**B**) parathyroid scintigraphy in a patient with a parathyroid adenoma of the left lower neck (*arrow*). The ^{201}Tl study was performed 4 days after the ^{99m}Tc-sestamibi study. The parathyroid adenoma-to-thyroid activity ratio is significantly increased with ^{99m}Tc-sestamibi.

oblique views or single-photon emission computed tomography (SPECT) imaging is added if necessary. Image processing, background subtraction methods, correction for patient motion, correction of scatter of ^{123}I into the ^{99m}Tc window (although small), and image normalization are similar to those used for ^{201}Tl in ^{201}Tl/^{99m}Tc-pertechnetate parathyroid scintigraphy. The advantages of ^{123}I as the radiopharmaceutical used for thyroid imaging include a better target-to-background ratio than that of ^{99m}Tc-pertechnetate and a more stable background within the thyroid during imaging. However, because of the relatively high cost of ^{123}I, its limited availability, and the significant delay between administration and imaging, ^{99m}Tc-pertechnetate is also used to outline the thyroid for subtraction studies. ^{99m}Tc-Pertechnetate is inexpensive and readily available. For parathyroid scintigraphy, ^{99m}Tc-pertechnetate can be injected either before or after ^{99m}Tc-sestamibi. If ^{99m}Tc-pertechnetate is injected intravenously before ^{99m}Tc-sestamibi, imaging is delayed slightly for 10 to 30 minutes. The patient is not moved, and ^{99m}Tc-sestamibi is injected immediately after thyroid imaging with ^{99m}Tc-pertechnetate. ^{99m}Tc-Pertechnetate can also be injected 2 to 3 hours after the administration of ^{99m}Tc-sestamibi. Subtraction of thyroid activity is performed in a manner similar to that for ^{123}I/^{99m}Tc-sestamibi.

Table 14.2 summarizes the results of ^{99m}Tc-sestamibi parathyroid scintigraphy in the detection of abnormal parathyroid glands with use of the dual-radiotracer approach. The overall sensitivity of 90% for the detection of parathyroid adenomas is higher than the sensitivity of ^{201}Tl/^{99m}Tc-pertechnetate scintigraphy by 10% to 15%. Most studies agree with this conclusion. Furthermore, Wei et al. (90) have reported the diagnostic accuracy to be similar for the two methods (^{123}I or ^{99m}Tc-pertechnetate). Sensitivity for the detection of hyperplastic glands is lower and depends on the scintigraphic criteria used to define hyperplastic parathyroid glands. A positive result for hyperplasia can be defined either by the presence of more than one focus of increased ^{99m}Tc-sestamibi uptake ("loose" criteria, without correlation of the number of glands found during surgical exploration) or by the presence of multiple foci of uptake corresponding exactly to the number of glands found at surgery ("strict" criteria).

Double-phase Parathyroid Scintigraphy

Based on the observations of Coakley and colleagues (74) that ^{99m}Tc-sestamibi washes out of parathyroid adenomas and hyperplastic glands at a slower rate than it does from the thyroid (differential washout), a preliminary study was conducted at our institution to evaluate ^{99m}Tc-sestamibi parathyroid imaging in the detection and localization of parathyroid adenomas in patients with proven hyperparathyroidism; in this study, the technical approach used was somewhat different from the one initially proposed

TABLE 14.2. SENSITIVITY OF ^{99m}TC-SESTAMIBI SCINTIGRAPHY IN DETECTION OF ABNORMAL PARATHYROID GLANDS: RESULTS WITH THE DUAL-RADIOTRACER APPROACH

Authors (ref)	Year	No. patients	Patient population	Technique	Sensitivity in detection of adenomas	Sensitivity in detection of multiglandular disease and/or hyperplastic glands
1—Coakley et al. (74)	1989	5	PH	^{123}I/MIBI	100% (4/4)	—
2—O'Doherty et al. (75)	1992	57	4 reoperations	^{123}I/MIBI	97% (39/40)	—
3—Thule et al. (76)	1994	14	PH	^{123}I/MIBI	93% (13/14)	—
4—Casas et al. (77)	1993	22	PH	^{123}I/MIBI	88% (14/16)	100% (5/5 patients)
5—Halvorson et al. (78)	1994	21	PH	^{123}I/MIBI	88% (14/16)	100% (5/5 patients)
6—Wei et al. (79)	1994	23	PH	Tc/MIBI	92% (12/13)	67% (6/9 patients)
7—Khan et al. (80)	1994	14	PH	Tc/MIBI	93% (13/14)	—
8—Hindie et al. (81)	1995	30	PH	^{123}I/MIBI	96% (26/27)	67% (2/3 patients) 62% (5/8 glands)
9—Bugis et al. (82)	1995	37	PH	^{123}I/MIBI	100% (7/7)	—
				Tc/MIBI	67% (10/15)	—
10—Chen et al. (83)	1995	35	reoperation	^{123}I/MIBI	76% (16/21)	50% (3/6 glands)
11—Johnston et al. (84)	1996	46	PH	Tc/MIBI	78% (28/36)	—
12—Borley et al. (85)	1996	56	PH	^{123}I/MIBI	94% (33/35)	—
13—Chesser et al. (86)	1997	18	TH	Tc/MIBI	—	82.6% (38/46 glands)
14—Hindie et al. (87)	1997	65	PH	^{123}I/MIBI	95% (56/59)	80% (12/15 patients)
15—Neumann et al. (88)	1997	15	PH	^{123}I/MIBI	88% (15/17)	—
Total					90% (300/334)	81% (30/37 patients) 77% (46/60 glands)

PH, primary hyperparathyroidism; TH, tertiary hyperparathyroidism; Tc, ^{99m}Tc-pertechnetate; ^{123}I, iodine 123; MIBI, ^{99m}Tc-sestamibi.

(91). As previously described, after Coakley et al. (74) substituted ^{99m}Tc-sestamibi for ^{201}Tl in the dual-radiotracer approach to parathyroid imaging, the drawbacks of a dual-radionuclide imaging procedure still remained, such as the relative injected activities of the tracers (related to the type of tracers and their order of injection), the use of computer subtraction techniques (with sensitivity possibly increased at the cost of decreased specificity), and computer alignment and display procedures.

Because we thought that a single-radiopharmaceutical study would potentially overcome the major drawbacks of a dual-radiotracer procedure, the behavior of ^{99m}Tc-sestamibi was initially evaluated at our institution in a few patients with parathyroid adenomas. After injection of 20 to 25 mCi of ^{99m}Tc-sestamibi (91–92), cervicothoracic images in the anterior view were obtained at different time intervals, ranging from 5 minutes to 10 hours (Fig. 14.3). This very preliminary study demonstrated that ^{99m}Tc-sestamibi is rapidly taken up by both thyroid and parathyroid parenchyma. However, as previously mentioned, thyroid uptake of ^{99m}Tc-sestamibi decreases significantly more rapidly than parathyroid adenoma uptake over time (1 to 3 hours after the injection). This thyroid–parathyroid differential washout of ^{99m}Tc-sestamibi provides the rationale for using ^{99m}Tc-sestamibi as a single radiotracer in a double-phase method of parathyroid imaging (Fig. 14.4).

With this approach, at least two sets of parathyroid images are obtained: the initial set at 5 to 10 minutes (early study) and the second set at 2 to 4 hours (delayed study) after the injection of 20 to 25 mCi of ^{99m}Tc-sestamibi. Because ^{99m}Tc-sestamibi is concentrated rapidly in the thyroid parenchyma, the initial set of images (early study) is called the "thyroid" phase of the study; the second set, obtained at 2 to 4 hours, is called the "parathyroid" phase because the washout of ^{99m}Tc-sestamibi from the parathyroid lesion is slower. For each set of images, planar imaging of the neck and upper portion of the thorax (including the mediastinum) is initially obtained in the anterior view with the patient supine and the head and neck extended and immobilized. Analogue and digital images are acquired with a preset time mode of 10 minutes per image by means of a scintillation camera with a large field of view. Comparative analysis of both the initial and delayed images is then performed (Figs. 14.5 and 14.6). A positive ^{99m}Tc-sestamibi study for the presence of parathyroid adenoma is defined as a focal area of increased uptake of radiotracer in a projection of the thyroid bed and surrounding areas or mediastinum that progressively increases with time, or a fixed uptake that persists on delayed imaging, in contrast to uptake in the surrounding normal thyroid tissue, which progressively decreases with time (differential washout analysis).

Since this initial report on double-phase ^{99m}Tc-sestamibi parathyroid imaging, several studies have been conducted in which the same approach was used (91–119) (Table 14.3). Most of these studies are relatively more recent than the studies of dual-radiotracer imaging. The overall sensitivity is 84% in the detection of parathyroid adenomas and approximately 60% in the evaluation of hyperplastic glands (depending again on the criteria used to define this condition) (Fig. 14.7). Specificity in the majority of the studies has been reported to be between 95% and 100%. As for the

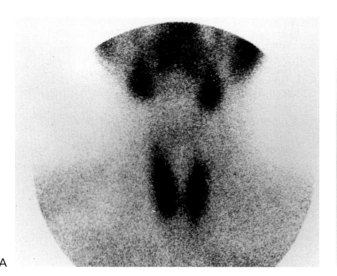
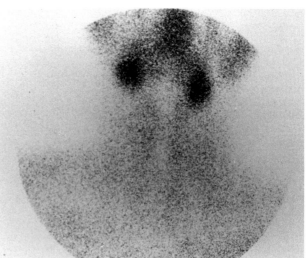

A

B

FIGURE 14.3. Normal results of ^{99m}Tc-sestamibi parathyroid scintigraphy with use of the dual-phase approach. In the early-phase study (**A**), performed 15 minutes after the injection, uniform thyroid uptake is seen without abnormal cervical uptake. On delayed imaging (**B**), obtained at 3 hours, no significant residual focus of uptake is apparent in the projection of the thyroid bed.

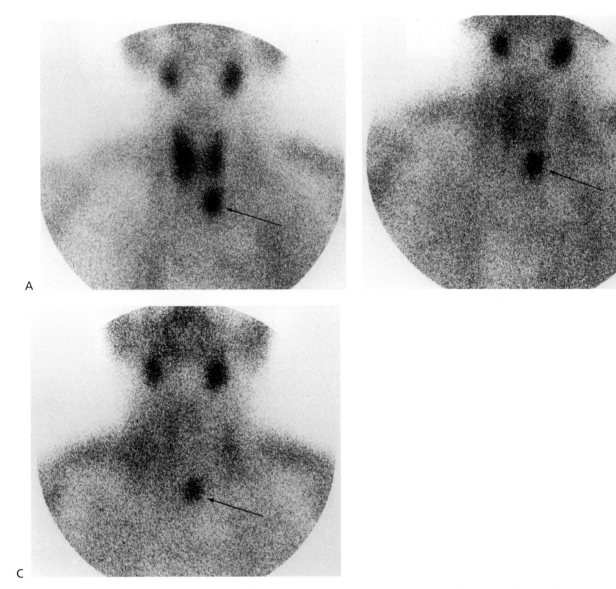

FIGURE 14.4. Serial parathyroid imaging obtained at 15 minutes (**A**), 2 hours (**B**), and 5 hours (**C**) after the injection of 25 mCi of ^{99m}Tc-sestamibi in a patient with a parathyroid adenoma of the left lower neck (*arrow*). Note the progressive thyroid washout over time, with concomitant relatively increased ^{99m}Tc-sestamibi uptake in the parathyroid lesion. This is an example of the differential thyroid–parathyroid lesion washout, which is the rationale for double-phase, single-radiotracer parathyroid scintigraphy with ^{99m}Tc-sestamibi.

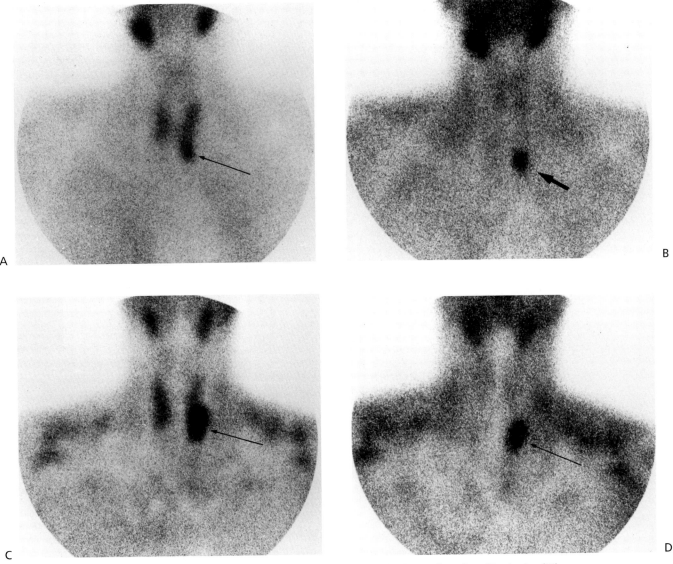

FIGURE 14.5. Parathyroid adenomas can be readily identified as early as 5 to 15 minutes ("thyroid" phase) after the injection of ^{99m}Tc-sestamibi. Early detection of parathyroid adenoma, which usually occurs with large or ectopic adenomas, is illustrated by the early (**A**) and (**C**) and delayed (**B**) and (**D**) images of two patients with a parathyroid adenoma of the left lower neck (*arrows*). Although the adenomas are seen on the early images, they are better visualized by combining both the early and delayed images.

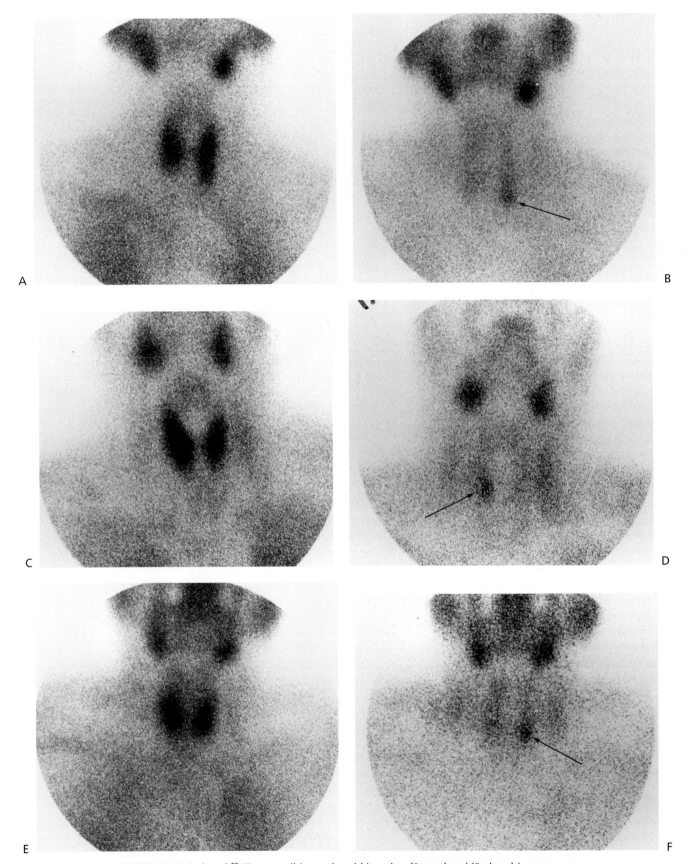

FIGURE 14.6. Delayed ^{99m}Tc-sestamibi parathyroid imaging ("parathyroid" phase) is more accurate in the detection of small parathyroid adenomas or lesions adjacent to the thyroid bed, as illustrated by the early images (**A**), (**C**), and (**E**) and corresponding delayed images (**B**), (**D**) and (**F**) of three patients in whom early imaging did not show significant parathyroid uptake because of predominant thyroid ^{99m}Tc-sestamibi uptake. Delayed imaging clearly demonstrated parathyroid adenomas (*arrows*).

A

B

C

D

E

F

TABLE 14.3. SENSITIVITY OF ⁹⁹ᵐTc-SESTAMIBI SCINTIGRAPHY IN THE DETECTION OF ABNORMAL PARATHYROID GLANDS: RESULTS WITH DOUBLE-PHASE STUDY

Authors (ref)	Year	No. patients	Patient population	Sensitivity in detection of adenomas	Sensitivity in detection of multiglandular disease and/or hyperplastic glands
1—Taillefer et al. (91)	1992	23	PH	90% (19/21)	0 (0/2 patients)
2—Joseph et al. (93)	1994	34	15 PH, 9 SH	80% (20/25)	67% (6/9 patients)
3—Billotey et al. (94)	1994	24	15 reoperations	83% (5/6)	84% (21/25 glands)
4—Bugis et al. (82)	1995	37	PH	60% (12/20)	—
5—Billy et al. (95)	1995	17	PH	83% (10/12)	75% (3/4 patients)
6—Lee et al. (96)	1995	39	1 reoperation	93% (28/30)	60% (18/30 glands)
7—Chen et al. (83)	1995	35	reoperation	64% (18/28)	45% (5/11 glands)
8—Caixas et al. (97)	1995	25	21PH, 4 SH	95% (20/21)	59% (10/17 glands)
9—Sofferman et al. (98)	1996	33	PH	91% (31/34)	—
10—Mazzeo et al. (99)	1996	73	PH	82% (28/34)	—
11—Light et al. (100)	1996	21	5 SH-TH, 3 reoperations	87% (13/15)	83% (5/6 patients) 44% (11/25 glands)
12—McHenry et al. (101)	1996	124	118 PH, 4 SH, 3 TH	74% (14/19)	—
13—Piga et al. (102)	1996	38	SH	100% (1/1)	44% (12/27 patients)
14—Perez-Monte et al. (103)	1996	47	14 reoperations	91% (31/34)	—
15—Neumann et al. (104)	1996	21	PH	43% (9/21)	—
16—Martin et al. (105)	1996	63	PH	82% (41/50)	82% (9/11 patients) 31% (9/29 glands)
17—Malhotra et al. (106)	1996	51	7 reoperations	100% (26/26)	56% (10/18 patients) 52% (36/69 glands)
18—Rauth et al. (107)	1996	21	PH	93% (13/14)	—
19—Irvin et al. (7)	1996	85	PH	88% (73/83)	—
20—Lee et al. (108)	1996	25	PH reoperation (17)	89% (16/18)	68% (13/19 glands)
21—Peeler et al. (109)	1997	25	reoperations	74% (14/19)	—
22—Blocklet et al. (110)	1997	55	34 PH, 21 SH	84% (27/32)	—
23—Staudenherz et al. (111)	1997	56	thyroid disease (50%)	78% (41/53)	—
24—Ishibashi et al. (112)	1997	11	3 PH, 8 SH	100% (3/3)	70% (14/20 glands)
25—Kézachian et al. (113)	1997	30	PH	89% (24/27)	67% (2/3 patients)
26—Bonjer et al. (114)	1997	27	6 reoperations	85% (23/27)	—
27—Carter et al. (115)	1997	16	PH	85% (11/13)	—
28—Shaha et al. (116)	1997	24	PH	85% (17/20)	—
29—Klieger et al. (117)	1998	37	PH	84% (21/25)	80% (8/10 patients)
30—Wei et al. (79)	1994	22	PH	84% (16/19)	—
31—Hindie et al. (118)	1998	30	PH	82% (22/27)	33% (1/3 patients)
32—Blanco et al. (119)	1998	41	31 PH 10 SH	92% (24/26)	63% (30/48 glands)
Total				84% (671/803)	60% (56/93 patients) 61% (167/273 glands)

PH, primary hyperparathyroidism; SH, secondary hyperparathyroidism; TH, tertiary hyperparathyroidism.

dual-radiotracer approach, it has generally been reported to be at least as good as or, most of the time, superior to other parathyroid imaging modalities. Since the introduction of the double-phase study and its widespread clinical use, individual variability has been noted, with a very rapid washout, like that of the thyroid, in some (sometimes large) adenomas causing a false-negative study result on delayed imaging (120–123) (Fig. 14.8). Fortunately, early imaging results are usually positive in large parathyroid adenomas. In these unusual cases, subtraction imaging can be more useful because it does not depend on the washout kinetics of the agent. On the other hand, many thyroid nodules will be mistaken for parathyroid lesions on subtraction imaging

(false-positives) but will not be falsely detected or less frequently seen on double-phase study. The specificity of both procedures, however, may be lower in geographic areas in which the incidence of thyroid nodules is significantly increased (111,124).

Various approaches can be used to avoid the false-positive results caused by thyroid nodules. Before the study, a routine palpation of the neck is performed to detect and locate nodules. When a persistent focus of increased uptake is seen in a patient with a palpable nodule in the projection of the thyroid bed on the delayed-phase image at 2 to 3 hours after the injection, a later image is obtained at approximately 5 to 6 hours. If late images are still inconclusive on the double-

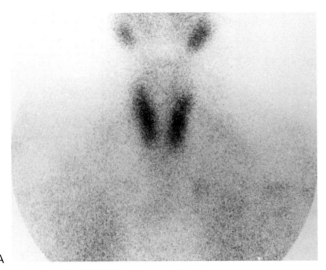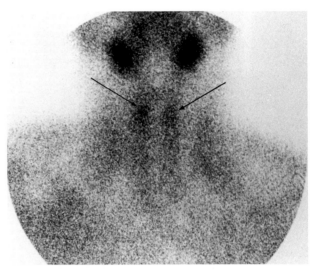

A   B

FIGURE 14.7. Early (**A**) and delayed (**B**) scintigraphy in a patient with histopathologically proven parathyroid hyperplasia. At least two foci of increased ⁹⁹ᵐTc-sestamibi uptake are seen in the upper lobes of the thyroid (*arrows*).

phase study, it is always possible to combine the two approaches to ⁹⁹ᵐTc-sestamibi parathyroid imaging by injecting ⁹⁹ᵐTc-pertechnetate after the delayed phase and looking for thyroid lesions or, ultimately, having the patient return for a ¹²³I thyroid study. SPECT may also be useful (125,126). Labeling with ⁹⁹ᵐTc and the relatively high dose of ⁹⁹ᵐTc-sestamibi administered provide optimal conditions for SPECT imaging. Although planar imaging gives satisfactory results, SPECT imaging is advantageous in this instance, and also when the lesion is barely seen on planar

imaging, deeply seated, or ectopic (88,127–129). However, at the present time, SPECT imaging is not considered part of routine ⁹⁹ᵐTc-sestamibi parathyroid scintigraphy. The use of pinhole collimators may also be of value.

Other technical methods have been proposed to improve the diagnostic accuracy of double-phase scintigraphy, such as factor analysis of dynamic structures and analysis of time–activity curves generated on regions of interest (94). Although an improvement in sensitivity was initially noted, these methods of parathyroid scintigraphy analysis are not

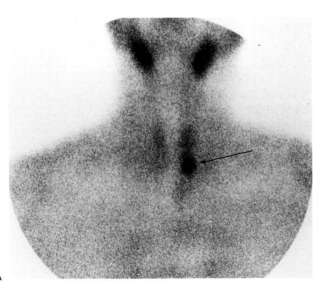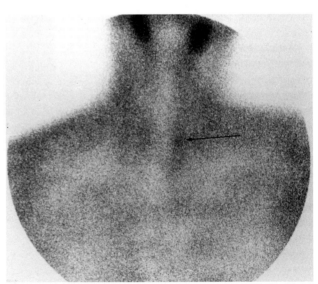

A   B

FIGURE 14.8. Patient with an obvious parathyroid adenoma of the left lower neck (*arrow*), seen on early imaging (**A**). On the delayed study, performed 3 hours later (**B**), only a faint persistent uptake appears at the site of the adenoma (*arrow*). This fast ⁹⁹ᵐTc-sestamibi washout is sometimes seen, especially in adenomas with a relatively small number of oxyphil cells.

TABLE 14.4. SENSITIVITY FOR DETECTION OF PARATHYROID ADENOMAS: COMPARISON BETWEEN ^{99m}Tc-SESTAMIBI SCINTIGRAPHY AND OTHER IMAGING MODALITIES

Authors (ref)	No. patients	No. adenomas	Patient population	^{99m}Tc-Sestamibi procedure	^{99m}Tc-Sestamibi	^{99m}Tc/^{201}Tl	US	CT	MRI
1—Bonjer et al. (114)	27	27	21 first surgery / 6 reoperation	double-phase	81% / 100% (6/6)	—	72% (13/18) / 50% (3/6)	—	—
2—Ishibashi et al. (112)	11	3	ectopic glands	double-phase	70% (14/20 glands)	—	—	40% (8/20)	60% (12/20)
3—Staudenherz et al. (123)	56	52	thyroid disease	double-phase	78%	64%	58%	—	—
4—Rauth et al. (107)	21	14	PH	double-phase	93% (13/14)	57% (8/14)	57% (8/14)	68% (13/19)	57% (8/14)
5—Peeler et al. (109)	25	25	reoperation	double-phase	74% (14/19)	50% (4/8)	45% (9/20)	68% (13/19)	—
6—Takami et al. (137)	41	24	26 PH / 15 SH	NA	92%	64%	88%	56%	—
7—Light et al. (100)	21	15	16 PH / 5 SH	double-phase	87% (13/15)	—	53% (8/15)	—	—
8—Mazzeo et al. (99)	73	66	PH	double-phase	82% (28/34)	62% (34/55)	85% (67/79)	—	—
9—Calxas et al. (97)	25	21	21 PH / 4 SH	double-phase	95% (20/21)	57% (4/7)	75% (6/8)	40% (4/10)	33% (1/3)
10—Billy et al. (95)	17	12	PH	double-phase	83% (10/12)	64% (9/14)	50% (6/12)	—	—
11—Khan et al. (80)	14	14	PH	MIBI/Tc	93% (13/14)	64% (9/14)	—	83%	—
12—Geatti et al. (138)	43	43	PH	MIBI/Tc	95% (40/42)	86% (36/42)	81%	25% (3/12)	0 (0/2)
13—Weber et al. (139)	14	10	reoperation	MIBI-^{123}I	88% (14/16)	17% (1/6)	—	42% (5/12)	33% (1/3)
14—McIntyre et al. (140)	42	31	reoperation	NA	86% (6/7)	67% (18/27)	27% (3/11)	42%	69%
15—Rodriguez et al. (141)	152	—	reoperation	double-phase	70%	60%	53%	20%	0
16—Thompson et al. (142)	44	—	37 reoperation	MIBI/Tc	79%	64%	59%	—	—
17—Casas et al. (77)	22	16	PH	MIBI/^{123}I	88% (14/16)	—	69% (11/16)	—	—
18—O'Doherty et al. (75)	57	40	PH	MIBI/^{123}I	97% (39/40)	92% (37/40)	—	—	—
19—Tallefer et al. (91)	23	21	PH	double-phase	90% (19/21)	75% (6/8)	—	—	—
20—Bergenfelz et al. (143)	39	36	PH	MIBI/Tc	86% (31/36)	—	47% (17/36)	—	—
21—Torregrosa et al. (144)	38	16	16 PH / 22 SH	double-phase	94% (15/16)	—	69% (11/16)	—	—
22—Ishibashi et al. (145)	20	9	9 PH / 11 SH	double-phase	100% (9/9)	—	78% (7/9)	—	100% (9/9)
23—Fayet et al. (146)	16	16	reoperation	double-phase	88% (14/16)	—	—	—	94% (15/16)
24—Lee et al. (108)	25	18	reoperation	double-phase	89% (16/18)	—	—	—	94% (17/18)

PH, primary hyperthyroidism; SH, secondary hyperthyroidism; Tc, ^{99m}Tc-pertechnetate; ^{123}I, iodine 123; MIBI, ^{99m}Tc-sestamibi.

widely used. Furthermore, a recent study comparing these methods with visual assessment showed the latter to be more efficient (110).

Results may differ from one study to another for several reasons. These include patient selection bias (surgery for patients with mild hyperparathyroidism or asymptomatic disease vs. tertiary referrals with an increased number of failed parathyroidectomies); imaging protocols and methods of data processing; criteria of interpretation; and type, size, location, and histology of the parathyroid lesion. The sensitivity of [99mTc]-sestamibi parathyroid scintigraphy is high in the detection of lesions weighing more than 500 mg but significantly decreases for lesions weighing less than 200 mg. Although sensitivity is higher in lesions with a large proportion of mitochondria-rich oxyphil cells, [99mTc]-sestamibi uptake can also be seen in lesions with a relatively low number of these cells.

The double-phase [99mTc]-sestamibi parathyroid imaging protocol is simple, accurate, and relatively less expensive than dual-radiotracer scintigraphy, and it avoids the drawbacks of a subtraction technique. There is no need for prolonged immobilization of the patient's head and neck. If necessary, the image acquisition time can also be shortened in case of musculoskeletal limitations or claustrophobia. The dual-radiotracer method may be more accurate in certain conditions. Modifications of the two original methods have produced a "hybrid" imaging protocol in which a double-phase approach is used in the initial study, followed by injection of [99mTc]-pertechnetate; this may be a useful and cost-effective method of performing [99mTc]-sestamibi parathyroid scintigraphy (130–136). Such a combination of the two "standard" [99mTc]-sestamibi parathyroid imaging protocols retains the advantages of each.

Although direct comparison between [99mTc]-sestamibi parathyroid scintigraphy and other parathyroid imaging modalities, such as [201Tl]/[99mTc]-pertechnetate scintigraphy, high-resolution ultrasonography, computed tomography, and magnetic resonance imaging, is relatively limited, it is clear from the medical literature that parathyroid imaging with [99mTc]-sestamibi represents an improvement over previously reported scintigraphic procedures. Furthermore, [99mTc]-sestamibi parathyroid imaging performed with either the dual-radionuclide or dual-phase imaging protocol compares favorably with the other imaging modalities (137–146) when the studies are performed and compared in the same patient population (Table 14.4).

Clinical Applications of [99mTc]-Sestamibi Parathyroid Scintigraphy

Most of the initial studies of [99mTc]-sestamibi parathyroid scintigraphy involved patients with a diagnosis of primary hyperparathyroidism who were undergoing a first parathyroidectomy. More recent studies have demonstrated the advantages of [99mTc]-sestamibi scintigraphy in the detection

of parathyroid lesions in patients with renal failure (and secondary or tertiary hyperparathyroidism), in second neck exploration for recurrent or persistent hyperparathyroidism, and in the identification of autotransplanted parathyroid tissue and parathyroid carcinoma (147–153) (Fig. 14.9). The identification of ectopic parathyroid adenomas, especially in the mediastinum, certainly represents one of the most interesting and clinically relevant applications of [99mTc]-sestamibi parathyroid scintigraphy (154–158). The excellent physical characteristics of the radiotracer and its slow washout from parathyroid tissue make it possible to obtain a clear delineation of mediastinal adenomas with either planar or SPECT imaging (Fig. 14.10). Up to 20% of parathyroids are ectopic, so patients and surgeons benefit from the preoperative localization of these lesions. Increased contrast resolution can be achieved with SPECT. Because [99mTc]-sestamibi has more favorable physical and biologic characteristics than [201Tl], and because [201Tl] has been shown to be more sensitive than ultrasonography, computed tomography, and magnetic resonance imaging in the detection of ectopic parathyroid lesions, it is likely that [99mTc]-sestamibi scintigraphy will be the preferred imaging modality in these cases.

Although the National Institutes of Health Consensus Development Conference Panel concluded in 1991 (before the clinical introduction of [99mTc]-sestamibi for parathyroid imaging) that preoperative localization of parathyroid lesions in patients without previous neck operation is rarely indicated and is not cost-effective (1), recent data on radionuclide parathyroid scintigraphy clearly demonstrate a clinical role for this imaging procedure. Several articles and presentations have indicated that [99mTc]-sestamibi parathyroid imaging

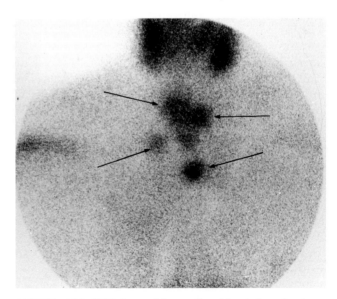

FIGURE 14.9. [99mTc]-Sestamibi parathyroid scintigraphy in a patient with parathyroid carcinoma and a few cervical metastases (*arrows*).

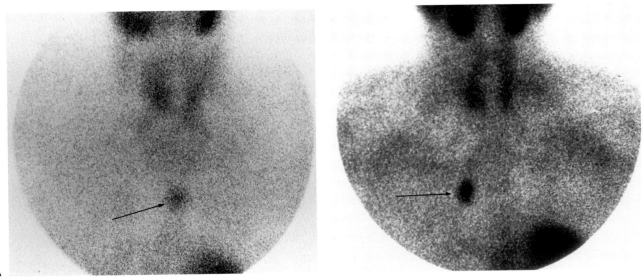

FIGURE 14.10. ^{99m}Tc-Sestamibi parathyroid scintigraphy in two patients with ectopic (mediastinal) parathyroid adenomas (*arrows*).

(with either the dual-radiotracer or double-phase approach) is sensitive and specific enough to localize a solitary parathyroid adenoma and can be used to guide the surgeon in performing a limited neck dissection. In a recent metaanalysis of the English medical literature performed during the last 10 years by Denham and Norman (5), ^{99m}Tc-sestamibi parathyroid scintigraphy had a sensitivity of 90.7% and a specificity of 98.8% in a group of 6,331 patients with an incidence of solitary parathyroid adenomas of 87% (slightly higher than the historically quoted 80% number). The authors evaluated the cost-effectiveness of preoperative ^{99m}Tc-sestamibi scintigraphy for primary hyperparathyroidism. Because one of the most costly aspects of parathyroid surgery is the time required for the surgeon to locate the normal and abnormal parathyroid glands, the authors compared the operative times for a standard bilateral neck exploration and for a ^{99m}Tc-sestamibi parathyroid imaging-guided limited exploration. The average operative time for a standard bilateral exploration in 15 articles regrouping a total of 753 patients was 109 ± 29 minutes (range, 87 to 148 minutes), whereas the average time for a limited dissection based on the results of a preoperative ^{99m}Tc-sestamibi study was 49 ± 5 minutes in four reported studies with a total of 143 patients. The difference between the two procedures is almost 50% (*p* < .0001). Furthermore, the average time spent by the patients in the recovery room after a unilateral neck exploration under monitored anesthesia (allowing same-day discharge and faster return to normal activities) was 30 minutes (range, 20 to 60 minutes), whereas the average was 82 minutes (range, 45 to 150 minutes) for those who underwent a bilateral neck exploration under general anesthesia (*p* < .05). When the cost of the operating room (per unit of time) and the recovery room were taken into consideration, the average savings per patient for the

limited exploration under local anesthesia were $650. These savings alone are sufficient to cover the cost of ^{99m}Tc-sestamibi parathyroid scintigraphy. Scintigraphy with ^{99m}Tc-sestamibi detects the 87% of patients with solitary adenomas with a sensitivity of 90%, so that 78% of patients with primary hyperparathyroidism could be candidates for a limited neck exploration. The authors showed that the additional cost for the remaining 22% of patients in whom preoperative scintigraphy would be of little or no benefit could also be absorbed by the potential savings from those undergoing a limited exploration. These data do not take into consideration the decreased number of second neck surgical explorations needed for adenomas missed on initial surgery (especially ectopic adenomas) because parathyroid scintigraphy was not used preoperatively. These failed initial operations would necessitate a more extensive and expensive preoperative workup.

Sofferman and Nathan (158) confirmed the cost justification of routine preoperative localization with ^{99m}Tc-sestamibi by analyzing five cases of ectopic adenoma (three remote mediastinal and two intrathyroidal adenomas) that probably would have been unidentifiable on routine surgery among a group of 59 patients with primary hyperparathyroidism who underwent preoperative ^{99m}Tc-sestamibi scintigraphy and ultrasonography. By taking into consideration the fact that a failed initial operation requires comprehensive imaging of the neck and thorax, including computed tomography and magnetic resonance imaging, which are mandatory to identify a likely ectopic adenoma with a high degree of confidence before a second exploration, their cost analysis showed some potential savings with the use of preoperative ^{99m}Tc-sestamibi scintigraphy. Accurate preoperative localization can increase operating room efficiency and reduce the number of frozen biopsy sections needed for histopathologic analysis. Considering the cost of failed surgery and the expenses incurred in prolonged exploration of an ectopic cervical or thoracic parathyroid adenoma, the authors concluded that the costs of ^{99m}Tc-sestamibi parathyroid scintigraphy and ultrasonography for routine preoperative localization in every patient with primary hyparparathyroidism undergoing a first neck exploration were virtually equivalent and therefore justified.

Based on the high level of diagnostic accuracy of new preoperative localizing procedures such as ^{99m}Tc-sestamibi parathyroid scintigraphy, a number of recent articles have questioned the dictum that all parathyroid glands must be examined either visually or histologically during neck exploration for parathyroidectomy. Taking advantage of the very high specificity of ^{99m}Tc-sestamibi (which is close to 98% to 100%), Norman et al. (6) performed a minimally invasive parathyroidectomy for primary hyperparathyroidism with a unilateral neck exploration through a 2.5-cm incision, which was extended as necessary. Only patients identified as having single-gland parathyroid disease on a high-quality ^{99m}Tc-sestamibi scintigraphy study were selected for minimal exploration. This selective approach allows one to avoid the 90% sensitivity of ^{99m}Tc-sestamibi scintigraphy, which is considered by some authors to be a limited advantage. They showed that unilateral neck exploration is highly efficacious and safe in these selected patients, and that this approach can be used without unnecessary risk of failure or complications. Furthermore, not only can the major potential complications associated with a bilateral neck exploration be reduced by the use of local anesthesia and limited dissection; cosmetic results are also greatly improved. However, the authors insist that high-quality preoperative ^{99m}Tc-sestamibi scintigraphy is mandatory for successful results.

To minimize operative intervention while maintaining the efficacy of a full neck exploration, the same group of authors (159) studied intraoperative radionuclide mapping performed with a hand-held gamma probe (the one used for sentinel node detection in patients with melanoma, breast cancer, or abdominal and pelvic cancers), as initially proposed by Gallowitsch et al. (160). Fifteen patients with primary hyperparathyroidism in whom a ^{99m}Tc-sestamibi scintigraphy demonstrated a single parathyroid adenoma were injected with ^{99m}Tc-sestamibi approximately 2.5 hours before a neck exploration. External radioactivity was measured with a hand-held gamma probe in four quadrants of the neck. A 2.0-cm incision was made according to the expected location of the adenoma, determined by preoperative scintigraphy and the probe. Dissection was performed until the source of increased counts (from the diseased glands) was found and the "background" counts in the neck reached equilibration. *Ex vivo* counting of the removed tissues was then performed to confirm the presence of radioactivity within the lesion. Intraoperative radionuclide mapping eliminates the problem of the few false-positive ^{99m}Tc-sestamibi scintigraphic studies suggesting that a

patient has a single parathyroid adenoma when hyperplasia or multiple adenomas are present. The authors also showed that the surgeon's exposure to radiation is minimal, with a cumulative radiation dose for their total of 15 patients of 1% of acceptable yearly exposure (which is 5 rem). The exposure hazard to pathology laboratory personnel is also acceptable; the parathyroid adenoma specimen contains only slightly more radioactivity than the natural background, with an exposure of 0.04 mR/h. Furthermore, the cryostat for frozen section studies and the instruments were not contaminated with radioactivity.

Bonjer et al. (161) came to the same conclusion that intraoperative radionuclide guidance is useful during parathyroid surgery. Using a hand-held gamma probe, they studied patients undergoing a first neck exploration for primary hyperparathyroidism, those undergoing reoperation for persistent or recurrent hyperparathyroidism, and patients with parathyroid cancers. Following preoperative administration of ^{99m}Tc-sestamibi, radioactivity in the neck was recorded after the thyroid gland had been retracted medially. Each quadrant of the neck was then investigated by placing the gamma probe at various angles on the thyroid, thymus, esophagus, and carotid space. The superior mediastinum was also scanned. With this technique, the sensitivity in identification of parathyroid tumors was 90.5% in first parathyroidectomies, 88.9% in reoperations for either persistent or recurrent hyperparathyroidism, and 100% in parathyroid cancer.

Irvin et al. (7,162) proposed the simultaneous use of preoperative ^{99m}Tc-sestamibi parathyroid scintigraphy and intraoperative monitoring of intact parathyroid hormone (iPTH) to provide the surgeon with quantitative assurance that all hyperfunctioning glands have been removed at the time of ambulatory parathyroidectomy for primary hyperparathyroidism. ^{99m}Tc-Sestamibi was administered 2 hours before the surgery. Samples for measuring iPTH levels were obtained from a peripheral vein after the induction of anesthesia but before incision and subsequent manipulation of the suspected hyperfunctioning gland, and again at up to 20 minutes after gland excision. With use of a modified commercially available iPTH assay, the results for each sample were quickly reported to the surgeon in approximately 10 minutes. The combination of removal of an abnormal gland with a subsequent decline in the iPTH level to 50% or less of the preoperative or preexcision level was taken as an indication that no other hyperfunctioning parathyroid tissue was present. Such monitoring of iPTH levels during the operation confirmed excision of all hyperfunctioning glands in 83 of 85 patients (98%) studied by the authors. For 57 of these 85 patients, the absence of limiting social or comorbid conditions also permitted consideration of parathyroidectomy in an ambulatory setting, with same-day discharge. This was successfully accomplished in 42 of them (74%). The combination of a shortened average procedure time and same-day discharge resulted in considerable cost savings.

OTHER RADIONUCLIDE IMAGING PROCEDURES

99mTc-Tetrofosmin

99mTc-Tetrofosmin, or 99mTc-1,2-*bis*[*bis*(2-ethoxyethyl)phos-phino]ethane, has recently been proposed as a new radio-pharmaceutical for radionuclide myocardial perfusion imaging. The physiologic and physical characteristics of 99mTc-tetrofosmin are similar to those of 99mTc-sestamibi, with avid mitochondrial uptake of the radiotracer (163). A preliminary study performed in 10 patients with hyper-parathyroidism and two normal subjects showed that the quality of both the raw and subtracted 99mTc-tetrofosmin images was superior to that of 201Tl images, similar to the observations reported with 99mTc-sestamibi (164). The authors concluded that on the basis of the diagnostic results (detection of 8 of 9 adenomas) and its favorable dosimetric characteristics, 99mTc-tetrofosmin is a suitable radiotracer for parathyroid scintigraphy. In a more recent study, 99mTc-tetrofosmin was directly compared with 99mTc-sestamibi for parathyroid scintigraphy (165). Sixteen patients with pri-mary hyperparathyroidism and a proven parathyroid ade-noma were prospectively studied with the two radiotracers. Planar imaging was performed between 5 minutes and 3 hours after the injection of 25 mCi (900 MBq) of 99mTc-tetrofosmin and 99mTc-sestamibi. The two studies were per-formed on different days. On early images, all the adeno-mas detected with 99mTc-sestamibi were equally well visualized with 99mTc-tetrofosmin and vice versa. However, on delayed imaging, the visualization of adenomas im-proved only in the 99mTc-sestamibi studies. The differential washout seen on 99mTc-sestamibi scintigraphy was never seen with 99mTc-tetrofosmin. The sensitivity of the two agents in the detection of parathyroid adenomas was 75% (12 of 16 adenomas). Therefore, in contrast to parathyroid imaging with 99mTc-sestamibi, delayed imaging with 99mTc-tetrofosmin has no diagnostic impact. Mansi et al. (166) compared the kinetics of 99mTc-sestamibi and 99mTc-tetro-fosmin in a case of surgically confirmed parathyroid ade-noma. The parathyroid adenoma-to-thyroid ratios were 1.57 and 3.00 for 99mTc-sestamibi at 20 and 120 minutes, respectively; the same ratios were 1.71 and 1.33 for 99mTc-tetrofosmin at 20 and 120 minutes, respectively. 99mTc-Tetrofosmin may be an alternative to 99mTc-sestamibi for parathyroid scintigraphy, but the number of studies reported so far with this new radiopharmaceutical is rela-tively limited. As seen in Table 14.5, five prospective stud-ies have indicated that the results of parathyroid scintigra-phy with 99mTc-sestamibi and 99mTc-tetrofosmin are comparable, although the uptake mechanism does not seem to be identical (165–170).

99mTc-Furifosmin (99mTc-Q12)

99mTc-Furifosmin, also known as 99mTc-Q12 or *trans*{1,2-*bis*[dihydro-2,2,5,5-tetramethyl-3-(2H)-furanone-4-methyl-ene-imino]ethane}*bis*[*tris*(3-methoxy-1-propyl)phos-phine]technetium(III)-99m, is another 99mTc-labeled radiopharmaceutical developed for radionuclide myocardial perfusion imaging. Because this compound shows similar characteristics to those of 99mTc-sestamibi and 99mTc-tetro-fosmin, it was reasonable to evaluate 99mTc-furifosmin as an agent for parathyroid scintigraphy. Aigner et al. (171) reported their initial experience using 99mTc-furifosmin scintigraphy in 10 patients with surgically proven parathy-roid adenomas. Patients were injected with 10 mCi (370 MBq) of 99mTc-furifosmin and images were obtained up to 300 minutes after injection. The mean retention half-time in the parathyroid adenomas was 1.27 hour, and the mean retention half-time in the thyroid gland was 1.05 hour. Parathyroid scintigraphy correctly identified all 10 adeno-mas. Two of their patients were also imaged with 99mTc-tetro-

TABLE 14.5. SENSITIVITY OF 99mTc-TETROFOSMIN SCINTIGRAPHY IN THE DETECTION OF ABNORMAL PARATHYROID GLANDS

Authors (ref)	Year	No. patients	Patient population	Technical aspects	Sensitivity in detection of Adenomas	Hyperplasias
1—Giordano et al. (157)	1996	10	PH	15–20 mCi, 5 min piv	88.9% (8/9)	—
2—Fjeld et al. (165)	1997	16	PH	25 mCi, 5 min to 3 h	75.0% (12/16)	—
3—Gallowitsch et al. (167)	1997	68	35 PH 13 SH	10 mCi, 5 and 45 min	69.2% (25/36) planar 94.4% (34/36) SPECT	38.5% (5/13) 61.5% (8/13)
4—Ishibashi et al. (168)	1997	26	7 PH 19 SH	20 mCi, 10 min and 2–3 h	100% (7/7)	73.3% (27/37)
5—Apostolopoulos et al. (169)	1998	45	27 PH 18 TH	10 mCi, 5 min ad 3 h + 99mTcO4	87.0% (20/23)	72.1% (49/68)
Total					79.1% (72/91)	68.6% (81/118)

PH, primary hyperparathyroidism; SH, secondary hyperparathyroidism; TH, tertiary hyperparathyroidism; SPECT, single-photon emission computed tomography; piv, postintravenous injection.

fosmin. In both cases, ^{99m}Tc-furifosmin provided better image contrast than ^{99m}Tc-tetrofosmin, with faster ^{99m}Tc-furifosmin thyroid clearance. This can be advantageous in patients with concomitant thyroid disease. Further comparative studies are necessary to establish which of the three radiotracers (^{99m}Tc-sestamibi, ^{99m}Tc-tetrofosmin, and ^{99m}Tc-furifosmin) is the most accurate for parathyroid scintigraphy.

Imaging Agents for Positron Emission Tomography

The compound 2-(fluorine 18)-fluoro-2-deoxy-D-glucose (FDG) has been shown to localize in abnormal parathyroid tissue. A recent study directly compared ^{99m}Tc-sestamibi and FDG-PET parathyroid imaging in 21 patients with primary hyperparathyroidism (172). The sensitivity in the preoperative localization of parathyroid adenomas was 43% (9 of 21) for ^{99m}Tc-sestamibi SPECT imaging and 86% (18 of 21) for FDG-PET studies; the specificity was 90% for ^{99m}Tc-sestamibi and 78% for FDG-PET. The poor sensitivity of ^{99m}Tc-sestamibi parathyroid scintigraphy in this study is quite surprising and does not correspond to results of previously reported studies. However, ^{18}F-FDG parathyroid imaging offers an interesting diagnostic alternative when it is available and accessible at a relatively low cost (173).

^{11}C-L-Methionine is another PET imaging radiopharmaceutical that has been used to detect parathyroid adenomas (174). The reported sensitivity was 85%.

CONCLUSIONS

If localization of affected parathyroid glands is required before a first parathyroidectomy or surgery for persistent or recurrent hyperparathyroidism, ^{99m}Tc-sestamibi scintigraphy (with either a dual-radiotracer or double-phase imaging protocol) is now recognized to be one of the most useful and accurate noninvasive methods to detect parathyroid adenomas; its sensitivity and specificity are both high. Although many authors do not advocate any preoperative localization procedure before a first parathyroidectomy, most agree that ^{99m}Tc-sestamibi parathyroid scintigraphy is certainly a useful guide for the surgeon (175–184). The high diagnostic accuracy and reliability of ^{99m}Tc-sestamibi parathyroid scintigraphy allow the surgeon to select the appropriate side for initial exploration with confidence and attempt a complete cure. In today's environment of managed care, sufficient data are now available to demonstrate the cost-effectiveness of routine, high-quality ^{99m}Tc-sestamibi parathyroid scintigraphy, even before a first neck exploration for hyperparathyroidism. Accurate and noninvasive preoperative localization of abnormal parathyroid tissue is certainly useful in the context of ambulatory parathyroidectomy.

REFERENCES

1. Consensus Development Conference Panel. Diagnosis and management of asymptomatic primary hyperparathyroidism: consensus development conference statement. *Ann Intern Med* 1991; 114:593–597.
2. Kaplan EL, Yashiro T, Salti G. Primary hyperparathyroidism in the 1990s: choice of surgical procedures for this disease. *Ann Surg* 1992;215:300–317.
3. Shaha AR, LaRosa CA, Jaffe BM. Parathyroid localization prior to primary exploration. *Am J Surg* 1993;166:289–293.
4. Casas AT, Burke GJ, Mansberger AR Jr, et al. Impact of technetium-99m-sestamibi localization on operative time and success of operations for primary hyperparathyroidism. *Am Surg* 1994; 60:12–16, discussion 16–17.
5. Denham DW, Norman J. Cost-effectiveness of preoperative sestamibi scan for primary hyperparathyroidism is dependent solely upon the surgeon's choice of operative procedure. *J Am Coll Surg* 1998;186:293–304.
6. Norman J, Chheda H, Farrell C. Minimally invasive parathyroidectomy for primary hyperparathyroidism: decreasing operative time and potential complications while improving cosmetic results. *Am Surg* 1998;64:391–396.
7. Irvin GL, Sfakianakis G, Yeung L, et al. Ambulatory parathyroidectomy for primary hyperparathyroidism. *Arch Surg* 1996; 131:1074–1078.
8. Clark OH, Dus QY. Primary hyperparathyroidism: a surgical perspective. *Endocrinol Metab Clin North Am* 1989;18: 701–714.
9. Levin KE, Clark OH. The reasons for failure in parathyroid operations. *Arch Surg* 1989;124:911–914.
10. Peck WW, Higgins CB, Fisher MR, et al. Hyperparathyroidism: comparison of MR imaging with radionuclide scanning. *Radiology* 1987;163:415–420.
11. Auffermann W, Gooding GAW, Okerlund MD, et al. Diagnosis of recurrent hyperparathyroidism: comparison of MR imaging and other imaging techniques. *Am J Roentgenol* 1988;150: 1027–1033.
12. Miller DL, Doppman JL, Sawker O, et al. Localization of parathyroid adenomas in patients who have undergone surgery, part I. Noninvasive imaging methods. *Radiology* 1987;162: 133–137.
13. Reading CC, Charbonneau JW, Janes EM, et al. High-resolution parathyroid sonography. *Am J Roentgenol* 1982;139:539–546.
14. Digiulio W, Lindenauer SM. Use of tolonium chloride in localization of parathyroid tissue. *JAMA* 1970;214:2302–2306.
15. Brennan MF, Doppman JL, Kurdy AG, et al. Assessment of techniques for preoperative parathyroid gland localization in patients undergoing reoperation for hyperparathyroidism. *Surgery* 1982; 91:6–11.
16. Sommer B, Welter HF, Splesberg F, et al. Computed tomography for localizing enlarged parathyroid glands in primary hyperparathyroidism. *J Comput Assist Tomogr* 1982;6:521–526.
17. Scheible W, Deutsch AL, Leopold GR. Parathyroid adenoma: accuracy of localization by high-resolution real-time sonography. *J Clin Ultrasound* 1981;9:325–330.
18. Stark DD, Moss AA, Gamsu G, et al. Magnetic resonance imaging of the neck II: pathologic findings. *Radiology* 1984;150: 455–461.
19. Doppman JL, Krudy AG, Marx SJ, et al. Aspiration of enlarged parathyroid glands for parathyroid hormone assay. *Radiology* 1983;148:31–35.
20. Sisson JC, Beierwalte WH. Radiocyanocobalamine (CO57B12) concentration in the parathyroid glands. *J Nucl Med* 1962;3: 160–162.
21. Potchen JE, Sodee DB. Selective isotope labeling of the human

parathyroid: a preliminary case report. *J Clin Endocrinol Metab* 1964;24:1125–1128.

22. Ferlin G, Conte N, Borsato N, et al. Parathyroid scintigraphy with [131]Cs and [201]Tl. *J Nucl Med Allied Sci* 1981;25:119–123.

23. Fukunaga M, Morita R, Yonekura Y, et al. Accumulation of ^{201}Tl chloride in a parathyroid adenoma. *Clin Nucl Med* 1979;4:229–230.

24. Ferlin G, Bursato N, Camerani M, et al. New perspectives in localizing enlarged parathyroid glands by technetium thallium subtraction scan. *Nucl Med* 1983;24:438–441.

25. Young AE, Gaunt JI, Croft DN, et al. Localization of parathyroid adenomas by thallium 201 and technetium 99m subtraction scanning. *Br Med J* 1983;286:1184–1186.

26. McCall A, Henkin R, Calendra D, et al. Routine use of the thallium technetium scan prior to parathyroidectomy. *Am Surg* 1987;53:380–384.

27. Stein BL, Wexler MJ. Preoperative parathyroid localization: a prospective evaluation of ultrasonography and thallium technetium scintigraphy in hyperparathyroidism. *Can J Surg* 1990;33:175–179.

28. Opelka FG, Brugham RA, Davies RS, et al. The role of dual radionuclide scintigraphy in the preoperative localization of abnormal glands. *Am Surg* 1988;54:240–242.

29. Ghandur Mnaymneh L, Cassady J, Hajianpour MA, et al. The parathyroid gland in health and disease. *Am J Pathol* 1986;125:292–299.

30. Gilmour JR, Martin WJ. The weight of the parathyroid glands. *J Pathol* 1937;44:431–462.

31. Grimelius L, Akerstrom G, Johannson H, et al. The parathyroid glands. In: Kovacs K, Asa S, eds. *Functional endocrine pathology.* Boston: Blackwell Science, 1990:375–395 (vol 1).

32. Akerstrom G, Malmaeus J, Bergstrom R. Surgical anatomy of human parathyroid glands. *Surgery* 1984;95:14–21.

33. Rosenblatt M, Kronenberg HM, Potts JT. Parathyroid hormone. Physiology, chemistry, biosynthesis, secretion, metabolism and mode of action. In: DeGroot LJ, ed. *Endocrinology.* Philadelphia: WB Saunders, 1989:848–891 (vol 2).

34. Fine E. Parathyroid imaging: its current status and future role. *Semin Nucl Med* 1987;17:350–359.

35. Hauty M, Swartz K, McClung M, et al. Technetium thallium scintiscanning for localization of parathyroid adenomas and hyperplasia: a reappraisal. *Am J Surg* 1987;153:479–486.

36. Basarab RM, Manni A, Harrison TS. Dual isotope subtraction parathyroid scintigraphy in the preoperative evaluation of suspected hyperparathyroidism. *Clin Nucl Med* 1985;10:300–314.

37. Borsato N, Zanco P, Camerani N, et al. Scintigraphy of the parathyroid glands with [201]Tl: experience with 250 operated patients. *Nucl Med* 1989;28:26–28.

38. Ferguson WR, Laird JD, Russel CFJ. Experience with technetium thallium subtraction imaging of parathyroid lesions. *J Nucl Med* 1984;25:19.

39. Fogelman I, McKillop JH, Bessent RG, et al. Successful localization of parathyroid adenoma by thallium 201 and technetium 99m subtraction scintigraphy: description of an improved technique. *Eur J Nucl Med* 1984;9:545–547.

40. Ling M, Okerlund M, O'Connel W, et al. Optimized dual isotope localization of parathyroid tumors: comparison of unprocessed, color comparison and subtraction techniques. *J Nucl Med* 1986;27:962.

41. Macfarlane SD, Hanelin LG, Taft DA, et al. Localization of abnormal parathyroid glands using thallium 201. *Am J Surg* 1984;148:7–12.

42. Okerlund MD, Sheldon K, Corpuz S, et al. A new method with high sensitivity and specificity for localization of abnormal parathyroid glands. *Ann Surg* 1984;200:381–387.

43. Park CH, Intenzo C, Cohen HE. Dual tracer imaging for localization of parathyroid lesions. *Clin* Nucl Med 1986;11:237–241.

44. Picard D, D'Amour P, Carrier L, et al. Localization of abnormal parathyroid gland(s) using Tl-201/iodine subtraction scintigraphy in patients with hyperparathyroidism. *Clin* Nucl Med 1987;12:60–64.

45. Percival RC, Blake GM, Urwin GH, et al. Assessment of thallium pertechnetate subtraction scintigraphy in hyperparathyroidism. *Br J Radiol* 1985;58:131–135.

46. Winzelberg GG, Hydovitz JD, O'Hara KR, et al. Prospective comparison of ^{201}Tl/Tc 99m pertechnetate parathyroid subtraction scintigraphy and high-resolution parathyroid ultrasonography in patients with suspected parathyroid adenomas. *Radiology* 1985;155:231–235.

47. Jones AG, Abrams MJ, Davison A, et al. Biological studies of a new class of technetium complexes: the *hexakis* (alkylisonitrile) technetium(II) cations. *Int J Nucl Med Biol* 1984;11:225–234.

48. Iskandrian A, Heo J, Kong B, et al. Use of technetium 99m isonitrile (RP30A) in assessing left ventricular perfusion and function at rest and during exercise in coronary artery disease and comparison with coronary arteriography and exercise thallium 201 SPECT imaging. *Am J Cardiol* 1989;64:270–275.

49. Kahn J, McGhie I, Akers M, et al. Quantitative rotational tomography with ^{201}Tl and ^{99m}Tc methoxyisobutylisonitrile: a direct comparison in normal individuals and patients with coronary artery disease. *Circulation* 1989;79:1282–1293.

50. Kiat H, Maddahi J, Roy L, et al. Comparison of technetium 99m methoxyisobutylisonitrile and thallium 201 for evaluation of coronary artery disease by planar and tomographic methods. *Am Heart J* 1989;117:1–11.

51. Taillefer R, Dupras G, Sporn V, et al. Myocardial perfusion imaging with a new radiotracer, technetium 99m hexamibi (methoxyisobutylisonitrile): comparison with thallium 201 imaging. *Clin Nucl Med* 1989;14:89–96.

52. Taillefer R, Lambert R, Dupras G, et al. Clinical comparison between thallium 201 and Tc 99m methoxyisobutylisonitrile (hexamibi) myocardial perfusion imaging for detection of coronary artery disease. *Eur J Nucl Med* 1989;15:280–286.

53. Wackers FJ, Berman DJ, Maddahi J, et al. Technetium 99m *hexakis* 2 methoxyisobutylisonitrile: human biodistribution, dosimetry, safety and preliminary comparison to thallium 201 for myocardial perfusion imaging. *J Nucl Med* 1989;30:301–311.

54. Aktolun C, Bayhan H, Kir M. Clinical experience with Tc 99m MIBI imaging in patients with malignant tumors: preliminary results and comparison with Tl 201. *Clin* Nucl Med 1992;17:171–176.

55. O'Tuama LA, Treves ST, Larar JN, et al. Thallium 201 versus technetium 99m MIBI SPECT in evaluation of childhood brain tumors: a within-subject comparison. *J Nucl Med* 1993;34:1045–1051.

56. Caner B, Kitapci M, Unlu M, et al. Technetium 99m MIBI uptake in benign and malignant bone lesions: a comparative study with technetium 99m MDP. *J Nucl Med* 1992;33:319–324.

57. Chiu ML, Kronange JF, Piwnica-Worms D. Effect of mitochondrial and plasma membrane potentials on accumulation of *hexakis* (2 methoxyisobutylisonitrile) technetium in cultured mouse fibroblasts. *J Nucl Med* 1990;31:1646–1653.

58. Piwnica-Worms D, Holman BL. Noncardiac applications of *hexakis* (alkylisonitrile) technetium 99m complexes. *J Nucl Med* 1990;31:1166–1167.

59. Crane P, Laliberté R, Heminway S, et al. Effect of mitochondrial viability and metabolism on technetium-99m-sestamibi myocardial retention. *Eur J Nucl Med* 1993;20:20–25.

60. Backus M, Piwnica-Worms D, Hockett D, et al. Microprobe

analysis of Tc-MIBI in heart cells: calculation of mitochondrial membrane potential. *Am J Physiol* 1993;265:178–187.

61. Sandrock D, Merino MJ, Norton JA, et al. Ultrastructural histology correlates with results of thallium 201/technetium 99m parathyroid subtraction scintigraphy. *J Nucl Med* 1993;34:24–29.

62. Lebrun J, Picard D, Morais J, et al. Étude comparative de la clairance du Tc99m sestamibi des nodules thyroïdiens et du tissu thyroïdien normal. *J Med Nucl Biophys* 1992;16:273.

63. Carpentier A, Jeannotte S, Verreault J, et al. Preoperative localization of parathyroid lesions in hyperparathyroidism: relationship between technetium-99m-MIBI uptake and oxyphil cell content. *J Nucl Med* 1998;39:1441–1444.

64. Mitchell BK, Cornelius EA, Zoghbi S, et al. Mechanism of technetium 99m-sestamibi parathyroid imaging and the possible role of p-glycoprotein. *Surgery* 1996;120:1039–1045.

65. Civelek AC, Durski K, Shafique I, et al. Failure of perchlorate to inhibit Tc 99m isonitrile binding by the thyroid during myocardial perfusion studies. *Clin Nucl Med* 1991;16:358–361.

66. Vattimo A, Bertelli P, Burroni L. Effective visualization of suppressed thyroid tissue by means of baseline ^{99m}Tc-methoxyisobutylisonitrile in comparison with ^{99m}Tc-pertechnetate scintigraphy after TSH stimulation. *J Nucl Biol Med* 1992;36:315–318.

67. Kao CH, Wang SJ, Liao SQ, et al. Quick diagnosis of hyperthyroidism with semiquantitative 30-minute technetium 99m methoxyisobutylisonitrile thyroid uptake. *J Nucl Med* 1993;34:71–74.

68. Kao CH, Lin WY, Wang SJ, et al. Visualization of suppressed thyroid tissue by Tc 99m MIBI. *Clin Nucl Med* 1991;16:812–814.

69. Osmanagaoglu K, Schelstraete K, Lippens M, et al. Visualization of parathyroid adenoma with Tc 99m MIBI in a case with iodine saturation and impaired thallium uptake. *Clin Nucl Med* 1993;18:214–216.

70. O'Driscoll CM, Baker F, Casey MJ, et al. Localization of recurrent medullary thyroid carcinoma with technetium 99m methoxyisobutylisonitrile scintigraphy: a case report. *J Nucl Med* 1991;32:2281–2283.

71. Balon HR, Fink Bennett D, Stoffer SS. Technetium 99m sestamibi uptake by recurrent Hürthle cell carcinoma of the thyroid. *J Nucl Med* 1992;33:1393–1395.

72. Briele B, Hotze A, Kropp J, et al. Vergleich von ^{201}Tl und ^{99m}Tc MIBI in der nachsorge des differenzierten schilddrusenkarzinoms. *Nucl Med* 1991;30:115–124.

73. Scott AM, Kostakoglu L, O'Brien JP, et al. Comparison of technetium 99m MIBI and thallium 201 chloride uptake in primary thyroid lymphoma. *J Nucl Med* 1992;33:1396–1398.

74. Coakley AJ, Kettle AG, Wells CP, et al. ^{99m}Tc-Sestamibi: a new agent for parathyroid imaging. *Nucl Med Commun* 1989;10:791–794.

75. O'Doherty MJ, Kettle AG, Wells P, et al. Parathyroid imaging with technetium 99m sestamibi: preoperative localization and tissue uptake studies. *J Nucl Med* 1992;33:313–318.

76. Thule P, Thakore K, Vansant J, et al. Preoperative localization of parathyroid tissue with technetium-99m sestamibi ^{123}I subtraction scanning. *J Clin Endocrinol Metab* 1994;78:77–82.

77. Casas AT, Bruke GJ, Sathyanarayana, et al. Prospective comparison of technetium-99m-sestamibi/iodine-123 radionuclide scan versus high-resolution ultrasonography for the preoperative localization of abnormal parathyroid glands in patients with previously unoperated primary hyperparathyroidism. *Am J Surg* 1993;166:369–373.

78. Halvorson DJ, Burke GJ, Mansberger AR Jr, et al. Use of technetium Tc 99m sestamibi and iodine 123 radionuclide scan for preoperative localization of abnormal parathyroid glands in primary hyperparathyroidism. *South Med J* 1994;87:336–339.

79. Wei JP, Burke GJ, Mansberger AR Jr. Preoperative imaging of abnormal parathyroid glands in patients with hyperparathyroid disease using combination Tc-99m-pertechnetate and Tc-99m-sestamibi radionuclide scans. *Ann Surg* 1994;219:568–572, discussion 572–573.

80. Khan A, Samtani S, Varma VM, et al. Preoperative parathyroid localization: prospective evaluation of technetium 99m sestamibi. *Otolaryngol Head Neck Surg* 1994;111:467–472.

81. Hindié E, Mellière D, Simon D, et al. Primary hyperparathyroidism: is technetium 99m-sestamibi/iodine-123 subtraction scanning the best procedure to locate enlarged glands before surgery? *J Clin Endocrinol Metab* 1995;80:302–307.

82. Bugis SP, Berno E, Rusnak CH, et al. Technetium-99m-sestamibi scanning before initial neck exploration in patients with primary hyperparathyroidism. *Eur Arch Otorhinolaryngol* 1995;252:149–152.

83. Chen CC, Skarulis MC, Fraker DL, et al. Technetium-99m-sestamibi imaging before reoperation for primary hyperparathyroidism. *J Nucl Med* 1995;36:2186–2191.

84. Johnston LB, Carroll MJ, Britton KE, et al. The accuracy of parathyroid gland localization in primary hyperparathyroidism using sestamibi radionuclide imaging. *J Clin Endocrinol Metab* 1996;81:346–352.

85. Borley NR, Collins RE, O'Doherty M, et al. Technetium-99m sestamibi parathyroid localization is accurate enough for scan-directed unilateral neck exploration. *Br J Surg* 1996;83:989–991.

86. Chesser AM, Carroll MC, Lightowler C, et al. Technetium-99m methoxyisobutylisonitrile (MIBI) imaging of the parathyroid glands in patients with renal failure. *Nephrol Dial Transplant* 1997;12:97–100.

87. Hindié E, Mellière D, Perlemuter L, et al. Primary hyperparathyroidism: higher success rate of first surgery after preoperative Tc-99m sestamibi-I-123 subtraction scanning. *Radiology* 1997;204:221–228.

88. Neumann DR, Esselstyn CB Jr, Go RT, et al. Comparison of double-phase 99mTc-sestamibi with 123-I-^{99m}Tc-sestamibi subtraction SPECT in hyperparathyroidism. *AJR Am J Roentgenol* 1997;169:1671–1674.

89. Greenspan BS, Brown ML, Billehay GL, et al. Procedure guideline for parathyroid scintigraphy. *J Nucl Med* 1998;39:1111–1114.

90. Wei JP, Burke GJ, Mansberger AR Jr. Prospective evaluation of the efficacy of technetium 99m sestamibi and iodine 123 radionuclide imaging of abnormal parathyroid glands. *Surgery* 1992;112:1111–1116, discussion 1116–1117.

91. Taillefer R, Boucher Y, Potvin C, et al. Detection and localization of parathyroid adenomas in patients with hyperparathyroidism using a single radionuclide imaging procedure with technetium-99m-sestamibi (double-phase study). *J Nucl Med* 1992;33:1801–1807.

92. Taillefer R. ^{99m}Tc-Sestamibi parathyroid scintigraphy. In: Freeman LM, ed. *Nuclear medicine annual 1995*. New York: Raven Press, 1995:51–79.

93. Joseph K, Loelcke V, Hoffken H, et al. Scintigraphy of parathyroid adenomas with ^{99m}Tc-sestamibi in an endemic goiter area. *Nuklearmedizin* 1994;33:93–98.

94. Billotey C, Aurengo A, Najean Y, et al. Identifying abnormal parathyroid glands in the thyroid uptake area using technetium-99m-sestamibi and factor analysis of dynamic structures. *J Nucl Med* 1994;35:1631–1636.

95. Billy HT, Rimkus DR, Hartzman S, et al. Technetium-99m-sestamibi single-agent localization versus high-resolution ultrasonography for the preoperative localization of parathyroid glands in patients with primary hyperparathyroidism. *Am Surg* 1995;61:882–888.

96. Lee VS, Wilkinson RH Jr, Leight GS Jr, et al. Hyperparathy-

roidism in high-risk surgical patients: evaluation with double-phase technetium-99m sestamibi imaging. *Radiology* 1995;197: 627–633.

97. Caixas A, Berna L, Piera J, et al. Utility of ^{99m}Tc-sestamibi scintigraphy as a first-line imaging procedure in the preoperative evaluation of hyperparathyroidism. *Clin Endocrinol* 1995; 43:525–530.

98. Sofferman RA, Nathan MH, Fairbank JT, et al. Preoperative technetium Tc-99m sestamibi imaging. Paving the way to minimal-access parathyroid surgery. *Arch Otolaryngol Head Neck Surgery* 1996;122:369–374.

99. Mazzeo S, Caramella D, Lencioni R, et al. Comparison among sonography, double-tracer subtraction scintigraphy, and double-phase scintigraphy in the detection of parathyroid lesions. *AJR Am J Roentgenol* 1996;166:1465–1470.

100. Light VL, McHenry CR, Jarjoura D, et al. Prospective comparison of dual-phase technetium-99m-sestamibi scintigraphy and high-resolution ultrasonography in the evaluation of abnormal parathyroid glands. *Am Surg* 1996;62:562–567, discussion 567–568.

101. McHenry CR, Lee K, Saadey J, et al. Parathyroid localization with technetium-99m-sestamibi: a prospective evaluation. *J Am Coll Surg* 1996;183:25–30.

102. Piga M, Bolasco P, Satta L, et al. Double-phase parathyroid technetium-99m-MIBI scintigraphy to identify functional autonomy in secondary hyperparathyroidism. *J Nucl Med* 1996;37: 565–569.

103. Perez-Monte JE, Brown ML, Shah AN, et al. Parathyroid adenomas: accurate detection and localization with Tc99m sestamibi SPECT. *Radiology* 1996;201:85–91.

104. Neumann DR, Esselstyn CB, MacIntyre WJ, et al. Comparison of FDG-PET and sestamibi-SPECT in primary hyperparathyroidism. *J Nucl Med* 1996;37:1809–1815.

105. Martin D, Rosen IB, Ichise M. Evaluation of single-isotope technetium 99m-sestamibi in localization efficiency for hyperparathyroidism. *Am J Surg* 1996;172:633–636.

106. Malhotra A, Silver CE, Deshpande V, et al. Preoperative parathyroid localization with sestamibi. *Am J Surg* 1996;172: 637–640.

107. Rauth JD, Sessions RB, Shupe SC, et al. Comparison of Tc-99m MIBI and Tl-201/Tc-99m pertechnetate for diagnosis of primary hyperparathyroidism. *Clin Nucl Med* 1996;21:602–608.

108. Lee VS, Spritzer CE, Coleman RE, et al. The complementary roles of fast spin-echo MR imaging and double-phase ^{99m}Tc-sestamibi scintigraphy for localization of hyperfunctioning parathyroid glands. *AJR Am J Roentgenol* 1996;167:1555–1562.

109. Peeler BB, Martin WH, Sandler MP, et al. Sestamibi parathyroid scanning and preoperative localization studies for patients with recurrent/persistent hyperparathyroidism or significant comorbid conditions. *Am Surg* 1997;63:37–46.

110. Blocklet D, Martin P, Schoutens A, et al. Presurgical localization of abnormal parathyroid glands using a single injection of technetium-99m methoxyisobutylisonitrile: comparison of different techniques, including factor analysis of dynamic structures. *Eur J Nucl Med* 1997;24:46–51.

111. Staudenherz A, Abela C, Niederle B, et al. Comparison and histopathological correlation of three parathyroid imaging methods in a population with a high prevalence of concomitant thyroid diseases. *Eur J Nucl Med* 1997;24:143–149.

112. Ishibashi M, Nishida H, Hiromatsu Y, et al. Localization of ectopic parathyroid glands using technetium-99m sestamibi imaging: comparison with magnetic resonance and computed tomographic imaging. *Eur J Nucl Med* 1997;24:197–201.

113. Kezachian B, Gray M, Bussière F, et al. Preoperative localization in primary hyperparathyroidism: value of Tc-99m-MIBI scintigraphy. *Rev Med Interne* 1997;18:21–25.

114. Bonjer HJ, Bruining HA, Valkema R, et al. Single radionuclide scintigraphy with ^{99m}technetium-sestamibi and ultrasonography in hyperparathyroidism. *Eur J Surg* 1997;163:27–32.

115. Carter WB, Sarfati MR, Fox KA, et al. Preoperative detection of sporadic parathyroid adenomas using technetium-99m-sestamibi: what role in clinical practice? *Am Surg* 1997;63: 317–321.

116. Shaha AR, Sarkar S, Strashun A, et al. Sestamibi scan for preoperative localization in primary hyperparathyroidism. *Head Neck* 1997;29:87–91.

117. Klieger P, O'Mara R. The diagnostic utility of dual-phase Tc-99m sestamibi parathyroid imaging. *Clin* Nucl Med 1998;23: 208–211.

118. Hindié E, Mellière D, Jeanguillaume C, et al. Parathyroid imaging using simultaneous double-window recording of technetium-99m-sestamibi and iodine-123. *J Nucl Med* 1998;39: 1100–1105.

119. Blanco I, Carril JM, Banzo I, et al. Double-phase Tc-99m sestamibi scintigraphy in the preoperative location of lesions causing hyperparathyroidism. *Clin Nucl Med* 1998;23:291–297.

120. Benard F, LeFebre B, Beuvon F, et al. Parathyroid scintigraphy: rapid washout of technetium 99m MIBI from a large parathyroid adenoma. *J Nucl Med* 1995;36:241–243.

121. Leslie WD, Riese KT, Dupont JO, et al. Parathyroid adenomas without sestamibi retention. *Clin Nucl Med* 1995;20:699–702.

122. Rantis PC Jr, Prinz RA, Wagner RH. Neck radionuclide scanning: a pitfall in parathyroid localization. *Am Surg* 1995;61: 641–645.

123. Staudenherz A, Telfeyan D, Steiner E, et al. Scintigraphic pitfalls in giant parathyroid glands. *J Nucl Med* 1995;36:467–469.

124. Koss WG, Brown MR, Balfour JF. A false-positive localization of a parathyroid adenoma with technetium-99m sestamibi scan secondary to a thyroid follicular carcinoma. *Arch Surg* 1996; 131:216–217.

125. Billotey C, Sarfati E, Aurengo A, et al. Advantages of SPECT in technetium-99m-sestamibi parathyroid scintigraphy. *J Nucl Med* 1996;37:1773–1778.

126. Schurrer ME, Seabold JE, Gurll NJ, et al. Sestamibi SPECT scintigraphy for detection of postoperative hyperfunctional parathyroid glands. *AJR Am J Roentgenol* 1996;166:1471–1474.

127. Chen CC, Holder LE, Scovill WA, et al. Comparison of parathyroid imaging with technetium-99m-pertechnetate/sestamibi, subtraction double-phase technetium-99m-sestamibi and technetium-99m-sestamibi SPECT. *J Nucl Med* 1997;38: 834–839.

128. Schurrer ME, Seabold JE, Gurll NJ, et al. Sestamibi SPECT scintigraphy for detection of postoperative hyperfunctional parathyroid glands. *AJR Am J Roentgenol* 1996;166:1471–1474.

129. Teigen LE, Kilgore EJ, Cowan RJ, et al. Technetium-99m-sestamibi SPECT localization of mediastinal parathyroid adenoma. *J Nucl Med* 1996;37:1535–1537.

130. Coakley AJ. Parathyroid imaging. *Nucl Med Commun* 1995;16: 522–533.

131. McBiles M, Lambert AT, Cote MG, et al. Sestamibi parathyroid imaging. *Semin Nucl Med* 1995;25:221–234.

132. Gordon BM, Gordon L, Hoang K, et al. Parathyroid imaging with ^{99m}Tc-sestamibi. *AJR Am J Roentgenol* 1996;167: 1563–1568.

133. Heath DA. Localization of parathyroid tumors. *Clin Endocrinol* 1995;43:523–524.

134. Mitchell BK, Kinder BK, Cornelius E, et al. Primary hyperparathyroidism: preoperative localization using technetium-sestamibi scanning. *J Clin Endocrinol Metab* 1995;80:7–10.

135. Takami H, Satake S, Nakamura K, et al. What are the indications for ^{99m}Tc-sestamibi scintigraphy in hyperparathyroidism? *Clin Endocrinol* 1996;45:121–122.

136. Shaha AR, LaRosa CA, Jaffe BM. Parathyroid localization prior to primary exploration. *Am J Surg* 1993;166:289–293.

136a. Wei JP, Burke GJ. Analysis of savings in operative time for primary hyperparathyroidism using localization with technetium 99m sestamibi scan. *Am J Surg* 1995;170:488–491.

137. Takami H, Satake S, Nakamura K, et al. Technetium 99m sestamibi scan is the useful procedure to locate parathyroid adenomas before surgery. *Am J Surg* 1996;172:93.

138. Geatti O, Shapiro B, Orsolon PG, et al. Localization of parathyroid enlargement: experience with technetium 99m methoxyisobutylisonitrile and thallium 201 scintigraphy, ultrasonography and computed tomography. *Eur J Nucl Med* 1994; 21:17–22.

139. Weber CJ, Vansant J, Alazraki N, et al. Value of technetium 99m-sestamibi iodine-123 imaging in reoperative parathyroid surgery. *Surgery* 1993;114:1011–1018.

140. McIntyre RC, Kumpe DA, Liechty D. Reexploration and angiographic ablation for hyperparathyroidism. *Arch Surg* 1994;129: 499–505.

141. Rodriguez JM, Tezelman S, Siperstein AE, et al. Localization procedures in patients with persistent or recurrent hyperparathyroidism. *Arch Surg* 1994;129:870–875.

142. Thompson GB, Mullan BP, Grant CS, et al. Parathyroid imaging with technetium-99m-sestamibi: an initial institutional experience. *Surgery* 1994;116:966–972, discussion 972–973.

143. Bergenfelz A, Tennvall J, Valdermarsson S, et al. Sestamibi versus thallium subtraction scintigraphy in parathyroid localization: a prospective comparative study in patients with predominantly mild primary hyperparathyroidism. *Surgery* 1997;121: 601–605.

144. Torregrosa JV, Palomar MR, Pons F, et al. Has double-phase ^{99m}TC-SESTAMIBI scintigraphy usefulness in the diagnosis of hyperparathyroidism? *Nephrol Dial Transplant* 1998;13[Suppl 3]:37–40.

145. Ishibashi M, Nishida H, Hiromatsu Y, et al. Comparison of technetium-99m-MIBI, technetium-99m-tetrofosmin, ultrasound and MRI for localization of abnormal parathyroid glands. *J Nucl Med* 1998;39:320–324.

146. Fayet P, Hoeffel C, Fulla Y, et al. Technetium-99m sestamibi scintigraphy, magnetic resonance imaging and venous blood sampling in persistent and recurrent hyperparathyroidism. *Br J Radiol* 1997;70:459–464.

147. Achong DM, Oates E. Tc-99m sestamibi uptake by parathyroid carcinoma. False-positive localization of parathyroid adenoma. *Clin* Nucl Med 1995;20:735.

148. Kitapci MT, Tastekin G, Turgut M, et al. Preoperative localization of parathyroid carcinoma using Tc-99m MIBI. *Clin* Nucl Med 1993;18:217–219.

149. Lightowler C, Carroll MJ, Chesser AM, et al. Identification of auto-transplanted parathyroid tissue by Tc-99m methoxyisobutylisonitrile scintigraphy. *Nephrol Dial Transplant* 1995;10: 1372–1375.

150. Majors JD, Burke GJ, Mansberger AR Jr, et al. Technetium Tc 99m sestamibi scan for localizing abnormal parathyroid glands after previous neck operations: preliminary experience in reoperative cases. *South Med J* 1995;88:327–330.

151. Stokkel MP, VanEck-Smith BL. Tc-99m MIBI in a patient with parathyroid carcinoma. What to expect from it. *Clin* Nucl Med 1996;21:142–143.

152. Perez-Monte JE, Brown ML, Clarke MR, et al. Parathyroid hyperplasia, thymic carcinoid and pituitary adenoma detected with technetium-99m-MIBI in MEN type I. *J Nucl Med* 1997; 38:1767–1769.

153. Sarfati E, Billotey C, Halimi B, et al. Early localization and reoperation for persistent primary hyperparathyroidism. *Br J Surg* 1997;84:98–100.

154. Berna L, Caixas A, Piera J, et al. Technetium-99m-methoxyisobutylisonitrile in localization of ectopic parathyroid adenoma. *J Nucl Med* 1996;37:631–633.

155. Caravalho J, Balingit AG, Rivera-Rodriguez JE, et al. Localization of an ectopic parathyroid adenoma by double-phase technetium-99m-sestamibi scintigraphy. *J Nucl Med* 1995;36:1840–1842.

156. Chiu NT, Cheng HM, Yao WJ. Tc-99m sestamibi scanning in the preoperative localization of mediastinal parathyroid adenomas. *Ann Nucl Med* 1995;9:157–159.

157. Giordano A, Meduri G, Corsello SM, et al. Detection of an intrathymic parathyroid adenoma by Tc-99m tetrofosmin: a comparison with Tl-201. *Clin* Nucl Med 1996;21:996–998.

158. Sofferman RA, Nathan MH. The ectopic parathyroid adenoma: a cost justification for routine preoperative localization with technetium Tc99m sestamibi scan. *Arch Otolaryngol Head Neck Surg* 1998;124:649–654.

159. Norman J, Chheda H. Minimally invasive parathyroidectomy facilitated by intraoperative nuclear mapping. *Surgery* 1997;122: 998–1004.

160. Gallowitsch HJ, Fellinger J, Kresnik E, et al. Preoperative scintigraphic and intraoperative scintimetric localization of parathyroid adenoma with cationic Tc-99m complexes and a hand-held gamma probe. *Nuklearmedizin* 1997;36:13–18.

161. Bonjer HJ, Bruining HA, Pols HAP, et al. Intraoperative nuclear guidance in benign hyperparathyroidism and parathyroid cancer. *Eur J Nucl Med* 1997;24:247–251.

162. Irvin GL, Prudhomme DL, DeRiso GT, et al. A new approach to parathyroidectomy. *Ann Surg* 1994;219:574–581.

163. Taillefer R. Technetium-99m furifosmin. In: Taillefer R, Tamaki N, eds. *New radiotracers in cardiac imaging.* Norwalk, CT: Appleton & Lange, 1999:101–112.

164. Giordano A, Meduri G, Marozzi P. Parathyroid imaging with ^{99m}Tc-tetrofosmin. *Nucl Med Commun* 1996;17:706–710.

165. Fjeld JG, Erichsen K, Pfeffer PF, et al. Technetium-99m-tetrofosmin parathyroid scintigraphy: a comparison with ^{99m}Tc-sestamibi. *J Nucl Med* 1997;38:831–834.

166. Mansi L, Rambaldi PF, Marino G, et al. Kinetics of Tc-99m sestamibi and Tc-99m tetrofosmin in a case of parathyroid adenoma. *Clin* Nucl Med 1996;21:700–703.

167. Gallowitsch HJ, Mikosch P, Kresnik E, et al. Technetium 99m tetrofosmin parathyroid imaging. Results with double-phase study and SPECT in primary and secondary hyperparathyroidism. *Invest Radiol* 1997;32:459–465.

168. Ishibashi M, Nishida H, Strauss HW, et al. Localization of parathyroid glands using technetium-99m-tetrofosmin imaging. *J Nucl Med* 1997;38:706–711.

169. Apostolopoulos DJ, Houstoulaki E, Giannakenas C, et al. Technetium-99m-tetrofosmin for parathyroid scintigraphy: comparison to thallium-technetium scanning. *J Nucl Med* 1998;39: 1433–1441.

170. Aigner RM, Fueger GF, Nicoletti R. Parathyroid scintigraphy: comparison of technetium-99m methoxyisobutylisonitrile and technetium-99m tetrofosmin studies. *Eur J Nucl Med* 1996;23: 693–696.

171. Aigner RM, Fueger GF, Wolf G. Parathyroid scintigraphy: first experiences with technetium(III)-99m-Q12. *Eur J Nucl Med* 1997;24:326–329.

172. Neumann DR, Esselstyn CB, MacIntyre WJ, et al. Comparison of FDG-PET and sestamibi-SPECT in primary hyperparathyroidism. *J Nucl Med* 1996;37:1809–1815.

173. Neumann DR, Esselstyn CB, Kim EY. Recurrent postoperative parathyroid carcinoma: FDG-PET and sestamibi-SPECT findings. *J Nucl Med* 1996;37:2000–2001.

174. Sundin A, Johansson C, Hellman P, et al. PET and parathyroid L-[carbon-11] methionine accumulation in hyperparathyroidism. *J Nucl Med* 1996;37:1766–1770.

175. Arkles LB, Jones T, Hicks RJ, et al. Impact of complementary parathyroid scintigraphy and ultrasonography on the surgical management of hyperparathyroidism. *Surgery* 1996;120: 845–851.

176. Hewin DF, Brammar TJ, Kabala J, et al. Role of preoperative localization in the management of primary hyperparathyroidism. *Br J Surg* 1997;84:1377–1380.

177. Huglo D, Nocaudie M, Lecomte-Houcke M, et al. Localisation préopératoire des lésions parathyroïdiennes par la scintigraphie ⁹⁹ᵐTc-sestamibi-iode-123. *Presse Med* 1996;25:2017–2021.

178. Jeanguillaume C, Ureña P, Hindié E, et al. Secondary hyperparathyroidism: detection with I-123-Tc-99m-sestamibi subtraction scintigraphy versus US. *Radiology* 1998;207: 207–213.

179. Mellière D, Hindié E, Voisin MC, et al. Hyperparathyroïdie primaire. Optimisation des résultats chirurgicaux par la scintigraphie au ⁹⁹ᵐTc-sestamibi pré-opératoire systématique. *Chirurgie* 1997;122:98–105.

180. O'Doherty MJ. Radionuclide parathyroid imaging [Editorial]. *J Nucl Med* 1997;38:840–841.

181. Petti GH, Kirk GA. Parathyroid imaging. *Otolaryngol Clin North Am* 1996;29:681–691.

182. Pons F, Torregrosa JV, Vidal-Sicart S, et al. Preoperative parathyroid gland localization with technetium-99m sestamibi in secondary hyperparathyroidism. *Eur J Nucl Med* 1997;24: 1494–1498.

183. Shen W, Sabanci U, Morita ET, et al. Sestamibi scanning is inadequate for directing unilateral neck exploration for first-time parathyroidectomy. *Arch Surg* 1997;132:969–976.

184. Sinha CK, Hamaker R, Hamaker RC, et al. Utility of preoperative radionuclide scanning for primary hyperparathyroidism. *Laryngoscope* 1997;107:753–758.

15

MEDULLARY CANCER OF THE THYROID: RADIOLABELED ANTIBODY THERAPY

MALIK E. JUWEID
DAVID M. GOLDENBERG

Medullary thyroid cancer (MTC) constitutes only about 10% of all thyroid cancers, but it has the second worst prognosis after the anaplastic type (1,2). Although the overall 10-year survival of patients with MTC has considerably improved with current surgical treatment (total thyroidectomy and central lymph node dissection) to 80% or more from a historical 50%, the prognosis of patients with MTC metastatic to distant organs (lungs, liver, or bone) remains very poor; only 30% survive 5 years (2–6). This is because the therapeutic modalities available to these patients are of limited effectiveness (6). Chemotherapy alone has not been very effective and is therefore not even attempted by many treating physicians. External beam radiation has no role in the setting of widespread metastatic disease, except for palliative purposes. For this reason, the search continues for new therapeutic modalities to be used alone or in combination in the management of patients with metastatic MTC.

Unlike differentiated thyroid cancers (DTCs), MTCs do not concentrate radioiodine (2). Nevertheless, the successful use of radioiodine for the treatment of DTC has stimulated the search for ways to deliver this, and possibly other therapeutic isotopes, to MTC cells in the hope of achieving similar therapeutic success. Monoclonal antibodies (mAbs) that target certain antigens expressed by MTC appeared to be a logical choice for this purpose. In addition to calcitonin, the classic tumor marker for MTC, carcinoembryonic antigen (CEA), has been shown to be expressed in 70% to 90% of MTCs, particularly when the disease is metastatic (7). In fact, CEA is theoretically a more suitable target for intravenously administered mAbs than calcitonin because it is expressed on the surface of MTC cells. The mostly intracellular biodistribution of calcitonin makes the *in vivo* administration of mAbs against it more difficult.

Whereas radiolabeled mAbs directed against CEA have been used to image MTC in humans for more than 15 years (8–12), it was not until 1995 that the use of murine [131]I-

labeled anti-CEA mAbs for MTC therapy was reported, albeit still in the context of exploratory or phase I studies that included patients with other CEA-producing cancers (13). Since then, radiolabeled mAb therapy for MTC has been developed further and now uses humanized mAbs, various therapeutic isotopes, and combined-modality approaches, some of which include conventional chemotherapy (13–21).

In this short chapter, we describe the clinical experience with radiolabeled mAbs, particularly against CEA, in the treatment of MTC. Recent developments in this approach, which hold promise for a more effective therapy, have been emphasized.

PILOT RADIOIMMUNOTHERAPY STUDIES IN MEDULLARY THYROID CANCER

The initial experience with radioimmunotherapy (RAIT) of MTC was first described by Juweid et al. (13,14). Eighteen patients with metastatic MTC were treated with two different types (the first-generation NP-4 and the second-generation, high-affinity MN-14) and forms (intact IgG or bivalent fragments) of murine ^{131}I-labeled anti-CEA mAbs. As stated earlier, these patients were treated in exploratory or phase I trials along with patients with other CEA-producing cancers. MTC patients negative for human anti-mouse antibodies (HAMA) received doses ranging from 46 to 77 mCi of ^{131}I-MN-14 IgG or 90 to 195 mCi of ^{131}I-MN-14 F(ab)$_2$ mAb, depending on the dose level they were entered into the various steps of the clinical trials. As in other RAIT studies in which nonmyeloablative doses of radiolabeled mAbs were used, red marrow suppression was the only observed dose-limiting toxicity noted (DLT) in these trials. Seven of 14 patients who could be assessed had moderate antitumor effects (minor responses or disease stabilization) for up to 26+ months, based on physical examination findings, computed tomography (CT), or tumor markers. The estimated mean tumor doses were relatively high compared with those in patients with other CEA-producing cancers; 11 and 18 cGy/mCi with ^{131}I-MN-14 F(ab)$_2$ and IgG, respectively. These studies also identified the bivalent fragment, [131]I-

M. E. Juweid: Department of Radiology, University of Iowa College of Medicine, Iowa City, Iowa 52242.

D. M. Goldenberg: Department of Microbiology and Immunology, New York Medical College, Valhalla, New York 10595; Garden State Cancer Center, Belleville, New Jersey 07109.

MN-14 F(ab)₂, as the ideal treatment agent because of its lower immunogenicity and higher tumor-to-marrow radiation absorbed dose ratio in comparison with the IgG form, and we proposed conducting MTC-specific phase I trials with this agent, preferably in patients with less advanced or bulky disease.

PHASE I/II TRIAL OF NONMYELOABLATIVE RADIOIMMUNOTHERAPY IN MEDULLARY THYROID CANCER WITH ¹³¹I-MN-14 F(AB)₂ ANTI-CARCINOEMBRYONIC ANTIGEN MONOCLONAL ANTIBODY

A phase I/II trial involving a total of 15 patients with metastatic MTC was completed with the murine ¹³¹I-MN-14 F(ab)₂ anti-CEA mAb (15). A unique feature of this study was that dose escalation was based on prescribed radiation absorbed doses to the red marrow; the initial dose was 140 cGy, escalated in 40-cGy increments until DLT (defined as grade 4 myelotoxicity of any duration or grade 3 myelotoxicity of > 2 weeks' duration) was reached. The "exact" radioactive amount given was determined by a tracer study, with the same mAb given 1 week before therapy. In this investigation, red marrow suppression was again the only DLT observed. The maximum tolerated dose (MTD) was determined to be 180 cGy to marrow, which corresponded to about 90 mCi/m² of the agent in patients with little complexing with CEA. Eleven patients were treated at this MTD. One of the 15 patients treated in this trial had a 45% decrease of tumor burden in the neck on CT, with dramatic improvement in the mass effect on the airways caused by tumor (Fig. 15.1).

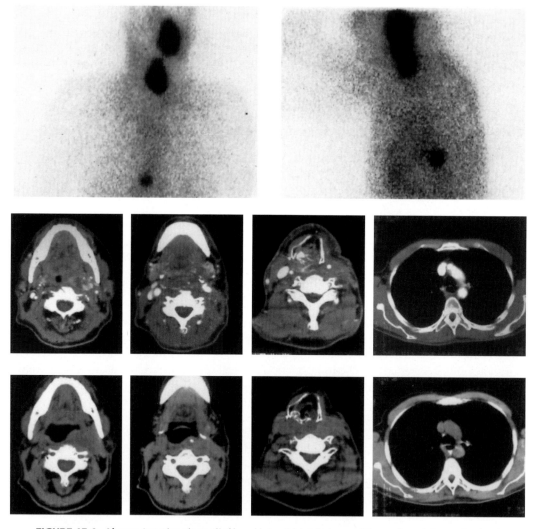

FIGURE 15.1.   Above: Anterior planar (*left*) and lateral (*right*) views of the neck and chest, obtained 9 days after the infusion of 8 mCi (1 mg) of ¹³¹I-MN-14 F(ab)₂, show tumor lesions in the left parapharyngeal space, hypopharynx, and right retrolaryngeal region, in addition to a lymph node metastasis in the posterior mediastinum (*arrows*). **Below:** Computed tomograms from the neck and mediastinum of the same patient obtained before (*above*) and 1 year after (*below*) therapy show a dramatic improvement in the mass effect on the airways caused by the tumor lesions in the neck, with a 45% reduction of overall tumor burden. The mediastinal lesion remains unchanged.

Seven patients had a 30% to 70% (median, 55%) decrease of tumor markers for 1 to 9+ months. Eleven of 12 assessable patients continued to have radiologically stable disease for 3+ to 26+ months (median, 12+ months). The estimated mean (± SD) tumor radiation absorbed dose was 24 ± 27 cGy/mCi (median, 17 cGy/mCi); the large standard deviation was primarily a consequence of different tumor sizes, both within the same patient and between patients. More favorable dosimetry was generally seen in relatively small tumors (≤ 3 cm), with doses approaching 100 cGy/mCi. Theoretical calculations showed the estimated median tumor dose at the marrow MTD to be 2,500 cGy. However, the dose to other critical organs (i.e., lung, kidney, and liver) at this MTD was still less than 500 cGy, and the estimated median tumor-to-lung, tumor-to-liver, and tumor-to-kidney radiation absorbed dose ratios were about 7, 8, and 5, respectively. Because radiation doses to these organs of up to 2,000 cGy (to kidney or lung) or 3,000 cGy (to liver) could be given without significant risk of DLT, tumor doses of up to 10,000 cGy would then be delivered if myelotoxicity were to be overcome to achieve this dose intensification. These considerations provided the rationale for dose escalation with autologous hematopoietic stem cell rescue (with either bone marrow or peripheral blood stem cells) in our subsequent trials, particularly in patients with advanced, rapidly progressing disease.

PHASE I/II TRIAL OF HIGH-DOSE RADIOIMMUNOTHERAPY WITH ^{131}I-MN-14 F(AB)$_2$ COMBINED WITH AUTOLOGOUS HEMATOPOIETIC STEM CELL RESCUE IN MEDULLARY THYROID CANCER

Our group has initiated a phase I/II trial of high doses of murine ^{131}I-MN-14 F(ab)$_2$ in combination with autologous hematopoietic stem cell rescue (AHSCR) in patients with metastatic MTC (16). Recognizing the potential risks of high-dose therapy and the fact that a substantial number of patients with metastatic MTC may unpredictably have relatively stable disease for a prolonged period of time, we entered only patients with clear evidence of disease progression before therapy into this trial. Autologous bone marrow (BM) (n = 5) or peripheral blood stem cells (PBSCs) (n = 7) were harvested in the 12 patients entered into the trial. Dose escalation was based on prescribed radiation doses to the critical organs (kidney, liver, and lung). Doses were started at 900 cGy to the kidney, not exceeding 1,200 cGy to liver and lung, and escalated in 300-cGy increments until DLT (defined as a grade 3 to 4 nonhematologic toxicity) was reached. Here again, the exact radioactive amount given was determined by a tracer study with the same mAb given 1 week before the start of therapy. Of the 12 patients, one was treated at 660, eight at 900, and three at 1,200 cGy to the kidney. Radioactivity ranged from 235 to 486 mCi of ^{131}I-MN-14 F(ab)$_2$. BM or PBSCs were given 1 to 2

weeks after therapy to all patients, when total-body radiation dose exposure was 2 mR/h or less. Expected grade 3 or 4 myelotoxicity was seen in 10 patients 2 to 5 weeks after therapy, but the duration of grade 4 myelotoxicity was 14 days or less in all patients. Only one of the 12 patients had DLT (grade 3 gastrointestinal toxicity at the 900-cGy level); otherwise, only mild grade 1 or 2 nonhematologic toxicity (gastrointestinal, cardiac, pulmonary, and hepatic) was noted, with no renal toxicity observed. One patient had a partial remission for 1 year, one a minor response for 3 months, and 10 stabilization of disease for 1 to 16 months after therapy. The median tumor dose delivered to the patients treated at only the first two dose levels planned (900 and 1,200 cGy) was approximately 3,900 cGy, and tumor doses ranged from 1,100 to as high as 74,000 cGy. As in the previous trial with nonmyeloablative doses of ^{131}I-MN-14 F(ab)$_2$, the median tumor-to-lung, tumor-to-liver, and tumor-to-kidney radiation dose ratios were 6, 4, and 5, respectively, and the median tumor dose at the presumed MTD (2,000 cGy to kidneys) was estimated to be approximately 9,400 cGy. Although the initial results of this study were encouraging, especially with regard to the potential for delivering high doses of radiation to tumors, it was discontinued in favor of a trial with humanized ^{90}Y-MN-14 (hMN-14) anti-CEA mAb combined with chemotherapy (see below). Preclinical studies in which the TT human MTC tumor model was used have shown better tumor-to-normal organ radiation absorbed dose ratios and better antitumor effects with ^{90}Y- than with ^{131}I-MN-14 (17). Because of this, plus the possibility of administering high, even myeloablative, doses of ^{90}Y-mAbs on a completely outpatient basis and the potential for immune effector function of the humanized form of MN-14 in comparison with the murine form, we have decided to use ^{90}Y-hMN-14 in our future trials of radiolabeled mAb therapy of MTC (18).

STUDIES OF EXPERIMENTAL THERAPY OF HUMAN MEDULLARY THYROID CARCINOMA

Several preclinical studies of MTC therapy were conducted by our group and others before novel therapy concepts were translated into clinical trials (17–19). For this purpose, a human MTC cell line, designated TT, is used. This model expresses CEA in addition to calcitonin and is therefore suitable for RAIT with anti-CEA mAbs. TT also expresses the general features of MTC; it is relatively slow-growing, chemoresistant, and radioresistant. For example, TT expresses the *MDR1* (multidrug resistance) gene and hence functions as a suitable model of doxorubicin-resistant MTC, as is the case in most patients with MTC. In preclinical studies performed by our group, more favorable tumor dosimetry and better antitumor effects were obtained with ^{90}Y-MN-14 anti-CEA mAb than with ^{131}I-MN-14 mAb (17). These studies also showed that the

MTD of ^{90}Y-MN-14 (i.e., the MTD of RAIT) could be combined with as much as 75% of the MTD of doxorubicin, even when given at the same time, and the MTD of doxorubicin could be combined with as much as 75% of the MTD of RAIT when doxorubicin was given 1 or 2 days after RAIT, but not at the same time (19). Administration of doxorubicin 1 or 2 days after RAIT was considered to be concurrent administration because more than 80% or 60% of the radiation dose from ^{90}Y-MN-14 is delivered 1 or 2 days after RAIT, respectively (i.e., after administering doxorubicin), a finding later confirmed in clinical studies. Giving doxorubicin 1 or 2 days after ther-

apy also did not appear to alter the biodistribution of radiolabeled mAb or tumor uptake of mAb, later confirmed in clinical studies. Most importantly, the combined-modality treatment appeared to be more effective than the MTD of RAIT and much more effective than the MTD of doxorubicin (Fig. 15.2). In addition, the toxicity of these combinations was not higher than that of the MTD of RAIT alone. The results of these studies laid the foundation for our clinical trial of RAIT with ^{90}Y-MN-14 (humanized form) combined with doxorubicin in the treatment of metastatic MTC.

PHASE I/II TRIAL OF HIGH-DOSE RADIOIMMUNOTHERAPY AND DOXORUBICIN COMBINED WITH PERIPHERAL BLOOD STEM CELL RESCUE IN PATIENTS WITH METASTATIC MEDULLARY THYROID CARCINOMA

Our group recently initiated a phase I/II trial of escalating doses of ^{90}Y-hMN-14 (0.75 mg/kg) and a fixed dose of doxorubicin (60 mg/m^2) given 24 hours after RAIT (20,21). Our intent in this trial is to administer high myeloablative doses of ^{90}Y-hMN-14, for the purpose of delivering high doses of radiation to tumors, in combination with doxorubicin chemotherapy. Hence, PBSCs were harvested in all patients and were reinfused when the ^{90}Y total-body activity (based on whole-body clearance of ^{111}In-hMN-14 as a surrogate for ^{90}Y-hMN-14) was 3 mCi/m^2 or less. All patients underwent a tracer study with ^{111}In-hMN-14 (6 mCi, 0.75 mg/kg) 1 week before RAIT to document tumor targeting of at least one known measurable tumor lesion and to estimate organ and tumor dosimetry with ^{90}Y-hMN-14. According to the recommendations of the Food and Drug Administration, dose escalation in this trial was based on body surface area; doses of ^{90}Y-hMN-14 were started at 20 mCi/m^2 and escalated in increments of 10 mCi/m^2 until DLT was reached. DLT was defined here as a grade 3 nonhematologic toxicity of more than 2 weeks' duration or a grade 4 nonhematologic toxicity of any duration except gastrointestinal toxicity and hyperbilirubinemia of up to 6 mg/dL, for which durations of 1 week and 10 days, respectively, were allowed. Fourteen patients have been treated to date (three at 20, three at 30, three at 40, and five at 50 mCi of ^{90}Y-hMN-14 per square meter). The blood pharmacokinetics of ^{111}In- and ^{90}Y-hMN-14 were seen to be very similar. Results of the ^{111}In-hMN-14 mAb scan were positive in all 14 patients treated, with nearly all disease sites 1 cm or larger in diameter detected. Doxorubicin did not appear to alter the biodistribution, tumor targeting, or dosimetry of ^{90}Y-hMN-14, as was demonstrated by a giving a second ^{111}In-hMN-14 injection together with ^{90}Y-hMN-14 1 week after the first ^{111}In-hMN-14 injection (Fig. 15.3). The estimated mean (± SD) tumor dose calculated for seven

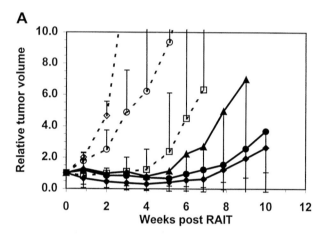

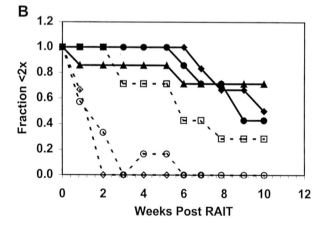

FIGURE 15.2. Growth of TT (human medullary thyroid carcinoma cell line) tumors in mice given various radioimmunotherapy and doxorubicin treatment regimens. Tumor-bearing mice were either left untreated (◇, n = 6); given a single injection of 60 mg of doxorubicin per square meter (○, n = 7) or 105 μCi of ^{90}Y-MN-14 (□, n = 6); or given 45 mg of doxorubicin per square meter 24 hours after 80 μCi of ^{90}Y-MN-14 (, n = 7), 60 mg of doxorubicin per square meter 24 hours after 80 μCi of ^{90}Y-MN-14 (♦, n = 6), or 45 mg of doxorubicin per square meter 24 hours after 104 μCi of ^{90}Y-MN-14 (●, n = 7). At the start of therapy, the mean tumor volume was 0.123 ± 0.086 cm^3 (range, 0.039 to 0.438 cm^3). **A:** Points represent the mean tumor size of the treatment groups. **B:** Points represent the fraction of mice in which tumors are less than two times the volume at the time of administration of ^{90}Y-MN-14.

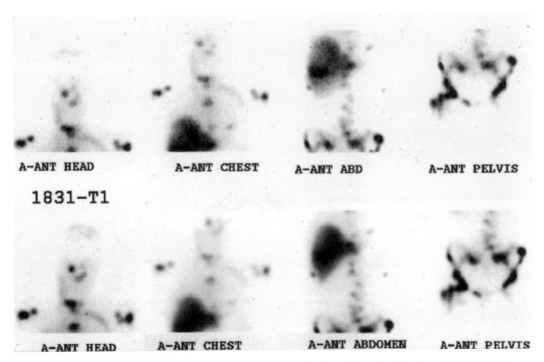

FIGURE 15.3. Above: Anterior planar views obtained 7 days after the injection of 5 mCi (0.75 mg/kg) of ^{111}In-hMN-14 in a patient with medullary thyroid carcinoma and multiple bony metastases. **Below:** Anterior planar views obtained in the same patient 7 days after the administration of 10 mCi (0.75 mg/kg) of ^{111}In-hMN-14 together with ^{90}Y-hMN-14, injected 24 hours before the administration of 60 mg of doxorubicin per square meter. The second injection of ^{111}In was given 7 days after the first injection.

patients to date ($n = 25$ tumors) is 51 ± 34 cGy/mCi, and the mean tumor-to-lung, tumor-to-kidney, and tumor-to-liver ratios are approximately 6, 7.5, and 5.0, respectively. PBSCs were reinfused 7 to 12 days after therapy in all patients. No grade 4 myelotoxicity was seen at 20 mCi of ^{90}Y-hMN-14 per square meter. Grade 4 neutropenia was seen in two of three patients treated at 30 mCi/m². Grade 4 neutropenia was observed in two of three patients treated at 40 mCi/m², and four patients treated at the dose level of 50 mCi/m² had a grade 4 neutropenia, with two patients also having a grade 4 thrombocytopenia. Most importantly, the duration of grade 4 neutropenia/thrombocytopenia was 8 days or less in all patients experiencing this condition, and the peripheral blood counts returned to normal levels (i.e., grade 0) within 2.5 to 7 weeks (median, 5.7 weeks) after therapy in all patients. Only one patient treated at 50 mCi/m² had a DLT (possibly treatment-related grade 4 toxicity). In other patients, only grade 1 or 2 nonhematologic toxicity (gastrointestinal and generally asymptomatic cardiopulmonary toxicity) was seen except in two, who had grade 3 nausea and vomiting for 1 and 5 days. No renal or hepatic toxicity has been observed to date. Of the 13 patients treated who are currently assessable for response, one had a partial response for 3 months, two had a minor response for 22+ and 11 months, and six had stable disease for 2, 2.5, 2.5, 6.5, 19+, and 5 months; the disease of four

patients progressed. Hence, the initial results of this trial demonstrate the feasibility of concurrent high-dose RAIT and chemotherapy in combination with PBSC rescue; rapid marrow reconstitution and relatively mild to moderate nonhematologic toxicity have been observed to date. Dose escalation continues to determine the MTD of this combination therapy.

CONCLUSIONS

Radiolabeled antibody therapy of MTC is still at a relatively early stage of development. Nevertheless, the results of clinical studies conducted to date indicate that this therapy, even when given at nonmyeloablative doses, is useful in the control of slowly progressing metastatic MTC. However, myeloablative doses appear to be required to achieve major responses in patients with aggressive disease. Preliminary data indicate that myeloablative RAIT combined with doxorubicin and PBSC rescue is feasible and may prove beneficial for the treatment of metastatic MTC. Future research should focus on combinations with other, potentially more effective chemotherapeutic agents and multiple-cycle therapy in an effort to perfect this multimodal approach to the treatment of a challenging, radioresistant and chemoresistant disease.

ACKNOWLEDGMENTS

We thank Dr. Robert Sharkey for supervising the radiolabeling facility and managing the clinical data, Dr. Rhona Stein for supervising the preclinical studies of MTC therapy, Tom Jackson for preparation and quality assurance of the labeled antibody, Clare Maccado for data management, Douglas Dunlop and Dion Yeldell for imaging and dosimetry assistance, and Enid Alston for help in the preparation of this manuscript.

This work has been supported in part by grant CA 66906 (Dr. Juweid) from the National Cancer Institute, National Institutes of Health; grants FD-R-001190 and FD-R-001555 from the Food and Drug Administration (Dr. Juweid); and grant CA 39841 (Dr. Goldenberg, Outstanding Investigator Grant) from the National Cancer Institute, National Institutes of Health.

REFERENCES

1. Robbins J, Merino MJ, Boice JD Jr, et al. NIH Conference. Thyroid cancer: a lethal endocrine neoplasm. *Ann Intern Med* 1991; 115:133–147.
2. Norton JA, Levin B, Jensen R. Cancer of the endocrine system. In: DeVita VT, Hellman S, Rosen SA, eds. *Cancer: principles and practice of oncology.* New York: JB Lippincott Co, 1989:1333–1435.
3. Rossi RL, Cady B, Meissner WA, et al. Nonfamilial medullary thyroid carcinoma. *Am J Surg* 1980;139:554–560.
4. Samaan NA, Schultz PN, Hickey RC. Medullary thyroid carcinoma: prognosis of familial versus sporadic disease and the role of radiotherapy. *J Clin Endocrinol Metabol* 1988;67:801–808.
5. Schroder S, Bocker W, Baisch H, et al. Prognostic factors in medullary thyroid carcinomas. Survival in relation to age, sex, stage, histology, immunocytochemistry and DNA content. *Cancer* 1988;61:806–816.
6. Cance WG, Wells SA Jr. Multiple endocrine neoplasia type IIa. *Curr Probl Surg* 1985;22:1.
7. Rougier PH, Calmettes C, Laplanche A, et al. The value of calcitonin and carcinoembryonic antigen in the treatment and management of non-familial medullary thyroid carcinoma. *Cancer* 1983;51:855–862.
8. Berche C, Mach JP, Lumbrosco JD, et al. Tomoscintigraphy for detecting gastrointestinal and medullary thyroid cancer: first clinical results using radiolabeled monoclonal antibodies against carcinoembryonic antigen. *Br Med J* 1982;285:1447–1451.
9. Reiners CH, Eilles CH, Spiegel W, et al. Immunoscintigraphy in medullary thyroid cancer using an [123]I- or ^{111}In-labelled monoclonal anti-CEA antibody fragment. *Nucl Med* 1986;25: 227–231.
10. Edington HD, Watson CG, Levine G, et al. Radioimmunoimaging of metastatic medullary carcinoma of the thyroid gland using an indium-111-labeled monoclonal antibody to CEA. *Surgery* 1988;104:1004–1010.
11. Vuillez JP, Peltier P, Caravel JP, et al. Immunoscintigraphy using ^{111}In-labeled F(ab')$_2$ fragments of anticarcinoembryonic antigen monoclonal antibody for detecting recurrences of medullary thyroid carcinoma. *J Clin Endocrinol Metab* 1992;74:157–163.
12. Juweid M, Sharkey RM, Behr T, et al. Improved detection of medullary thyroid carcinoma with radiolabeled antibodies to carcinoembryonic antigen. *J Clin Oncol* 1996;14:1209–1217.
13. Juweid M, Sharkey RM, Behr T, et al. Targeting and initial radioimmunotherapy of medullary thyroid carcinoma with ^{131}I-labeled monoclonal antibodies to carcinoembryonic antigen. *Cancer Res* 1995;55:5946–5951.
14. Juweid M, Sharkey RM, Behr T, et al. Radioimmunotherapy of medullary thyroid carcinoma with ^{131}I-labeled anti-CEA antibodies. *J Nucl Med* 1996;37:905–911.
15. Juweid M, Hajjar G, Swayne LC, et al. Phase I/II trial of ^{131}I-MN-14 F(ab)$_2$ anti-carcinoembryonic antigen monoclonal antibody in the treatment of patients with metastatic medullary thyroid carcinoma. *Cancer* 1999;85:1828–1842.
16. Juweid M, Hajjar G, Stein, et al. Initial experience with high-dose radioimmunotherapy of metastatic medullary thyroid carcinoma using ^{131}I-MN-14 F(ab)$_2$ anti-carcinoembryonic antigen (CEA) monoclonal antibody and autologous hematopoietic stem cell rescue (AHSCR). *J Nucl Med* 2000;41:93–103.
17. Stein R, Juweid M, Mattes MJ, et al. Carcinoembryonic antigen as a target for radioimmunotherapy of human medullary thyroid cancer. Antibody processing, targeting, and experimental therapy with [131]I- and ^{90}Y-labeled mAbs. *Cancer Biother Radiopharm* 1999;14: 37–47.
18. Stein R, Juweid M, Goldenberg DM. Effects of unlabeled anti-CEA on the growth of medullary thyroid cancer xenografts. *Proc Am Assoc Cancer Res* 1999;40:18.
19. Stein R, Juweid M, Zhang C-H, et al. Assessment of combined radioimmunotherapy and chemotherapy for treatment of medullary thyroid cancer. *Clin Cancer Res* 1999;5:3199S–3206S.
20. Juweid M, Rubin A, Hajjar G, et al. Preclinical and clinical findings support concurrent RAIT and chemotherapy in patients with medullary thyroid cancer (MTC). *Proceedings of the American Society of Clinical Oncology* 1999;18:407A(abst).
21. Juweid M, Rubin A, Hajjar G, et al. First clinical results of combined RAIT and chemotherapy in patients with medullary thyroid cancer (MTC). *Program and Abstracts of the Endocrine Society 81st Annual Meeting* 1999;P2-726(abst).

16

POSITRON EMISSION TOMOGRAPHY IMAGING

ABDULAZIZ AL-SUGAIR
R. EDWARD COLEMAN

An estimated 180,000 new cases of lung cancer will be diagnosed in the United States this year. Lung cancer accounts for approximately 25% of all cancer deaths. The overall 5-year survival rate remains at 14% and has not changed in several decades (1). The diagnosis and treatment of lung cancer are major health problems globally.

New diagnostic and treatment strategies are needed to improve the survival rates of patients with lung cancer. The current approach of demonstrating anatomic and morphologic changes has proved insensitive for characterizing this malignancy. Moreover, more invasive approaches of tissue sampling by bronchoscopy, percutaneous needle biopsy, thoracoscopy, and open lung biopsy have limitations. Because physiologic and biochemical alterations occur before gross structural and anatomic changes, the need for a functional method for early detection has emerged.

The combined approach of ^{18}F-2-fluoro-2-deoxyglucose positron emission tomography (FDG-PET) and computed tomography (CT) has made a major impact in the diagnosis and staging of lung cancer. FDG-PET imaging provides accurate characterization of lesions that are indeterminate by conventional imaging, accurate staging of the mediastinum, accurate detection of distant metastatic disease, and prognostic information at the time of diagnosis. Multiple studies worldwide have demonstrated that FDG-PET has a major role in the diagnosis and staging of lung cancer, and its application is cost-effective. The use of PET in oncology has been increasing dramatically. The ability of PET to differentiate tumor cells from normal cells relies on alterations in the metabolism of various substrates within tumor cells, in which glycolysis and protein synthesis are enhanced and amino acid transport and incorporation are increased (2–3). Tumor cells have low levels of glucose-6-phosphatase and high levels of hexokinase

(4). These processes result in trapping of FDG-6-phosphate within tumor cells and provide the basis for FDG-PET tumor imaging. Similarly, increased amino acid incorporation into tumors has been demonstrated, and several radiolabeled amino acids, such as ^{11}C-methionine, ^{11}C-leucine, and ^{11}C-thymidine, have been investigated and show promising results in the differential diagnosis of indeterminate nodules and in the determination of the response of lung cancer to radiotherapy (3–5).

Camera-based PET devices are now available at many centers. In addition, there are now more than three times the number of camera-based PET devices than dedicated PET devices in the United States, and the number of camera-based PET scanners is increasing rapidly. The major advantage of these devices is that they can be used in both general nuclear medicine and PET imaging. The use of thicker sodium iodide crystals than in conventional gamma cameras has improved their sensitivity in the detection of annihilation radiation without affecting ^{99m}Tc radiopharmaceutical image quality.

IMAGING WITH ^{18}F-FLUORODEOXYGLUCOSE

To minimize the competitive inhibition of FDG uptake by serum glucose, a minimum of 4 hours of fasting is recommended before ^{18}F-FDG is injected. In patients with a history of glucose intolerance, a serum glucose level is obtained before FDG is administered. In our facility, if the serum glucose level is below 200 mg/dL, FDG is administered. If the serum level is 200 mg/dL or higher, the study is delayed until the serum glucose level is below 200 mg/dL. Although the effect of diabetes mellitus and elevated serum glucose levels has not been carefully studied, administering insulin at the same time as FDG leads to an increased accumulation of FDG in skeletal muscle and less accumulation in tumors (Fig. 16.1). It is essential that the blood sugar level

A. Al-Sugair: Department of Radiology, King Faisal Specialist Hospital and Research Centre, Riyadh, Saudi Arabia.

R. E. Coleman: Department of Radiology, Duke University Medical Center, Durham, North Carolina 27710.

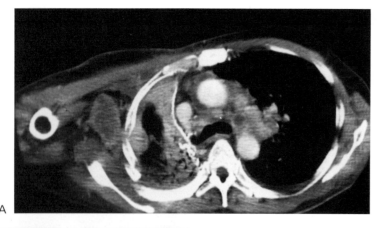

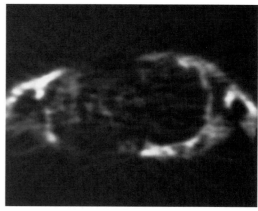

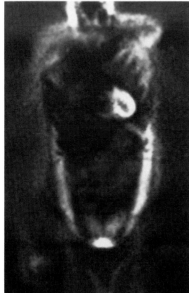

FIGURE 16.1. A: Computed tomography of the chest in a diabetic patient with a history of prior surgical resection for non-small cell lung cancer demonstrates an abnormal right upper lobe opacity with precarinal lymph node. **B:** Transaxial image through the right upper lobe lesion reveals faint accumulation of FDG, suggestive of malignancy. This patient had a recurrence of malignancy. **C:** Whole-body positron emission tomography after administration of FDG shows most of the FDG to be intramuscular because of insulin administration at approximately the same time.

of a diabetic patient who undergoes FDG-PET be monitored and controlled before FDG is administered. With dedicated PET scanners, the administered dose of FDG is 0.145 µCi/kg, to a maximum of 20 mCi. Sodium iodide-based PET scanners cannot acquire data accurately at high count rates if more than 4 mCi is in the body at the time of imaging; thus, lower doses (5 to 6 mCi) of ^{18}F-FDG are administered, or the delay between FDG administration and imaging is lengthened.

Most patients being evaluated for a lung nodule or for staging require a whole-body FDG scan. Attenuation-corrected whole-body images should be performed for more accurate detection of lesions. However, the role of attenuation is still being determined. When a PET scanner with a 15-cm axial field of view is used, 10 or more bed positions are required for a whole-body scan of an average adult. If 8-minute emission scans and 10-minute transmission scans

were performed at 10 bed positions, a 3-hour imaging study would be required. Segmentation of transmission scans is becoming available that permits transmission scans to be performed in 1 to 2 minutes per bed position. Furthermore, most institutions use 4 minutes per bed position for emission acquisition in performing whole-body scans. Thus, whole-body attenuation-corrected scans can be obtained in approximately 1 hour with these new techniques.

In patients with lung cancer, our technique for performing a whole-body study with the General Electric Advance scanner (General Electric Medical Systems, Milwaukee, Wisconsin) begins 30 minutes after FDG injection with a 4-minute brain scan in the three-dimensional (3D) acquisition mode. The system is switched to 2D acquisition mode and non–attenuation-corrected scans are obtained for 4 minutes per bed position from the base of the brain through the middle of the thighs. The acquisition can be extended below the midthigh level if the presence of a lesion in the lower extremities is known or suspected. An attenuation-corrected scan is performed using 3 minutes for the transmission scan at each bed position.

IMAGE INTERPRETATION

Images obtained with FDG-PET can be interpreted qualitatively, semiquantitatively, or quantitatively. Quantification of glucose metabolic rates has not been used clinically. For qualitative interpretations, areas of abnormality are detected by comparison with background activity. For the characterization of lung nodules, the intensity of accumulation in the nodule is compared with mediastinal and cardiac blood pool intensities on the attenuation-corrected images. A greater intensity of accumulation in the nodule than in the blood pool indicates a malignant lesion. If the intensity of the accumulation in the nodule is the same as or less than the activity in the mediastinal blood pool, a benign lesion is likely. The non-attenuation images should also be reviewed, but the criteria for characterizing a nodule as malignant are based on the attenuation-corrected images.

Semiquantitative parameters may be used to characterize lesions as benign or malignant on the attenuation-corrected FDG image. This semiquantitative parameter is the *standardized uptake ratio* (SUR) and is referred to as the *standardized uptake value* (SUV) (6,7). The SUR normalizes the amount of FDG accumulation in a region of interest (ROI) according to the total injected dose and patient's body weight. An ROI is placed on the abnormality on an attenuation-corrected image and the mean activity (mCi/mL) is measured. The decay-corrected activity is then used to compute the SUR by the following formula:

$$SUR = \frac{Mean\ ROI\ Activity\ (mCi/mL)}{Injected\ Dose\ (mCi)/Body\ Weight\ (g)}$$

The use of lean body weight instead of actual body weight has been advocated by some investigators. Correction for serum glucose has been also suggested. SUR values are time-dependent, and the time of acquisition after FDG injection must be standardized for the value to be useful. Most of the data in the literature have used the image obtained 45 to 60 minutes after FDG administration.

EVALUATION OF FOCAL PULMONARY OPACITIES

FDG-PET has been used to characterize indeterminate focal pulmonary opacities, which primarily consist of solitary pulmonary nodules (8,9). Approximately 130,000 patients are identified each year in the United States with solitary pulmonary nodules. These lesions are usually identified on plain radiographs obtained during either routine screening or preoperative evaluation. Further radiographic evaluation is often recommended for characterization of the lesion with serial chest radiography or computed tomography (CT) of the chest. In the past, plain chest radiography and serial chest radiography were the most common imaging modalities used to differentiate malignant from benign nodules (Fig. 16.2). Now, CT is frequently used to characterize suspect lesions present on chest radiography. The two main radiographic criteria that are used to distinguish benign from malignant solitary nodules are based on the presence of lateral, concentric, or stippled calcification, as seen on chest radiography or CT, and stability of the nodule for more than 2 years (10). If the nodule is not definitely benign by its characteristics on CT, the nodule is labeled as indeterminate and requires further evaluation (11,12) (Figs. 16.3 and 16.4).

Multiple studies (4,13–26) have demonstrated the significant advantages of characterizing solitary pulmonary nodules with FDG-PET. The reported sensitivity and specificity of FDG-PET in differentiating benign from malignant lesions have been uniformly high. When an SUR cutoff value of 2.5 or higher is used to indicate malignancy, the difference between the values of malignant (6.8 ± 3.7) and benign (1.5 ± 0.9) lesions is significant ($p < .0001$) (13).

The sensitivity and specificity of FDG-PET for characterizing focal pulmonary opacities in our initial report of 51 patients were found to be 100% and 89%, respectively (13). An SUR value of 2.5 or higher was considered indicative of malignancy. Results of analysis of the accumulation of FDG in a focal lung lesion are not significantly different according to whether the SUR or visual analysis is used. When 89 patients underwent evaluation of indeterminate solitary pulmonary nodules in a multicenter prospective study, a sensitivity of 92% and specificity of 90% were found, in comparison with a sensitivity of 98% and a specificity of 68% for visual analysis. The results for visual analysis were slightly higher, but not statistically significant. Furthermore, the accuracy of PET does not differ according to whether nodules 1.5 cm or less in diameter or nodules larger than 1.5 cm in diameter are being evaluated (27,28). A recent phantom study by Coleman et al. (29) demonstrated the detection of a 6-mm-diameter nodule in a realistic chest phantom that was scanned by a dedicated PET imaging device with attenuation correction.

False-positive results have been reported to occur in some inflammatory and infectious processes, such as tuberculosis, histoplasmosis, Wegener's granulomatosis (Fig. 16.5), and fungal disease (5,10,26). Most chronic or indolent inflammatory processes and most acute infectious processes do not exhibit significant FDG accumula-

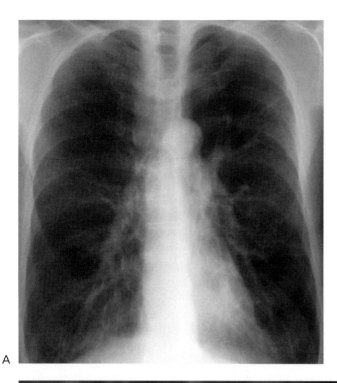

A

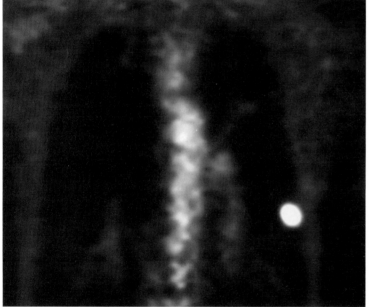

B

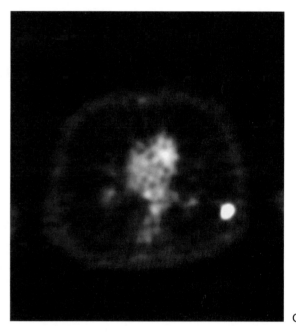

C

FIGURE 16.2. A: Newly diagnosed 1.5-cm-diameter smoothly marginated nodule in the left lower lung on posteroanterior chest roentgenography. This nodule was not seen on a prior study. **B,C:** Coronal and transaxial images obtained with positron emission tomography after administration of FDG demonstrate hypermetabolism in a peripherally located nodule in the left lower lobe. Wedge resection of the left lower lobe revealed non-small cell lung cancer.

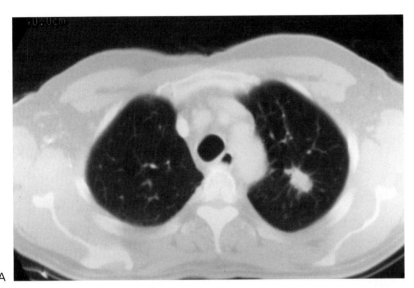
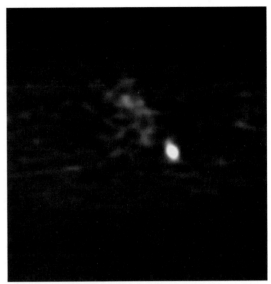

A

B

FIGURE 16.3. A: Computed tomography demonstrates a 2-cm-diameter spiculated nodule in the left upper lobe. **B:** Positron emission tomography after administration of FDG demonstrates a solitary focus of hypermetabolism in the left upper lobe, corresponding to the CT abnormality. Resection of the left upper lobe revealed squamous cell carcinoma.

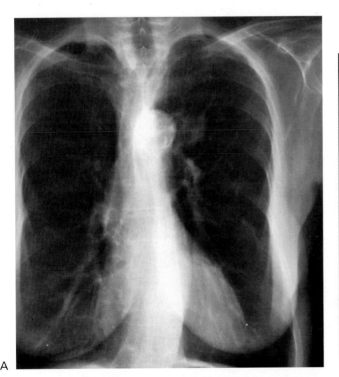
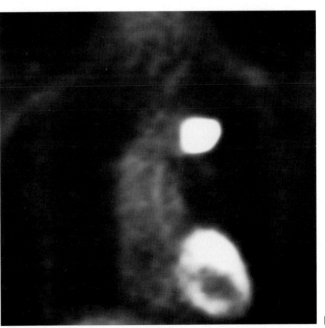

A

B

FIGURE 16.4. A: Left upper lobe opacity measuring 2.5 cm seen on posteroanterior chest radiography. **B:** Coronal image obtained with positron emission tomography after administration of FDG demonstrates a solitary focus of increased ^{18}F-FDG accumulation in the left upper lobe, consistent with neoplasm. The primary adenocarcinoma was completely resected.

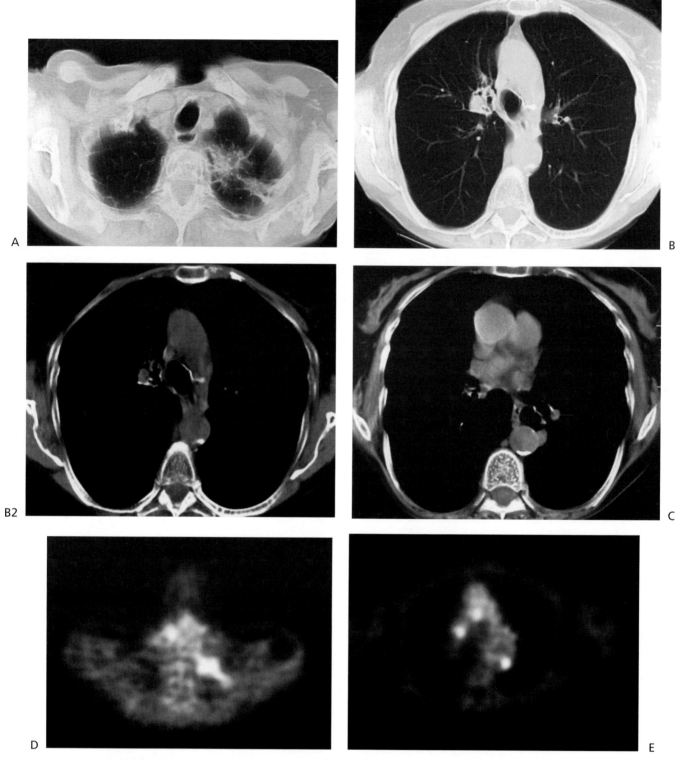

FIGURE 16.5. A: Computed tomography of the lungs demonstrates a poorly defined left apical opacity. **B1,B2:** Ill-defined right suprahilar opacity seen on lung and soft-tissue windows. **C:** Lymph node 1 cm in diameter in the periaortic region, seen on computed tomography. **D:** Transaxial positron emission tomography (*PET*) demonstrates abnormally increased accumulation of FDG in the apical region of the left lung. Biopsy findings in this region were consistent with Wegener's granulomatosis. **E:** Multiple foci of increased ^{18}F-FDG metabolism in the transaxial plane in the right suprahilar, precarinal, and periaortic regions.

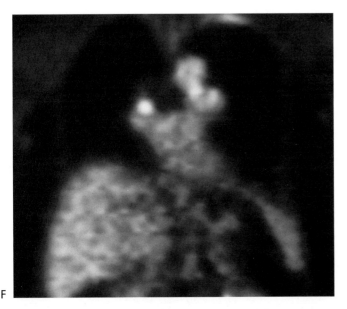

F

FIGURE 16.5. (*continued*) F: Coronal view obtained with ¹⁸F-FDG-PET demonstrates hypermetabolism in the apical and suprahilar abnormalities.

tion (Fig. 16.6). For this reason, the specificity of PET in the evaluation of focal pulmonary opacities remains high.

False-negative results of PET studies have been reported in tumors with relatively low levels of metabolic activity, such as carcinoid and bronchioloalveolar cell carcinoma (24,30) (Fig. 16.7). Another potential cause for a false-negative study is the size of the nodule. The accuracy of FDG-PET in characterizing nodules less than 6 mm in size has not been determined.

Evaluation of a solitary pulmonary nodule with FDG-PET obviates the need for invasive tissue sampling in patients with lesions that are not metabolically active, and patients who have benign nodules on PET are spared surgi-

cal intervention. However, nodules that accumulate FDG require a biopsy (27). The cost savings of FDG-PET in the evaluation of solitary pulmonary nodules represent the prevention of unnecessary thoracotomies (31).

In addition to its diagnostic value, FDG-PET imaging provides prognostic information. A significantly shorter median survival, of approximately 13 months, was observed in patients who had a lung cancer with an SUR of 10 or higher than in patients with an SUR value of less than 10, whose median survival was 25 months. Multivariate analysis demonstrated that PET results provide prognostic information independently of other clinical and imaging findings (25).

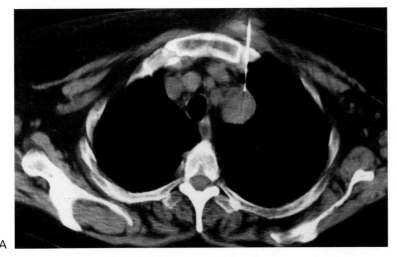
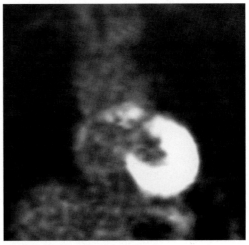

A

B

FIGURE 16.6. A: Computed tomography demonstrates 3 x 3-cm mass within the supraaortic region, suspected of being primary bronchogenic carcinoma. However, biopsy revealed a benign process. **B:** Coronal image obtained with positron emission tomography after administration of FDG demonstrates no FDG metabolism corresponding to the supraaortic mass identified on chest computed tomography.

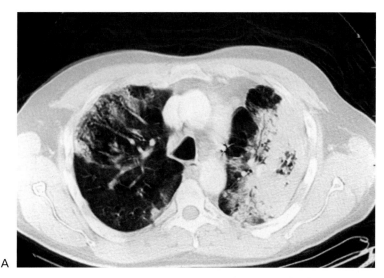
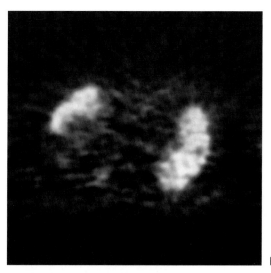

A

B

FIGURE 16.7. A: Computed tomography demonstrates diffuse bilateral infiltrates. **B:** Positron emission tomography after administration of FDG demonstrates abnormally increased FDG metabolism bilaterally in the lungs. The infiltrative lung masses were in keeping with the diagnosis of bronchoalveolar cell carcinoma.

STAGING OF LUNG CANCER

The mediastinum is the most common site for metastases in a patient who has bronchogenic carcinoma (Fig. 16.8). Because the criteria used for the diagnosis of metastatic disease in mediastinal nodes is size-dependent, the low accuracy of CT and magnetic resonance imaging (MRI) in staging the mediastinum is not surprising. In a prospective evaluation of 100 patients with non-small cell lung cancer who underwent staging by mediastinoscopy and CT, the sensitivity and specificity of mediastinoscopy were 89% and 100%, respectively, and the sensitivity and specificity of CT were 63% and 57%, respectively, for mediastinal lymph node metastases. This study found that 24% of normal sites contained metastases (32).

A study by Patz et al. (32a) demonstrated a statistically significant increase in accuracy for FDG-PET in comparison with CT in determining the nodal (N) status of disease. In 42 patients with newly diagnosed bronchogenic carcinoma, the sensitivity and specificity of PET imaging for detecting mediastinal nodal station metastases were 92% and 100%, respectively, whereas for CT, the sensitivity and specificity were 58% and 80%, respectively. For hilar and mediastinal thoracic nodal station metastases, the sensitivity and specificity of PET imaging were 83% and 82%, respectively, and for CT, they were 43% and 85%, respectively (33).

A unique advantage of FDG-PET over the combined use of other routine studies is in the staging of distant metastases (M status). It has been reported that about 40% of patients with newly diagnosed lung cancer present with distant disease (34). The accuracy of clinical evaluation and laboratory results in these patients is low, about 50% (35,36). Clearly, better methods are needed to screen for distant foci and multisystem involvement in patients with newly diagnosed lung cancer (Fig. 16.9).

In a recent report of 100 patients who underwent staging of non-small cell lung cancer with FDG-PET, PET was superior to conventional imaging in detecting metastases to bone, lung, adrenal gland, and liver (37).

The sensitivity and specificity of PET in detecting brain metastases were 60% and 99%, respectively, and positive and negative predictive values were 75% and 97%, respectively, in comparison with 100% sensitivity, specificity, positive predictive value, and negative predictive value for conventional imaging (37). The value of FDG-PET in detecting skeletal metastatic disease is limited (Fig. 16.10). In a recent study of 299 patients with possible bone metastases, PET results were compared with results of bone scanning in patients with lung cancer. Results of FDG-PET were significantly more likely than results of bone scans to be normal when skeletal metastatic disease was absent. The sensitivity and specificity of PET were 75% and 82%,

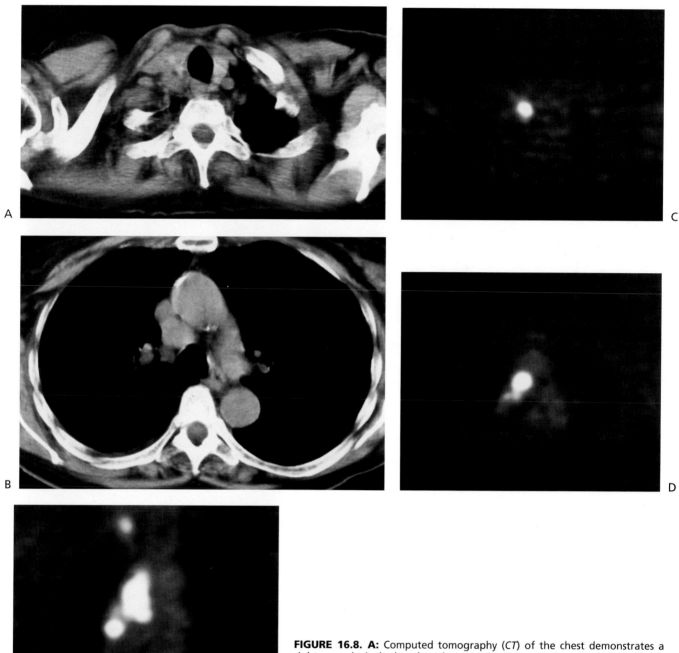

FIGURE 16.8. A: Computed tomography (*CT*) of the chest demonstrates a right supraclavicular lymph node measuring 1.2 cm in diameter. **B:** Right para-tracheal lymph node measuring 1.6 x 1.2 cm in diameter. **C:** Increased FDG metabolism in right supraclavicular region, corresponding to CT abnormality. **D:** Increased FDG metabolism in the right paratracheal and precarinal regions and in the right upper lobe on transaxial images obtained with FDG positron emission tomography (*PET*). **E:** Coronal FDG-PET demonstrates right perihilar mass and lymph node metastases. Mediastinoscopy confirmed the diagnosis of metastatic non-small cell lung cancer.

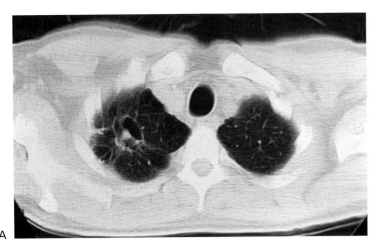

A

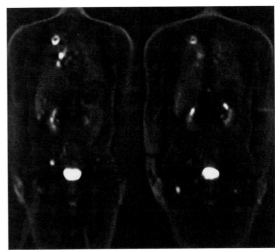

C

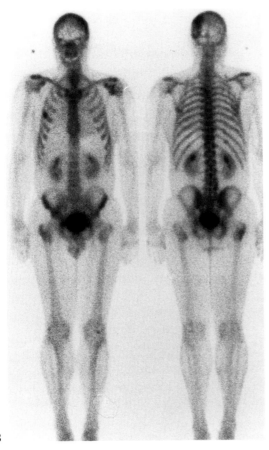

B

FIGURE 16.9. A: Computed tomography demonstrates a cavitary lesion in the right upper lobe with a nodular component and spiculation. **B:** Whole-body bone scan demonstrates increased tracer accumulation in *1*, right fourth rib anteriorly; *2*, proximal right femur; *3*, posterior skull on the left. **C:** Whole-body positron emission tomography after administration of FDG demonstrates the following areas of abnormal FDG accumulation: *1*, right upper lobe with central photopenia, suggestive of central necrosis; *2*, right hilar region; *3*, liver; *4*, lower thoracic spine, proximal femora bilaterally, and right and left ilia. The findings are consistent with metastases.

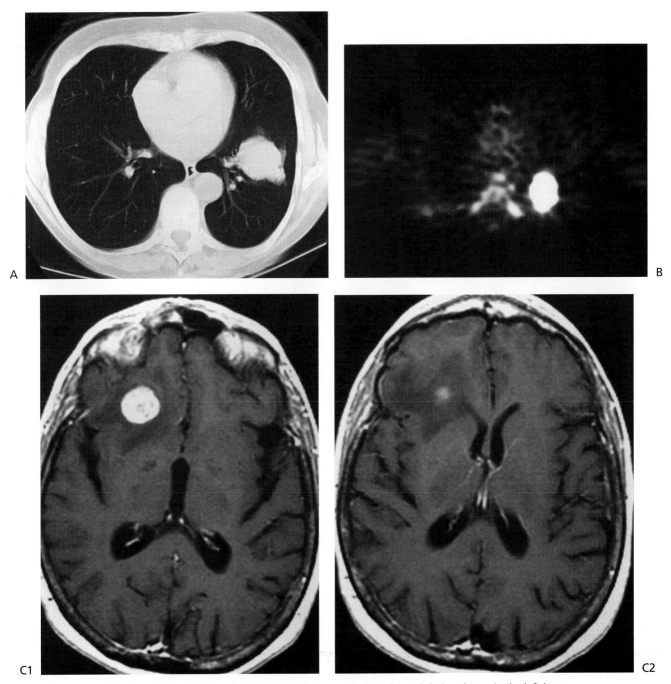

FIGURE 16.10. **A:** Computed tomography demonstrates a large, lobulated mass in the left lower lobe. This was in keeping with secondary metastases to the lung. **B:** Transaxial image obtained with positron emission tomography after administration of FDG shows intense hypermetabolism in the left lower lobe mass. **C1:** Magnetic resonance imaging of the brain demonstrates a 1.8 x 1.9-cm mass in the right frontal lobe. **C2:** Mild mass effect on the anterior horn, with vasogenic edema and minimal midline shift. *(continued)*

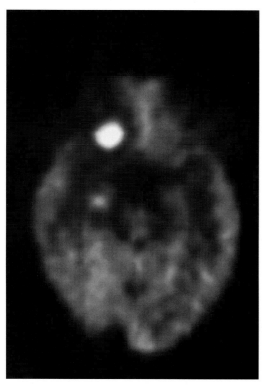

FIGURE 16.10. (*continued*) D: FDG-PET of the brain demonstrates two foci of FDG hypermetabolism in the right frontal lobe, consistent with metastases.

respectively, and the sensitivity and specificity of bone scan were 96% and 85%, respectively (38).

DETECTION OF PERSISTENT OR RECURRENT DISEASE

Multiple studies have demonstrated the superiority of PET over conventional imaging in monitoring recurrence and predicting response to therapy before the initiation of treatment (39–44). A recent study by Ichija et al. (40) evaluated the usefulness of FDG-PET in predicting and assessing response to radiation therapy in 30 patients with untreated lung cancer who underwent an FDG scan before therapy. Twenty patients underwent scanning posttherapy. Lesions with higher tumor-to-muscle ratios (> 7) on the pretherapy study showed better early response than those with lower ratios. However, the relapse rate was also higher in lesions with higher uptake (> 10) on the pretherapy study and in lesions with higher uptake on posttherapy study.

Monitoring the progress of patients after the induction of chemotherapy or radiation has been a difficult task. PET is more accurate than conventional imaging in predicting downstaging and clinical outcome after the induction of chemotherapy (40). Although FDG-PET identifies changes in tumor glucose uptake, studies have shown an increased uptake of FDG in tissue after radiation. Radiation pneumonitis does accumulate FDG and can be confused with recurrent tumor after therapy.

COST-EFFECTIVENESS

Gambhir et al. (31) have shown that a combined strategy of CT and PET is cost-effective in the staging of non-small cell lung cancer because it reduces the probability that a patient with unresectable disease will undergo an unnecessary attempt at curative surgery. The study evaluated the expected costs and projected life expectancy. When CT and PET were compared with the alternate strategy of CT alone, the savings of the combination strategy were $1,154 per patient, without loss of life expectancy. The estimated yearly savings for an estimated 85,000 patients (based on national cancer statistics) is $98 million per year. ^{18}F-FDG-PET is cost-effective in that it prevents patients with unresectable disease from undergoing unnecessary surgery.

REIMBURSEMENT

As of January 1, 1998, the Health Care Financing Administration (HCFA), which administers Medicare in the United States, has adopted a policy to pay for FDG-PET in the evaluation of indeterminate solitary pulmonary nodules up to 4 cm in diameter and in the initial staging of pathologically diagnosed non-small cell lung cancer. Many other third-party payers have similar policies. The reimbursement rate for the technical component, which includes the cost of radiopharmaceuticals, is approximately $1,900.

REFERENCES

1. Boring CC, Squires TS, Tung T. Cancer statistics. *Cancer* 1992;42:19–43.
2. Smith TAD. FDG uptake, tumor characteristics, and response to therapy: a review. *Nucl Med Commun* 1998;19:97–105.
3. Wahl R. *Principles and Practice of Oncology.* 1997;1:5–8.
4. Kubota K, Matsuzawa T, Fujiwara T, et al. Differential diagnosis of lung tumor with positron emission tomography: a prospective study. *J Nucl Med* 1990;31:1927–1932.
5. Kubota K, Yamada S, Ishiwata K, et al. Positron emission tomography for treatment evaluation and recurrence detection compared with CT in long-term follow-up cases of lung cancer. *Clin Nucl Med* 1992;17:877–881.
6. Strauss LG, Dimitrakopoulou AD, Haberkorn U, et al. PET follow-up studies to evaluate tumor perfusion and metabolism in patients with small cell carcinoma of the lung. *Radiology* 1992;5:139P.
7. Slosman DO, Spiliopoulos A, Couson F, et al. Satellite PET and

lung cancer: a prospective study in surgical patients. *Nucl Med Commun* 1993;14:955–961.

8. Stoller JK, Ahmad M, Rice TW. Solitary pulmonary nodule. *Cleve Clin J Med* 1988;55:68–74.

9. Lowe VJ, Coleman RE. Application of PET in oncology imaging. In: Sandler MP, Coleman RE, Wackers FJ, et al., eds. *Diagnostic nuclear medicine*, 3rd ed. Baltimore: Williams & Wilkins, 1995;1293–1308.

10. Dewan NA, Gupta NC, Redepennig L, et al. Diagnostic efficacy of PET-FDG imaging in solitary pulmonary nodules; potential role in evaluation and management. *Chest* 1993;104:997–1002.

11. Mori K, Saitov Y, Tominaga K, et al. Small nodular lesions in the lung periphery: new approach to diagnosis with CT. *Radiology* 1990;177:843–849.

12. Kuriyama K, Tateishi R, Doi O, et al. Prevalence of air bronchograms in small peripheral carcinomas of the lung on the thin-section CT: comparison with benign tumors. *AJR Am J Roentgenol* 1991;156:921–924.

13. Patz EF, Lowe VJ, Hoffman JM, et al. Focal pulmonary abnormalities: evaluation with [18F] fluorodeoxyglucose PET scanning. *Radiology* 1993;188:487–490.

14. Lowe VJ, Hoffman JM, DeLong DM, et al. Semiquantitative and visual analysis of FDG-PET images in pulmonary abnormalities. *J Nucl Med* 1994;35:1771–1776.

15. Wahl RL, Quint LE, Greenough RL, et al. Staging of mediastinal non-small cell lung cancer with FDG-PET, CT, and fusion images: preliminary prospective evaluation. *Radiology* 1994;191:371–377.

16. Dehdashti F, Griffeth LK, McGuire AH, et al. FDG-PET evaluation of suspicious pulmonary and mediastinal masses. *J Nucl Med* 1992;32:961P.

17. Hunter GJ, Fischman AJ, Alpert NM, et al. Quantitative [18F] FDG-PET in the monitoring and management of response to lung cancer therapy. *Radiology* 1992;185:186P.

18. Knopp MV, Bischoff H, Ostertag H, et al. Clinical application of FDG-PET for staging of bronchogenic carcinoma. *J Nucl Med* 1993;34:21P.

19. Khonsary SA, Mandelkern MA, Brown CV, et al. PET-FDG scanning in pulmonary mass lesions. *Clin Nucl Med* 1993;19:922.

20. Berlangieri SU, Scott AM, Knight S, et al. Mediastinal lymph node staging in non-small cell lung carcinoma: comparison of [18F]-FDG positron emission tomography with surgical pathology. *Eur J Nucl Med* 1994;21:62S.

21. Weber W, Romer W, Ziegler S, et al. Clinical value of F-18-FDG PET in solitary pulmonary nodules. *Eur J Nucl Med* 1995;22:775.

22. Paulus P, Benoit TH, Bury TH, et al. Positron emission tomography with 18F-fluoro-deoxyglucose in the assessment of solitary pulmonary nodules. *Eur J Nucl Med* 1995;22:775.

23. Baum R P, Rust M, Strassmann O, et al. Whole-body positron emission tomography PET with 2-[18F]-fluorodeoxyglucose for preoperative staging of lung cancer: influence on patients' management. *Eur J Nucl Med* 1995;22:775.

24. Duhaylongsod FG, Lowe VJ, Patz EF, et al. Detection of primary and recurrent lung cancer by means of F-18 fluorodeoxyglucose positron emission tomography FDG PET. *J Thorac Cardiovasc Surg* 1995;110:130–140.

25. Ahuja V, Coleman RE, Herndon J, et al. Prognostic significance of FDG-PET imaging in patients with non-small cell lung cancer. *Cancer* 1998;83:918–924.

26. Strauss LG, Conti PS. The application of PET in clinical oncology. *J Nucl Med* 1991;32:623–648.

27. Lowe VJ, Fletcher JW, Gobar L, et al. Prospective investigation of PET in lung nodules. *J Clin Oncol* 1998;16:1075–1084.

28. Lowe VJ, Duhaylongsod FG, Patz EF, et al. FDG-PET and lung malignancy—a retrospective study of pulmonary and PET analysis. *Radiology* 1997;202:435–439.

29. Coleman RE, Laymon CE, Turkington TG. FDG imaging of lung nodules: a phantom study comparing SPECT, camera-based PET and dedicated PET. *Radiology* 1999;210:823–827.

30. Higashi K, Seki H, Tanigushi M, et al. Bronchioalveolor carcinoma: false negative results in FDG-PET. *J Nucl Med* 1997;38:79(abst).

31. Gambhir SS, Hoh CG, Phelps ME, et al. Decision tree sensitivity analysis for cost-effectiveness of FDG-PET in the staging and management of non-small cell lung carcinoma. *J Nucl Med* 1996;37:1428–1436.

32. Gdeedo A, Vanschill P, Cathouts B, et al. Prospective evaluation of computed tomography and mediastinoscopy in mediastinal lymph node staging. *Eur Respir J* 1997;103:1547–1551.

32a. Patz EF, Lowe VJ, Goodman P, et al. Thoracic nodal staging with PET imaging with FDG patients with bronchogenic carcinoma. *Chest* 1995;108:1617–1621.

33. Lowe VJ, Fletcher JW, Gobar L, et al. Prospective investigation of positron emission tomography in lung nodules. *J Clin Onc* 1998;16:1075–1084.

34. Landis SH, Murray T, Bolden S, et al. Cancer statistics. *CA Cancer J Clin* 1998;48:629.

35. Salvatierra A, Baamonde C, Llamas J, et al. Extrathoracic staging of bronchogenic carcinoma. *Chest* 1990;97:1052–1058.

36. Quinn DL, Ostrow LB, Porter DK, et al. Staging of non-small cell bronchogenic carcinoma. *Chest* 1988;989:270–275.

37. Marom E, McAdams H, Erasmus J, et al. Staging non-small cell lung cancer with whole body positron emission tomography. *Radiology* 1999;3:803–809.

38. Al-Sugair A, Delong D, Coleman RE. Relative diagnostic efficacy of 18FDG-PET and bone scan scintigraphy for detection of osseous metastases in primary or secondary lung cancer. *J Nucl Med* 1999;40:20P.

39. Hebert M, Lowe V, Hoffman J, et al. Positron emission tomography in the pretreatment evaluation and follow-up of non-small cell lung cancer patients treated with radiotherapy. *Am J Clin Oncol* 1996;19:416–421.

40. Ichija Y, Kuwabara Y, Sasaki M, et al. A clinical evaluation of FDG-PET to assess the response in radiation therapy for bronchogenic carcinoma. *Ann Nucl Med* 1996;10:193–200.

41. Vansteenkiste J, Stoobants S, DeLyn P, et al. Prognostic significance of FDG-PET after induction chemotherapy in stage IIIA-N2 non-small cell lung cancer (N2-NSCLC): analysis of 13 cases. *Proc Am Soc Clin Oncol* 1998;16:75.

42. Patz EF Jr, Lowe VJ, Hoffman JM, et al. Persistent or recurrent bronchogenic carcinoma: detection with PET and 2-[18F]-fluoro-2-deoxy-D-glucose. *Radiology* 1994;191:379–382.

43. Inoue T, Kim EE, Komaki R, et al. Detecting recurrent or residual lung cancer with FDG-PET. *J Nucl Med* 1995;36:788–793.

44. Kim EE, Chung SK, Haynie TP, et al. Differentiation of residual or recurrent tumors from post treatment changes with F-18 FDG PET. *Radiographics* 1992;12:269–279.

Nuclear Oncology: Diagnosis and Therapy, edited by I. Khalkhali, J. Maublant, and S.J. Goldsmith, Lippincott Williams & Wilkins, Philadelphia © 2001

17

LABELED PEPTIDE SCINTIGRAPHY

HIRSCH HANDMAKER
JAY E. BLUM

Lung cancer has reached epidemic proportions globally. It is now the most common cause of cancer deaths among both men and women in the United States and in most countries throughout the world (1,2). Progress has been made in the earlier detection of lung cancer at the potentially curable stage of the pulmonary nodule (3). In the United States, 130,000 new solitary pulmonary nodules (SPNs) are found each year, estimated as 1 in each 500 chest roentgenograms and accounting for approximately 20% of all newly diagnosed lung cancers (4,5). Notably, only a fraction of patients with SPN, estimated in various series at 28% to 39%, are ultimately found to have a malignant neoplasm (6,7). Consequently, the clinical problem regarding the indeterminate nature of many lesions identified by conventional morphologic techniques, either chest roentgenography or computed tomography (CT), is significant. This lack of specificity results in a burden of expense and patient morbidity related to the need to perform more invasive procedures, such as CT-guided biopsy, to confirm or exclude malignancy. Indeed, a definitive diagnosis is not always obtained even with CT-guided biopsy. For example, Sheiman et al. (8) reported that 4 of 32 patients (13%) with lung lesions who underwent a CT-guided core biopsy had false-negative results. The emergence of new algorithms for evaluating patients at high risk for lung cancer, highlighted by the study of the pioneering Early Lung Cancer Action Project (ELCAP), will only increase the number of potentially evaluable nodules (3). Unfortunately, until recently, most noninvasive radiographic methods or minimally invasive procedures, such as bronchoscopy, have resulted in a high percentage of indeterminate diagnoses (9–15). Even the recently presented results of a multicenter trial of lung nodule enhancement at CT had significant morphologic constraints on the study population (16). These circumstances have led to the investigation of other noninvasive methods

to provide a better characterization of abnormalities detected on chest roentgenography and CT, particularly SPN.

Radiopharmaceuticals and nuclear medicine procedures have become increasingly popular for this purpose, most notably ^{18}F-fluorodeoxyglucose positron emission tomography (FDG-PET). The relatively limited availability of dedicated PET scanners and the expense of this procedure, however, have limited the widespread adoption of this technique. The efficacy of gamma camera-based systems for FDG imaging, although these are somewhat more available and less expensive than dedicated PET scanners, remains largely unproven at the present time, especially in characterizing smaller lung lesions (< 2 cm) (17). Such systems are still significantly less available than conventional single-photon emission computed tomography (SPECT) systems, which are deployed in virtually all nuclear medicine facilities throughout the world. As a result, the most desirable radiopharmaceuticals for characterizing lung lesions are those that can be readily, reliably, and economically detected by conventional SPECT systems.

Early work by various investigators (18–21) suggested that the nonspecific tracer gallium ^{67}Ga citrate could be employed to image lung cancer of all types. They reported that ^{67}Ga is taken up by more than 90% of these tumors. Because ^{67}Ga binds to serum transferrin, ferritin, and tissue lactoferrin and is engulfed by leukocytes, it is of little value in distinguishing malignant pulmonary masses from masses related to benign inflammatory processes, a crucial issue in evaluating patients with lung lesions. ^{67}Ga has other limitations; multiple photopeaks (all outside the 140-keV energy range for optimized contemporary SPECT systems), relatively slow clearance from the blood stream, and the dose limitations imposed by dosimetry considerations result in relatively low-contrast image resolution, so that it is difficult to depict lesions smaller than 3 cm. Hence, ^{67}Ga has been of only limited value the detection and characterization of lung cancer.

Another nonspecific tracer, thallium ^{201}Tl chloride, has been investigated for the evaluation of lung lesions. The rationale for the use of this cardiac imaging agent is the

H. **Handmaker:** Healthcare Technology Group, Phoenix, Arizona 85016.
J. E. **Blum:** Pulmonary Division, CIGNA HealthCare of Arizona, Phoenix, Arizona 85006; Department of Medicine, University of Arizona College of Medicine, Tuscon, Arizona 85724.

"upregulation" in malignant tissues, relative to normal or inflammatory cells, of the sodium–potassium pump and adenosine triphosphatase activity of the membrane transport systems (22,23). In a comparison of ^{201}Tl-SPECT with FDG-PET in 33 patients, Higashi et al. (24) found that in all but the patients with small lesions (< 2 cm), the sensitivity of ^{201}Tl-SPECT was comparable with that of FDG-PET. Both ^{201}Tl and FDG-PET failed to detect bronchoalveolar carcinoma in two patients. This series did not include any patients without proven malignancy, so no statement about specificity can be made. Although ^{201}Tl does reliably detect pulmonary malignancies, it is also taken up by inflammatory cells, so that its specificity is reduced significantly (25). Image quality is inferior to that obtained with ^{99m}Tc-labeled compounds, which is a result of its low-energy photons and the relatively low dose administered. Although SPECT imaging with ^{201}Tl improves lesion detectability, the usefulness of this agent is reduced for small lesions. ^{99m}Tc-Sestamibi and ^{99m}Tc-tetrofosmin have also been investigated to image lung cancer (26–28). Studies comparing ^{201}Tl and ^{99m}Tc-sestamibi in two series of 45 and 37 patients with primary lung cancer reported comparable sensitivities, in the order of 96% to 98%, for the two tracers in patients with relatively large lung masses (29,30). No patients with benign lung masses were evaluated. An earlier publication, comparing ^{99m}Tc-sestamibi with FDG-PET and CT in 19 patients with proven lung cancer, concluded that SPECT with ^{99m}Tc-sestamibi and FDG-PET are equally successful in detecting primary lesions (31). ^{99m}Tc-Sestamibi is less reliable than ^{201}Tl and FDG-PET in detecting malignancy in patients who are undergoing chemotherapy and radiotherapy, presumably because of alterations in binding of the mono-ionic cation in intracellular protein, multidrug resistance factor, and alterations in P-glycoprotein (32).

Two radiopharmaceuticals originally described for renal imaging, ^{99m}Tc-glucoheptonate (GH) (33) and ^{99m}Tc-dimercaptosuccinic acid (DMSA), have also been studied in patients with lung cancer. Vorne et al. (34) reported the correct identification of 23 of 26 primary lung cancers, and only one false-positive in eight benign lesions evaluated with ^{99m}Tc-GH. In an early study with DMSA, Kao et al. (35) reported poor sensitivity (43%), specificity (70%), and accuracy (48%) in detecting lung cancer. However, a later study, by Hirano et al. (36), reported a sensitivity of approximately 90% in patients with a variety of lung cancers. Atasever (37) reported the correct identification of 33 of 36 lung malignancies with the use of DMSA; one lung abscess also demonstrated increased uptake.

Critical analysis of the investigations discussed to this point suggests the commonality of low sensitivity for small lesions (< 2 cm) and poor specificity with failure to distinguish between inflammatory and neoplastic processes. Study designs also failed to included more than a small number of benign lesions. As such, FDG-PET has emerged as the "gold standard" for the noninvasive detection and characterization of lung masses, its practical limitations of limited availability and cost notwithstanding.

In the course of evaluating a new class of radiopharmaceuticals to image neuroendocrine and non-neuroendocrine tumors, Kwekkeboom et al. (38) reported encouraging results in imaging small cell and non-small cell lung cancers with [^{111}In-DTPA-D-Phe[1]]octreotide (Octreoscan). The efficacy of Octreoscan has been well established in the detection and localization of neuroendocrine tumors, and it has received approval from the Food and Drug Administration for this indication.

This compound is a synthetic peptide analogue of the primarily downregulatory hormone somatostatin, and it has the ability to bind to somatostatin-type receptors (SSTRs) expressed in a variety of human tissues, including neuroendocrine tissue. Five SSTR subtypes have been identified to date. Despite this ubiquity of SSTR distribution in normal human tissue, many neoplasms, including small cell cancers, bind somatostatin analogues more avidly than granulomatous or other non-neoplastic tissue does (39–42). Blum et al. and Fujita et al. (43–45) have suggested the presence of SSTRs in non-small cell cancer, and clinical studies have supported the phenomenon of SSTR overexpression or more avid somatostatin binding in these cancers. The exploitation of this phenomenon of overexpression of SSTR or increased somatostatin binding in abnormal tissue has broad implications. A functional approach to the diagnosis of malignancy utilizing the biologic rather than the morphologic properties of tissue is now feasible. This is somewhat analogous to the improved elucidation that radioastronomy offers in comparison with the more conventional optical approach in celestial investigations. The relatively long half-life of indium (2.8 days), which limits the amount of dose that can be administered, and its less-than-optimal imaging properties in comparison with nuclides like 99mTc, which limit the evaluation of smaller nodules, were considered impediments to the evaluation of lung cancer in large populations.

Depreotide is a small synthetic peptide (molecular weight of 1,358) with a somatostatin-binding domain and the ability to form a stable ligand with ^{99m}Tc, so that imaging characteristics are improved and cost is lower in comparison with ^{111}In-octreotide (46,47). Additionally, because of the relatively short half-life of 6 hours, clearance is rapid, and optimal dosing is possible, along with the production of high-contrast SPECT image resolution. Favorable reports led to the investigation of a ^{99m}Tc-labeled SSTR compound, ^{99m}Tc-depreotide (NeoTect™, or P829) (46). In early trials, this small peptide radiopharmaceutical demonstrated increased localization in a variety of malignancies, including breast cancer, lung cancer, melanoma, and lymphoma (48). The novel nature of depreotide was manifested not only by its limited degree of cross-reactivity with SSTR on neuroendocrine tumors but also by its avid binding to non-small cell lung cancer (49).

The real utility of ^{99m}Tc-depreotide in the rapid, cost-effective and noninvasive evaluation of lung cancer had to be elucidated. Blum et al. (43) reported preliminary results with ^{99m}Tc-depreotide in a prospective study of 30 patients with significant risk factors for primary lung cancer and solitary pulmonary nodules (SPNs) in which they compared scintigraphy with "gold standard" tissue histologic examination. The excellent reliability of ^{99m}Tc-depreotide in the noninvasive evaluation and characterization of SPN was demonstrated by a sensitivity of 93% and specificity of 88%. The series was also significant in that it included 18 patients with subsequently proven benign disease, so that a major shortcoming of prior studies evaluating radiopharmaceuticals in imaging SPN and lung cancer was overcome; Food and Drug Administration approval of ^{99m}Tc-depreotide for this indication was subsequently granted. Indeed, the only two false-positive determinations in the study were in two patients with coccidioidomycosis and atypical tuberculosis. Interestingly, during follow-up, the lesions of both patients regressed on plain radiography, which suggested that imaging of active but subclinical granulomatous disease with ^{99m}Tc-depreotide led to the false-positive determinations. Furthermore, in this series, nodules smaller than 2 cm were consistently correctly characterized as malignant. The only false-negative study in this series was on a repeated study positive in the region of malignancy; one of the investigators felt the initial study was inadequate based on the unusually high background distribution of activity.

In this relatively small study, pneumothoraces related to CT-guided biopsy developed in four patients with lesions correctly characterized as benign by ^{99m}Tc-depreotide, which further indicates the potential favorable socioeconomic impact of a cost-effective, accurate, noninvasive technique for SPN evaluation. Figures 17.1 and 17.2 are examples of two patients from this study. The area of abnormality on plain film and CT is compared with the corresponding region on ^{99m}Tc-depreotide planar and transaxial SPECT. In Fig. 17.1, a benign process (coccidioidomycosis) is correctly characterized by the absence of tracer uptake. In Fig. 17.2, a malignant process (adenocarcinoma) demonstrates intense tracer uptake.

Further confirmation of this method of differentiating SPNs with a benign cause from malignant SPNs was obtained in a much larger, multiinstitutional trial comprising 114 patients with SPN; the diagnosis of all these patients was subsequently confirmed by tissue analysis. In this series, Blum and colleagues (45) reported a sensitivity for ^{99m}Tc-depreotide scintigraphy of 96.6% and a specificity of 73.1%, figures that compare quite favorably with the figures widely published for FDG-PET (50–52). Malignant lesions correctly identified by ^{99m}Tc-depreotide ranged from 0.8 to 6.0 cm in size, so that the problems involved in detecting small nodules with methods discussed previously were overcome. ^{99m}Tc-Depreotide correctly identified the

only bronchoalveolar carcinoma in this series. FDG-PET in a previous series had failed to identify this tumor type (24). Conceivable explanations include the relatively low metabolic activity of this frequently indolent tumor and the independence of SSTR expression or uptake from cellular metabolism.

Also in this series, small cell and non-small cell cancers, including adenocarcinomas, squamous cell cancers, carcinoid tumors, large cell cancers, and Hodgkin's lymphomas, were correctly characterized. Of the 88 nodules found to be compatible with malignancy on histologic examination, 85 were correctly characterized. The three false-negative determinations involved small ($\leq$ 2 cm) adenocarcinomas. One of these lesions was determined to be a solitary metastasis from a colonic primary tumor, and the ability of depreotide to bind with this type of cytologic process has not been elucidated (53). Conceivably, the small size of the other two lesions could have led to interference by osseous structures in the background, such as ribs.

False-positive results were obtained for 7 of 26 benign lesions, all of which were granulomatous processes. Both FDG-PET and ^{99m}Tc-depreotide SPECT have been shown to yield false-positive results in 15% to 27% of patients with SPN, primarily those with active inflammatory disease, especially granulomatous diseases such as coccidioidomycosis, sarcoidosis, and tuberculosis (54,55). Although the concept of increased metabolic activity in active granulomatous processes accounts for false-positivity in FDG-PET studies, the phenomenon in ^{99m}Tc-depreotide studies is less well characterized. Reports of significant ^{111}In-octreotide activity in Graves' disease, sarcoidosis, and tuberculosis (56) suggest the possibility of somatostatin overexpression or increased binding in activated lymphocytes.

In this multiinstitutional study, the participants were patients considered to be at risk for primary lung cancer, and as such they were at least 35 years of age (57). The single exception was a 33-year-old patient with a 5.5-cm mass, worrisome for malignancy on the basis of size alone. ^{99m}Tc-Depreotide correctly characterized this lesion as benign. Histologically, it proved to be a fibroma. This case is reviewed in Fig. 17.3. Figure 17.4 demonstrates the high-resolution delineation of a non-small cell malignancy from a patient in this multiinstitutional study.

Gambhir et al. (58) have concluded that SPECT with ^{99m}Tc-depreotide would be more favorable than FDG-PET in the evaluation of SPNs over a range of probability of malignancy of 20% to 70% (58). At probabilities below 20%, radiographic follow-up was calculated to be most efficacious. At probabilities above 70%, direct thoracotomy was most cost-effective. In the broad range of probabilities applicable to ^{99m}Tc-depreotide, the annual cost savings in the United States with the utilization of a strategy of CT plus ^{99m}Tc-depreotide in the evaluation of SPN were projected to be $51 million. In this strategy, lesion identification by CT is followed by evaluation with ^{99m}Tc-depreo-

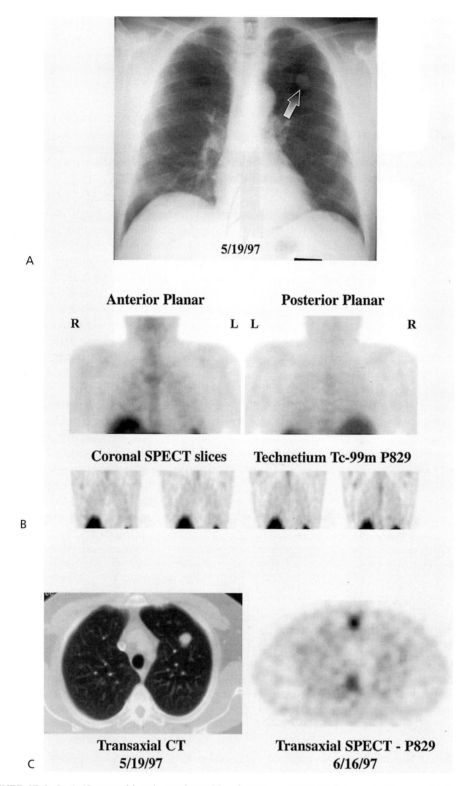

FIGURE 17.1. A: A 42-year-old male smoker with asbestos exposure and a newly diagnosed left upper lobe solitary pulmonary nodule (*SPN*) on plain film. **B:** ^{99m}Tc-Depreotide planar and single-photon emission computed tomography (*SPECT*) images show normal biodistribution and no increased uptake of tracer in the region corresponding to the SPN. **C:** Transaxial computed tomography and corresponding transaxial ^{99m}Tc-depreotide SPECT show no abnormal tracer uptake in the region corresponding to the SPN. Diagnosis: coccidioidomycosis. [From Blum JE, Handmaker H, Rinne NA. The utility of a somatostatin-type receptor binding peptide radiopharmaceutical (P829) in the evaluation of solitary pulmonary nodules. *Chest* 1999;115:224–232, with permission.]

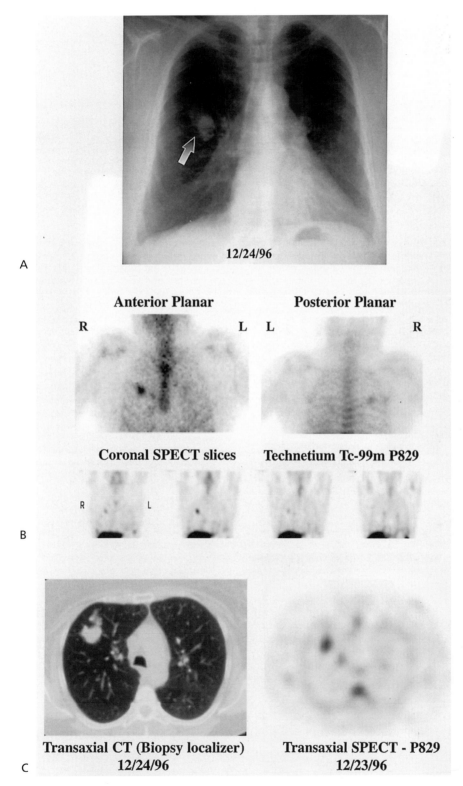

FIGURE 17.2. A: A 57-year-old woman with a significant history of tobacco intake and a newly diagnosed right upper lobe solitary pulmonary nodule (*SPN*) on plain film. **B:** ^{99m}Tc-Depreotide planar single-photon emission computed tomography (*SPECT*) image demonstrates focal tracer uptake in the region corresponding to the SPN. **C:** Transaxial computed tomography and corresponding ^{99m}Tc-depreotide SPECT images demonstrate tracer uptake in the region corresponding to the SPN. Diagnosis: adenocarcinoma of the lung. [From Blum JE, Handmaker H, Rinne NA. The utility of a somatostatin-type receptor binding peptide radiopharmaceutical (P829) in the evaluation of solitary pulmonary nodules. *Chest* 1999;115:224–232, with permission.]

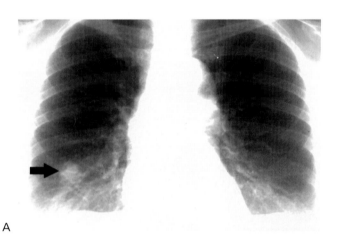

A

B

FIGURE 17.3. **A:** Computed tomographic (*CT*) image of a 33-year-old male nonsmoker with a 5.5-cm mass lesion in the apex of the left lung. **B:** Imaging with ⁹⁹ᵐTc-depreotide reveals no abnormal radiopharmaceutical activity in the region of the CT abnormality, consistent with a benign process. Diagnosis: benign fibroma. [From Blum JE, Handmaker H, Lister-James J, et al. A multicenter trial with a somatostatin analog, ⁹⁹ᵐTc-depreotide, in the evaluation of solitary pulmonary nodules. *Chest* 2000;117:1232–1238, with permission.]

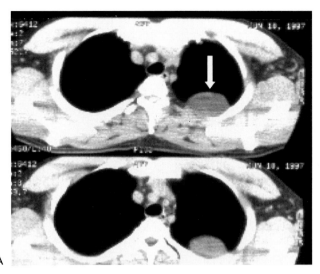

A

Figure 17.4. A: A 77-year-old female smoker with a newly diagnosed 2-cm nodule of the right middle lobe on plain film. **B:** Corresponding transaxial computed tomographic image. **C:** Corresponding transaxial ⁹⁹ᵐTc-depreotide image demonstrates intense tracer uptake. **D:** Corresponding ⁹⁹ᵐTc-depreotide coronal image also demonstrates intense tracer uptake. **E:** Corresponding sagittal ⁹⁹ᵐTc-depreotide single-photon emission computed tomography (*SPECT*) delineation of the presence of a process expressing somatostatin-type receptors. Diagnosis: non-small cell cancer of the lung. [From Blum JE, Handmaker H, Lister-James J, et al. A multicenter trial with a somatostatin analog, ⁹⁹ᵐTc-depreotide, in the evaluation of solitary pulmonary nodules. *Chest* 2000;117: 1232–1238, with permission.]

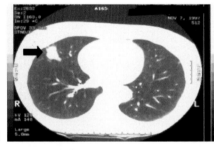

B

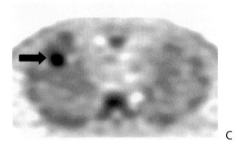

C

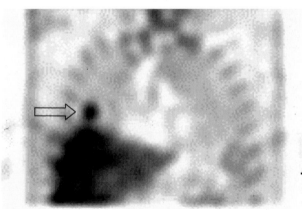

D

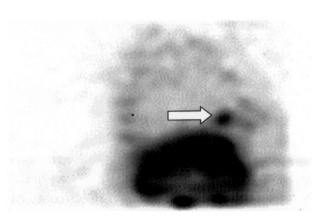

E

tide. The problem of very small nodules identified on CT was addressed by the ELCAP study, which demonstrated the safety of serial CT evaluation in patients with nodules smaller than 1 cm (3). A study combining the now proven improved sensitivity of the ELCAP CT screening (3) with a logical strategy of ^{99m}Tc-depreotide SPECT for lesions larger than 1 cm is currently under way.

No studies have been reported of the use of ^{99m}Tc-depreotide in staging or follow-up after therapeutic interventions in lung cancer patients, and therefore the published reliability of FDG-PET for these purposes makes it the preferred noninvasive technique (59).

The rationale of functional imaging procedures, whether based on the increased glucose metabolism in malignant tissue (FDG-PET) or receptor binding of a small peptide radiopharmaceutical (SPECT with ^{99m}Tc-depreotide), will lead to improved accuracy in the preoperative diagnosis of pulmonary malignancies and will reduce the number of biopsies and surgical resections performed on patients with benign lesions. The concept of exploitation of the biologic rather than the morphologic properties of abnormal tissue for characterization is coming of age. SSTR-binding radiopharmaceuticals offer the additional promise that with a simple exchange of a therapeutic isotope, such as ^{188}Re or ^{90}Y, for the diagnostic radioisotope ^{99m}Tc, internal administration of an agent for targeted therapy could provide an alternative for external beam radiotherapy or surgery for these now largely fatal malignancies.

REFERENCES

1. Travis W, Lubin J, Ries L, et al. United States lung carcinoma incidence trends. *Cancer* 1996;10:151–172.
2. Valanis BG. Epidemiology of lung cancer: a worldwide epidemic. *Semin Oncol Nurs* 1996;12:251–259.
3. Henschke CI, McCauley DI, Yankelevitz DF, et al. Early Lung Cancer Action Project: overall design and findings from baseline screening. *Lancet* 1999;354:99–105.
4. Good C, Wilson T. The solitary circumscribed pulmonary nodule: study of 7 years. *JAMA* 1958;166:210–215.
5. Stoller JK, Ahmad M, Rice TW. Solitary pulmonary nodule. *Cleve Clin J Med* 1988;55:68–74.
6. Siegelman S, Khouri N, Leo F, et al. Solitary pulmonary nodules: CT assessment. *Radiology* 1986;160:307–312.
7. Katz S, Peabody J, Davis E. The solitary pulmonary nodule. *Dis Mon* 1961;7:3–38.
8. Sheiman RG, Fey C, McNicholas M, et al. Possible causes of inconclusive results on CT-guided thoracic and abdominal core biopsies. *AJR Am J Roentgenol* 1998;170:1603–1607.
9. Viggiano R, Swenson S, Rosenew E. Evaluation and management of solitary and multiple pulmonary nodules. *Clin Chest Med* 1992;13:83–94.
10. Dewan N, Shehan C, Reeb S, et al. Likelihood of malignancy in a solitary pulmonary nodule. *Chest* 1997;112;416–422.
11. Garland L. Studies on the accuracy of diagnostic procedures. *Am J Roentgenol* 1959;82:25–53.
12. Yamashita K, Matsunobe S, Tsuda T, et al. Solitary pulmonary nodule: preliminary study of evaluation with incremental dynamic CT. *Radiology* 1995;194:399–405.
13. Swenson S, Brown L, Colby T, et al. Pulmonary nodules: CT evaluation of enhancement with iodinated contrast material. *Radiology* 1995;194:393–398.
14. Frey WC, Arendt WF, Williams JB, et al. Evaluation of the solitary pulmonary nodule by dynamic spiral CT. *Chest* 1998;114 [Suppl]:305S–306S.
15. Rafanan AL, Mehta AC. Role of bronchoscopy in the evaluation of a solitary pulmonary nodule. *Mediguide Pulm Med* 1998;5:1–6.
16. Swensen SJ, Viggiano RW, Midthun DE, et al. Lung nodule enhancement at CT: multicenter study. *Radiology* 2000;214:73–80.
17. Worsley DF, Celler A, Adam MJ, et al. Pulmonary nodules: differential diagnosis using ^{18}F-fluorodeoxyglucose single-photon emission computed tomography. *AJR Am J Roentgenol* 1997;168:771–774.
18. Edwards CL, Hayes RL. Scanning malignant neoplasms with gallium-67. *JAMA* 1970;212:1182.
19. DeLand FM, Sauerbrunn BJL, Boyd C. ^{67}Ga citrate in untreated primary lung cancer: preliminary report of a cooperative group. *J Nucl Med* 1974;15:408.
20. Siemsen JK, Grebe SF, Sargenet EN. Gallium-67 scintigraphy of pulmonary diseases as a complement to radiography. *Radiology* 1976;118:371.
21. Bekerman C, Hoffer PB, Bitran JD. The role of gallium-67 in the clinical evaluation of cancer. *Semin Nucl Med* 1984;4:296–323.
22. Tonami N, Shuke N, Yokoyama K, et al. Thallium-201 single photon emission computed tomography in the evaluation of suspected lung cancer. *J Nucl Med* 1989;30:997–1004.
23. Schweil AM, McKillop JH, Milroy R, et al. Mechanism of ^{201}Tl uptake in tumours. *Eur J Nucl Med* 1989;15:376–379.
24. Higashi K, Nishikawa T, Seki H, et al. Comparison of fluorine-18-FDG PET and thallium-201 SPECT in evaluation of lung cancer. *J Nucl Med* 1998;39:9–15.
25. Sahweil A, Milroy R, McKillop JH. Thallium-201 chloride in the staging of lung cancer. Abstract presented at the British Nuclear Medicine Annual Meeting, London, April 13–15, 1987.
26. Hassan IM, Sahweil A, Constantinides C, et al. Uptake and kinetics of Tc-99m *hexakis* 2-methoxy isobutyl isonitrile in benign and malignant lesions in the lungs. *Clin Nucl Med* 1989;14:333–340.
27. Aktolun C, Bayhan H, Kir M. Clinical experience with Tc-99m MIBI imaging in patients with malignant tumors: preliminary results and comparison with Tl-201. *Clin Nucl Med* 1992;17:171–176.
28. LeBouthillier G, Taillefer R, Lamber R. Detection of primary lung cancer with ^{99m}Tc-sestamibi. *J Nucl Med* 1993;34:140P.
29. Nishiyama Y, Kawasadi Y, Yamamoto Y, et al. Technetium-99m-MIBI and thallium-201 scintigraphy of primary lung cancer. *J Nucl Med* 1997;38:1358–1361.
30. Kashitani N, Makihara S, Maeda T, et al. Thallium-201-chloride and technetium-99m-MIBI SPECT of primary and metastatic lung carcinoma. *Oncol Rep* 1999;6:127–133.
31. Wang H, Maurea S, Mainolfi C, et al. Tc-99m MIBI scintigraphy in patients with lung cancer: comparison with CT and fluorine-18 FDG PET imaging. *Clin Nucl Med* 1997;22:243–249.
32. Hassan IM, Sahweil A, Constantinides C, et al. Uptake and kinetics of Tc-99m *hexakis* 2-methoxy isobutyl isonitrile in benign and malignant lesions in the lungs. *Clin Nucl Med* 1989;14:333–340.
33. Xie C, Li Y, Zhang C, et al. Clinical value of lung scintigraphy with Tc-99m gluconate in distinguishing benign from malignant lung diseases. *Clin Nucl Med* 1992;17:887–893.
34. Vorne M, Sakki S, Jarvi K, et al. Tc-99m glucoheptonate in detection of lung tumors. *J Nucl Med* 1982;23:250–254.

35. Kao CH, Wang SJ, Wey SP, et al. Using technetium-99m(V) dimercaptosuccinic acid to detect malignancies from single solid masses in the lungs. *Eur J Nucl Med* 1992;19:890–893.

36. Hirano T, Otake H, Yoshida I, et al. Primary lung cancer SPECT imaging with pentavalent technetium-99m-DMSA. *J Nucl Med* 1995;36:202–207.

37. Atasever T, Gundogdu C, Vural G, et al. Evaluation of pentavalent Tc-99m DMSA scintigraphy in small cell and nonsmall cell lung cancers. *Nuklearmedizin* 1997;36:223–227.

38. Kwekkeboom DJ, Kho GS, Lamberts SW, et al. The value of octreotide scintigraphy in patients with lung cancer. *Eur J Nucl Med* 1994;21:1106–1113.

39. Reubi J, Torhorst J. The relationship between somatostatin, epidermal growth factors and steroid hormone receptors in breast cancer. *J Med Chem* 1967;19:1133–1141.

40. Raynor K, Reisine T. Somatostatin receptors. *Neurobiology* 1992;16:273–289.

41. Reubi J, Maurer R, von Werder K, et al. Somatostatin receptors in human endocrine tumors. *Cancer Res* 1987;47: 551–558.

42. Virgolini I, Yang Q, Li S, et al. Cross-competition between vasoactive intestinal peptide and somatostatin for binding to tumor cell membrane receptors. *Cancer Res* 1994;54:690–700.

43. Blum JE, Handmaker H, Rinne NA. The utility of a somatostatin-type receptor binding peptide radiopharmaceutical (P829) in the evaluation of solitary pulmonary nodules. *Chest* 1999;115: 224–232.

44. Fujita T, Yamaji Y, Sato M, et al. Gene expression of somatostatin receptor subtypes, SSTR1 and SSTR2, in human lung cancer cell lines. *Life Sci* 1994;55:1797–1806.

45. Blum JE, Handmaker H, Lister-James J, et al. A multicenter trial with a somatostatin anal^{og}, 99m*Tc-depreotide (NeoTect), in the evaluation of solitary pulmonary nodules.* Chest 2000;117: 1232–1238.

46. Vallabhajosula S, Moyer BR, Lister-James J, et al. Preclinical evaluation of technetium-99m-labeled somatostatin receptor-binding peptides. *J Nucl Med* 1996;37:1016–1022.

47. Virgolini I, Pangerl T, Bischof C, et al. Somatostatin receptor expression in human tissues: a prediction for diagnosis and treatment of cancer? *Eur J Clin Invest* 1997;27:645–647.

48. Handmaker H, Mohler K, Dann R, et al. Oncoscintigraphy of neuroendocrine and non-neuroendocrine tumors with a novel ssr binding peptide, technetium Tc-99m P829: preliminary experience in 39 patients. *Clin Nucl Med* 1997;22:350(abst).

49. Virgolini I, Leimer M, Handmaker H, et al. Somatostatin receptor subtype specificity and *in vivo* binding of a novel tumor tracer, ^{99m}Tc-P829. *Cancer Res* 1998;58:1850–1859.

50. Patz EF, Lowe VJ, Hoffman JM, et al. Focal pulmonary abnormalities: evaluation with F-18 fluorodeoxyglucose PET scanning. *Radiology* 1993;188:487–490.

51. Gupta NC, Maloof J, Gunel E. Probability of malignancy in solitary pulmonary nodules using fluorine-18-FDG and PET. *J Nucl Med* 1996;37:943–948.

52. Lowe V, Fletcher J, Gobar L, et al. Prospective investigation of positron emission tomography in lung nodules. *J Clin Oncol* 1998;16:1075–1084.

53. Reubi JC, Krenning E, Lamberts SWJ, et al. *In vitro* detection of somatostatin receptors in human tumors. *Metabolism* 1992;41 [Suppl 2]:104–110.

54. Lewis PJ, Salama A. Uptake of fluorine-18-fluorodeoxyglucose in sarcoidosis. *J Nucl Med* 1994;35:1647–1649.

55. Strauss LG. Fluorine-18 deoxyglucose and false-positive results: a major problem in the diagnostic of oncological patients. *Eur J Nucl Med* 1996;23:1409–1415.

56. Krenning E, Kwekkeboom D, Bakker W. Somatostatin receptor scintigraphy with [^{111}In-DPTA-D-Phe^{1}]- and [^{123}I-Tyr^{3}]-octreotide: the Rotterdam experience with more than 1,000 patients. *Eur J Nucl Med* 1993;20:716–731.

57. Cummings S, Lillington G, Richard R. Estimating the probability of malignancy in solitary pulmonary nodules. *Am Rev Respir Dis* 1986;134:449–452.

58. Gambhir S, Shepherd J, Handmaker H, et al. Cost-effective analysis modeling for the role of a somatostatin analog—Tc99m depreotide (NeoTect)—scintigraphy in the evaluation of patients with a solitary pulmonary nodule. *J Nucl Med* 1999; 40[Suppl]: 57 P.

59. Wahl RL, Quint LE, Greenough RL, et al. Staging of mediastinal non-small cell lung cancer with FDG PET, CT, and fusion images: preliminary prospective evaluation. *Radiology* 1994;191:371–377.

18

SCINTIMAMMOGRAPHY WITH SINGLE-PHOTON TRACERS

JOHN R. BUSCOMBE
IRAJ KHALKHALI

BREAST CANCER

The incidence of breast cancer has slowly risen during the past 40 years, and in most developed nations, breast cancer now kills more women than any other form of cancer (1). Rates vary with culture and geographic location. Among white Americans, the incidence is approximately 89/100,000 per year, whereas in the United Kingdom, it is lower, at 56/100,000 per year. Even in the countries with the lowest incidence, the lifetime risk for breast cancer is about 1 in 12. It is predicted that in the year 2000, 1.4 million new cases of breast cancer will be diagnosed worldwide (2).

The incidence of the disease in women under 40 appears to have increased. It is not apparent whether this increase represents a real change or is related to earlier discovery by patients as a result of increased awareness.

A genetic component is significant in breast cancer—that is, the risk for breast cancer is increased in women whose mother or sister has been affected. Women with the genes *BRCA1* and *BRCA2* appear to be at a higher risk. These genes are not specific for breast cancer; women carrying them are also at higher risk for other forms of cancer, such as cancer of the ovary. In many families of patients with breast cancer who do not carry the genes, the incidence is nonetheless much greater than in the general population.

The disease itself is complex. Several histologic varieties have been described. Invasive ductal breast cancer tends to be more aggressive than other types and occurs in a younger age group. The prognosis may be linked to various factors, such as nuclear pleomorphism or the Ki-67 status, but the two most important prognostic factors are the size of the tumor at diagnosis (those smaller than 10 mm having a

good prognosis) and the presence or absence of axillary lymph node involvement. The prognosis is best if a patient with minimal disease seeks treatment early.

It may not be possible for a patient or even a trained surgeon to palpate a very small tumor. Therefore, physicians rely on imaging to detect small, possibly curable cancers. At present, the imaging method of choice is mammography. The evidence is clear that during 10 to 15 years, this technique has resulted in as much as a 20% decrease in deaths from breast cancer (3).

Because early diagnosis and accurate staging are essential, an accurate and cost-effective imaging method is needed for patients with breast cancer.

CONVENTIONAL IMAGING OF THE BREAST

Mammography is the principal imaging method to detect breast cancer. It is optimized to image soft-tissue densities. If compression is inadequate, particularly of a breast that is very glandular, breast masses may not be recognized, as they sometimes overlie one another. Two views of each breast are normally obtained, a craniocaudal view and a mediolateral view.

The interpretation of the mammogram requires skill. The results of between 4% and 40% of mammograms are reported as normal in the presence of cancer (4). Many factors affect these figures. The major factor is the type of patients studied; this has varied greatly among trials. The best figures are derived from large groups of patients seen in screening programs. Problems arise when denser breasts are imaged. In a recent series of women with palpable breast masses who were subsequently found to have cancer, the results of 45% of the mammograms were reported as negative or equivocal for cancer (5).

Although breast cancer is less common in younger patients, it remains the major cause of cancer death in younger women, and the incidence of breast cancer appears to be rising in younger women. The main problem

J. R. Buscombe: Department of Nuclear Medicine, Royal Free Hospital, London NW 2 QG, United Kingdom.

I. Khalkhali: Department of Radiology, University of California, Los Angeles School of Medicine, Los Angeles, California 90095; Breast Imaging and Outpatient Radiology Services, Harbor-UCLA Medical Center, Torrance, California 90502.

in interpreting mammograms in younger women is that breast tissue is normally dense at this age. Also, some evidence suggests that the development of breast cancer is more likely in women with denser breasts (6).

The site of the cancer can lead to additional problems. Most missed tumors are deep. Thirty-seven percent of subareolar tumors may be missed. In addition, scarring from a previous biopsy may make it more difficult to identify small tumors (7).

The size of any cancer is critical, particularly noncalcified cancers, in which the diagnosis depends on the interpretation of subtle changes in architecture (8). This has been improved by the use of digital mammography. In the absence of calcification, however, identifying small (< 5 mm) tumors remains a problem. Some cancer types, such as lobular cancer, do not always contain calcium and do not cause classic architectural changes in the breast. Up to 22% of lobular cancers may be mammographically silent (9).

Having two readers interpret a mammogram has been shown to reduce the rate of false-negative results of mammography by half, but it leads to further expense (10). The use of objective reporting regimes, such as the American College of Radiologists breast imaging reporting and data system (BI-RADS), has been proposed as a method to provide more consistency and help reduce the rate of false-negative studies.

In a recent review of 2,600 screening mammograms, 302 cancers were subsequently identified by histologic analysis. Of these, between 21% and 27% were reported as normal or benign by different radiologists (11). Only 21% were reported as positive for cancer, the majority being reported as equivocal. The level of agreement on reporting was good, however, with agreements in the range of 78% to 90%. The fact that cancers were missed consistently by a number of radiologists would suggest that the failure to detect about 15% of cancers despite double reads of mammograms was reader-, not method-, dependent.

It is often necessary to act on the report of an equivocal result as though it were positive for cancer, so that a significant number of patients with "positive" studies undergo further investigation even though they do not have cancer. This reduces the positive predictive value (PPV) of mammography. In a study by Kerlikowske et al. (11), the PPV for two readers was only 12.6%; most reports described findings as "equivocal, requiring further interpretation."

It has been recognized for many years that in younger women, or women with denser breasts, the PPV of mammography is likely to be lower than in older women, who tend to have fatty breasts. The reported PPV of mammography for women under 40 is 12%; for women over 79, it is 46%. The PPV does not change abruptly with menopause but improves gradually with age (12). It is not clear how these figures will change as more patients take perimenopausal hormone (estrogen) replacement therapy. It is expected that the PPV for women in their fifties and sixties on hormone replacement therapy will be similar to that for younger women. This is of some concern because women in their fifties and sixties taking hormone replacement therapy are included in European national screening programs. In most of these European programs, approximately 25% of women have dense breasts on mammography (13).

Breast density appears to be the major factor affecting the PPV of mammography. The use of new and better film formulations and the application of zoom and digitalization have improved the quality of mammography, with a subsequent increase in PPV. In Nijmegen, The Netherlands, in 1982, the PPV of standard mammography in women with dense breasts was 29%; in women with fatty breasts, it was 52%. With the use of newer techniques of mammography 15 years later, the PPV of mammography in dense breasts is 59%, and in fatty breasts the PPV has improved to 72% (14).

Although the accuracy of performing mammography and reporting results has improved significantly, especially with the use of optimal imaging methods, double reading, and objective reporting criteria, the results of a significant number of studies are still reported as negative in the presence of cancer; likewise, in younger women, a positive result may not mean cancer. To help improve the certainty of the results of breast imaging, new methods of diagnosing breast cancer to complement mammography are required.

ULTRASONOGRAPHY

Breast ultrasonography has proved useful as an additional test when the results of mammography are doubtful. Doppler techniques, based on changes in blood flow caused by tumor angiogenesis, help to identify malignancy. A sensitivity of 82% and a specificity of 81% were recorded in a group of patients with palpable masses (15). Clearly identifying a lesion as cancer may be difficult with the use of ultrasonography alone. In a group of 18 patients with cancer but clinically benign breast masses, two masses were identified by ultrasonography as cancer, one was reported as normal, and the remaining 15 were reported as indeterminate (16). Unfortunately, ultrasonography appears to be no more accurate than mammography in cases in which mammography is problematic. Tumor pathology affected the sensitivity of ultrasonography in 63 patients with lobular breast cancer; the sensitivity of ultrasonography was 78%, and for mammography it was 81% (17). In patients with dense breasts, in whom mammography is least accurate, no additional information regarding the presence of cancer could be gained by adding ultrasonographic examination to mammography (18). Ultrasound is operator-dependent, so that it is difficult to conduct blinded trials.

MAGNETIC RESONANCE IMAGING

The use of magnetic resonance imaging (MRI) of the breast has been restricted by the high capital cost of the equipment required and by the lack of a generally accepted protocol for imaging the breast and interpreting results.

The best results appear to be obtained with the use of a special breast coil and Gd-DTPA (gadolinium-diaminetriamine pentaacetic acid) contrast (19). Although imaging can be rapid, extensive analysis of the data is required, as the rate of Gd-DTPA uptake and washout is calculated to improve the specificity of the technique. Results can be impressive. Of 239 breast cancers imaged with MRI, 200 were identified. It was noted, however, that among the cancers not identified there were eight ductal carcinomas *in situ*, which suggests that MRI is effective for mass lesions (20). Many images must be obtained in three different planes. Up to 300 individual images may be generated. These factors increase both the technical requirements and the time radiologist must put in. Until standard imaging protocols can be agreed on for the instruments of the various manufacturers, it will be difficult to set standards for image quality and reporting. In the best hands, breast MRI can have a sensitivity of more than 90%, but specificity may be much lower (21). It has been noted that the appearance of fibroadenomas varies greatly. For example, in one series of 21 patients, 11 of whom had adenomas, gadolinium enhancement was good, similar to that seen in cancer, but in nine cases no enhancement change was noted (22). In elderly patients, enhancement was less common. For them, however, mammography is more accurate, and therefore MRI is not normally indicated.

SCINTIMAMMOGRAPHY WITH ^{99m}TC-MIBI

^{99m}Tc-MIBI (methoxyisobutylisonitrile) was developed from a class of pharmaceuticals used primarily for myocardial perfusion mapping. As ^{201}Tl could be used to image tumors, it was suggested that the uptake of ^{99m}Tc-MIBI might be increased in cancer cells relative to surrounding normal tissues because of the differential metabolic activity in cancer and normal cells. *In vitro* tests in cancer cell lines confirmed that the uptake of ^{99m}Tc-MIBI is similar to, and often better than, that of ^{201}Tl. Breast imaging was also performed, but the results were poor because small breast tumors could not be seen when overlying the heart and liver, in both of which activity was significantly greater than in the nearby tumor. Successful imaging was achieved by placing the patient in a prone position on a couch with a cutout, with the breast suspended and thereby separated from the intrathoracic and intraabdom-

inal regions of activity. The contralateral breast was compressed against the imaging board by the patient's weight and was therefore removed from the field of view (23) (Fig. 18.1).

In the first reported series in which ^{99m}Tc-MIBI was used, the sensitivity and specificity were 80% and 90%, respectively, a significant improvement in comparison with the results of previous, supine studies (24) (Table 18.1). The results of this study demonstrated a high sensitivity and specificity for the method in identifying breast cancer. Only two small cancers were missed, both of which were invasive ductal carcinomas smaller than 1 cm; this might have been related to the resolution of the gamma camera, although six cancers smaller than 1 cm were identified. Prior mammography was an entry criterion, and all scans were read with clinical knowledge of the mammography results. A significant proportion of women had dense breasts on mammography, but the results were not compared.

A similar study was performed in Canada in 65 women (25). All mammograms were reported with clinical knowledge, and scintimammography was reported blind. In 47 of these women, breast cancer was subsequently proven on biopsy. In addition, the authors reported imaging the axillary lymph nodes (Table 18.2). The four false-negative cases in this study were all ductal carcinomas smaller 0.7 cm; one was microscopic and found during surgery serendipitously.

Most of these trials, however, comprise tightly controlled groups of patients with a single site and have a single reader. More useful information on the technique is gleaned from a multicenter trial. The largest of these was performed in the United States and enrolled 673 patient, 286 of whom had palpable masses (26). The results of this study (Table 18.3) confirmed that the technique can be used at multiple centers. Consistent results were obtained even when many people performed the procedures and reported the results blinded to clinical knowledge.

A further interesting detail emerged when the effect of breast density on the results of the study was analyzed. The overall results were divided according to whether the images were of fatty or dense tissue (26). The results were similar. Unlike both ultrasonography and mammography, scintimammography is not affected by breast density, and its accuracy is the same in patients with dense breasts as in those with fatty breasts (Table 18.4).

Scintimammography is a robust technique that can be used successfully by centers with training. Results differ little among centers, which is not the case with other breast-imaging techniques, such as ultrasonography and MRI. The results of blind reporting of scintimammography indicate consistent interpretation. When the readers of 70 scintimmamograms were blinded, interobserver agreement was 97% (κ = .90) (27). All these features indi-

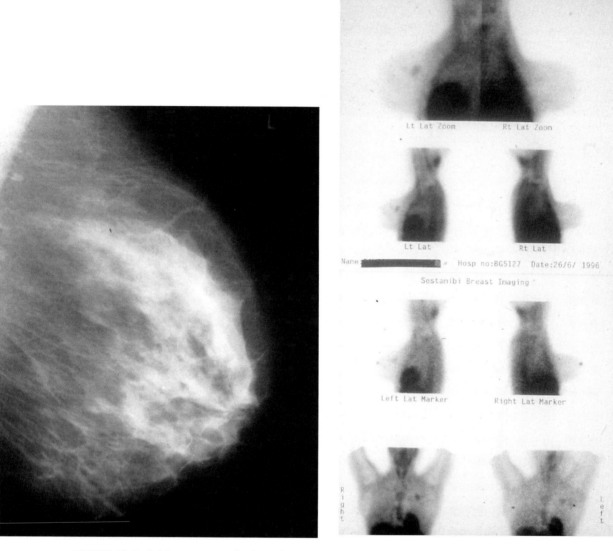

A   B

FIGURE 18.1. **A:** Mammogram of a dense breast in a 39-year-old woman with "lumpy" breasts. Results of previous biopsies and mammograms were all negative. **B:** Scintimammography with ^{99m}Tc-MIBI (methoxyisobutylisonitrile) identifies a single lesion in the left breast on the left lateral and anterior view. Ultrasonographically directed core biopsy of this area identified a 10-mm invasive ductal carcinoma.

TABLE 18.1. RESULTS IN 100 WOMEN UNDERGOING SCINTIMAMMOGRAPHY

	Sensitivity	Specificity	PPV	NPV
scintimammography	93.7%	87.8%	76.9%	97%

PPV, positive predictive value; NPV, negative predictive value.
From Khalkhali I, Cutrone J, Mena I, et al. Technetium-99m sestamibi scintimammography of breast lesions: clinical and pathological follow-up. *J Nucl Med* 1995;36:1784–1789, with permission.

TABLE 18.2. RESULTS OF SCINTIMAMMOGRAPHY IN IMAGING PRIMARY BREAST CANCER AND AXILLARY LYMPH NODES IN 64 WOMEN

Site of disease	Sensitivity (%)	Specificity (%)
Breast	91.5	94.5
Axillary lymph nodes	84.2	90.9

From Taillefer R, Robidoux A, Lambert R, et al. Technetium-99m sestamibi prone scintimammography to detect primary breast cancer and axillary lymph node involvement. *J Nucl Med* 1995;36:1758–1765, with permission.

TABLE 18.3. RESULTS OF U.S. MULTICENTER TRIAL OF 673 PATIENTS

	Sensitivity (%)	Specificity (%)	PPV (%)	NPV (%)
Palpable	95	74	77	94
Nonpalpable	72	86	70	87
Overall	85	81	74	90

From Khalkhali I, Villanueva-Meyer S, Edell L, et al. Diagnostic accuracy of Tc-99m sestaMIBI breast imaging in breast cancer detection. *J Nucl Med* 1996;37:74P, with permission.

TABLE 18.4. IMPACT OF BREAST DENSITY ON ACCURACY OF SCINTIMAMMOGRAPHY IN 673 PATIENTS

Breast type	Sensitivity (%)	Specificity (%)	PPV (%)	NPV (%)
Fatty	84	82	76	88
Dense	86	80	72	91

PPV, positive predictive value; NPV, negative predictive value. From Khalkhali I, Villanueva-Meyer S, Edell L, et al. Diagnostic accuracy of Tc-99m sestaMIBI breast imaging in breast cancer detection. *J Nucl Med* 1996;37:74P, with permission.

cate that scintimammography is a reliable technique that can be used widely in patients with nondiagnostic results on mammography.

OTHER RADIOPHARMACEUTICALS

Bone-seeking Radiopharmaceuticals

It may be possible to identify primary breast tumors with the use of ^{99m}Tc-diphosphonate. Accumulation of tracer in the 3-hour bone image was thought to be the result of microcalcification, local breast edema, or tumor necrosis. It was evaluated if early (10 to 15 minutes after injection of ^{99m}Tc-diphosphonate) imaging of the breast was effective. Good results have been claimed for the method. It may be as sensitive as ^{99m}Tc-MIBI scintimammography in finding cancers larger than 10 mm (28).

The patients selected for this study all had known carcinoma of the breast, and as a consequence they had a 100%

pretest probability for a breast neoplasm. This was therefore not a fair test of the method. It is not known how the method would perform in a group of patients suspected of having cancer but with a lower pretest probability.

The relative activity of ^{99m}Tc-diphosphonate in tumor in comparison with surrounding tissue appears to be less than that of ^{99m}Tc-MIBI (29). This method may be useful in patients with known breast cancer when it is necessary to determine the extent of disease. It can be performed as part of a bone scan with little additional cost.

[99m]Tc-Tetrofosmin

This radiopharmaceutical is similar to ^{99m}Tc-MIBI. It was also developed initially for myocardial perfusion imaging. In a series of patients with primary breast cancer, initial results were similar to those with ^{99m}Tc-MIBI (30), although uptake was lower than that of ^{99m}Tc-MIBI in breast cancer cell cultures (31).

Most of the work performed so far has assessed sensitivity and specificity in groups of highly selected patients. Formal phase III trials have not yet been undertaken. It is also not known whether the factors affecting uptake and efflux of ^{99m}Tc-MIBI also affect ^{99m}Tc-tetrofosmin. Further laboratory and clinical data are needed before the routine use of ^{99m}Tc-tetrofosmin can be recommended.

COMPARISON OF SCINTIMAMMOGRAPHY AND MAMMOGRAPHY

The comparison of radiographic mammography and ^{99m}Tc-MIBI scintimammography is complex because the findings of radiographic mammography are often used to select the patients to be studied with scintimammography. If a study uses an equivocal or nondiagnostic radiographic mammogram as an entry criterion, it will preselect those patients in whom radiographic mammography is at a disadvantage. In one study, the patients were selected more objectively based on criteria of symptomatic breasts and no previous imaging. The patients underwent mammography, scintimammography, and gadolinium-enhanced breast MRI before any suspect areas were removed by biopsy. The sensitivity of the two methods was similar, but the specificity of ^{99m}Tc-MIBI scintimammography was higher (21) (Figs. 18.2 and 18.3; Table 18.5).

A study from Israel compared scintimammography and mammography in 61 palpable tumors and 24 nonpalpable tumors. The nonpalpable tumors were smaller than the palpable tumors; their mean size was 1.34 cm, compared with 2.57 cm for the palpable tumors (32). The results for scintimammography are presented in Table 18.6 and for mammography in Table 18.7.

These results appear not to be as good as those obtained in the studies of Khalkhali et al. (26) and Taillefer et al. (25).

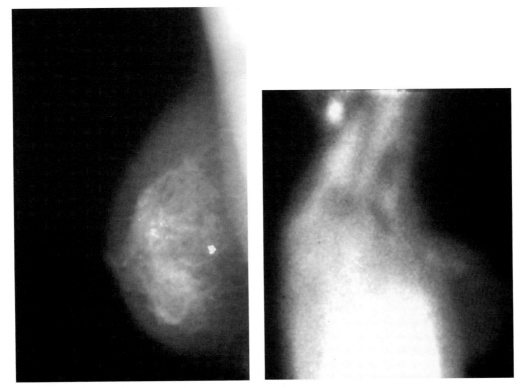

FIGURE 18.2. A 67-year-old woman with a breast mass. **Left:** Mammography shows a small but dense breast not thought to harbor cancer. **Right:** Scintigraphy with ^{99m}Tc-MIBI (methoxy-isobutylisonitrile) demonstrates a multicentric invasive ductal carcinoma.

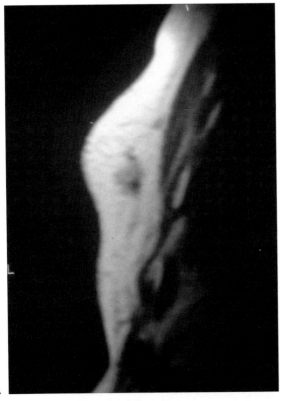

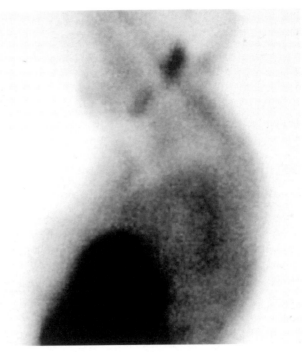

A

B

FIGURE 18.3. A 70-year-old woman with a left-sided breast lump at presentation. **A:** Unenhanced magnetic resonance imaging (T$_1$-weighted) shows an area of low signal corresponding to the lump. **B:** The ^{99m}Tc-MIBI (methoxyisobutylisonitrile) scan shows uptake of tracer in a 14-mm invasive ductal carcinoma.

TABLE 18.5. SENSITIVITY AND SPECIFICITY OF THREE DIFFERENT BREAST IMAGING TECHNIQUES IN 43 PATIENTS WITH PALPABLE BREAST MASSES THOUGHT CLINICALLY TO BE BREAST CANCER

Method	Sensitivity (%)	Specificity (%)
Scintimammography	91	62
Mammography	95	10
MRI	91	15

MRI, magnetic resonance imaging.
From Palmedo H, Grunwald F, Bender H, et al. Scintimammography with technetium-99m methoxyisobutylisonitrile: comparison with mammography and magnetic resonance imaging. *Eur J Nucl Med* 1996;23:940–946, with permission.

Unfortunately, because not all patients underwent both studies, the validity of the comparison is reduced. In patients with palpable tumors, the accuracy of scintimammography was much higher than that of mammography. This is even more surprising because the readers of all the mammograms had full clinical knowledge, whereas the readers of the scintimammograms were all blinded. Selection of the patients with nonpalpable lesions was based on suspect findings on mammography, which further skewed the results. In a comparison of the two techniques, careful assessment of patient selection and the methodology is necessary.

The authors did note that scintimammography was able to differentiate cancerous from noncancerous lesions in those patients whose results on mammography were described as indeterminate. Similar results were obtained by Khalkhali et al. (26); cancer was correctly identified in 32 of the 150 patients with very dense breast or uninterpretable mammograms.

It is clear then that scintimammography is able to demonstrate the presence or absence of cancer when results of the radiographic mammogram is indeterminate. In a report from the United Kingdom, the authors studied 74 lesions suspected of being breast cancer for which the mammogram was reported as either indeterminate, equivocal, or at variance with clinical findings (33). The nature of any abnormality on either mammography or scintimammography was confirmed

TABLE 18.6. RESULTS OF SCINTIMAMMOGRAPHY IN 85 WOMEN WITH 30 PALPABLE MASSES AND 55 NONPALPABLE MASSES SUSPECTED OF BEING BREAST CANCER

Tumor	Sensitivity (%)	Specificity (%)	PPV (%)	NPV (%)
Palpable	95.1	75	89.4	76.3
Nonpalpable	54.2	93.6	86.7	72.5

PPV, positive predictive value; NPV, negative predictive value.
From Mekhmandarov S, Sandbank J, Cohen M, et al. Technetium-99m-MIBI scintimammography in palpable and nonpalpable breast lesions. *J Nucl Med* 1998;39:86–91, with permission.

TABLE 18.7. RESULTS OF MAMMOGRAPHY IN 82 WOMEN WITH 32 PALPABLE MASSES AND 50 NONPALPABLE MASSES SUSPECTED OF BEING BREAST CANCERS

Tumor	Sensitivity (%)	Specificity (%)	PPV (%)	NPV (%)
Palpable	90.1	57.1	85.9	66.6
Nonpalpable	95.5	32.1	52.5	90.0

PPV, positive predictive value; NPV, negative predictive value.
From Mekhmandarov S, Sandbank J, Cohen M, et al. Technetium-99m-MIBI scintimammography in palpable and nonpalpable breast lesions. *J Nucl Med* 1998;39:86–91, with permission.

by surgical biopsy within 14 days of the imaging. The sensitivity of scintimammography, with the readers blinded, was 89%, and it was 70% for mammography, with the readers having full knowledge of the clinical features. Specificities of the two methods were similar. This again demonstrates that scintimammography provides unique and accurate information regarding the presence and site of breast cancer in patients with indeterminate or uncertain results on mammography.

The authors graded the reports according to five levels of certainty: grade 1, definitely normal; grade 2, possibly normal; grade 3, equivocal; grade 4, probably cancer; grade 5, definitely cancer. Only grades 1 and 5 indicate some degree of certainty; the remaining grades indicate a degree of uncertainty. With radiographic mammography, 42% of results were graded 2 to 4. With scintimammography, the reports of only 20% of the patients were graded 2 to 4. Not only were the results of scintimammography more accurate than mammography, but the decision of whether or not cancer was present was made with a greater degree of certainty.

Complementary, Not Competitive

The above data provide clear evidence that ^{99m}Tc-MIBI scintimammography is useful in identifying breast cancer in patients with unclear results on radiographic mammography or ultrasonography. Although the number of such patients is small (about 20% of those considered for surgery), it does include many who are premenopausal, the very group in which the results mammography are difficult to interpret because of the poor PPV associated with dense breasts (34). In addition, this group has had the largest increase in incidence of breast cancer. Being able to identify breast cancer accurately and determine its extent is most useful. Women who take estrogen-based hormone replacement therapy or herbal medicines (which contain estrogen-like substances) are more likely to have dense breasts, even in their fifties and sixties. This is the age group toward which most mammographic screening programs are targeted.

The breast may have been compromised by previous surgery or placement of a prosthesis, both of which make the usual triple assessment by physical examination, radiographic mammography, and ultrasonography difficult. The specificity of ^{99m}Tc-MIBI is not 100%. False-positive rates as high as 40% have been recorded, although most centers achieve a specificity of at least 80% (8,10,11). False-positive uptake can be seen in fibrocystic disease and fibroadenomas with epithelial hyperplasia and also in tumor phyllodes (33).

Although comparisons of the two methods are published, in clinical practice, a combination of mammography and scintimammography often results in an improved accuracy, better than that of either method alone.

It is possible to predict the effective use of the technique with use of a receiver–operator characteristic (ROC) curve. In a study of 120 patients with suspected primary breast cancer whose radiographic mammograms were difficult to interpret, five degrees of certainty were used to identify ROC curves for mammography, scintimammography, and a combination thereof. The sensitivity of a combination of radiographic mammography and scintimammography was 98%, significantly better than that of either mammography or scintimammography alone ($p < .05$). This was achieved while a specificity of 80% was maintained (35). Although these data provide only a mathematical model, they show that adding scintimammography in cases in which the results of mammography are doubtful significantly affects the ability to detect breast cancer.

In Spain, a group looked at the additional use of ^{99m}Tc-MIBI scintimammography in patients with nonpalpable breast lesions (36). The initial mammograms were divided into three groups. In one group, the mammograms of 46 patients indicated a high probability of malignancy; 36 of these patients had histologically confirmed cancer, and the remaining 10 had benign disease. The results of scintimammography were positive in 30 of the patients with cancer, and three of the studies were false-positive. In another group, 31 mammograms indicated an intermediate probability of cancer; four of these patients had cancer, and all were identified by ^{99m}Tc-MIBI. Finally, there was one cancer, found only on ^{99m}Tc-MIBI imaging, in the group whose mammograms indicated a low probability of cancer (Table 18.8). With a combination of mammography and ^{99m}Tc-scintimammography, all the breast cancers were correctly identified, whereas with mammography alone, five of 40 patients (12.5%) would have been missed. (In Europe, a mammogram that indicates a medium risk does not automatically qualify the patient for a breast biopsy.)

When both mathematical models and patient data are analyzed, it is clear that scintimammography provides useful adjunctive information in the diagnosis of breast cancer and should be used when the results of mammography are equivocal or negative and at variance with the clinical findings.

CLINICAL USES OF SCINTIMAMMOGRAPHY
General

In recent years, because of the advent of fine-needle aspiration cytology and the histopathologic sampling of nonpalpable breast lesions with the use of stereotactic techniques, the diagnosis and management of breast lesions have been dramatically altered (37). Part of the alteration depends solely on institutional experience. For instance, if an experienced cytopathologist is available, many groups opt to incorporate this useful technique in their practice for breast diagnosis. Generally, clinicians have different guidelines for the workup and management of "palpable" and "nonpalpable" breast lesions.

Management of Palpable Breast Lesions

The palpable breast mass is one of the most common diagnostic challenges confronting clinicians. The goal is to determine appropriate therapy based on the "triple test" of physical examination, mammography, and fine-needle aspiration cytology. When the mass is malignant, the patient is offered therapeutic options and appropriate therapy begins. The problem arises when the fine-needle aspiration specimen is nondiagnostic or hypocellular. The subsequent course depends on institutional experience. If the results of fine-needle aspiration are not diagnostic, a core needle biopsy can be performed to obtain tissue. The negative predictive value of negative results on all three basic component tests is 99% (38).

Mammography and ultrasonography have limitations in the dense breast, and some uncertainty exists in reporting the results of anatomic breast imaging. Other imaging studies are available to prevent unnecessary excisional biopsy.

TABLE 18.8. NUMBER OF BREAST CANCERS FOUND BY SCINTIMAMMOGRAPHY DEPENDING ON THE RESULTS OF MAMMOGRAPHY

Probability of cancer on mammogram	No. of patients in each group	No. of cancers present in each group	No. of cancers seen on scintimammography
Low	20	1	1
Medium	31	4	4
High	46	36	30

From Prats E, Aisa F, Abas MD, et al. Mammography and Tc-99m MIBI scintimammography in suspected breast cancer. J Nucl Med 1999;40:296–301, with permission.

One such method is ultrasonography. Ultrasonography can differentiate solid masses from cysts with a high degree of accuracy. Although it cannot categorize lesions as benign or malignant, classic cysts are virtually always benign and do not mandate surgery or cytologic examination of an aspirate. Fine-needle aspiration can alleviate symptoms caused by cysts. With ultrasonographic guidance, complete aspiration is possible. When the lesion is clearly seen, ultrasonography can guide the biopsy device to the area of interest and increase the yield.

Ultrasonography has been used to guide the placement of small-gauge needles for fine-needle aspiration, large needles for core biopsy, vacuum-assisted core biopsy devices, radiocolloid for sentinel lymph node biopsy, and to guide wire localization for subsequent excisional biopsy.

Although it is less commonly performed at present, pneumocystography has found a role in the management of breast cysts. Pneumocystography is performed as an adjunct to breast cyst aspiration. Use of this technique decreases the incidence of cyst recurrence and rules out the presence of an associated solid component in the wall of a questionable cyst, which occurs in 0.2% of breast cysts. The incidence of recurrence is markedly decreased when cysts are insufflated with air after aspiration (37).

Scintimammography with ^{99m}Tc-MIBI can be useful in the further evaluation of patients with palpable masses. Although establishing a tissue diagnosis of a palpable mass is a straightforward exercise, scintimammography is useful in assessing the remainder of breast tissue when mammography is of limited use, as in cases of dense breast parenchyma and implants. In addition, given the high reported sensitivity of scintimammography, even if the palpable abnormality is malignant, scintimammography helps in preoperative planning. In this setting, scintimammography may identify multifocal or multicentric carcinoma and provide some indication of the axillary node status (Figs. 18.4 and 18.5).

In cases of biopsy-proven malignancy, scintimammography has been used to assess the axillary nodal basin for metastatic disease. Waxman (39) found a sensitivity and specificity of 79% and 80%, respectively, in predicting the

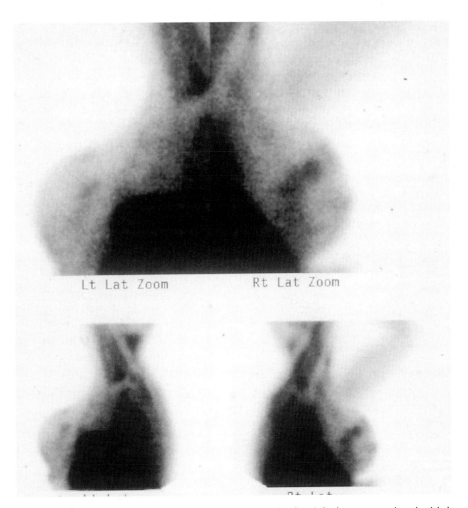

FIGURE 18.4. Patient with a large, palpable carcinoma in the right breast associated with lymphedema and axillary swelling. ^{99m}Tc-MIBI (methoxyisobutylisonitrile) scintimammography identifies extensive, multicentric cancer throughout the right breast and an unexpected second primary in the left breast. This tumor was not seen on mammography.

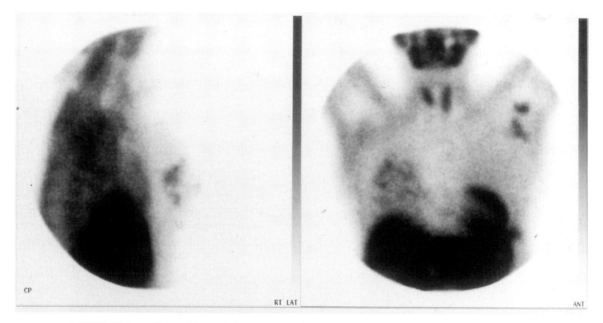

FIGURE 18.5. Patient with small breasts and a palpable mass on the right side suspected of being cancerous. Scintimammography with ^{99m}Tc-MIBI (methoxyisobutylisonitrile) identified a large mass with axillary uptake, proven on biopsy to be a papillary carcinoma. However, close inspection of the anterior image revealed uptake by the nipple and faint uptake in the axilla. Biopsy revealed a coexistent invasive ductal carcinoma with lymph node metastases.

presence of nodal metastases. Although the results of preliminary studies with MIBI and other agents are encouraging, this noninvasive means of surveying the axilla does not replace nodal dissection at the present time.

Scintimammography is also helpful in cases of an isolated axillary mass. At the Harbor-University of California Medical Center in Los Angeles, a woman had an isolated axillary mass, normal findings on mammography, and no palpable breast abnormality at presentation. Detection of an abnormal focus of uptake on scintimammography allowed wire localization with a cobalt 57-tipped needle and excisional biopsy, based on which the diagnosis of primary breast carcinoma was made.

Nonpalpable Lesions

With screening through routine mammography now more prevalent, particularly in northern Europe (Sweden, The Netherlands, Norway, the United Kingdom, and now Ireland have publicly funded national screening programs), clinicians today encounter a greater number of nonpalpable breast lesions. These abnormalities are seen as a mass, a cluster of microcalcifications, asymmetric density, or architectural distortion. The lesions can be sampled for histologic diagnosis by either stereotactic or needle-localized excisional biopsy. Traditionally, tissue was removed by a wire-

guided excisional biopsy. At Harbor-UCLA Medical Center, mammographically detected lesions are now either sampled with needle localization or excised with stereotactic techniques. Standard core biopsy, vacuum-assisted core biopsy, and biopsy with the advanced breast biopsy instrument (ABBI) and other techniques are used widely for tissue sampling of nonpalpable breast lesions. At Harbor-UCLA, ABBI is used for breast lesions that are highly suspect for malignancy (category 5 according to the BI-RADS) (40) and are less than 15 mm in their greatest dimension. A specimen removed intact provides important staging information (T stage) in cases of small malignant masses. Additionally, if the lesion is removed with negative margins, repeated excision may not be necessary. Given the maximum dimension of the ABBI device (20 mm), lesions much larger than 15 mm that are highly suspect on mammogram cannot be removed *in toto*, and the less invasive vacuum-assisted biopsy technique is used for such lesions.

Ultrasonography plays a role in the management of nonpalpable as well as palpable masses. When detected by mammography, BI-RADS category 0 lesions (insufficiently visualized for adequate assessment) can be further studied with ultrasonography. Lesions that are probably benign can also be assessed. Ultrasonography can reassure both clinician and patient that the lesion appears to be benign if cystic and can help guide minimally invasive biopsy if the lesion is solid.

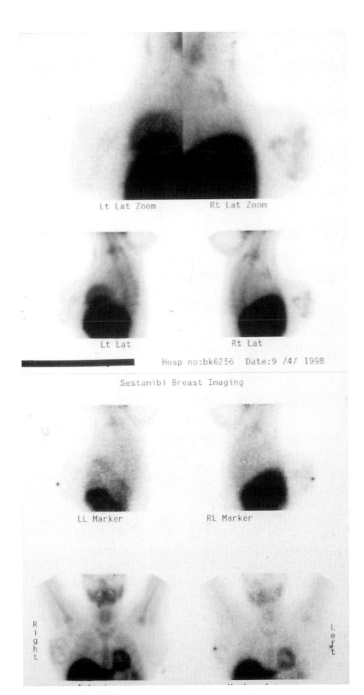

Lt Lat Zoom   Rt Lat Zoom

Lt Lat   Rt Lat

Hosp no:bk6256 Date:9 /4/ 1998

Sestamibi Breast Imaging

LL Marker   RL Marker

FIGURE 18.6. A 32-year-old woman with anemia and a palpable mass in the right axilla at presentation. Biopsy showed adenocarcinoma of the breast. No breast lump could be palpated. Multiple mammograms and ultrasonography with biopsy failed to identify a breast cancer, but ^{99m}Tc-MIBI (methoxyisobutylisonitrile) showed a multicentric tumor in the right breast. Note the humeral bone marrow seen bilaterally in the anterior view. Cancer in the bone marrow caused the presenting anemia.

If malignancy is detected by stereotactic core biopsy, the patient can undergo a mastectomy, or the mass can be excised by needle localization. Wire placement is facilitated by a small clip left in the biopsy bed during the original procedure. Other lesions, such as atypical ductal hyperplasia, are also widely excised in this manner. Mammographic lesions that are very close to the chest wall, located peripherally in the breast, or otherwise inaccessible to the stereotactic device are removed by the standard needle-localized excisional biopsy technique.

Occasionally, a lesion is not well characterized by either mammography or ultrasonography. In these instances, other methods, such as MRI, positron emission tomography, or computed tomography can be used to characterize the lesion and guide wire placement for excisional biopsy. At Harbor-UCLA, we commonly use scintimammography with ^{99m}Tc-MIBI to guide biopsy procedures. When the lesion is seen only with scintimammography, tissue sampling has been problematic. With use of a new technique, we have been able to perform MIBI-localized biopsies in six patients, with demonstration of malignancy in 50% (41).

When the patient has evidence of axillary disease clinically but no clinical or radiologic evidence of a primary breast cancer (so-called TxN1M), scintimammography and MRI can help identify the primary breast lesion. The Royal Free Hospital group in the United Kingdom has identified a primary breast lesion in two such patients. Localization of the tumor can be improved with the use of single-photon emission computed tomography (SPECT) or a radiolabeled agent (Fig. 18.6). Because this is a rare situation, no series of the use of either technique has been published.

Determining the Extent of Disease

With scintimammography, it is possible to identify additional sites of tumor not seen on routine mammography. This may help in identifying multifocal or multicentric disease and in planning appropriate surgery (Figs. 18.7 and 18.8) and will become more important as more patients undergo breast-conserving surgery. In younger patients, especially those with positive genetic markers for breast cancer, it has been possible to identify mammographically negative bilateral cancer. In the first series of 150 suspected primary breast cancers, three patients had unsuspected bilateral breast cancer (S. P. Parbhoo, *personal communication*).

Detecting Lymph Node Disease

Locoregional lymph node involvement in the axilla has a major bearing on the prognosis of breast cancer. In patients with invasive primary breast cancer, axillary node dissection is a routine procedure but is often associated

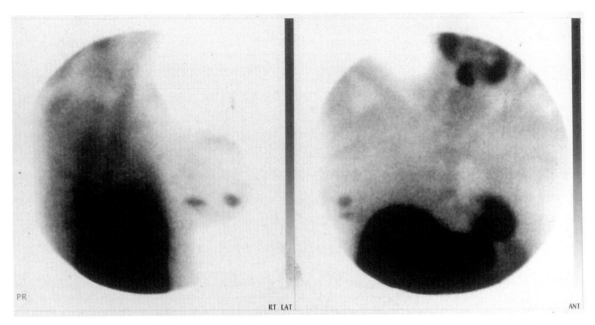

FIGURE 18.7. Small breast cancer in the right breast was identified with mammography. Scinti-mammography shows a second, radiologically occult tumor close to the chest wall.

with significant morbidity. The ability of ^{99m}Tc-MIBI scintimammography to predict accurately the presence of axillary lymph node involvement avoids unnecessary axillary dissection (Fig. 18.9 and Table 18.9).

Planar ^{99m}Tc scintimammography was found to have a sensitivity of 84% and a specificity of 91% for axillary

lymph node disease (25). Higher rates of accuracy were obtained when SPECT was performed, but this finding has not been confirmed in other studies. The value of SPECT remains unclear. It appears to provide better localization of tumors in the breast, which is of particular use if the lesions are nonpalpable (42).

Despite the accuracy of ^{99m}Tc-MIBI scintimammography for the detection of axillary lymph nodes, it is not sufficient to eliminate axillary dissection when the results of imaging are negative. Because the axilla is imaged in the standard imaging protocol, abnormal lymph node uptake of ^{99m}Tc-MIBI should be identified and evaluated (Fig. 18.10).

Detecting Recurrent Disease

The frequency of local recurrence of breast carcinoma remains small, less than 5%, but it may increase with the trend toward breast-conserving surgery (43). Accordingly, early identification and assessment of recurrence should be of clinical benefit. The interpretation of radiographic mammography may be difficult because of previous surgery or effects of radiotherapy on breast density. Recent work has shown that the sensitivity of ^{99m}Tc-MIBI is similar in finding recurrent cancer within the breast to its sensitivity in detecting primary breast cancer (44). ^{99m}Tc-MIBI identifies recurrence in other adjacent tissues not seen on radiographic mammography. It has been observed, however, that the uptake of ^{99m}Tc-MIBI is much less intense than in primary cancers. This is proba-

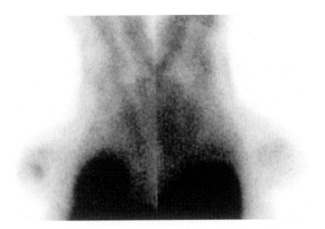

FIGURE 18.8. Woman found to have a mass in the left breast 3 weeks post partum. Mammography and ultrasonography showed reactive breast tissue. Scintigraphy with ^{99m}Tc-MIBI (methoxy-isobutylisonitrile) revealed active uptake in breast tissue and focal uptake in the left breast at the site of a ductal carcinoma. (Radiation protection point: Breast feeding is suspended for 6 hours after injection of ^{99m}Tc-MIBI.)

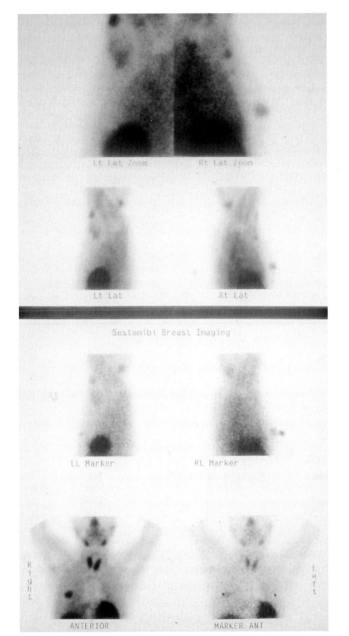

FIGURE 18.9. A 47-year-old man with a palpable right axillary lymph node at presentation. Scintimammography showed an extensive primary cancer, best seen on the anterior view.

bly related to the fact that local recurrence within the breast consists not of a tight mass of cells, but rather diffuse islands and sheets of cells within the breast tissue itself.

As with primary breast cancer, a combined approach is useful. In the only series published on the use of ^{99m}Tc-MIBI and radiographic mammography in recurrent breast cancer, the sensitivity of radiographic mammography was 50%, and it was 70% for ^{99m}Tc-MIBI. The combination of both techniques found all patients with recurrent breast cancer.

TABLE 18.9. INDICATIONS FOR SCINTIMAMMOGRAPHY

Diagnostic: which patients?
Under 50 with nondiagnostic mammogram but palpable mass
Dense, "lumpy" breasts with nondiagnostic mammogram
Taking postmenopausal hormone replacement therapy or herbal medicines with dense mammogram
Previous breast surgery distorting anatomy, including breast prosthesis
Raised levels of breast tumor markers but no palpable mass
Strong family history of breast cancer, carrying genetic marker, and further diagnostic information needed
Axillary disease found but no evidence of primary (TxN1M)

Determining extent of disease: which patients?
Suspected multifocal/multicentric or bilateral disease (this should include most young women with breast cancer)
Possible axillary lymph node involvement (ipsilateral and contralateral)
Clinical extent of disease at variance with other imaging results
Determining sites for biopsy (including ultrasonographically guided)
Finding residual disease after excision biopsy
Finding recurrent disease in breast or locoregional tissues

Modified from Buscombe JR, Cwikla JB, Thakrar DS, et al. Scintimammography: a review. *Nucl Med Rev* 1999;2:36–41, with permission.

CONCLUSIONS

At present, ^{99m}Tc-MIBI is the only radiotracer approved for breast imaging. ^{99m}Tc-MIBI scintimammography provides essential information when the results of standard radiologic investigations are equivocal or nondiagnostic. Additional indications include assessment of the extent of

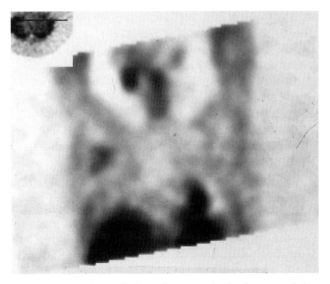

FIGURE 18.10. Coronal slices of a prone single-photon emission computed tomographic study showing a right-sided axillary lymph node.

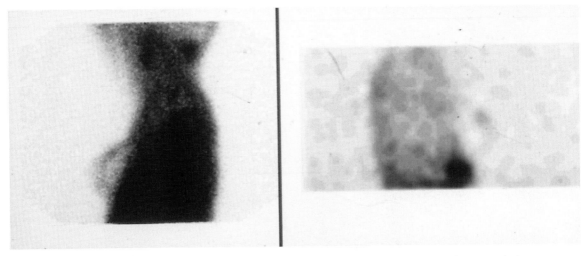

FIGURE 18.11. Planar and single-photon emission computed tomographic (*SPECT*) prone scintimammography in a 32-year-old woman with a cosmetic breast prosthesis. The planar view is unremarkable, but the sagittal SPECT slice shows an area of focal uptake overlying the prosthesis. A 4-mm invasive ductal carcinoma was confirmed at surgery.

cancer and the identification of locally recurrent disease (Fig. 18.11).

REFERENCES

1. Kelsey JL. Gammon MD. The epidemiology of breast cancer. *Cancer* 1991;41:146–165.
2. Broeders MJ, Verbeck AL. Breast cancer epidemiology and risk factors. *Q J Nucl Med* 1997;41:179–188.
3. Frisell J, Eklund G, Hellstrom L, et al. Randomized study of mammography screening—preliminary report on mortality in the Stockholm trial. *Breast Cancer Res Treat* 1991;18:49–56.
4. Huynh PT, Jarolimek AM, Daye S. The false-negative mammogram. *Radiographics* 1998;18:1137–1154.
5. Olivetti L, Bergonzini R, Vanoli C, et al. Is mammography useful in the detection of breast cancer in women 35 years of age or younger? *Radiol Med (Torino)* 1998;95:161–164.
6. Byng JW, Yaffe MJ, Jong RA, et al. Analysis of mammographic density and breast cancer risk from digitized mammograms. *Radiographics* 1998;18:1587–1598.
7. Bird RE, Wallace TW, Yankaskas BC. Analysis of cancers missed at screening mammography. *Radiology* 1992;184:613–617.
8. Martin JE, Moskowitz M, Milbrath JR, Breast cancer missed by mammography. *Am J Radiol* 1979;132:737–739.
9. Wallis MG, Walsh MT, Lee JR. A review of false negative mammography in a symptomatic population. *Clin Radiol* 1991;44:13–15.
10. Thurfjell EL, Lindgren JA. Population-based mammography screening in Swedish clinical practice: prevalence and incidence screening in Uppsala County. *Radiology* 1994;193:351–357.
11. Kerlikowse K, Grady D, Barclay J, et al. Variability and accuracy in mammographic interpretation using the American College of Radiology Breast Imaging Reporting and Data System. *J Natl Cancer Inst* 1998;90:1801–1809.
12. Kopans BD, Moore RH, McCarthy KA, et al. Positive predictive value of breast biopsy performed as a result of mammography: there is no abrupt change at age 50 years. *Radiology* 1986;200:357–360.
13. Jackson VP, Hendrick RE, Feig SA, et al. Imaging of the radiographically dense breast. *Radiology* 1993;188:297–301.
14. van Gils CH, Otten JD, Verbeek AL, et al. Effect of mammographic density on breast screening programmes: a study in Nijemegen, The Netherlands. *J Epidemiol Community Health* 1998;52:267–271.
15. Peters-Engl C, Medl M, Leodolter S. The use of colour-coded and spectral Doppler ultrasound in the differentiation of benign and malignant breast lesions. *Br J Cancer* 1995;71:137–139.
16. Lister D, Evans AJ, Burrell HC, et al. The accuracy of breast ultrasound in the evaluation of clinically benign discrete, symptomatic breast lumps. *Clin Radiol* 1998;53:490–492.
17. Rissanen TJ, Makarainen HP, Apaja-Sarkkinen MA, et al. Mammography and ultrasound in the diagnosis of contralateral breast cancer. *Acta Radiol* 1995;36:358–366.
18. Maestro C, Cazenove F, Marcy PY, et al. Systematic ultrasonography in asymptomatic dense breasts. *Eur J Radiol* 1998;26:254–256.
19. Kaiser WA, Zeitler E. MR imaging of the breast: fast imaging sequences with and without Gd-DTPA. Preliminary observations. *Radiology* 1989;170:681–686.
20. Rieber A, Merkle E, Zeitler H, et al. Doubtful mammographic findings: the value of negative MR mammography for tumor exclusion. *Rofo Fortschr Geb Rontgenstr Neuen Bildgeb Verfahr* 1997;167:392–398.
21. Palmedo H, Grunwald F, Bender H, et al. Scintimammography with technetium-99m methoxyisobutylisonitrile: comparison with mammography and magnetic resonance imaging. *Eur J Nucl Med* 1996;23:940–946.
22. Hochman MG, Orel SG, Powell CM, et al. Fibroadenomas: MR imaging appearances with radiologic–histopathologic correlation. *Radiology* 1997;204:123–129.
23. Khalkhali I, Mena I, Jouann E, et al. Prone scintimammography in patients with suspicion of carcinoma of the breast. *J Am Coll Surg* 1994;31:1166–1167.
24. Khalkhali I, Cutrone J, Mena I, et al. Technetium-99m-sestamibi scintimammography of breast lesions: clinical and pathological follow-up. *J Nucl Med* 1995;36;1784–1789.
25. Taillefer R, Robidoux A, Lambert R, et al. Technetium-99m sestamibi prone scintimammography to detect primary breast can-

cer and axillary lymph node involvement. *J Nucl Med* 1995;36:1758–1765.

26. Khalkhali I, Villaneuva-Meyer S, Edell L, et al. Diagnostic accuracy of Tc-99m sestaMIBI breast imaging in breast cancer detection. *J Nucl Med* 1996;37:74P.

27. Tolmos J, Cutrone JA, Wong B, et al. Scintimammographic analysis of non-palpable breast lesions previously identified on conventional mammography. *J Natl Cancer Inst* 1998;90:846–849.

28. Piccolo S, Lastoria S, Mainolfi C, et al. Technetium-99m- methylene diphosphonate scintimammography to image primary breast cancer. *J Nucl Med* 1995;36:718–724.

29. Barlow RV, McCool D, Thakrar DS, et al. Quantification of uptake of Tc-99m sestamibi and MDP in suspected breast tumors. *Nucl Med Commun* 1996;17:296–297.

30. Rambaldi PF, Mansi L, Procaccini E, et al. Breast cancer detection with Tc-99m tetrofosmin. *Clin Nucl Med* 1995;20:703–705.

31. de Jong M, Bernard BF, Breeman WA, et al. Comparison of uptake of 99mTc-MIBI, 99mTc-tetrofosmin and 99mTc-Q12 into human breast cancer cell lines. *Eur J Nucl Med* 1996;23:1361–1366.

32. Mekhmandarov S, Sandbank J, Cohen M, et al. Technetium-99m-MIBI scintimammography in palpable and non-palpable breast lesions. *J Nucl Med* 1998;39:86–91.

33. Cwikla JB, Buscombe JR, Kelleher SM, et al. Comparison of accuracy of scintimammography and x-ray mammography in the diagnosis of primary breast cancer in patients selected for surgical biopsy. *Clin Radiol* 1998;53:274–280.

34. Kopans DB. The positive predictive value of mammography. *AJR Am J Roentgenol* 1992;158:521–526.

35. Cwikla JB, Buscombe JR, Parbhoo SP, et al. Prediction of the utility of combined mammography and scintimammography in suspected primary breast cancer using ROC curves. *J Nucl Med* 1998;39:138P.

36. Prats E, Aisa F, Abos MD, et al. Mammography and Tc-99m MIBI scintimammography in suspected breast cancer. *J Nucl Med* 1999;40:296–301.

37. Taber L, Pentek Z, dean PB. Diagnostic and therapeutic value of breast cyst puncture and pneumocystography. *Radiology* 1981;141:659–665.

38. Butler JA, Vargas HI, Worthen N, et al. Accuracy of combined clinical–mammographic–cytologic diagnosis of dominant breast masses. A prospective study. *Arch Surg* 1990;125:893–895.

39. Waxman AD. The role of (99m)Tc methoxyisobutylisonitrile in imaging breast cancer. *Semin Nucl Med* 1997;27:40–54.

40. Baker JA, Kornguth PJ, Floyd CE. Breast imaging reporting and data system standardized mammography lexicon: observer variability in lesion description. *AJR Am J Roentgenol* 1996;166:773–778.

41. Vargas HI. Presentation to the Society of Surgical Oncology, 1997.

42. Buscombe JR, Cwikla JB, Thakrar DS, et al. Prone SPECT scintimammography. *Nucl Med Commun* 1999;20:237–245.

43. Saphner T, Tormey DC, Gray RJ. Annual hazard rates of recurrence for breast cancer after primary therapy. *Clin Oncol* 1996;14:2738–2746.

44. Cwikla JB, Buscombe JR, Kelleher SM, et al. Use of Tc-99m MIBI in the assessment of patients with recurrent breast cancer. *Nucl Med Commun* 1998;19:649–655.

45. Buscombe JR, Cwikla JB, Thakrar DS, et al. Scintimammography: a review. *Nucl Med Rev* 1999;2:36–41.

Nuclear Oncology: Diagnosis and Therapy, edited by I. Khalkhali, J. Maublant, and S.J. Goldsmith, Lippincott Williams & Wilkins, Philadelphia © 2001

19

POSITRON EMISSION TOMOGRAPHY IMAGING

LEE P. ADLER
GEORGE BAKALE

The clinical use of 2-deoxy-2-fluoro-D-glucose labeled with fluorine 18 (hereafter denoted simply as FDG) stems from the seminal studies of glucose metabolism of Warburg in the 1930s (1), from which it was recognized that malignant masses generally exhibit an enhanced rate of glucose metabolism relative to normal tissues. FDG was first applied to studies of glucose metabolism by Som et al. (2) in 1980 and subsequently by others; from these studies, a better understanding of the preferential uptake of FDG in malignant tumors has emerged. The accumulation of FDG is enhanced in tumor cells relative to normal tissues for the following reasons: (a) Glucose transport to tumors is enhanced relative to normal tissue; (b) the increased concentration of hexokinase in tumors generally enhances the metabolic rate; and (c) FDG is phosphorylated by cancer cells but is not further metabolized, which results in the accretion of FDG in tumors. The first point is especially pertinent to breast cancer because of its overexpression of the erythrocyte-type Glut-1 glucose transporter, which was reported by Brown and Wahl (3). These factors combine to yield median tumor-to-nontumor uptake ratios above 10 at 1 hour after intravenous injection of FDG (e.g., see reference 4). Another reason for the widespread use of FDG is the relatively long half-life of ^{18}F (109 minutes), which allows imaging to be performed for a longer period than is possible with ^{11}C, ^{13}N, or ^{15}O, with half-lives of 20, 10, and 2 minutes, respectively. The longer half-life of ^{18}F also facilitates the application of mathematical models for FDG metabolism, which improves the delineation of malignancies.

HISTORICAL DEVELOPMENT OF APPLICATION OF POSITRON EMISSION TOMOGRAPHY TO BREAST CANCER

Carcinoma of the breast is the most common solid tumor malignancy among women in the United States. The use of the optimal means available to detect breast cancer early and alleviate its devastating effects is warranted. Early detection reduces the morbidity and mortality of breast cancer when malignancies are found and excised before they spread to other sites. Mammography is a major component of efforts at early detection. The contribution of mammography to decreases in morbidity and mortality has been well documented in numerous surveys (5–7). However, like any primary screening tool, mammography frequently yields false-positive results, which lead to the performance of a large number of unnecessary biopsies with their associated morbidity (8–10). More importantly, mammography detects macroscopic anatomic changes in tissues surrounding the tumor site, in contrast to positron emission tomography (PET), which monitors the biochemical changes in the microenvironment of the site of carcinogenesis that invariably precede detectable morphologic changes. This unique attribute of PET to identify regions of enhanced metabolic activity complements mammography and other imaging modalities based on structural anatomic changes (computed tomography, magnetic resonance imaging, and ultrasonography). Numerous comparisons of PET with mammography and the other imaging techniques have been made.

Positron emission tomography with fluorodeoxyglucose (FDG-PET) was first applied to breast imaging 16 years ago by Beany et al. (11) in their studies of blood flow and oxygen consumption in the tumors of breast cancer patients. In 1991, Wahl et al. (12) used FDG-PET to screen 10 patients with primary breast cancers ranging in size from 3.2 to 12 cm and identified all patients correctly, including two whose mammographic results were negative because of

L. P. Adler: Section of Nuclear Medicine, Division of Radiologic Sciences, Wake Forest University Baptist Medical Center, Winston-Salem, North Carolina 27157.

G. Bakale: Department of Radiology, Case Western Reserve University, University Hospitals of Cleveland, Cleveland, Ohio 44106.

dense parenchyma. Soon thereafter, Tse et al. (13) used whole-body FDG-PET to evaluate 14 patients with newly discovered breast masses and correctly identified 8 of 10 cancers, for a sensitivity of 80%. No abnormal FDG uptake was noted in the four patients whose lesions were found to be benign, for a specificity of 100%. The eight correct positive and four correct negative responses yielded an overall accuracy of 86% (12/14). The basis and methodology of PET imaging are depicted in Figures 19.1 and 19.2, respectively.

METHODOLOGY

Since the cursory studies of breast cancer by Beany et al. (11), PET imaging of breast neoplasms has advanced to provide well-delineated images of FDG avidity with good resolution (Figs. 19.3–19.5). Details of the protocol are described in the figure legends. PET imaging can be enhanced by scanning the patient in the prone position.

RESULTS

Application of Positron Emission Tomography to Breast Cancer

Results of FDG-PET studies are summarized in Table 19.1 (14–21). In a total of 259 lesions studied, the overall sensitivity of FDG-PET in identifying primary breast cancer was 92%, the specificity was 94%, and the accuracy was 92% (14–21). Although these results are encouraging, caution

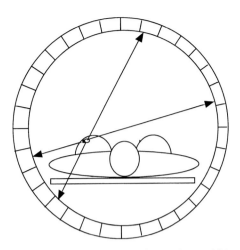

FIGURE 19.2. Schematic diagram of a patient within a single ring of a positron emission tomography (*PET*) scanner that detects the occurrence of two annihilation events. Modern PET cameras are comprised of approximately 50 such rings (half real and half virtual), which produce an equal number of cross-sectional slices through patients.

should be exercised in comparing results from different patient populations for which selection bias may exist in preliminary investigations such as these.

In the study by Dehdashti et al. (17), FDG was compared with ^{18}F-estradiol (FES) to determine whether the labeled hormone would yield results concordant with the estrogen receptor (ER) status of the tumor and perhaps offer advantages over FDG in detecting primary breast cancer with PET. The FES-ER concordance was high (88%), but the primary breast cancers of 18 of the 24 patients were FES-negative, so that the sensitivity of FES was only 25%.

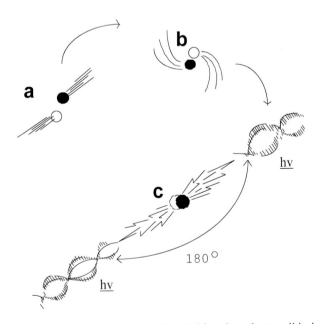

FIGURE 19.1. A: A positron (*white circle*) and an electron (*black circle*) approach each other. **B:** They are drawn together by coulombic forces. **C:** They undergo an annihilation reaction, which results in the production of two photons moving in nearly opposite directions.

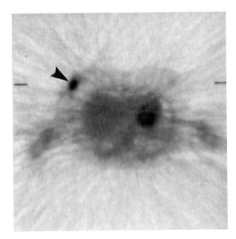

FIGURE 19.3. Transaxial plane of an attenuation-corrected positron emission tomographic (*PET*) image illustrating fluorodeoxyglucose (*FDG*) localization in a primary breast mass (*arrowhead*), found to be grade 3 infiltrating ductal breast carcinoma. The larger area of FDG uptake (*arrow*) represents cardiac activity. (Reprinted from Adler et al. Axillary lymph node metastases: screening with [F-18] 2-deoxy-2-fluoro-D-glucose (FDG) PET. *Radiology* 1997;203:323–332, with permission.)

TABLE 19.1. SUMMARY OF RESULTS OF STUDIES USING FDG-PET TO IDENTIFY PRIMARY BREAST CANCER

Study (reference)	No. lesions	Sensitivity (%) (positive scans for malignancies)	Specificity (%) (negative scans for benign lesions)	Accuracy (%) (correctly positive and negative for total lesions)
Wahl et al. 1991 (12)	10	10/10 = 100	—	10/10 = 100
Tse et al. 1992 (13)	14	8/10 = 80	4/4 = 100	12/14 = 86
Adler et al. 1993 (14)	35	26/27 = 96	8/8 = 100	34/35 = 97
Nieweg et al. 1993 (15)	19	10/11 = 91	8/8 = 100	18/19 = 95
Hoh et al. 1993 (16)	20	15/17 = 88	1/3 = 33	16/20 = 80
Dehdashti et al. 1995 (17)	32	21/24 = 88	8/8 = 100	29/32 = 91
Avril et al. 1996 (18)	67	33/36 = 92	30/31 = 97	63/67 = 94
Scheidhauer et al. 1996 (19)	30	21/23 = 91	6/7 = 86	27/30 = 90
Kole et al. 1997 (20)	13	10/10 = 100	2/3 = 67	12/13 = 92
Palmedo et al. 1997 (21)	19	12/13 = 92	6/6 = 100	18/19 = 95
TOTAL	**259**	**166/181 = 92%**	**73/78 = 94%**	**239/259 = 92%**

FDG-PET, positron emission tomography with fluorodeoxyglucose.

In an earlier study by the same group, a ^{18}F-substituted analogue of another breast hormone, 16α-ethyl-19-norprogesterone (FENP), was studied. Results correlated poorly with progesterone receptor status (22). Scheidhauer et al. (19) used a streamlined PET protocol with a total patient examination time of less than 70 minutes, including FDG administration. This group concluded that "FDG-PET showed a higher accuracy than clinical examination, mammography and ultrasonography." Kole et al. (20) used ^{11}C-tyrosine in addition to FDG to image 13 patients and found an enhanced uptake of both tracers in all of 10 malignant breast masses. The specificity of the labeled tyrosine was 100%, whereas a false-positive result was reported for FDG in one of three benign tumors.

These data suggest that PET may be the noninvasive imaging modality needed to reduce the large number of breast biopsies with negative results that are performed each year, estimated to be as high as two of every three cases (23). It must be recognized, however, that PET must compete with less expensive imaging techniques, one of the most promising of which is scintimammography with ^{99m}Tc-2-*hexakis*-2-methoxyisobutylisonitrile (MIBI). Palmedo et al. (21) compared FDG-PET and scintimammography with MIBI in the same patients. The sensitivity (92%) and specificity (100%) were the same for both modalities in detecting primary breast cancers; however, PET also correctly identified axillary metastases in 5 of 12 patients.

Another potential application of FDG-PET is to assist surgeons in visualizing breast lesions preoperatively by combining orthogonal and volume-rendered images constructed from simultaneously obtained emission and transmission scans. These combined displays provide an image of body contours in which FDG-avid hot spots are evident, which facilitates the localization of lesions (24). A portable PET unit weighing less than 50 kg and specifically designed for breast imaging would significantly reduce the cost of breast PET and make the technique more widely available (25). Such a dedicated breast-imaging device has been developed, and the technique, positron emission mammography (PEM), has been evaluated in clinical trials (26). In early studies, PEM appeared to be at least as accurate as conventional PET in identifying breast lesions, and scanning was performed at a fraction of the cost.

Evaluation of Axillary Lymph Nodes by Positron Emission Tomography

Although PET appears to have distinctive advantages relative to other imaging modalities in diagnosing primary breast cancer, its greatest potential value is in the locoregional staging of newly discovered breast cancer. All patients with breast carcinoma except those with microscopically invasive or minimally invasive tumors currently undergo axillary lymph node dissection (ALND). Whether the practice should continue has been debated intensely (29,30), and this issue is the focus of increasing attention (31). The root of the debate stems from the significant inherent morbidity of ALND, which includes the development of seroma and arm edema, a decreased range of motion, and neurologic impairment, in addition to the costs associated with the required hospitalization, general anesthesia, and 1 to 2 weeks of postoperative drain care (32). Most breast cancer patients are subjected to ALND and are thus at risk for these complications, but only 25% to 30% of patients who undergo ALND are found to have metastases (23). Clearly, a noninvasive screening technique is needed to reduce the large number of ALND with negative results that are currently performed (31).

In Fig. 19.4, an extensive accumulation of FDG is seen in the axillary lymph nodes of a patient with breast cancer. In

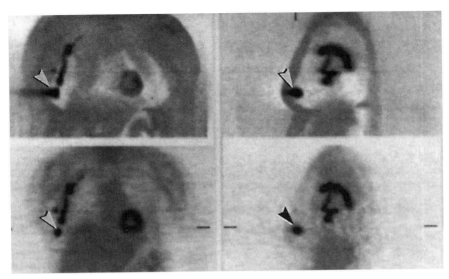

FIGURE 19.4. Coronal (*left*) and sagittal (*right*) planes of positron emission tomographic images illustrating fluorodeoxyglucose localization in a primary breast mass (*arrowheads*) and the right axillary lymph nodes (*arrows*), found to be malignant. Upper scans are not corrected for attenuation; lower scans are corrected. (Reprinted from Adler et al. Axillary lymph node metastases: screening with [F-18] 2-deoxy-2-fluoro-D-glucose (FDG) PET. *Radiology* 1997;203:323–332, with permission.)

contrast to this example of extensive nodal metastasis, subtle foci of increased activity in the axilla must be carefully identified in Fig. 19.5. As indicated in a recent review by Strauss et al. (32), achieving the sensitivity needed to identify such foci may result in a lower specificity in patients without metastases because of enhanced FDG uptake in processes such as inflammation, which may be incorrectly identified as metastases. Despite this caveat, however, several studies have demonstrated that FDG-PET is a promising technique to identify metastasis to the axilla (13–16,19,33–38) (Table 19.2).

Caution should be exercised in drawing conclusions from the results listed in Table 19.2 because these are data pooled from different studies with differing selection criteria. In the early studies, the prevalence of disease is usually

high. It appears, however, from the overall sensitivity and specificity in the 10 studies of 88% and 82%, respectively, that FDG-PET is an efficacious means to screen breast cancer patients noninvasively for possible metastases to axillary lymph nodes. These same data reveal study-to-study fluctuations of high sensitivity coupled with low specificity and vice versa, which indicate that the boundary between positive and negative interpretations of scans is not well defined. The studies by Utech et al. (36) and Adler et al. (14,34) sacrifice specificity to minimize the number of false-negative scans obtained, whereas Avril et al. (35) and Crippa et al. (38) report nine false-negative scans among the 51 patients with metastasis to the axilla but only five false-positive scans among 72 benign cases.

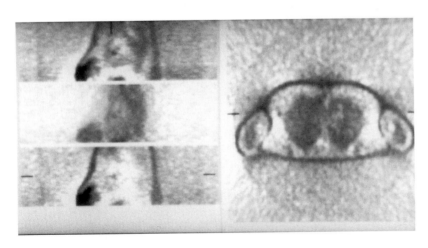

FIGURE 19.5. Positron emission tomography in a 49-year-old woman with newly diagnosed grade 2 infiltrating ductal breast cancer. A small focus of fluorodeoxyglucose enhancement is evident in the right axilla (*arrows*). This focus of activity represents metastasis of a solitary lymph node among the 21 that were dissected. (Reprinted from Adler et al. Axillary lymph node metastases: screening with [F-18] 2-deoxy-2-fluoro-D-glucose (FDG) PET. *Radiology* 1997;203:323–332, with permission.)

**TABLE 19.2. SUMMARY OF RESULTS OF STUDIES
USING FDG-PET TO IDENTIFY AXILLARY LYMPH NODE INVOLVEMENT
IN BREAST CANCER PATIENTS**

Study (reference)	No. ALNDs	Sensitivity (%) (positive scans for malignancies)	Specificity (%) (negative scans for benign lesions)	Accuracy (%) (correctly positive and negative for total lesions)
Wahl et al. 1991 (33)	8	5/5 = 100	2/3 = 68	7/8 = 88
Tse et al. 1992 (13)	10	4/7 = 57	3/3 = 100	7/10 = 70
Nieweg et al. 1993 (15)	5	5/5 = 100	—	5/5 = 100
Hoh et al. 1993 (16)	14	6/9 = 68	5/5 = 100	11/14 = 79
Adler et al. 1996 (14)	52	19/20 = 95	21/32 = 66	40/52 = 77
Avril et al. 1996 (35)	51	19/24 = 79	26/27 = 96	45/51 = 88
Scheidhauer et al. 1996 (19)	18	9/9 = 100	8/9 = 89	17/18 = 94
Utech et al. 1996 (36)	124	44/44 = 100	60/80 = 75	104/124 = 84
Bender et al. 1997 (37)	75	28/32 = 88	42/43 = 98	70/75 = 93
Crippa et al. 1998 (38)	72	23/27 = 85	41/45 = 91	64/72 = 89
TOTAL	**429**	**162/182 = 88%**	**208/247 = 82%**	**370/429 = 83%**

FDG-PET, positron emission tomography with fluorodeoxyglucose.

The ambiguous boundary between positive and negative interpretations raises the question of risk versus benefit: How many false-positive scans that result in needless ALNDs should be equated with a false-negative scan that precludes a needed ALND and results in metastasis and loss of life? This question in turn raises the issues of how the cost-effectiveness of breast cancer management can be optimized and how PET can impact most beneficially in this area, issues that were addressed by the ICP Breast Cancer Task Force several years ago (39). The task force compared the conventional breast cancer algorithm for candidates for breast-conservation therapy (BCT), which includes a partial mastectomy and ALND, with a modification that involves applying FDG-PET to identify those patients least likely to benefit from ALND (i.e., those with a negative result on PET) (39). The savings with use of the protocol that included FDG-PET instead of the conventional algorithm were estimated to be $1,611 per patient in this 1994 study. For cancer cases in the United States, annual savings of $160 million were projected. For the 208 patients in Table 19.2 who had negative PET results and no metastases, the savings were more than $330,000. Perhaps more significant than the estimated cost savings was the related projection made by the Breast Cancer Task Force that for each patient with a false-negative PET result who would therefore fail to have an appropriate ALND, 33 patients would avoid a needless ALND and thereby avoid the morbidity associated with this procedure. A somewhat analogous cost–benefit analysis was recently reported for MIBI screening of patients with abnormal results on mammography and nonpalpable breast masses, and significant cost savings were also projected (40). Direct comparison between the 1994 PET and the 1997 MIBI studies is difficult, however, because of numerous differences in assumptions and patient costs in the two analyses.

Avril et al. (35) reported that among the 23 patients in their study with primary tumors larger than 2 cm in diameter, the sensitivity and specificity of axillary PET were 94% and 100%, respectively. This result was the basis for a suggestion that a prudent course of action would be to use PET imaging in the preoperative staging of cancer only for patients with primary tumors larger than 2 cm, who account for more than half of breast cancer patients. For those T1a patients in whom ALND is precluded based on staging decisions independent of PET results, Crippa et al. (38) recommend follow-up PET to identify potential axillary relapse noninvasively. Avril et al. (35) suggest that the low sensitivity of PET in imaging malignant lymph nodes less than 1 cm in diameter is a consequence of the partial volume effect, in which FDG uptake by objects smaller than twice the spatial resolution of the scanner cannot be imaged accurately. Efforts to circumvent this limitation include the development of dedicated scanners in which the source-to-detector distance affecting resolution is greatly reduced in comparison with that in conventional generic PET scanners (41), and recently published computational methods compensate for this effect (42).

Computed tomography (CT) and magnetic resonance imaging (MRI) have been compared with FDG-PET in 63 of 75 patients. Bender et al. (37) found the sensitivity of CT/MRI to be 89% (17/19) and the specificity 86% (38/44). No direct comparisons of ultrasonography and FDG-PET in the evaluation of breast masses have been made. Whereas FDG had a sensitivity of 89% and a specificity of 86% in the evaluation of 158 axillary lymph nodes in 45 breast cancer patients, Feu et al. (43) reported both a sensitivity and a specificity of 84% using ultrasound detection. Likewise, [99mTc]-MIBI scintimammography has not been directly compared with FDG-PET imaging. Tolmus reports a sensitivity of 75% and a specificity of 82% for the detection of axillary lymph node metastases in 31 breast patients (44).

SUMMARY

In summary, FDG-PET successfully identifies malignant breast masses with an accuracy greater than that of other noninvasive imaging modalities. FDG-PET also identifies axillary lymph node metastases more accurately than other noninvasive imaging modalities. The challenge, however, is to decide between the use of FDG-PET and the widespread use of invasive sampling, of both the primary breast mass and the regional axillary lymph nodes. Lymphoscintigraphy has recently provided a means to identify the sentinel lymph node, which may reduce the morbidity of ALND. Currently, FDG-PET provides a reasonable alternative to ALND. It remains to be determined whether the considerable reduction in morbidity is sufficient to justify the replacement of lymph node sampling.

REFERENCES

1. Warburg O. *The metabolism of tumors.* New York, Richard R. Smith, 1931.
2. Som P, Atkins HL, Bandoypadhyay D, et al. A fluorinated glucose analog, 2-fluoro-2-deoxy-D-glucose (F-18): nontoxic tracer for rapid tumor detection. *J Nucl Med* 1980;21:670–675.
3. Brown RW, Wahl RL. Overexpression of GLUT-1 glucose transport in human breast cancer: an immunohistocmeical study. *Cancer* 1993;72:2979–2985.
4. Wahl RL, Hutchins GD, Buchsbaum DJ, et al. ^{18}F-2-deoxy-2-fluoro-D-glucose (FDG) uptake into human tumor xenografts: feasibility studies for cancer imaging with PET. *Cancer* 1991;67:1544–1550.
5. Shapiro S, Venet W, Strax P. Ten- to fourteen-year effect of screening on breast cancer mortality. *J Natl Cancer Inst* 1982;69:349–355.
6. Tabar L, Faberberg CJG, Grad A, et al. Reduction in mortality from breast cancer after mass screening with mammography. Randomized trial from the Breast Cancer Screening Working Group of the Swedish National Board of Health and Welfare. *Lancet* 1985;1:829–832.
7. Rodes N, Lopez M, Pearson D. The impact of breast cancer screening on survival: a 5- to 10-year follow-up study. *Cancer* 1986;57:581–585.
8. Elmore JG, Barton MB, Mocieri VM, et al. Ten-year risk of false-positive screening mammograms and clinical breast exams. *N Engl J Med* 1998;338:1089–1096.
9. Ellman R, Angeli N, Christians A, et al. Psychiatric morbidity associated with screening for breast cancer. *Br J Cancer* 1989;62:781–784.
10. Gram IT, Lund E, Slenker SE. Quality of life following a false-positive mammogram. *Br J Cancer* 1990;62:1018–1022.
11. Beaney RP, Lammertsma AA, Jones T, et al. Positron emission tomography for *in vivo* measurement of regional blood flow, oxygen utilization and blood volume in patients with breast carcinoma. *Lancet* 1984;1:131–134.
12. Wahl RL, Cody RL, Hutchins GD, et al. Primary and metastatic breast carcinoma: initial clinical evaluation with PET with the radiolabeled glucose analogue 2-[F-18]-fluoro-2-deoxy-D-glucose. *Radiology* 1991;179:765–770.
13. Tse NY, Hoh CK, Hawkins RA, et al. The application of positron emission tomographic imaging with fluorodeoxyglucose to the evaluation of breast disease. *Ann Surg* 1992;216:27–34.
14. Adler LP, Crowe JP, Al-Kaisi NK, et al. Evaluation of breast masses and axillary lymph nodes with [F-18] 2-deoxy-2-fluoro-D-glucose PET. *Radiology* 1993;187:743–750.
15. Nieweg OE, Kim EE, Wong WH, et al. Positron emission tomography with fluorine 18-deoxyglucose in the detection and staging of breast cancer. *Cancer* 1993;71:3920–3925.
16. Hoh CK, Hawkins RA, Glaspy JA, et al. Cancer detection with whole-body PET using 2-[^{18}F] fluoro-2-deoxy-D-glucose. *J Comput Assist Tomogr* 1993;17:582–589.
17. Dehdashti F, Mortimer JE, Siegel BA, et al. Positron tomographic assessment of estrogen receptors in breast cancer: comparison with FDG-PET and *in vitro* receptor assays. *J Nucl Med* 1995;36:1766–1774.
18. Avril N, Dose J, Janicke F, et al. Metabolic characterization of breast tumors with positron emission tomography using F-18. *J Clin Oncol* 1996;14:1848–1857.
19. Scheidhauer K, Scharl A, Pietrzyk U, et al. Qualitative [^{18}F]FDG positron emission tomography in breast cancer: clinical relevance and practicability. *Eur J Nucl Med* 1996;23:618–623.
20. Kole AC, Nieweg OE, Pruim J, et al. Standardized uptake value and quantification of metabolism for breast cancer imaging with FDG and L-[1-^{11}C} tyrosine. *J Nucl Med* 1997;38:692–696.
21. Palmedo H, Bender H, Grunwald F, et al. Comparison of fluorine-18 fluorodeoxyglucose positron emission tomography and technetium methoxyisobutylisonitrile scintimammography in the detection of breast tumors. *Eur J Nucl Med* 1997;24:1138–1145.
22. Dehdashti F, McGuire AH, Van Brocklin HF, et al. Assessment of 21-[^{18}F]fluoro-16α-ethyl-19-norprogesterone as a positron-emitting radiopharmaceutical for the detection of progestin receptors in human breast carcinomas. *J Nucl Med* 1991;32:1532–1537.
23. Meyer JS. Sentinel lymph node biopsy: strategies for pathologic examination of the specimen. *J Surg Oncol* 1998;69:212–218.
24. Pietrzyk U, Scheidhauer K, Scharl A, et al. Presurgical visualization of primary breast carcinoma with PET emission and transmission imaging. *J Nucl Med* 1995;36:1882–1884.
25. Thompson CJ, Murthy K, Weinberg IN, et al. Feasibility study for positron emission mammography. *Med Phys* 1994;21:529–538.
26. Weinberg IN, Majewski S, Weisenberger A, et al. Preliminary results for positron emission mammography: real-time functional breast imaging in a conventional mammography gantry. *Eur J Nucl Med* 1996;23:804–806.
27. White RE, Vezeridis MP, Konstadoulakis M, et al. Therapeutic options and results for the management of minimally invasive carcinoma of the breast: influence of axillary dissection for treatment of T1a and T1b lesions. *J Am Coll Surg* 1996;183:575–582.
28. Cady B. The need to reexamine axillary lymph node dissection in invasive breast cancer. *Cancer* 1994;73:505–508.
29. (a) Cady B. Case against axillary lymphadenectomy for most patients with infiltrating breast cancer. *J Surg Oncol* 1997;66:7–10; (b) Jamali FR, et al. Role of axillary dissection in mammographically detected breast cancer. *Surg Oncol Clin N Am* 1997;6:343–358.
30. Cady B. Dilemmas in breast disease. *Breast J* 1995;2:121–124.
31. Moore MP, Kinne DW. Is axillary lymph node dissection necessary in the routine management of breast cancer? Yes. In: De Vita VT, Hellman S, Rosenberg SA, eds. *Important advances in oncology.* Philadelphia: Lippincott–Raven Publishers, 1996:245–250.

32. Strauss LG. Fluorine-18 deoxyglucose and false-positive results: a major problem in the diagnostics of oncological patients. *Eur J Nucl Med* 1996;23:1409–1415.

33. Wahl RL, Cody RL, August D. Initial evaluation of FDG-PET for the staging of the axilla in newly diagnosed breast cancer patients. *J Nucl Med* 1991;32:981.

34. Adler LP, Faulhaber PF, Schnur KC, et al. Axillary lymph node metastases: screening with [F-18] 2-deoxy-2-fluoro-D-glucose (FDG) PET. *Radiology* 1997;203:323–332.

35. Avril N, Dose J, Janicke F, et al. Assessment of axillary lymph node involvement in breast cancer patients with positron emission tomography using radiolabeled 2-(fluorine-18)-fluoro-2-deoxy-D-glucose. *J Natl Cancer Inst* 1996;88:1204–1209.

36. Utech CI, Young CS, Winter PF. Prospective evaluation of fluorine-18 fluoro-deoxyglucose positron emission tomography in breast cancer for staging of the axilla related to surgery and immunochemistry. *Eur J Nucl Med* 1996;23:1588–1593.

37. Bender H, Kerst J, Palmedo H, et al. Value of ^{18}F-fluoro-deoxyglucose positron emission tomography in the staging of recurrent breast carcinoma. *Anticancer Res* 1997;17:1687–1692.

38. Crippa F, Agresti R, Sefegni E, et al. Prospective evaluation of fluorine-18-FDG PET in presurgical staging of the axilla in breast cancer. *J Nucl Med* 1998;39:4–8.

39. ICP Breast Cancer Task Force (LP Adler, Chair, 1994). *Clinical applications and economic implications of PET in the assessment of axillary lymph node involvement in breast cancer.*

40. Hillner BE. Decision analysis: MIBI imaging of nonpalpable breast abnormalities. *J Nucl Med* 1997;38:1772–1778.

41. Williams MB, Pisano ED, Schnall MD, et al. Future directions in imaging of breast diseases. *Radiology* 1998;206:297–300.

42. Chen CH, Muzic RF, Nelson AD, et al. A nonlinear spatially variant object-dependent system model for prediction and correction of partial volume effect in PET. *IEEE Trans Med Imaging* 1998;17:214–227.

43. Feu J, Tressara F, Fabregas R. Metastatic breast carcinoma in axillary lymph nodes: *in vitro* US detection. *Radiology* 1997;205:831–835.

44. Tolmos J, Khalkhali I, Vargas H, et al. Detection of axillary lymph node metastasis of breast carcinoma with technetium-99m sestamibi scintimammography. *Ann Surg* 1997;63:850–853.

Nuclear Oncology: Diagnosis and Therapy, edited by I. Khalkhali, J. Maublant, and S.J. Goldsmith, Lippincott Williams & Wilkins, Philadelphia © 2001

20

LYMPHOSCINTIGRAPHY AND LYMPHATIC MAPPING

CLAUDIA G. BERMAN
NORMAN J. BRODSKY

THE NATURE OF THE PROBLEM

The average American woman today carries a one-in-eight lifetime risk for the development of cancer of the breast and approximately a 3% risk for dying of this disease. Annual mortality rates are in the vicinity of 21 deaths per 100,000 women in the United States and Canada. The highest mortality rates, 25 to 26 deaths per 100,000 women per year, are reported from Denmark, The Netherlands, and the United Kingdom. The lowest, 6 to 7 deaths per 100,000 women per year, are observed in urban China and Japan (1). Although explanations for these disparities have been offered, their causes are not known.

Also unexplained is the recent trend of declining mortality in the higher-risk countries but increasing mortality in the lower-risk countries, both in Europe and Asia (2,3). For example, the age-adjusted breast cancer death rate in the United States dropped by 6.8% between 1989 and 1993 (4). The improvement in the death rate in these countries continues (5).

Although any explanation(s) for this declining mortality remain speculative at this time, a likely partial explanation is the trend to diagnosis at an earlier stage. Indeed, a meta-analysis of randomized mammographic screening studies shows a 33% decrease in breast cancer mortality for women between 50 and 69 years of age undergoing mammographic surveillance in comparison with women who are not (6). It may well be that the increasing popularity of and technical improvements in mammography during recent years account in large part for the increase in the proportion of patients in the United States presenting with more curable stage 0 and stage I disease, from 42.5% in 1985 to 56.2% in 1995 (7,8). Moreover, it appears likely that improve-

ments in adjuvant treatment are increasing the rescue of some of these patients with surreptitious adenopathy accompanied by lethal micrometastatic disease. The most recent statistics from the National Cancer Data Base show 10-year relative survival rates of 88% for stage I (small primary, node-negative) disease, 66% for stage II (predominantly node-positive) disease, 36% for stage III (regionally extensive) disease, and 7% for stage IV (metastatic or inflammatory carcinoma) disease (9).

It has long been established that the presence of axillary metastatic adenopathy is the dominant predictor of mortality risk in cancer of the breast (10). Valagussa and colleagues (11), for example, reporting on the survival of 716 consecutive patients treated with radical mastectomy, found the 10-year survival for node-negative patients to be 80%. Among node-positive patients, it was 38%. For those with four or more positive nodes, it was 24%, whereas for those with one to three positive nodes, it was 50%.

One would expect this evident correlation between axillary nodal tumor burden and risk for relapse to continue, with progressively lesser amounts of axillary nodal disease reflecting a progressively lesser risk for distant metastatic relapse, but it has been difficult to prove it for micrometastatic disease thus far. The American Joint Committee on Cancer (AJCC) staging system for breast carcinoma currently assigns nodal tumor deposits with a cross section of less than 2 mm to a special category, N1a, which carries a prognosis equivalent to that of N0 disease (12).

In an exhaustive review of the literature on the significance of micrometastatic disease, Yeatman and Cox (13) demonstrated that the reports negating the increased relapse risk of patients with axillary nodal micrometastasis are as a rule retrospective, and almost without exception have poor statistical power. To the contrary, the few prospective studies with large numbers of patients and employing more meticulous pathologic techniques have demonstrated an increased relapse risk in patients with micrometastic nodal disease. For example, de Mascarel (14) and colleagues prospectively examined the lymph nodes of 1,680 patients by means of a technique ("serial macroscopic sectioning") in which each lymph node is

C. G. Berman: Department of Radiology, University of South Florida; Department of Radiology, H. Lee Moffitt Cancer Center and Institute, Tampa, Florida 33612.

N. J. Brodsky: Department of Radiology, University of South Florida, Tampa, Florida, 33612; Department of Radiation Oncology, Lykes Cancer Center, Clearwater, Florida 34616.

sectioned into 1.5-mm slices and each slice is then examined microscopically. They identified 120 patients with a single micrometastatic nodal deposit. During 7 years of follow-up, both disease-free survival (*p* = .005) and overall survival (*p* = .0369) were decreased in these patients in comparison with the survival rates of the node-negative patients in the study. Similarly, Friedman and colleagues (15) prospectively examined 1,153 axillary specimens with use of the "serial macroscopic sectioning" technique. They found that 18% of their patients harbored a single peripheral sinus micrometastasis and 3.5% of them had a single nodal parenchymal micrometastasis. The relative risk for relapse among patients with micrometastasis at either site was 1.7 (*p* = .05) in comparison with the N0 patients in their study group.

This issue is of particular relevance to the evolving role of sentinel lymph node (SLN) biopsy in the management of breast cancer. Specifically, it is anticipated that SLN biopsy, while simplifying the technique and diminishing the morbidity of axillary node sampling, will permit a much more exhaustive pathologic examination of the true high-risk node(s). The presumption is that many of the patients who are node-negative on traditional pathologic examination and eventually relapse will be accurately identified by more elaborate pathologic examination as node-positive, often with micrometastatic disease that is potentially curable by adjuvant systemic therapy. It is hoped, therefore, that SLN biopsy will improve the resolution of axillary dissection as a diagnostic tool in determining whether a patient should receive chemotherapy and, if so, what type.

The recognition of the strong link between metastatic axillary adenopathy and risk for disease relapse, and the availability of chemotherapeutic agents having a significant palliative effect in patients with overt metastatic disease, led to the first trials of adjuvant combination chemotherapy delivered to node-positive patients following mastectomy (16,17). The initial successful results of these trials have been maintained through extended periods of follow-up. In turn, these have led to trials of adjuvant chemotherapy (and hormonal therapy) in successively earlier stages of disease in the hope of protecting the diminishing, but still significant, cohort of patients at each stage who are at risk for death from breast cancer metastasis (18).

Exhaustive statistical "metaanalysis" of these studies has consistently shown reductions in risk for relapse, particularly in the early years following treatment, and in risk for death 5 years and more beyond treatment. The reductions in relative risk, in comparison with patients not receiving adjuvant chemotherapy, are in the vicinity of one fourth to one third. In women under 50 years of age, the absolute reduction in mortality at 10 years is in the vicinity of 7% for node-negative patients and 11% for node-positive patients (19). In women 50 to 69 years of age, the absolute reduction in mortality at 10 years is in the vicinity of 2% to 3% for both node-negative and node-positive patients. These benefits translate, in women under age 50, to 10-year survivals of 78% versus 71% in node-negative women and 53% versus 42% in node-positive women. For women 50 to 69 years of age, 10-year survivals are 49% versus 46% in node-positive women and 69% versus 67% in node-negative women.

In a prescient and still highly relevant editorial published in conjunction with the first four (positive) adjuvant trials of systemic therapy in patients with node-negative breast cancer, William McGuire (20) discussed the problems that have been raised again by the most recent metaanalysis. Simply put, are the material resources and toxicity that the adjuvant treatment of so many (node-negative patients) entails worth the small (statistical) gains? In their most recent report, the Early Breast Cancer Trialists' Group analyze what they term a "hypothetical" cohort of particularly low-risk, node-negative patients, who are much more frequently seen in today's environment of early mammographic diagnosis than was the case when the studies with 10-year follow-up that they are now analyzing were accruing patients (19). According to their analysis of this "hypothetical" group of node-negative patients with tumors of subcentimeter size, now commonly seen in clinical practice, among those more than 50 years of age, 100 must be treated to benefit a single patient. For patients younger than 50 years, it is necessary to treat 25 to benefit one. The therapeutic gains, however, quickly double and triple for patients with larger tumors, but still a substantial majority of these patients are subjected to substantial morbidity and cost for no possible benefit. It is this analysis that lays the basis for the present practice of considering systemic therapy for N0 patients with primary tumors larger than 1 cm in the greatest dimension. What is clear, however, is that even in this medium-risk group, more patients are treated than need to be treated. At the same time, treatment is withheld from the small minority of low-risk patients who are destined to die of breast cancer. Would a more accurate method of metastatic node identification allow us to identify better the small proportions of patients among these large groups who, unknown to us today, are at greater risk?

The problem can also be considered from the "opposite" perspective of higher-risk groups of node-negative patients with truly large primary tumors or tumors characterized by adverse traits (e.g., HER-2/*neu* overexpression), for which chemotherapy is usually recommended. Overexpression of HER-2/*neu* gene or receptor protein is seen in 25% to 50% of breast cancers and is associated with the development of aggressive visceral metastatic disease (21). This association is far stronger in node-positive than in node-negative patients (22). Unfortunately, methotrexate-based chemotherapy appears to be ineffective in patients with these tumors, so that these patients must undergo more toxic Adriamycin-based treatment. Here too, a more accurate method for identifying axillary nodal disease offers the prospect of exposing fewer patients to toxic but unnecessary treatment (23).

It is to be hoped, but remains to be proved, that SLN biopsy techniques will help to supply some answers in these very different groups of patients with node-negative breast cancer whose postoperative management is so strongly hampered by our ignorance of their true risk for the development of distant metastatic disease (24,25).

AXILLARY NODE SAMPLING

The staging of patients with carcinoma of the breast must include some procedure to allow the most accurate possible evaluation of critical axillary nodal tissue. Clinical examination of the axillary nodes is notoriously inaccurate. Consistently, 25% to 30% of patients are found to have false-positive, palpable, but benign lymph nodes or false-negative, impalpable, but malignant lymph nodes (26,27). Given the unreliability of physical examination, a surgical procedure to retrieve axillary nodes for pathologic examination is a necessity. The evolution of these surgical procedures follows our changing understanding of the biology of breast cancer and reflects the competing needs of obtaining adequate and appropriate tissue for reliable pathologic examination and minimizing the long-term morbidity of the procedure.

In modern surgical practice, the axilla has been divided into three levels according to the lower and upper margins of the pectoralis minor muscle. Surgical studies have established that although higher level (level III) involvement carries a worse prognosis because of the typically large number of nodes containing metastatic disease in such patients (28), the progression of axillary nodal disease appears to be stepwise, from proximal to distal. Distal node involvement without the involvement of more proximal axillary nodes is uncommon (29). Most notably, Rosen and colleagues (30) examined the levels of malignant axillary nodes found among a group of 1,228 patients undergoing axillary dissection as part of mastectomy. They found that only 3% of the 508 patients with malignant adenopathy had disease that "skipped" an axillary level. Of these, half had disease in level II only.

These observations were made simultaneously with the publication of a series of randomized surgical trials that showed equivalent survival and equivalent local control in patients with early-stage breast cancer despite progressively less radical surgical procedures. The most extreme circumstance tested involved the randomization of women to radical mastectomy versus "extended" radical mastectomy (31). The former procedure requires removal of the breast, both pectoralis muscles, and the entire contents of the axilla *en bloc*. The latter adds to this the removal of internal mammary nodes. The impetus for such a study was the recognition that internal mammary node metastasis can occur in the absence of axillary node metastasis. In a review of 7,070 patients in whom both axillary and internal mammary node basins were examined pathologically, Morrow and Foster (32) found approximately a 5% incidence of adenopathy restricted to the internal mammary drainage. Based on this, they recom-

mended a policy of internal mammary node biopsy in patients with medially and centrally located tumors or in patients with large lateral tumors in whom frozen section of the clinically most suspect axillary node failed to identify malignant adenopathy. Their goal was to increase the detection of node metastasis to select node-positive patients for systemic therapy. In contrast, the randomized study asked whether extended radical mastectomy directly improved patient outcomes versus radical mastectomy. It did not and was more morbid, and it has been essentially discarded from clinical practice. The value of the approach of Morrow and Foster, however, of sampling internal mammary nodes as part of a staging strategy has not been tested in a randomized study. The advent of the new technologies comprising SLN biopsy techniques will almost certainly lead to the consideration of such studies in the near future.

The need for radical mastectomy versus modified radical mastectomy was tested in two further randomized, prospective studies published during the same period. Modified radical mastectomy differs from radical mastectomy in that the pectoralis major and usually the pectoralis minor muscle are spared, and a less aggressive approach to axillary dissection is used (33,34). No difference in survival or local control was demonstrated between radical mastectomy and modified radical mastectomy among nearly 1,000 women enrolled in the two studies (35,36). What does distinguish these two surgical procedures, however, is the incidence and severity of postoperative morbidity. It is clear, both from the medical literature and the widespread clinical consensus among physicians managing these patients, that radical mastectomy produces far more frequent and severe problems of compromised shoulder mobility, arm swelling, and dysesthesias than the modified procedure does (37,38). Radical mastectomy as a consequence is now rarely performed (39).

The final "nails in the coffin" for regionally extensive surgery for early-stage cancer of the breast have been a series of randomized studies undertaken by the National Surgical Adjuvant Breast and Bowel Project. In their B-04 study, women with clinically node-negative breast cancer were randomized to one of three groups: (a) radical mastectomy, (b) simple mastectomy without axillary node dissection followed clinically, or (c) simple mastectomy without axillary node dissection irradiated prophylactically. Although 18% of their patients who did not receive axillary treatment did require subsequent axillary dissection for relapse, both survival and ultimate local control were equivalent in the three groups (40). From this point forward, it became clear that from a therapeutic perspective, no immediate dissection of the clinically negative axilla is necessary. Therefore, the optimal axillary surgical procedure is the minimal and least morbid one capable of providing the needed diagnostic and staging information. The subsequent B-06 trial proved the same point in regard to surgical treatment of the breast primary lesion itself (41).

Reports of morbidity from the local treatment of breast cancer are difficult to analyze and compare because of differences between definitions of morbidity and methods of measuring it, and also differences between combinations and details of surgery, systemic therapy, and radiation that patients receive (42). For example, Larson and colleagues (42), describing a group of patients treated with lumpectomy and irradiation and separate axillary dissection, reported an incidence of arm edema ranging from 5% to 37% at 6 years' follow-up. Predictors of arm edema included the surgeon's perception of the extensiveness of dissection (a "full" dissection with stripping of the axillary vein being particularly morbid), the number of lymph nodes removed, and the dose of radiation, if any, delivered to the axilla. Most patients had mild edema. A detailed quantitative description of edema is not presented. In general, despite these uncertainties, an overall risk for arm edema in the range of 5% to 10% for the currently prevalent axillary dissection techniques appears realistic (43). The incidence of seroma and short-term shoulder dysfunction is somewhat higher. Dysesthesias of the upper chest wall and facing medial proximal arm are also characteristic and, like the above, vary in severity and chronicity with the extent of axillary dissection performed (44).

BREAST LYMPHOSCINTIGRAPHY

Lymphoscintigraphy was first introduced into breast cancer management as a means of visualizing flow through lymphatic trunks that could not be cannulated for contrast lymphography (45,46). The studies were evaluated from the same perspective as lymphographic studies would be, with enlargement of nodes or apparent obstruction to flow through lymphatic trunks considered as indicators of the presence of tumor (47). Extensive investigations of internal mammary nodes and axillary nodes in patients with breast cancer were undertaken by Ege (48), who elaborated on techniques utilizing subcostal injections or injections into the finger webbing of ^{198}Au, first described by Rossi and Ferri (49) and by Schenk (50). Ege's technique involved the injection of 500 μCi of ^{99m}Tc-antimony sulfide colloid, in a volume no greater than 0.3 mL, superficial to the posterior tendinous sheath of the anterior rectus muscle just below its subcostal insertion. An initial injection on the side of the malignancy was followed 3 hours later by a second, contralateral injection. The delay allowed for the demonstration of crossover flow. The injection of both sides provided a control to help evaluate excess or skipped uptake, both signs of malignant nodal disease, on the side of the malignancy. A lateral image was obtained at 6 hours to aid in planning radiation or biopsy and to identify mediastinal communications (51). These early investigators viewed such techniques as potential substitutes for surgical biopsy of nodes. Lymphoscintigraphy, it was hoped, would circumvent the need

for the surgical pathologic diagnosis of internal mammary and even axillary nodal basins in the staging of breast cancer, with its associated morbidity (52,53). Not surprisingly, systematic, surgically controlled testing of this imaging strategy showed that it lacks the sensitivity and specificity to supersede pathologic diagnosis (54).

Probably the first report of the use of lymphoscintigraphy to identify the paths of lymphatic drainage from the breast, as opposed to the anatomic location of a group of lymph nodes adjacent to the breast, was published in 1972 by Vendrell-Torne and associates (55) as a study of lymphatic drainage pathways in the intact, normal breast. They mapped the paths of colloidal ^{198}Au drainage from injected sites in the four quadrants of the breast and the subareolar region. No attempt to visualize the first draining lymph node was made. They established the presence of unexpected, sometimes multiple pathways of drainage to axillary, internal mammary, and supraclavicular nodal basins in a significant minority of their subjects. These variant pathways of lymphatic drainage were observed from injected sites in all five of the specified regions in these normal and otherwise undisturbed breasts.

The definitive elaboration of this earlier work, performed in patients with cancer of the breast, was presented by Uren and colleagues (56). They used ^{99m}Tc-antimony sulfide colloid with a 3- to 12-nm particle size to study 34 patients, among them two men, who had breast carcinoma. Injections of 0.05 to 0.1 mL of radiocolloid were placed at the four quadrants at the periphery of each patient's tumor by means of a tuberculin syringe with a 25-gauge needle. A 0.05-mL air bubble was positioned in the syringe above the tracer injectate and introduced after the tracer to ensure delivery of the precise dose at each injection site. A waterproof dressing was applied to the trunk with a window cut to accommodate the area to be injected so as to minimize the risk for skin contamination. Injections were placed within 2 to 3 mm of the tumor margin. The depth of injection (and precise position of the tumor) was determined in each case by high-resolution ultrasonography. Activity varied from 2.5 to 7.0 MBq per injection. All studies were performed before excision of the tumor. The tumor and adjacent injection sites were subsequently excised within 1 week.

All scans were obtained with a digital camera that had a large, rectangular field of view and a low-energy, high-resolution collimator. Each view was collected during 10 minutes. Imaging was performed immediately after injection so that the enhancement capability of the digital camera could aid in identifying faint pathways of early drainage. Scanning was repeated at 2.5 hours in all patients. In patients with no nodal visualization, a second scan was obtained at 4 hours. Images were obtained in an anterior view of the chest and axilla in all patients. A lateral or oblique view was added to assess the depth of axillary sentinel nodes. Immediate scanning was performed to identify lymph channels draining the tumor. Delayed scanning was performed to

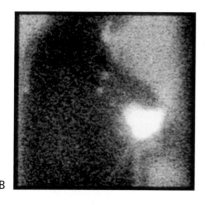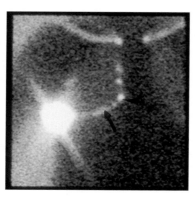

A,B

FIGURE 20.1. A: The right lateral chest lymphoscintigram shows uptake in the right axilla (*arrowheads*) from an outer quadrant breast cancer. **B:** The anterior chest lymphoscintigram shows an afferent lymphatic channel (*small arrow*) that crosses the midline and drains into a sentinel lymph node in the right internal mammary chain (*arrowhead*).

locate persistent uptake in nodes. The sentinel node was considered to be the first node to take up colloid on the immediate scan or the node with the most activity on the delayed scan.

Conventional wisdom, noting that most breast carcinomas arise within the upper outer quadrant, holds that nodal drainage will be to the axilla and that only the most medial tumors will drain to the internal mammary chain. Among the 34 patients of Uren and colleagues, ipsilateral axillary node drainage was confirmed in 29 (85%) and was the only drainage site in 18 of the 34 (53%). The multiplicity and variability of drainage patterns were unexpected, however, and confirmed the unpredictability of drainage patterns previously described by Vendrell-Torne et al. (55). In 28% of patients with outer quadrant tumors, unexpected drainage to internal mammary nodes was noted (Fig. 20.1), and 33% of inner quadrant tumors had axillary drainage. Thus, one third of patients with lateralized tumors had drainage that crossed the midline of the breast. Twenty percent of patients with upper quadrant tumors had direct drainage to supraclavicular or infraclavicular nodes (Fig. 20.2). In one patient, an intransit intramammary node, lying in the breast parenchyma between the primary lesion and the axilla, was discovered. This in-transit lymph node was in fact the SLN and contained metastatic disease. Standard axillary dissection would not have identified this node and, by implication, the patient's need for systemic adjuvant therapy.

Immediate scans were able to identify lymph channels in only 7 of the 34 patients (21%). This was a potential drawback only in patients with internal mammary node drainage because multiple nodal uptake candidates for SLN designation were characteristically present on delayed scans in the internal mammary but not the axillary or periclavicular basins. In three patients, no migration of tracer from the injection site was seen. In one of them, gross chest wall and axillary tumor masses were present.

THE SENTINEL LYMPH NODE

In 1954, Hultborn and colleagues (57) first described radiocolloid injection with imaging of lymph channels and lymph nodes as a method to aid in the examination of mastectomy specimens in the pathology laboratory. Their technique involved preoperative injection of the breast parenchyma with colloidal ^{198}Au and postoperative *ex vivo* imaging of the radical or extended radical mastectomy specimen. The gamma camera image directed the pathologist's dissection of the operative specimen. They also utilized a gamma probe to aid node localization in indistinctly visualized specimens. Their discussion quite remarkably presages the present-day thinking driving the development of lymphoscintigraphically guided sentinel node staging of breast carcinoma. They recognized a typical pattern of visualization of some but not all

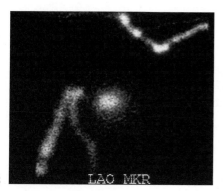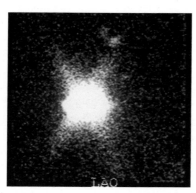

A,B

FIGURE 20.2. A: This anterior "marker" view of the chest shows the body contour outlined with a "hot" technetium marker. **B:** The anterior view of the chest without marking shows an infraclavicular sentinel lymph node (*arrowhead*) that is hidden on the marker view.

axillary nodes, which, they concluded, "probably indicates a segmental arrangement of the lymph drainage from the breast to the axilla," or, in our jargon, drainage of each specific segment of breast parenchyma by one of a number of sentinel nodes, any one of which must first be embolized by tumor from its parenchymal segment before the succeeding node(s) higher up the lymph node chain can become site(s) of metastasis.

Cabanas (58) is usually credited with the first clinical proposal of a sentinel node biopsy technique. His method was developed to avoid unnecessary and highly morbid groin dissections in patients with penile carcinoma and was premised on the existence of a sentinel node that would predict the nodal status of the remainder of the nodal drainage basin. He used lymphography of the lymphatics adjacent to the dorsal vein of the penis to identify this node, which was generally in the vicinity of the superficial epigastric vein. The lymphographic technique, however, was cumbersome and exacting and did not gain popularity.

Dye Technique

Our contemporary concept of breast SNL localization and biopsy, adapted from earlier work with melanoma, was developed and first tested by Giuliano and colleagues (59) at the John Wayne Cancer Institute at Saint John's Hospital and Health Center in Santa Monica, California. They reported their results in 174 early-stage breast cancer patients undergoing axillary dissection, either as part of a modified radical mastectomy or in conjunction with lumpectomy. After induction of general anesthesia, 1% isosulfan blue vital dye was injected into the breast mass and the immediately surrounding breast tissue with a 25-gauge needle. After the first 20 patients, the dose was standardized to 3 to 5 mL. Larger volumes were used for tumors farther from the axilla and smaller volumes for primary lesions close to the axilla so as to avoid flooding of the axilla by the dye. Similarly, the delay between injection and commencement of axillary dissection was standardized at 5 minutes after the first 20 cases. A transverse incision was made just below the hair-bearing region of the axilla, and blunt dissection was performed until a blue-stained lymphatic or node was encountered. Dissection was carried distally as necessary to reach a node and proximally if possible to ensure that the first stained node was in fact excised. Thereafter, axillary dissection was completed to include levels I and II and at least some level III nodes. If grossly involved metastatic nodes were present, a complete level III node dissection was performed. Standard hematoxylin and eosin pathology techniques were employed for the initial evaluation; however, false-negative sentinel nodes were retrospectively examined by cytokeratin immunohistochemical techniques.

Among this group of 174 patients, the SLN was successfully identified in 114 (65.5%). In these patients, the pathologic status of the SLN accurately predicted the pathologic status of the whole axilla as determined by standard axillary dissection with an accuracy of 95.6%. The authors noted a distinct learning curve, with all their false-negative studies falling within the first half of their series. Among the five false-negative cases, three were found on reexamination not to have contained lymph nodes, one remained false-negative, and one was reassigned as positive by virtue of a positive result on immunohistochemical cytokeratin examination.

As the technique has been perfected, it is now recommended that the dye be injected into the aspect of the tumor volume facing the axilla (60). Injection of the skin, the subfascial region, or a biopsy cavity *per se* must be avoided or reliable patterns of lymphatic flow will not to be produced. Firm manual compression of the breast over the injection site with use of a gentle rotating motion is now recommended and must be begun immediately after injection and continued until axillary dissection is commenced to achieve optimal dye filling of the lymphatics. It is recommended that for high upper outer quadrant primary lesions dissection commence after a 3-minute massage following the injection. Lower inner quadrant lesions should be massaged for 7 to 10 minutes to allow dye to reach the axilla before node dissection is commenced. For all other regions, a 5-minute massage/delay appears optimal. Giuliano further recommends that during axillary dissection, the subcutaneous tissue be dissected by electrocautery without regard to transection of fine superficial subcutaneous lymphatics, should they be stained. Meticulous care, however, is required once the clavipectoral fascia is reached so that hemostasis is optimized, the blue-stained lymph vessel is identified and preserved, and the path to the lymph nodes of interest, both proximal and distal, can be traced (61).

Complications of this procedure appear to be related to the dissection alone. When the pathologic results of sentinel node sampling are negative, complications are minimal. Typically, patients have blue-tinged urine and feces for up to 2 days following the procedure. Additionally, a blue tinge to the breast skin near the injection site may develop; when the injection is performed after a lumpectomy has been completed, this discoloration may persist for some months. Allergic reactions occur in up to 1.5% of patients and usually are of a wheal-and-flare type overlying the injection site, with pruritus and sometimes blue hives of the hands, neck, abdomen, and intertriginous areas. These usually respond to intravenous diphenhydramine. Anaphylactoid reactions have also been reported with isosulfan blue, but these have not (yet) occurred in a sentinel node biopsy series. Isolated hypotension occurring one-half hour after injection has been described in one patient. It has been postulated that more severe adverse reactions may occur when isosulfan blue is mixed in a syringe with local anesthetic, which causes the dye to precipitate. Obviously, this must be avoided (62–64).

Gamma Probe Technique

Krag and associates (65,66) were the first to introduce radiocolloid localization for SLN identification and biopsy in patients with breast cancer. The report of their pilot study describes the procedure in 22 patients, three with clinically positive axillae, who underwent levels I, II, and III axillary dissection following completion of the sentinel node procedure. The total dose of radiocolloid (^{99m}Tc-sulfur colloid) administered was 0.4 mCi in a total volume of 0.5 mL of normal saline solution. Injection was performed from 1 to 9 hours before the initiation of axillary dissection. Radiocolloid was injected along a 180-degree arc at the periphery of the tumor or biopsy cavity facing the axilla. Five 0.1-mL injections were placed. Before incision, the axilla was scanned with a hand-held gamma detector. The practical cutoff points for identifying a sentinel node were 30 counts in 10 seconds through the skin or 25 counts in 10 seconds *ex vivo* in the resected specimen. In the event that multiple candidates were obtained, the node with the highest count was designated the sentinel node. By these criteria, sentinel nodes were isolated from 19 of the 22 patients before completion of the axillary dissection. Standard hematoxylin and eosin pathologic evaluation was performed on all nodal material. Among the 18 evaluable patients, seven had some metastatic axillary adenopathy. All these had positive sentinel nodes. In three patients, only the sentinel node contained tumor. In three of the patients, the sentinel node was found in an unusually lateral and inferior location and might have been missed in a standard axillary dissection. The mean 10-second counts for SLNs were 296 through the skin before incision and 899 *ex vivo* in the resected nodal tissue.

This initial success led promptly to a multicenter validation study undertaken by a group of 11 surgeons, by design practicing in a variety of settings (67). The technique was altered to deliver a ^{99m}Tc-sulfur colloid activity of 1.0 mCi in a volume of 4.0 mL. It was hoped that this increased volume would enhance sentinel node localization. Between 30 minutes and 8 hours before surgery, the radiocolloid suspension was injected in equally divided aliquots at the four clock quadrants (3, 6, 9, and 12 o'clock) into the breast tissue surrounding the primary tumor or biopsy cavity. Using the hand-held gamma probe, the surgeon first outlined the diffusion zone of radioactivity immediately surrounding the injected volume. Next, the axilla was examined, and all sites of activity producing more than 25 counts in 10 seconds were marked on the skin. Dissection was then carried down to each of these sites, and as much tissue was resected as was necessary to return the background counts to less than 10% of the highest "hot spot" count. Axillary dissection of levels I and II nodes was then performed. Level III nodes were removed if deemed suspect by the surgeon. Standard hematoxylin and eosin pathologic examination was performed on all specimens.

Among the 443 patients entered into the study, sentinel nodes were identified in 413 (93%). Nodal malignancy was found in 114 patients. Positive and negative predictive values and overall accuracy were quite high—100%, 96%, and 97%, respectively. Even though all 11 surgeons had gone through a training period and performed at least five procedures before operating on the patients in the study, considerable variability among results was seen. Three surgeons had no false-negative results. One had a 28.6% rate of false-negatives. Most fell in the 10% to 17% range. Similar variability (but no correlation) was seen in the surgeons' ability to find sentinel nodes.

Approximately 93% of the patients had only one "hot spot." Patients with multiple hot spots tended to have internal mammary sentinel nodes. Only 4.3% of sentinel nodes, however, were in the internal mammary region; 89% of sentinel nodes were in the level I axilla, and 4.0% were in level II axilla or elsewhere.

The authors noted that all their known false-negative studies were in patients with primaries in the lateral breast and proposed further increases in the diluent volume used for radiocolloid injection in an effort to improve sentinel node visibility. Alternatively, the use of blue dye was suggested as a supplementary tool. They suggested that internal mammary node involvement might be understated because of "shine-through" from radioactivity in the nearby medial primaries. They noted poorer results in studies performed after large excisions. They also found, contrary to our experience, a lower sensitivity in older patients.

The overriding concern raised by this important report, however, must be the 11% false-negative rate. Clearly, this will not do for life-and-death decision making. The authors have given much thought to the potential explanations for these false-negative studies. Studies continue in efforts to reduce the frequency of false-negative results. One possible explanation from our experience is the surgical learning curve.

We have analyzed outcomes to generate a set of learning curves for five surgeons principally performing combined dye–radiocolloid sentinel node biopsy procedures (69). The high initial failure rate that was noted declines precipitously after the first 20 cases are completed. The learning curve representing the mean of five surgeons' performances indicates that 23 cases must be completed to achieve a 90% success rate, and 53 cases to reach a 95% success rate. The most effective remedy for the high false-negative rate seen in the multicenter validation study is practice.

Combined Dye and Gamma Probe Technique with Augmented Pathologic Examination

Technique of Injection and Scanning

At the H. Lee Moffitt Cancer Center and Research Institute, we have combined vital dye and radiocolloid mapping with augmented pathologic examination in the hope of maximizing the capabilities of the SLN approach. Because hours are typically required for intense SLN uptake, we usually inject radiocolloid approximately 2 to 4 hours before scheduled surgery. The transport of blue dye is much quicker, so blue dye is injected in the operative suite just before incision of the axilla.

If the tumor is palpable, six peripheral injections are performed at the depth of the tumor. Care is taken not to inject into the tumor, as this appears to impede lymphatic flow during the course of the study. It also makes the tumor radioactive, which complicates processing frozen sections in a routine and timely manner. If the tumor has already been excised, a seroma cavity is usually present and palpable. This is handled for injection purposes as if it were the tumor itself. Care should be taken not to inject the radiopharmaceutical into the seroma cavity, as this will impede lymphatic flow. Also, if the seroma cavity is disrupted, as is likely during surgery, spillage of radioactive material will occur, and possibly contamination.

With impalpable lesions that have been only mammographically identified, we inject circumferentially around the lesion, approximately 1 cm from the localization wire. This is a departure from our earlier practice of injecting through the localization needle, which we have discontinued because radiopharmaceutical has been lost or wicked out through the localization needle, resulting in a significant loss of dose and, more importantly, substantial skin contamination, which complicates the detection of lymph nodes with the hand-held gamma probe.

The use of ultrasonography is encouraged during all injection procedures, but especially when the tumor or seroma is not palpable. Ultrasonography allows precise injection at the correct depth and through the shortest distance of tissue. It also obviates any concern of creating a pneumothorax. Additionally, ultrasonographic localization of the needle is advantageous. When localization is performed with the mammographic technique, the distal tip of the wire can be identified by ultrasonography to allow for a simple injection. If the patient has small breasts or the lesion is superficial, the patient can be taken out of mammographic compression and the injection can be performed at the correct depth with the patient supine and the arm raised over the head. If the patient has large breasts or the lesion is deep, the patient can be injected while in the mammographic grid. Injections are made circumferentially at the approximate depth of the tumor.

A dose of 450 μCi of ^{99m}Tc-sulfur colloid, previously passed through a 0.2-μm filter, is used in most cases. This provides a particle size that has been found to be nearly optimal for traversing lymphatics. If the particle is too small, it is taken up to some extent in the capillaries, so that the target-to-background ratio is poor. If the particle is too large, it tends to linger *in situ* and increase the amount of injection site artifact. If the location of the lesion is extremely medial

or extremely lateral, the dose is reduced to 250 μCi to limit artifacts related to the injection site, which can potentially mask sentinel lymph nodes and result in false-negative studies. As a rule, we use freshly prepared radiocolloid to minimize clumping, which effectively increases the particle size.

The radiopharmaceutical should be well shaken just before the injection. The ideal volume of diluent is a matter of controversy. In a randomized study comparing 2-mL and 6-mL injections, we found no difference in the SLN-to-background uptake ratio for the two volumes. Accordingly, the use of 2 mL of diluent is advocated. Intuitively, this is more physiologic; also, less "blooming" and artifact related to the injection site activity is noted when the injection with the greater specific activity is used. All doses are divided so that six injections can be performed. Injections are made circumferentially so that internal mammary drainage, if present, will be identified.

Massaging the breast for 3 to 5 minutes after injection of the radiopharmaceutical is highly beneficial. It enables earlier visualization of the SLN and more uptake of the radiopharmaceutical within the SLN. The number of lymph nodes identified is not increased following breast massage. Imaging can be performed immediately, but usually the lymph nodes are more clearly visualized after a delay, which allows the radiopharmaceutical to traverse through the afferent lymphatics. Therefore, if an SLN is not identified on immediate imaging, imaging should be repeated after a 2- to 4-hour delay.

The patient is placed in a supine position beneath the gamma camera. A scintillation camera with a large field of view and a high-resolution collimator are used. The window is set for the 140-Kev energy peak of ^{99m}Tc. The patient's arm is extended above the head, and the hand is placed under the head to optimize axillary exposure. The patient is imaged in lateral, anterior, and oblique projections. Every effort is made to remove the injection site from the field of view, or to position the injection site away from the draining lymph node groups. This can be achieved by having the patient imaged while standing, by taping the breast out of the field of view, or by applying a lead shield. Cine-imaging can be helpful, but because the lymphatic flow is slower than with cutaneous lesions, it is usually neither necessary nor helpful. The persistence scope is used to identify accumulations of the radiopharmaceutical corresponding to the lymph nodes.

Images are acquired during 8 to 10 minutes to ensure a high count density. Internal mammary and supraclavicular lymph nodes can be tattooed or marked on the skin in the anterior projection, and the axillary lymph nodes are tattooed or marked with the patient in the lateral position with the arm above the head. The patient can be imaged on a cobalt flood source to define the body contour. Alternatively, the body contour and landmarks can be demonstrated with use of a ^{99m}Tc marker. Imaging is performed immediately after injection and subsequently, following a 2- to 4-hour delay, just before removal to the surgical suite.

As a generality, we prefer the longest practical delay between injection and axillary surgery so as to maximize the target-to-background ratio. Delays beyond the range of 12 to 14 hours, however, begin to pose problems with radionuclide decay. Cases scheduled for the early morning can successfully be injected with the radiopharmaceutical the afternoon before surgery. In the operative suite, the surgeon first scans the axilla and the tattooed sites to identify areas of high activity. The primary tumor site is injected with 5 to 10 mL of isosulfan blue vital dye. The technique is similar to that used for the radiopharmaceutical injection.

In our institution, surgeons have been able to locate 94% of all SLNs within a 5-cm circle in the low axilla. The center of this circle is defined by the intersection of two lines: a line tangential to the axillary hairline, anterior to posterior, and a line through the central axilla that cuts the hairline into halves. The great majority of the remaining SLNs are found in level II. The circle described is most useful as a starting point for identifying the SLN with the hand-held gamma probe. Incision is made over the suspected SLN site. Dissection should initially proceed perpendicularly toward the chest wall rather than cephalad. Once the clavipectoral fascia is penetrated, the lateral thoracic vein is identified. The point where the lateral branch of the third intercostal nerve crosses the vein defines the center of the region wherein most SLNs are found (69). Dissection follows the blue-stained afferent lymphatics to the sentinel lymph node. Particular care is taken to avoid spillage of blood or lymphatic fluid. Sentinel lymph nodes are defined as any blue node or any node with three times the number of *in vivo* background counts per minute or more (*ex vivo*, 10 times the counts per minute of a nonsentinel node). After initial excision, the gamma probe is returned to the axillary bed. Dissection is continued so long as the lymph node bed has more than 150% of background counts.

Pathologic Examination of the Sentinel Lymph Node

A crucial element in our studies is the pathology protocol developed to maximize the retrieval of information from the sentinel nodes that are removed (70). The goals are to minimize the need for repeated hospitalization and anesthesia and to maximize the sensitivity of sentinel node pathologic evaluation such that the fewest possible micrometastases are missed. Clearly, to avoid the need for repeated hospitalization, it is necessary to inform the surgeon of the presence of a malignant sentinel node at the time of the sentinel node procedure. Full axillary dissection can then be completed as an extension of the same procedure. At our institution, we have developed an intraoperative imprint cytology technique, or touch preparation (71). Nodes larger than 5 mm are serially sectioned at 2- to 3-mm intervals to maximize the surface area available for intraoperative imprint cytology. Cross sections are then imprinted on clean, noncoated, charged glass slides, which are air dried in preparation for Diff-Quik staining. With interpretation, the turnaround time for this procedure is about 16 minutes. Results of studies are reported as positive, negative, or indeterminate. Indeterminate readings are most likely in cases of low tumor volume or of lobular or low-grade ductal carcinoma. The pathology department has recently been able to adapt a cytokeratin immunostaining procedure that has helped to identify many negative and positive studies within the indeterminate group (*unpublished data*). All sentinel nodes, in particular those remaining in the negative or indeterminate groups, are fixed in formalin, and the ^{99m}Tc label is allowed to decay a minimum of 10 half-lives, after which the nodes are prepared for permanent section. The initial section from nodes failing to show malignancy is stained with both hematoxylin and eosin and cytokeratin immunostain. Care is taken to examine the subcapsular lymphatic sinuses, which most typically harbor the micrometastatic tumor cell clusters, and also the medullary sinuses and follicular areas. The pathologists have described a diffuse single-cell parenchymal metastatic pattern typical of metastatic lobular carcinoma, in which hematoxylin and eosin staining is almost always negative but cytokeratin immunostaining is positive.

If the node remains negative, one to three 5-μm-thick specimens taken at 50-μm intervals per block are stained with hematoxylin and eosin. In our institutional experience, the intraoperative imprint cytology method confirmed 100% of grossly malignant SLNs. The false-negative rate was 8.3% among 291 grossly negative SLNs. The false-positive rate was 0.3%. Our permanent section technique, including cytokeratin immunostaining, has identified micrometastasis in 41 of 385 hematoxylin and eosin-negative SLNs (10.6%). Because metastatic disease was identified in 134 of 385 patients whose SLNs were examined, our augmented technique alone identified 30.6% of patients in need of more aggressive therapy (72).

Results of Combined Injection Method with Augmented Pathology

With the use of these evolving techniques, we now have data from 700 breast cancer patients, three fourths of whom were treated with lumpectomy and one fourth with mastectomy (73). A total of 186 phase I patients underwent axillary lymph node dissection following the sentinel node biopsy procedure. Of these, 120 had negative findings on SLN pathology, and only one of them was found to have metastasis elsewhere in the axilla on review of the formal axillary lymph node dissection. This constitutes a false-negative rate of 0.83%, with a 95% confidence interval of 0.02% to 4.6%. Among these phase I patients, we achieved an SLN identification rate of 92%. All patients in whom an SLN was not identified had medial lesions and possibly no axillary nodal drainage of their tumors. Thirty-two percent of our patients, all of whom had benign findings on axillary physical examination, were found on pathology to have axillary metastases, consistent with the known and expected incidence for this clinical group. Importantly, all patients with axillary metastasis had metastatic disease within the SLN. In two thirds of patients with axillary metastasis, the SLN was the only site of metastatic disease. The average yield of sentinel nodes was 2.03 per patient.

Among the remaining 514 patients, axillary node dissection was performed only in those with positive sentinel node biopsy results or in whom no sentinel node could be found. Among the 368 remaining patients with negative findings on sentinel node pathology but no follow-up axillary dissection, no axillary relapses have occurred during a mean follow-up of 20 months.

Overall, we were successful in identifying and excising sentinel nodes in 95% of our patients. Blue dye identified the sentinel node in 76.1%. Radiocolloid identified the sentinel node in 90.1%. Among the 35 patients in whom a sentinel node was not found, metastasis was identified in eight (22.8%). Of the 95% of patients in whom SLN imaging was successful, 176 (26.5%) harbored nodal metastatic disease.

Among the 700 patients enrolled in the study, the T-stage distribution was 21.4%, 5.7%, 22.3%, 32.4%, 15.8%, and 2.3% for stages Tis, T1a, T1b, T1c, T2, and T3, respectively. The corresponding instances of nodal metastatic disease were Tis, 7.6%; T1a, 12.8%; T1b, 23.5%; T1c, 29.8%; T2, 46.7%; and T3, 92.3%. The significant percentage of patients with carcinoma apparently *in situ* who are found to have nodal metastatic disease is surprising and of concern. Most of these patients underwent initial biopsy at outside institutions; we have not been able to categorize these patients in detail with regard to such parameters as tumor size, subtype, extent of microinvasion, and nuclear grade. Clarification of these data requires significant attention.

Controversies

Systematic evaluation of the technical variables involved in SLN developmental studies is urgently needed. It is of particular importance that techniques reflect an approach that is practical for the community setting if this technology is to become useful in clinical practice. As a particular caution, SLN techniques useful in melanoma have not been shown to be useful in breast carcinoma.

Many investigators have been successful with an array of radiotracers and techniques in melanoma studies (74). This is probably because of the particular richness of cutaneous lymphatics and because the intradermal injection forces the eluant into the lymphatics under pressure. These factors are absent in the breast.

We continue to favor ^{99m}Tc-sulfur colloid over ^{99m}Tc-human serum albumin as the preferred imaging agent. The tendency of human serum albumin to pass rapidly through multiple lymph nodes raises the risk that SLNs will be passed through and second-echelon nodes mistakenly sampled. The frequent labeling of six to eight lymph nodes during our attempts to use human serum albumin supports this concern. Additionally, the labeling of so many nodes requires a much more extensive and potentially morbid surgical sampling.

Although ^{99m}Tc-antimony trisulfide is widely used in Europe, Australia, and Canada, it is not available in the United States. This agent is popular because its distribution of particle sizes is nearly ideal for lymph node uptake and sequestration. ^{186}Re-Colloid is also widely used in Europe with great success. However, ^{99m}Tc-sulfur colloid can be prepared to provide a comparable range of particle sizes. Alazraki et al. (75) have studied the effects of duration of heating and elution time, in addition to filtration of the colloid, in an effort to optimize the particle size distribution of the ^{99m}Tc-sulfur colloid injectate. This group has had excellent results in melanoma studies with their preparation. Whether this preparation will prove advantageous in breast carcinoma is not known. Of note, we and others have had comparable results in our melanoma series with less rigorously prepared radiolabeled agents. Indeed, Krag and colleagues (76), in their multicenter validation study of breast SLN biopsy, have used unfiltered ^{99m}Tc-sulfur colloid and obtained a sensitivity of 89%.

We believe that it is probably desirable to remove at least some of the larger particles. Because the larger particles tend to deposit in and around the injection site, excluding them from the injectate will diminish the confounding effects of lingering activity at the primary site. The relatively high false-negative SLN detection rate described in the study of Krag et al. (76), in which all false-negatives occurred in patients with laterally situated breast primaries, may have been the consequence of high residual activity in injection sites obscuring lesser activity in the nearby SLN. Similarly, the frequent failure to identify SLNs in medially placed tumors may be caused by residual activity in the medial primary sites obscuring internal mammary node activity. These missed internal mammary SLNs cannot be scored as false-negatives because no "control" dissections of the internal mammary node basin were performed to prove that nodes were present and were missed. Indeed, we suspect that the 1,000-μCi injection dose of Krag et al. is comparable to our 450-μCi dose and the 400-μCi doses of others, with the greater part of the 600-μCi discrepancy retained not in the nodes but in the primary and its surroundings. In our practice, axillary tail primaries are injected with only 250 μCi so that the likelihood that the SLN will be "outshone" and obscured by activity in the primary site is absolutely minimized.

Other groups of patients have been identified by the Multicenter Validation Study as likely to have false-negative results on radiocolloid SLN biopsy. These include elderly women, in whom fat that has replaced lymph nodes may retard radiocolloid uptake, and women who have undergone excisional biopsy before SLN dissection. We have not seen poorer results in elderly women and cannot explain why this has been the experience in the Multicenter Validation Study. We have also studied the effect of prior excisional biopsy on the results of radiocolloid SLN examination (77). In our experience, prior excisional biopsy did not alter the success rate of SLN lymphoscintigraphy but did increase the mean number of SLNs harvested from approximately two to approximately three. We have found, however, an adverse impact on SLN sensitivity among patients who have gone on to mastectomy and breast reconstruction. Presumably, this group includes many patients with (relatively) larger biopsy cavities in whom breast conservation would be unsatisfactory. Hence our suspicion that the larger the postlumpectomy cavity, the greater the likelihood of a false-negative SLN study.

Two noteworthy innovations proposed to simplify the method and improve results in breast SLN detection have been questioned recently by Uren and associates (78). We share the concerns they have raised. One of these strategies is to increase the volume of injected diluent to improve the performance of breast SLN lymphoscintigraphy. Our concern is that the use of large volumes, which disrupt the mechanism and pattern of lymph flow, is not physiologic and will lead to false-positive studies. Obviously, we do not agree with Uren's group that the six 1-mL aliquots used in our department transgress the nonphysiologic threshold. Parenthetically, we have compared total injectate volumes of 2 mL versus 6 mL in a blinded, randomized study in our department and found no difference in performance between the two, and no statistically significant difference in the count ratios of SLN to background (79).

The other innovation that causes us concern is injection of the skin overlying the tumor to track the lymphatic flow and locate the SLN(s). Given the rich dermal and subdermal lymphatic network and the high rate of lymphatic fluid flow, this should identify the most easily visualized nodes and certainly the most easily accessed site for injection and lymphatic mapping. Our concern is that it may not be the most accurate. Veronesi and colleagues (80) have described the use of subdermal injections and reported a false-negative SLN rate of 5.4%. This is less accurate than the results obtained at the John Wayne Cancer Institute and at our institution in more than 700 patients (< 1% false-negative SLNs) and raises in our minds the concern that this discrepancy may be a consequence of what we perceive to be a substantial but nevertheless incomplete overlap in drainage patterns between breast parenchyma and overlying skin.

Perhaps the most challenging investigations in this area have been undertaken by Borgstein et al. (81). In a pilot study, he describes a group of 33 patients who underwent peritumoral radiocolloid injection followed a day later by intradermal injection of 0.5 mL of Patent Blue V dye, 2.5% solution, into the skin immediately overlying the tumor. A variety of breast tumor sizes and locations were included in the study. They found a 100% concordance in SLN delineation between blue dye and radiocolloid, ^{99m}Tc-colloidal albumin in this case. No false-negatives were reported. In a follow-up study, he and his associates describe two groups of breast SLN patients, each also undergoing radiocolloid peritumoral injection (82). The day after the radiocolloid injection, 0.5 to 1.0 mL of Patent Blue V dye was injected into the skin overlying the tumor (first 68 patients) or into the skin lateral to the areola, without regard to tumor site (succeeding 85 patients). They found a 91% concordance between radiotracer and blue dye in the first group and a 96% concordance in the second group. Dye failed to identify a "hot" (radioactive) SLN in 8% of their first patient group and 3% of their second patient group. The difference, they suggest, may be attributable to a learning curve for the surgeons. They cite evidence that the breast and its overlying skin develop from the same ectodermal region and that their lymphatics therefore drain as a single biologic unit. They argue that their findings reflect the underlying biology of the breast and its skin rather than a rich but incomplete interchange between adjacent lymphatic networks.

Based on our clinical experience, we remain cautious about this approach. In our estimation, this approach is nonphysiologic and presupposes that lymphatic flow from skin corresponds to that from the underlying tumor. In our extensive experience with melanoma lymphoscintigraphy, for example, we have never seen a clear case of internal mammary uptake from a mammary skin site. Indeed, melanoma SLNs are commonly found in the ipsilateral or contralateral supraclavicular or jugular basins, or even the contralateral axilla. Among our more than 700 SLN patients injected at the tumor site, we have seen crossover to the contralateral axilla only once. We suspect that the frequent presence of two or even three SLNs in patients injected in the skin overlying the tumor probably reflects drainage from a different, and much richer, lymphatic system than that of the underlying breast (tumor) (83,84). It will require a substantial clinical effort to put this controversy to rest. To conduct a study with an 80% likelihood of recognizing a 5% discrepancy between two approaches to injection will require randomization of 424 patients (85). We are also in the process of performing parallel studies designed to provide a better understanding of the approaches presented by Veronesi et al. (80) and Borgstein et al. (81).

One innovation for which we share the general enthusiasm, however, is the increasingly popular use of massage of the injection site. We massage the site for 3 to 5 minutes immediately after injection and have found that this does shorten the time to localization and improves the target-to-background ratio. We are in the process of accumulating data to quantify these effects.

CONCLUSIONS

Preoperative breast lymphoscintigraphy directs the surgeon to the site of the SLN, thereby minimizing the operative time

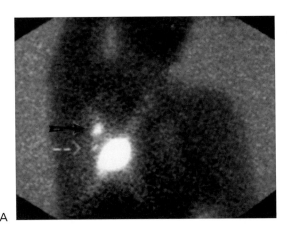
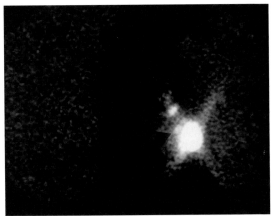

A

B

FIGURE 20.3. A: The right anterior oblique chest lymphoscintigram is the only way to identify an in-transit intramammary lymph node (*broken arrow*). The axillary lymph node (*arrow*) is also present. **B:** The right lateral chest lymphoscintigram shows the in-transit intramammary lymph node (*arrowhead*) near the injection site in the breast parenchyma and also the axillary lymph node (*arrow*).

and extent of dissection and the likelihood of late morbidity. Because our data show that a particular surgeon must perform a number of procedures (53 cases to achieve a 95% success rate) to become truly proficient, it is likely that a longer apprenticeship than has hitherto been required is likely to improve the accuracy of the procedure. Preoperative lymphoscintigraphy may also be helpful in the training process. Identification of in-transit intramammary lymph nodes (Fig. 20.3) can be accomplished only with the use of lymphoscintigraphy, which identifies a subset of patients inadequately examined by standard axillary dissection techniques. Two thirds of patients with medial tumors have no discernible flow to the axilla (Fig. 20.4). The use of lymphoscintigraphy may obviate the need for axillary dissection in these patients altogether. At a minimum, identification of internal mammary SLNs (Fig. 20.5) allows for rational radiotherapeutic planning in patients who might not otherwise be recognized to be potential candidates for this therapy.

Two complementary methodologies are available for lymphatic mapping to identify SLNs in patients with breast carcinoma. Blue dye gives the surgeon important visual clues and should be used as an adjunct to radiocolloid. In particular, blue dye is often useful as a backup in the 10% of cases that fail to show evidence of radiopharmaceutical uptake.

Many questions remain regarding the optimal methods for performing these procedures. The site of injection, the volume of injectate, and the ideal particle size and activity of the radiocolloid all remain uncertain. Nevertheless, the combined use of vital blue dye and radiocolloid lymphoscintigraphy and lymphatic mapping appears to be a practical technique for identifying SLNs, so that selective lymphadenectomy can be performed in patients with carcinoma of the breast. It reduces morbidity and improves the diagnostic yield.

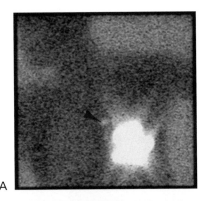

A

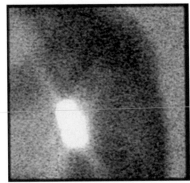

B

FIGURE 20.4. A: Anterior chest lymphoscintigraphy shows uptake in the ipsilateral internal mammary chain (*arrowhead*) in a medial quadrant tumor. **B:** The left lateral chest lymphoscintigram shows no definite afferent drainage to the axilla, as is the case with two thirds of medial tumors.

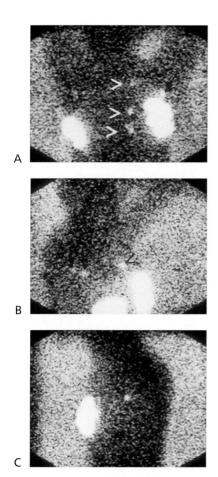

FIGURE 20.5. Anterior chest (**A**), right anterior oblique chest (**B**), and left lateral chest (**C**) lymphoscintigrams from a patient with bilateral breast cancers show left internal mammary uptake (*arrowheads*) and bilateral axillary drainage (*arrows*).

REFERENCES

1. Mettlin C. Global breast cancer mortality statistics. *CA Cancer J Clin* 1999;49:138–144.
2. La Vecchia C, Negri E, Levi F, et al. Age, cohort-of-birth, and period-of-death trends in breast cancer mortality in Europe [Letter]. *J Natl Cancer Inst* 1997;89:732–734.
3. Nagata C, Kawakami N, Shimizu H. Trends in the incidence rate and risk factors for breast cancer in Japan. *Breast Cancer Res Treat* 1997;44:75–82.
4. Chu KC, Tarone RE, Kessler L, et al. Recent trends in U.S. breast cancer incidence, survival and mortality rates. *J Natl Cancer Inst* 1996;88:1571–1579.
5. Wingo PA, Ries LA, Rosenberg HM, et al. Cancer incidence and mortality, 1973–1995: a report card for the U.S. *Cancer* 1998;82:1197–1207.
6. Fletcher WE, Black W, Harris R, et al. Report of the International Workshop on Screening for Breast Cancer. *J Natl Cancer Inst* 1993;85:1644–1656.
7. Bland KI, Menck HR, Scott-Conner CE, et al. The National Can-

cer Data Base 10-year survey of breast cancer treatment at hospitals in the United States. *Cancer* 1998;83:1262–1273.
8. American Cancer Society. Mammographic guidelines 1983. Background statement and update of cancer-related check-up guidelines for breast cancer detection in asymptomatic women ages 40–49. *CA Cancer J Clin* 1983;33:254.
9. Fremgen AM, Bland KI, McGinnis LS Jr, et al. Clinical highlights from the National Cancer Data Base, 1999. *CA Cancer J Clin* 1999;49:145–158.
10. Ferguson D, Meier P, Karrison T, et al. Staging of breast cancer and survival rates: an assessment based on 50 years of experience with radical mastectomy. *JAMA* 1970;248:1337–1341.
11. Valagussa P, Bonadonna G, Veronesi U. Patterns of relapse and survival following radical mastectomy: analysis of 716 consecutive patients. *Cancer* 1978;41:1170–1178.
12. American Joint Committee on Cancer. *Cancer staging manual*, 5th ed. Philadelphia: Lippincott–Raven Publishers, 1997:171–178.
13. Yeatman TJ, Cox CE. The significance of breast cancer lymph node micrometastases. *Surg Oncol Clin N Am* 1999;8:481–496.
14. de Mascarel I, Bonichon F, Coindre JM, et al. Prognostic significance of breast cancer axillary lymph node micrometastases assessed by two special techniques: reevaluation with longer follow-up. *Br J Cancer* 1992;66:523–527.
15. Friedman S, Bertin F, Mouriesse H, et al. Importance of tumor cells in axillary node sinus margins ("clandestine" metastases) discovered by serial sectioning in operable breast carcinoma. *Acta Oncol* 1988;27:483–487.
16. Bonadonna G, Brusamolino E, Valagussa P. Combination chemotherapy as an adjuvant treatment in operable breast cancer. *N Engl J Med* 1976;294:405–410.
17. Fisher B, Carbone P, Economou SG. L-Phenylalanine mustard (L-PAM) in the management of primary breast cancer: a report of early findings. *N Engl J Med* 1975;292:117–122.
18. Bonadonna G. Evolving concepts in the systemic adjuvant treatment of breast cancer. *Cancer Res* 1992;52:2127–2137.
19. Early Breast Cancer Trialists' Group. Polychemotherapy for early breast cancer: an overview of the randomised trials. *Lancet* 1998;352:930.
20. McGuire WL. Adjuvant therapy of node-negative breast cancer. *N Engl J Med* 1989;320:525–527.
21. Kallionieme OP, Holli K, Visakorpi T, et al. Association of c-erB-2 protein overexpression with high rate of cell proliferation, increased risk of visceral metastasis and poor long-term survival in breast cancer. *Int J Cancer* 1991;49:650.
22. Noguchi M, Koyasaki N, Ohta N, et al. C-erB-2 oncoprotein expression versus internal mammary lymph node metastases as additional prognostic factors in patients with axillary lymph node-positive breast cancer. *Cancer* 1992;69:2953.
23. Munster PN, Hudis CA. Adjuvant therapy for resectable breast cancer. *Hematol Oncol Clin North Am* 1999;13:391–413.
24. Dowlatshahi K, Fan M, Bloom K, et al. Occult metastases in the sentinel lymph nodes of patients with early stage breast carcinoma: a preliminary study. *Cancer* 1999;86:990–996.
25. Allred DC, Elledge RM. Caution concerning micrometastatic breast carcinoma in sentinel lymph nodes. *Cancer* 1999;86:905–907.
26. Schottenfeld D, Nash A, Robbins G, et al. Ten-year results of the treatment of primary operable breast cancer. *Cancer* 1976;38:1001–1007.
27. Bucalossi P, Veronesi U, Zingo L, et al. Enlarged mastectomy for breast cancer: review of 1213 cases. *Am J Roentgenol Radium Ther Nucl Med* 1971;111:119–122.
28. Smith J, Gamez-Araujo J, Gallager H, et al. Carcinoma of the breast. *Cancer* 1977;39:527–532.

29. Veronesi U, Rilke F, Luini R. Distribution of axillary node metastases by level of invasion. An analysis of 539 cases. *Cancer* 1987; 59:682–687.

30. Rosen P, Lesser M, Kinne D. Discontinuous or "skip" metastases in breast carcinoma: analysis of 1228 axillary dissections. *Ann Surg* 1983;187:276–283.

31. Veronesi U, Valagussa P. Inefficacy of internal mammary node dissection in breast cancer surgery. *Cancer* 1981;47:170–175.

32. Morrow M, Roster RS Jr. Staging of breast cancer: a new rationale for internal mammary node biopsy. *Arch Surg* 1981;116:748–751.

33. Baker R, Montague A, Childs J. A comparison of modified radical mastectomy to radical mastectomy in the treatment of operable breast cancer. *Ann Surg* 1979;189:553–559.

34. Bland KI. Enhancing the accuracy for predictors of axillary nodal metastasis in T1 carcinoma of the breast: role of selective biopsy with lymphatic mapping [Editorial]. *J Am Coll Surg* 1996;183: 262–264.

35. Turner L, Swindell R, Bell W. Radical versus modified radical mastectomy for breast cancer. *Ann R Coll Surg Engl* 1981;63:239–243.

36. Maddox W, Carpenter J, Laws H. A randomized prospective trial of radical mastectomy versus modified radical mastectomy in 311 breast cancer patients. *Ann Surg* 1983;198:207–212.

37. Say C, Donegan W. A biostatistical evaluation of complications from mastectomy. *Surg Gynecol Obstet* 1974;138:370–376.

38. Aitken D, Minton J. Complications associated with mastectomy. *Surg Clin North Am* 1983;63:1331–1352.

39. Robinson G, Van Heerden J, Payne WEA. The primary surgical treatment of carcinoma of the breast. A changing trend toward modified radical mastectomy. *Mayo Clin Proc* 1976;51: 433–442.

40. Fisher B, Redmond C, Fisher E. Ten-year results of a randomized clinical trial comparing radical mastectomy and total mastectomy with or without radiation. *N Engl J Med* 1985;312:674–681.

41. Fisher B, Redmond C, Poisson R, et al. Eight-year results of a randomized clinical trial comparing total mastectomy and lumpectomy with and without radiation in the treatment of breast cancer. *N Engl J Med* 1989;320:822–828.

42. Larson D, Weinstein M, Goldberg I, et al. Edema of the arm as a function of the extent of axillary surgery in patients with stage I–II carcinoma of the breast treated with primary radiotherapy. *Int J Radiat Oncol Biol Phys* 1986;12:1575–1582.

43. Siegel B, Mayzel K, Love S. Level I and II axillary dissection in the treatment of early stage breast cancer. *Arch Surg* 1990;125: 1144–1147.

44. Pezner R, Patterson M, Hill L. Arm edema in patients treated conservatively for breast cancer: relationship to patient age and axillary node dissection technique. *Int J Radiat Oncol Biol Phys* 1986;12: 2079–2083.

45. Sherman AI, Ter-Pogossian M. Lymph node concentration of radioactive colloidal gold following interstitial injection. *Cancer* 1953;6:1238–1240.

46. Matsuo S. Studies on the metastasis of breast cancer lymph nodes—II. Diagnosis of metastasis to internal mammary nodes using radiocolloid. *Acta Med Okayama* 1974;28:361–371.

47. Croll MN, Brady LW, Dadparvar S. Implications of lymphoscintigraphy in oncologic practice: principles and differences *vis-à-vis* other imaging modalities. *Semin Nucl Med* 1983;13:4–8.

48. Ege GN. Internal mammary lymphoscintigraphy. The rationale, technique, interpretation and clinical application: a review based on 848 cases. *Radiology* 1976;118:101–107.

49. Rossi R, Ferri O. La visualizzazione della catena mammaria internal con ¹⁹⁸Au. Presentazione di una nuova metodica: la linfoscintigrafia. *Minerva Med* 1966;57:1151–1155.

50. Schenk P. Scintigraphisce darstellung des parasternalen lymphsystems. *Strahlentherapie* 1966;130:504–508.

51. Ege GN. Lymphoscintigraphy—techniques and applications in the management of breast carcinoma. *Semin Nucl Med* 1983;13:26–34.

52. Dionne L, Friede J, Blais R. Internal mammary lymphoscintigraphy in breast carcinoma—a surgeon's perspective. *Semin Nucl Med* 1983;13:35–41.

53. Mclean RG, Ege GN. Prognostic value of axillary lymphoscintigraphy in breast carcinoma patients. *J Nucl Med* 1986;27:1116–1124.

54. Noguchi M, Michigishi T, Nakajima K, et al. The diagnosis of internal mammary node metastases of breast cancer. *Int Surg* 1993; 78:171–175.

55. Vendrell-Torne E, Setoain-Quinquer J, Domenech-Torne FM. Study of normal lymphatic drainage using radioactive isotopes. *J Nucl Med* 1972;13:801–805.

56. Uren RF, Howman-Giles RB, Thompson JF, et al. Mammary lymphoscintigraphy in breast cancer. *J Nucl Med* 1995;36:1775–1780.

57. Hultborn KA, Larsson LG, Ragnhult I. The lymph drainage from the breast to the axillary and parasternal lymph nodes studied with the aid of colloidal Au-198. *Acta Radiol* 1954;43:52–64.

58. Cabanas RM. An approach for the treatment of penile carcinoma. *Cancer* 1977;39:456–466.

59. Giuliano AE, Kirgan DM, Guenther JM, et al. Lymphatic mapping and sentinel lymphadenectomy for breast cancer. *Ann Surg* 1994;220:391–401.

60. Haigh PI, Giuliano AE. The technique of intraoperative lymphatic mapping and sentinel lymphadenectomy in breast cancer using blue dye alone. In: Whitman ED, Reintgen D, eds. *Radioguided surgery*. Austin, TX: Landes Bioscience, 1999, pp.83–89.

61. Cox CE, Bass SS, Reintgen DS. Techniques for lymphatic mapping in breast carcinoma. *Surgncol Clin N Am* 1999;8:447–468.

62. Product insert: lymphazurin 1% (isosulfan blue). Norwalk, CT: United States Surgical Corporation, 1997.

63. Hietala SO, Hirsch JI, Faunce HF. Allergic reaction to patent blue violet during lymphography. *Lymphology* 1977;10:158–160.

64. Longnecker SM, Guzzardo MM, Van Voris LP. Life-threatening anaphylaxis following subcutaneous administration of isosulfan blue 1%. *Clin Pharmacol* 1985;4:219–221.

65. Alex JC, Krag DN. Gamma-probe guided localization of lymph nodes. *Surg Oncol* 1993;2:137–143.

66. Krag DN, Weaver DL, Alex JC, et al. Surgical resection and radiolocalization of the sentinel lymph node in breast cancer using a gamma probe. *Surg Oncol* 1993;2:335–340.

67. Krag D, Weaver D, Ashikaga T, et al. The sentinel node in breast cancer. A multicenter validation study. *N Engl J Med* 1998;339: 941–946.

68. Cox CE, Bass SS, Boulware D, et al. Implementation of a new surgical technology: outcome measures for lymphatic mapping of breast carcinoma. *Ann Surg Oncol* 1999;6:553–561.

69. Cox CE, Bass SS, Reintgen DS. Techniques for lymphatic mapping in breast carcinoma. *Surg Oncol Clin N Am* 1999;8:447–468.

70. Ku NNK. Pathologic examination of sentinel lymph nodes in breast cancer. *Surg Oncol Clin N Am* 1999;8:469–479.

71. Cox C, Ku NNK, Nicosia S, et al. Touch preparation cytology of breast lumpectomy margins. *Arch Surg* 1991;126:490.

72. Ku NNK. Pathologic examination of sentinel lymph nodes in breast cancer. *Surg Oncol Clin N Am* 1999;8:469–479.

73. Bass SS, Dauway E, Mahatme A, et al. Lymphatic mapping with sentinel lymph node biopsy in patients with breast cancer < 1 cm (T1a–T1b). *Am Surg* 1999;65:857–862.

74. Glass EC, Essner R, Morton DL. Kinetics of three lymphoscintigraphic agents in patients with cutaneous melanoma. *J Nucl Med* 1998;39:1185–1190.

75. Alazraki NP, Eshima D, Eshima LA, et al. Lymphoscintigraphy, the sentinel node concept, and the intraoperative gamma probe in melanoma, breast cancer, and other potential cancers. *Semin Nucl Med* 1997;27:55–67.

76. Krag D, Weaver D, Ashikaga T, et al. The sentinel node in breast cancer: a multicenter validation study. *N Engl J Med* 1998;339: 941–946.

77. Bass SS, Pendas S, Ku N, et al. Diagnostic accuracy of sentinel node mapping in patients with breast cancer following excisional vs nonexcisional biopsy. *Surg Forum* 1998;49:406–408.

78. Uren RF, Thompson JF, Howman-Giles R. Correspondence. *Lancet* 1998;352:1472.

79. Berman C, Williamson M, Giuliano R, et al. Comparison of 2 cc vs 6 cc of radiopharmaceutical diluent in injections for breast lymphatic mapping. *Eur J Nucl Med* 1999;26[Suppl S1]:S66.

80. Veronesi U, Zurrida S, Galimberti V. Consequences of sentinel node in clinical decision making in breast cancer and prospects for future studies. *Eur J Surg Oncol* 1998;24:93–95.

81. Borgstein PJ, Meijer S, Pijpers R. Intradermal blue dye to identify the sentinel lymph node in breast cancer. *Lancet* 1997;349: 1668–1669.

82. Borgstein PJ, Meijer S, Pijpers R, et al. Lessons learned from an *in vivo* study of functional lymphatic anatomy in breast carcinoma. Echoes from the past and the peri-areolar blue dye method. In: *The sentinel node concept: consequences of lymphatic tumour spread in melanoma and breast cancer.* Amsterdam, The Netherlands: Academisch Proefschrift, Free University of Amsterdam, 1999, pp. 67–89.

83. Veronesi U, Paganelli G, Galimberti V, et al. Sentinel-node biopsy to avoid axillary dissection in breast cancer with clinically negative lymph-nodes. *Lancet* 1997;349:1864–1867.

84. Veronesi U. Correspondence. *Lancet* 1997;350:809.

85. Lachin J. Introduction to sample size determination and power analysis for clinical trials. *Control Clin Trials* 1981;2:93–113.

21

MONOCLONAL ANTIBODY IMAGING

LAMK M. LAMKI
BRUCE B. BARRON

Several radiolabeled monoclonal antibodies (mAbs) that are potentially useful in breast cancer imaging are commercially available in the United States or are available through a research protocol. None of these agents, however, have been approved by the Food and Drug Administration specifically for breast imaging. Although breast cancer radioimmunoscintigraphy has been in use for some time, breast imaging with monoclonal antibodies has not yet found its niche in clinical practice. Some very useful monoclonal antibodies to breast cancer have been tested clinically, but their role in patient management has not been defined. Some of the newer radiolabeled antibodies have a potential clinical role. In the late 1980s and early 1990s, serious work on breast cancer immunoscintigraphy began (1–22) with studies of breast-specific antibodies. It was observed that less specific anti-CEA (carcinoembryonic antigen) mAbs could react also with breast cancer. Improvement in radiolabeling techniques and success with ^{99m}Tc labeling opened new doors for breast cancer immunoscintigraphy.

To develop mAbs to breast cancer, antigens had to be identified that were more abundant in breast cancer than in normal breast tissue. In addition, the density of such antigens had to low in benign breast tumors and inflammatory breast tissues in comparison with the density in malignant lesions. To date, the greatest success has been achieved with CEA (23). Most breast cancers can produce CEA, even though the serum levels of CEA are normal. Tumor-associated glycoprotein (TAG-72) is also of great interest. Other antigens found to be usable include epithelial antigens, milk fat globule membranes, cell surface receptors, oncogene products, and cytokeratin epidermal growth factor receptors EGF-R and HER-2/*neu*

(15,24–42). The development of mAbs to these antigens and their current role will be discussed. Multiple target epitopes of tumor-associated antigens such as CEA and TAG-72 have been identified. Thus, several different mAbs can be identified that react with the same antigen (43,44). Common antibodies besides anti-CEA include B72.3 against TAG-72 and antibodies to HMFG1 (human milk fat globulin) and HMFG2, BM-2, and EGF-R.

TARGET ANTIGENS AND THEIR ANTIBODIES

Antigens Used

Numerous antigens have been discovered in breast cancer cells. A large number of these have been successfully labeled. Many of the trials have yielded mediocre results.

The most commonly tested antigen is CEA, found on the surface of the tumor cells. TAG-72, reactive with the pancarcinoma antibody B72.3, is also found in a majority of breast cancers, in addition to other tumors. Neither CEA nor TAG-72 is therefore specific for breast cancer. Antigens located in other parts of the breast tissue can also be expressed in breast cancer. The polymorphic breast epithelial antigen (mucin) has proved useful in tumor detection. The *MUC1* gene product, known as polymorphic epithelial mucin, is a transmembrane high-molecular-weight glycoprotein expressed by breast, pancreatic, ovarian, and other cancer types. Numerous antibodies have been developed against this antigen, most being reactive to an immunodominant tandem repeat sequence (45,46). Certain glycolipids that are altered during malignant transformation have also been used. More recently, antibodies against the growth factor receptors EGF-R and HER-2/*neu* have been studied (45).

Additionally, Thomsen Friedenreich antigen, which is a tumor-associated glycoconjugate, and human milk fat glob-

L.M. Lamki and B.B. Barron: Department of Radiology, University of Texas–Houston Medical School; Division of Nuclear Medicine; Memorial-Hermann Hospital, Houston, Texas 77030.

ulin (HMFG) have been evaluated. Antibodies include HMFG1, HGMF2, SM3, DF3, 12H12, BM-2, BM-7, EBA-1, and MA5. In general, the sensitivity and specificity found for primary and metastatic disease have been modest, in the range of 50% to 90% (45).

An antibody against EGF-R has been developed. The antigen is a transmembrane glycoprotein with an intracellular tyrosine kinase domain and has been implicated in controlling breast cancer growth (47). Using the mAb or egf/r3 that recognizes EGF-R, Ramos-Suzarte et al. (48) detected 88.9% (16/18) of breast cancers, although it was not specific for breast carcinoma.

Antibodies: IgG, Fragments, and Subfragments

Initial work with breast immunoscintigraphy was based on intact antibodies (usually IgG and rarely IgM) labeled with ^{111}In or ^{131}I (49–52). However, with the development of techniques for labeling with ^{99m}Tc, it became more attractive to explore the use of fragments of the IgG mAb (53–56). The biologic half-life of the whole IgG was suitable for ^{131}I and ^{111}In radiolabels, but the shorter half-life of ^{99m}Tc was a better match for the shorter biologic half-life of the fragments of IgG (Fig. 21.1; see also Color Plate 3 following p. 350). The whole IgG antibody can be enzymatically digested *in vitro* to produce Fab, Fab', or F(ab')$_2$ fragments. The use of fragments rather than the intact antibody is now universally accepted as a better choice for diagnostic purposes (57–62). Intact antibodies are more immunogenic, with a resultant high incidence of human anti-mouse antibodies (HAMAs) (63). The Fc fragment is removed from the IgG (by pepsin or papain action) (Fig. 21.1) to

result in Fab, Fab', or F(ab')$_2$ fragments, or by genetic engineering. In either case, the absence of the Fc portion in these fragments reduces significantly the immunogenicity of the mAb used, and the incidence of HAMAs is significantly lower. Other advantages of fragments include a shorter interval between injection and imaging, lower background activity, and better lesion contrast.

The biodistribution of fragments is also different from that of the intact IgG. Intact antibody is more likely to be localized and metabolized in the liver. Fragments and subfragments are more desirable, therefore, in a search for liver metastases. The long half-life of the whole IgG antibody is poorly suited for ^{99m}Tc and better suited for labeling with a less ideal isotope (e.g., ^{111}In or ^{131}I). However, more rapid clearance of fragments from the bloodstream results in low background imaging. They also have greater penetrating capacity than the intact IgG (64). The fragments themselves differ; Fab and Fab' are monovalent, whereas (Fab')$_2$ is divalent, with twice the capacity to bind antigen. However, the sensitivity of (Fab')$_2$ is not significantly better than that of Fab or Fab'.

CLINICALLY USED MONOCLONAL ANTIBODIES IN BREAST CANCER

Anti-CEA Antibodies

A useful antibody for breast cancer is anti-CEA, initially studied as a polyclonal product and more recently as an mAb. CEA is a tumor-associated antigen that was first discovered by Gold and Freedman (65). Since then, at least two CEAs have been described, the classic one being

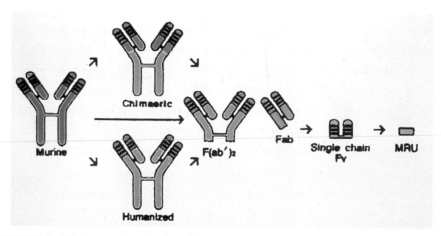

FIGURE 21.1. Efforts to reduce the size of the monoclonal antibody component led to the development of chimeric (humanized) antibodies and progressively smaller molecules, such as the molecular recognition unit (MRU). (See also Color Plate 3 following p. 350.) (Reprinted from Rodwell JD. Engineering monoclonal antibodies. *Nature* 1989;342:99–100, with permission of Macmillan and Company.)

the 200-kd molecule (66). The other form has a molecular weight of 180 kd and has been given various names, including meconium antigen, normal cross-reactive antigen II, normal fecal antigen, and CEA-low. Thus, the CEA molecule is a glycoprotein having molecular mass of between 180,000 and 200,000 d (67,68). It was initially considered to be a fetal antigen because it was found at high tissue levels in the fetal gastrointestinal tract, but more sensitive assays have since then detected CEA in the normal adult colon. The CEA content in normal colon is approximately 1 μg/g. In colon cancer, it is typically in the range of 5 to 10 μg/g of tumor. When CEA is secreted by cancer cells into the extracellular fluid, it gains access to the blood, and serum CEA levels are normally in the range of 0 to 2.5 ng/mL. These values may be elevated with cigarette smoking and other lung injury, acute nonmalignant chronic inflammatory conditions of the gastrointestinal tract (69), breast cancer, and lung cancer. CEA levels may climb to above 15 ng/mL in patients with metastatic disease. In 1980, a National Institutes of Health consensus panel concluded that serum CEA levels may be of value in the management of patients with lung, breast, and colon cancer (70). In an imaging study with a ^{99m}Tc-CEA intact IgG, Lind et al. (71) evaluated 46 women with suspected breast cancer or recurrence. They found a sensitivity of 83% and a specificity of 69% in patients who had only slightly elevated blood levels of CEA. In these patients, only 5 of 30 positive cases were positive for CEA by immunohistologic analysis.

Many of the earlier discrepancies, especially those related to immunohistologic analysis, were a consequence of poorly characterized antibodies, some of which reacted with nonspecific cross-reactive antigens (NCAs) related to CEA molecules (45). One NCA antibody in particular has shown expression in 40% of breast cancer cells in 44% of the specimens examined.

In 1978, Goldenberg and Larson (72) were highly impressed by the specificity of the affinity-purified ^{131}I-labeled anti-CEA goat antibody IgG given to patients with advanced cancer. However, because of significant blood pool activities seen with these antibodies, a nonspecific blood pool marker such as ^{99m}Tc-albumin was used for computer subtraction of background to improve the specificity further. Early work with ^{131}I-labeled antibodies demonstrated a resolution of 2 cm for CEA-producing neoplasms (66), and occult neoplasms were also detected. In the 1980s, a series of CEA murine monoclonal antibodies were developed and characterized, including the NP series of antibodies (43,73,74). Patients were initially evaluated with use of an ^{131}I-labeled NP-2 antibody. Although most of the early investigations were concerned with evaluation for colorectal carcinoma, the same antibodies have the potential to image breast neoplasms, both occult and primary. When anti-CEA antibody is used to detect colon or

breast cancer, it identifies occult lesions up to 2 years before they become clinically obvious or are detected by other imaging technique (75).

Another anti-CEA antibody, designated as NP-4, demonstrated even greater specificity for CEA. It is now approved by the Food and Drug Administration and is currently commercially available as CEA-Scan (arcitumomab) for colon cancer. During early clinical trials, it was also referred to as IMMU-4. However, it has not yet been approved by the Food and Drug Administration for the diagnostic detection of breast cancer, only for colon cancer. Numerous clinical studies have been performed to evaluate this agent for breast cancer detection (40, 76–82). Arcitumomab, previously called IMMU-4, is an anti-CEA antibody of the IgG1 class, specific for the 200,000-d CEA molecule. Initially, the whole antibody was labeled with ^{131}I and images were not obtained for 24 hours or longer after injection. Wahl et al. (61) found that earlier imaging could be obtained if antibody fragments were used instead of the whole antibody. This antibody has excellent specificity; it is nonreactive with blood and vascular elements and does not cross-react with "normal cross-reactive antigens" but is specific for the 200,000-d form of CEA. It does not complex significantly with circulating CEA. The Fab' fragment is derived from the intact IgG by pepsin cleavage, which produces F(ab')$_2$, and further action of papain at the hinge region results in Fab' (Fig. 21.1). Currently, the commercially available anti-CEA antibody (arcitumomab) is an Fab' fragment.

Results of early phase II studies evaluating this antibody in breast cancer were promising, showing a 71.4% sensitivity for known lesions. A recently concluded phase III study at M. D. Anderson Cancer Center was undertaken to determine whether results of imaging with this antibody could alter management and whether metastatic occult lesions or axillary lymph nodes could be found. At our center, it had a sensitivity of 93% to 100% for primary lesions and an 83% sensitivity overall (Figs. 21.2–21.8; see also Color Plates 4 and 5 following p. 350). Unknown (occult) lesions were also detected. Two of four unknown lymph nodes were confirmed, one of which took 2 years to become clinically evident. Three of five occult breast lesions were confirmed. This antibody was also helpful in identifying previously undetected liver and lung metastases in two of the patients. In this study, 7 of 15 patients were either downstaged or upstaged based on imaging data. No primary tumor was missed. In fact, a 4-mm lesion was found in the contralateral breast of one patient (Fig. 21.6). These results were similar to those of a study performed by Nabi et al. (74), in which 5 of 5 palpable lesions were detected and only 2 of 8 nonpalpable cancers, for a positive predictive value of 78% in the M. D. Anderson study. Of the 8 nonpalpable masses, 7 were smaller than 1 cm. The negative predictive value was 100% for patients deter-

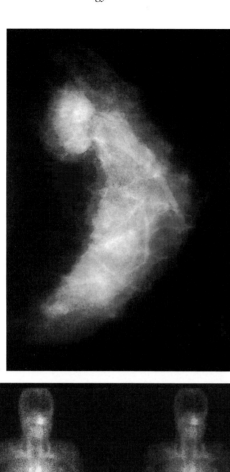

A

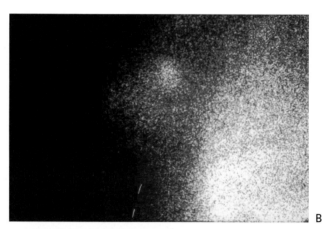

B

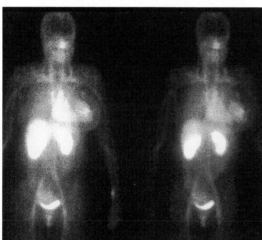

A

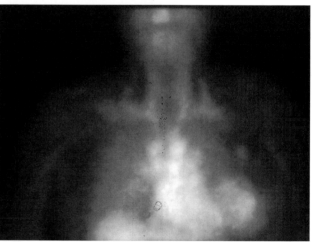

B

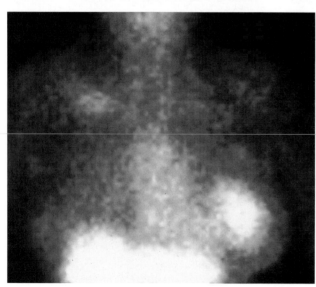

C

FIGURE 21.2. A: Mammogram showing primary tumor in the left upper breast. **B:** Scintimammogram showing uptake in the left breast, corresponding to the abnormal lesion on mammography. The right breast (not shown) was normal. (Reprinted from Lamki M, Barron BJ. Radiolabeled antibodies. In: Taillefer R, Khalkhali I, Waxman AD, et al., eds. *Radionuclide imaging of the breast.* 1998. New York: Marcel Dekker Inc, with permission.)

FIGURE 21.3. A: Anterior whole-body image 4 hours after injection of ^{99m}Tc-anti-carcinoembryonic antigen antibody demonstrating physiologic uptake of tracer in the blood pool, liver, and kidneys and abnormal uptake in the left breast. (Reprinted from Lamki M, Barron BJ. In: Taillefer R, Khalkhali I, Waxman AD, et al., eds. *Radionuclide imaging of the breast.* New York: Marcel Dekker Inc, with permission.) **B:** Anterior planar image of the chest obtained 4 hours after injection demonstrating diffuse abnormal uptake in the region of the tumor in the left breast. In addition, a small focal area of uptake is seen in the axilla, corresponding to an involved lymph node. (Reprinted from Lamki M, Barron BJ. Radiolabeled antibodies. In: Taillefer R, Khalkhali I, Waxman AD, et al., eds. *Radionuclide imaging of the breast.* 1998. New York: Marcel Dekker Inc, with permission.) **C:** This 24-hour planar image of the chest shows persistent abnormal uptake in the left breast. In addition, uptake noted in the right supraclavicular region was thought to represent an abnormal lymph node. However, this lymph node was not clinically detectable for 2 years after injection.

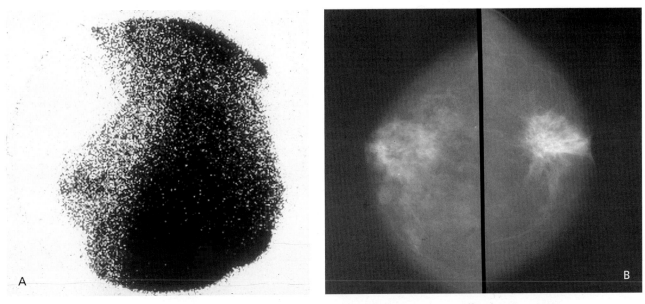

FIGURE 21.4. A: Planar scintimammogram taken 24 hours after injection of ^{99m}Tc-arcitumomab demonstrating extensive area of abnormal tracer accumulation. **B:** Bilateral mammogram showing a left spiculated mass with nipple retraction, consistent with carcinoma. (Reprinted from Lamki M, Barron BJ. Radiolabeled antibodies. In: Taillefer R, Khalkhali I, Waxman AD, et al., eds. *Radionuclide imaging of the breast.* 1998. New York: Marcel Dekker Inc, with permission.)

mined to have benign disease, such as fibrocystic changes, ductal hyperplasia, and fibroadenoma.

The difference between these studies is that single-photon emission computed tomography (SPECT) was performed on all patients in the first study and not in the study of Nabi et al. All primary tumors were detected by SPECT (100% sensitivity) (Figs. 21.4–21.7), whereas only 14 of 15 were positive by planar images (93% sensitivity). In addition, 7 of 7 known positive lymph nodes were detected by

SPECT, whereas only 5 of 7 were seen on planar images. SPECT has clearly improved the sensitivity in our study. These two studies offer hope that ^{99m}Tc-arcitumomab is a potential agent for the detection of nodal disease in addition to primary disease (74,77).

A variety of anti-CEA mAbs have been studied by other investigators on both sides of the Atlantic. Lind et al. (36) in 1991 utilized preoperative intravenous administration of ^{99m}Tc-labeled IgG anti-CEA in 45 women

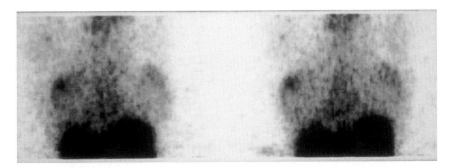

FIGURE 21.5. Planar coronal images obtained 24 hours after injection demonstrating bilateral breast uptake, which was thought to be the result of hormonal therapy. (Reprinted from Lamki M, Barron BJ. Radiolabeled antibodies. In: Taillefer R, Khalkhali I, Waxman AD, et al., eds. *Radionuclide imaging of the breast.* 1998. New York: Marcel Dekker Inc, with permission.)

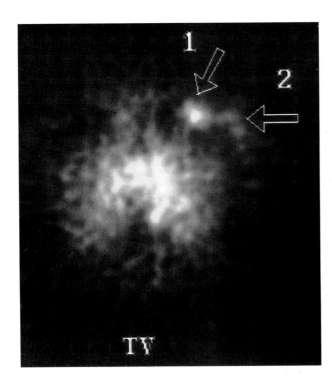

FIGURE 21.6. A 4-hour tomographic image in the transverse plane demonstrating a focal area of abnormal uptake in the left breast. (See also Color Plate 4 following p. 350.)

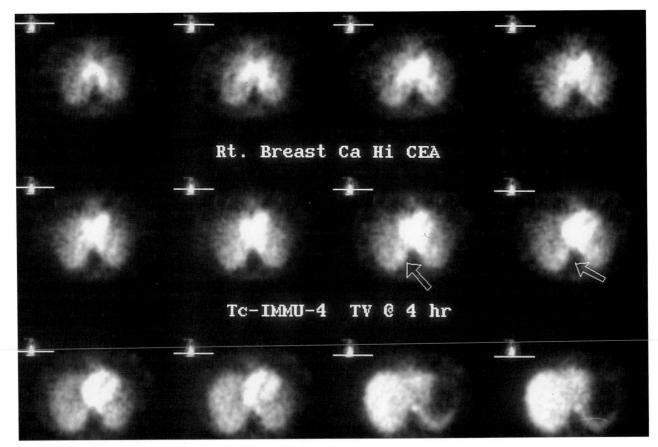

FIGURE 21.7. Transverse sections of the lungs of a 40-year-old woman with breast cancer and brain metastasis. Focal areas of increased activity in the posterior aspect of the slices correspond to multiple pulmonary metastases. (Reprinted from Lamki M, Barron BJ. Radiolabeled antibodies. In: Taillefer R, Khalkhali I, Waxman AD, et al., eds. *Radionuclide imaging of the breast*. 1998. New York: Marcel Dekker Inc, with permission.)

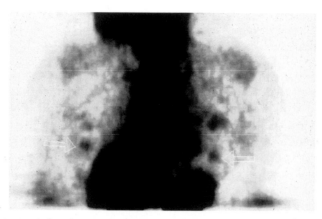

FIGURE 21.8. Coronal slice showing bilateral nipple uptake (lower lesions). In addition, a focal area of abnormal uptake seen above the left nipple corresponds to the primary. Another lesion, which measured 4 mm, was detected above the right nipple. (See also Color Plate 5 following p. 350.) (Reprinted from Lamki M, Barron BJ. Radiolabeled antibodies. In: Taillefer R, Khalkhali I, Waxman AD, et al., eds. *Radionuclide imaging of the breast.* 1998. New York: Marcel Dekker Inc, with permission.)

with breast cancer. A sensitivity of 82% was obtained, with the smallest detectable lesion by SPECT being 7 mm. Only 17% of patients with breast cancer had elevated CEA levels detectable in serum, which supports the notion that expression of tumor markers such as CEA in tumors does not necessarily result in detectable serum levels. Haseman et al. (67) used ^{111}In-labeled intact murine IgG anti-CEA mAb ZCE-25 to detect occult lesions in 140 patients who had negative or equivocal findings on CT. This antibody is an intact murine IgG1 antibody with a high affinity for CEA. A number of patients had a history of prior murine antibody injections, and their adverse reaction rate was 18%, in comparison with 1% for patients with no prior exposure. Liver metastases were diagnosed with SPECT in 19 of 19 patients. Seventeen of these were "hot" lesions. The number of breast cancer patients in this series, however, was extremely small. In this study, 75 of 95 patients with occult cancer (disease not detected by CT) were correctly identified. This further supports the utility of anti-CEA mAb imaging of cancer patients to search for occult disease. Nabi et al. (40) studied patients with another ^{99m}Tc-labeled anti-CEA fragment, CYT-380, to evaluate its utility in detecting lymph node involvement and residual disease after excisional biopsy. Radioimmunoscintigraphy demonstrated positive localization in 4 of 4 primary carcinomas, with the smallest lesion seen being 1 cm in size. In two patients with prior definitive surgery, no abnormal uptake was noted. Two small axillary lymph nodes were not detected in one patient. CYT-380 was useful in ruling out the presence of involved lymph nodes and residual disease after excisional biopsy. However, smaller nodes have been detected with ^{99m}Tc-arcitumomab and SPECT imaging. At this point, given the small number of patients imaged with CYT-380, an accurate comparison is not possible (40). Riva et al. (83) used monoclonal anti-CEA antibody

FO23C5 injected intraperitoneally. The sensitivity and specificity for identifying hepatic metastases were improved after intraperitoneal injection. De Castiglia et al. (54) and Duran et al. (55) separately reported using B2C114, an anti-CEA antibody, in the detection of murine mammary carcinoma. Detection of these tumors was good, although not any better than with the labeled fragments.

The above brief review of the literature reflects the current interest in anti-CEA antibodies, which is based on the fact that patients with recurrent disease often present with elevated serum CEA levels, negative or equivocal CT findings, and a prior history of a CEA-producing tumor. This situation poses a difficult challenge for the oncologist and the radiologist. Scanning with monoclonal anti-CEA antibodies can contribute significantly to the accurate diagnosis of these difficult cases. Earlier detection of metastases or recurrence permits early therapeutic intervention—surgical or conservative, whichever is more relevant. In patients with breast cancer, identification of nodal involvement or of satellite breast lesions may preclude or modify surgical intervention and also help in timing chemotherapy and radiation therapy.

B72.3 Antibodies (Anti-TAG-72)

Besides antibodies to CEA, antibodies to other breast cancer antigens, such as TAG and breast epithelial antigen (mucin), have proved successful. The B72.3 mAb is one such antibody in an IgG subclass, which reacts with a 200,000- to 400,000-d TAG-72 antigen (17). With immunohistologic methods, up to 80% of human breast cancers have been found to be reactive with the antibody B72.3 (84).

We ran the early clinical trials of this antibody for breast cancer and obtained very good results for the primary lesion

(Fig. 21.9–21.11, see also Color Plate 6 following p. 350). Two milligrams of the antibody were labeled with 5 mCi of ^{111}In by means of the site-directed GYK-DTPA (diethylenetriamine pentaacetic acid) method (at the carbohydrate moiety). The antibody is now approved by the Food and Drug Administration and commercially available in the United States under the tradename OncoScint and the generic name satumomab, but only for the investigation of colon cancer and ovarian cancer, not breast cancer. Using this antibody, we imaged patients up to 96 hours after injection of the ^{111}In-labeled intact IgG mAb. We acquired special axillary views from both anterior and oblique perspectives and with the patient's arms raised and lowered for the best view of axillary lymph nodes (Fig. 21.12), in addition to anterior, lateral, and oblique views of the breast and the whole body. The planar spot views were acquired by using a 125 x 125 matrix or 256 x 256 matrix for 7 to 10 minutes each. SPECT is acquired for 360 degrees with dual-head gamma cameras. Typically for SPECT, we use 30 seconds per stop for 64 stops in a stop-and-shoot technique. Blood samples are taken before injection of antibody to screen for HAMA levels and to assess pharmacokinetics. In the research setting, the HAMA test was also repeated at 1 week and at 1 month or as called for

by individual protocols. However, new studies involving fragments of the antibody are about to be started in Great Britain (85). The use of fragments should result in a lower incidence of HAMA than we had with the intact IgG. It is also hoped that the sensitivity of the fragments will be better for the detection of axillary nodes.

We have used ^{111}In-B72.3 mAb in 16 patients to detect and stage breast cancer (86). Doses of 0.2, 2, or 20 mg of the antibody were ^{111}In-GYK-DTPA-labeled with 5 mCi of indium. The 2-mg dose was optimal. The pancarcinoma antibody is a murine mAb of the IgG class directed against the TAG-72 antigen. It has been shown to react with 80% of needle biopsy aspirates of breast cancer but not with normal tissue (67,79). Other cancers also express TAG-72 antigen, including 96% of small cell cancers of the lung, 100% of epithelial ovarian cancers, and 80% of colon cancers, among others. Of the 16 patients in our study, 14 were found to have primary breast cancer at the time of surgery. All 14 primary breast lesions were detected with ^{111}In-B72.3 (100% sensitivity). Normal nipple was visualized in about half of the patients and may have been related to timing of the procedure relative to the menstrual cycle. Seven patients had proven axillary lymph

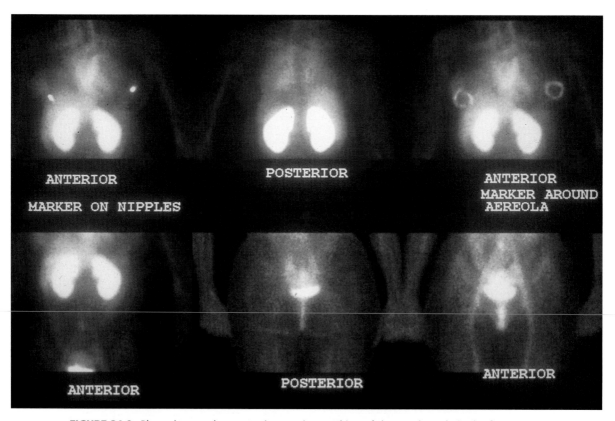

FIGURE 21.9. Planar images demonstrating routine marking of the areola and nipples for correlation with findings. (Reprinted from Lamki M, Barron BJ. Radiolabeled antibodies. In: Taillefer R, Khalkhali I, Waxman AD, et al., eds. *Radionuclide imaging of the breast.* 1998. New York: Marcel Dekker Inc, with permission.)

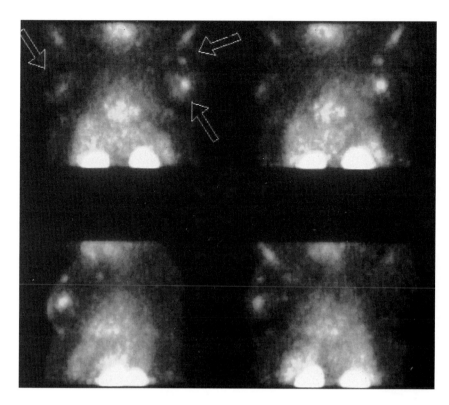

FIGURE 21.10. Tomographic images demonstrating bilateral axillary lymph nodes in addition to the left breast mass. (See also Color Plate 6 following p. 350.) (Reprinted from Lamki M, Barron BJ. Radiolabeled antibodies. In: Taillefer R, Khalkhali I, Waxman AD, et al., eds. *Radionuclide imaging of the breast.* 1998. New York: Marcel Dekker Inc, with permission.)

node metastases that were not detected by radioimmunoscintigraphy. This is in contrast to the higher percentage of lymph node metastases detected by the IMMU-4 anti-CEA antibody fragment labeled with ^{99m}Tc. Although the sensitivity of the B72.3 mAB in our laboratory was 100% for detection of the primary tumor (14/14), the negative findings in axillary nodes were a major setback in that study. We did not detect the four patients' proven axillary lymph nodes metastases. Two benign breast lesions

were not detected by the radioimmunoimaging, in keeping with good specificity. The size of the primary lesions ranged from 1.2 to 2.5 cm, and the size of the lymph nodes resected was 0.3 to 1.5 cm. Three occult lesions were discovered, and all were confirmed. Three distant metastatic lesions, one each to the skin, bone, and lymph node (Fig. 21.13), were detected that were previously not known. All these were found to be true positives on subsequent follow-up of these patients. Two of the 12 patients tested for

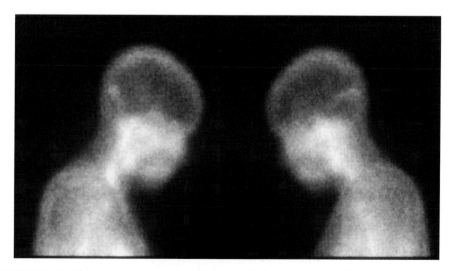

FIGURE 21.11. Planar images demonstrating a subtle increase of activity in the right parietal region, consistent with a brain metastasis in this region.

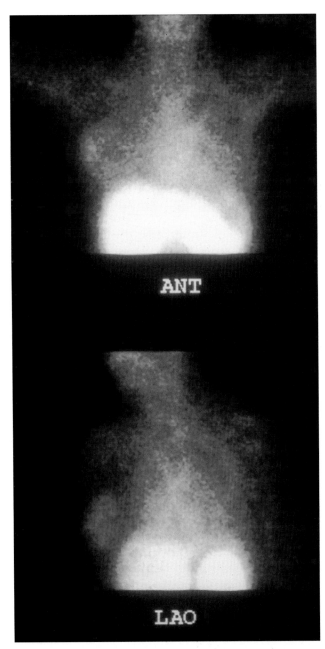

FIGURE 21.12. In this 36-year-old woman who had undergone mastectomy for a left breast mass, uptake in the right breast was both focal and diffuse. The patient opted for a right mastectomy. Inflammatory ductal ectasia was found on biopsy. (Reprinted from Lamki M, Barron BJ. In: Taillefer R, Khalkhali I, Waxman AD, et al., eds. *Radionuclide imaging of the breast.* New York: Marcel Dekker Inc, with permission.)

HAMA had a positive response. HAMA incidence is actually higher in other studies.

Other antibodies have been produced against a variety of TAGs (87–89). One of them, B6.2, has been used by several investigators. They consist of cell surface glycoproteins and glycolipids altered during malignant transformation (80). However, results with these antibodies are not any better than results with the original B72.3 (OncoScint) that we

tested. Fragments of this antibody may have a potential role and will be tested in the near future.

Other Monoclonal Antibodies Used for Breast Cancer

Human milk fat globulin antigens are found in a number of epithelial tumors. Antibodies to HMFG have been used in several clinical trials for a variety of tumors (20,41,42, 90–93). Early clinical imaging with these antibodies was performed by Epenetos et al. (94) and then by Kalofonos et al. (91). Rosner et al. (20) were able to demonstrate successful imaging in five of five patients with ^{99m}Tc-anti-CEA antibody and in five of seven with anti-HMFG labeled with ^{123}I. They concluded that anti-HMFG may be potentially useful as a diagnostic agent for the evaluation of primary or recurrent breast cancer. Several other workers have studied the anti-HMFG and anti-mucin antibodies for breast imaging. Brummendorf et al. (26,95) obtained good tumor-to-background ratios when they used ^{99m}Tc-radiolabeled anti-mucin antibodies in mice to image human mammary cancer xenografts (26). Athanassiou et al. (39) used an antibody targeting HMFG1 or HMFG2. Injecting this labeled antibody subcutaneously for immunolymphoscintigraphy or intravenously did not result in good tumor localization. Conversely, Nabi et al. (40), studying 13 patients with ^{123}I-HMFG1, identified recurrences in three of three patients: bone metastases in one patient and primary operable cancer in two. A lesion measuring 0.8 cm was not detected by the scan. Major et al. (90) investigated another labeled antibody directed against the epithelial membrane antigen MA5. Variable degrees of uptake were noted in those primary lesions or metastases larger than 3 cm, whereas smaller lesions were not detected. Expression of a limited amount of antigen at the tumor surface may explain the lack of significant uptake. Kramer et al. (21) investigated ^{111}In-(MX-DTPA)-BrE-3, an antibody detected against another breast epithelial mucin found in HMFG, in 15 patients. The expression of the epitope recognized by this antibody was first checked by means of immunohistochemical staining of previously obtained tumor specimens. Seventy-two separate sites of disease were identified by conventional diagnostic modalities. These included 43 skeletal, 7 chest wall, 8 lymph node, 6 liver, and 8 other lesions. Overall, 62 (86%) of the lesions, including 2 of 6 liver metastases, 3 of 4 lung metastases, and 7 of 8 lymph node metastases, were detected by ^{111}In-BrE-3. In addition, 39 of 43 skeletal lesions were detected (91% sensitivity). Radiation dosimetry performed for this agent showed that the liver and spleen received the highest doses, as expected for an ^{111}In-labeled whole antibody. The doses were 1.30 ± 0.46 rads/mCi and 1.48 ± 0.85 rads/mCi, respectively. The average whole-body dose was 0.45 ± 0.11 rads/mCi. The

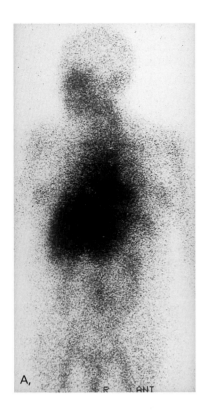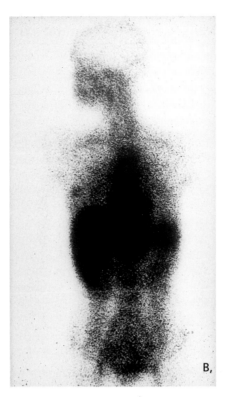

FIGURE 21.13. A,B: Total-body images of two different patients given ^{111}In-labeled B72.3 intact whole IgG antibody. Images were taken at 48 hours after injection. Note the blood pool and heavy distribution of radiolabeled antibody in the liver, in addition to some activity in the bowel. The blood pool typically does not clear until well after 96 hours. Note normal breast uptake in (A) and focal, intense, increased uptake in the right breast from cancer in (B). (Reprinted from Lamki M, Barron BJ. In: Taillefer R, Khalkhali I, Waxman AD, et al., eds. *Radionuclide imaging of the breast*. New York: Marcel Dekker Inc, with permission.)

ability of this antibody to detect skeletal and lymph node metastases is encouraging and may have a future application in therapy. The antibody was also ester-labeled with ^{90}Y for therapeutic trials.

Besides the anti-CEA (arcitumomab, CEA-Scan) and B72.3 (satumomab, OncoScint) antibodies, other antibodies have been used successfully for breast cancer imaging. The anti-mucin and anti-HMFG antibodies discussed above are not yet marketed. Other antibodies directed against a variety of antigens (Table 21.1) have been studied. The antibody 170H.82 appears to have a good detection rate and lower false-negative rate for soft-tissue lesions. In the studies of McEwan et al. (52,96), 6 of 7 breast lesions and 17 of 19 lymph node metastases were correctly detected. Detection of bone metastases was also good, a finding not supported by most other investigators. For this antibody, a 9% HAMA response has been reported.

Two antibodies against Thomsen Friedenreich antigen, a tumor-associated glycoconjugate, have been evaluated. This antigen is expressed on the cell surface early in the malignant transformation of cells or even in a preneoplastic phase. The antibodies 155HF and 170H.82 were labeled with ^{111}In, and 170H.82 has also been labeled with ^{99m}Tc and used in 15 patients with an overall sensitivity of 90% to 96%. McEwan et al. (97) used this antibody in patients with primary or metastatic breast cancer, and 25 of 32 soft-tissue metastatic sites were detected but only 1

of 5 bone metastases. In further studies by McEwan et al., 18 of 20 breast lesions, 36 of 40 lymph nodes, and 23/28 bone metastases were detected. A sensitivity of 90% for the localization of soft-tissue disease and a specificity of 93% were reported (97). In a recent trial involving the ^{99m}Tc-labeled anti-CA-15-3 antibody SM3, while planar imaging was unsuccessful, but axillary node involvement was correctly determined in 11 of 13 patients; 6 of 7 results were true-negatives and 5 of 6 were true-positives. This antibody also has potential for the early detection of breast cancer and for presurgical staging (18). Few reports have been published on antibodies that target protooncogene products such as ICR. Allan et al. (38) used the gene product of c-*erb* B-2 (98) as the target antigen. Epenetos et al. (94) used ^{123}I-labeled tumor-associated monoclonal antibodies to ovarian, breast, and gastrointestinal tumors (94). Rosner et al. (78) proposed using this antibody to screen for potential lesions and indeterminate mammograms before biopsy, in the same way that ^{99m}Tc-sestamibi is currently used clinically. This has the potential to reduce the number of unnecessary biopsies performed in 75% of women who have abnormal results on conventional mammography but do not have cancer. Monoclonal antibodies are used to detect not only the primary breast tumor or axillary nodes but also distant metastases (e.g., liver, lung, bone marrow, brain, and soft tissue). Most investigators have been more successful in imaging the primary tumor than in imaging metastases, as has already been discussed

TABLE 21.1. BREAST CANCER ANTIGENS AND THEIR RADIOLABELED ANTIBODIES USED FOR BREAST IMMUNOSCINTIGRAPHY

Antibody	Antigen	Isotope	Comments (investigators)
Carcinoembryonic antigen			
Bw431/26	CEA	^{99m}Tc	Intact Fab (Lind, Kairemo)
CYT-380	CEA	^{99m}Tc	Fragment (Nabi, Rosner)
BC2C114	CEA	^{99m}Tc	Intact IgG (Duran)
Arcitumomab	CEA	^{99m}Tc	Fragment (Goldenberg, Barron, Nabi, Tumor)
ZCE-25	CEA	^{111}In	Intact IgG (Patt, Haseman)
ZCE-25	CEA	^{111}In	Fragment (Lamki)
MN-14	CEA	^{131}I	IgG intact fragment (Goldenberg)
IORCEA1	CEA	^{99m}Tc	IgG intact (Duran)
NP-2	CEA	^{131}I	Polyclonal goat (Deland)
Tumor-associated glycoprotein			
B72.3	TAG-72	^{111}In	Intact IgG (Lamki, Thor)
155HF	TAG	^{111}In	Intact fragment (Longenecker, Springer, MacLean, McEwan)
170H.82	Thomsen Friedenreich Ag (TAG)	^{111}In, ^{99m}Tc	Intact IgG (Longenecker, Springer, MacLean, McEwan)
B6.2	TAG-72	^{125}I	Intact IgG (Stephens, Thor, Nieroda)
Epithelial mucin			
12H12	Mucin glycoprotein TAG-12	^{99m}Tc, ^{125}I, ^{131}I	Intact IgG (Brummendorf)
BM-2	Mucin glycoprotein TAG-12	^{99m}Tc	Fragment (Brummendorf)
Anti-HMFG1	Mucin/breast epithelial	^{123}I	Intact IgG to human milk fat globule (Taylor-Papadimitriou, Burchell, Major, Arklie, Rosner)
Anti-HMFG1	Mucin/epithelial	^{111}In	Fragment (Kalofonos)
Anti-HMFG2	Mucin/epithelial	^{123}I	Fragment (Espenetos)
MA5	Mucin/epithelial	^{111}In	Intact IgG (Major)
SM3	CA-15-3	^{99m}Tc	Fragment (Granowski)
BM-7	Mucin	^{99m}Tc	Intact IgG (Brummendorf)
BrE-3 (HMFG1)	Mucin, BEM*	^{111}In	*Breast epithelial mucin, intact IgG (Kramer)
Miscellaneous antigens			
3C6F9	37-kd surface Ag	^{123}I	IgG2a ILS (Mandeville)
RCC-1	Membrane/cytoplasm	^{131}I	Intact IgG (Tjandra)
Anti-c-*erb* B-2	p185	^{99m}Tc	Ag is a gene product of protooncogene p185 (Allan, Mangili)
3E1.2	Membrane/cytoplasm	^{131}I	IgM (Tsandra)
34BE12	Keratins 1.5.10 and 14		(Joshi, Lee) No imaging
4D5	p185 HER-2/*neu* oncogene		(De Santes) No imaging
7c2	p185 HER-2/*neu* oncogene		Fragment (Kennedy) No imaging
16.88* (human)	CTA 16.88 keratin	^{111}In	Intact IgM for lymphoscintigraphy (Pecking)
		^{99m}Tc	(*Same as antibody 88 BV 59)
EBA-1	Nonspecific	^{111}In	Intact and F(ab')$_2$ (Yemul)
BW250/183	Granulocyte/myelocyte	^{99m}Tc	For bone marrow, fragment (Korpii-Tommola)

in the sections on specific antibodies. Korpi-Tommola et al. (99) used the two most popular mAbs to investigate breast cancer metastases in bone marrow. Several other workers have detected distant metastases with a variety of mAbs and techniques (100–106), but no convincing large series has shown that antibody staging of breast cancer is a valid clinical trial.

Mangili et al. (104) used immunohistochemical staining to determine whether multiple different antibodies could lead to improved imaging detection. The authors evaluated CEA, c-*erb* B-2 protein, and TAG-72 expression in 100 cases of breast cancer with FO23C5 anti-CEA, B72.3 anti-TAG-72, and anti-c-*erb* B-2 protein mAbs. The results showed immunoreactivity for c-*erb* in 39 of 99 cases, B72.3 in 41 of 100 cases, and CEA in 15 of 100 cases. Multifocal lesions demonstrated positivity for c-*erb* in 6 of 16, B72.3 in 11 of 16, and anti-CEA in 1 of 16 cases. For lymph node metastases, the immunoreactivity was positive for c-*erb* in 12 of 33, B72.3 in 21 of 33, and CEA in 8 of 33 cases. When all three antibodies were considered together, the sensitivity improved to 60% for primary tumors, 78% in lymph nodes, and 81.2% in multifocal lesions.

Immunolymphoscintigraphy

Another important diagnostic advance utilizing immunoscintigraphy is the detection of metastatic breast cancer, especially in regional lymph nodes. Most women in whom breast cancer is diagnosed do not have clinical evidence of lymph node metastases. However, approximately 30% with clinical stage I have occult lymph node metastases. Detection of lymph node metastases is a major challenge for the imaging community. Fewer antibody imaging studies have been performed to detect breast cancer spread to lymph nodes than have been to detect the spread of other cancers, such as colon or prostate. Most of the older studies (107,108) involved either intravenous or subcutaneous injection of the radiolabeled mAb, and in general variable results were reported. The subcutaneous route of administration and even direct injection into the lymphatics has been used. The advent of labeled antibodies had stirred interest in this technique. One of the earliest studies was performed by DeLand et al. (142), who studied nine patients with an ^{131}I-anti-CEA goat antibody. Interdigital injection of the antibody resulted in axillary accumulation in all eight patients with surgically confirmed disease. The ninth patient had no uptake and no axillary disease. This result provided the impetus for future work. Studies involving radiolabeled antibodies 3E1.2 (106) and 3C6F9 (109) reported similar results. Kairemo et al. (58) studied breast cancer patients with a ^{99m}Tc-labeled anti-CEA mAb, Bw431/26, which had a sensitivity of 90% and a specificity of 88% for lymphoscintigraphic detection of axillary metastases.

Lymph node scintigraphy after intravenous injection of labeled antibody has identified lymph node involvement (110). Various researchers have attempted injection into the lymphatic system to improve detection. Some nonspecific uptake in hyperplastic lymph nodes has been discovered.

Tjandra et al. (111) evaluated ^{131}I-labeled antibodies injected interdigitally to evaluate involved axillary lymph nodes. The antibodies used, 3E1.2 (IgM) and RCC-1 (IgG), react strongly with the membrane and cytoplasm of breast carcinomas in approximately 90% of cases, and very little cross-reactivity with normal breast tissue is noted. Forty patients with clinically suspected breast cancer were studied prospectively (36 of 40 eventually proved to have breast cancer). At 16 to 24 hours after injection, anterior scintigrams were taken of the chest and axillae. Lymph nodes that were resected were processed and 6-μm sections were stained. HAMA antibodies developed in one patient who received 3E1.2 and one who received RCC-1. The axillary node status was correctly predicted in only 41% (9/22) of patients in the preoperative scan and in 59% of patients (13/22) in the preoperative clinical assessment. These results were not promising, as better prediction can be obtained after intravenous injection of antibodies such as ^{99m}Tc-IMMU-4. Lymphoscintigraphy performed with ^{131}I-RCC-1 resulted in a sensitivity of 86% and a specificity of 92% (69,75,111,112).

Other antibodies nonspecifically localize in normal lymph nodes. Pecking et al. (103) injected an ^{111}In-labeled human antibody against cytoplasmic antigen, CTA 16.88, directly into mammary glands. At the same time, ^{111}In-CTA 16.88 was injected subcutaneously into juxtaareolar sites. Although CTA-16.88 was detected in all the primary tumors and involved lymph nodes tested, it was also detected in 89% of nodes with follicular hyperplasia. Overall, radioimmunolymphoscintigraphy had a sensitivity of 72.7%, a specificity of 80.4%, and an accuracy of 77.7%.

The detection rates of involved lymph nodes with radioimmunolymphoscintigraphy appear to be very good. However, this technique is not accepted by oncologists.

BREAST CANCER IMMUNOSCINTIGRAPHY: FUTURE PROSPECTS

Potential Clinical Role

Because of the potential risk of HAMA formation or adverse reaction to the protein component and its debatable clinical role, immunoscintigraphy is currently not recommended as a primary method for screening or diagnosing primary breast cancer.

Radiolabeled mAbs against tumor-associated antigens can indeed detect primary and metastatic tumors but may miss critical areas. TAG-72 is a good example; its detection of primary tumors is excellent, although it falls short in detecting involved lymph nodes (16). The agent that seems to be the

TABLE 21.2. HUMAN ADULT ORGAN DOSIMETRY ESTIMATES FOR ^{99m}TC ANTI-CEA AND ^{111}IN B72.3

Organ/tissue	^{99m}Tc Arcitumomab		^{111}In Satumomab	
	Rad/20 mCi	mGy/740 MBq	Rad/5 mCi	mGy/185 MBq
Total body	0.340	3.404	2.7	27
Red marrow	0.736	7.360	12	120
Lung	0.572	5.720	4.9	49
Liver	0.770	7.700	15	150
Spleen	1.176	11.760	16	160
Kidney	7.424	74.240	9.7	97
Urinary bladder	1.232	12.320	2.8	28
Ovaries	0.568	5.680	2.9	29
Testes	0.330	3.300	1.4	14
Breast	0.112	1.120	—	—
Bone surfaces	0.588	5.880	3.3	33
Thyroid	0.208	2.080	1.5	15
Small intestine	0.416	4.160	3.0	30
Upper large intestine	0.408	4.080	3.1	31
Lower large intestine	0.346	3.460	2.5	25
Uterus	—	—	2.7	27
Pancreas	—	—	3.7	37
Other tissues	—	—	2.3	23

CEA, carcinoembryonic antigen.

best compromise for detecting primary and metastatic lesions, including lymph nodes, is ^{99m}Tc-arcitumomab (CEA-Scan). This antibody is now commercially available for colon cancer but can be used for breast cancer at the discretion of the physician. The big question is: What is the relative role of this and the anti-TAG antibody OncoScint (satumomab)? The dosimetry of the ^{99m}Tc-labeled antibody is better than the one labeled with ^{111}In (Table 21.2). Although radioimmunodetection has a definite potential in the management of breast cancer, no consensus has been reached. No approved antibody accurately stages lymph nodes. Surgical sampling of nodes is still needed, as the recurrence rate after radiotherapy of nodes is still 3% (100). In patients with suspect mammographic abnormalities or inconclusive mammographic findings (e.g., dense or fatty breasts), mAbs could be used for scintimammography, as ^{99m}Tc-sestamibi is, to separate benign from malignant lesions. Many clinicians believe that patients should not be subjected to this testing because of the possibility that HAMAs or allergic reactions will develop. No studies have demonstrated the role of this agent in screening scintimammography. Based on our experience, the sensitivity for detection of primary tumors is very good. In fact, several lesions that were detected by this scan did not become clinically evident for 2 months to 2 years afterward. This fact was also noted by Kramer et al. (21) when they used the BrE-3 antibody. The potential problem is nonspecificity. A trial similar to the ^{99m}Tc-sestamibi breast trial would be helpful in defining the role of this and other labeled antibodies before biopsy and in presurgical evaluation for multifocal disease.

Another issue is related to the utility of these agents in accurately staging disease before radical or sparing surgery is performed. Again, in our experience, radiolabeled antibodies have detected unsuspected multifocal disease in several patients, so that surgery was postponed to allow the initiation of adjuvant chemotherapy. Immunoscintigraphy might play an important role in defining multicentric disease systemically or in clarifying mammographic findings locally. It might also help identify the extent of disease (e.g., carcinoma *in situ*), so that surgery could possibly be avoided or the approach modified. Radioimmunoscintigraphy may be helpful in forewarning the surgeon of what to expect regarding axillary involvement.

A third consideration is the usefulness of radiolabeled antibodies to determine the adequacy of chemotherapy and a patient's response before surgery is performed, especially regarding lymph node involvement. If the response to chemotherapy is good, based on a reduction of tracer localization on a follow-up scan, the surgeon is more likely to agree to perform a curative operation. On the other hand, if the scan does not show any improvement, further chemotherapy or a switch of therapeutic agents may be desired.

The last unexplored area involves the use of radiolabeled antibodies to look for occult metastases in someone with a rising CEA level or as part of routine follow-up imaging. Radiolabeled anti-CEA has been fairly successful in finding occult tumors in patients with a history of colon cancer (2,3,57). Its utility in detecting occult breast metastases has not been adequately studied, nor has the potential of these agents to find the primary lesion in patients with adenocarcinoma of unknown origin.

Complementary Roles of Mammography and Immunoscintigraphy

Preliminary evidence suggests that ^{99m}Tc-arcitumomab (CEA-Scan) can disclose tumors missed by mammography (56,77). Mammography effectively detects nonpalpable breast carcinoma, but it cannot always reliably differentiate benign from malignant lesions. As a result, a substantial number of breast biopsies are performed in patients with benign conditions. CEA-Scan may prove more specific than ^{99m}Tc-sestamibi. Rosner et al. (79) evaluated the utility of ^{99m}Tc-arcitumomab in 72 patients with nonpalpable, indeterminate, or suspect mammographic lesions. Among 13 cases of early, nonpalpable primary breast cancer, six were detected by scintigraphy, and seven results were false-negative. These seven had subtle uptake that was not believed to be significant. Among the 59 patients with benign disease, 57 had negative scans, and two had false-positive results, for a specificity of 97%, which is better than the 75% reported for mammography. The false-negative rate in patients with low-probability, indeterminate mammograms was 4.1%, versus 10.2% for mammography (79). Scintigraphy can also help differentiate between benign abnormal hyperplasia with atypia and carcinoma, so that its specificity is higher than that of mammography (57). Unfortunately, this potential cannot be widely utilized because the antibody is not approved by the Food and Drug Administration for this use in the United States.

A recent evaluation of labeled arcitumomab (CEA-Scan) demonstrated its ability to image both palpable and nonpalpable breast lesions. Results indicate that arcitumomab can complement mammography by providing a high specificity and positive predictive value, useful in deciding when a patient with an abnormal result on a mammogram should proceed directly to definitive surgery without an intermediate biopsy.

In one study, arcitumomab was compared with mammography in 59 patients who had indeterminate mammographic lesions. In 41 patients with low-probability mammograms, scintigraphy disclosed three cancers not detected on mammography. Two false-positive results were also obtained. Mammography yielded five false-negative studies, versus two for the antibody scan. In the patients with suspect or highly suspect mammograms, there were eight true-positive cases and 10 false-positives, compared with three and zero for scintigraphy. Ninety percent of this group had nonmalignant disease on biopsy. With the use of scintigraphy, 75% of the patients would have been spared an unnecessary biopsy because of the true-negative finding on the antibody study. In addition, a higher positive predictive value for cancer was noted for scintigraphy than for mammography. This finding would allow direct surgical resection to be undertaken, with biopsy bypassed. The results suggest a paradigm in which a patient with an antibody-positive lesion and an abnormal, highly suspect mammogram in addition to abnormal, low-probability mammogram should proceed to biopsy or lumpectomy (45).

REFERENCES

1. Lamki L. Radiommunoscintigraphy of cancer: problems, pitfalls and prospects. In: Freeman L, ed. *Nuclear medicine annual*. New York: Raven Press, 1990:113–150.
2. Lamki LM, Patt YZ, Rosenblum MG, et al. Metastatic colorectal cancer: radioimmunoscintigraphy with a stabilized In-111-labeled F(ab')$_2$ fragment of an anti-CEA monoclonal antibody. *Radiology* 1990;174:147–151.
3. Patt YZ, Lamki LM, Shanken J, et al. Imaging with indium-111-labeled anticarcinoembryonic antigen monoclonal antibody ACE-025 of recurrent colorectal or CEA-producing cancer in patients with rising serum carcinoembryonic antigen and occult metastases. *J Clin Oncol* 1990;8:1246–1254.
4. Doerr RJ, Abdel-Nabi H, Merchant B. Indium-111 ACE 025 immunoscintigraphy in occult recurrent colorectal cancer with elevated carcinoembryonic antigen level. *Arch Surg* 1990;125:226–229.
5. Abdel-Nabi H, Doerr RJ, Chan HW. Safety and role of repeated administration of In-111-labeled anticarcinoembryonic antigen monoclonal antibody ACE 025 in the postoperative follow-up of colorectal carcinoma patients. *J Nucl Med* 1992;33:14–22.
6. Divgi CR, McDermott K, Johnson DK. Detection of hepatic metastases from colorectal carcinoma using indium-111 (^{111}In)-labeled monoclonal antibody (mAb): MSKCC experience with mAb ^{111}In-C110. *Nucl Med Biol* 1991;18:705–710.
7. Doerr RJ, Abdel-Nabi H, Baker JM, et al. Detection of primary colorectal cancer with indium-111 monoclonal antibody B72.3. *Arch Surg* 1990;125:1601–1605.
8. Lamki LM, Zukiwski AA, Shanken LJ, et al. Radioimaging of melanoma using ^{99m}Tc-labeled Fab fragment reactive with a high-molecular-weight melanoma antigen. *Cancer Res* 1990;50 [Suppl]:904s–908s.
9. Murray JL, Lamki LM, Rosenblum MG. Radioimmunoimaging of malignant melanoma with monoclonal antibodies. In: Nathanson L, ed. *Cancer treatment and research. Malignant melanoma: biology, diagnosis, and therapy*. Boston: Kluwer Academic Publishers, 1988:123–153.
10. Murray JI, Lamki LM, Shanke LJ, et al. Immunospecific saturable clearance mechanisms for indium-111 labeled anti-melanoma monoclonal antibody 96.5 in humans. *Cancer Res* 1998;48:4417–4422.
11. Lamki L, Murray JL, Rosenblum M, et al. Effect of unlabelled monoclonal antibody (MoAb) on biodistribution of 111-indium labelled MoAb. *Nucl Med Commun* 1988;9:553–564.
12. Mardirossian G, Wu C, Rusckowski M, et al. The stability of ^{99m}Tc directly labelled to an Fab' antibody via stannous ion and mercaptoethanol reduction. *Nucl Med Commun* 1992;13:503–512.
13. Wahl RL, Swanson NA, Johnson JW, et al. Clinical experience with Tc-99m-labeled (N2S2) anti-melanoma antibody fragments and single-photon emission computed tomography. *Am J Physiol Imag* 1992;7:48–58.
14. Crippa F, Buraggi GL, Di Re E, et al. Radioimmunoscintigraphy of ovarian cancer with the Mov18 monoclonal antibody. *Eur J Cancer* 1991;27:724–729.

15. Kim EE, Podoloff DA, Moulopoulos I, et al. Magnetic resonance imaging, positron emission tomography and radioimmunoscintigraphy of breast cancer. *Cancer Bull* 1993;45:500–505.

16. Lamki L, Buzdar AU, Singletary SE, et al. Indium-111-labeled B72.3 monoclonal antibody in the detection and staging of breast cancer: a phase I study. *J Nucl Med* 1991;32:1326–1332.

17. Colcher D, Horan-Hand P, Nuti J, et al. A spectrum of monoclonal antibodies reactive with human mammary tumors. *Proc Natl Acad Sci U S A* 1981;78:3199–3203.

18. Granowska M, Biassoni L, Carroll MJ, et al. Breast cancer ^{99m}Tc SM3 radioimmunoscintigraphy. *Acta Oncol* 1996;35:319–321.

19. Murray JL, Macey DJ, Grant EJ, et al. Enhanced TAG-72 expression and tumor uptake of radiolabeled monoclonal antibody CC49 in metastatic breast cancer patients following alpha-interferon treatment. *Cancer Res* 1995;55[23 Suppl]:5925s–5928s.

20. Rosner D, Nabi H, Wild L, et al. Diagnosis of breast carcinoma with radiolabeled monoclonal antibodies (MoAbs) to carcinoembryonic antigen (CEA) and human milk fat globulin (HMFG). *Cancer Invest* 1995;13:573–582.

21. Kramer EL, DeNardo SJ, Liebes L, et al. Radioimmunolocalization of breast cancer using BrE-3 monoclonal antibody. *Adv Exp Med Biol* 1994;353:181–192.

22. Peterson JA, Ceriani RL. Breast mucin and associated antigens in diagnosis and therapy. *Adv Exp Med Biol* 1994;353:1–8.

23. Steinstrasser A, Oberhausen E. Anti-CEA labeling kit BW 431/26: results of the European multicenter trial. *Nuklearmedizin* 1995;34:232–242.

24. Christian RB, Couto JR, Peterson JA, et al. Cloning and expression of cDNAs encoding the variable domains of the antibreast carcinoma antibody Mc5'. *Hybridoma* 1996;15:155–158.

25. Allan SM, Dean CJ, Eccles S, et al. Clinical radioimmunolocalization with a rat monoclonal antibody directed against c-erbB-2. *Cell Biophysics* 1994;24/25:93–98.

26. Brummendorf TH, Kaul S, Schuhmacher J, et al. Immunoscintigraphy of human mammary carcinoma xenografts using monoclonal antibodies 12H12 Bs BM-2 labeled with ^{99m}Tc and radioiodine. *Cancer Res* 1994;54:4162–4168.

27. Yemul S, Leon JA, Pozniakoff T, et al. Radioimmunoimaging of human breast carcinoma xenografts in nude mouse model with ^{111}In-labeled new monoclonal antibody EBA-1 and F(ab')$_2$ fragments. *Nucl Med Biol* 1993;20:325–335.

28. Lind P, Hans-Jurgen G, Mikosch P, et al. Radioimmunoscintigraphy with Tc-99m-labeled monoclonal antibody 170H.82 in suspected primary, recurrent, or metastatic breast cancer. *Clin Nucl Med* 1997;22:30–34.

29. Witters LM, Kumar R, Chinchilli VM, et al. Enhanced antiproliferate activity of the combination of tamoxifen plus HER-2. *New Antibody Breast Cancer Res Treatment* 1997;42:1–5.

30. DiGiovanna MP, Carter D, Flynn SD, et al. Functional assay for Her-2/neu demonstrates active signalling in a minority of Her-2/neu overexpressing invasive human breast tumors. *Br J Cancer* 1996;74:802–806.

31. Tosi E, Valota O, Canevari S, et al. Anti-idiotypic response to antigrowth factor receptor monoclonal antibodies. *Eur J Cancer* 1996;32A:498–505.

32. Charpin C, Bonnier P, Devictor B, et al. Immunodetection of Her-2/neu protein in frozen sections evaluated by image analysis: correlation with overall and disease-free survival in breast carcinomas. *Anticancer Res* 1993;13:603–612.

33. DeSantes K, Slamon D, Anderson SK, et al. Radiolabeled antibody targeting of the Her 2/neu oncoprotein. *Cancer Res* 1996;52:1916–1923.

34. Merino MJ, Monteagudo C, Neumann RD. Monoclonal antibodies for radioimmunoscintigraphy of breast cancer. *Int J Radiat Appl Instr B Nucl Med Biol* 1991;18:437–443.

35. DeNardo SJ, O'Grady LF, Macey DJ, et al. Quantitative imaging of mouse L-6 monoclonal antibody in breast cancer patients to develop a therapeutic strategy. *Int J Radiat Appl Instr B Nucl Med Biol* 1991;18:621–631.

36. Lind P, Smola MG, Lechner P, et al. The immunoscintigraphy use of Tc-99m-labelled monoclonal anti-CEA antibodies (BW 431-26) in patients with suspected primary, recurrent and metastatic breast cancer. *Int J Cancer* 1991;47:865–869.

37. Thor A, Edgerton SM. Monoclonal antibodies reactive with human breast or ovarian carcinoma: *in vivo* applications. *Semin Nucl Med* 1989;4:295–308.

38. Allan SM, Dean C, Fernando I, et al. Radioimmunolocalisation in breast cancer using the gene product of c-erbB2 as the target antigen. *Br J Cancer* 1993;67:706–712.

39. Athanassiou A, Pectasides B, Pateniotis K, et al. Immunoscintigraphy with ^{131}I-labelled HMFG2 and HMFG1 F(ab')$_2$ in the pre-operative detection of clinical and subclinical lymph node metastases in breast cancer patients. *Int J Cancer* 1988;3[Suppl]:89–95.

40. Nabi HA, Rosner D, Ortman-Nabi J, et al. Immunoscintigraphy of breast cancers with I-123 HMFG1 and 99m-Tc anti-CEA (CYT-380) monoclonal antibodies: initial clinical results and literature review. *Tumor Targeting* 1995;1:223–231.

41. Taylor-Papadimitriou J, Peterson JA, Arklie J, et al. Monoclonal antibodies to epithelium-specific components of the human milk fat globule membrane: production and reaction with cells in culture. *Int J Cancer* 1981;28:17–21.

42. Burchell J, Durbin H, Taylor-Papadimitriou J. Complexity of expression of antigenic determinants, recognized by monoclonal antibodies HMFG1 and HMFG2 in normal and malignant human mammary epithelial cells. *J Immunol* 1983;131:508–513.

43. Primus FJ, Newell KD, Blue A, et al. Immunological heterogeneity of carcinoembryonic antigen: antigenic determinants on carcinoembryonic antigen distinguished by monoclonal antibodies. *Cancer Res* 1983;43:686–692.

44. Reynoso G, Chu TM, Haloyoke D, et al. Carcinoembryonic antigen in patients with different cancers. *JAMA* 1972;220:361–365.

45. Goldenberg DM, Nabi HA. Breast cancer imaging with radiolabeled antibodies. *Semin Nucl Med* 1999;29:46–48.

46. Price MR, Rye PD, Petrakou E, et al. Summary report on the ISOBM TD-4 Workshop: analysis of 56 monoclonal antibodies against the MUCI mucin. *Tumor Biol* 1998;19[Suppl 1]:1–20.

47. Sledge GW Jr. Implications of the new biology for therapy in breast cancer. *Semin Oncol* 1996;23:76–81.

48. Ramos-Suzarte M, Rodriquez N, Oliva J, et al. 99m-Tc-labeled antihuman epidermal growth factor receptor antibody in patients with tumors of epithelial origin: part III. Clinical trials safety and diagnostic efficacy. *J Nucl Med* 1999;40:768–775.

49. GL DeNardo, SJ DeNardo, LF O'Grady, et al. Fractionated radioimmunotherapy of B-cell malignancies with ^{131}I lym-1. *Cancer Res* 1990;50[3 Suppl]:1014s–1016s.

50. Goldenberg DM, Horowitz JA, Sharky RM, et al. Targeting dosimetry and radioimmunotherapy of B-cell lymphomas with iodine-131 labeled LL2 monoclonal antibody. *J Clin Oncol* 1991;9:548–564.

51. Nabi HA, Erb DA, Cronin VR. Superiority of SPECT to planar imaging in the detection of colorectal carcinomas with ^{111}In monoclonal antibodies. *Nucl Med Commun* 1995;16:631–639.

52. McEwan AJB, McLean GD, Hooper HR, et al. MoAb 170H.82: an evaluation of a novel panadenocarcinoma monoclonal antibody labelled with Tc-99m and In-111. *Nucl Med Commun* 1992;13:11–19.

53. Griffiths GL, Goldenberg DM, Jones AL, et al. Radiolabeling of monoclonal antibodies and fragments with technetium and rhenium. *Bioconjug Chem* 1992;3:91–99.

54. De Castiglia SG, Duran A, Fiszman G, et al. 99mTc direct labeling of anti-CEA monoclonal antibodies: quality control and preclinical studies. *Nucl Med Biol* 1995;22:367–372.

55. Duran AP, Asurmendi S, D'Orio E, et al. Direct labeling of monoclonal antibodies with ^{99m}Tc and radioimmunodetection of a murine mammary carcinoma with ^{99m}Tc-B2C114. *J Nucl Biol Med* 1994;38[4 Suppl 1]:33–37.

56. Gulec SA, Serafini AN, Sfakianakis GN, et al. CEA-Scan in diagnosis and staging of breast cancer. *J Nucl Med* 1996;37[Suppl 5]:238P(abst).

57. Goldenberg DM, Juweid M, Dunn RM, et al. Cancer imaging with radiolabeled antibodies: new advances with technetium-99m-labeled monoclonal antibody Fab' fragments, especially CEA-Scan and prospects for therapy. *J Nucl Med Technol* 1997;25:18–23.

58. Kairemo KJ. Immunolymphoscintigraphy with Tc-99m-labelled monoclonal antibody (BW 431/26) reacting with carcinoembryonic antigen in breast cancer. *Cancer Res* 1990;50[3 Suppl]:949s–954s.

59. Hansen HJ, Jones AL, Sharkey RM, et al. Pre-clinical evaluation of an instant Tc-99m labeling kit for antibody imaging. *Cancer Res* 1990;50[3 Suppl]:794s–798s.

60. Schultes BC, Reinsberg J, Wagner U, et al. Idiotypic cascades after injection of the monoclonal antibody OC125: a study in the mouse model. *Cell Biophysics* 1994;24/25:259–266.

61. Wahl RL, Parker CW, Philpott GW. Improved radioimaging and tumor localization with monoclonal F(ab')₂. *J Nucl Med* 1983;24:316–325.

62. Pinsky CM, Sasso NL, Mojsiak JZ, et al. Results of a multicenter phase III clinical trial of ImmuRaid-CEA-Tc-99m imaging of patients with colorectal cancer. *Proc Am Soc Clin Oncol* 1991;10:136(abstr).

63. Torres G, Berna L, Estorch M, et al. Preexisting human anti-murine antibodies and the effect of immune complexes on the outcome of immunoscintigraphy. *Clin Nucl Med* 1993;18:477–481.

64. Larson SM, Carrasquillo JA, Krohn KA, et al. Localization of 131I-labeled p97-specific Fab fragment in human melanoma as a basis for radiotherapy. *J Clin Invest* 1983;72:2101–2114.

65. Gold P, Freedman SO. Demonstration of tumor-specific antigens in human colon carcinomata by immunological tolerance and adsorption techniques. *J Exp Med* 1965;21:439–462.

66. Krupey J, Wilson T, Freedman SO, et al. The preparation of purified carcinoembryonic antigen of the human digestive system from large quantities of tumor tissue. *Immunochemistry* 1972;9:617–622.

67. Haseman MK, Brown DW, Keeling CA, et al. Radioimmunodetection of occult carcinoembryonic antigen-producing cancer. *J Nucl Med* 1992;33:1750–1756.

68. Chung JK, Jang JJ, Lee DS, et al. Tumor concentration and distribution of carcinoembryonic antigen measured by *in vitro* quantitative autoradiography. *J Nucl Med* 1994;35:1499–1505.

69. Hansen HJ, Snyder JJ, Miller E, et al. Carcinoembryonic antigen (CEA) assay. A laboratory adjunct in the diagnosis and management of cancer. *Hum Pathol* 1974;5:139–147.

70. Goldenberg DM, Neville AM, Carter AC, et al. CEA (carcinoembryonic antigen): its role as a marker in the management of cancer. *J Cancer Res Clin Oncol* 1981;101:239–242.

71. Lind P, Smola MG, Lechner P, et al. The immunoscintigraphic use of Tc-99m labelled monoclonal anti-CEA antibodies (BW 431/26) in patients with suspected primary, recurrent and metastatic breast cancer. *Int J Cancer* 1991;47:865–869.

72. Goldenberg DM, Larson SM. Radioimmunodetection in cancer identification. *J Nucl Med* 1992;33:803–814.

73. Stramignoni D, Bowen R, Atkinson BM, et al. Differential reactivity of monoclonal antibodies with human colon adenocarcinomas and adenomas. *Int J Cancer* 1981;31:543–552.

74. Nabi HA, Rosner D, Erb D, et al. Evaluation of suspicious mammographic findings with CEA-Scan and correlation with histopathological results. *J Nucl Med* 1996;37[Suppl]:238P(abst).

75. Barron B, Lamki LM, Pinero S, et al. Clinical use of Tc-99m anti-carcinoembryonic antigen antibody in the evaluation of the breast. *Radiology* 1994;193(P):424.

76. Lamki L, Kim EE, Haynie TP. Tumor immunoscintigraphy using monoclonal antibodies. In: Roth J, ed. *Monoclonal antibodies in cancer: advances in diagnosis and treatment.* Mount Kisco, New York: Futura Publishing, 1986:259–288.

77. Barron B, Lamki L, Pinero S, et al. Clinical utility of Tc-99m-anti-CEA antibody (IMMU-4) in the evaluation of breast cancer. *Clin Nucl Med* 1994;19:267(abst).

78. Rosner D, Abdel-Nabi H, Panaro V, et al. Immunoscintigraphy (IS) may reduce the number of surgical biopsies in women with benign breast disease (BBD) and indeterminate mammograms: a novel approach. *Proc Am Soc Clin Oncol* 1996;15:102(abst).

79. Rosner D, Abdel-Nabi H, Panaro V, et al. Carcinoembryonic antigen immunoscintigraphy may reduce the number of surgical biopsies in women with mammographically abnormal, non-palpable, benign breast disease. *Proc Am Soc Clin Oncol* 1996;15:102(abst).

80. Nabi HA. Antibody imaging in breast cancer. *Semin Nucl Med* 1997;27:30–39.

81. Harwood SJ, Abdel-Nabi H. The use of monoclonal antibodies for radioscintigraphic detection of cancer. *J Pharm Proc* 1994;7:93–116.

82. Nabi HA, Seldin D, Barron B, et al. CEA-SCAN radioimmunodetection of primary breast lesions: results of phase II multicenter trial. *Eur J Nucl Med* 1995;22(P).

83. Riva P, Marangolo M, Tison V, et al. Treatment of metastatic colorectal cancer by means of specific monoclonal antibodies conjugated with iodine-131: a phase II study. *Int J Radiat Appl Instr B Nucl Med Biol* 1991;18:109–119.

84. Nuti M, Teramato YA, Marian-Constantini R, et al. A monoclonal antibody (B72.3) defines patterns of distribution of a novel tumor-associated antigen in human mammary carcinoma cell populations. *Int J Cancer* 1982;29:539–545.

85. Britton K. Personal communication.

86. Goldenberg DM, Kim EE, DeLand FM, et al. Radioimmunodetection of cancer with radioactive antibodies to carcinoembryonic antigen. *Cancer Res* 1980;40:2984–2992.

87. Hayes BF, Zalutsky MR, Kaplan W, et al. Pharmacokinetics of radiolabeled monoclonal antibody B6.2 in patients with metastatic breast cancer. *Cancer Res* 1986;46:3957–3163.

88. Thor A, Ohuchi N, Szpak CA, et al. Distribution of oncofetal antigen tumor-associated glycoprotein-72 defined by monoclonal antibody B72.3. *Cancer Res* 1986;46:3118–3124.

89. Nieroda CA, Mojzisik C, Sardi A, et al. Staging of carcinoma of the breast using a hand-held gamma detecting probe and monoclonal antibody B72.3. *Surg Gynecol Obstet* 1989;169:35–40.

90. Major P, Wang TQ, Ishida M, et al. Breast cancer imaging with mouse monoclonal antibodies. *Eur J Nucl Med* 1989;15:655–660.

91. Kalofonos HP, Sakier JM, Hatzistylianou M, et al. Kinetics, quantitative analysis and radioimmunolocalization using indium-111-HMFG1 monoclonal antibody in patients with breast cancer. *Br J Cancer* 1989;59:939–942.

92. McKenzie IF, Xing PX. Mucins in breast cancer: recent immunological advances. *Cancer Cells* 1990;2:75–78.

93. Arklie J, Taylor, Papadimitrious J, et al. Differentiation antigens expressed by epithelial cells in the lactating breast are also detectable in breast cancer. *Int J Cancer* 1981;28:23–29.

94. Epenetos A, Britton KE, Mather S, et al. Targeting of I-123-labeled tumor-associated monoclonal antibodies to ovarian, breast and gastrointestinal tumors. *Lancet* 1982;2:999–1005.

95. Brummendorf TH, Kaul S, Schulmacher J, et al. Immunoscintigraphy of breast cancer xenografts. 99m-Tc-labeled anti-mucin monoclonal antibodies BM-7 and 12H12. *Nuklearmedizin* 1995; 34:197–202.

96. McEwan AJB, McLean GD, Goldberg L, et al. Tc-99m-170H.82 (TRUSCINT), a new monoclonal antibody for imaging breast cancer: a preliminary analysis. *J Nucl Med* 1993;34: 213P(abstr).

97. McEwan A, MacLean GD, Golberg L, et al. Evaluating radioimmunoscintigraphy in patients with breast cancer. *Eur J Nucl Med* 1994;21:748P(abstr).

98. De Santes K, Slamon D, Anderson SK, et al. Radiolabeled antibody targeting of the HER-2/neu oncoprotein. *Cancer Res* 1992; 52:1916–1923.

99. Korpi-Tommola ET, Kairemo KJ, Jekunen AP, et al. Double-tracer dosimetry of organs in assessment of bone marrow involvement by two monoclonal antibodies. *Acta Oncol* 1996;35:357–365.

100. Fisher B, Redmond C, Fisher ER, et al. Ten-year results of a randomized clinical trial comparing radical mastectomy and total mastectomy with or without radiation. *N Engl J Med* 1985;312: 674–681.

101. Tijandra JJ Sacks NP, Thompson CH, et al. The detection of axillary lymph node metastases from breast cancer by radiolabelled monoclonal antibodies: a prospective study. *Br J Cancer* 1989;59:296–302.

102. Stephens AD, Punja U, Sugarbaker PH. False-positive lymph nodes by radioimmunoguided surgery: report of a patient and analysis of the problem. *J Nucl Med* 1993;34:804–808.

103. Pecking AP, Lokiec FM. Pre-operative immunolymphoscintigraphy with human monoclonal antibody (16.88 lilo) to assess the nodal involvement in breast cancer. In: Cluzan RV, Peckign AP, Loklec FM, eds. *Progress in lymphology XIII*. Excerpta Medica, Amsterdam: 1992:307–311.

104. Mangili F, Sassi I, DiRocco M, et al. Breast carcinoma detection with a combination of radiolabeled monoclonal antibodies: promising results from immunohistochemical studies. *Cancer* 1996;78:2334–2339.

105. Lind P, Lechner P, Kuttnig M, et al. Differentiation in a patient with follicular thyroid and breast cancer. *Nuklearmedizin* 1990; 29:278–281.

106. Thompson CH, Lichtenstein M, Stacker SA, et al. Immunoscintigraphy for detection of lymph node metastases from breast cancer. *Lancet* 1984;2:1245–1247.

107. Rombi G, Cossu F, Melis G. MoAb-labeled liposomes in breast cancer cell targeting: therapeutics and diagnostic use of polyspecific artificial carriers. *Ann N Y Acad Sci* 1993;698:429–435.

108. Mackworth-Young CG. The Michael Mason Prize essay: antiphospholipid antibodies and disease. *Br J Rheumatol* 1995;34: 1009–1030.

109. Mandeville R, Patiesky N, Philipp K, et al. Immunolymphoscintigraphy of axillary lymph node metastases in breast cancer patients using monoclonal antibodies: first clinical findings. *Anticancer Res* 1986;6:1257–1263.

110. Nabi HA, Goldenberg DM, Lamki L, et al. The role of carcinoembryonic antigen (CEA) imaging in the diagnosis of breast cancer. *Eur J Nucl Med* 1998;25:872.

111. Tjandra JJ, Russell IS, Collins JP, et al. Immunolymphoscintigraphy for the detection of lymph node metastases from breast cancer. *Cancer Res* 1989;49:1600–1608.

112. Carrasquillo JA, Sugarbaker P, Colcher D. Radioimmunoscintigraphy of colon cancer with iodine-131 labeled B72.3 monoclonal antibody. *J Nucl Med* 1988;29:1022–1030.

113. DeLand F, Kim E, Corgan R, et al. Axillary lymphoscintigraphy in radioimmunodetection of carcinoembryonic antigen in breast cancer. *J Nucl Med* 1979;20:1243–1250.

114. Longnecker BM, Willans DJ, Maclean GD, et al. Monoclonal antibodies and synthetic tumor-associated glycoconjugates in the study of Thomson-Friedenreich-like and Tn-like antigens on human cancers. *J Natl Cancer Inst* 1987;78:489–496.

115. Granowski M, Biassoni L, Carroll MJ, et al. Breast cancer 99mTc SM3 radioimmunoscintigraphy. *Acta Oncol* 1996;35:319–321.

116. Joshi MG, Lee AD, Pedersen CA, et al. The role of immunocytochemical markers in the differential diagnosis of proliferative and neoplastic lesions of the breast. *Mod Pathol* 1996;9:57–67.

117. Kennedy MJ. Metastatic breast cancer. *Curr Opin Oncol* 1996;8: 485–490.

118. Korpi-Tommola ET, Kairemo KJ, Jekunen AP, Niskanen EO, Savolainen SE. Double-tracer dosimetry of organs in assessment of bone marrow involvement by two monoclonal antibodies. *Acta Oncologia* 1996;35:357–365.

22

RADIONUCLIDE THERAPY

SALLY J. DeNARDO
PABLO J. CAGNONI
JEFFREY Y.C. WONG
CAROL RICHMAN

Breast cancer is the second most common cause of cancer death in women in the United States. Approximately 180,000 new cases are expected per year. Although some patients can be cured by initial treatment and many receive temporary palliation with currently available therapy, approximately 44,000 women die of the disease each year (1). Improved treatment strategies are urgently needed, particularly for patients with metastatic disease, whose the average survival is less than 2 years (2). The purpose of this chapter is to provide the most significant results of studies of systemically administered tumor-targeting radionuclide therapy as radioimmunotherapy (RIT) for breast cancer. This represents a new modality for the care of patients with breast cancer and an opportunity to develop innovative strategies for combined-modality therapy.

Single-agent RIT has been proved to deliver effective systemic, tumor-targeted radiation therapy in hematologic malignancies, particularly non-Hodgkin's lymphoma. Although promising, RIT has been less effective for solid tumors, in part because they are less radiosensitive. However, the radiosensitivity of breast cancer has been demonstrated by the observation that conservative surgery followed by external beam radiation therapy to microscopic residual disease in the breast produces the same 8- to 10-year regional control and disease-free and overall survival rates as modified radical mastectomy in patients with early-stage disease (3–6). The radiosensitivity of normal tissues has prevented the administration of similar doses of external beam radiation therapy to the entire body as part of combined-modality therapy for metastatic breast cancer. The therapeutic index of systemically administered, tumor-targeted RIT has been enhanced during the past decade, so

that between three and 50 times the highest radiation dose to normal tissue can now be delivered to tumor deposits throughout the body (Fig. 22.1). With the current RIT agents in clinical trials for breast cancer, the delivery of 2,000 to 4,000 rads to metastatic tumors per cycle of therapy has increasingly become a reality when autologous peripheral blood marrow stem cell support is used (Table 22.1). This makes combined-modality therapy with RIT for breast cancer a realistic and compelling goal. The major dose-limiting effect is myelosuppression; other toxicities have been minimal. Dose-escalation studies have not

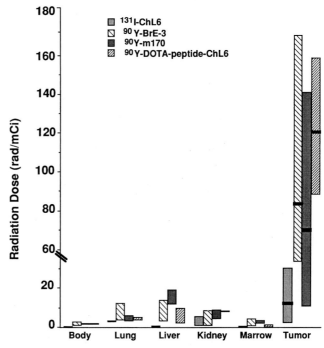

FIGURE 22.1. Radiation dose (rad/mCi) to normal organs and tumors in patients with breast cancer who received ¹³¹I-ChL6, ⁹⁰Y-MX-DTPA-BrE-3, ⁹⁰Y-2IT-BAD-m170, or ⁹⁰Y-DOTA-peptide-ChL6. Therapeutic indices of the newer radiopharmaceuticals can be compared.

S. J. DeNardo and C. Richman: Departments of Internal Medicine and Radiology, University of California, Davis, Sacramento, California 95816.

P. J. Cagnoni: Bone Marrow Transplant Program, University of Colorado, Denver, Colorado 80220.

J. Y. C. Wong: Division of Radiation Oncology, City of Hope National Medical Center, Duarte, California 91010.

TABLE 22.1. CLINICAL BREAST CANCER TRIALS IN WHICH RESPONSE RATES HAVE BEEN REPORTED FOR RADIOIMMUNOTHERAPY

Antigen target	Radiolabeled antibody	Number of therapy cycles	Cumulative tumor dose (rad)	Response
L6 glycoprotein	^{131}I-ChL6 (11,37)[a]	1–4	200–7,000	4/10 PR 2/10 MR
MUC-1 peptide	^{90}Y-mBrE-3 (10)[a]	1	100–2,500	1/6 PR 1/6 MR
MUC-1 peptide	^{90}Y-mBrE-3 (28)[b]	1	500–1,100	4/8 PR
MUC-1 peptide	^{90}Y-hBrE-3 (29)[b,d]	1	NA	2/9 PR 1/9 M 1/9 SD
CEA	^{90}Y-cT84.66 (21)[c,d]	1	NA	1/6 MR 1/6 SD
MUC-1 sugar	^{90}Y-m170 (30)[a,d]	1–3	500–8,200	1/4 PR 1/4 MR 1/4 SD

[a]University of California Davis, Sacramento, California.
[b]University of Colorado, Denver, Colorado.
[c]City of Hope, Duarte, California.
[d]Current studies in progress, peripheral blood stem cell support.
PR, partial response (a decrease in the sum of the products of all tumor dimensions by at least 50%, or all tumor volumes by at least 70%); MR, minor response (30–50% reduction in tumor volume, or 50–70% reduction in the sum of the products of all tumor dimensions); M, mixed response; SD, stable disease; NA, not available.

reached levels of second-organ toxicities (Table 22.1). In fact, a total dose to metastatic breast cancer tumor as high as 11,200 rad was delivered to one patient in three cycles of ^{131}I-ChL6 multicycle therapy with stem cell support (150 mCi/m^2), while the highest dose to a normal organ, a total of 3,100 rad to lung, produced no evidence of toxicity (7).

Phase I/II trials of RIT specifically for breast cancer have reported clinically relevant (though transient) response rates of 30% to 60% in heavily treated patients. The highest dose to a normal organ is to liver, lung, or kidney, depending on the antigen target, antibody or antibody fragment, radionuclide, and method of attachment. All play a role in the pharmacokinetics, dosimetry, therapeutic index, toxicity, and efficacy of this treatment modality. However, the clinical impact of RIT on the management and cure of breast cancer also depends on identification of the optimal sequence and timing of combined synergistic therapies.

MOLECULAR TARGETS

Theoretically, an ideal target for radionuclide therapy of metastatic breast cancer would be tumor-specific and generously expressed on all the breast cancer cells of all breast cancer patients. It would not be released into the circulation, and when bound by the RIT antibody, it would internalize the targeted therapy and/or trigger cell responses that would sensitize the tumor cell to radiation. Although such ideal tumor-specific targets for RIT have yet to be found, useful cancer cell targets have been identified. Studies of

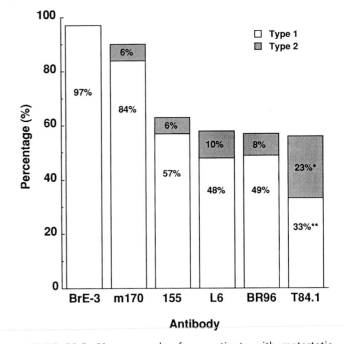

FIGURE 22.2. Biopsy samples from patients with metastatic breast carcinoma staining with antibody on immunopathology as a percentage of samples positive by Mattes type 1 or 2 criteria (12,13). Samples in which 75% or more of the tumor cells in the section showed strong brown staining of the cytoplasm were considered type 1. Staining of 50% to 74% of the tumor cells represented type 2. *Staining of biopsy samples for carcinoembryonic antigen was evaluated in a separate study (14) and reported as the percentage of cells staining in the biopsy sample; staining of 15% or more of the cells designated 113 of 202 (56%) biopsy samples positive; more than 90% of the cells stained in 33% of these samples.

pharmacokinetics in patients have provided evidence that truly cancer-specific target molecules are not necessary to deliver effective RIT (8–11). Oncofetal antigens such as carcinoembryonic antigen (CEA) represent possible RIT targets for breast cancer. Others can be grouped by associated characteristics: the MUC-1 molecule on human milk fat globules (HMFG); related epithelial membrane antigens (EMA); integral membrane glycoprotein triggers of cell growth (i.e., L6); growth factor receptors (i.e., EGF); and oncogene products (i.e., HER-2/*neu*). Many of these antigen targets are found to be pancarcinoma targets and therefore may be useful for several tumor types. However, as noted by Mattes et al. (12) and Howell et al. (13), the antibodies in earlier breast cancer trials frequently targeted epitopes found only on a low percentage of breast cancer cells. Although other factors influence effective RIT, the presence of available antigen target is crucial (Fig. 22.2).

Carcinoembryonic Antigen Target

Expression of CEA has been reported in 10% to 95% of breast cancers. First described by Gold and Freedman in 1965, CEA was thought to be a specific marker for colon adenocarcinoma. However, subsequent studies demonstrated CEA expression in other human adenocarcinomas that are not of gastrointestinal origin, including the surface membrane of breast cancer cells. The reported percentages of breast cancers expressing CEA on immunohistopathologic analysis have ranged from as low as 1.9% to as high as 95%. In immunohistochemistry studies of the incidence of CEA expression performed with a well-characterized monoclonal antibody (mAb), T84.66, having high affinity and specificity for a CEA epitope that lacks cross-reactivity with any of the known proteins of the CEA gene family, 56% of 202 breast cancer tumors had the CEA epitope on more than 15% of the tumor cells; 33% of these tumors demonstrated staining of more than 90% of cells (14) (Fig 22.2).

Many anti-CEA antibodies have been used for radioimmunolocalization and for phase I/II therapy trials in patients with various cancers (15–17). NP-4 belongs to the murine IgG1 subclass and is specific for CEA, reacting with a class III peptide epitope of the CEA molecule. Phase I/II dose-escalation studies of tumor-targeted ^{131}I-NP-4 therapy have been reported in a mixed adenocarcinoma patient group with some therapeutic responses noted, including responses in breast cancer (18).

More extensive therapy studies in breast cancer have been performed with T84.66, also developed as a murine IgG1 but with high specificity and affinity for a different epitope of the CEA molecule (14,19). T84.66 does not cross-react with any other molecule of the large CEA gene family and has been classified in the Gold I group according to its epitope reactivity (14,19). A chimeric form (mouse–human mAb) has been used in clinical studies for the scintigraphic detection of mammary breast cancer and in current phase I/II therapy

trials (20). The maximum tolerated dose for ^{90}Y-DTPA-cT84.66 was defined at 22 mCi/m^2 by grade 3 reversible myelosuppression. The most recent trial evaluates the administration of higher activities of ^{90}Y-DTPA-cT84.66 with autologous peripheral blood stem cell support after therapy in patients with CEA-expressing metastatic breast cancer (21). Six patients demonstrated tumor imaging and received a single cycle of ^{90}Y-cT84.66 at 15 mCi/m^2 (three patients) and 22.5 mCi/m^2 (three patients). All patients demonstrated blood count recovery after their stem cell reinfusion. One patient demonstrated stable disease for 4 months, one had a minor response with improvement of the bone scan and reduction of an ovarian metastasis and malignant pleural effusion for 14 months, one had a reduction in bone pain for 1 month, and a fourth patient had resolution of bone pain for 3 months. Preliminary results from this ongoing phase I trial are promising and suggest the potential for antitumor effects of stem cell-supported ^{90}Y-cT84.55 therapy in CEA-producing breast cancer (21) (Table 22.1).

MUC-1 Antigen Target

MUC-1 mucins are large, complex glycoproteins comprising a polypeptide core with multiple oligosaccharide side chains in *O*-linkage to serine or threonine residues. The mature molecule is anchored within the cell surface by a characteristic transmembrane domain, but most of the mucin is expressed extracellularly in an elongated form extending far beyond most other cell surface-expressed macromolecules (22). In malignant cells, the expression of MUC-1 is elevated, and its orientation within the tissue is no longer polarized at apical surfaces. MUC-1 mucins released from their surface location may therefore have access to the circulation. Measurements of these molecules in the blood are used to provide a guide to tumor burden, and sequential determinations reflect disease recurrence and progression or response to therapy (e.g., CA-15-3).

Several antibodies have been found to react with MUC-1 epitopes seldom found in blood or normal tissues. Sixteen research groups participated in a recent workshop in which the reactivity and specificity of 56 mAbs against MUC-1 mucin were investigated with a diverse panel of target antigens and MUC-1 mucin-related synthetic peptides and glycopeptides (22). The majority of antibodies (34/56) defined epitopes located within the 20-amino acid tandem repeat sequence of the MUC-1 mucin protein core. Evidence was found of the involvement of carbohydrate residues in the epitopes for 16 of the remaining 22 antibodies. The MUC-1 protein core is known to contain variable numbers of the 20-amino acid tandem repeat sequence PDTRPAPG-STAPPAHGVTSA (23). Many antibodies bind rather simple linear peptide motifs of only a few residues in this MUC-1 protein core. This is particularly important because in the malignant cell, aberrant glycosylation may lead to truncated or incomplete oligosaccharide side chains that may be new epitopes or that may expose *de novo* cancer-related determinants within the MUC-1 core. Antibodies to both the peptide core and the aberrant sugar residues have been studied in clinical trials for imaging and therapy of breast cancer (9,10,24–27). Two of these, which demonstrated high levels of staining on most breast cancer biopsy specimens (13) (Fig. 22.2), provided excellent RIT tumor targeting on performed imaging studies *in vivo*. Pharmacokinetics, dosimetry, and therapy trials of radioimmunoconjugates to these antigens in patients with metastatic breast cancer are described below (10,28–30) (Table 22.1).

BrE-3 antibody, a murine IgG1 mAb, reacts with an epitope on the tandem repeat of the peptide core of MUC-1 (31). Immunopathology studies of metastatic breast cancer biopsy specimens demonstrated a vigorous reaction of BrE-3 with more than 75% of the cells of more than 95% of the breast cancers (13,31) (Fig. 22.2). Results of initial studies of nuclear imaging and pharmacokinetics suggested that therapeutic radiation could be effectively targeted to breast cancer on this BrE-3 antibody (9). Therefore, a dose-escalation study was initiated to determine the maximum tolerated dose with ^{90}Y-MX-DTPA-BrE-3 (10) (Fig. 22.3; see also Color Plate 7 following p. 350). In three of six patients, objective evidence of response to therapy lasted for 3 to 8 weeks. Of three patients in a 6.25 mCi/m^2 group, one had a partial response (PR) in a liver metastasis (Fig. 22.4). In a 9.25 mCi/m^2 group, one patient had a temporary reduction in skin lesions and arm swelling, and another had a measurable reduction in liver tumor that did not meet the criteria for PR. Although patients in this study received only a

single, modest dose of ^{90}Y, a decrease in measurable disease was observed in three of six patients, although it lasted only briefly. The therapy was well tolerated, and the therapeutic index (tumor-to-normal organ radiation ratio) was considered good (10) (Fig. 22.1). The data suggested that multiple cycles of ^{90}Y-MX-DTPA-BrE-3 or higher doses could result in more frequent and durable responses.

Because the limiting toxicity was myelosuppression, a phase I trial to explore the use of a single high dose of ^{90}Y-BrE-3 and autologous peripheral blood stem cell support was initiated. Nine women with heavily pretreated disease were enrolled (28). All the patients had tumors positive for BrE-3 by immunostaining and were treated with one dose of ^{90}Y (15 mCi/m^2, three patients; 20 mCi/m^2, six patients). ^{111}In-BrE-3 (5 mCi) was given simultaneously for imaging. The only toxicity noted was hematologic. Grade 4 platelet toxicity requiring transfusion support developed in four patients. Grade 4 white blood cell toxicity was seen in two patients that resolved in 3 to 9 days. All hematologic nadirs occurred approximately 25 days after treatment. Objective PRs were noted in four of eight (50%) evaluable patients with measurable tumors (four of the total of nine patients). Because antibodies to the BrE-3 mouse antibody (human antimonoclonal antibodies, or HAMAs) developed rapidly in most patients, such that more than one dose of therapy could not be considered, a humanized BrE-3 was developed.

The framework amino acids of BrE-3 were mutated from murine to human with the exception of the amino acids judged by computer modeling to be important in antigen binding. The humanized V_L and V_H frameworks are, respectively, 93% and 90% identical to the corresponding human frameworks (28). A pharmacokinetic/dosimetry study, performed in seven patients wherein ^{90}Y dosimetry was calculated from ^{111}In-MX-DTPA-hBrE-3, demonstrated 70 ± 31 rad/mCi to tumor and 21 ± 12 rad/mCi to liver (32). A phase I study was then initiated of a single dose of ^{90}Y-MX-DTPA-hBrE-3 followed by granulocyte colony-stimulating factor (G-CSF)-mobilized autologous peripheral blood stem cell (PBSC) support in patients with refractory metastatic breast cancer (29). ^{111}In-MX-DTPA-h-BrE was co-injected for imaging and dosimetry purposes. Nine patients have been treated and analyzed who represent the first three cohorts. Patients received 10 mCi/m^2 (n = 3), 20 mCi (n = 3), or 33 mCi (n = 3) of ^{90}Y-MX-DTPA-hBrE-3 followed 14 days later by PBSC support. No nonhematologic, noninfectious toxicities were seen in any of the patients despite the fact that seven of the nine had previously failed autologous stem cell transplant. Radiation absorbed dose estimates for ^{90}Y in the first two patients, extrapolated from ^{111}In, were 2.81 and 2.94 rad/mCi for the whole body (29). Of the nine patients, four had measurable disease. Responses in these patients were one PR (liver lesion), one PR (nodes and chest wall PR with stable liver disease), one mixed response, and one stable dis-

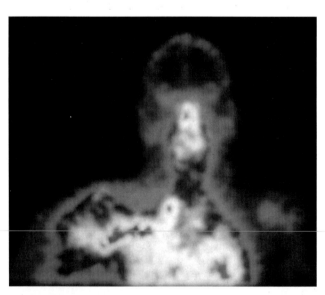

FIGURE 22.3. Nuclear medicine scintigram showing tumor targeting of radioimmunotherapy in a breast cancer patient with metastases in right subclavical and cervical lymph nodes and left and right anterior chest wall. The image was obtained 48 hours after therapy with ^{111}In/^{90}Y-BrE-3 monoclonal antibody (MUC-1 antigen target) (10). Excellent tumor uptake is demonstrated. (See also Color Plate 7 following p. 350.)

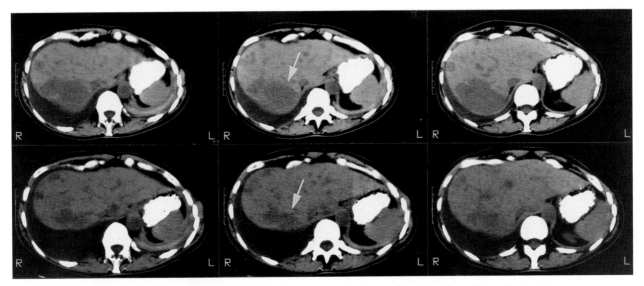

FIGURE 22.4. Computed tomography of a patient demonstrating regression of breast cancer in the liver after therapy with ^{90}Y-BrE-3 (10). CT sections in the upper row were obtained before therapy, and those in the lower row, 5 weeks after therapy. *Arrow* indicates shrinking lesion.

ease (Table 22.1). Of the five without measurable disease, three had a clinical improvement in bone pain (29). Dose escalation will continue until the maximum tolerated dose with PBSC support is reached.

Another anti MUC-1 mAb, 170H.82, was derived against a synthetic asialo GM1 terminal disaccharide associated with the cell membrane and is related to the Thomsen Friedenreich antigen (33). ^{99m}Tc and ^{111}In radioimmunoconjugates of 170H.82 (m170) are effective for imaging primary and metastatic breast cancer and have been shown to detect lesions less than 1 cm in size with an overall clinical accuracy of 92% (34). Of 99 metastatic breast cancer biopsy specimens, 89 (90%) demonstrated abundant staining with m170 (13) (Fig. 22.2).

Dosimetry data from ^{111}In-2IT-BAD-m170 pharmacokinetics studies have been utilized to determine the maximum dose of ^{90}Y-2IT-BAD-m170 that can be administered without exceeding normal organ limits. Limits have been set at a total of 800 rad to normal organs other than marrow for each of three cycles of therapy for level 1, and at 1,000 rad to normal organs other than marrow for level 2. Sufficient PBSCs are harvested and frozen before therapy for infusion after each dose. The mean and range of calculated radiation doses (rad/mCi) for all studies ($n = 10$) are as follows: whole body, 2.2 (2.1 to 2.4); liver, 17.4 (12.7 to 22.2); lung, 6.3 (4.8 to 7.2); kidney, 8.1 (6.3 to 11.5); marrow, 3.3 (1.9 to 4.4); and tumors ($n = 33$), 81.1 (14.1 to 141.5). With 800 rads to liver, lung, or kidney per therapy cycle used as the limit to the injected dose of ^{90}Y, the liver has been the calculated dose-limiting organ. Of the six patients who initiated the study, four have proceeded from dosimetry to treatment; with injected doses of 37 to 57 mCi (20 to 33 mCi/m^2) of ^{90}Y (level 1), one of these had a

PR, one had measurable tumor reduction but less than a PR, one had stable disease for more than 1 month, and one cannot yet be evaluated (Table 22.1). PBSC support prevented prolonged myelosuppression. The therapeutic responses, coupled with an absence of significant adverse sequelae, suggest that this dosimetry-based approach combined with PBSC support may lead to meaningful therapy when higher doses of ^{90}Y are reached (30,35).

L6 Antigen Target

The L6 cell surface antigen, which is highly expressed on lung, breast, colon, and ovarian carcinomas, is a 24-kd surface protein. The predicted L6 peptide sequence is 202 amino acids long and contains three predicted amine terminus hydrophobic transmembrane regions, which are followed by a hydrophilic region containing two potential N-linked glycosylation sites and a carboxyl terminus hydrophobic transmembrane region. The L6 antigen is related to a number of cell surface proteins with similar predicted membrane topology that have been implicated in cell growth. Two other members of this family of proteins, CD63 (ME491) and CO-029, are also highly expressed on tumor cells (36). L6 antigen was also found to be expressed in human vascular endothelium but could be covered by an infusion of nonradioactive L6 mAb, so that subsequent radiolabeled L6 mAb could reach tumor cells (8,37,38).

The chimeric version of L6 (ChL6) labeled with ^{131}I was administered in up to four monthly cycles to patients with metastatic breast cancer who had failed standard therapy. Ten patients with metastatic breast cancer reactive with L6 by immunohistopathology (13) received an imaging dose of ^{131}I-ChL6, which was followed 24 hours later by a therapy dose of ^{131}I-ChL6 (20 to 70 mCi/m^2). The tumor radiation dose was 120 to 3,700 rad per therapy cycle, five to 30 times higher than the whole-body dose. Therapy resulted in minimal acute or subacute toxicity. Dose-limiting toxicities were neutropenia and thrombocytopenia. Six of 10 patients had clinically measurable tumor responses, and five had responses that lasted more than 1 month (1.5 to 5 months) (11,37). Three additional patients were treated at a dose of 150 mCi/m^2 with PBSC support after each dose. Hematologic toxicity was modest, with thrombocytopenia resolving after a maximum duration of 7 days. Significant nonhematologic toxicity was not observed. Two of three patients treated with a dose of 150 mCi/m^2 received only a single cycle of RIT because of the development of HAMAs. The third patient, treated with cyclosporin A to prevent HAMA formation, completed all three therapy cycles. She received cumulative radiation doses to the lungs and tumor of 3,100 and 11,200 cGy, respectively. For 9 months, she had a reduction in bone pain, a decline in serum tumor markers, and decreased tumor uptake on PET scan, in addition to improved performance status and no toxicity (39).

Because ^{131}I-ChL6 RIT demonstrated therapeutic promise for patients with breast cancer, a novel means of attachment of radioactivity was developed to enhance further this potential for therapy. The radioimmunoconjugate consists of a macrocyclic chelator, DOTA (tetraazacyclododecane-N,N',N'',N'''-tetraacetic acid), which tightly binds [90]Y. This is then linked to the mAb ChL6 by an intrahepatic catabolizable peptide (40,41) (Fig. 22.5). Thus, ^{90}Y-DOTA-peptide-ChL6 was designed to minimize the radiation dose to critical normal tissues, particularly the liver. The initial patient received two therapeutic doses of ^{90}Y-DOTA-peptide-ChL6 and showed regression of tumors and tumor markers (42). In comparison with earlier ^{131}I-ChL6 dosimetry, dosimetry in five studies with ^{111}In/^{90}Y-DOTA-peptide-ChL6 demonstrated excellent tumor targeting and a greatly enhanced therapeutic index (42) (Figs. 22.1 and 22.6; see also Color Plate 8 following p. 350). Further development of such cleavable radioactivity linkages specific for enzymes in hepatic and renal cell metabolic pathways should allow chelated radioactivity to be excreted more rapidly without

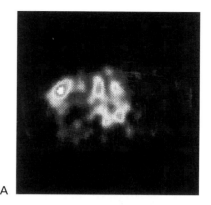

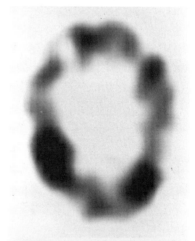

A

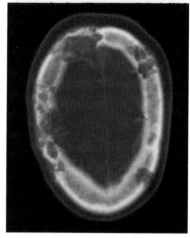

B

FIGURE 22.6. A: Single-photon emission computed tomographic (*SPECT*) image of the midchest area of a patient with metastatic breast cancer 72 hours after injection of 4 mCi of ^{111}In-DOTA-peptide-ChL6. Uptake in metastatic lesions is seen in the anterior and posterior mediastinal lymph nodes and a large right anterior tumor mass in the lung. **B:** SPECT (*upper*) and cross-sectional CT (*lower*) of a patient 3 days after infusion of ^{111}In-DOTA-peptide-ChL6 reveals multiple skull metastases. Uptake of ^{111}In is remarkable because antibody uptake in skeletal metastases is often less intense than in soft-tissue tumors. (See also Color Plate 8 following p. 350.)

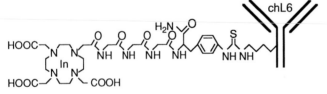

FIGURE 22.5. ChL6 antibody conjugated with [111]In- or ^{90}Y-DOTA-peptide isothiocyanate (62). This creates a prototype linkage that is meant to be catabolized rapidly in the liver but not in tumor, so that a lower hepatic radiation dose and higher therapeutic index are obtained. Initial studies in patients have been promising (42).

affecting tumor targeting. The therapeutic index calculated from this prototype radioimmunoconjugate represents a major step forward for therapeutic enhancement.

HER-2/*neu* Antigen Target

The *neu* oncogene was discovered during transfection experiments. It was subsequently shown to encode a transmembrane phosphoglycoprotein bearing extensive structural homology to the epidermal growth factor receptor. A viral oncogene encoding a truncated representation of the epidermal growth factor receptor, the human homologue of *neu*, was identified and designated c-*erb* B-2, or HER-2. The oncogene was also isolated from MAC117, a human mammary carcinoma cell line, where it was found to be amplified 5- to 10-fold. Several studies have now documented that amplification of the HER-2/*neu* gene occurs in approximately 25% to 35% of breast and ovarian adenocarcinomas and is uniformly associated with augmented expression of the oncogene protein p185. Moreover, amplification and overexpression of HER-2/*neu* have been correlated with a poor response to primary therapy and decreased survival.

The use of recombinant humanized mAb HER-2 in patients with metastatic breast cancer overexpressing HER-2/*neu* has resulted in objective, although transient, clinical responses. Currently, an anti-HER-2/*neu* mAb (Herceptin) is approved by the Food and Drug Administration for advanced breast cancer and is in clinical use as "naked antibody" therapy.

Radioactive anti-HER-2/*neu* mAbs are considered attractive agents for radioimmunodiagnosis and radioimmunotherapy for the 25% to 35% of breast cancers that are positive for HER-2/*neu*. Because some antibodies to HER-2/*neu* can be internalized, effective strategies for retarding the intracellular catabolism of ^{131}I or the use of radioactive metals (e.g., ^{90}Y, ^{67}Cu) may be necessary to optimize clinical utility.

TAG-72 Antigen Target

The widely described murine monoclonal antibody B72.3 targets TAG-72 and was derived from immunization of a nude mouse with tumor extract obtained from a patient with breast cancer. TAG-72 (tumor-associated glycoprotein) is expressed by the vast majority of adenocarcinomas (43). After careful study in human xenograft mouse models, antibodies to the TAG-72 antigen, particularly B72.3 and ChB72.3, were evaluated in patients. Dosimetry data derived from ^{111}In-B72.3 pharmacokinetics studies in patients with breast cancer suggested that maximum tumor uptake would be only 0.004% ID/g (injected dose per gram of tumor) (44). Therapy studies were conducted in two groups of patients with colon cancer with the human IgG4 chimeric version of this mAb (^{131}I-ChB72.3). A slight response in one of 24 patients

was documented, but a high incidence of HAMA development interrupted therapy (45,46).

A newer antibody to a different epitope of TAG-72, CC49 tagged with lutetium 177 (^{177}Lu), demonstrated improved tumor uptake in mouse biodistributions. CC49 is a murine IgG1 mAb. Immunohistochemical and immunocytochemical techniques have demonstrated preferential expression of TAG-72 in breast, gastrointestinal, and ovarian adenocarcinomas in comparison with normal tissues, except for the secretory endometrium. At doses below the median lethal dose (LD$_{50}$) of 400 to 500 μCi with ^{177}Lu-CC49, a high rate of complete tumor regression was achieved in mouse therapy studies (47). A ^{131}I-CC49 imaging/dosimetry study was conducted in women with metastatic breast cancer to evaluate the use of interferon alfa to enhance TAG-72 antigen expression and tumor uptake of ^{131}I-CC49 (48). A therapy study was then performed comparing the combination of interferon alfa followed by RIT and of RIT followed by interferon alfa (49). Treatment with interferon alfa was found to enhance TAG-72 expression in tumors by 46%, and the uptake of ^{131}I-CC49 in tumors of these patients was also significantly increased. One partial and two minor tumor responses were seen in the 15 treated patients (49).

ACUTE AND SUBACUTE TOXICITY

With most mAb infusions, little or no toxicity occurs. Infrequent mild fever or nausea are reported. Mild hypotension or hypertension are occasionally reported in the studies of RIT with nonbiologically active antibodies. Mild to moderate clinical toxicity has been anticipated and reported with the use of biologically active mAbs or immune targeting molecules with or without other biologic response modifiers (i.e., interleukin 2, IL-6, tumor necrosis factor) as part of the RIT (37,50–52). It is not surprising that activation of complement, the triggering of normal immune effector cell responses, and the stimulation of other inflammatory mechanisms can cause clinical symptoms. In these instances, fever, chills, urticaria, nausea, headache, hypotension, tachycardia, and muscle aches may frequently be expected, as reported with the ChL6 infusions. These are generally mild (grade 1 to 2), respond to oral antipyretic and antihistamine medications, and are dose rate-related. These responses are clearly different from acute hypersensitivity reactions or delayed hypersensitivity reactions, which are almost never seen but must always be anticipated.

INTERMEDIATE AND DELAYED TOXICITY

The main forms of toxicity associated with RIT in patients with metastatic breast cancer are thrombocytopenia and neutropenia (11,53). When ^{131}I-mAb is administered intravenously, most of the marrow radiation dose is from radio-labeled antibodies in the circulation unless tumor cells in the marrow increase the marrow cell dose by a "bystander" effect. Thus, radiolabeled antibodies with a longer circulation time deliver substantially more radiation to the marrow and produce more myelosuppression per injected dose than radiolabeled antibodies with more rapid blood clearance. It should be noted, however, that in the stem cell-supported breast cancer RIT studies, radiation doses that would be expected to cause second-organ toxicity have not yet been been reached in dose-escalation trials.

BIOLOGIC EFFECTS ON THERAPEUTIC RESPONSE

The L6 and ChL6 antibodies were chosen for study in RIT because of their antibody-dependent cellular cytotoxicity (ADCC) and complement-dependent cytotoxicity (CDC) activity *in vitro*; it was thought that some inflammatory response at the tumor site could occur and in turn enhance delivery of radioimmunoconjugate via increased vascular permeability. This hypothesis was based on experience with lymphoma patients who received therapy with ^{131}I-Lym-1, a mouse IgG2a biologically active mAb. In several of these lymphoma patients, redness, warmth, and tenderness developed in superficial tumors within 3 to 6 hours of infusion, and these symptoms seemed to be associated with good tumor uptake and response (54).

Imaging (pharmacokinetics) studies with ^{131}I-L6 demonstrated that a vascular target could be coated with 150 to 200 mg of unlabeled L6. That enabled a subsequent dose of ^{131}I-L6 to reach extravascular breast cancer metastases in quantities that allowed tumor visualization by imaging (8). A dose of 50 to 100 mg of L6 or ChL6 also activates the classic complement cascade, with a decrease in C3 and C4. However, soluble IL-2 receptor (IL-2R) is not released in amounts above preinfusion baseline levels unless 150 mg or more of L6 or ChL6 is infused. Furthermore, in those patients who underwent imaging and received only 50 or 100 mg of L6, IL-2R was not released, even 4 to 5 hours after the end of infusion. All but one patient receiving more than 150 mg of L6 or ChL6 had an increased IL-2R level within that time frame (37). The exceptional patient was the only one whose tumor progressed during the first month after therapy. In these patients, the rise in serum IL-2R was dose- and time-dependent, and likely an intermediate cytokine was released from cells at extravascular sites. The rise in IL-2R levels during therapy correlated directly with the subsequent therapeutic response. Among the nine patients who underwent sequential imaging and received therapy doses, six had metastatic disease in superficial areas distinct from blood pool structures. Uptake in these tumors 24 hours after injection of the initial dose of ^{131}I-ChL6 (imaging) was compared with that in each tumor

24 hours after the second ^{131}I-ChL6 injection. Even before correction for coincidence for the therapy doses, mean tumor uptake was almost doubled in five of the six patients in comparison with uptake of the imaging dose (37).

HUMAN ANTIMONOCLONAL ANTIBODIES

After exposure to antibodies containing foreign proteins, HAMAs may develop. A HAMA response usually results in rapid clearance of the therapeutic antibodies from the circulation, so that tumor uptake is reduced. The development of an HAMA response varies considerably among patients. Imaging with very small amounts of antibody (1 to 2 mg) seldom elicits HAMAs after one dose. Chimeric and humanized mAbs in moderate doses also elicit a smaller HAMA response. In general, HAMA responses are less frequent in patients who are immunosuppressed. HAMAs develop in approximately half of immunocompetent patients after a single dose of 5 to 50 mg of intact murine antibodies; this rate increases to approximately 90% in patients who receive three doses or more of antibody fragments (55). HAMAs can be detected in some patients as soon as 1 week after the administration of murine antibodies and may persist for months or years, so that tumor targeting with subsequent antibody infusions is precluded.

In the presence of HAMAs, the worldwide experience has generally been that multiple infusions seldom cause clinical problems if the infusion is given slowly. However, serial therapy is frequently terminated when an HAMA response develops because the therapeutic agent is no longer able to reach its target. On the other side of the coin, multiple investigators have suggested that with the more common HAMA response, antibodies are sometimes elicited to the immune reactive region of the initial mAb and then to those of the anti-idiotype antibodies, so that a cascade capable of creating effective antitumor antibody titers is initiated. This suspicion has led individual investigators to postulate that some delayed tumor responses are in fact a response to this "vaccine"-like effect of the initial antibody injection.

On the other hand, several investigators have successfully administered modest doses of cyclosporin A orally once or twice a day for 1 to 2 weeks after a mAb infusion to prevent HAMA formation, with minimal or no toxicity (39,56,57). In clinical trials in breast cancer patients receiving [131]I- or ^{90}Y-DOTA-peptide-ChL6 and cyclosporin A "prophylaxis," four of four patients remained HAMA-negative after up to six exposures to antibody (39,42). This result is in contrast to the 100% HAMA response observed without cyclosporin A in patients receiving intensive-dose ChL6 RIT and supports the ability of cyclosporin A to facilitate fractionated RIT. The rate of clearance of the antibody may dicate the duration of cyclosporin A prophylaxis required to prevent an HAMA response (35).

PERIPHERAL BLOOD STEM CELL TRANFUSIONS

In a breast cancer trial reported by Richman et al. (7,39), PBSC transfusions were prophylactically administered to patients who had been treated with ^{131}I-ChL6 once the level of radioactivity in the blood had decreased below 1 µCi/mL and the dose to circulating cells from blood and whole body was calculated to be around 5 rad based on dosimetry data of 11 patients. The dose equivalent constant of ^{90}Y is four to five times greater than that of ^{131}I; therefore, a blood level of less than 0.25 µCi of ^{90}Y per milliliter was utilized for reinfusion of PBSCs. PBSCs were selected because they are particularly well suited to ameliorating thrombocytopenia. In the previously mentioned studies by Schrier et al. (28) and Cagnoni et al. (29), patients prophylactically received either autologous marrow or PBSCs 15 days after ^{90}Y-BrE-3 to minimize the risk for life-threatening neutropenia or thrombocytopenia. In all the above studies, G-CSF was given after the PBSCs in an effort to shorten the neutropenic period. In the three current studies listed in Table 22.1, PBSCs harvested after G-CSF stimulation are being given several days after the injected radioactive dose, when the radiation dose that the infused stem cells will receive is considered low enough not to affect engraftment (35,58).

PRECLINICAL STUDIES OF RADIOIMMUNOTHERAPY AND TAXOL SYNERGY STUDIES

Novel, synergistic, multimodality therapy is needed for breast cancer to combat the molecular mechanisms, genetic mutations, and epigenetic abnormalities that protect the cancer from therapeutic interventions. Work with the aggressive human breast cancer model HBT3477 exemplifies the study of RIT of breast cancer with such mechanisms (i.e., mutant, nonfunctional p53 and a high level of expression of *bcl2*) (Fig. 22.7). Taxol (paclitaxel) has been shown to have efficacy in ovarian and breast cancers because it stabilizes microtubule formation, which results in mitotic block, *bcl2* dysfunction,

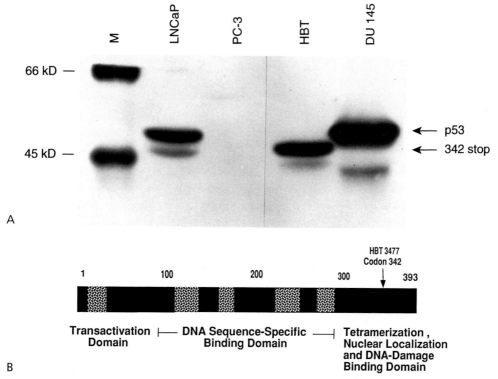

FIGURE 22.7. A: Western blot analysis of the mutational status of p53 protein. The loss of 52 amino acids from the carboxyl terminus of the *p53* transcript results in a truncated nonfunctional p53 protein (48.2 kd). *Lane 1*, high-molecular-weight marker; *lane 2*, LNCaP cell line; *lane 3*, PC-3 cell line; *lane 4*, HBT3477 xenograft tumors; *lane 5*, DU 145 cell line. In the HBT3477, the p53 protein made from the gene with a stop mutation migrates to the predicted lower-molecular-weight position. **B:** The *p53* gene map shows where the *p53* mutation is located (codon 342) in the HBT3477 cell line. The majority of mutations occur within the conserved region (*black and white pattern*) of *p53*. The mutation shown here deletes the part of the p53 protein involved in the detection of and response to DNA damage (i.e., from radiation) (63).

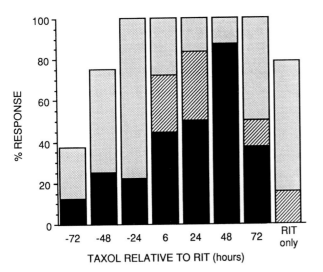

FIGURE 22.8. Effect of radioimmunotherapy (*RIT*) and Taxol synergy in treating human breast cancer as xenografts in mice. Mice were treated with Taxol (600 μg) from 72 hours before to 72 hours after treatment with ⁹⁰Y-DOTA-peptide-ChL6 (260 μCi). Response categories were cure (*black*), complete response (*crosshatch*), and partial response (*grey*). RIT (260 μCi) alone resulted in no cures. Taxol alone had no effect. Comparatively, cures were achieved in all groups receiving combined RIT/Taxol. A response was achieved in 100% of tumors when Taxol was administered 24 hours before RIT or later. The maximum cure rate (88%) was achieved when Taxol was given 48 hours after RIT (59,61).

and activation of apoptosis (59,60). Taxol may be even more effective in the presence of mutant *p53*. Because mutations of *p53* are frequent in breast cancer, the potential synergism between Taxol and ⁹⁰Y-ChL6 was assessed in the HBT3477 breast cancer model. Because the sequence, timing, and dose of these agents could be critical for synergy, a modified response surface approach was used to evaluate the therapeutic combination. Statistically, no tumor response occurred in mice receiving ChL6 or Taxol alone. In mice receiving ⁹⁰Y-ChL6 alone, 79% (15/19) of tumors responded, although none was cured. When Taxol was administered 24 to 72 hours before ⁹⁰Y-ChL6, again 79% (23/29) of tumors responded, but 21% were cured. When Taxol was given 24 hours after ⁹⁰Y-ChL6, 50% of these anaplastic breast cancer xenografts were cured, and Taxol given 48 hours after RIT resulted in an 88% cure rate. Taxol given with ⁹⁰Y-ChL6 did not substantially increase toxicity (Fig. 22.8). In conclusion, Taxol appears to be synergistic with ⁹⁰Y-DOTA-peptide-ChL6 in this human breast cancer model (59,61).

SUMMARY

Radioimmunotherapy with systemically administered mAbs linked to high-energy, beta-emitting radionuclides is a promising approach for treating metastatic cancer. Because of the selective biologic concentration of the antibody and therefore the radionuclide in tumor tissue, this modality can deliver substantial doses of radiation to tumors while minimizing the concomitant exposure of normal tissue. In addition, multiple metastases throughout the body can be targeted in a single treatment. Although excellent results have been reported for RIT in advanced hematologic malignancies, success in solid tumors has been limited. However, pilot clinical trials using the murine and chimeric antibody L6, which targets a variety of adenocarcinoma cell types, have yielded objective responses in approximately half of the patients with predominantly chemotherapy-refractory breast cancer, with minimal toxicity. Similar antitumor responses have been reported after a single cycle of a moderate dose of ⁹⁰Y linked to BrE-3, and higher doses as ⁹⁰Y-BrE-3, ⁹⁰Y-cT84.66, or ⁹⁰Y-m170 with PBSC support.

The purpose of this chapter has been to provide an overview of strategies that appear promising for RIT in breast cancer. It is apparent that combination therapy is required. Biodegradable peptide linkers between the chelated metal and the antibody have been shown to improve the therapeutic index. However, clinical impact on the management and cure of metastatic breast cancer will ultimately depend on the identification of synergistic therapies based on the following facts: (a) Continuous, low-dose radionuclide therapy acts through apoptosis, and (b) apoptosis is often blocked in breast cancer metastasis because of abnormal molecular biology in breast cancer cells that results in ineffective p53 and increased expression of *bcl2*. Agents such as paclitaxel (Taxol) are particularly attractive as synergistic agents for RIT because of cell cycle arrest in the radiosensitive G2M phase and p53-independent apoptosis. Optimal sequence and timing in combined-modality treatment with RIT will be critical to achieve maximum synergy and minimize toxicity.

ACKNOWLEDGMENTS

This work was supported by National Institutes of Health grants PO1-CA-47829 (University of California Davis), PO1-CA-43904 (City of Hope), and RO3 CA-77131-01 (University of Colorado), and Department of Education grant DE FG-03-84ER60233 (University of California Davis). Special thanks to Jeannette Peacock for help in preparing the chapter.

REFERENCES

1. Landis SH, Murray T, Bolden S, et al. Cancer statistics. *CA Cancer J Clin* 1998;48:6–29.
2. Sledge GW, Antman KH. Progress in chemotherapy for metastatic breast cancer. *Semin Oncol* 1992;19:317–332.
3. Fisher B, Redmond C, Poisson R, et al. Eight-year results of a randomized clinical trial comparing total mastectomy and lumpectomy with or without irradiation in the treatment of breast cancer. *N Engl J Med* 1989;320:822–828.
4. Lichter AS, Lippman ME, Danforth DNJ, et al. Mastectomy ver-

sus breast-conserving therapy in the treatment of stage I and II carcinoma of the breast: a randomized trial at the National Cancer Institute. *J Clin Oncol* 1992;10:976–983.

5. Sarrazin D, Le MG, Arriagada R, et al. Ten-year results of a randomized trial comparing a conservative treatment to mastectomy in early breast cancer. *Radiother Oncol* 1989;14:177–184.

6. van Dongen JA, Bartelik H, Fentiman IS, et al. Randomized clinical trial to assess the value of breast-conserving therapy in stage I and II breast cancer: EORTC 10801 trial. *Monogr Natl Cancer Inst* 1992;11:15–18.

7. Richman CM, Schuermann TC, Wun T, et al. Peripheral blood stem cell mobilization for hematopoietic support of radioimmunotherapy in patients with breast carcinoma. *Cancer* 1997;80:2728–2732.

8. DeNardo SJ, O'Grady LF, Macey DJ, et al. Quantitative imaging of mouse L-6 monoclonal antibody in breast cancer patients to develop a therapeutic strategy. *Int J Radiat Appl Instr B* 1991;18:621–631.

9. Kramer EL, DeNardo SJ, Liebes L, et al. Radioimmunolocalization of breast carcinoma using BrE-3 monoclonal antibody: phase I study. *J Nucl Med* 1993;34:1067–1074.

10. DeNardo SJ, Kramer EL, O'Donnell RT, et al. Radioimmunotherapy for breast cancer using indium-111/yttrium-90 BrE-3: results of a phase I clinical trial. *J Nucl Med* 1997;38:1180–1185.

11. DeNardo SJ, O'Grady LF, Richman CM, et al. Radioimmunotherapy for advanced breast cancer using I-131-ChL6 antibody. *Anticancer Res* 1997;17:1745–1752.

12. Mattes MJ, Major PP, Goldenberg DM, et al. Patterns of antigen distribution in human carcinomas. *Cancer Res* 1990;50[Suppl]:880–884.

13. Howell LP, DeNardo SJ, Levy N, et al. Immunohistochemical staining of metastatic ductal carcinomas of the breast by monoclonal antibodies used in imaging and therapy: a comparative study. *Int J Biol Markers* 1995;10:126–135.

14. Esteban JM, Felder B, Ahn C, et al. Prognostic relevance of carcinoembryonic antigen and estrogen receptor status in breast cancer patients. *Cancer* 1994;74:1575–1583.

15. Goldenberg DM. New developments in monoclonal antibodies for cancer detection and therapy. *CA Cancer J Clin* 1994;44:43–64.

16. Sharkey RM, Goldenberg DM, Murthy S, et al. Clinical evaluation of tumor targeting with a high-affinity, anticarcinoembryonic antigen-specific, murine monoclonal antibody, MN-14. *Cancer* 1993;71:2082–2096.

17. Nabi HA. Antibody imaging in breast cancer. *Semin Nucl Med* 1997;27:30–39.

18. Behr TM, Sharkey RM, Juweid ME, et al. Phase I/II clinical radioimmunotherapy with an iodine-131-labeled anti-carcinoembryonic antigen murine monoclonal antibody IgG. *J Nucl Med* 1997;38:858–870.

19. Wagener C, Yang HJ, Crawford FG, et al. Monoclonal antibodies for carcinoembryonic antigen and related antigens as a model system: a systematic approach for the determination of epitope specificities of monoclonal antibodies. *J Immunol* 1983;130:2308–2315.

20. Neumaier M, Shively L, Chen FS, et al. Cloning for the genes for T84.66, an antibody that has a high specificity and affinity for carcinoembryonic antigen, and expression of chimeric human-mouse T84.66 gene in myeloma and Chinese hamster ovary cells. *Cancer Res* 1990;50:2128–2134.

21. Wong JYC, Somlo G, Odom-Maryon T, et al. Initial results of a phase I trial evaluating ^{90}yttrium (^{90}Y)-chimeric T84.66 (cT84.66) anti-CEA antibody and autologous stem cell support in CEA-producing metastatic breast cancer. *Cancer Biother Radiopharm* 1998;13:314(abst).

22. Price MR, Rye PD, Petrakou E, et al. Summary report on the ISOBM TD-4 workshop: analysis of 56 monoclonal antibodies against the MUC1 mucin. *Tumour Biol* 1998;19:1–20.

23. Fontenot JD, Tjandra N, Bu D, et al. Biophysical characterization of one-, two-, and three-tandem repeats of human mucin (MUC-1) protein core. *Cancer Res* 1993;53:5386–5394.

24. Granowska M, Biassoni L, Carroll MJ, et al. Breast cancer ^{99m}Tc SM3 radioimmunoscintigraphy. *Acta Oncol* 1996;35:319–321.

25. Baum RP, Brummendorf TH. Radioimmunolocalization of primary and metastatic breast cancer. *Q J Nucl Med* 1998;42:33–42.

26. Major PP, Dion AS, Williams CJ, et al. Breast tumor radioimmunodetection with a 111-In-labeled monoclonal antibody (MA5) against a mucin-like antigen. *Cancer Res* 1990;50:927s–931s.

27. Buckman R, De Angelis C, Shaw P, et al. Intraperitoneal therapy of malignant ascites associated with carcinoma of ovary and breast using radioiodinated monoclonal antibody 2G3. *Gynecol Oncol* 1992;47:102–109.

28. Schrier DM, Stemmer SM, Johnson T, et al. High-dose ^{90}Y Mx-diethylenetriaminepentaacetic acid (DTPA)-BrE-3 and autologous hematopoietic stem cell support (AHSCS) for the treatment of advanced breast cancer: a phase I trial. *Cancer Res* 1995;55:5921s–5924s.

29. Cagnoni PJ, Ceriani RL, Cole WC, et al. Phase I study of high-dose radioimmunotherapy with 90-Y-hu-BrE-3 followed by autologous stem cell support (ASCS) in patients with metastatic breast cancer. *Cancer Biother Radiopharm* 1998;13:328.

30. Richman CM, DeNardo SJ, O'Donnell RT, et al. Dosimetry-based therapy in metastatic breast cancer patients using ^{90}Y MAB 170H.82 with autologous stem cell support and cyclosporin A. *Cancer Biother Radiopharm* 1998;13:314(abst).

31. Blank EW, Pant KD, Chan CM, et al. A novel anti-breast epithelial mucin MoAb (BrE-3). *Cancer* 1992;5:38–44.

32. Kramer EL, Liebes L, Wasserheit C, et al. Initial clinical evaluation of radiolabeled MX-DTPA humanized BrE-3 antibody in patients with advanced breast cancer. *Clin Cancer Res* 1998;4:1679–1688.

33. MacLean GD, McEwan A, Noujaim A, et al. Two novel monoclonal antibodies have potential for gynecologic cancer imaging. *Antibody Immunoconjug Radiopharm* 1991;4:297–308.

34. McEwan AJB, MacLean GD, Hooper H, et al. MAb 170H.82: an evaluation of a novel panadenocarcinoma monoclonal antibody labeled with ^{99m}Tc and with ^{111}In. *Nucl Med Commun* 1992;13:11–19.

35. Richman CM, DeNardo SJ, O'Donnell RT, et al. Dosimetry-based therapy in metastatic breast cancer patients using ^{90}Y Mab 170H.82 with autologous stem cell support and cyclosporin A. *Clin Cancer Res* 1999;5:3243–3248.

36. Marken JS, Schieven GL, Hellstrom I, et al. Cloning and expression of the tumor-associated antigen L6. *Proc Natl Acad Sci U S A* 1992;89:3503–3507.

37. DeNardo SJ, Mirick GR, Kroger LA, et al. The biologic window for chimeric L6 radioimmunotherapy. *Cancer* 1994;73[Suppl]:1023–1032.

38. DeNardo SJ, O'Grady LF, Hellstrom I, et al. Dose-dependent human biokinetics of L-6 MoAb. *J Nucl Med* 1989;30:907(abst).

39. Richman CM, DeNardo SJ, O'Grady LF, et al. Radioimmunotherapy for breast cancer using escalating fractionated doses of ^{131}I-labeled chimeric L6 antibody with peripheral blood progenitor cell transfusions. *Cancer Res* 1995;55[Suppl]:5916–5920.

40. Meares CF, McCall MJ, Deshpande SV, et al. Chelate radiochemistry: cleavable linkers lead to altered levels of radioactivity in the liver. *Int J Cancer* 1988;2[Suppl]:99–103.

41. DeNardo SJ, Zhong G-R, Salako Q, et al. Pharmacokinetics of chimeric L6 conjugated to indium-111 and yttrium-90-DOTA-peptide in tumor-bearing mice. *J Nucl Med* 1995;36:829–836.

42. DeNardo SJ, Richman CM, Goldstein DS, et al. Yttrium-

90/indium-111-DOTA-peptide-chimeric L6: Pharmacokinetics, dosimetry and initial results in patients with incurable breast cancer. *Anticancer Res* 1997;17:1735–1744.

43. Schlom J, Molinolo A, Simpson JF, et al. Advantage of dose fractionation in monoclonal antibody-targeted radioimmunotherapy. *J Natl Cancer Inst* 1990;82:763–771.

44. Khazaeli MB, Saleh MN, Liu TP, et al. Pharmacokinetics and immune response of ^{131}I-chimeric mouse/human B72.3 (human gamma 4) monoclonal antibody in humans. *Cancer Res* 1991;51:5461–5466.

45. Meredith RF, Bueschen AJ, Khazaeli MB, et al. Phase I trial of iodine-131-chimeric B72.3 (human IgG4) in metastatic colorectal cancer. *J Nucl Med* 1992;33:23–29.

46. Meredith RF, Khazaeli MB, Liu T, et al. Dose fractionation of radiolabeled antibodies in patients with metastatic colon cancer. *J Nucl Med* 1992;33:1648–1653.

47. Schlom J, Siler K, Milenic DE, et al. Monoclonal antibody-based therapy of a human tumor xenograft with a 177-lutetium-labeled immunoconjugate. *Cancer Res* 1991;51:2889–2896.

48. Murray JL, Macey DJ, Grant EJ, et al. Enhanced TAG-72 expression and tumor uptake of radiolabeled monoclonal antibody CC49 in metastatic breast cancer patients following alpha-interferon treatment. *Cancer Res* 1995;55:5925s–5928s.

49. Macey DJ, Grant EJ, Kasi LP, et al. Effect of recombinant alpha-interferon on pharmacokinetics, biodistribution, toxicity, and efficacy of ^{131}I-labeled monoclonal antibody CC49 in breast cancer: a phase II trial. *Clin Cancer Res* 1997;3:1547–1555.

50. Goodman GE, Hellstrom I, Brodzinsky L, et al. Phase I trial of murine monoclonal antibody L6 in breast, colon, ovarian and lung cancer. *J Clin Oncol* 1990;8:1083–1092.

51. Goodman GE, Hellstrom I, Yelton DE, et al. Phase I trial of chimeric (human-mouse) monoclonal antibody L6 in patients with non-small-cell lung, colon, and breast cancer. *Cancer Immunol Immunother* 1993;36:267–273.

52. Ziegler LD, Palazzolo P, Cunningham J, et al. Phase I trial of murine monoclonal antibody L6 in combination with subcutaneous interleukin-2 in patients with advanced carcinoma of the breast, colorectum, and lung. *J Clin Oncol* 1992;10:1470–1478.

53. DeNardo SJ. Radioimmunotherapy in the treatment of metasta-tic breast cancer: an overview. In: Goldenberg DM, ed. *Cancer therapy with radiolabeled antibodies.* Boca Raton, FL: CRC Press, 1995:189–201.

54. DeNardo SJ, DeNardo GL, O'Grady LF, et al. Treatment of B cell malignancies with I-131 Lym-1 monoclonal antibodies. *Int J Cancer* 1988;3[Suppl]:96–101.

55. Sears HF, Atkinson B, Mattis J, et al. Phase I clinical trial of monoclonal antibody in treatment of gastrointestinal tumors. *Lancet* 1982;1(8275):762–765.

56. Ledermann JA, Begent RH, Massof C, et al. A phase I study of repeated therapy with radiolabelled antibody to carcinoembryonic antigen using intermittent or continuous administration of cyclosporin A to supress the immune response. *Int J Cancer* 1991;47:659–664.

57. Weiden PL, Wolf SB, Breitz HB, et al. Human anti-mouse antibody suppression with cyclosporin A. *Cancer* 1994;73:1093–1097.

58. Press OW, Eary JF, Appelbaum FR, et al. Treatment of relapsed B cell lymphomas with high-dose radioimmunotherapy and bone marrow transplantation. In: Goldenberg DM, ed. *Cancer therapy with radiolabeled antibodies.* Boca Raton, FL: CRC Press, 1995:229–237.

59. DeNardo SJ, Kukis DL, Kroger LA, et al. Synergy of Taxol and radioimmunotherapy with yttrium-90-labeled chimeric L6 antibody: efficacy and toxicity in breast cancer xenografts. *Proc Natl Acad Sci U S A* 1997;94:4000–4004.

60. Marangolo M, Emiliani E, Rosti G, et al. Paclitaxel and radiotherapy in the treatment of advanced non-small cell lung cancer. *Semin Oncol* 1996;23:31–34.

61. DeNardo SJ, Richman CM, Kukis DL, et al. Synergistic therapy of breast cancer with Y-90-chimeric L6 and paclitaxel in the xenografted mouse model: development of a clinical protocol. *Anticancer Res* 1998;18:4011–4018.

62. Li M, Meares CF. Synthesis, metal chelate stability studies, and enzyme digestion of a peptide-linked DOTA derivative and its corresponding radiolabeled immunoconjugates. *Bioconjug Chem* 1993;4:275–283.

63. Winthrop MD, DeNardo SJ, Muenzer JT, et al. p53-independent response of a human breast cancer xenograft to radioimmunotherapy. *Cancer* 1997;80[Suppl]:2706–2712.

23

POSITRON EMISSION TOMOGRAPHY IMAGING

CARL K. HOH

In this chapter, the applications of positron emission tomography (PET) in esophageal, gastric, and pancreatic cancer are reviewed. In other tumors, PET has been found to be useful in staging disease, differentiating post-therapy changes from residual tumor, restaging disease at the time of recurrence, and evaluating the response to chemotherapy. Although patients with such cancers typically have a poor prognosis, some applications of this technology are potentially useful in diagnostic and therapeutic algorithms for management.

ESOPHAGEAL CANCER

Most patients with esophageal carcinoma have advanced disease at the time of initial diagnosis (1). Knowing the stage of disease, however, is important in planning local (surgery and/or radiation) and systemic (chemotherapy) therapy. Important factors in selecting appropriate treatment and determining the prognosis include the extent of local tumor invasion, tumor size, lymph node involvement, and presence of metastases at the time of diagnosis.

Patients usually have advanced disease at the time of initial diagnosis for several reasons. Because of the unconfined anatomic space of the esophagus and its ability to distend to compensate for a partially obstructed lumen, a tumor may grow for several years without causing symptoms. Esophageal cancer is characterized by extensive local growth, lymph node metastases, and invasion of local adjacent structures. The blood supply to the esophagus comes from three sources, which divide into minute branches before arriving at the esophageal mucosa. This rich plexus of vessels allows various portions of the esophagus to be mobilized and remain viable. The venous drainage of the esophagus is also rather direct, via the azygous and hemiazygous systems and the intercostal veins. In the more superior portion of the esophagus, the venous drainage is to the cervical veins, whereas the inferior portion drains to the inferior phrenic veins.

The lymphatic drainage of the esophagus is quite extensive; typically, it is to three major regions. The upper third of the esophagus drains to the internal jugular, cervical, and supraclavicular areas. Lymphatic drainage from the mucosal to the submucosal and muscular layers through a complex plexus of channels allows lymphatic fluid, and therefore tumor, to spread from one portion of the esophagus to other portions, and also throughout the thorax. In addition, the lymphatic plexus allows tumors in any portion of the esophagus to drain into the nodal basins in the supraclavicular and cervical regions. These may be palpable on physical examination.

Patients with the best chance for cure have early, superficial lesions that can be completely removed surgically. Even with the newer surgical techniques, however, and postoperative management, the morbidity and postoperative mortality associated with esophageal resection are still relatively high. Even patients whose tumors are thought to have been completely resected have poor rates of long-term survival because of undetected metastatic disease at the time of surgery (2). Autopsy studies have shown that distant metastatic disease is almost always present at the time of death. When the patient presents with dysphagia from carcinoma of the esophagus, subclinical metastatic disease is probably already present (3).

The perfect imaging technology for esophageal cancer (and for most tumors) must identify and measure the size of the primary lesion, detect and determine the extent of local disease with reference to invasion to other anatomic structures, and detect distant metastatic disease. For esophageal cancer, the evaluation of the primary lesion includes determining the length of the lesion, which is correlated with the extent of involvement of adjacent structures and is inversely related to survival. Because ultimate long-term survival depends on complete resection of the tumor, detection of unsuspected metastatic disease is clinically important in esophageal cancer. The current recommendations for preoperative clinical staging are chest

C. K. Hoh: Department of Radiology, University of California, San Diego; Department of Nuclear Medicine, University of California, San Diego Medical Center, San Diego, California 92103.

roentgenography, barium swallow, and computed tomography (CT) of the chest and upper abdomen, which includes the liver and adrenal glands. CT allows the detection of vascular and bronchial invasion. It is relatively insensitive, however, for detecting abdominal lymph node metastases and small liver metastases. Bronchoscopy is mandatory for patients with a lesion in the middle to upper third of the esophagus. A bone scan should be performed in patients reporting bone pain. Conventional imaging techniques may help to confirm the presence of the lesion and potentially allow the biopsy of indeterminate lesions. However, because of the large number of patients who later develop recurrence, the negative predictive value of current imaging methods is low.

For PET with fluorodeoxyglucose (FDG-PET) to have an impact on survival, it must be effective in detecting metastatic lesions at the time of the initial diagnosis (Figs. 23.1 and 23.2). This depends on the tumor biology and the imaging technology. Important factors in the tumor biology include the size of metastatic lesions and the metabolic characteristics of the tumor at the time of initial diagnosis. The important technical factor is the resolution of PET imaging or coincidence imaging systems. Because the confirmation and detection of micrometastatic disease is possi-

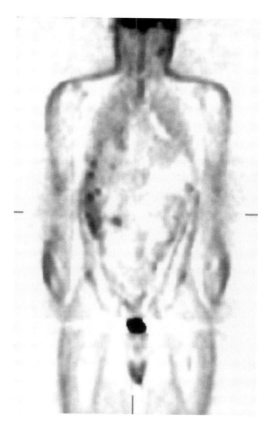

FIGURE 23.2. Coronal whole-body fluorodeoxyglucose (*FDG*) image in a patient with a history of esophageal carcinoma. Multiple foci of increased FDG activity in the liver are consistent with metastatic disease.

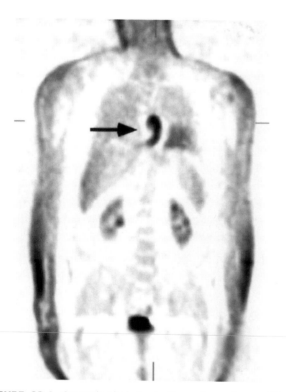

FIGURE 23.1. Coronal whole-body fluorodeoxyglucose (*FDG*) image in a patient with adenocarcinoma of the distal esophagus. The image was acquired without attenuation correction. The primary lesion is clearly shown with intense FDG accumulation (*arrow*). No evidence of metastatic disease was seen. The patient received induction chemotherapy, and on surgical resection, all 13 sampled lymph nodes were negative for tumor.

ble only by histology, and because biopsy of all suspect lesions on FDG-PET is impossible, even if these metabolic lesions can be correlated with an anatomic lesion on CT or magnetic resonance imaging (MRI), it is ultimately impossible to determine the absolute accuracy of FDG-PET. The natural progression of disease and the findings on close clinical and imaging follow-up are more indirect parameters used to assess accuracy.

Only a limited number of studies have addressed the ability of PET to stage esophageal cancer. The largest study comprised 36 patients with biopsy-proven, newly diagnosed carcinoma of the esophagus who had undergone FDG-PET during the preoperative evaluation (4). FDG-PET was able to identify the primary tumor in all patients. More importantly, in a subset of 29 patients who underwent curative surgery, an evaluation of nodal metastatic disease was possible. In this subset, the sensitivity of CT for detecting nodal disease was 28% and its specificity was 73%, whereas for PET the sensitivity was 72% and the specificity was 82%. In this study, false-positive PET results were caused by the presence of granulomatous disease, and false-negatives results were obtained when nodal metastases were less than 1 cm in diameter or close to the primary tumor. CT was incorrect in assessing these and other sites. The investigators stated that PET could potentially contribute to the staging of esophageal carcinoma by detecting small (not microscopic) metastatic lesions or extensive local lymph node disease not detected by conventional imaging techniques. Based on the identification of such lesions, the disease could be staged as inoperable. Among 36 patients, PET imaging would have diverted four patients from surgery, whereas CT findings would have diverted only one patient.

A smaller but prospective study also investigated FDG-PET as a means of detecting metastatic disease in patients with esophageal tumors and compared its results with surgical and histologic findings (5). In this study, all 26 patients underwent PET and CT for staging. The sensitivity of both CT and PET was high in detecting the primary lesions (81% and 96%, respectively); however, neither CT nor PET could accurately assess the extent of esophageal wall invasion. Among 13 patients with nodal metastases, CT detected only five (sensitivity, 38%). However, no CT findings were false-positive for nodal disease; all patients in whom CT demonstrated an enlarged node (short axis > 1 cm) were confirmed to have nodal metastases (specificity, 100%). The sensitivity and specificity of PET were high for lymph node metastases (92% and 88%, respectively). In the evaluation of resectability, PET was correct in 23 of 26 patients (accuracy, 88%), whereas CT was correct in 17 of 26 patients (accuracy, 65%). The overall accuracy for resectability when both CT and PET results were used was 92%, whereas for CT alone it was 65% and for PET alone it was 88%.

The approach to staging of disease has traditionally been based on the anatomic parameters of lesion size, depth of invasion, and presence of nodal or distant metastases; these are important indicators of prognosis because surgical resection is the only potentially curative treatment. With PET, a numeric parameter for the metabolic activity of the tumor is also available. The biologic significance of this metabolic parameter, its use in the management of treatment, and its relationship to clinical outcome are unknown. One publication has looked at this metabolic parameter in 48 patients with esophageal carcinoma (6). In this study, dynamic FDG-PET imaging was performed so that the continuous changes in tracer activity in plasma and in tumor could be measured and used to calculate the tracer kinetics. In addition, the standardized uptake value (SUV) was determined. SUV is a ratio of tracer activity in the tumor to estimated tracer activity distributed throughout the body. The investigators found that certain parameters in the tracer kinetic model (k_3) and the SUV correlated well with tumor cellular hexokinase activity ($p < 0.05$). The investigators found a diagnostic accuracy of 98.3% when an SUV threshold of 2.0 was used to differentiate benign from malignant esophageal lesions. They also found that patients with a preoperative SUV above 7.0 had a worse prognosis than patients with a preoperative SUV below 7.0.

GASTRIC CANCER

Gastric cancer was the leading cause of cancer death in the United States at the beginning of the 20th century; however, the incidence of the disease has dropped significantly, to only 2% of all new cancers (7). In the Far East, the incidence of stomach cancer can be as high as 48/100,000. Nevertheless, the mortality rate in patients with gastric cancer remains unchanged (8).

The arterial and venous supply to the stomach is very extensive. The venous drainage is ultimately through the portal system, which is why the liver is the primary site of metastatic spread. The lymphatic drainage of the stomach, like that of the esophagus, is also extensive. It includes six perigastric lymph node groups and second-echelon nodes consisting of hepatic, left gastric, splenic hilum, celiac, and periaortic nodes. This distribution can lead to involvement of the intrathoracic lymph channels and the presence of tumor in a left supraclavicular node (Virchow's node). It is for this reason that an imaging technology capable of providing a comprehensive evaluation of nodal disease in the upper to middle torso is important in the staging of gastric cancer (Fig. 23.3). Because micro-

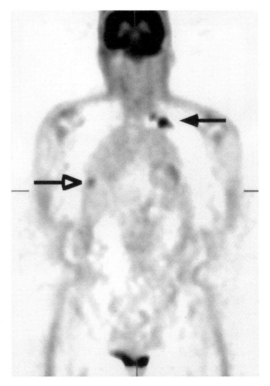

FIGURE 23.3. Coronal whole-body fluorodeoxyglucose image from a patient who had undergone subtotal gastrectomy for gastric carcinoma 1 month before positron emission tomography. Increased FDG activity in the liver (*open arrow*), supraclavicular area (*solid arrow*), and periaortic area (not shown on this image plane), corresponds to liver metastases and enlarged periaortic nodes seen on recent computed tomography.

TABLE 23.1. DETECTION OF PANCREATIC CANCER

Reference	n	Sensitivity (%)	Specificity (%)	PPV (%)	NPV (%)	Accuracy (%)
Bares et al. 1994 (11)	40	92	84	93	85	90
Friess et al. 1995 (12)	80	94	88	92	90	91
Inokuma et al. 1995 (15)	46	94	82	94	64	85
Stollfuss et al. 1995 (13)	73	95	90	95	95	93
Ho et al. 1996 (14)	14	100	67	80	100	86
Zimny et al. 1997 (18)	106	85	84	93	71	85
Diederichs et al. 1998 (19)	171					
Glucose <130 mg/dL	152	86	78	Not reported	Not reported	
Glucose >130 mg/dL	19	42	86	Not reported	Not reported	
Frohlich et al. 1999 (24)	168	68	95	65	95	91
Imdahl et al. 1999 (21)	48	96	100	100	95	98

metastatic disease cannot be detected, current imaging techniques can detect nodal disease (if of sufficient size) but cannot exclude nodal disease.

No large studies have specifically applied PET in the staging of gastric cancer. One study used PET to detect the response to chemotherapy in patients with esophageal and gastric cancer (9). In this study, 14 patients with various stages of either esophageal or gastric cancer were imaged with PET and CT before and after two to three cycles of chemotherapy. Clinical response was measured by changes in weight and dysphagia scores. Changes in tracer uptake were seen in all tumors after chemotherapy. A 30% reduction in FDG activity was noted in six patients, whereas a reduction in tumor size was shown in only four of these six by CT. Prolonged survival in a patient with advanced disease who had a large reduction in FDG activity after therapy suggests that PET may have a role in patients receiving palliative chemotherapy. A technique capable of predicting a favorable response to potentially toxic chemotherapy would be clinically helpful in determining which patients might benefit from continuing therapy. It is reasonable to expect that the metabolic characteristics of a tumor will change before any measurable reduction in tumor size is noted.

PANCREATIC CANCER

Approximately 28,000 patients die of pancreatic cancer annually in the United States. Pancreatic cancer is the fourth most common cause of cancer-related death for men and the fifth most common cause in women (7). The presenting symptoms of pancreatic cancer are weight loss, jaundice, pain, and dyspepsia; however, more than 80% of patients at the time of presentation cannot be cured with surgical resection (10). Surgical cure is possible only with very early diagnosis. Detection of extrapancreatic disease is important, especially in older patients, who can than be

spared a major surgical procedure. Pancreatic cancer is usually diagnosed after the identification of a pancreatic mass on ultrasonography or CT and percutaneous biopsy of the lesion. Other techniques used include endoscopic retrograde cholangiopancreatography, endoscopic ultrasonography, and laparoscopy. Laparoscopy identifies peritoneal implants and studding of tumor on the liver, which can be missed by CT.

The lymphatic drainage of the pancreas is associated with its surface and anatomic borders via the celiac, preaortic, and superior mesenteric nodal groups. Because of the extensive lymphatic drainage around the pancreas, metastatic drainage can be directed to any surrounding nodal groups. Patients who are surgical candidates for potential cure are those whose tumor remains within the pancreatic capsule (Fig. 23.4). Stage II disease with invasion into the duodenum or peripancreatic soft tissue is not surgically resectable. This is also true for stage III (lymph node involvement) and stage IV disease (distant metastasis). Therefore, the potential applications of PET would be in differentiating a malignant pancreatic mass from a benign mass and determining the presence of metastatic disease.

During the last few years, several reports have been published on the use of FDG-PET to characterize a pancreatic mass and detect metastases from pancreatic cancer. In one of the earlier studies addressing both of these issues, results were encouraging in 40 patients (11) (Table 23.1). The FDG-PET results were compared with results of CT and ultrasonography. In the detection of pancreatic malignancies, the sensitivity of PET was high (92%); however, its specificity was lower (84%) than that of the other techniques. False-positive results were said to be secondary to retroperitoneal fibrosis and pancreatitis. However, for the detection of lymph nodes involved by tumor, PET had a sensitivity of 76%, which was superior to that of both CT (17%) and ultrasonography (6%).

In three other studies (12–14), similar results were found. Thirty-two patients with chronic pancreatitis were evaluated, and 28 were correctly identified by FDG-PET to have benign lesions (12). These authors found no major difficulty in differentiating pancreatic carcinoma from chronic pancreatitis. The mean SUV was found to be significantly higher in patients with pancreatic carcinoma (3.09 ± 2.18) than in those with chronic pancreatitis (0.87 ± 0.56), (*p* < .001). In another study (13), 73 patients with pancreatic lesions (pancreatic cancer vs. chronic pancreatitis) underwent both CT and PET. In this study, an SUV threshold of 1.53 resulted in a sensitivity and specificity of 93% for tumor detection. Visual interpretation had a slightly higher sensitivity (95%) but a lower specificity (90%). The sensitivity and specificity of CT were 80% and 74%, respectively. The third study reported 12 patients with indeterminate masses on CT and two patients with typical findings of malignancy (14). PET was able to identify the malignant lesion in all eight patients when an SUV cutoff of 2.5 was used. This same SUV correctly identified four of the six patients with benign lesions.

Some investigators, however, have reported a significant number of false-positive cases when using FDG-PET in patients with pancreatitis (15,16). In the differentiation of mass-forming pancreatitis from pancreatic cancer, results were less encouraging (16). In this study, PET was compared with MRI in 15 patients with pancreatic cancer and nine patients with mass-forming pancreatitis. Although the dose uptake ratio differed significantly (*p* < .05) between pancreatic cancer and mass-forming pancreatitis (4.64 ± 1.94 vs. 2.84 ± 2.22), overlap was sufficient to limit the diagnostic utility of this method.

Although more recent studies continue to report a high sensitivity and specificity for the detection of pancreatic cancer (88% and 83%, respectively) (17), these studies also encountered false-positive results in patients with pancreatitis. The authors reported a range of SUVs with some overlap between malignant and benign lesions. For malignant lesions, the SUV ranged from 1.0 to 10.1, whereas for benign lesions it ranged from 0 to 5.8.

Because of the relatively frequent false-negative results in certain patients with pancreatic cancer, the relationship between a patient's metabolic state and the detectability of pancreatic cancer has been examined. In a series of 106 patients, the results of FDG-PET were false-negative in 11 patients, 10 of whom had elevated levels of serum glucose (18). The authors concluded that the diagnostic accuracy of PET examinations is very dependent on serum glucose levels. Similar results were also found in another study (19), in which detectability rates dropped from 86% to 42% when the plasma glucose level went above 130 mg/dL.

The biologic cause of the reduced detectability appears to be related to several factors involved in FDG uptake by pancreatic cancer. The glucose transporter Glut-1 is essential in FDG uptake by the tumor. Tumor cellularity has a significant influence on the SUV only in the presence of increased Glut-1 (20).

Some of the differences in results may be related to the time at which the acquisition or analysis is performed. In one study, when the SUV analysis was performed 90 to 120 minutes after injection (21), the investigators found an improved ability to differentiate pancreatic cancer (SUV > 4.0) from chronic pancreatitis (SUV between 3.0 and 4.0).

The application of FDG-PET in the current clinical management of a patient with a pancreatic mass requires further refinement. Because FDG-PET activity in a pancreatic mass cannot be considered diagnostic, the diagnosis of pancreatic cancer still requires tissue examination. FDG-PET may be considered in patients with indeterminate findings on CT. At present, a negative or a positive FDG-PET result cannot entirely exclude or confirm a diagnosis.

However, FDG-PET may have a role in the staging of pancreatic cancer. Detection of liver metastasis is important because if it is present, the patient cannot be cured by

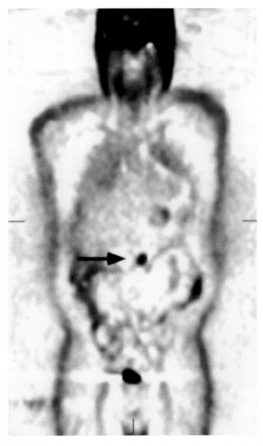

FIGURE 23.4. Coronal whole-body fluorodeoxyglucose (*FDG*) image from a patient who had undergone a Whipple procedure 6 months earlier for pancreatic cancer. The patient at the time of positron emission tomography complained of back pain and was noted to have a rising level of CA-19-9. Results of recent abdominal computed tomography were negative. The FDG image shows a relatively intense focus of tumor activity in the midline of the abdomen at the level of the kidneys (*arrow*).

surgery (22,23). One study found PET to be reliable in the detection of liver metastases larger than 1 cm (24). False-positive results were caused by intrahepatic cholestasis. Quantitative indices such as the SUV and tumor-to-liver ratio were of limited value. The tumor-to-liver ratio was 2.3 ± 1.1 for malignant lesions and 1.9 ± 0.3 for false-positive lesions. As discussed earlier, the ability of FDG-PET to detect nodes involved by tumor was better than that of CT or ultrasonography (11), so that a guided lymph node biopsy might confirm the presence of metastases and obviate an unnecessary morbid surgical procedure.

Patients with pancreatic cancer have also undergone FDG-PET for "metabolic staging." A high glycolytic rate, reflected by the rate of FDG uptake, has been shown to be associated with a more aggressive tumor and a worse prognosis. In a study with 14 patients, the prognosis was worse in patients with high tumor SUVs (≥ 3.0) than in those with a low SUVs (< 3.0) (25). Patients with high SUVs had a mean survival of 5 months, whereas those with low SUVs had a mean survival of 14 months.

Tracers other than ^{18}F-FDG have been investigated for imaging pancreatic cancer. An early PET study of pancreatic cancer used ^{11}C-methionine in 85 patients (26). PET with ^{11}C-methionine was more sensitive and specific than CT in detecting pancreatic lesions by showing a metabolic defect; however, it was unable to distinguish between benign and malignant pancreatic lesions.

In summary, the sensitivity of FDG-PET in detecting primary pancreatic cancer appears to range from 85% to 100%, and the specificity from 67% to 90%. Glucose levels should be controlled to avoid decreasing tumor detectability. Imaging interpretation and SUV analysis should be based on a delayed scan (60 to 90 minutes) after injection of FDG. A potential role for FDG-PET in pancreatic cancer may be in the evaluation of patients with equivocal findings on CT or percutaneous biopsy for whom laparotomy would be the next step. Because false-positive results can be caused by pancreatitis, benign mucinous cystic tumors, and serous cystadenomas, a percutaneous or laparoscopic biopsy may still be needed to confirm the diagnosis. After the confirmation of pancreatic cancer by percutaneous biopsy, a promising role of FDG-PET is in detecting metastatic lymph nodes or liver disease and identifying patients who would not benefit from pancreatectomy.

CONCLUSIONS

The ability of FDG-PET to detect the primary tumor appears promising in esophageal, gastric, and pancreatic cancers. However, the presence of high levels of FDG activity as a result of inflammation of the pancreatitis can cause false-positive interpretations. The lymphatic drainage patterns in all three of these tumors are unpredictable, but the correlation of high rates of metabolic activity in tumor-involved lymph nodes with CT findings has the potential to stage disease more accurately before surgical intervention. The level of FDG activity in these tumors may also provide an additional prognostic parameter in determining therapeutic options.

REFERENCES

1. Roth JA, Putnam JB, Lichter AS, et al. Cancer of the esophagus. In: DeVita VT, Hellman S, Rosenberg SA, eds. *Cancer principles and practice of oncology*, 4th ed. Philadelphia: JB Lippincott Co, 1993:776–817.
2. Mantravadi R, Ladd T, Briele H, et al. Carcinoma of the esophagus: sites of failure. *Int J Radiat Oncol Biol Phys* 1982;8:1987.
3. Arbito A, Straus M, Granklin G, et al. Infusional chemotherapy and cyclic chemotherapy for inoperable esophageal and gastric cardia carcinoma. *Am J Clin Oncol* 1983;6:195.
4. Flanagan FL, Dehdashti F, Seigel BA, et al. Staging of esophageal cancer with ^{18}F-fluorodeoxyglucose positron emission tomography. *AJR Am J Roentgenol* 1997;168:417–424.
5. Kole AC, Plukker JT, Nieweg OE, et al. Positron emission tomography for staging of oesophageal and gastroesophageal malignancy. *Br J Surg* 1998;78:521–527.
6. Fukunaga T, Okazumi S, Koide Y, et al. Evaluation of esophageal cancers using fluorine-18-fluorodeoxyglucose PET. *J Nucl Med* 1998;39:1002–1007.
7. Landis SH, Murray T, Bolden S, et al. Cancer statistics 1998. *CA Cancer J Clin* 1998;48:6–30.
8. Alexander HR, Kelsen DP, Tepper JE. Cancer of the stomach. In: DeVita VT, Hellman S, Rosenberg SA, eds. *Cancer principles and practice of oncology*, 4th ed. Philadelphia: JB Lippincott Co, 1993:818–848.
9. Couper GW, McAteer D, Wallis F, et al. Detection of response to chemotherapy using positron emission tomography in patients with oesophageal and gastric cancer. *Br J Surg* 1998;85:1403–1406.
10. Warshaw AL, del Fernandez C. Pancreatic carcinoma. *N Engl J Med* 1992;326:455–465.
11. Bares R, Klever P, Hauptmann S, et al. F-18 fluorodeoxyglucose PET *in vivo* evaluation of pancreatic glucose metabolism for detection of pancreatic cancer. *Radiology* 1994;192:79–86.
12. Friess H, Langhans J, Ebert M, et al. Diagnosis of pancreatic cancer by 2[^{18}F]-fluoro-2-deoxy-D-glucose positron emission tomography. *Gut* 1995;36:771–777.
13. Stollfuss JC, Gatting G, Griess H, et al. 2-(fluorine-18)-fluoro-2-deoxy-D-glucose PET in detection of pancreatic cancer: value of quantitative image interpretation. *Radiology* 1995;195:339–344.
14. Ho CL, Dehdashti F, Griffeth LK, et al. FDG-PET evaluation of indeterminate pancreatic masses. *J Comput Assist Tomogr* 1996;20:363–369.
15. Inokuma T, Tamaki N, Torizuka T, et al. Evaluation of pancreatic tumors with positron emission tomography and F-18 fluorodeoxyglucose: comparison with CT and US. *Radiology* 1995;195:345–352.
16. Kato T, Fukatsu H, Ito K, et al. Fluorodeoxyglucose positron emission tomography in pancreatic cancer: an unsolved problem. *Eur J Nucl Med* 1995;22:32–39.
17. Keogan MT, Tyler D, Clark L, et al. Diagnosis of pancreatic carcinoma: role of FDG PET. *AJR Am J Roentgenol* 1998;171:1565–1570.
18. Zimny M, Bares R, Fass J, et al. Fluorine-18 fluorodeoxyglucose

positron emission tomography in the differential diagnosis of pancreatic carcinoma: a report of 106 cases. *Eur J Nucl Med* 1997;24: 678–682.

19. Diederichs CG, Staib L, Glatting G, et al. FDG PET: elevated plasma glucose reduces both uptake and detection rate of pancreatic malignancies. *J Nucl Med* 1998;39:1030–1033.
20. Higashi T, Tamaki N, Torizuka T, et al. FDG uptake, GLUT-1 glucose transporter and cellularity in human pancreatic tumors. *J Nucl Med* 1998;39:1727–1735.
21. Imdahl A, Nitzsche E, Krautmann F, et al. Evaluation of positron emission tomography with 2-[18F]fluoro-2-deoxy-D-glucose for the differentiation of chronic pancreatitis and pancreatic cancer. *Br J Surg* 1999;86:194–199.
22. Brennan MF, Kinsella TJ, Casper ES. Cancer of the pancreas. In:

DeVita VT, Hellman S, Rosenberg SA, eds. *Cancer principles and practice of oncology*, 4th ed. Philadelphia: JB Lippincott Co, 1993: 849–882.
23. Tempero M, Hoffman J, Willet C, et al. NCCN practice guidelines for pancreatic cancer. *NCCN Proc Oncol* 1997;11:41–55.
24. Frohlich A, Diederichs CG, Staib L, et al. Detection of liver metastases from pancreatic cancer using FDG PET. *J Nucl Med* 1999;40:250–255.
25. Nakata B, Chung YS, Nishimura S, et al. 18F-fluorodeoxyglucose positron emission tomography and the prognosis of patients with pancreatic adenocarcinoma. *Cancer* 1997;79:695–699.
26. Syrota A, Duquesnoy N, Paraf A, et al. The role of positron emission tomography in the detection of pancreatic disease. *Radiology* 1982;143:249–253.

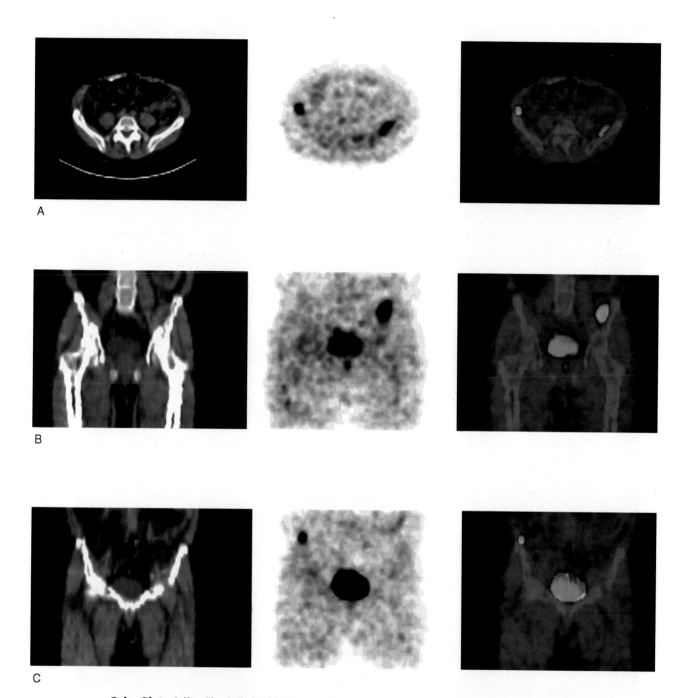

Color Plate 1 (See Fig. 1-6). In this 51-year-old patient with poorly differentiated non-small cell lung cancer who had previously undergone chemotherapy and radiotherapy, computed tomography of the chest detected a new lesion in the lower lobe of the left lung. The patient was referred for an ¹⁸F-fluorodeoxygluclose (*FDG*) coincidence study for restaging. Transmission and emission tomographic images (first and second columns) are displayed. The third column represents "fusion" images of the simultaneously displayed first and second columns. On the ¹⁸F-FDG images, two areas of abnormal uptake are apparent, one on either side of the pelvis. The combined image localizes one area in the right ilium. This finding was confirmed on bone scintigraphy. The other area of increased uptake is localized in the soft tissues adjacent to the left ilium. Magnetic resonance imaging confirmed the presence of a mass in the left iliac muscle. (Images courtesy of Dr. Ora Israel, Rambam Medical Center, Haifa, Israel.)

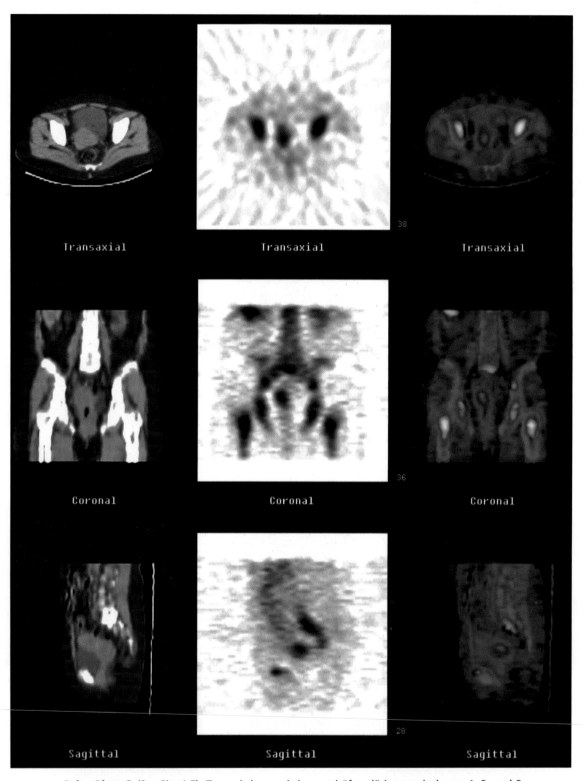

Transaxial	Transaxial	Transaxial
Coronal	Coronal	Coronal
Sagittal	Sagittal	Sagittal

Color Plate 2 (See Fig. 1-7). Transmission, emission, and "fused" images (columns 1, 2, and 3, respectively) from a patient who underwent ^{67}Ga scintigraphy after resection of the uterine cervix with the unexpected histopathologic finding of diffuse mixed large and small cell non-Hodgkin's lymphoma. Pelvic activity in residual tumor in the uterus is demonstrated to be distinct from bladder and rectal activity. It is likely that the ^{67}Ga activity in the pelvis would have been interpreted as physiologic without the improved anatomic localization available with fusion imaging. (Images courtesy of Dr. Ora Israel, Rambam Medical Center, Haifa, Israel.)

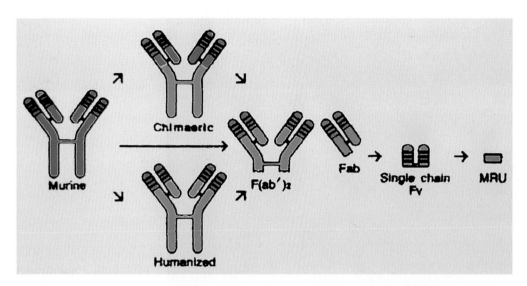

Color Plate 3 (See Fig. 21-1). Efforts to reduce the size of the monoclonal antibody component led to the development of chimeric (humanized) antibodies and progressively smaller molecules, such as the molecular recognition unit (MRU). (Reprinted with permission of Macmillan and Company.)

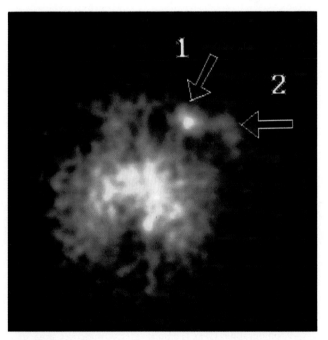

Color Plate 4 (See Fig. 21-6). A 4-hour tomographic image in the transverse plane demonstrating a focal area of abnormal uptake in the left breast.

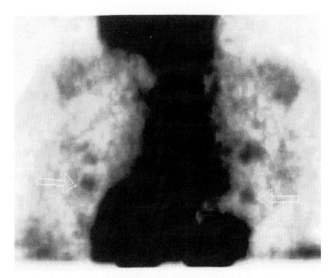

Color Plate 5 (See Fig. 21-8). Coronal slice showing bilateral nipple uptake (lower lesions). In addition, a focal area of abnormal uptake seen above the left nipple corresponds to the primary. Another lesion, which measured 4 mm, was detected above the right nipple. (Reprinted from Lamki M, Barron BJ. In: Taillefer R, Khalkhali I, Waxman AD, et al., eds. *Radionuclide imaging of the breast*. New York: Marcel Dekker Inc, with permission.)

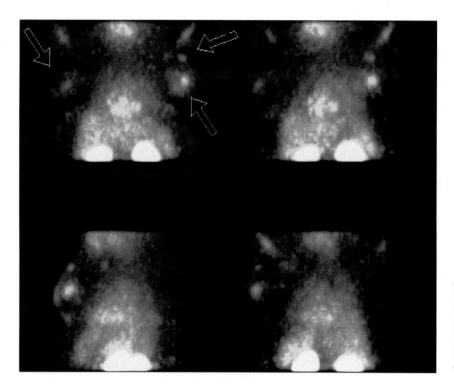

Color Plate 6 (See Fig. 21-10). Tomographic images demonstrating bilateral axillary lymph nodes in addition to the left breast mass. (Reprinted from Lamki M, Barron BJ. In: Taillefer R, Khalkhali I, Waxman AD, et al., eds. *Radionuclide imaging of the breast.* New York: Marcel Dekker Inc, with permission.)

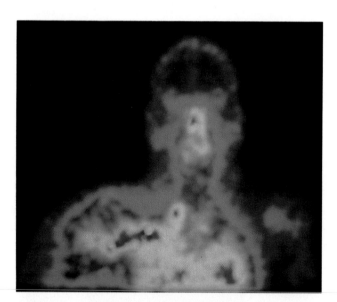

Color Plate 7 (See Fig. 22-3). Nuclear medicine scintigram showing tumor targeting of radioimmunotherapy in a breast cancer patient with metastases in right subclavical and cervical lymph nodes and left and right anterior chest wall. The image was obtained 48 hours after therapy with ^{111}In/^{90}Y-BrE-3 monoclonal antibody (MUC-1 antigen target) (10). Excellent tumor uptake is demonstrated.

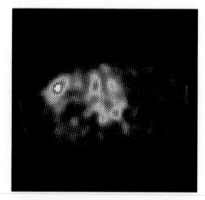

Color Plate 8 (See Fig. 22-6A). Single-photon emission computed tomographic (*SPECT*) image of the midchest area of a patient with metastatic breast cancer 72 hours after injection of 4 mCi of ^{111}In-DOTA-peptide-ChL6. Uptake in metastatic lesions is seen in the anterior and posterior mediastinal lymph nodes and a large right anterior tumor mass in the lung.

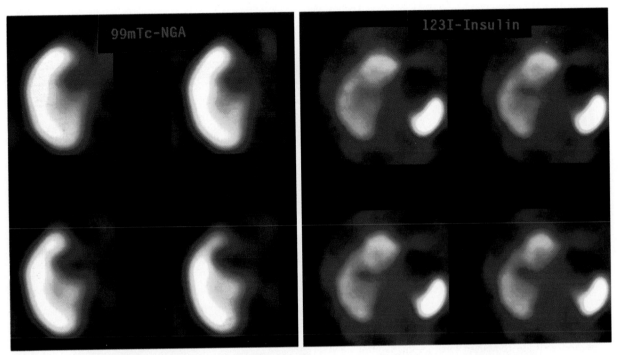

Color Plate 9 (See Fig. 27-1). Hepatocellular cancer. ^{99m}Tc-NGA (galactosyl neoglycoalbumin) scintigraphy shows a significant cold spot (*left panel*) in the left lobe of the liver (single-photon emission computed tomography, transverse view) with a corresponding accumulation in the lesion of ^{123}I-Tyr-(A14)-insulin (*right panel*).

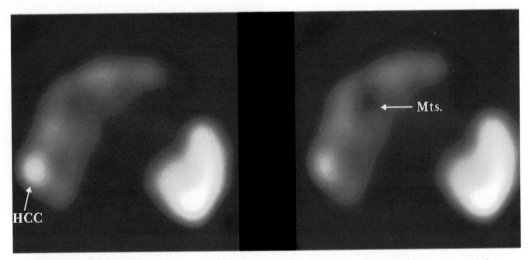

Color Plate 10 (See Fig. 27-2). Visualization of a hepatocellular cancer (*HCC*) lesion and of a colonic adenocarcinoma metastasis in a patient by ^{123}I-Tyr-(A14)-insulin scintigraphy (single-photon emission computed tomography, transverse view). Whereas HCC shows a significantly increased accumulation of ^{123}I-Tyr-(A14)-insulin, no accumulation of tracer is seen over the colonic adenocarcinoma metastasis.

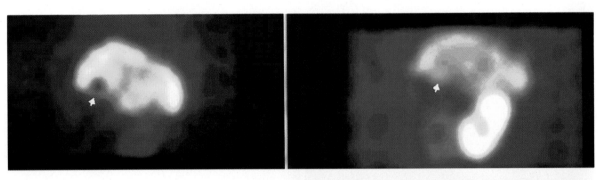

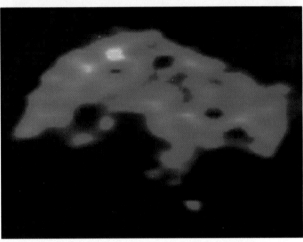

Color Plate 11 (See Fig. 27-4). 99mTc-NGA (galactosyl neoglycoalbumin) scintigraphy (*left upper panel*; single-photon emission computed tomography, sagittal view) in a patient with hepatocellular cancer (*HCC*) demonstrates no accumulation of tracer in the lesion seen on magnetic resonance imaging (see Figure 27-4, left lower panel). After administration of 123I-Tyr-(A14)-insulin, accumulation is seen over the lesion (*right upper panel*), as HCC expresses insulin receptors. Positron emission tomography with 18F-fluorodeoxyglucose (*right lower panel*) in the same patient reveals a cold spot over the lesion.

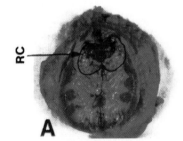 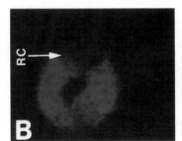 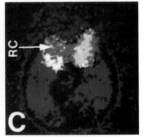

Color Plate 12 (See Fig. 30-3). **A:** Kidney placed on gamma camera. Note the tumor (*RC, arrow*) in the upper pole. **B:** Image of the kidney; the blue area represents distribution of 99mTc-human serum albumin. Note that the distribution of albumin in the tumor is relatively low. **C:** Distribution of 131I is limited to tumor, confirming selective uptake of radiolabeled antibody.

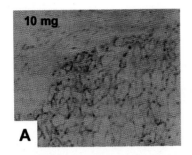

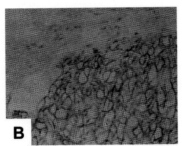

10 mg

A

B

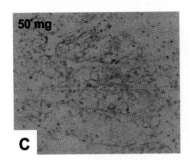

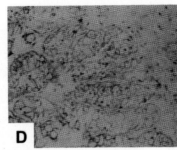

50 mg

C

D

Color Plate 13 (See Fig. 30-4). Immunohistochemistry, without exogenous antibody, of a 5-μm slice from a kidney tumor excised 7 days after administration of 10 mg of mG250 (**A**); the targeting of mG250 administered a week before surgery is demonstrated, although all antigen sites are not targeted, as shown by the addition of exogenous antibody (**B**). Increasing the administered dose to 50 mg does not result in an appreciable increase in targeting of available antigen sites, as shown in comparable slices (**C,D**).

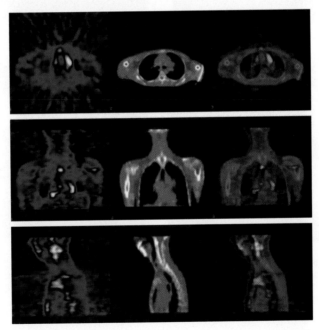

Color Plate 14 (See Fig. 36-1). Imaging of a patient with Hodgkin's disease with combined transmission and ^{67}Ga emission tomography (Hawkeye, Elgems, GE, Haifa, Israel). Abnormal uptake of ^{67}Ga in sites of mass on computed tomography (*CT*). The regions of mass on CT are larger than the areas of ^{67}Ga uptake, which indicates fibrosis in the tumor mass.

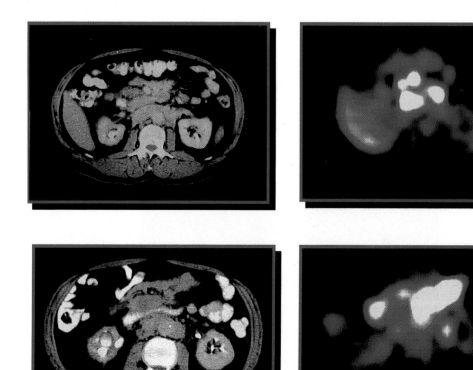

Color Plate 15 (See Fig. 38-4). Computed tomography (*CT, left*) and single-photon emission computed tomography (*SPECT, right*) from the same patient show focal accumulation of ^{111}In on SPECT in the tumor marker, which is apparent on CT. (Images courtesy of C. White, IDEC Pharmaceuticals, San Diego, California.)

24

POSITRON EMISSION TOMOGRAPHY IMAGING: DIAGNOSIS AND MANAGEMENT

DOMINIQUE DELBEKE
PETER E. VALK

In 1996, approximately 133,500 new cases of colorectal carcinoma were diagnosed in the United States; 54,900 patients died of their neoplasm that same year. In about 70% of patients, the disease is deemed resectable, and they undergo surgery with an expectation of cure. However, only two thirds of these patients are cured by resection. Recurrence is noted in the remaining one third of these patients in the first 2 years after resection. Of all the patients with recurrent cancer, only about 25% can be cured (1). Some of these patients have a recurrence limited to a regional site amenable to surgical resection and potential cure. For example, about 14,000 patients per year present with isolated liver metastases at their first recurrence (2), and about 20% of these patients die with metastases exclusively to the liver. Hepatic resection is the only curative therapy in these patients, but it is associated with a mortality of 2% to 7% (3) and has the potential for significant morbidity. Early detection and prompt treatment of recurrences may lead to a cure in up to 25% of patients (1). However, the size and number of hepatic metastases and the presence of extrahepatic disease affect the prognosis. The poor prognosis of patients with extrahepatic metastases is believed to be a contraindication to hepatic resection (4). Therefore, accurate noninvasive detection of inoperable disease with imaging modalities plays a pivotal role in selecting patients who would benefit from surgery.

METHODOLOGY

Methods of Diagnosing and Staging Recurrence

Serum levels of carcinoembryonic antigen (CEA) may be used to monitor patients for recurrence with a sensitivity of 59% and specificity of 84%, but this marker does not localize recurrent lesions (5). Barium studies have been used to detect local recurrence with an accuracy in the range of 80%. However, barium studies have been reported to be only 49% sensitive and 85% specific for overall recurrence (6).

The rapid advances in imaging technologies are a challenge for both radiologists and clinicians, who must integrate these technologies for optimal patient care and outcome at minimal cost. Because of new developments in computed tomography (CT), magnetic resonance imaging (MRI), and ultrasonography (US), images of improved quality make possible better lesion detection, characterization, and relationship to vascular structures. CT has been the conventional imaging modality used to localize recurrence, with an accuracy of 25% to 73% (7), but it fails to demonstrate hepatic metastases in up to 7% of patients and underestimates the number of lobes involved in up to 33% of patients. In addition, metastases to the peritoneum, mesentery, and lymph nodes are commonly missed on CT, and the results of efforts to differentiate postsurgical changes from tumor recurrence are often equivocal (8–12). Among patients with negative findings on CT, 50% are found to have nonresectable lesions at the time of exploratory laparotomy. CT portography (superior mesenteric arterial portography) is more sensitive (80% to 90%) than CT (70% to 80%) for the detection of hepatic metastases (13–15), but its considerable rate of false-positive findings lowers the positive predictive value (16).

In patients undergoing exploration for recurrent colorectal cancer, the presence of adhesions or the limitations of surgical exposure (transverse upper abdominal incision for liver resection) often preclude detailed operative staging.

Although functional imaging does not replace anatomic imaging, because of limitations related to resolution and lack of landmarks, functional imaging can be of tremendous help in identifying malignant lesions that are not seen on anatomic imaging or in characterizing lesions with an equivocal appearance. Both anatomic and functional images provide

D. Delbeke: Department of Radiology and Radiological Sciences, Vanderbilt University, Nashville, Tennessee 37232.

P.E. Valk: Department of Molecular and Medical Pharmacology, University of California Los Angeles School of Medicine, Los Angeles, California 90095; Northern California PET Imaging Center, Sacramento, California 95816.

complementary information, and in many circumstances registration of both sets of images is necessary for correct interpretation. Registration can be performed visually, although various computerized methods are becoming more readily available.

Functional imaging with single-photon emitters used in the detection and staging of malignancies has well-known limitations. Radioimmunoscintigraphy is limited by difficulties with antigen modulation and variable depiction of tumor and nontumor cells, and also by physiologic hepatic and bowel excretion. For the imaging of colorectal carcinoma, the Food and Drug Administration has currently approved two antibodies: (a) B72.3 (OncoScint) targets the tumor-associated glycoprotein (TAG-72) and is labeled with ^{111}In, and (b) CEA-Scan, comprised of monoclonal antibody Fab' fragments labeled with ^{99m}Tc, targets the tumor marker CEA. Phase III clinical trials have demonstrated that both antibodies are superior to CT in the detection of extrahepatic metastases but not of liver metastases because of high levels of liver background activity (Table 24.1). Imaging with intact monoclonal antibodies requires that delayed images be obtained several days later, a major disadvantage in clinical management (17).

[18]F-Fluorodeoxyglucose (^{18}F-FDG) is used to evaluate glucose metabolism. Is the most commonly used tracer in oncology, with a practical half-life of 110 minutes. The tumor-to-background contrast ratio of ^{18}F-FDG is a relatively high in most malignant lesions, and the good resolution of ^{18}F-FDG images accounts for the high reported sensitivity and specificity of [18]FDG imaging.

Glucose metabolism is increased in tumor cells (18), in part because of increased glucose transporter proteins and increased intracellular hexokinase and phosphofructokinase, which promote glycolysis (19–21). Positron emission tomography with the glucose analogue ^{18}F-FDG ([18]FDG-PET) can be used to exploit the metabolic differences between benign and malignant cells for imaging purposes (22,23). Although variations in uptake are known to exist among tumor types, elevated uptake of ^{18}F-FDG has been demonstrated in various malignant primary tumors, including colorectal carcinoma. [18]FDG imaging has been investigated for the differentiation of benign from malignant lesions, staging of malignant lesions, detection of malignant recurrence, and monitoring of therapy.

Technical Considerations in Imaging with Fluorodeoxyglucose

Current PET systems provide for the correction of soft-tissue attenuation, which is measured by transmission scanning with use of an external positron source. The detectors are calibrated with an external source of known activity (also [68]Ge). Subsequently, the true count rate can be determined in a region of interest identified on the images. Dynamic imaging of an organ or lesion of interest after injection of ^{18}F-FDG and dynamic arterial blood sampling to determine both tissue and plasma tracer concentrations over time allow the actual metabolic rate to be quantified by means of tracer kinetic modeling. This approach is time-consuming, cumbersome, and more invasive than obtaining a static image after the radiopharmaceutical concentration has reached a plateau—usually 60 minutes after intravenous administration of ^{18}F-FDG. In oncology, true quantification of metabolism is usually not performed because tumor kinetics are generally not known, dynamic imaging is not possible over the entire body, and determination of the metabolic rate offers no diagnostic advantage over PET imaging. Static imaging of the entire body offers the advantage of detecting unsuspected lesions in addition to evaluating a specific lesion. Static [18]FDG-PET images can be evaluated visually or semiquantitatively with use of the standard uptake value (SUV) or a lesion-to-background ratio. The SUV is the measured activity in the lesion in microcuries per milliliter divided by injected dose, expressed as millicuries per kilogram of body weight. Semiquantitative evaluation provides a more objective report of uptake in a lesion than does visual image interpretation. However, it most cases, visual interpretation is sufficient for clinical needs. Modifications of the SUV that may improve the semiquantitative evaluation of [18]FDG uptake include normalizing the dose to the body surface area (24) or lean body weight (25) instead of the total weight of the patient, which may be significant because the concentration of [18]FDG is higher in muscle tissue than in fat.

NORMAL DISTRIBUTION OF FLUORODEOXYGLUCOSE

Fluorodeoxyglucose is an analogue of glucose and is used as a tracer of glucose metabolism. Therefore, the distribution of ^{18}F-FDG is not limited to malignant tissue. [18]FDG enters cells by the same transport mechanism as glucose and is phosphorylated within the cells by a hexokinase to form [18]FDG-6-phosphate ([18]FDG-6-P). As [18]FDG competes with glucose for intracellular transport, [18]FDG uptake is significantly influenced by plasma glucose levels; the uptake decreases when the plasma glucose level is elevated (26–28). For oncologic imaging, the patient should be in the fasting state (4 hours). To interpret [18]FDG images, one must be familiar with the normal distribution of ^{18}F-FDG, physio-

TABLE 24.1. RADIOIMMUNOSCINTIGRAPHY: PHASE III CLINICAL TRIALS FOR COLORECTAL CARCINOMA

Sensitivity	Conventional imaging (%)	OncoScint scintigraphy (%)	CEA-Scan scintigraphy (%)
Extrahepatic	32–57	66–74	55–69
Liver	64–84	41	63

logic variations, and benign conditions in which ^{18}FDG accumulates (29–31).

Some physiologic variations are important in the interpretation of ^{18}FDG imaging in colorectal carcinoma. Uptake in the gastrointestinal tract is variable from patient to patient, and uptake along the esophagus is common, especially in the distal portion and in the presence of esophagitis; the esophagus is best identified on sagittal views. The wall of the stomach is usually faintly seen and can be used as an anatomic landmark, but occasionally the uptake can be relatively intense. Uptake in the cecum of many patients may be related to abundant lymphoid tissue in the intestinal wall, among other factors. When marked activity is present in the bowel, recurrence at the anastomotic site can be masked. Uptake is also usually seen at colostomy sites.

Fluorodeoxyglucose is filtered by the glomerulus and is not reabsorbed, so that the reader should be aware of accumulation of ^{18}FDG in the renal collecting system. Keeping the patient well hydrated to promote diuresis can reduce this, and administration of diuretics (20 mg of furosemide intravenously 20 minutes after administration of ^{18}FDG) may also be helpful. High levels of bladder activity can result in positive and negative pelvic image artifacts if images are not corrected for tissue attenuation. Attenuation correction and iterative image reconstruction avoid such artifacts, and bladder catheterization is not needed.

In the resting state, accumulation of ^{18}FDG in the muscular system is low, but after exercise, ^{18}FDG accumulates to a significant degree in selected muscular groups, so that the interpreter can be misled. Hyperventilation may induce uptake in the diaphragm, and stress-induced muscle tension is often seen in the trapezius and paraspinal muscles. Muscle relaxants such as benzodiazepines (5 to 10 mg of diazepam orally 30 to 60 minutes before administration of ^{18}FDG) may be helpful in these tense patients.

Inflammation in general can cause ^{18}FDG uptake severe enough to be confused with malignancy, especially granulomatous inflammation, including tuberculosis, sarcoidosis, histoplasmosis, and aspergillosis, among other forms (32). In the early healing phase, sites of surgical intervention demonstrate ^{18}FDG uptake.

In conclusion, to avoid misinterpretation of ^{18}FDG images, it is critical to standardize the environment of the patient during the uptake period; to examine the patient for postoperative sites, tube placement, and stomata; and to know the history of the invasive procedure and any therapeutic interventions. In addition, a 4-hour fasting period is recommended during which no beverages with sugar are consumed and no intravenous dextrose is administered; a 12-hour fasting period is better if the chest is being evaluated to prevent myocardial uptake. Drinking water should be encouraged to keep the patient hydrated and promote diuresis, which will decrease activity in the renal collecting system and bladder.

IMAGING WITH FLUORODEOXYGLUCOSE POSITRON EMISSION TOMOGRAPHY IN THE DETECTION AND STAGING OF RECURRENT COLORECTAL CARCINOMA

Three indications for functional imaging have been established in patients with known or suspected recurrent colorectal carcinoma: (a) a rising serum level of CEA in the absence of a known source; (b) an equivocal lesion on conventional imaging; and (c) preoperative staging before curative resection of recurrent disease. A number of studies have demonstrated the role of ^{18}FDG-PET as a functional imaging modality to detect colorectal carcinoma (33–50). In Table 24.2, the accuracy, sensitivity, and specificity of ^{18}FDG-PET

TABLE 24.2. COMPARISON OF POSITRON EMISSION TOMOGRAPHY AND COMPUTED TOMOGRAPHY FOR STAGING RECURRENT COLORECTAL CARCINOMA

Author (reference)	Year	No. patients	CT Sensitivity (%)	CT Specificity (%)	CT Accuracy (%)	PET Sensitivity (%)	PET Specificity (%)	PET Accuracy (%)
Yonekura et al. (33)	1982	3	—	—	—	100	100	100
Strauss et al. (34)	1989	29	—	—	—	100	100	100
Ito et al. (35)	1992	15	—	—	—	100	100	100
Gupta et al. (36)	1993	16	60	100	65	90	66	87
Falk et al. (37)	1994	16	47	100	56	87	67	83
Schiepers et al. (38)	1995	76	—	—	65–93	—	—	95–98
Vitola et al. (39)	1996	24	86	100	76	90	100	93
Ogunbiyi et al. (41)	1997	58	—	—	66	—	—	95
Delbeke et al. (40)	1997	61	79	58	76	93	89	92
Ruhlmann et al. (42)	1997	59	—	—	—	100	67	—
Valk et al. (43)	1999	155	69	96	—	93	98	—
TOTAL		512	47–86	58–100	56–93	87–100	66–100	83–100

TABLE 24.3. SENSITIVITY OF POSITRON EMISSION TOMOGRAPHY AND COMPUTED TOMOGRAPHY BY SITES OF TUMOR RECURRENCE

Site	PET	CT	Difference (95% confidence interval)
Liver	54/57 (95%)	48/57 (84%)	11% (−1–22%)
Pelvis	30/31 (97%)	21/31 (68%)	29% (9–49%)
Abdomen	22/28 (79%)	13/28 (46%)	33% (11–54%)
Retroperitoneum	12/12 (100%)	7/12 (58%)	42% (10–74%)
Lungs	16/17 (94%)	16/17 (94%)	0% (−19–19%)
Other[a]	12/12 (100%)	4/12 (33%)	67% (36–98%)
TOTAL	146/157 (93%)	109/157 (69%)	24% (16–32%)

[a]Other sites: hila and mediastinum, 4; bone, 4; abdominal wall, 2; adrenal glands, 2.

and CT are compared for a variety of anatomic locations and clinical indications.

Valk et al. (43) compared the sensitivity and specificity of PET and CT for specific anatomic locations and found PET to be more sensitive than CT in all locations except the lung, where the two modalities were equivalent (Table 24.3). The largest difference between PET and CT was found in the abdomen, pelvis, and retroperitoneum, where more than one third of lesions positive on PET were negative by CT. PET was more specific than CT at all sites except the retroperitoneum, but the differences were smaller than the differences in sensitivity (Table 24.4). Lai et al. (47), in their study of 34 patients, found ^{18}FDG-PET to be especially useful to detect retroperitoneal and pulmonary metastases.

Several studies have compared PET and CT to differentiate scar from local recurrence (Table 24.5, Fig. 24.1). For that purpose, PET is clearly more accurate (range, 90% to 100%) than CT (range, 48% to 65%), and the results of CT are equivocal in most cases. Table 24.6 presents the findings of studies that have compared the accuracy rates of PET and CT in the detection of liver metastases. Overall, PET was more accurate than CT. However, most of these studies suffer from a major limitation, which is that PET was performed prospectively, whereas CT was reviewed retrospectively and performed at various institutions, so that quality was variable.

Vitola et al. (39) and Delbeke et al. (40) reported a comparison of ^{18}FDG with CT and CT portography to detect both hepatic and extrahepatic metastases. CT portography, which is more invasive and more costly than PET or CT alone, is regarded as the most effective means of determining the resectability of hepatic metastases by imaging. PET had a higher accuracy (92%) than CT (78%) or CT portography (80%) in detecting liver metastases, and although the sensitivity of ^{18}FDG-PET (91%) was lower than that of CT portography (97%), the specificity of ^{18}FDG-PET was much higher, particularly at postsurgical sites.

In addition, whole-body PET imaging made it possible to identify metastatic disease in the chest, abdomen, or pelvis and guided subsequent CT examination of these regions to evaluate the exact anatomic location and potential resectability of any extrahepatic lesions. Outside the liver, ^{18}FDG-PET was especially helpful in detecting nodal involvement, differentiating local recurrence from postsurgical changes, and evaluating the malignancy of indeterminate pulmonary nodules—indications for which CT has known limitations. PET changed the surgical management of 28% of patients, either by identifying a resectable metastasis or by demonstrating unresectable extrahepatic disease

TABLE 24.4. SPECIFICITY OF POSITRON EMISSION TOMOGRAPHY AND COMPUTED TOMOGRAPHY BY SITES OF TUMOR RECURRENCE

Site	PET	CT	Difference (95% confidence interval)
Liver	58/58 (100%)	55/58 (95%)	5% (−1–12%)
Pelvis	81/84 (96%)	76/84 (90%)	6% (−2–13%)
Abdomen	87/87 (100%)	85/87 (98%)	2% (−2–6%)
Retroperitoneum	103/103 (100%)	103/103 (100%)	0
Lungs	97/98 (99%)	94/98 (96%)	3% (1–5%)
Other	103/104 (99%)	101/104 (98%)	1% (−1–1%)
TOTAL	529/534 (99%)	514/534 (96%)	3% (1–5%)

TABLE 24.5. 18FDG-PET TO DETECT LOCAL RECURRENCE

Author (reference)	Year	No. Patients	Accuracy of PET (%)	Accuracy of CT (%)
Strauss et al. (34)	1989	29	100	E
Ito et al. (35)	1992	15	100	E
Falk et al. (37)	1994	16	93	60
Beets et al. (46)	1994	8/35	63[a]	E
Schiepers et al. (38)	1995	76	95	65
Ogunbiyi et al. (41)	1997	21/58	90	48

[a]Sensitivity.
18FDG-PET, positron emission tomography with fluorodeoxyglucose; CT, computed tomography; E, equivocal.

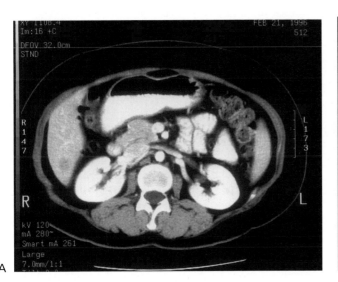

A

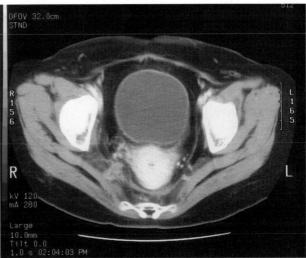

B

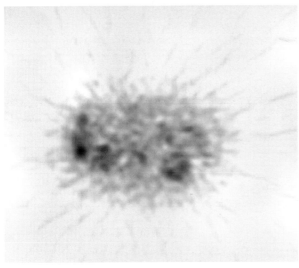

C

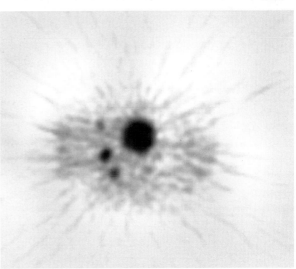

D

FIGURE 24.1. A 32-year old woman who had undergone resection of a rectal carcinoma 2 years earlier was found to have a solitary lesion in the right lobe of the liver on computed tomography (*CT*) (**A**). CT showed minor abnormalities in the pelvis that were considered to be consistent with postsurgical change (*right*) (**B**). Fluorodeoxyglucose positron emission tomography (with attenuation correction) showed (**C**) the liver lesion and (**D**) foci of recurrent tumor in the pelvis. Clinical and CT follow-up confirmed pelvic recurrence.

TABLE 24.6. ¹⁸FDG-PET TO DETECT HEPATIC METASTASES

Author (reference)	Year	No. Patients	Sensitivity/specificity PET (%)	Sensitivity/specificity CT (%)
Schiepers et al. (38)	1995	76	98ᵃ	93ᵃ
Vitola et al. (39)	1996	24	90/100	86/58
Delbeke et al. (40)	1997	61	91/95	81/60
Ogunbiyi et al. (41)	1997	58	95/100	74/85
Valk et al. (43)	1999	115	95/100	84/95

ᵃ*Accuracy.
¹⁸FDG-PET, positron emission tomography with fluorodeoxyglucose; CT, computed tomography.

that was not suspected clinically and was negative or equivocal on CT. PET changed the management by initiating surgery in one third and precluding surgery in two thirds of the patients.

Flanagan et al. (48) reported the use of ¹⁸FDG-PET in 22 patients with unexplained elevation of the serum CEA level after resection of colorectal carcinoma and no abnormal findings on conventional workup, including CT. The sensitivity and specificity of PET for tumor recurrence were 100% and 71% respectively. Valk et al. (43) reported a sensitivity of 93% and a specificity of 92% in a similar group of 18 patients. In both studies, PET correctly demonstrated tumor in two thirds of patients with rising CEA levels and negative findings on CT (Fig. 24.2).

Only one study has addressed the utility of ¹⁸FDG-PET in the staging of primary colorectal cancer. Abdel-Nabi and al. (50) evaluated ¹⁸FDG-PET for staging patients with known or suspected primary colorectal carcinomas. In 48 patients, ¹⁸FDG-PET imaging identified all primary carcinomas (Fig. 24.3). They found ¹⁸FDG and CT to have equally poor sensitivity (29% for both) for detecting local lymph node involvement. ¹⁸FDG-PET was, however, superior to CT for detecting liver metastases; it had a sensitivity and specificity of 88% and 100%, respectively, compared with 38% and 97% for CT.

The greater sensitivity of PET than of CT in the diagnosis and staging of recurrent tumor is based on two factors: (a) PET detects abnormal tumor metabolism before changes become apparent on anatomic imaging, and (b) global, whole-body imaging can be performed, so that tumor can be diagnosed when it occurs in unusual and unexpected sites. Detection of unsuspected distant recur-

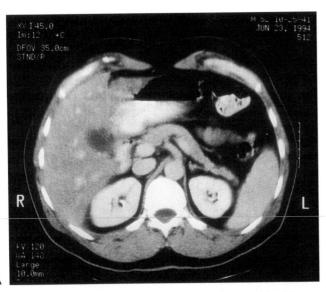
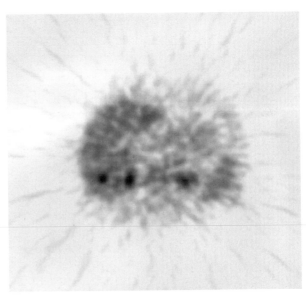

FIGURE 24.2. A 52-year-old man with a history of colon carcinoma was found to have elevated serum levels of carcinoembryonic antigen. **A:** Computed tomography (*CT*) of the pelvis and abdomen showed no abnormality in the liver or elsewhere. **B:** Fluorodeoxyglucose positron emission tomography (with attenuation correction) demonstrated a metastatic focus in the corresponding image section. (More medially, excreted activity is seen in the renal collecting system.) Two other liver foci were seen in other image sections. CT repeated 13 weeks later showed interim development of low-attenuation lesions at the sites of abnormal ¹⁸FDG uptake.

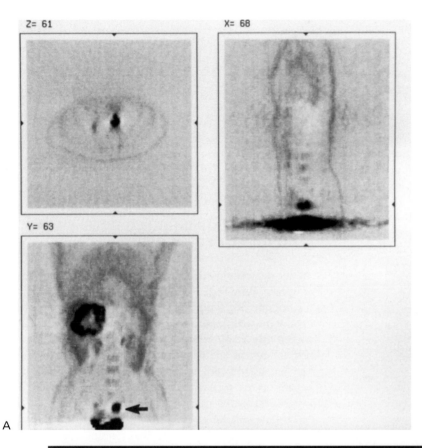

A

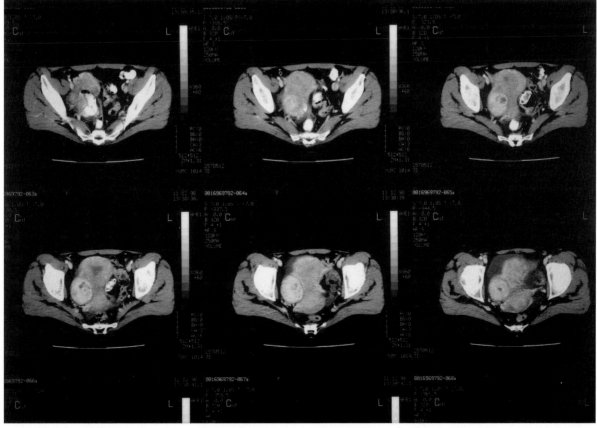

B

FIGURE 24.3. A 37-year-old woman presented with abdominal pain and was found to have a large mass in the liver on computed tomography (*CT*). She had no history of malignant disease. Liver biopsy showed metastatic, poorly differentiated adenocarcinoma. **A:** Transverse (*upper left*), coronal (*lower*), and sagittal (*upper right*) fluorodeoxyglucose positron emission tomography (*¹⁸FDG-PET*) (without attenuation correction) demonstrated the liver lesion and also showed a focus of uptake in the pelvis. **B:** CT of the pelvis showed only normal-appearing colon in the area of ¹⁸FDG-PET abnormality. Subsequent colonoscopy demonstrated a small carcinoma in the sigmoid colon.

rence by PET in patients undergoing preoperative staging has been reported (40,43,46,47,49) (Table 24.7). In a total of 249 patients, PET demonstrated tumor at unsuspected sites in 66 (26%).

Unnecessary surgery is avoided when PET demonstrates nonresectable tumor negative by CT in patients with known recurrence. With PET, earlier evaluation for treatment is possible because recurrence is detected while the patient is still CT-negative. Whether PET can also reduce the rate of repeated recurrence by making it possible to excise residual tumor at surgery or can improve the resectability rate by detecting tumors earlier remains to be determined.

Including [18]FDG-PET in the evaluation of patients with recurrent colorectal carcinoma has been shown to be cost-effective in a study based on clinical evaluation of effectiveness with modeling of costs (43), and in a study based on decision analysis (51). In both studies, all costs were calculated according to Medicare reimbursement rates and a cost of $1,800 for a PET scan. In a management algorithm in which recurrence at more than one site was treated as nonresectable, Valk et al. (43) evaluated cost savings in 78 patients undergoing preoperative staging of recurrent colorectal carcinoma. This study, which was limited to preoperative patients, demonstrated potential savings of $3,003 per patient resulting from the diagnosis of nonresectable tumor by PET. Gambhir et al. (51) used a quantitative decision tree model combined with sensitivity analysis to evaluate cost-effectiveness in all patients with recurrent colorectal cancer. The conventional strategy for detection of recurrence and determination of resectability by means of CEA levels and CT was compared with the conventional strategy plus PET for all patients presenting with suspected recurrence. The assumptions included prevalence of resectable disease of 3%, sensitivity of 65% and specificity of 45% for CT, and sensitivity of 90% and specificity of 85% for PET. An incremental saving of $220 per patient was demonstrated for the conventional strategy plus PET without any loss of life expectancy.

Based on these data, all patients facing resection of recurrent or metastatic colorectal carcinoma should undergo [18]FDG-PET preoperatively. If limited liver metastases are seen, CT portography should be performed to evaluate resectability and to look for small metastases that are beyond the resolution capability of PET. If extrahepatic foci are present on the PET images (with or without liver metastases), a CT of the corresponding region of the body should be performed for anatomic evaluation. This approach allows for the more accurate selection of patients who would benefit from surgery than is possible with conventional imaging approaches. More importantly, patients will be identified who would not benefit from laparotomy and liver resection because of unrecognized extrahepatic recurrence.

LIMITATIONS OF IMAGING WITH FLUORODEOXYGLUCOSE

Tumor detectability depends on both lesion size and degree of uptake. False-negative results may be obtained when partial volume averaging leads to an underestimation of the uptake in small lesions (< 1 cm), or when necrotic lesions with a thin viable rim are present, which are classified as benign instead of malignant (52). In the experience of Vitola et al. (39), for example, in approximately half of the hepatic lesions smaller than 1 cm, [18]FDG uptake could easily be identified visually.

In some inflammatory lesions, mainly those that are granulomatous, [18]FDG uptake is high, presumably because of the presence of activated macrophages, and they can be mistaken for malignant tumors (32). Inflammation related to recent surgery or placement of drainage tubing and catheters can also be misleading. [18]FDG uptake normally present in the gastrointestinal tract can occasionally be difficult to differentiate from uptake in a malignant lesion (40,43), but the linear pattern of uptake that is characteristic of the bowel is usually easily recognizable and best seen on coronal views. The clinical history, physical examination findings, pattern of uptake, and correlation with anatomic features seen by CT are more helpful in avoiding false-positive interpretations than is semiquantitative evaluation by SUV.

FLUORODEOXYGLUCOSE IMAGING TO MONITOR THERAPY OF COLORECTAL CARCINOMA

Positron emission tomography with fluorodeoxyglucose has been used successfully to monitor therapy in colorectal carcinoma. [18]FDG-PET differentiates local recurrence from scarring after prior radiation therapy (34,35), but it has also been shown that [18]FDG uptake may be increased immediately after radiation by inflammatory changes without residual viable tumor (53). The time course of [18]FDG uptake after radiation has not been studied systematically; it is, however, generally accepted that 6 months or more after radiation, [18]FDG uptake indicates tumor recurrence. Findlay et al. (54)

TABLE 24.7. DETECTION OF UNSUSPECTED METASTASES IN PREOPERATIVE STAGING

Author (reference)	Year	No. Patients	Detection of unsuspected metastases (%)
Beets et al. (46)	1994	16	25 (4/16)
Lai et al. (47)	1996	34	32 (11/34)
Delbeke et al. (40)	1997	61	28 (17/61)
Valk et al. (43)	1999	78	32 (25/78)
Flamen et al. (49)	1999	103	15 (9/60)
TOTAL		292	26 (66/249)

monitored liver metastases following chemotherapy with 5-fluorouracil in 18 patients. By comparing ^{18}FDG uptake before and 4 to 5 weeks after the commencement of therapy, they were able to discriminate responders from nonresponders. Regional therapy to the liver by chemoembolization can also be monitored with ^{18}FDG-PET (55). ^{18}FDG uptake decreased in responding lesions, and the presence of residual uptake can help in guiding further regional therapy.

SUMMARY

The evaluation of patients with known or suspected recurrent colorectal carcinoma is now an accepted clinical indication for imaging with ^{18}FDG-PET. ^{18}FDG-PET does not replace imaging modalities such as CT for preoperative anatomic evaluation but is indicated as the initial test for the diagnosis and staging of recurrence and for the preoperative staging of known recurrence that is considered to be resectable. PET imaging is valuable to differentiate changes following treatment from recurrent tumor and benign from malignant lymph nodes, and to monitor therapy. The addition of ^{18}FDG-PET to the evaluation of these patients reduces overall treatment costs by accurately identifying patients who will and will not benefit from surgical procedures.

REFERENCES

1. August DA, Ottow RT, Sugarbaker PH. Clinical perspectives on human colorectal cancer metastases. *Cancer Metastasis Rev* 1984;3:303–324.
2. Foster JH, Lundy J. Liver metastases. *Curr Probl Surg* 1981;18:158–202.
3. Holm A, Bradley E, Aldrete J. Hepatic resection of metastases from colorectal carcinoma: morality, morbidity and pattern of recurrence. *Ann Surg* 1989;209:428–434.
4. Hughes KS, Simon R, Songhorabodi S, et al. Resection of liver for colorectal carcinoma metastases: a multi-institutional study of indications for resection. *Surgery* 1988;103:278–288.
5. Moertel CG, Fleming TR, McDonald JS, et al. An evaluation of the carcinoembryonic antigen (CEA) test for monitoring patients with resected colon cancer. *JAMA* 1993;270:943–947.
6. Chen YM, Ott DJ, Wolfman NT, et al. Recurrent colorectal carcinoma: evaluation with barium enema examination and CT. *Radiology* 1987;163:307–310.
7. Sugarbaker PH, Grianola FJ, Dwyer S, et al. A simplified plan for follow-up of patients with colon and rectal cancer supported by prospective studies of laboratory and radiologic test results. *Surgery* 1987;102:79–87.
8. Steele G Jr, Bleday R, Mayer R, et al. A prospective evaluation of hepatic resection for colorectal carcinoma metastases to the liver: Gastrointestinal Tumor Study Group protocol 6584. *J Clin Oncol* 1991;9:1105–1112.
9. Granfield CAJ, Charnsangaveg C, Dubrow RA, et al. Regional lymph node metastases in carcinoma of the left side of the colon and rectum: CT demonstration. *AJR Am J Roentgenol* 1992;159:757–761.
10. Charnsangavej C, Whitley NO. Metastases to the pancreas and peripancreatic lymph nodes from carcinoma of the right colon: CT findings in 12 patients. *AJR Am J Roentgenol* 1993;160:49–52.
11. McDaniel KP, Charnsangavej C, Dubrow R, et al. Pathways of nodal metastases in carcinoma of the cecum, ascending colon and transverse colon: CT demonstration. *AJR Am J Roentgenol* 1993;161:61–64.
12. Moss AA. Imaging of colorectal carcinoma. *Radiology* 1989;170:308–310.
13. Soyer P, Levesque M, Elias D, et al. Detection of liver metastases from colorectal cancer: comparison of intraoperative US and CT during arterial portography. *Radiology* 1992;183:541–544.
14. Nelson RC, Chezmar JL, Sugarbaker PH, et al. Hepatic tumors: comparison of CT during arterial portography, delayed CT and MR imaging for preoperative evaluation. *Radiology* 1989;172:27–34.
15. Small WC, Mehard WB, Langmo LS, et al. Preoperative determination of the resectability of hepatic tumors: efficacy of CT during arterial portography. *AJR Am J Roentgenol* 1993;161:319–322.
16. Peterson MS, Baron RL, Dodd GD III, et al. Hepatic parenchymal perfusion detected with CTPA: imaging–pathologic correlation. *Radiology* 1992;183:149–155.
17. Suckler LS, DeNardo GL. Trials and tribulations: oncological antibody imaging comes to the fore. *Semin Nucl Med* 1997;27:10–29.
18. Warburg O. Versuche und uberledbeudem carcinomgewebe (methoden). *Biochem Z* 1923;142:317–333.
19. Flier JS, Mueckler MM, Usher P, et al. Elevated levels of glucose transport and transporter messenger RNA are induced by rats or *src* oncogenes. *Science* 1987;235:1492–1495.
20. Monakhov NK, Neistadt EI, Shaylovskii MM, et al. Physiochemical properties and isoenzyme composition of hexokinase from normal and malignant human tissues. *J Natl Cancer Inst* 1978;61:27–34.
21. Knox WE, Jamdar SC, Davis PA. Hexokinase, differentiation, and growth rates of transplanted tumors. *Cancer Res* 1970;30:2240–2244.
22. Som P, Atkins HL, Bandoypadhayay D, et al. A fluorinated glucose analog, 2-fluoro-2-deoxy-2-D-glucose [^{18}F]: nontoxic tracer for rapid tumor detection. *J Nucl Med* 1980;21:670–675.
23. Gallagher BM, Fowler JS, Gutterson NI, et al. Metabolic trapping as a principle of radiopharmaceutical design: some factors responsible for the biodistribution of [^{18}F]2-deoxy-2-fluoro-D-glucose. *J Nucl Med* 1978;19:1154–1161.
24. Kim CK, Gupta NC, Chandramouli B, et al. Standardized uptake values of ^{18}FDG: body surface area correction is preferable to body weight correction. *J Nucl Med* 1994;35:164–167.
25. Zasadny KR, Wahl RL. Standard uptake values of normal tissues at PET with 2-[fluorine-18]-fluoro-deoxy-D-glucose: variations with body weight and a method for correction. *Radiology* 1993;189:847–850.
26. Lindholm P, Minn H, Leskinen-Kallio S, et al. Influence of the blood glucose concentration on ^{18}FDG uptake in cancer—a PET study. *J Nucl Med* 1993;34:1–6
27. Langen KJ, Braun U, Kops ER, et al. The influence of plasma glucose levels on fluorine-18-fluorodeoxyglucose uptake in bronchial carcinomas. *J Nucl Med* 1993;34:355–359.
28. Diedrichs CG, Staib L, Glatting G, et al. Elevated plasma glucose reduces both uptake and detection rate of pancreatic malignancies. *J Nucl Med* 1998;39:1030–1033.
29. Cook GJR, Fogelman I, Maisey MN. Normal physiological and benign pathological variants of 18-fluoro-2-deoxyglucose positron emission tomography scanning: potential for error in interpretation. *Semin Nucl Med* 1996;26:308–314.
30. Engel H, Steinert H, Buck A, et al. Whole body PET: physiological and artifactual fluorodeoxyglucose accumulations. *J Nucl Med* 1996;37:441–446.

31. Bakheet SM, Powe J. Benign causes of 18-FDG uptake on whole body imaging. *Semin Nucl Med* 1998;28:352–358.

32. Kubota R, Yamada S, Kubota K, et al. Intratumoral distribution of fluorine-18-fluorodeoxyglucose *in vivo*: high accumulation in macrophages and granulocytes studied by microautoradiography. *J Nucl Med* 1992;33:1972–1980.

33. Yonekura Y, Benua RS, Brill AB, et al. Increased accumulation of 2-deoxy-2[18F]fluoro-D-glucose in liver metastases from colon carcinoma. *J Nucl Med* 1982;23:1133–1137.

34. Strauss LG, Clorius JH, Schlag P, et al. Recurrence of colorectal tumors: PET evaluation. *Radiology* 1989;170:329–332.

35. Ito K, Kato T, Tadokoro M, et al. Recurrent rectal cancer and scar: differentiation with PET and MR imaging. *Radiology* 1992;182:549–552.

36. Gupta NC, Falk PM, Frank AL, et al. Pre-operative staging of colorectal carcinoma using positron emission tomography. *Nebr Med J* 1993;78:30–35.

37. Falk PM, Gupta NC, Thorson AG, et al. Positron emission tomography for preoperative staging of colorectal carcinoma. *Dis Colon Rectum* 1994;37:153–156.

38. Schiepers C, Penninckx F, De Vadder N, et al. Contribution of PET in the diagnosis of recurrent colorectal cancer: comparison with conventional imaging. *Eur J Surg Oncol* 1995;21:517–522.

39. Vitola JV, Delbeke D, Sandler MP, et al. Positron emission tomography to stage metastatic colorectal carcinoma to the liver. *Am J Surg* 1996;171:21–26.

40. Delbeke D, Vitola JL, Sandler MP, et al. Staging recurrent metastatic colorectal carcinoma with PET. *J Nucl Med* 1997;38:1196–1201.

41. Ogunbiyi OA, Flanagan FL, Dehdashti F, et al. Detection of recurrent and metastatic colorectal cancer: comparison of positron emission tomography and computed tomography. *Ann Surg Oncol* 1997;4:613–620.

42. Ruhlmann J, Schomburg A, Bender H, et al. Fluorodeoxyglucose whole-body positron emission tomography in colorectal cancer patients studied in routine daily practice. *Dis Colon Rectum* 1997;40:1195–1204.

43. Valk PE, Abella-Columna E, Haseman MK, et al. Whole-body PET imaging with F-18-fluorodeoxyglucose in management of recurrent colorectal cancer. *Arch Surg* 1999;134:503–511.

44. Kim EE, Chung SK, Haynie TP, et al. Differentiation of residual or recurrent tumors from post-treatment changes with F-18 18FDG-PET. *Radiographics* 1992;12:269–279.

45. Vogel SB, Drane WE, Ros PR, et al. Prediction of surgical resectability in patients with hepatic colorectal metastases. *Ann Surg* 1994;219:508–516.

46. Beets G, Penninckx F, Schiepers C, et al. Clinical value of whole-body positron emission tomography with [18F]fluorodeoxyglucose in recurrent colorectal cancer. *Br J Surg* 1994;81:1666–1670.

47. Lai DT, Fulham M, Stephen MS, et al. The role of whole-body positron emission tomography with [18F]fluorodeoxyglucose in identifying operable colorectal cancer. *Arch Surg* 1996;131:703–707.

48. Flanagan FL, Dehdashti F, Ogunbiyi OA, et al. Utility of 18FDG PET for investigating unexplained plasma CEA elevation in patients with colorectal cancer. *Ann Surg* 1998;227:319–323.

49. Flamen P, Stroobants S, Cutsem EV, et al. Additional value of whole-body positron emission tomography with fluorine-18-2-fluoro-2-deoxy-D-glucose in recurrent colorectal cancer. *J Clin Oncol* 1999;17:894–901.

50. Abdel-Nabi H, Doerr RJ, Lamonica DM, et al. Staging of primary colorectal carcinomas with fluorine-18 fluorodeoxyglucose whole-body PET: correlation with histopathologic and CT findings. *Radiology* 1998;206:755–760.

51. Gambhir SS, Valk P, Shepherd J, et al. Cost-effective analysis modeling of the role of 18FDG-PET in the management of patients with recurrent colorectal cancer. *J Nucl Med* 1997;38:90P.

52. Hoffman EJ, Huang SC, Phelps ME. Quantitation in positron emission computed tomography: effect of object size. *J Comput Assist Tomogr* 1979;3:299–308.

53. Haberkorn U, Strauss LG, Dimitrakopoulou A, et al. PET studies of fluorodeoxyglucose metabolism in patients with recurrent colorectal tumors receiving radiotherapy. *J Nucl Med* 1991;31:1485–1490.

54. Findlay M, Young H, Cunningham D, et al. Noninvasive monitoring of tumor metabolism using fluorodeoxyglucose and positron emission tomography in colorectal cancer liver metastases: correlation with tumor response to fluorouracil. *J Clin Oncol* 1996;14:700–708.

55. Vitola JV, Delbeke D, Meranze SG, et al. Positron emission tomography with F-18-fluorodeoxyglucose to evaluate the results of hepatic chemoembolization. *Cancer* 1996;78:2216–2222.

25

RADIOLABELED ANTIBODY DETECTION AND THERAPY

DAVID M. GOLDENBERG

Cancers of the digestive organs comprise the second highest number of new cancer cases and deaths annually in the United States and Western Europe, estimated at 228,000 new cases and 130,000 deaths in the United States in 1998 (1). Colorectal cancer alone is the fourth most frequent tumor and the second leading cause of death among cancers in men and women, and accounted for about 132,000 new cases in the United States in 1998 (1). About 36,000 cases (27%) were confined to the rectum, with the remainder occurring in the colon. It was anticipated that pancreatic cancer, in the same year, would be diagnosed in 29,000 and would kill 28,900 Americans, and that the incidence and mortality rates of liver and intrahepatic biliary duct cancers would be 14,000 and 13,000, respectively (1). More than any other types of cancer, digestive tract tumors, particularly colorectal neoplasms, have been the focus of immunologic analysis to define tumor-associated antigens and develop tumor-localizing antibodies (2,3).

The two prototype cancer-associated antigens of the digestive system are carcinoembryonic antigen (CEA) and alpha-fetoprotein (AFP). CEA was first described by Gold and Freedman in 1965 (4), and although it is not a diagnostic marker for cancer when measured in serum assays, it has a proven use in monitoring disease activity (5,6). AFP has gained a similar role in primary liver malignancy and certain germ cell tumors of the testis and ovary (7–9). Both antigens served as the first selective targets for localizing antibodies, which have been shown to detect tumors expressing these markers, and they may also prove to be opportune targets for antibody-based therapy. This chapter is not intended to be a comprehensive review of the extensive literature on antibody agents reported to image or treat gastrointestinal cancers, but rather to summarize the current status of applications and indications, in addition to future prospects. A number of reviews are available elsewhere (2,3, 5,10–17).

D. M. Goldenberg: Department of Microbiology and Immunology, New York Medical College, Valhalla, New York 10595; Garden State Cancer Center, Belleville, New Jersey 07109.

RADIOLABELED ANTIBODIES

Radiolabeled antibodies are a relatively new class of imaging and therapeutic agents (10,13,14–18,19); commercial products have been introduced only in the past 7 years. External imaging to disclose foci of increased radioactivity after injection of radioactive antibodies has been termed radioimmunodetection (RAID) or radioimmunoscintigraphy (RIS) (18–21). The same principle of targeting radionuclides to cancers by specific antibodies is being investigated as radioimmunotherapy (RAIT) (13,14,16).

The procedure of RAID involves not only the broad disciplines of nuclear medicine and immunology but also such specific topics as image processing, enhancement, and instrumentation; radiochemistry; immunochemistry; antibody development, purification, and reengineering; antibody pharmacology and pharmacokinetics; and host–tumor interactions (10,11). The requirements for successful RAID involve an understanding of the nature, location, and distribution of the antigen to be targeted; the class, character, form, and targeting properties of the antibody developed; the properties of the radiolabel and the nature and effects of the labeling method; the administration and metabolic processing of the antibody and its label; and the imaging system used to disclose both targeted and nontargeted radioactivity. Ultimately, image resolution depends on the target-to-nontarget (T/NT) ratio. In RAIT, however, the T/NT ratio is important only for selectivity; also required is the delivery of a high radiation dose within a time frame that will allow sufficient radioactivity to be deposited (13,14,16).

The ideal tumor antigen for antibody targeting should have the following attributes:

1. It should be tumor-specific, with high T/NT ratios.
2. It should be uniformly distributed on tumor cells.
3. Expression on tumor cells should be dense, allowing high rates of accretion and a long residence time.
4. It should be highly accessible to the antibody.
5. It should not be modulated after antibody binding, or reexpressed after binding.

6. It should not circulate, so that no complexation with the injected antibody occurs.

7. It should not elicit any untoward host reactions, such as immune or other responses after complexation.

Unfortunately, no tumor antigen target has fulfilled all these criteria, especially the first three. Usually, the target antigens are only quantitatively increased in tumor, and often they are also present in the circulation, as CEA and AFP are. Nevertheless, truly cancer-distinct antigens have not been required for RAID and RAIT to be successful, and the availability of pancarcinoma antibodies, or antibodies that target antigens that are quantitatively increased in many different cancer types, permits such reagents to be used in many cancer patients, so that so-called individual or "private" specificity for cancer antigens is not needed. Also, even though many candidate cancer antigens are shed into the circulation, the amount of complexation with the injected antibodies does not appear to preclude successful targeting if the proper dose of antibody is used (21–23). Another problem often referred to is tumor heterogeneity in the expression of the candidate target molecule. This is more theoretical than actual, as targeting has been achieved even when only a small percentage of the cells contain the target antigen, and the issue of what is or is not expressed is very much a function of the sensitivity of the method used to detect antigen expression. Indeed, a general discordance has been noted between *in vitro* methods of detecting antigens expressed in tumors or released into the circulation and the targeting of tumors *in vivo* by antibody localization (22,24); thus, the predictability of such *in vitro* tests of tumor localization by radioactive antibodies is poor.

Many factors other than the antigen target influence RAID and RAIT, including the antibody and its form, the label, and the nature and location of the tumor within the host, as mentioned above and described in greater detail elsewhere (10,16). The antibody form, whether it is an intact IgG or a fragment, influences targeting and retention in the tumor, and the radiolabel used for imaging or therapy influences the timing, count statistics, therapeutic potential, and side effects (23,25,26).

GENERAL CLINICAL FINDINGS OF RADIOIMMUNODETECTION

Since the late 1970s, when ^{131}I-labeled polyclonal antibodies against CEA were used to image diverse CEA-expressing cancers (18,20), many different isotopes, antibodies, and imaging protocols have been used to image various cancers in different stages (10,11,15). Accordingly, a diversity of clinical results has been obtained. In the first phase of the development of this technology, ^{131}I-labeled whole IgG antibodies, first polyclonal and then monoclonal, were studied. This was followed with ^{111}In-labeled antibodies, ^{123}I-labeled antibody F(ab')[2] and Fab' fragments, and then ^{99m}Tc-labeled antibody

Fab' fragments (11,19). More recently, studies to achieve higher T/NT ratios have involved various pretargeting procedures, including bispecific antibodies and biotin–avidin conjugates (27–29). These many efforts, involving literally thousands of patients in retrospective and prospective studies, clearly showed the utility of RAID in disclosing unknown tumor sites (thus upstaging disease), and RAID proved to be superior or complementary to other available imaging modalities. On the basis of these studies, the two most prominent indications for RAID are (a) the confirmation of sites of cancer first revealed by conventional radiologic methods, the basis of which may be more anatomic than functional, and (b) the detection of occult tumors. The major use of RAID has been in the evaluation of patients who have been treated or are being followed after surgery, radiotherapy, or chemotherapy. The presence of a functional marker of a neoplasm allows RAID to distinguish between a viable recurrence and variations in tissue density revealed by diagnostic roentgenography, ultrasonography, computed tomography (CT), and magnetic resonance imaging (MRI). For example, post-therapy fibrotic lesions are detected by these conventional radiologic methods as density changes consistent with a mass, but not as a functional neoplasm that can be identified by targeting a marker substance produced by viable cells. In certain circumstances in which conventional radiologic methods are unreliable, such as CT in abdominal and retroperitoneal regions, particularly in the assessment of normal-sized lymph nodes, RAID can detect occult recurrent or metastatic tumors (12,21,30–32).

The role of RAID in initial diagnosis and staging is still under study in different tumor types with diverse reagents. If performed before surgery, RAID could alter management if more extensive disease is shown to be present and extensive surgery is contraindicated. In the postsurgical setting, in which surveillance may be critical to early identification of potentially treatable recurrences and metastases, RAID may be useful as an adjunct to other diagnostic tests, aiding in the choice of therapy. These issues are discussed below, as data are available, for each gastrointestinal tumor of interest.

The question of the specificity of RAID, which diffentiates it from most other imaging modalities because RAID targets functional markers associated with malignancy, can be addressed in several ways. Most studies have recorded the true-negative rate, based on other diagnostic modalities and outcome, from which specificity is derived, and in some studies, this can be above 90% (11,15,25,31,32). In the early years of RAID, our own group determined specificity with the use of normal goat IgG, and it was found that very large tumors could be imaged with the irrelevant IgG, whereas a few benign lesions, such as empyema and diverticulosis, were imaged nonspecifically with the antibody (21). Studies have found that benign lesions can also be imaged, particularly with certain ^{111}In-labeled preparations (e.g., OncoScint), such as degenerative joint disease, abdominal aneurysms, postoperative bowel adhesions, and local inflammatory lesions, including bowel disease or scars secondary to surgery or radiation (33). This can be a function of the antigen being targeted or the metabolism of the radionuclide. Clinically, the smaller the tumor, the more likely that the imaging result is true-positive, yet very small tumors, below 1 cm in diameter, can be missed with current nuclear cameras and imaging methods. Hence, improvements in image resolution are still desired for RAID, which could come from pretargeting, bispecific antibody systems (29). Although positron emission tomography with fluorodeoxyglucose (FDG-PET) is currently very popular as a sensitive imaging method for disclosing small, malignant lesions, it is not without limitations (34,35). The combination of PET radionuclides and cameras with antibodies is receiving attention as a means to combine the sensitivity of PET with the specificity of certain anticancer antibodies (36–39). Indeed, the combination of pretargeting, bispecific antibodies, and PET may prove to be the optimal approach.

Most antibody-based imaging agents require single-photon emission computed tomographic (SPECT) imaging to provide superior resolution, even for lesions smaller than 1 cm. However, the nuclear reader requires experience in interpreting these images, which must be acquired with the best count statistics and filters if artifacts are to be avoided. Optimal statistics and a reduction in artifacts are achieved with multiple-head detectors. As a general rule, as many projections as the matrix size should be acquired. In most cases, 120 steps of 30 to 40 seconds each in a 128 matrix are appropriate. Optimal filtering is achieved when the major vascular landmarks have sharp edges and the background activity is visualized well. Planar images also have reduced contrast in comparison with other nuclear imaging studies, such as bone scans. For this reason, timed acquisitions of 10 minutes each or slow whole-body scans of 10 cm/min are best. When planar images are made, training and experience are required to read foci of often reduced contrast. Therefore, it is recommended that these scans be read aggressively, as lesions on RAID scans can be subtle and are frequently missed by other imaging modalities.

It should be appreciated that different murine antibody products result in different levels of immune response. This is based on varying inherent immunogenicity in the antibodies, different antibody forms, and different protein doses administered. For example, the intact IgG of OncoScint, given as a 1-mg injectate, has been found to result in an elevated human anti-mouse antibody (HAMA) titer in about 40% of patients (40). Likewise, with the whole anti-CEA IgG antibody labeled with ^{99m}Tc, BW 431/26, the HAMA response rate was 30% (25). In addition to presenting a risk for anaphylaxis, particularly on readministration of a murine protein, elevated HAMA levels have been found to interfere with *in vitro* immunoassays that utilize murine antibodies, so that a case can be mismanaged because of an erroneously elevated CEA or other blood analyte value (41,42). To circumvent this problem, small antibody fragments (43) or fully human antibodies have been developed as imaging agents (44).

ANTIBODY IMAGING (RADIOIMMUNODETECTION) OF COLORECTAL CANCER

As with almost all other cancers, patients die of metastases, so early diagnosis of curatively resectable disease remains the goal of any diagnostic imaging method. In colorectal cancer, 15% to 20% of patients present with distant metastases (1), and 30% to 50% of patients treated by potentially curative surgery relapse (45). Up to 25% of recurrences are at the site of the primary tumor that is resected, indicating incomplete excision (46). Because 80% of relapses are detected within 2 years of surgery (46), it is likely in such cases that disseminated cells or micrometastases are already present at the time of initial surgery. Metastases usually occur in the liver, peritoneal cavity, pelvis, retroperitoneum, and lungs, and are frequently multifocal. Some metastases, such as about 15% to 30% of those in the lung or liver, are curatively resectable, especially when they represent a limited number of sites in an organ. Thus, the challenge is to find all disease at the initial operation, and to find metastases early, when salvage surgery is most likely to be successful. Unfortunately, current methods of preoperative evaluation and selection do not identify about 35% of patients who are found to have additional hepatic or extrahepatic metastases at exploratory laparotomy. To reduce the spread of disease that is micrometastatic or involves disseminated cells, a systemic adjuvant therapy is required. Likewise, systemic therapy is needed when metastases are not resectable.

Thus, the role of RAID in primary colorectal cancer is to detect synchronous colorectal and extracolorectal malignancy. In patient follow-up after surgical resection, its role is to identify recurrence or spread early enough that successful therapeutic interventions can be undertaken, including resection of metastases.

Two antibody-based imaging agents for colorectal cancer have been approved: CEA-Scan (arcitumomab; Immunomedics, Morris Plains, New Jersey) in the United States, Canada, and Europe, and OncoScint CR/OV (satumomab pendetide; Cytogen Corporation, Princeton, New Jersey) in the United States and Europe. CEA-Scan is a murine antibody Fab' fragment against CEA that is labeled with 25 mCi (925 MBq) of technetium ^{99m}Tc pertechnetate (47). OncoScint is a whole murine IgG molecule against the TAG-72 antigen originally derived from breast cancer (48) and is labeled with 4.3 mCi (159 MBq) of ^{111}In (40).

As an Fab' fragment, CEA-Scan targets CEA-expressing cancers very rapidly, so that imaging can be performed within a few hours, and is cleared from the body via the urinary system; hence, the kidneys and urinary bladder are "hot" (32,43). OncoScint, as an intact antibody three times the molecular size of a monovalent fragment, requires longer (2 to 7 days) to localize adequately for imaging; its metabolic activity in the liver is considerable, also because indium accretes in this organ (40,49,50). Thus, with one agent, detection of tumor deposits on or near the kidneys can be difficult, whereas liver metastases are difficult to detect with the other (unless a negative image is sufficient for diagnosis, which is then not true antibody uptake, but a defect). Because the major site of spread of colorectal cancer is the liver, this is a severe limitation for OncoScint, which is why its indication is for imaging extrahepatic abdominal and pelvic tumors, where it is superior to CT (50).

In contrast, within 5 hours of administration, CEA-Scan is equivalent to CT for imaging liver metastases, and it is superior to CT for imaging the extrahepatic abdomen and pelvis (43). Another distinction between the products involves safety. As an intact murine IgG, OncoScint produces an HAMA response in about 40% of patients after a single injection of the 1-mg dose (40,50), whereas the 1-mg dose of the Fab' of CEA-Scan is virtually without a HAMA response after one or two injections (43,51). Because antibody-based therapeutics are developing, this difference may prove to be important in terms of allowing a patient without HAMAs to receive murine or murine–human chimeric antibodies therapeutically. HAMAs can affect antibody targeting and pharmacokinetics (23,24).

Several studies with either agent have demonstrated clinical utility. In the case of CEA-Scan, single-institution studies have shown high rates of sensitivity, specificity, and accuracy for detecting colorectal cancer as primary lesions or as metastases to the liver, abdomen, and pelvis, with sensitivity and specificity in the range of 80% to 90% (32,52–55). In one such prospective study, Lechner et al. (32) reported that CEA-Scan correctly detected 28 of 29 primary colorectal cancers and 12 of 12 recurrent tumors, and that RAID influenced treatment planning in every third primary colorectal cancer patient and was superior to CT in the detection of early recurrences. In a multicenter prospective trial comparing CEA-Scan with CT and CEA-Scan plus CT with CT alone in the detection of colorectal cancer in patients suspected or confirmed to have metastases or recurrence, Moffat et al. (43) reported that CEA-Scan was statistically more sensitive than conventional diagnostic imaging methods (mostly CT) for imaging colorectal tumor sites, and also disclosed occult tumors missed by other methods. Of 178 patients in whom surgery confirmed the presence of cancer, CEA-Scan detected at least one lesion that had been missed by conventional imaging methods in 60 patients (34%). CEA-Scan was complementary to CT in detecting liver metastases, and statistically superior to conventional imaging modalities in the extrahepatic abdomen and pelvis. Most importantly, it was found that 154 of 157 lesions positive by both CEA-Scan and conventional diagnostic imaging methods proved to be malignant, so that the positive predictive

value for cancer was 98%, which was significantly higher than the positive predictive value of conventional diagnostic tests without CEA-Scan (only 66%). Thus, when results with CEA-Scan and another diagnostic test, such as CT, are both positive, a therapeutic decision can be made without the need of a confirmatory tissue diagnosis. On a lesion basis, CEA-Scan had a sensitivity of 60% for lesions 1 cm in size or smaller, 70% for lesions larger than 1 cm, and 80% for tumors larger than 2 cm. The overall accuracy of the agent, based on an analysis by anatomic site, was 83%. The incidence of potentially adverse events was less than 1.2%. Minor side effects included transient eosinophilia, fever, minor gastrointestinal upset, headache, bursitis, pruritus, and subdermal induration (each in only one patient). Fewer than 1% (two patients) had an increase in the HAMA titer. In more recent studies, however, an HAMA response rate of less than 0.3% has been observed after a single injection, and no HAMA increase has been found after at least two injections (51).

The clinical utility of these findings was evaluated and reported by Hughes et al. (56), who performed a blinded analysis of 209 patients with known or suspected colorectal cancer given CEA-Scan. In this study, the accuracy of CEA-Scan alone and combined with CT was compared with that of CT for predicting abdominopelvic tumor resectability by correlating the results with surgical and histopathologic findings. The analysis showed CEA-Scan to be more accurate than CT for assessing resectability status, both in all patients undergoing evaluation for curative abdominopelvic resection of colorectal cancer and in a subset of patients with suspected or proven liver metastases. The additional use of CEA-Scan with CT potentially doubled the number of patients who could be spared the cost, morbidity, and mortality of unnecessary abdominopelvic surgery and increased the number of those with disease potentially resectable for cure by 40%. Thus, at the current time, CEA-Scan, if applied properly with careful SPECT imaging, can be used in the following settings: (a) presurgical evaluation of extent of disease, (b) follow-up examination of sites of recurrence or spread, and (c) possibly systematic surveillance of patients with resected colorectal cancer for recurrence or metastasis.

On the basis of predictive values of CEA-Scan and CT scans, a clinical paradigm was proposed by Hughes et al. (56) for managing patients with potentially resectable or inoperable colorectal cancer (Fig. 25.1). The important finding is that when both imaging modalities indicate resectability, the surgeon should operate, whereas when both indicate nonresectability, the predictive values indicate that no surgery need be performed.

The potential use of CEA-Scan in the postoperative monitoring of disease is suggested by a recent study by Lechner et al. (57), who found CEA-Scan used intensively in the follow-up of patients with resected rectal cancer to be more reliable for detecting recurrence than monitoring of blood CEA lev-

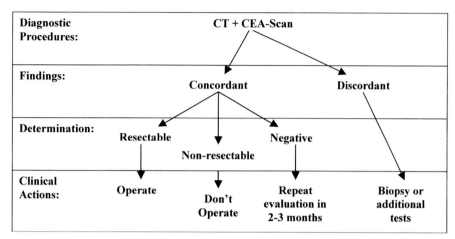

FIGURE 25.1. Suggested patient management paradigm for use of CEA-Scan in conjunction with computed tomography in patients presenting with metastatic colorectal carcinoma.

els or other diagnostic procedures. The therapeutic benefit of serial imaging with CEA-Scan during a 5-year follow-up was demonstrated by 6 of 16 (37.5%) patients with recurrence who underwent potentially curative second-look surgery, compared with 6 of 69 (8.7%) patients from a comparable population studied during the previous 6-year period. Although only a small number of patients were involved in their study, these authors suggest that inclusion of CEA-Scan in the intensive surveillance of patients with resected rectal cancer makes it possible to detect tumor recurrence at a stage when surgical salvage therapy is more likely to be successful, and that monitoring with CEA-Scan is more likely to detect recurrence than monitoring of blood CEA titers (57).

An example of a colorectal cancer recurrence identified exclusively by CEA-Scan, but missed by CT and FDG-PET, is provided in Fig. 25.2.

Another issue is whether blood CEA levels need to be elevated before CEA-Scan or another such diagnostic test is used. It was found that the lesions of patients with metastatic disease could be revealed by CEA-Scan even when their blood CEA titers were not elevated (21,25,43). Conversely, an elevated blood CEA titer is a reliable sign of disease activity and should therefore be an indication of the presence of a CEA-producing tumor. This is sufficient reason to use CEA-Scan if other methods are not revealing. Indeed, in the follow-up study by Lechner et al. (57), CEA-Scan was more sensitive than monitoring of blood CEA for identifying tumor recurrence after surgery, and the rate of potentially curative salvage surgery was higher than when CEA-Scan was not used in an intensive follow-up monitoring scheme. This agrees with the findings of Patt et al. (58), who observed that occult colorectal cancers in patients with rising blood CEA titers could be identified by RAID with CEA antibodies, including CEA-Scan, and such identification led to potentially complete tumor resection in about one third of the cases.

An earlier CEA imaging test introduced in Europe involved direct labeling of intact CEA whole IgG with ^{99m}Tc (59). Clinical trials showed excellent imaging results, but the rates of nonspecific liver imaging were higher, and elevated HAMA titers were found in about one third of the patients (25,59–61).

OncoScint preceded CEA-Scan in pivotal clinical trials and practice, and in many ways this agent created some prejudices against antibody imaging agents in general, as discussed above, because of poor results with liver imaging and the development of a HAMA response to an intact murine IgG. By contrast, CEA-Scan (containing an Fab' fragment instead of intact IgG) evokes a HAMA response in only a small fraction (< 1%) of patients. Nevertheless, many studies support the clinical utility of OncoScint in the management of patients with colorectal cancer. In a multicenter trial of OncoScint compared with CT in 155 patients with colorectal cancer, RAID proved to be superior to CT in the extrahepatic abdomen and pelvis but was statistically inferior to CT for liver metastases (50). In the pivotal multicenter trial, OncoScint detected occult disease in 12% of presurgical colorectal cancer patients (62). OncoScint had a statistically greater sensitivity than CT for detecting extrahepatic abdominal and pelvic tumors, but it was statistically inferior in the liver (50).

After injection of OncoScint intravenously, radioactivity is prominent in the blood pool and large vessels, especially in the thorax, bladder, bone marrow, and soft tissues at 24 hours, and declines gradually during the next 72 to 96 hours. The best contrast is obtained at 96 and 144 hours, but activity in the liver remains "hot," so that "cold" defects are produced when a mass lesion is present. This makes the differentiation of liver metastases from benign lesions extremely difficult (40,49,50,62,63). Low levels of radioactivity are seen in the large bowel in about 50% to 60% of patients, presumably because of targeting of TAG-72 in the

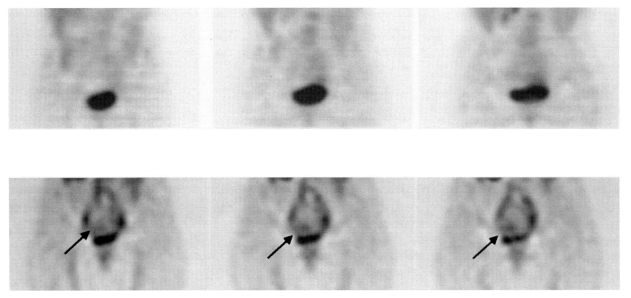

FIGURE 25.2. This 44-year-old woman had an adenocarcinoma of the right side of the colon resected in May 1998. She also had a hysterectomy in December 1998. Chemotherapy was started in August 1998, and the treatment was continued at the time the CEA-Scan study was performed in June 1999. The blood level of carcinoembryonic antigen in May 1999 was 38 ng/mL. The patient had no physical symptoms of recurrence, and results of computed tomography were unrevealing. Whole-body positron emission tomography with fluorodeoxyglucose (*FDG- PET*) in June 1999 did not show any evidence of disease in the abdomen or pelvis at 50 minutes after injection of ^{18}F-FDG. The CEA-Scan images show a large focus of disease in the right side of the pelvis near the bladder (*arrows*), confirmed by surgery to be metastatic adenocarcinoma of the colon. (Case provided by Joseph Machac, M.D., Department of Nuclear Medicine, Mt. Sinai Medical Center, New York, New York.)

normal mucosa. Mild cathartics or laxatives may be helpful in eliminating this activity from the lumen of the bowel, but the mucosa may still be radioactive. Serial imaging can be helpful to differentiate between specific and nonspecific foci of activity, as the latter may move with time. Although results in individual patients vary, radioactivity may also be seen in the bowel, blood pool, kidneys, urinary bladder, male genitalia, and breast nipples in women.

Low rates (6%) of antibody-related adverse reactions were reported, the most frequent being transient fever and itching that resolved spontaneously (62). Following a single intravenous administration of 1 mg of OncoScint, a positive HAMA titer develops in about 40% of patients. When 68 patients received multiple injections of OncoScint about 6 months apart, adverse effects were seen in 3.7%. Elevated HAMA titers were seen in 36% of patients following initial or repeated infusions, and these returned to normal levels in 21% of patients. Patients with a HAMA response had a much more rapid clearance of the radioconjugate and an altered metabolism, with marked deposition of radioactivity in the liver and bone marrow. Thus, OncoScint injections should be repeated in patients proven to be without HAMA elevations, as scan interpretations can be affected. As mentioned previously, elevated HAMA levels can alter

the results of murine-based *in vitro* immunoassays, such as for CEA or CA-125 (41,42).

RADIOIMMUNODETECTION OF PANCREATIC CANCER

It is estimated that 29,000 new cases of pancreatic cancer develop annually in the United States, with an annual mortality of 28,900 (1). These statistics suggest that symptomatology and initial diagnosis come too late for salvage surgery in almost all cases. Therefore, RAID studies can be used either for the initial differential diagnosis in a patient presenting with symptoms suggestive of this malignancy, or for assessing the extent of disease at various times during management.

Antibodies purported to be specific for pancreatic carcinoma have rarely been used for targeting this neoplasm because of a paucity of antibodies truly specific for this tumor type (2). Pancarcinoma antibodies, therefore, such as 17-1A, 19.9, and CEA, are frequently used (2,11). CEA antibodies probably have been studied more than any others to image pancreatic carcinoma. In our own experience with CEA antibodies, among 29 patients with pancreatic cancer who underwent 31 RAID studies (126 sites) with diverse CEA antibodies labeled with ^{131}I, a sensitivity of 81%, specificity of 94%, and accuracy of 86% were achieved (2). Because sites of spread in the abdomen, pelvis, liver, and chest were included, few data are available on the role of RAID in the detection of primary pancreatic cancer. It should be mentioned, however, that SPECT was not used in these early studies, which were thus at a disadvantage for disclosing small abdominal lesions. Nevertheless, a sensitivity of 79% was achieved in the abdomen when both primary and recurrent pancreatic tumors were included (2).

Other antibodies for the imaging or therapy of pancreatic cancer are under development. Gold et al. (64) described a MUC-1 variant recognized by the PAM4 antibody that appears to show selectivity for pancreatic carcinomas. A pilot clinical trial showed successful targeting of pancreatic cancer with radiolabeled PAM4 (65). Recently, a murine–human chimeric monoclonal antibody, Nd2, was labeled with ^{111}In and studied in 19 patients suspected of having pancreatic carcinoma (66). On the basis of surgery, 12 of 14 (85.7%) of the cancer patients were imaged, and liver metastases were found correctly in one case. Of the five patients with pancreatitis, four had true-negative results by RAID. None of the patients had an anti-chimeric antibody response. These preliminary results suggest that the antibody may be able to differentiate malignancy from pancreatitis.

RADIOIMMUNODETECTION OF HEPATOCELLULAR CANCER

Primary tumors of the liver comprise one of the most common cancers worldwide, with an annual incidence of about 1 million cases (67). In the United States, the incidence of liver and intrahepatic bile duct cancers is low (13,900), but these are extremely aggressive neoplasms that cause 13,000 deaths annually (1). Etiologic factors include ingestion of dietary carcinogens, and an association with hepatitis has been noted, but the biology of the disease may differ in different populations. It is still not clear whether cirrhosis is a predisposing factor for or a consequence of the factors that cause hepatocellular cancer (HCC). A test that could differentiate these two pathologies would be helpful in defining the progression of cirrhosis to HCC.

Most RAID studies for HCC and hepatoblastoma have been performed with antibodies against AFP, which is a functional serum marker for these and certain germ cell tumors of the testis and ovary (7–9). Occasionally, other tumors, such as gastrointestinal (gastric, pancreatic, and biliary tract cancers) and lung cancers, are found to produce AFP (7). AFP can be increased in the serum of adults with hepatitis and cirrhosis (9). Some patients with HCC have normal AFP blood titers, like colorectal cancer patients with normal CEA titers; therefore, elevation of the blood

marker is not a prerequisite for RAID with AFP antibodies. Since the early 1980s, several AFP antibody reagents labeled with ^{131}I have been used with planar imaging to detect various neoplasms expressing this marker (68–70). Even with high titers of AFP in the blood, successful tumor targeting could be demonstrated by RAID (68–70).

In a recent study in which a ^{99m}Tc-labeled anti-AFP monoclonal antibody Fab' reagent (AFP-Scan; Immunomedics) was used, 25 consecutive patients with a history of HCC were examined by planar and SPECT imaging at 6 and 24 hours after intravenous injection of 1 mg labeled with 925 MBq (25 mCi) of [99m]Tc (71). In 20 patients, specific binding of the Fab' antibody to the primary tumor was noted, whereas in four who presented with elevated serum AFP levels, no specific targeting was found and no malignant lesions were evident by CT or biopsy. In five of six patients with normal serum AFP levels, focal uptake was demonstrated. In this study, diagnostically relevant information was provided in all patients by the 24-hour scans, especially with SPECT. The earlier images were less revealing because of a more homogeneous liver uptake of the radiolabeled Fab'. When AFP-Scan was compared with CT in this series, the former showed a higher sensitivity (95% vs. 63%) and specificity (67% vs. 17%), and the overall accuracy was 88% for AFP-Scan versus 52% for CT. AFP-Scan appeared to differentiate between HCC and benign lesions or nodular changes associated with cirrhosis; CT did not. No HAMA responses were found after use of this product, nor were other significant adverse clinical or laboratory findings observed. Thus, RAID with ^{99m}Tc-anti-AFP Fab' was capable of targeting primary HCC in most patients and even revealed extrahepatic metastatic spread during the whole-body planar scanning performed in one patient. At the present time, it appears that this agent also may have an important use in defining viable liver cancer after therapy, and in determining whether a patient is a candidate for liver transplantation by revealing the presence or absence of extrahepatic spread. However, the product is not available yet commercially.

INTRAOPERATIVE RADIOIMMUNODETECTION OF CANCER

Because of the demonstrated ability of radiolabeled antibody preparations to bind to cancer sites in the body, surgeons attempted to use targeted radioactivity and an intraoperative probe to guide cancer resection procedures, a method termed *radioimmunoguided surgery* (72–74). In the initial studies, performed mostly in patients with colorectal cancer, ^{125}I was conjugated to a whole IgG, usually against the TAG-72 antigen (a pancarcinoma marker) (48). These investigations showed that targeted radioactivity could be detected with a sensitive gamma radiation probe during surgery. However, when whole IgG was used, a delay of about 20 days was required to clear the blood pool and nontargeted radioactivity before tumor could be detected, and the use of ^{125}I as the label precluded presurgical imaging. The results showed uptake in some areas that later failed to be cancerous on histopathology. Whether this is a specificity problem or a reflection of a method that is more sensitive than histopathology remains to be determined by using tests more sensitive for cancer and cancer markers. Nevertheless, use of the reagent improved the intraoperative staging of disease (72–74).

To obviate the need to wait more than 20 days between injection of the radiolabeled compound and surgery, Lechner et al. (75) used ^{99m}Tc-conjugated anti-CEA Fab' (CEA-Scan) in patients with colorectal cancer. They operated on patients 24 hours after injecting the CEA-Scan. Tumor could be found when the mean tumor-to-background ratio was above 1.5; primary tumors were correctly identified in all 20 patients, and disease, usually involving additional lymph nodes, was upstaged in 7 of the 20 patients (35%). As in the studies of Martin et al. (72–74), false-negative and false-positive findings occurred that could mostly be attributed to the presence of nodes near major vessels. Later operating times, such as between 24 and 48 hours, are being evaluated currently, and results are encouraging because nonspecific blood pool activity decreases with time (A. Chevinsky, *personal communication*, 1999). The feasibility of using ^{99m}Tc-labeled antibodies in a short time frame after injection has been confirmed by others (76). Avidin–biotin pretargeting methods have also been applied to intraoperative scintimetry (77).

As with RAID, intraoperative probe detection of tumor radioactivity requires that reagents, probes, and procedures be standardized, and that prospective studies be performed to correlate results with those of other sensitive tests for tumor detection, including molecular probes. The initial results from several groups, however, are sufficiently encouraging to warrant an intensive investigation of this application of radiolabeled antibodies. Colorectal surgery, even when thought to be complete, is clearly inadequate (tumor eventually recurs in one third of patients), and better methods of preoperative and intraoperative staging are needed. This may prove to be a really unique opportunity to make use of currently available radiolabeled antibodies, as PET imaging agents do not appear to be applicable in this setting. RAID could be used to define the extent of disease preoperatively, and then the residual activity from the same injection could be used by the surgeon during exploratory laparotomy to define tumor margins, nonpalpable lymph nodes, and other sites of spread that may have been suspected or missed by external imaging studies.

RADIOIMMUNOTHERAPY OF GASTROINTESTINAL CANCERS

The logical extension of using antibodies as targeting agents for cancer is to use similar antibodies to deliver therapeutic doses of radiation, a method referred to as *radioimmunotherapy* (RAIT) (13,14,16). Although RAIT has been investigated in many different tumor types and with various antibodies and labels, most studies have again involved patients with colorectal cancer and CEA antibodies labeled with [131]I. However, ^{90}Y, ^{125}I, [188]Re, ^{64}Cu, and ^{177}Lu labels are also of considerable interest currently (14,16,26,78–84). When CEA antibodies labeled with ^{131}I were studied in various CEA-expressing tumor types, the highest rad doses delivered were to colorectal and medullary thyroid cancers, corresponding to the higher level of CEA in these tumors than in the many others evaluated (23,24). It was also found that tumor size is inversely proportional to the radiation dose delivered; the smaller the tumor, the higher the dose accreted (23,24,85,86). However, murine anti-CEA antibodies did cause complicating HAMA responses after 2 or more doses, and the major dose-limiting toxicity was myelosuppression (23,24,85). Therefore, a phase I trial of escalating single doses of the ^{131}I-labeled humanized anti-CEA antibody hMN-14 (CEA-Cide; Immunomedics) was undertaken in patients with drug-refractory colorectal cancer and small-volume (≤ 2.5 cm) metastases (87). Even with clearly suboptimal doses given in a dose-escalation trial, an overall 60% response rate was achieved, including an 18% objective tumor response rate, with very minor adverse effects and no anti-human antibody (HAHA) responses (87). These results are quite consistent with the findings of studies in animals of human colonic cancer xenografts treated with single-dose radioiodinated anti-CEA antibodies, in which improved survival and cure rates, in comparison with those in untreated or drug-treated animals, were obtained (25,87–91). In other preclinical studies, RAIT has been found to enhance the antitumor effects of standard chemotherapy (92,93) or external beam radiotherapy (94–97) in human colonic carcinoma xenograft models. Thus, the prospects of nonmyeloablative and myeloablative (with autologous peripheral blood stem cell grafting) RAIT, alone or in combination with chemotherapy or other forms of therapy, are challenging. Although most of the emphasis has been put on metastatic colorectal cancer, the evaluation of RAIT in an adjuvant setting, particularly in rectal carcinoma, and in other gastrointestinal malignancies, such as pancreatic, gastric, and hepatocellular carcinomas, is indicated.

In addition to the use of novel isotopes and chelates, different antigen-targeting antibodies, and human or humanized forms of antibodies, improvements in RAIT are being sought by reengineering antibodies as single (98) or multivalent fragments (99), single-chain binding proteins (100,101), and vasoactive agent or cytokine combinations (102–104).

A major problem in both targeting and therapy has been concomitant radioactivity in the blood pool. In therapy, this results in bone marrow toxicity, derived from the circulating antibody, as was addressed in the very first publication of the clinical results of RAID more than 20 years ago (21). More recent efforts to reduce blood pool and nontargeted radioactivity have involved various pretargeting methods in which the targeting antibody is separated from the delivery of radioactivity, or in which antibodies against the primary antibody or the chelate of the antibody are injected as a clearance step (27,28,105–109). Each method has its own merits and limitations, but one of most promising currently involves a so-called affinity-enhancement system, in which the first targeting dose of a bispecific antibody is separated from the second dose of a bivalent hapten carrying the diagnostic or therapeutic radioactivity, given 2 to 4 days later. A few hours after the second dose of radioactivity is administered, very selective tumor images, with little background activity, can be obtained (108).

CONCLUSIONS

Although the use of radiolabeled antibodies for cancer detection and therapy has been studied for more than two decades, these techniques are still evolving as less immunogenic and more specific antibody-targeting agents and improved procedures, radiolabels, cameras, and supportive procedures to mitigate myelotoxicity during high-dose RAIT are introduced. As external irradiation has found its place in cancer therapy as an adjunct to surgery and chemotherapy, it is likely that more systemic and tumor-targeted irradiation will be combined with other therapy modalities. RAIT is a continuum of preoperative, intraoperative, and postoperative tumor detection methods in which radiolabeled antibodies are used. Another decade may well be required before disease management algorithms involving these reagents and procedures for cancer detection, staging, and therapy are established, as each agent and approach will require careful, prospective, multicenter trials (110). Given the better reception for therapeutics than for imaging agents to date (111), it is reasonable to predict that radiolabeled antibodies will gain an important role in the evolving biologic therapies of cancer, and that this will ultimately stimulate a greater interest in use of the approach for diagnostic imaging.

REFERENCES

1. Landis SH, Murray T, Bolden S, et al. Cancer statistics, 1998. *CA Cancer J Clin* 1998;48:6–29.
2. Goldenberg DM. Imaging and therapy of gastrointestinal cancers with radiolabeled antibodies. *Am J Gastroenterol* 1991;86:1392–1401.
3. Welt S, Ritter G. Antibodies in the therapy of colon cancer. *Semin Oncol* 1999;26:683–690.
4. Gold P, Freedman SO. Specific carcinoembryonic antigens of the human digestive system. *J Exp Med* 1965;122:467–481.
5. Gold P, Goldenberg NA. The carcinoembryonic antigen (CEA): past, present, and future. *McGill Med J* 1997;3:46–66.
6. Goldenberg DM, Neville AM, Carter AC, et al. Carcinoembryonic antigen: its role as a marker in the management of cancer.
7. National Institutes of Health Consensus Development Conference. *Ann Intern Med* 1981;94:407–409.
8. McIntire KR, Waldmann TA, Moertel CG, et al. Serum α-fetoprotein in patients with neoplasms of the gastrointestinal tract. *Cancer Res* 1975;35:991–996.
9. Norgaard-Pedersen B, Albrechtsen R, Teilum G. Serum alpha-fetoprotein as a marker for endodermal sinus tumor (yolk sac tumour) or a vitelline component of "teratocarcinoma." *Acta Pathol Microbiol Scand* 1975;83:573–589.
10. Wepsic HT, Kirkpatrick A. Alpha-fetoprotein and its relevance to human disease. *Gastroenterology* 1979;77:787–796.
11. Goldenberg DM, ed. *Cancer imaging within radiolabeled antibodies.* Norwall, MA: Kluwer Academic Publishers, 1990.
12. Goldenberg DM, Larson SM. Radioimmunodetection in cancer identification. *J Nucl Med* 1992;33:803–814.
13. Goldenberg DM, Goldenberg H, Sharkey RM, et al. Imaging of colorectal carcinoma with radiolabeled antibodies. *Semin Nucl Med* 1989;19:262–281.
14. Goldenberg DM. Targeting of cancer with radiolabeled antibodies: prospects for imaging and therapy. *Arch Pathol Lab Med* 1988;112:580–587.
15. Goldenberg DM. Future role of radiolabeled antibodies in oncologic diagnosis and therapy. *Semin Nucl Med* 1989;19:332–339.
16. Larson SM. Clinical radioimmunodetection 1978–1988: overview and suggestions for standardization of clinical trials. *Cancer Res* 1990;50:892–898.
17. Goldenberg DM, ed. *Cancer therapy with radiolabeled antibodies.* Boca Raton, FL: CRC Press, 1995.
18. DeNardo GL, O'Donnell RT, Kroger LA, et al. Strategies for developing effective radioimmunotherapy for solid tumors. *Clin Cancer Res* 1998;5:3219s–3225s.
19. Goldenberg DM. Immunodiagnosis and immunodetection of colorectal cancer. *Cancer Bull* 1978;30:213–218.
20. Goldenberg DM. Clinical radioimmunodetection: the second decade. In: Goldenberg DM, ed. *Cancer imaging with radiolabeled antibodies.* Norwall, MA: Kluwer Academic Publishers, 1990:3–9.
21. Goldenberg DM, DeLand F, Kim E, et al. Use of radiolabeled antibodies to carcinoembryonic antigen for the detection and localization of diverse cancers by external photoscanning. *N Engl J Med* 1978;298:1384–1388.
22. Goldenberg DM, Deland FH, Bennett SJ, et al. Radioimmunodetection of cancer with radioactive antibodies to carcinoembryonic antigen. *Cancer Res* 1980;40:2984–2992.
23. Primus FJ, Bennett SJ, Kim EE, et al. Circulating immune complexes in cancer patients receiving goat radiolocalizing antibodies to carcinoembryonic antigen. *Cancer Res* 1980;40:497–501.
24. Behr TM, Sharkey RM, Juweid ME, et al. Factors influencing the pharmacokinetics, dosimetry, and diagnostic accuracy of radioimmunodetection and radioimmunotherapy of carcinoembryonic antigen-expressing tumors. *Cancer Res* 1996;56:1805–1816.
25. Lind P, Lechner P, Arian-Schad K, et al. Anti-carcinoembryonic antigen immunoscintigraphy (technetium-99m-monoclonal antibody BW 431/26) and serum CEA levels in patients with suspected primary and recurrent colorectal carcinoma. *J Nucl Med* 1991;32:1319–1325.
26. Behr TM, Sharkey RM, Juweid ME, et al. Variables influencing tumor dosimetry in radioimmunotherapy of CEA-expressing cancers with anti-CEA and antimucin monoclonal antibodies. *J Nucl Med* 1997;38:409–418.
27. Sharkey RM, Blumenthal RD, Behr TM, et al. Selection of radioimmunoconjugates for the therapy of well-established or micrometastatic colon carcinoma. *Int J Cancer* 1997;29:477–485.
28. Goodwin DA, Mears CF, McCall MJ, et al. Pre-targeted

immunoscintigraphy of murine tumors with 111-indium-labeled bifunctional haptens. *J Nucl Med* 1988;29:226–234.

28. Paganelli G, Malcovati M, Fazio F. Monoclonal antibody pretargeting techniques for tumour localization: the avidin–biotin system. *Nucl Med Commun* 1991;12:211–234.

29. Le Doussal J-M, Chetanneau A, Gruaz-Guyon A, et al. Bispecific monoclonal antibody-mediated targeting of an indium-111-labeled DTPA dimer to primary colorectal tumors: pharmacokinetics, biodistribution, scintigraphy and immune response. *J Nucl Med* 1993;34:1662–1671.

30. Goldenberg DM, Kim EE, Bennett SJ, et al. Carcinoembryonic antigen radioimmunodetection in the evaluation of colorectal cancer and in the detection of occult neoplasms. *Gastroenterology* 1983;84:524–532.

31. Bischof-Delaloye A, Delaloye B, Buchegger F, et al. Clinical value of immunoscintigraphy in colorectal carcinoma patients: a prospective trial. *J Nucl Med* 1989;30:1646–1656.

32. Lechner P, Lind P, Binter G, et al. Anticarcinoembryonic antigen immunoscintigraphy with a ^{99m}Tc-Fab′ fragment (Immu 4) in primary and recurrent colorectal cancer. A prospective study. *Dis Colon Rectum* 1993;36:930–935.

33. Abdel-Nabi HH, Chan H-W, Doerr RJ. Indium-labeled anti-colorectal carcinoma monoclonal antibody accumulation in non-tumored tissues in patients with colorectal carcinoma. *J Nucl Med* 1990;31:1975–1979.

34. Shreve PD, Anzai Y, Wahl RL. Pitfalls in oncologic diagnosis with FDG PET imaging: physiologic and benign variants. *Radiographics* 1999;19:61–77.

35. Abdel-Nabi H, Doerr RJ, Lamonica DM, et al. Staging of primary colorectal carcinomas with fluorine-18 fluorodeoxyglucose whole-body PET: correlation with histopathologic and CT findings. *Radiology* 1998;206:755–760.

36. Westera G, Reist HW, Buchegger F, et al. Radioimmuno positron emission tomography with monoclonal antibodies: a new approach to quantifying *in vivo* tumour concentration and biodistribution for radioimmunotherapy. *Nucl Med Commun* 1991;12:429–437.

37. Philpott GW, Schwarz SW, Anderson CJ, et al. Radioimmuno PET: detection of colorectal carcinoma with positron-emitting copper-64-labeled monoclonal antibody. *J Nucl Med* 1995;36:1818–1824.

38. Klivenyi G, Schuhmacher J, Patzelt E, et al. Gallium-68 chelate imaging of human colon carcinoma xenografts pretargeted with bispecific anti-CD44V6/anti-gallium chelate antibodies. *J Nucl Med* 1998;39:1769–1776.

39. Griffiths GL, Goldenberg DM, Roesch F, et al. Radiolabeling of an anti-carcinoembryonic antigen antibody Fab′ fragment (CEA-Scan) with the positron-emitting radionuclide, Tc-94m. *Clin Cancer Res* 1998;5:3001s–3003s.

40. Maguire RT, Schmelter RF, Pascucci VL, et al. Immunoscintigraphy of colorectal adenocarcinoma: results with site-specifically radiolabeled B72.3 (^{111}In-CYT-103). *Antibody Immunoconjug Radiopharm* 1989;2:257–269.

41. Hansen HJ, LaFontaine G, Newman ES, et al. Solving the problem of antibody interference in commercial "sandwich"-type immunoassays of carcinoembryonic antigen. *Clin Chem* 1989;35:46–150.

42. Hansen HJ, Sullivan CL, Sharkey RM, et al. HAMA interference with murine monoclonal antibody-based immunoassays. *J Clin Immunoassays* 1993;16:294–299.

43. Moffat FL Jr, Pinsky CM, Hammershaimb L, et al. Clinical utility of external immunoscintigraphy with the IMMU-4 technetium-99m Fab′ antibody fragment in patients undergoing surgery for carcinoma of the colon and rectum: results of a pivotal, phase III trial. *J Clin Oncol* 1996;14:2295–2305.

44. Wolff BG, Bolton J, Baum R, et al. Radioimmunoscintigraphy of recurrent, metastataic, or occult colorectal cancer with technetium Tc 99m 88BV59H21-2V67-66 (HumaSPECT-Tc), a totally human monoclonal antibody. Patient management benefit from a phase III multicenter study. *Dis Colon Rectum* 1998;41:953–962.

45. Steele G Jr. Follow-up plans after treatment of primary colon and rectum cancer. *World J Surg* 1991;15:583–588.

46. Galandiuk S, Wieland HS, Moertel CG, et al. Patterns of recurrence after curative resection of carcinoma of the colon and rectum. *Surg Gynecol Obstet* 1992;174:27–32.

47. Hansen HJ, Jones AL, Sharkey RM, et al. Preclinical evaluation of an "instant" ^{99m}Tc-labeling kit for antibody imaging. *Cancer Res* 1990;50:794s–798s.

48. Colcher D, Hand HP, Nuti M, et al. A spectrum of monoclonal antibodies reactive with human mammary tumor cells. *Proc Natl Acad Sci U S A* 1981;78:3199–3203.

49. Patt YZ, Lamki LM, Shanken J, et al. Imaging with indium 111-labeled anticarcinoembryonic antigen monoclonal antibody ZCE-025 of recurrent colorectal or carcinoembryonic antigen-producing cancer in patients with rising serum carcinoembryonic antigen levels and occult metastases. *J Clin Oncol* 1990;8:1246–1254.

50. Collier BD, Nabi H, Doerr RJ, et al. Immunoscintigraphy performed with In-111-labeled CYT-103 in the management of colorectal cancer: comparison with CT. *Radiology* 1992;185:179–186.

51. Wegener WA, Petrelli N, Serafini A, et al. Safety and efficacy of arcitumomab imaging in colorectal cancer following repeat administrations. *J Nucl Med* 2000;41:1016–1020.

52. Goldenberg DM, Goldenberg H, Sharkey RM, et al. Clinical studies of cancer radioimmunodetection with carcinoembryonic antigen monoclonal antibody fragments labeled with ^{123}I or ^{99m}Tc. *Cancer Res* 1990;50:909s–921s.

53. Podoloff DA, Patt YZ, Curley SA, et al. Imaging of colorectal carcnoma with technetium 99m radiolabeled Fab′ fragment (Immu4) in primary and recurrent colorectal cancer: a prospective study. *Dis Colon Rectum* 1993;36:930–935.

54. Moffat FL Jr, Vargas-Cuba RD, Serafini AN, et al. Radioimmunodetection of colorectal carcinoma using technetium-99m labeled Fab′ fragments of the IMMU-4 anti-carcinoembryonic antigen monoclonal antibody. *Cancer* 1994;73:836–845.

55. Behr TM, Goldenberg DM, Scheele JR, et al. Klinische Relevanz der Immunszintigraphie mit 99m Tc-markierten Anti-CEA-Fab′-Fragmenten in der Nachsorge des kolorektalen Karzinoms: Chirurgische Resektabilitäts-Beurteilung aus der Kombination mit konventioneller Bildgebung. *Deutsch Med Wochenschr* 1997;122:463–470.

56. Hughes K, Pinsky CM, Petrelli NJ, et al. Use of carcinoembryonic antigen radioimmunodetection and computed tomography for predicting the resectability of recurrent colorectal cancer. *Ann Surg* 1997;226:621–631.

57. Lechner P, Lind P, Goldenberg DM. Can postoperative surveillance with serial CEA immunoscintigraphy detect resectable rectal cancer recurrence and potentially improve tumor-free survival? *J Am Coll Surg* 2000 (in press).

58. Patt YZ, Pdoloff DA, Curley S, et al. Monoclonal antibody imaging in patients with colorectal cancer and increasing levels of serum carcinoembryonic antigen. Experience with ZCE-025 and IMMU-4 monoclonal antibodies and proposed directions for clinical trials. *Cancer* 1993;71:4293–4297.

59. Steinstrasser A, Oberhausen E. Anti-CEA labelling kit BW 431/26. Results of the European multicenter trial. *Nuklearmedizin* 1995;34:232–242.

60. Baum RP, Hertel A, Lorenz M, et al. ^{99m}Tc-labeled anti-CEA monoclonal antibody for tumour immunoscintigraphy: first clinical results. *Nucl Med Commun* 1989;10:345–352.

61. Zwas ST, Goshen E, Rath P, et al. Detection efficiency of colorectal carcinoma recurrence using technetium pertechnetate anti-carcinoembryonic antigen monoclonal antibody BW431/26. *Cancer* 1995;76:215–222.

62. Doerr RJ, Abdel-Nabi H, Krag D, et al. Radiolabeled antibody imaging in the management of colorectal cancer: results of a multicenter clinical study. *Ann Surg* 1991;214:118–124.

63. Grossman SJ, Krag DN, Mitchell EP. Immunoscintigraphy performed with In-111-labeled CYT-103 in the management of colorectal cancer: comparison with CT. *Radiology* 1992;185:179–186.

64. Gold DV, Lew K, Maliniak R, et al. Characterization of monoclonal antibody PAM4 reactive with a pancreatic cancer mucin. *Int J Cancer* 1994;57:204–210.

65. Mariani G, Milea N, Bacciardi D, et al. Initial tumor targeting, biodistribution, and pharmacokinetic evaluation of the monoclonal antibody PAM4 in patients with pancreatic cancer. *Cancer Res* 1995;55:5911s–5915s.

66. Sawada T. Preoperative clinical radioimmunodetection of pancreatic cancer by ^{111}In-labeled chimeric monoclonal antibody Nd2. *Jpn J Cancer Res* 1999;90:1179–1186.

67. Muir CL. Cancer incidence in five continents. *IARC Sci Publ* 1992;5:25–30.

68. Goldenberg DM, Kim EE, DeLand FH, et al. Clinical studies on the radioimmunodetection of tumors containing alpha-fetoprotein. *Cancer* 1980;45:2500–2505.

69. Kim EE, DeLand FH, Nelson MO, et al. Radioimmunodetection of cancer with radiolabeled antibodies to α-fetoprotein. *Cancer Res* 1980;40:3008–3012.

70. Goldenberg DM, Goldenberg H, Ford EH, et al. Imaging of primary metastatic liver cancer with I-131 monoclonal and polyclonal antibodies against alpha-fetoprotein. *J Clin Oncol* 1987;5:1827–1835.

71. Dresel S, Kirsch CM, Tatsch K, et al. Detection of hepatocellular carcinoma with a new alpha-fetoprotein antibody imaging kit. *J Clin Oncol* 1997;15:2683–2690.

72. Martin W Jr, Thurston MO. The use of monoclonal antibodies (MAbs) and the development of an intraoperative hand-held probe for cancer detection. *Cancer Invest* 1996;4:560–571.

73. Arnold MW, Young DM, Hitchcock CL, et al. Staging of colorectal cancer: biology vs. morphology. *Dis Colon Rectum* 1998;41:1482–1487.

74. Martin EW JR, Thurston MO. Intraoperative radioimmunodetection. *Semin Surg Oncol* 1998;15:205–208.

75. Lechner P, Lind P, Binter G. Tc-99m-labeled anti-CEA antibodies in intraoperative diagnosis of colorectal cancer. *Nuklearmedizin* 1995;34:8–14.

76. Moffat FL Jr, Vagas-Cuba RD, Serafini AN, et al. Preoperative scintigraphy and operative probe scintimetry of colorectal carcinoma using technetium-99m-88BV59. *J Nucl Med* 1995;36:738–745.

77. Paganelli G, Stella M, Zito F, et al. Radioimmunoguided surgery using iodine-125-labeled biotinylated monoclonal antibodies and cold avidin. *J Nucl Med* 1994;35:1970–1975.

78. Sharkey RM, Kaltovich FA, Shih LB, et al. Radioimmunotherapy of human colonic cancer xenografts with ^{90}Y-labeled monoclonal antibodies to carcinoembryonic antigen. *Cancer Res* 1988;48:3270–3275.

79. Wong JYC, Williams LE, Yamauchi DM, et al. Initial experience evaluating ^{90}Yttrium-radiolabeled anti-carcinoembryonic antigen chimeric T84.66 in a phase I radioimmunotherapy trial. *Cancer Res* 1995;55:5929s–5934s.

80. Welt S, Scott AM, Divgi CR, et al. Phase I/II study of iodine 125-labeled monoclonal antibody A33 in patients with advanced colon cancer. *J Clin Oncol* 1996:14:1787–1797.

81. Meredith RF, Khazaeli MB, Plott WE, et al. Initial clinical evaluation of iodine-125-labeled chimeric 17-1A for metastatic colon cancer. *J Nucl Med* 1995;36:2229–2233.

82. Connett JM, Buettner TL, Anderson CJ. Maximum tolerated dose and large tumor radioimmunotherapy studies of ^{64}Cu-labeled monoclonal antibody 1A3 in a colon cancer model. *Clin Cancer Res* 1999;5:3207s–3212s.

83. Mulligan T, Carrasquillo JA, Chung Y, et al. Phase I study of intravenous Lu-labeled CC49 murine monoclonal antibody in patients with advanced adenocarcinoma. *Clin Cancer Res* 1995;1:1447–1454.

84. Juweid M, Sharkey RM, Swayne LC, et al. Pharmacokinetics, dosimetry and toxicity of rhenium-188-labeled anti-carcinoembryonic antigen monoclonal antibody, MN-14, in gastrointestinal cancer. *J Nucl Med* 1998;39:34–42.

85. Juweid ME, Sharkey RM, Behr T, et al. Radioimmunotherapy of patients with small-volume tumors using iodine-131-labeled anti-CEA monoclonal antibody NP-4 F(ab')$_2$. *J Nucl Med* 1996;37:1504–1510.

86. Dunn RM, Juweid M, Sharkey RM, et al. Can occult metastases be treated by radioimmunotherapy? *Cancer* 1997;80:2656–2659.

87. Behr TM, Salib A, Liersch T, et al. Radioimmunotherapy of small volume disease of colorectal cancer metastatic to the liver: preclinical evaluation in comparison to standard chemotherapy and initial results of a phase I clinical study. *Clin Cancer Res* 1999;5:3232s–3241s.

88. Blumenthal RD, Sharkey RM, Kashi R, et al. Comparison of therapeutic efficacy and host toxicity of two different ^{131}I-labelled antibodies and their fragments in the GW-39 colonic cancer xenograft model. *Int J Cancer* 1989;44:292–300.

89. Buchegger F, Pfister C, Fournier K, et al. Ablation of human colon carcinoma in nude mice by ^{131}I-labeled monoclonal anti-carcinoembryonic antigen antibody F(ab')$_2$ fragments. *J Clin Invest* 1989;83:1449–1456.

90. Saga T, Sakahara H. Nakamoto Y, et al. Radioimmunotherapy for liver micrometastases in mice: pharmacokinetics, dose estimation, and long-term effect. *Jpn J Cancer Res* 1999;90:342–348.

91. Mahteme H, Lovqvist A, Graf W, et al. Adjuvant ^{131}I-anti-CEA-antibody radioimmunotherapy inhibits the development of experimental colonic carcinoma liver metastases. *Anticancer Res* 1998;18:843–848.

92. Tschmelitsch J, Barendswaard E, Williams C Jr, et al. Enhanced antitumor activity of combination radioimmunotherapy (^{131}I-labeled monoclonal antibody A33) with chemotherapy (fluorouracil). *Cancer Res* 1997;1:57:2181–2186.

93. Kinuya S, Yokoyama K, Tega H, et al. Efficacy, toxicity and mode of interaction of combination radioimmunotherapy with 5-flourouracil in colon cancer xenografts. *J Cancer Res Clin Oncol* 1999;125:630–636.

94. Roberson PL, Buchsbaum DJ. Reconciliation of tumor dose response to external beam radiotherapy versus radioimmunotherapy with ^{131}iodine-labeled antibody for a colon cancer model. *Cancer Res* 1995;55:5811s–5816s.

95. Vogel CA, Galmiche MC, Buchegger F. Radioimmunotherapy and fractionated radiotherapy of human colon cancer liver metastases in nude mice. *Cancer Res* 1997;57:447–453.

96. Sun LQ, Vogel CA, Mirimanoff RO, et al. Timing effects of combined radioimmunotherapy and radiotherapy on a human solid tumor in nude mice. *Cancer Res* 1997;57:1312–1319.

97. Barendswaard EC, O'Donoghue JA, Larson SM, et al. ^{131}I radioimmunotherapy and fractionated external beam radiotherapy: comparative effectiveness in a human tumor xenograft. *J Nucl Med* 1999;40:1764–1768.

98. Behr TM, Memtsoudis S, Sharkey RM, et al. Experimental studies on the role of antibody fragments in cancer radioimmunotherapy: influence of radiation dose and dose rate on toxicity and anti-tumor efficacy. *Int J Cancer* 1998;31;77:787–795.

99. Casey JL, Pedley RB, King DJ, et al. Dosimetric evaluation and radioimmunotherapy of anti-tumour multivalent Fab' fragments. *Br J Cancer* 1999;81:972–980.

100. Begent RHJ, Verhaa MJ, Chester KA, et al. Clinical evidence of efficient tumor targeting based on single-chain Fv antibody selected from a combinatorial library. *Nat Med* 1996;2:979–984.

101. Pavlinkova G, Booth BJ, Batra SK, Colcher D. Radioimmunotherapy of human colon cancer xenografts using a dimeric single-chain Fv antibody construct. *Clin Cancer Res* 1999;5: 2613–2619.

102. Khawli LA, Miller GK, Epstein AL. Effect of seven new vasoactive immunoconjugates on the enhancement of monoclonal antibody uptake in tumors. *Cancer* 1994;73:824–831.

103. Pedley RB, Boden JA, Boden R, et al. Ablation of colorectal xenografts with combined radioimmunotherapy and tumor blood flow-modifying agents. *Cancer Res* 1996;56:3293–3300.

104. Meredith RF, Khazaeli MB, Plott WE, et al. Phase II study of dual ^{131}I-labeled monoclonal antibody therapy with interferon in patients with metastatic colorectal cancer. *Clin Cancer Res* 1996; 2:1811–1818.

105. Blumenthal RD, Sharkey RM, Snyder D, et al. Reduction by anti-antibody administration of the radiotoxicity associated with ^{131}I-labeled antibody to carcinoembryonic antigen in cancer radioimmunotherapy. *J Natl Cancer Inst* 1989;81:194–199.

106. Sandström P, Johansson A, Ullén A, et al. Idiotypic–anti-idiotypic antibody interactions at experimental radioimmunotargeting. *Clin Cancer Res* 1999;5:3073s–3088s.

107. Goodwin DA, Meares CF. Pretargeting. General principles: October 10–12, 1996. *Cancer* 1997;80:2675–2680.

108. Barbet J, Kraeber-Bodere F, Vuillez J-P, et al. Pretargeting with the affinity enhancement system for radioimmunotherapy. *Cancer Biother Radiopharm* 1999;14:153–166.

109. Casey JL, King DJ, Pedley RB, et al. Clearance of yttrium-90 labelled anti-tumour antibodies with antibodies raised against the 12N4 DOTA macrocycle. *Br J Cancer* 1998;78:1307–1312.

110. Bischof Delaloye A, Delaloye B. Immunoscintigraphy in cancer care. *Cancer* 1994;73:900–904.

111. Goldenberg DM. New developments in monoclonal antibodies for cancer detection and therapy. *CA Cancer J Clin* 1994;44: 27–42.

26

SCINTIGRAPHY AND RADIONUCLIDE THERAPY

MARION DE JONG
ROELF VALKEMA
WOUT A. P. BREEMAN
WILLEM H. BAKKER
PETER P. M. KOOIJ
THEO J. VISSER
STAN PAUWELS
ERIC P. KRENNING

SOMATOSTATIN, SOMATOSTATIN ANALOGUES, AND SOMATOSTATIN RECEPTORS

Because somatostatin and its analogues (and their receptors) are the most frequently discussed and used of all peptides in relation to neuroendocrine tumor scintigraphy and radionuclide therapy, their application is the main focus of this chapter.

Somatostatin (SST14) is a cyclic disulfide-containing peptide hormone comprising 14 amino acids (Fig. 26.1). It is present in the hypothalamus, cerebral cortex, brain stem, gastrointestinal tract, and pancreas. Somatostatin was isolated and characterized in 1973 (1). Somatostatin receptors (SSTRs) have been identified in the gastrointestinal tract and central nervous system, and on many cells of neuroendocrine origin, including the somatotropes of the anterior pituitary gland, C cells in the thyroid, and D cells of the pancreatic islets (1,2). Non-neuroendocrine cells, such as lymphocytes (3), possess these receptors also. In the central nervous system, somatostatin acts as a neurotransmitter, and its hormonal activities

M. de Jong, R. Valkema, W. A. P. Breeman, W. H. Bakker, and P. P. M. Kooij: Department of Nuclear Medicine, Erasmus Medical Center Rotterdam, 3015 GD Rotterdam, The Netherlands.

T. J. Visser: Department of Internal Medicine, Erasmus Medical Center Rotterdam, 3015 GD Rotterdam, The Netherlands.

S. Pauwels: Department of Nuclear Medicine, Catholic University of Louvain, 10200 Brussels, Belgium.

E. P. Krenning: Departments of Nuclear Medicine and Internal Medicine, Erasmus Medical Center Rotterdam, 3015 GD Rotterdam, The Netherlands.

include inhibition of the release of growth hormone, insulin, glucagon, and gastrin (4).

The general inhibitory effect of somatostatin on hormone secretion of various glands led to the consideration of possible beneficial effects of somatostatin in the treatment of diseases based on gland hyperfunction or overproduction of hormones by tumors originating in endocrine tissue. However, the tetradecapeptide SST14 is unsuitable for routine treatment because it has a very short half-life of approximately 3 minutes after intravenous administration as a consequence of rapid enzymatic degradation. In recent years, successful efforts have been undertaken to synthesize somatostatin analogues that are more resistant to enzymatic degradation. The molecule has been modified but its biologic activity preserved by introducing D-amino acids and shortening the molecule to the bioactive core sequence; the somatostatin analogue octreotide, containing eight amino acids, is the result (Fig. 26.1). At present, octreotide is widely used in the treatment of symptoms caused by neuroendocrine tumors, such as growth hormone-producing pituitary adenomas and gastroenteropancreatic tumors (5–7). The biology and clinical application of somatostatin and somatostatin analogues have been described extensively (6–9).

Peptide receptor scintigraphy with radioactive somatostatin-analogues, initially with [^{123}I-Tyr^3]octreotide and more recently [^{111}In-DTPA^0]octreotide (OctreoScan) (10–14), appeared to be a sensitive and specific technique to demonstrate the presence and abundance of SSTRs on various tumors *in vivo*.

Somatostatin receptors are structurally related integral membrane glycoproteins. Recently, five different human somatostatin receptor types have been cloned, and splice variants have been reported. All subtypes bind SST14 and

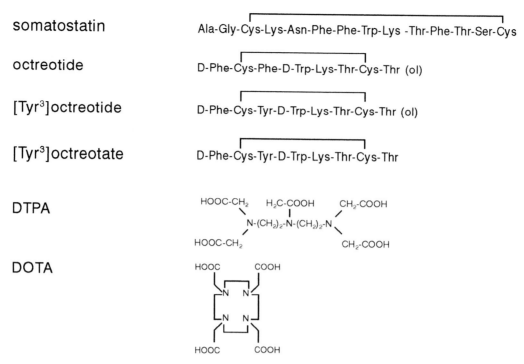

FIGURE 26.1. Structures of somatostatin, octreotide, [Tyr³]octreotide, [Tyr³]octreotate, diethylenetriamine pentaacetic acid (*DTPA*), and tetraazacyclododecane tetraacetic acid (*DOTA*).

SST28 (a polypeptide of 28 amino acids with SST14 at its carboxyl terminus) with high affinity, whereas the affinities of numerous somatostatin analogues for the five different subtypes differ considerably (15–18). Octreotide binds with a high affinity to SSTR2 (human somatostatin receptor type 2) and a relatively high affinity to SSTR5, but this analogue has a relatively low affinity for SSTR3 and shows no binding to SSTR1 and SSTR4 (15–19). Octreotide scintigraphy is therefore based on the visualization of (an) octreotide-binding somatostatin receptor(s), SSTR2 and SSTR5.

Internalization of Radiolabeled Somatostatin Analogues

The ligand–receptor complex is internalized via invagination of the plasma membrane in a process of receptor-mediated endocytosis whereby cell surface receptors capture their ligands from the extracellular milieu (20,21). The resulting intracellular vesicles, termed *endosomes*, rapidly acidify, causing the ligand to dissociate from the receptor. The ligand is delivered to the lysosome (22), and the receptor recycles back to plasma membrane. The whole process takes approximately 15 minutes (20), and a single receptor can deliver numerous ligand molecules to the lysosomes.

Equivocal data have been described with respect to cellular internalization of the SST14–receptor complex. This process has been demonstrated in rat anterior pituitary cells

and in rat islet cells (23–30), whereas other investigators have found that [¹²⁵I-Tyr¹]SST14 and [¹²⁵I-Tyr¹¹]SST14 are not significantly internalized by GH₄C₁ rat pituitary cells and RINm5F insulinoma cells, respectively, probably because of degradation of these radioligands at the cell surface (31,32). We have studied the internalization and degradation of radiolabeled [DTPA⁰]octreotide in the SSTR-positive rat pancreatic tumor cell lines CA20948 and AR42J and in the SSTR-negative human anaplastic thyroid tumor cell line ARO and detected internalization of the radiopharmaceutical *in vitro*, in accordance with the findings of Andersson et al. (33), and found this process to be receptor-specific and temperature-dependent (34). Earlier, we reported *in vitro* studies in which AtT20 mouse pituitary tumor cells were used to detect internalization of [¹²⁵I-Tyr³]octreotide (35).

Receptor-mediated internalization of [¹¹¹In-DTPA⁰]octreotide results in degradation to the final radiolabeled metabolite ¹¹¹In-DTPA-D-Phe in the lysosomes. This metabolite is not capable of passing through lysosomal or other cell membrane(s) (36) and therefore remains in the lysosomes.

Internalization of [¹¹¹In-DTPA⁰]octreotide is essential for successful scintigraphy and radionuclide therapy of tumors, as various radionuclides suitable for radiotherapy (e.g., those emitting conversion and Auger electrons) are only a few nanometers to micrometers from their target, the nuclear DNA.

Effect of Dose and Specific Activity on the Biodistribution of [¹¹¹In-DTPA⁰]Octreotide in Tissues Positive for Somatostatin Receptors

In *in vitro* experiments involving saturable processes (i.e., radioimmunoassays and receptor binding studies), the signal-to-background ratio is often improved by lowering the mass of the radiotracer or by increasing its specific radioactivity. In previous studies (13), we reported the visualization of SSTR-positive tumors in rats by gamma camera scintigraphy with the use of [¹¹¹In-DTPA⁰]octreotide. In those studies, the administered mass of peptide and the radioactive dose were such that more than 90% of the ligand was unlabeled. Theoretically, the presence of unlabeled [DTPA⁰]octreotide will have a negative effect on the percentage uptake of [¹¹¹In-DTPA⁰]octreotide in SSTR-positive tissues because of competition with the unlabeled peptide for the same receptor. After the first labeling of [¹¹¹In-DTPA⁰]octreotide in 1989, the composition of the commercially available ¹¹¹InCl₃ was improved so that the specific radioactivity could be increased up to 740 MBq of ¹¹¹In per microgram of [DTPA⁰]octreotide. We hypothesized that the target-to-background ratio would be optimal for receptor scintigraphy at the lowest possible mass of peptide with the highest specific radioactivity, so that sensitivity of the imaging technique would be higher. This hypothesis was investigated in rats. Also, because several reports (37,38) suggested a positive effect of prior administration of unlabeled peptide on the percentage uptake of the radioactive counterpart, the effects of administration of the unlabeled ligand were studied in rats and in patients. The results of these investigations indicated that, contrary to what was expected, the percentage uptake of [DTPA⁰]octreotide in octreotide receptor-positive tissues is not optimal at the lowest possible dose of the highest specific radioactivity. The uptake expressed as a percentage of the administered dose is a bell-shaped function of the injected mass, being optimal between 0.5 and 5 μg of [¹¹¹In-DTPA⁰]octreotide (39). This implies that the sensitivity of receptor scintigraphy to detect SSTR-positive tumors can be improved by varying the mass of the radiopharmaceutical, which has now been confirmed in patients (40). Findings in patients indicate that when a standard dose of 220 MBq of ¹¹¹In is coupled to less than 5 μg of [DTPA⁰]octreotide, the quality of scintigraphy is decreased and uptake in tumors is significantly reduced (40).

METHODOLOGY

Chemistry of [DTPA⁰]Octreotide

The N-α-diethyleletriame pentaacetic acid (DTPA) derivative of octreotide was synthesized by Sandoz (Basel, Switzerland). The protected [ε-t-butyloxy-carbonyl-Lys⁵]octreotide was used as the starting material, which was available by the reaction of octreotide with di-t-butyl-dicarbonate [(Boc)₂O] in dimethylformamide. DTPA was coupled to the selectively protected octreotide in the form of its dianhydride. Purification of the product was achieved by silica gel chromatography to separate the wanted [DTPA⁰-ε-Boc-Lys⁵]octreotide from the contaminating double-substituted DTPA-derivative and unreacted starting material. Deprotecting with trifluoroacetic acid and subsequent sequential purification yielded homogeneous [DTPA⁰]octreotide (also called [DTPA-D-Phe¹]octreotide) as lyophilisate. The purity was checked by reverse-phase high-performance liquid chromatography. Structure and amino acid composition were proved by means of nuclear magnetic resonance, fast atom bombardment mass spectrometry, and amino acid analysis (12).

Radiolabeling

[DTPA⁰]Octreotide and ¹¹¹InCl₃ (DRN 4901, 370 MBq/mL in HCl, pH 1.5 to 1.9) are from Mallinckrodt Medical (Petten, The Netherlands). The kit preparation of a patient dose consists of addition of 222 MBq (6 mCi) of ¹¹¹InCl₃ to freeze-dried [DTPA⁰]octreotide.

Quality Control

Thirty minutes after the start of this procedure, quality control is performed by instant thin-layer chromatography with silica gel and 0.1 M sodium citrate, pH 5, as eluent. Under these conditions, indium citrate and indium chloride migrate along with the solvent front, whereas peptide-bound ¹¹¹In stays near the origin.

SCINTIGRAPHY WITH [¹¹¹IN-DTPA⁰]OCTREOTIDE

Methods

The preferred dose of ¹¹¹In-labeled octreotide (at least 10 μg of the peptide) is about 200 MBq. With such a dose, it is possible to perform single-photon emission computed tomography (SPECT), which may increase the sensitivity to detect octreotide receptor-expressing tissues and provides a better anatomic delineation than planar views. Planar and SPECT images are obtained with a gamma camera with a large field of view that is equipped with a medium-energy parallel-hole collimator. Pulse height analyzer windows are centered over both ¹¹¹In photon peaks (172 and 245 keV) with a window width of 20%. Data from both windows are added to the acquisition frames. Acquisition parameters for planar images (spot views) (anterior and posterior views are necessary) with a single-head camera with analogue imaging are as follows: (a) images of head/neck (also from lateral): 300,000 preset counts or 15 minutes per view at 24 hours and 15 minutes of preset time (about 200,000 counts) at 48 hours after injection; (b) images of the remainder of the body with separate images of the chest (including as little as possible of the liver and spleen), shoulders and axillae (with arms upraised to detect metastases in the armpits), and upper (including liver/spleen and kidneys) and lower abdomen: 500,000 counts or 15 minutes; with single- and dual-head cameras with digital imaging: (i) 256 x 256 word matrix, (ii) 15 minutes preset time images, and (iii) digital images of upper and lower abdomen viewed at both low- and high-intensity settings, and those of other parts of the body viewed at a level optimized for low-radioactivity structures. For SPECT images the acquisition parameters are as follows: (a) single-head camera: (i) 60 projections, (ii) 64 x 64 word matrix, (iii) *at least* 45 to 60 seconds acquisition time per projection; (b) dual-head camera: (i) 60 steps of 6 degrees each, (ii) 64 x 64 matrix, (iii) *at least* 30 seconds acquisition time per step; (c) triple-head camera: (i) 40 steps of 3 degrees each, (ii) 64 x 64 word matrix, (iii) *at least* 30 seconds acquisition time per step (45 seconds for SPECT of the head). SPECT analysis is performed with a Wiener or Metz filter on original data. The filtered data are reconstructed with a Ramp filter. When the counting time to obtain these "preset" counts for the planar views is short, especially when tissues with relatively high accumulation (e.g., abdominal organs) are included in the field of view or tumor types are being scanned in which the receptor density is low (as in both breast cancer and lymphomas), additional images with a longer counting time (15 minutes per planar view) are necessary to visualize small lesions or lesions with low SSTR density. The above-mentioned counting times per projection for planar imaging with a single-head camera also imply an appropriate (long) duration of whole-body planar scintigraphy with a dual-head camera (e.g., at least approximately 40 minutes from head to pelvis or a maximum speed of 3 cm/min). In general, the more counts collected, the better the results to detect or localize tissue(s) expressing ligand–receptor complexes. The importance of SPECT of the chest for breast cancer (primary and metastases) versus planar imaging is not known at the moment. Chiti et al. (41) compared planar imaging with SPECT in patients with breast cancer. In our view, however, the acquisition times used, 5 and 10 minutes at 4 and 24 hours after injection, are too short for planar imaging of breast cancer. Our results have been obtained with planar imaging only. However, our impression is that SPECT of the chest, including iterative reconstruction, might improve the sensitivity for breast cancer detection. Iterative reconstruction improves the quality of the images by reducing background noise and reconstruction artifacts.

Planar and SPECT studies are preferably performed 24 hours after injection of the radiopharmaceutical. Planar studies after 24 and 48 hours can be carried out with the same protocol. Repeated scintigraphy after 48 hours is indicated, especially when 24-hour scintigraphy shows accumulation in the abdomen, to exclude radioactive bowel content.

Dosimetry

The effective dose equivalent of 222 MBq of [^{111}In-DTPA^0]octreotide (about 16 mSv) is comparable with values for other ^{111}In-labeled radiopharmaceuticals and is acceptable in view of the clinical indications. Furthermore, these radiation doses have to be compared with the values of commonly used imaging techniques for these clinical indications (e.g., CT chest, 7 to 11 mSv) (42,43).

General Results

Somatostatin receptor imaging with [^{111}In-DTPA^0]octreotide makes it possible to visualize the primary and metastatic sites of a variety of neuroendocrine tumors, such as carcinoids, islet cell tumors, and paragangliomas (12,14,42, 43). Figure 26.2 is a flow diagram for the use of [^{111}In-DTPA^0]octreotide scintgraphy of neuroendocrine tumors. The *in vitro* demonstration of high-affinity binding sites for somatostatin on these tumors validates the significance of *in vivo* tumor visualization (12). A positive SSTR scan closely predicts a beneficial effect of long-term octreotide therapy on hormonal hypersecretion by these tumors (44).

The efficacy of scintigraphy with [^{111}In-DTPA^0]octreotide was evaluated in the European Multicenter Trial in 350 patients with a histologically or biochemically proven gastroenteropancreatic tumor (43). Tumor sites were detected by conventional imaging methods in 88%, whereas results of SSTR scintigraphy were positive in 80%. The highest success rates of SSTR scintigraphy were observed with glucagonomas (100%), vipomas (88%), carcinoids (87%) and nonfunctioning islet cell tumors (82%). The low detection rate (46%) noted for insulinomas is related to the lower incidence of SSTR2 on insulinoma cells. However, the overall 80% sensitivity is somewhat lower than the 88% obtained at the Erasmus University Rotterdam in 130 patients with gastroenteropancreatic tumors. This may be related to important differences in scanning procedures, such as the amount of radioligand administered (minimal dose of 200 MBq of ^{111}In and at least 10 μg of peptide at the Erasmus University Rotterdam), the duration of the acquisition, and the use of SPECT (with a triple head camera at the Erasmus University Rotterdam). The fact that abdominal SPECT was not systematically performed in all patients in the European Multicenter Trial may explain the only 73% rate of positive scans in gastrinoma patients, compared with the 90% to 100% sensitivity reported in other studies. In the European Multicenter Trial, a total of 388 sites were

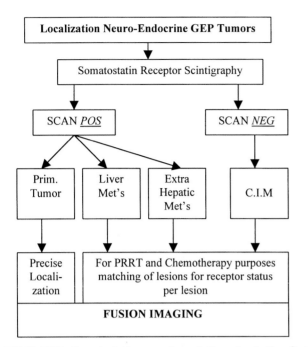

Localization Neuro-Endocrine GEP Tumors

Somatostatin Receptor Scintigraphy

SCAN *POS*   SCAN *NEG*

Prim. Tumor   Liver Met's   Extra Hepatic Met's   C.I.M

Precise Locali-zation   For PRRT and Chemotherapy purposes matching of lesions for receptor status per lesion

FUSION IMAGING

FIGURE 26.2. Somatostatin receptor scintigraphy is the first imaging modality performed to localize and map sites of neuroendocrine tumors, except insulinomas. Conventional imaging modalities are a combination of ultrasonography, computed tomography, magnetic resonance imaging, and angiography. Peptide receptor radionuclide therapy is administered only to patients with peptide receptor-positive lesions, whereas chemotherapy is administered only in cases of dedifferentiated or anaplastic forms of neuroendocrine tumors, which are somatostatin receptor-negative. See text for imaging protocol of somatostatin receptor scintigraphy. (From Krenning EP, Kwekkeboom DJ, Pauwels S, et al. Somatostatin receptor scintigraphy. In: Freeman LM, ed. *Nuclear medicine annual.* New York: Raven Press, 1995:1–50.).

visualized with conventional imaging methods in 308 of the 350 patients. In addition to 297 known localizations, SSTR scintigraphy revealed 166 unsuspected lesions. Forty percent of these unsuspected lesions were subsequently confirmed as true-positive findings based on the results of additional imaging procedures or histology obtained during the 1-year follow-up period. The clinical relevance of detecting additional tumor sites depends on the clinical status of the patient. The demonstration of an unsuspected lesion in a patient with known metastatic spread usually has little impact on management. In contrast, the detection of unsuspected tumor sites in patients with a single known lesion or without any known lesion is important, in that it may affect selection for curative surgery, which remains the treatment of choice for patients with this type of tumor. In the cohort of 350 patients studied, 42 had no lesion detected by conventional imaging methods, and 178 were known to have a single tumor localization before the study. Results of SSTR scintigraphy were positive in 11 of the 42 patients (25%), and 12 of 16 lesions revealed by SSTR scintigra-

phy were further confirmed as true-positives. SSTR scintigraphy demonstrated multiple tumor sites in 62 of the 178 patients (35%), and 60% of these lesions were confirmed by follow-up (at 1 year) procedures. A reply to an impact questionnaire was obtained for 235 patients. Overall, the scintigraphic findings led to management changes in 40% of the 235 patients.

In a prospective study, Gibril et al. (45) compared the sensitivity of SSTR scintigraphy with that of computed tomography (CT), magnetic resonance imaging (MRI), ultrasonography, and selective angiography in the detection of primary and metastatic gastrinomas. They concluded that SSTR scintigraphy is the single most sensitive method for imaging either primary or metastatic liver lesions in patients with Zollinger-Ellison syndrome. The same group studied the effect of SSTR scintigraphy on clinical management based on the data of this comparative study (45,46). Because this technique altered management of 47% of the patients, they concluded that SSTR scintigraphy should be the initial imaging modality for patients with gastrinomas, based on its superior sensitivity, high specificity, simplicity, and cost-effectiveness. Furthermore, it is likely that this conclusion can be extended to other pancreatic endocrine tumor syndromes, with the exception of insulinomas (46).

Recently, Gibril et al. studied the specificity (or occurrence of false-positive results) of SSTR scintigraphy and its effect on management in 146 patients with Zollinger-Ellison syndrome (47). It was concluded that false-positive localization occurs in 1 of 10 patients with Zollinger-Ellison syndrome. However, when the diseases or circumstances that cause false-positive localizations are thoroughly understood and the findings are considered within the clinical context, the percentage of patients in whom false-positive localizations result in altered management can be reduced to below 3%, and the correct diagnosis can be made in almost every case.

Cases

Case 1

Figure 26.3 shows a [^{111}In-DTPA^0]octreotide scintigram of a patient with neuroendocrine tumor in the pancreas. Parts A and B show spot views obtained at 24 and 48 hours after injection of the radioligand. Note the physiologic accumulation in the thyroid gland, liver, spleen, kidneys, and urinary bladder, and the bowel radioactivity. The latter has disappeared at 48 hours after injection, except in the region of the hepatic flexure. The tumor is visible between the kidneys at both time points. Part C shows transverse (upper two panels) and coronal (lower two panels) SPECT views of the upper abdomen in the same patient at 24 hours after injection. The tumor is clearly visible medial and ventral to the kidneys. Bowel radioactivity is apparent ventral to the kidneys and tumor.

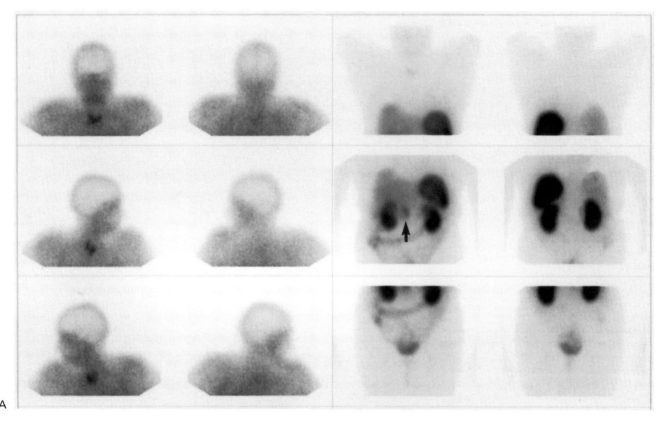

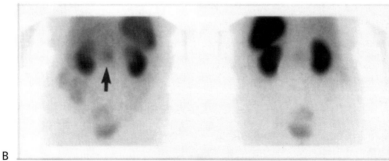

FIGURE 26.3. [¹¹¹In-DTPA⁰]Octreotide scintigram of a patient with neuroendocrine tumor in the pancreas. **A,B:** Spot views obtained 24 and 48 hours after injection of the radioligand. Note physiologic accumulation in the thyroid gland, liver, spleen, kidneys, and urinary bladder, and bowel radioactivity. The latter has disappeared at 48 hours after injection except in the region of the hepatic flexure. The tumor is visible between the kidneys at the two time points.

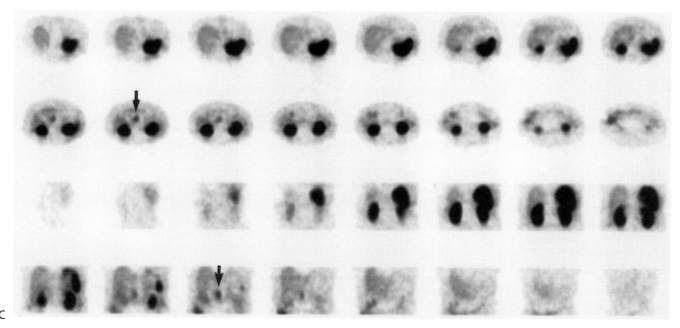

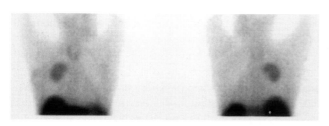

FIGURE 26.3. (continued) C: Transverse (*upper two panels*) and coronal (*lower two panels*) single-photon emission tomographic views of the upper abdomen in the same patient 24 hours after injection. The tumor is clearly visible medial and ventral to the kidneys. Also, bowel radioactivity is apparent ventral to the kidneys and tumor.

Case 2

Figure 26.4 shows a 24-hour [^{111}In-DTPA^0]octreotide scintigram of a 69-year-old patient with slowly progressive disease since 1995 in the posterior segment of the right upper lobe of the lung based on chest roentgenography. Bronchoscopy did not reveal any abnormality. The positive [^{111}In-DTPA^0]octreotide scintigram identifies a carcinoid tumor. The patient declined surgery.

Case 3

Figure 26.5 shows a 24-hour [^{111}In-DTPA^0]octreotide scintigram (planar and transverse SPECT) of a 70-year-old patient

FIGURE 26.4. Twenty-four-hour [^{111}In-DTPA^0]octreotide scintigram of a 69-year-old patient with slowly progressive disease in the posterior segment of the right upper lobe of the lung since 1995, according to chest roentgenograms. Bronchoscopy did not reveal any abnormality. The positive [^{111}In-DTPA^0]octreotide scintigram points to a carcinoid. The patient refused surgery.

with nonspecific abdominal symptoms. Ultrasonography revealed a solitary lesion in the uncinate process of the pancreas, 22 x 25 mm, confirmed by CT (22 x 27 mm). [^{111}In-DTPA^0]Octreotide scintigraphy showed a solitary lesion 35 mm in diameter (*arrow*). At surgery, two lesions adjacent to each other, 2 and 1 cm in diameter, were removed. On immunohistochemistry, the neuroendocrine tumors were negative for the presence of insulin, gastrin, and somatostatin.

Case 4

In Fig. 26.6, 24-hour [^{111}In-DTPA^0]octreotide scintigraphy in a 33-year-old patient demonstrates SSTRs in the many metastases of a neuroendocrine tumor (positive for chromogranin on immunohistochemistry). Three months after the [^{111}In-DTPA^0]octreotide scintigram, CT demonstrated progressive disease. Despite chemotherapy, the patient died 3 months later.

RADIONUCLIDE THERAPY WITH [^{111}IN-DTPA^0]OCTREOTIDE

General Considerations

Historically, targeted radionuclide therapy with ^{131}I was first used to treat well-differentiated thyroid carcinoma. This technique exploits the property of thyroid cells to concentrate iodide (48). Radiopharmaceutical treatment with

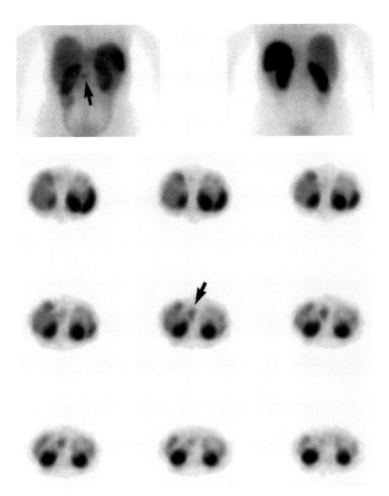

FIGURE 26.5. Twenty-four-hour [^{111}In-DTPA^0]octreotide scintigram [planar image (*left*) and transverse single-photon emission computed tomographic image (*right*)] of a 70-year-old patient with nonspecific abdominal symptoms. Ultrasonography revealed a 22 x 25-mm solitary lesion in the uncinate process of the pancreas, confirmed by computed tomography (22 x 27 mm). [^{111}In-DTPA^0]Octreotide scintigraphy shows a solitary lesion 35 mm in diameter (*arrow*). At surgery, two lesions adjacent to each other were removed, with diameters of 2 and 1 cm. The neuroendocrine tumors on immunohistochemistry were negative for insulin, gastrin, and somatostatin.

the iodo compound ^{131}I-MIBG (metaiodobenzylguanidine), which is preferentially taken up by catecholamine-synthesizing cells of the sympathetic nervous tissues and produces antiproliferative effects in neuroblastomas and pheochromocytomas, is a well-established technique (49).

As soon as the success of peptide receptor scintigraphy for tumor visualization became clear, the next logical step was to try to label the peptides with radionuclides emitting alpha or beta particles, or Auger or conversion electrons, and use them for radiotherapy.

A (mono-energetic) conversion electron arises when the atomic nucleus transfers energy to one of its surrounding electrons, enabling it to leave the atom (50). The resulting vacancy is filled by electrons from higher orbitals, which may result in emission of an Auger electron (51). In addition, Auger electrons may arise when vacancies in the electron orbitals are caused by electron capture, in which an orbital electron is captured by the nucleus.

It is well known that *in vivo* effects often differ from the calculated estimated dose, largely because of the current shortcomings of microdosimetry. For instance, nonhomogeneity of receptors throughout the target, potential internalization of the ligand, and (sub)cellular localization of the radionuclide are unknown factors. Because the energy of conversion and Auger electrons is usually less than that of beta particles, their linear energy transfer (LET) and consequently their cell-killing probability is larger than that of beta particles. When a radionuclide with a high LET is located within a few nanometers of the DNA, its radiotoxicity is very high. Therefore, the heterogeneity of radionuclide deposition is most serious for short-range alpha emitters and Auger emitters and less serious for long-range beta emitters.

The frequently mentioned potential use of ^{131}I-labeled somatostatin analogues for radiotherapy was evaluated. This was done with special attention given to radiochemistry and the technical aspects of producing radiotherapeutic pharma-

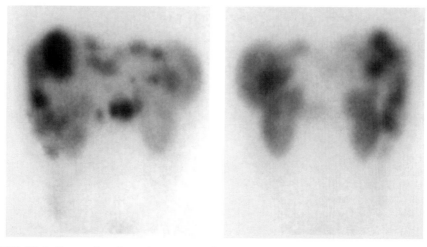

FIGURE 26.6. Twenty-four-hour [111In-DTPA0]octreotide scintigram of a 33-year-old patient shows the localization and presence of somatostatin receptors in multiple metastases of a neuroendocrine tumor (immunohistochemistry positive for chromogranin). Three months after the [111In-DTPA0]octreotide scintigram, computed tomography demonstrated progressive disease, and despite chemotherapy, the patient died 3 months later.

ceuticals. In the presence of 370 MBq of ^{131}I, somatostatin analogues showed extensive radiolytic damage in aqueous solution with a half-life of only 1 hour (52). Consequently, we concluded that intact monoiodinated ^{131}I-labeled peptides would be very hard to obtain, especially if a dose of more than 3,700 MBq of ^{131}I-labeled peptide were required.

A new perspective for patients with SSTR-positive tumors is peptide receptor radionuclide therapy (PRRT) with [^{111}In-DTPA^0]octreotide. After internalization of the radiopharmaceutical in the tumor cells, the radioactive ligand is close to the nucleus. Because ^{111}In emits not only gamma rays, which are visualized with SSTR scintigraphy, but also short-range Auger electrons, an effect on tumor cell proliferation can be expected (53–55).

Methods

The typical dose of [^{111}In-DTPA^0]octreotide per administration is 6,000 to 7,000 MBq of ^{111}In incorporated in 40 to 50 µg of [DTPA^0]octreotide. Doses are given at least 2 weeks apart, with a goal of administering eight doses. In a few patients, this has been increased to approximately 20 doses. Radionuclide therapy with [^{111}In-DTPA^0]octreotide was begun after witnessed informed consent and approval by the medical ethics committee had been obtained. Measurement of the usual hematologic and chemical parameters of bone marrow, liver, kidney, and endocrine pancreatic (glucose or hemoglobin A$_{1c}$) function before and between all doses served to monitor side effects. Pituitary function (free thyroxine, luteinizing hormone and follicle-stimulating hormone in postmenopausal women, testosterone in men) was assessed before and 4 weeks after the fourth and eight doses of [^{111}In-DTPA^0]octreotide. Additionally, possible effects on (a) the endocrine activity of the tumors or their production of specific serum markers, and (b) tumor size (CT or MRI) were investigated. Testing of pituitary–adrenal axis function (metyrapone test) before and after eight doses and long-term follow-up at 3- to 4-month intervals was performed if feasible.

Dosimetry

Tumor uptake in patients before the start of treatment with [^{111}In-DTPA^0]octreotide was scored visually on scintigrams obtained 24 hours after injection of a diagnostic dose (220 MBq) of [^{111}In-DTPA^0]octreotide. The scoring grades used were 4, intense; 3, clear (higher than liver uptake); 2, clear but faint (lower than or equal to liver uptake); 1, equivocal; 0, no accumulation. Patients were also scanned 3 and 7 days after each administration of the radiotherapeutic dose. Percentage uptake of the administered dose in the total body and in the most prominent tumor was calculated. Uptake decreased slowly or remained the same if the interval between successive doses was less than 1 month. In patients who had six or more doses of 6,000 to 7,000 MBq of [^{111}In-DTPA^0]octreotide with maximal intervals of 1 month between administrations, uptake in the tumor was still clearly visible after the last administration. Typical radiation doses to tissues with doses of 6,000 to 7,000 MBq of [^{111}In-DTPA^0]octreotide are as follows: kidneys, 300 to 1,400 cGy, depending on the relative biologic effectiveness (1 to 20) for Auger electrons; spleen, 200 cGy; liver, 50 cGy; bone marrow, 13 cGy (target organ for gamma photons); thyroid gland, 25 cGy; pituitary, 70 cGy. The critical organs are the kidneys and spleen. With these doses, the estimated tumor radiation doses for a 10-g tumor (assumptions of 1% uptake, effective half-life equal to the physical half-life) are 1,700 and 6,700 cGy (for Auger electrons with relative biologic effec-

TABLE 26.1. CHARACTERISTICS OF PATIENTS TREATED WITH [^{111}IN-DTPA-D-PHE^1]OCTREOTIDE

	No.	Grade 2	Grade 3	Grade 4
Carcinoid	10	1 (P)	6 (2*,	
Neuroendocrine tumor	7	1 (R)	P,2S,R)	3 (2*,S)
Gastrinoma	1		3 (2*,P)	3
Vipoma	1		1 (S)	(P,S,R)
Glucagonoma	1			
Medullary thyroid	4	4		1 (R)
carcinoma	2	(1*,2P,S)		1 (R)
Papillary thyroid	1	2 (1*,S)		
carcinoma	2			
Glomus tumor	1	2 (P,S)		1 (R)
Pheochromocytoma		1 (1*)		
Leiomyosarcoma				
TOTAL	21 (+9*)	8 (+3*)	6 (+4*)	7 (+2*)
Positive effect (S + R)	67%	50%	67%	86%

*<<20 GBq and/or no FU.
DTPA, diethylenetriamine pentaacetic acid; P, progression; S, stable; R, reduction in tumor size.

tiveness values of 1 and 20, respectively), and for a 100-g tumor (1% uptake), they are 250 and 750 cGy, respectively.

The high rate of uptake in the kidneys is a problem during radionuclide therapy with the radiolabeled octapeptide [^{111}In-DTPA^0]octreotide. Small peptides in the blood plasma are filtered through the glomerular capillaries in the kidneys and subsequently are almost completely reabsorbed (about 90%) by the proximal tubular cells via carrier-mediated endocytosis. After degradation in the tubule cell lysosomes, the labeled degradation products are "trapped" (36) and emit high levels of radiation to the kidneys, thereby reducing the sensitivity of scintigraphy to detect small tumors in the perirenal region and limiting radionuclide therapy. We showed that renal uptake of [^{111}In-DTPA^0]octreotide in rats could be reduced about 50% by a single intravenous administration of 400 mg of L- or D-lysine per kilogram (56,57). This is in agreement with the findings of other reports (58). The membranes of renal tubular cells contain negatively

charged sites. It is believed that positively charged residues of peptides or proteins bind to these sites and that the binding process can be inhibited by administering the positively charged amino acid lysine (both D- and L-lysine). We are currently testing the effects of infusions of L-lysine on renal uptake and estimates of radiation absorbed dose.

Results

Thirty patients with end-stage disease have been treated with [^{111}In-DTPA^0]octreotide (Table 26.1). Twenty-one received a total cumulative dose of at least 20 GBq of [^{111}In-DTPA^0]octreotide. Of the nine patients treated with a total dose lower than 20 GBq, seven had to stop prematurely because of progressive disease despite treatment with [^{111}In-DTPA^0]octreotide, and two have not yet concluded the first course of four doses. Tumor scores in the seven patients with very progressive disease were 2 (*n* = 3), 3 (*n* = 2), or 4

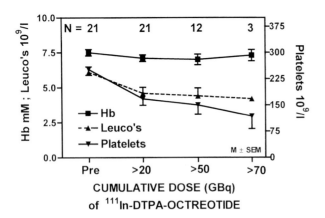
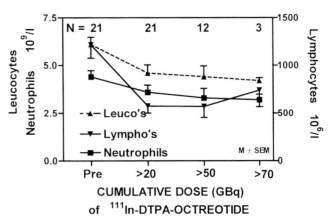

FIGURE 26.7. Course of hemoglobulin and blood cells during peptide receptor radionuclide treatment with the indicated cumulative doses of [^{111}In-DTPA^0]octreotide. *N*, number of patients (mean ± standard error of the mean).

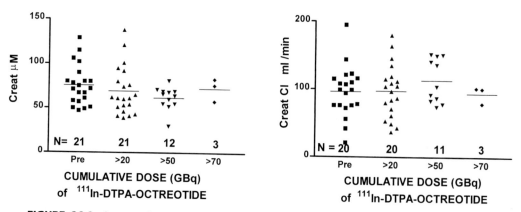

FIGURE 26.8. Course of serum creatinine and creatinine clearance during peptide receptor radionuclide treatment with the indicated cumulative doses of [^{111}In-DTPA^0]octreotide. *N*, number of patients.

($n = 2$). High, multiple radiotherapeutic doses of [^{111}In-DTPA^0]octreotide were given to 21 patients, up to total cumulative doses of 22 to 30 GBq, and to 12 patients, up to 50 to 60 GBq per patient. Three patients received maximum doses of 75 GBq. No major side effects were noticed in the first patient after a cumulative dose of 25 GBq and a follow-up interval of 2 years, which is so far the longest follow-up period. In the other patients, no major clinical side effects were observed.

Figure 26.7 shows the course of hemoglobin and blood cells during radionuclide therapy with [^{111}In-DTPA^0]octreotide. A transient effect on the number of white blood cells is observed, and an even greater effect on platelets. Renal func-

tion was monitored by measurements of serum creatinine and creatinine clearance (Fig. 26.8). If there is any effect on the kidney function, it is of no clinical relevance to date. Remarkably, average kidney function in the seven patients with creatinine clearance values between 21 and 80 mL/min before radionuclide therapy did not significantly change after cumulative doses of 20 to 30 GBq ($n = 4$) and 50 to 60 GBq ($n = 3$) with a maximum follow-up period of 2 years. Endocrine parameters of pituitary and pancreatic function during treatment cycles and follow-up after treatment with [^{111}In-DTPA^0]octreotide did not change either.

Impressive antiproliferative effects have been noted. An example is shown in Fig. 26.9. All 21 patients who subse-

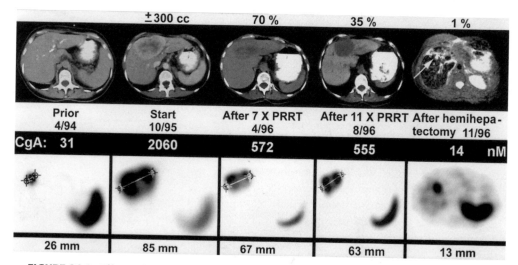

FIGURE 26.9. Effects of peptide receptor radionuclide therapy with [^{111}In-DTPA^0]octreotide in a patient with a hepatic metastasis of a neuroendocrine tumor, administered according to the described protocol. **Upper panel:** Transverse computed tomograms, except for 11/96 (magnetic resonance image). **Lower panel:** Transverse slices of ^{111}In-DTPA^0]octreotide single-photon emission computed tomograms. Also indicated are the chromogranin levels measured in the serum. The decline in tumor size (300 mL) was 30% after seven courses of treatment, and 65% after 11 courses. After 11 courses of treatment, the option of hemihepatectomy became feasible, and this procedure was carried out. A lesion 9 mm in diameter (magnetic resonance imaging) was left *in situ* at the cutting edge.

quently received a total cumulative dose of at least 20 GBq of ^{111}In-labeled [DTPA[0]]octreotide had progressive disease before the start of [^{111}In-DTPA[0]]octreotide therapy—that is, an unequivocal increase in tumor volume according to CT or MRI. In eight patients, treatment resulted in stable disease, and in another six patients it resulted in actual tumor shrinkage. Thus, an antiproliferative effect was noted in 14 of 21 patients with progressive disease who received an adequate dose of at least 20 GBq of [^{111}In-DTPA[0]]octreotide.

A response to treatment with [^{111}In-DTPA[0]]octreotide, based on antiproliferative effects and a lowering of tumor marker levels in serum and urine, was observed when (a) the cumulative therapeutic dose of [^{111}In-DTPA[0]]octreotide was at least about 20 GBq, and (b) tumor uptake was at least grade 2 (for stabilization of disease) and grade 3 or 4 (for reduction in tumor size) (Table 26.1). The observed responses to this radionuclide therapy are in agreement with those expected after internalization of [^{111}In-DTPA[0]]octreotide into tumor cells and an antiproliferative effect induced by electrons (59,60). In the clinical phase I study of therapy with [^{111}In-DTPA[0]]octreotide, only end-stage patients with (neuroendocrine) tumors expressing a homogeneous distribution of SSTRs and preferably a high accumulation of the radioligand were included. Based on our results with [^{111}In-DTPA[0]]octreotide scintigraphy, and given a relatively high accumulation of the radioligand in the tumor, it is anticipated that patients with gastroenteropancreatic metastatic tumors and paragangliomas, 30% of patients with malignant lymphomas, and 40% of those with small cell lung cancers may be candidates for this kind of treatment.

FUTURE TRENDS

New Somatostatin Analogues

Several reports have been published on binding to SSTRs *in vitro* of another somatostatin analogue, the octapeptide RC-160, with a structure very similar to that of octreotide (61–64). It has been reported that the affinity of RC-160 is higher than that of octreotide for SSTRs in human breast, ovarian, exocrine pancreatic, prostatic, and colonic cancer (61–63), which can be explained by the difference in binding between octreotide and RC-160 for SSTR4 [50% inhibitory concentration (IC$_{50}$) values of > 1,000 and 45 nM, respectively] (18). The binding of RC-160 to an SSTR subtype that does not bind octreotide offers a potential alternative to octreotide as a therapeutic radionuclide carrier ligand.

In our experiments, [^{111}In-DTPA[0]]RC-160 did not appear to have any advantages over [^{111}In-DTPA[0]]octreotide as a radiopharmaceutical for SSTR scintigraphy, despite the fact that [^{111}In-DTPA[0]]RC-160 demonstrates specific high-affinity binding to various SSTR-positive organs (65–67). Unlike radioiodinated RC-160, which crosses the blood–brain barrier, [^{111}In-DTPA[0]]RC-160 and [^{111}In-DTPA[0]]octreotide did not cross the blood–brain barrier in our exper-

iments. Compared with [^{111}In-DTPA[0]]octreotide, the main disadvantage of [^{111}In-DTPA[0]]RC-160 is its relatively low tumor-to-blood (background) ratio, implying poorer tumor detection *in vivo*.

We have recently evaluated and compared other ^{111}In-chelator–peptide constructs in terms of binding to octreotide receptors on mouse pituitary tumor cell membranes and internalization in rat pancreatic tumor cells. Biodistribution in tumor-bearing rats was also investigated. [DTPA[0],Tyr[3]]octreotide and [DTPA[0],Tyr[3]]octreotate (structures shown in Fig. 26.1) were tested. In octreotate, the carboxyl terminus threoninol has been replaced with the native amino acid threonine. Residues of Phe were replaced with Tyr to increase the hydrophilicity of the peptides. Furthermore, [DTPA[0],Tyr[3]]octreotate, with the carboxyl terminus threonine, was synthesized to investigate the effects of an additional negative charge on clearance and cellular uptake. [DOTA[0],Tyr[3]]octreotide was also synthesized (by Novartis and Professor H. Mäcke of Basel, Switzerland) and tested, as this compound provides stable radiolabeling with both ^{111}In and [90]Y (DOTA is tetraazacyclododecane tetraacetic acid). [90]Y emits beta particles; the maximum energy of the electrons is 2.3 MeV, and their mean range in tissue is a few millimeters. Radiolabeling and quality control procedures were mostly as described for [DTPA[0]]octreotide; for radiolabeling of [DOTA[0],Tyr[3]]octreotide, the mixture was heated for 25 minutes at 100°C.

In studies of receptor binding performed *in vitro*, all unlabeled compounds showed high levels of specific binding for the SSTRs, with IC$_{50}$ values in the low nanomolar range. [DOTA[0],Tyr[3]]octreotide showed the highest affinity of the compounds tested (68). Comparison of specific internalization of the ^{111}In-labeled compounds in two SSTR-positive cell lines showed that internalized radioactivity was by far the highest after incubation with [^{111}In-DTPA[0],Tyr[3]]octreotate (68). Also, in biodistribution experiments in SSTR2-positive CA20948 tumor-bearing rats, uptake in the SSTR2-expressing organs and tumor of ^{111}In-labeled [DTPA[0],Tyr[3]]octreotide, [DOTA[0],Tyr[3]]octreotide, and [DTPA[0],Tyr[3]]octreotate was significantly higher than that of [^{111}In-DTPA[0]]octreotide at the time points tested. [^{111}In-DTPA[0],Tyr[3]]octreotate showed the highest uptake in the SSTR2-positive organs of the ^{111}In-labeled peptides tested, also in agreement with results in the *in vitro* internalization studies. Uptake of this ^{111}In-labeled peptide in the SSTR2-positive target organs represented mostly specific binding to the octreotide receptors, as uptake was decreased to less than 7% of control by pretreatment of the rats with 0.5 mg of unlabeled octreotide. Clearance from the blood was rapid. We concluded that ^{111}In-labeled [DTPA[0],Tyr[3]]octreotide and [DTPA[0],Tyr[3]]octreotate and their DOTA-coupled counterparts are most promising for scintigraphy and radionuclide therapy of octreotide receptor-positive tumors in humans (68).

The first two human radionuclide therapy trials with [^{90}Y-DOTA[0],Tyr[3]]octreotide have started recently (69,70). Based on assumptions of 1% uptake, effective half-life equal to the physical half-life, and a similar biodistribution of [111]In- and ^{90}Y-labeled peptide, the estimated tumor radiation dose after an administered dose of 3.7 GBq of ^{90}Y-labeled peptide will be 16,500 cGy (10 g, 1% uptake) to 1,800 cGy (100 g, 1% uptake). Estimated tissue doses are 2,400 cGy for the kidneys, 150 cGy for the liver, and 1,400 cGy for the spleen. Because of the long path length of the therapeutic electrons, tumors with an inhomogeneous cellular distribution of SSTRs may respond in a favorable way to this treatment because of better a cross-fire effect in comparison with [111]In.

New Peptide Analogues Other than Somatostatin Analogues

Receptors for vasoactive intestinal peptide (VIP), a 28-amino acid neuroendocrine mediator, have been found in many tumors (71). VIP receptor scintigraphy might become a sensitive tool to detect primary tumors and their metastases. VIP receptor scintigraphy with ^{123}I-VIP has been reported (72). The theoretical application of VIP receptor scintigraphy based on results of autoradiography studies is very broad. However, some drawbacks to its possible use for peptide receptor scintigraphy are the requirements for in-house labeling with [123]I (expense and personnel logistics) and the intense accumulation of ^{123}I-VIP in lung during the first hours after injection. In our view, further use of this agent requires a chelated VIP analogue to allow for easier radiolabeling.

Receptor scintigraphy with ^{111}In-labeled DTPA-chelated substance P has mostly been performed in patients with autoimmune diseases (73). Substance P, an undecapeptide, belongs to a family of compounds known as *tachykinins*. This peptide acts as a neurotransmitter in the central nervous system. It has vasodilator potency and increases vascular permeability. Furthermore, it affects immune response and angiogenesis. Receptor autoradiography studies with radiolabeled substance P have shown positivity for the presence of substance P receptors in different tumor samples (74). In most tumors, the distribution of substance P receptors is nonhomogeneous. The role of substance P receptors in neuroendocrine tumors and the application of radiolabeled substance P ligands have not been established.

Bombesin is a high-affinity ligand for the gastrin-releasing peptide receptor. The gastrin-releasing peptide receptor has been found to be expressed in several tumors and tumor cell lines, including those of lung, prostate, and pancreas (75). The development of chelated bombesin/gastrin-releasing peptide analogues for use in nuclear medicine is in progress.

Cholecystokinin B, or gastrin, is another peptide of potential interest. Recently, the presence of cholecystokinin B (gastrin) receptors was demonstrated in more than 90% of medullary thyroid cancers. In addition, it has been identified in a high percentage of small cell lung cancers, stromal ovarian cancers, astrocytomas, and several other tumor types (76). Unlike SSTR expression in other neuroendocrine tumors, SSTR expression is rather low in medullary

thyroid cancer and completely absent in clinically aggressive forms (77,78). Therefore, the cholecystokinin B receptor represents a new and promising target for tumor scintigraphy and radionuclide therapy.

The so-called amino acid sequences in the complementarity-determining regions of the variable domains of monoclonal antibodies have been suggested as candidates for use in radiolabeled form for scintigraphy (79).

COMPARISON WITH OTHER MODALITIES

Scintigraphy with ^{111}In-DTPA[0]octreotide has been shown to localize well-differentiated and slowly growing neuroendocrine tumors (see above), whereas increased uptake of fluorodeoxyglucose (^{18}F-FDG) is associated with malignancy. Adams et al. (80,81) compared the effectiveness of positron emission tomography with ^{18}F-FDG (FDG-PET) and ^{111}In-DTPA[0]octreotide scintigraphy in detecting malignant neuroendocrine tumors in two studies. It was concluded that PET imaging of gastroenteropancreatic tumors reveals increased glucose metabolism only in undifferentiated gastroenteropancreatic tumors with high rates of proliferative activity. In assessing these tumors, FDG-PET should be performed if the results of ^{111}In-DTPA[0]octreotide scintigraphy are negative.

SUMMARY

Radiolabeled peptides are new ligands used for scintigraphy of neuroendocrine tumors. Their future application in tumor scintigraphy should be to indicate prognosis, not solely to assess localization, because other powerful alternatives are already available. An exception might be the demonstration or localization of recurrence, as it is questionable whether more sensitive technique(s) exist(s) to detect the recurrence of disease in an early phase. Peptide receptor radionuclide therapy in which radionuclides with appropriate particle ranges are used may become a new treatment modality. One might consider the use of radiolabeled somatostatin analogues in an adjuvant setting after surgery for SSTR-positive tumors to eradicate occult metastases, and to detect cancer recurrence at a later stage. Studies to find compounds that upregulate the tumor density of SSTRs *in vivo* have not been successful to date. The use of radiosensitizers may enhance the biologic effect of peptide receptor radionuclide therapy.

REFERENCES

1. Reubi J-C, Maurer R. Autoradiographic mapping of somatostatin receptors in the rat CNS and pituitary. *Neuroscience* 1982;15:1183–1193.
2. Patel YC, Amherdt M, Orci L. Quantitative electron microscopic autoradiography of insulin, glucagon and somatostatin binding on islets. *Science* 1982;217:1155–1156.
3. Sreedharan SP, Kodama KT, Peterson KE, et al. Distinct subset

of somatostatin receptors on cultured human lymphocytes. *J Biol Chem* 1989;264:949–953.

4. Brazeau P. Somatostatin: a peptide with unexpected physiologic activities. *Am J Med* 1986;81:8–13.

5. Lamberts SWJ, Uitterlinden P, Verschoor L, et al. Long-term treatment of acromegaly with the somatostatin analogue SMS 201-995. *N Engl J Med* 1985;313:1576–1580.

6. Lamberts SWJ. The role of somatostatin in the regulation of anterior pituitary hormone secretion and the use of its analogs in the treatment of human pituitary tumors. *Endocr Rev* 1988;9: 417–436.

7. Lamberts SWJ, Krenning EP, Reubi JC. The role of somatostain and its analogues in the diagnosis and treatment of tumors. *Endocr Rev* 1991;12:450–482.

8. Schally AV. Oncological applications of somatostatin analogues. *Cancer Res* 1988;48:6977–6985.

9. Kvols LK, Moertel CG, O'Connell MJ, et al. Treatment of malignant carcinoid syndrome. Evaluation of a long-acting somatostatin analogue. *N Engl J Med* 1986;315:663–666.

10. Krenning EP, Bakker WH, Breeman WAP, et al. Localization of endocrine-related tumours with radioiodinated analogue of somatostatin. *Lancet* 1989;1:242–245.

11. Bakker WH, Krenning EP, Breeman WAP, et al. Receptor scintigraphy with a radioiodinated somatostatin analogue: radiolabeling, purification, biologic activity, and *in vivo* application in animals. *J Nucl Med* 1990;31:1501–1509.

12. Bakker WH, Albert R, Bruns C, et al. [^{111}In-DTPA-D-Phe^1]octreotide, a potential radiopharmaceutical for imaging of somatostatin receptor-positive tumors: synthesis, radiolabeling and *in vitro* validation. *Life Sci* 1991;49:1583–1591.

13. Bakker WH, Krenning EP, Reubi J-C, et al. *In vivo* application of [^{111}In-DTPA-D-Phe^1]octreotide for detection of somatostatin receptor-positive tumors in rats. *Life Sci* 1991;49:1593–1601.

14. Krenning EP, Kwekkeboom DJ, Bakker WH, et al. Somatostatin receptor scintigraphy with [^{111}In-DTPA-D-Phe^1]- and [^{123}I-Tyr^3]-octreotide: the Rotterdam experience with more than 1,000 patients. *Eur J Nucl Med* 1993;20:716–731.

15. Bell GI, Riesine T. Molecular biology of somatostatin receptors. *Trends Neurosci* 1993;16:34–38.

16. Yamada Y, Kagimoto S, Kubota A, et al. Cloning, functional expression and pharmacological characterization of a fourth (hSSTR4) and a fifth (hSSTR5) human somatostatin receptor subtype. *Biochem Biophys Res Commun* 1993;195:844–852.

17. Bruno JF, Berelowitz M. Somatostatin receptors: orphan that found family and function. *Mol Cell Neurosci* 1993;4:307–309.

18. Patel YC, Greenwood MT, Panetta R, et al. The somatostatin receptor family. Mini review. *Life Sci* 1995;57:1249–1265.

19. Kubota A, Yamada Y, Kagimoto S, et al. Identification of somatostatin receptor subtypes and an implication for the efficacy of somatostatin analogus SMS 201–995 in treatment of human endocrine tumors. *J Clin Invest* 1994;93:1321–1325.

20. Schwarz AL, Fridovich SE, Lodish HF. Kinetics of internalization and recycling of the asialoglycoprotein receptor in hepatoma cell line. *J Biol Chem* 1982;257:4230–4237.

21. Weigel PH. Mechanisms and control of glyoconjugate turnover. In: Allen HJ, Kisaulis EC, eds. *Glycoconjugates: composition, structure and function.* New York: Marcel Dekker Inc, 1992, pp.421–497.

22. Duncan JR, Welch MJ. Intracellular metabolism of indium-111-DTPA-labeled receptor targeted proteins. *J Nucl Med* 1993;34: 1728–1738.

23. Morel G, Mesguich P, Dubois MP, et al. Ultrastructural evidence for endogenous somatostatin-like immunoreactivity in the pituitary gland. *Neuroendocrinology* 1983;36:291–299.

24. Morel G, Pelletier G, Heisler S. Internalization and subcellular distribution of radiolabeled somatostatin-28 in mouse anterior pituitary tumor cells. *Endocrinology* 1986;119:1972–1979.

25. Morel G, Leroux P, Pelletier G. Ultrastructural autoradiographic localization of somatostatin-28 in the rat anterior pituitary gland. *Endocrinology* 1985;116:1615–1619.

26. Amherdt M, Patel YC, Orci L. Binding and internalization of somatostatin, insulin, and glucagon by cultured rat islet cells. *J Clin Invest* 1989;84:412–417.

27. Draznin B, Sherman N, Sussman K, et al. Internalization and cellular processing of somatostatin in primary cultures of rat anterior pituitary cells. *Endocrinology* 1985;117:960–966.

28. Mentlein R, Buchholz C, Krisch B. Binding and internalization of gold-conjugated somatostatin and growth hormone-releasing hormone in cultured rat somatotropes. *Cell Tissue Res* 1989;258: 309–317.

29. Steiner C, Dahl R, Sherman N, et al. Somatostatin receptors are biologically active before they are inserted into the plasma membrane. *Endocrinology* 1986;118:766–772.

30. Sussman KE, Mehler PS, Leitner JW, et al. Role of the secretion vesicle in the transport of receptors: modulation of somatostatin binding to pancreatic islets. *Endocrinology* 1982;111:316–323.

31. Presky DH, Schonbrunn A. Receptor-bound somatostatin and epidermal growth factor are processed differently in GH$_4$C$_1$ rat pituitary cells. *J Cell Biol* 1986;102:878–888.

32. Sullivan SJ, Schonbrunn A. The processing of receptor-bound [^{125}I-Tyr^{1}1]somatostatin by RINm5F insulinoma cells. *J Biol Chem* 1986;261:3571–3577.

33. Andersson P, Forssel-Aronsson E, Johanson V, et al. Internalization of In-111 into human neuroendocrine tumor cells after incubation with indium-111-DTPA-D-Phe^{1}octreotide. *J Nucl Med* 1996;37:2002–2006.

34. De Jong M, Bernard HF, de Bruin E, et al. Internalization of radiolabeled [DTPA^0]octreotide and [DOTA^0,Tyr^3]octreotide: peptides for somatostatin receptor-targeted scintigraphy and radionuclide therapy. *Nucl Med Commun* 1998;19:283–288.

35. Hofland LJ, van Koetsveld PM, Waaijers M, et al. Internalization of the radioiodinated somatostatin analogue [^{125}I-Tyr^3]octreotide by mouse and human pituitary tumor cells: increase by unlabeled octreotide. *Endocrinology* 1995;136:3698–3706.

36. Duncan JR, Stephenson MI, Wu HP, et al. Indium-111-diethylenetriaminepentaacetic acid-octreotide is delivered *in vivo* to pancreatic tumor cell, renal, and hepatocyte lysosomes. *Cancer Res* 1997;57:659–671.

37. Dörr U, Wurm K, Höring E, et al. Diagnostic reliability of somatostatin receptor scintigraphy during continuous treatment with different somatostatin analogs. *Hormone Metabolic Res* 1992;27:36–43.

38. Dörr U, Räth U, Sautter-Bihl M-L, et al. Improved visualization of carcinoid liver metastases by indium-111 pentetreotide scintigraphy following treatment with cold somatostatin analogue. *Eur J Nucl Med* 1993;20:431–433.

39. Breeman WAP, Kwekkeboom DJ, Kooij PPM, et al. Effect of dose and specific activity on tissue distribution of In-111-pentetreotide in rats. *J Nucl Med* 1995;36:623–627.

40. Kooij PPM, Kwekkeboom DJ, Breeman WAP, et al. The effects of specific activity on tissue distribution of [^{111}In-DTPA-D-Phe^1]octreotide in humans. *J Nucl Med* 1994;35:226P.

41. Chiti A, Agresti R, Maffioli LS, et al. Breast cancer staging using technetium-99m sestamibi and indium-111 pentetreotide single-photon emission tomography. *Eur J Nucl Med* 1997;24:192–196.

42. Krenning EP, Bakker WH, Kooij PPM, et al. Somatostatin receptor scintigraphy with [^{111}In-DTPA-D-Phe^1]-octreotide in man: metabolism, dosimetry, and comparison with [^{123}I-Tyr^3]-octreotide. *J Nucl Med* 1992;33:652–658.

43. Krenning EP, Kwekkeboom DJ, Pauwels S, et al. Somatostatin receptor scintigraphy. In: Freeman LM, ed. *Nuclear medicine annual.* New York: Raven Press, 1995:1–50.

44. Lamberts SWJ, Hofland LJ, van Koetsveld PH, et al. Parallel *in*

vivo and *in vitro* detection of functional somatostatin receptors in human endocrine pancreatic tumors: consequences with regards to diagnosis, localization and therapy. *J Clin Endocr Metab* 1990;71: 566–574.

45. Gibril F, Reynolds JC, Doppman JL, et al. Somatostatin receptor scintigraphy: its sensitivity compared with that of other imaging methods in detecting primary and metastatic gastrinomas. *Ann Intern Med* 1996;125:26–34.

46. Termanini B, Gibril F, Reynolds JC, et al. Value of somatostatin receptor scintigraphy: a prospective study in gastrinoma of its effect on clinical management. *Gastroenterology* 1997;112:335–347.

47. Gibril F, Reynolds JC, Chen CC, et al. Specificity of somatostatin receptor scintigraphy: a prospective study and effects of false-positive localizations on management in patients with gastrinomas. *J Nucl Med* 1999;40:539–553.

48. Wheldon TE. Targeting radiation to tumours. *Int J Radiat Biol* 1994;65:109–116.

49. Hoefnagel CA. *The clinical use of ¹³¹I-meta-iodobenzylguanidine (MIBG) for the diagnosis and treatment of neural crest tumours* [Thesis]. University of Amsterdam, 1989.

50. Bambynek W, Craseman B, Fink RW. X-ray fluorescence yields, Auger and Coster-Kronig transition probabilities. *Rev Phys* 1972; 44:716–813.

51. Auger P. Sur l'effet photoélectrique composé. *J Phys Radium* 1925; 6:205.

52. Bakker WH, Breeman WAP, van der Pluijm ME, et al. Iodine-131 labelled octreotide: not an option for somatostatin receptor therapy. *Eur J Nucl Med* 1996;23:775–781.

53. Krenning EP, Kooij PPM, Bakker WH, et al. Radiotherapy with a radiolabeled somatostatin analogue, [¹¹¹In-DTPA-D-Phe¹]-octreotide. A case history. *Ann N Y Acad Sci* 1994;733:496–506.

54. Krenning EP, Kooij PPM, Pauwels S, et al. Somatostatin receptor: scintigraphy and radionuclide therapy. *Digestion* 1996;57:57–61.

55. Krenning EP, de Jong M, Kooij PPM, et al. Radiolabelled somatostatin analogue(s) for peptide receptor scintigraphy and radionuclide therapy. *Ann Oncol* 1999;10:S23.

56. De Jong M, Rolleman EJ, Bernard HF, et al. Inhibition of renal uptake of indium-111 DTPA-octreotide *in vivo*. *J Nucl Med* 1996; 37:1388–1392.

57. Bernard HF, Krenning EP, Breeman WAP, et al. D-Lysine for reduction of renal [¹¹¹In-DTPA⁰,D-Phe¹]octreotide and [⁹⁰Y-DTPA⁰,D-Phe¹,Tyr³]octreotide uptake. *J Nucl Med* 1997;38:1929–1933.

58. Hammond PJ, Wade AF, Gwilliam ME, et al. Amino acid infusion blocks renal tubular uptake of an indium-labelled somatostatin analogue. *Br J Cancer* 1993;67:1437–1439.

59. Fjalling M, Andersson P, Forssell-Aronsson E, et al. Systemic radionuclide therapy using indium-111-DTPA-D-Phe¹-octreotide in midgut carcinoid syndrome. *J Nucl Med* 1996;37:1519–1521.

60. McCarthy KE, Lemen L, Espenan G, et al. Dose-escalation of indium-111 pentetreotide (Somatother): toxicity and clinical response. *Clin Nucl Med* 1999;24:213.

61. Srkalovic G, Cai R-Z, Schally AV. Evaluation of receptors for somatostatin in various tumors using different analogs. *J Clin Endocrinol Metab* 1990;70:661–669.

62. Liebow C, Reilly C, Serrano M, et al. Somatostatin analogues inhibit growth of pancreatic cancer by stimulating tyrosine phosphatase. *Proc Natl Acad Sci U S A* 1989;86:2003–2007.

63. Pinski J, Milovanovic TY, Hamaoui A, et al. Biological activity and receptor binding characteristics to various human tumors of acetylated somatostatin receptors. *Proc Soc Exp Biol Med* 1992;200: 49–56.

64. Reubi JC, Schaer C, Waser B, et al. Expression and localization of somatostatin receptor SSTR1, SSTR2, and SSTR3 messenger RNAs in primary human tumors using *in situ* hybridization. *Cancer Res* 1994;54:3455–3459.

65. Breeman WAP, Hofland LJ, Bakker WH, et al. Radioiodinated somatostatin analogue RC-160: preparation, biological activity, *in vivo* application in rats and comparison with [¹²³I-Tyr³]octreotide. *Eur J Nucl Med* 1993;20:1089–1094.

66. Breeman WAP, Hofland LJ, van der Pluijm M, et al. A new radiolabeled somatostatin analogue [¹¹¹In-DTPA-D-Phe¹]RC-160: preparation, biological activity, receptor scintigraphy in rats and comparison with [¹¹¹In-DTPA-D-Phe¹]octreotide. *Eur J Nucl Med* 1994;21:328–335.

67. Breeman WAP, Hagen PM van, Kwekkeboom DJ, et al. Somatostatin receptor scintigraphy using [¹¹¹In-DTPA⁰]RC-160 in humans: a comparison with [¹¹¹In-DTPA⁰]octreotide. *Eur J Nucl Med* 1998;25:182–186.

68. De Jong M, Breeman WAP, Bakker WH, et al. Comparison of ¹¹¹In-labeled somatostatin-analogs for tumor scintigraphy and radionuclide therapy. *Cancer Res* 1998;58:437–441.

69. Otte A, Jermann E, Behe M, et al. Dotatoc: a powerful new tool for receptor-mediated radionuclide therapy. *Eur J Nucl Med* 1997; 24:792–795.

70. Otte A, Mueller-Brand J, Dellas S, et al. Yttrium-90 labeled somatostatin analogue for cancer treatment. *Lancet* 1998;351: 417–418.

71. Reubi JC. *In vitro* identification of vasoactive intestinal peptide receptors in human tumors: implication for tumor imaging. *J Nucl Med* 1995;36:1846–1853.

72. Virgolini I, Raderer M, Kurtaran A, et al. Vasoactive intestinal peptide-receptor imaging for the localization of intestinal adenocarcinomas and endocrine tumors. *N Engl J Med* 1994;331: 1116–1121.

73. VanHagen PM, Breeman WAP, Reubi JC, et al. Visualization of the thymus by substance P receptor scintigraphy in man. *Eur J Nucl Med* 1996;23:1508–1513.

74. Hennig IM, Laissue JA, Horisberger O, et al. Substance-P receptors in human primary neoplasms: tumoral and vascular localization. *Int J Cancer* 1995;61:786–792.

75. Markwalder R, Reubi JC. Gastrin-releasing peptide receptors in the human prostate: relation to neoplastic transformation. *Cancer Res* 1999;59:1152–1159.

76. Reubi JC, Schaer JC, Waser B. Cholecystokinin (CCK)-A and CCK-B/gastrin receptor in human tumors. *Cancer Res* 1997;57: 1377–1386.

77. Reubi JC, Chayvialle JA, Franc B, et al. Somatostatin receptors and somatostatin content in medullary thyroid carcinomas. *Lab Invest* 1991;64:567–573.

78. Kwekkeboom DJ, Reubi JC, Lamberts SWJ, et al. *In vivo* somatostatin receptor imaging in medullary thyroid carcinoma. *J Clin Endocrinol Metab* 1993;76:1413–1417.

79. Sivolapenko GB, Douli V, Pectasides D, et al. Breast cancer imaging with radiolabeled peptide from complementarity-determining region of antitumour antibody. *Lancet* 1995;346:1662–1666.

80. Adams S, Baum R, Rink T, et al. Limited value of fluorine-18 fluordeoxyglucose positron emission tomography for the imaging of neuroendocrine tumours. *Eur J Nucl Med* 1998;25:79–83.

81. Adams S, Baum RP, Hertel A, et al. Metabolic (PET) and receptor (SPET) imaging of well- and less well-differentiated tumours: comparison with the expression of the Ki-67 antigen. *Nucl Med Commun* 1998;19:641–647.

27

PRIMARY HEPATIC TUMORS: RECEPTOR IMAGING AND DIFFERENTIAL DIAGNOSIS

IRENE J. VIRGOLINI
AMIR KURTARAN

EPIDEMIOLOGY OF PRIMARY HEPATIC TUMORS

Tumors of the liver are among the most common malignancies in the world. In high-incidence countries such as China or Korea, the annual death rates are as high as 23/100,000 to 150/100,000, whereas in low-incidence countries such as the United States, the annual death rate is about 2/100,000 (1). In Asia and Africa, the high incidence rates have been associated with high rates of chronic hepatitis B carriage or hepatitis C virus infection, but ethnic factors also appear to be important (2,3). A large variety of hepatic carcinogens have been intensively investigated. For example, data on aflatoxin B1 (a product of *Aspergillus* fungus) contamination of foodstuffs correlate well with incidence rates reported for Africa and China (4). A considerable body of literature exists on the hepatic carcinogenicity of anabolic steroids, and on the role of estrogens in the induction of benign hepatic adenomas (5). Furthermore, a strong association of hepatocellular cancer (HCC) with underlying cirrhosis has been long recognized (6).

From 85% to 95% of all tumors of the liver are malignant epithelial neoplasms. From 6% to 12% are benign and are also largely of epithelial origin. About 1% to 3% are malignant mesenchymal tumors (7). Many other tumors have a propensity to metastasize to the liver or the adjacent biliary tree as a result of hematogenous spread through the portal vein or hepatic artery. The most frequent tumors that metastasize to the liver include melanomas and gallbladder, colon, pancreas, lung, and breast carcinomas (7). Metastatic tumors are often peripheral and multiple, whereas primary hepatic tumors are more often central and solitary.

THE HEPATOCYTE AND ITS TARGET RECEPTORS FOR SCINTIGRAPHY

The liver is the largest organ of the body (with the exception of the skin) and is responsible for gathering, transforming, and accumulating metabolites, and for neutralizing and eliminating toxic substances. The liver epithelial cell, the hepatocyte, is at the same time a cell with endocrine and exocrine functions. The hepatocyte synthesizes proteins for its own maintenance and various other proteins for export, such as albumin, prothrombin, or fibrinogen of the blood plasma. In addition to the hepatocytes, the liver contains reticuloendothelial cells, known as Kupffer's cells, that are active in the phagocytosis and metabolism of a variety of particles and macroaggregates. Most interestingly, the liver is able to increase its numbers of cells after surgical removal or after damage by toxins or disease. Several molecular signals regulate liver cell growth (8). Mitogens producing hepatocyte proliferation include HGF (hepatocyte growth factor), EGF (epidermal growth factor), TGF-α (transforming growth factor-α) and FGF (fibroblast growth factor). Growth inhibitory substances have also been identified, such as IL-1α (interleukin 1α) and retinoic acid.

The Asialoglycoprotein Receptor (Hepatic Binding Protein)

In 1968, Morell and colleagues (9) discovered a liver cell surface receptor specific for asialoglycoproteins. This surface receptor, also called *hepatic binding protein* (HBP), is hepatocyte-specific. Based on the significant role of the receptor in hepatic physiology, Vera et al. (10,11) pro-

I. J. Virgolini: Departments of Experimental Nuclear Medicine and Internal Medicine, Lainz Hospital of the City of Vienna, A-1130 Vienna, Austria.

A. Kurtaran: Department of Nuclear Medicine, Vienna University Hospital, A-1090 Vienna, Austria.

posed this receptor as a basis for hepatic imaging. A series of analogue ligands of asialoglycoproteins have evolved. One ligand is obtained by attaching a galactosyl unit to human serum albumin (HSA); the resulting galactosyl neoglycoalbumin (NGA) can be radiolabeled with ^{99m}Tc (10–15). After binding at the hepatocyte membrane, the ligand–receptor complex is internalized and transported to hepatic lysosomes, where the ligand is degraded and catabolized. The receptor is subsequently recycled to the cell surface (16,17). ^{99m}Tc-NGA follows the same pathway as the native ligand–receptor complex. Another ligand analogue, ^{99m}Tc-human serum galactosyl albumin (GSA), is now commercially available for routine clinical use in Japan (18,19). These two agents differ in the number of galactose groups attached to the serum albumin molecule. Both ^{99m}Tc-NGA and ^{99m}Tc-GSA have proved clinically useful in patients with liver disease.

The principal of NGA/GSA receptor binding is a second-order reaction, demonstrated by saturability of the reaction. Hence, hepatic uptake is sensitive to alterations in the HBP receptor concentration and is dose-dependent, affinity-dependent, and hepatic plasma flow-dependent. Healthy liver tissue is an efficient and active system for the removal of desialylated glycoproteins from the circulation. In patients with chronic liver disease, such as hepatitis or cirrhosis, the binding of desialylated glycoproteins to the HBP receptors is thought to be inhibited by another heterologous population of glycoproteins (20). Clinical studies have shown that the hepatic uptake of ^{99m}Tc-NGA/GSA gives a fairly good indication of the residual functional liver capacity (21–24). Other studies have shown that the densities of HBP receptors are reduced by *in vitro* chemical hepatocellular injury (25). In the case of ^{99m}Tc-NGA, receptor binding can be subdivided into high-affinity and low-affinity sites (15). Receptor-mediated binding and subsequent cellular endocytosis do not occur in HCC (21,24) or metastatic tumors (26) because the receptors are lost during malignant dedifferentiation.

The Hepatocyte Insulin Receptor

Insulin stimulates a growth response in a variety of cell types. Autoradiographic studies have demonstrated that insulin binds to hepatocytes and, to a lesser extent, to the hematopoietic cells of the liver (27). With the use of ^{123}I-/^{131}I-labeled insulin, a new dimension is added to the *in vivo* study of insulin kinetics and metabolism in both diabetic and nondiabetic subjects (28). In recent years, hepatoma cell lines have been used as models for the study of insulin–insulin receptor interactions. In hepatoma, a remarkably higher number of specific ^{123}I-Tyr-(A14)-insulin receptors was identified. Whereas normal liver tissue

binds about 3 pmol of ^{123}I-Tyr-(A14)-insulin per milligram of protein (K_d, 5 nM), hepatoma tissue binds about 1,500 pmol of ^{123}I-Tyr-(A14)-insulin per milligram of protein (K_d, 5 nM) (27). Hence, insulin appears to be a specific growth factor for hepatoma cells. Based on these *in vitro* studies, radiolabeled insulin has been suggested as a potential imaging agent for the noninvasive visualization of hepatoma (26–32).

Other Hepatocyte Receptors

A large variety of other hepatocyte receptors have been described. Receptors for somatostatin (SST) and vasoactive intestinal peptide (VIP) are overexpressed on certain secondary hepatic malignancies, but not on primary hepatomas. In fact, ^{123}I-VIP has proved useful for the visualization of metastatic spread from colorectal or pancreatic cancer (33,34). Long-acting SST analogues that preferentially bind to neuroendocrine tumors, such as radiolabeled octreotide (35) or lanreotide (36), may be clinically useful for the differentiation of certain liver lesions (37). Radiolabeled lanreotide, however, does not bind to HCC *in vivo* (38).

METHODOLOGY FOR SCINTIGRAPHIC IMAGING

NGA/GSA Receptor Scintigraphy

^{99m}Tc-NGA or ^{99m}Tc-GSA (approximately 50 nmol; 150 to 200 MBq of ^{99m}Tc) should be injected as a slow intravenous bolus. Planar and single-photon computed tomographic (SPECT) images are to be obtained with a general-purpose low-energy collimator (140 keV). Planar images of the liver should be obtained (anterior, posterior, and right lateral) with a matrix of 256 x 256 pixels. Three hundred to five hundred kilocounts should be acquired. SPECT images should be obtained with a matrix of 128 x 128 pixels, 360 degrees, 6 degrees per step, 60 seconds per step. SPECT imaging is recommended for precise correlation of suspected lesions with results of computed tomography (CT) and magnetic resonance imaging (MRI). The imaging procedures can be performed 10 minutes after the injection. Delayed acquisitions are not necessary.

Insulin Receptor Scintigraphy

Insulin radioiodinated at the tyrosine in position A14 [^{123}I-Tyr-(A14)-insulin] is the most frequently used insulin radioligand (27). The specific activity of ^{123}I-Tyr-(A14)-insulin should be about 150 MBq/10 μg (i.e., 1 IU). Product identity and radiochemical purity above 98% should be established by high-performance liquid chromatography. Patients must receive thyroid gland blockade. After slow intravenous bolus injection, planar images of the liver in anterior, posterior, and right lateral views (256 x 256 matrix, 300 kilocounts) are obtained at 10 minutes after the injection. Images should be obtained with gamma camera that has a large field of view and is equipped with a low-energy, general-purpose collimator. SPECT imaging should be performed with the following parameters: matrix of 64 x 64 pixels, 45 to 60 seconds per projection, 360 degrees, 6 degrees per step.

RESULTS

NGA/GSA Receptor Scintigraphy

Immediately after injection, ^{99m}Tc-NGA/GSA generates a hepatic image. In subjects with normal liver function, the liver is the exclusive site of tracer uptake, which exceeds 95% of the injected dose as early as 10 minutes after injection. The main excretory route of radioactivity is the biliary system; urinary excretion is low (21–24).

The last 15 years have demonstrated that ^{99m}Tc-NGA/GSA scintigraphy is useful for the differentiation of focal liver masses. Liver uptake can be remarkably delayed and reduced in patients with a variety of liver diseases, reflecting the functional status of the hepatocyte. As receptor-mediated binding and subsequent cellular endocytosis do not occur in HCC or metastatic tumors, a lack of receptor binding of ^{99m}Tc-NGA/GSA is anticipated. HCC lesions and metastatic tumor spread from adenocarcinomas are therefore demonstrated as focal defects (cold spots) (27). Benign nodules, such as focal nodular hyperplasia (FNH) (39) and adenomatous hyperplasia (40), and macroregenerating nodules (24) contain normal functioning hepatocytes and exhibit "normal" or increased tracer uptake.

In our own more recent studies, ^{99m}Tc-NGA scintigraphy was prospectively applied to differential diagnosis in 125 patients with focal liver lesions (27,39). Final diagnosis of the lesions was obtained histopathologically. Sixty-five patients had HCC, 15 had FNH, and the remaining 35 had metastatic spread from gastrointestinal carcinomas. All HCC lesions were identified as focal defects (cold spots) on ^{99m}Tc-NGA scintigrams, which indicated the absence of HBP receptors (21) (Fig. 27.1; see also Color Plate 9 following p. 350). Likewise, all metastatic lesions showed up as cold spots on ^{99m}Tc-NGA scintigrams, which indicated the lack of HBP receptors (Fig. 27.2; see also Color Plate 10 following p. 350). In contrast, all lesions of FNH (Fig.3) showed a normal or increased accumulation of ^{99m}Tc-NGA (38). In fact, initial studies at the University of Vienna (22) had already indicated that kinetic modeling (24) estimates normal *in vivo* receptor densities in patients with FNH, and nearly normal densities in patients with liver fibrosis. A distinction between metastases and HCC by ^{99m}Tc-NGA/GSA scintigraphy alone is not possible.

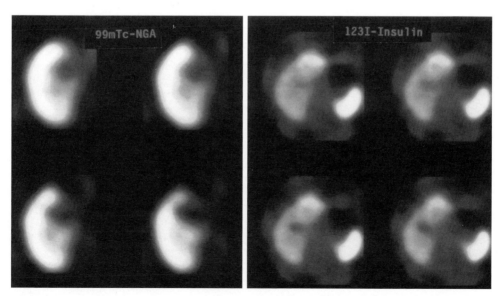

FIGURE 27.1. Hepatocellular cancer. ^{99m}Tc-NGA (galactosyl neoglycoalbumin) scintigraphy shows a significant cold spot (*left panel*) in the left lobe of the liver (single-photon emission computed tomography, transverse view) with a corresponding accumulation in the lesion of ^{123}I-Tyr-(A14)-insulin (*right panel*). (See also Color Plate 9 following p. 350.)

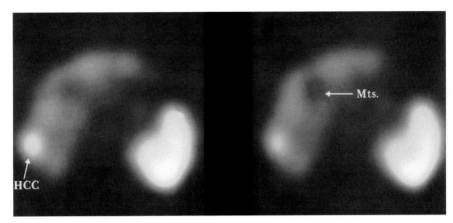

FIGURE 27.2. Visualization of a hepatocellular cancer (*HCC*) lesion and of a colonic adenocarcinoma metastasis in a patient by ^{123}I-Tyr-(A14)-insulin scintigraphy (single-photon emission computed tomography, transverse view). Whereas HCC shows a significantly increased accumulation of ^{123}I-Tyr-(A14)-insulin, no accumulation of tracer is seen over the colonic adenocarcinoma metastasis. (See also Color Plate 10 following p. 350.)

Insulin Receptor Scintigraphy for the Differential Diagnosis of Hepatic Lesions

After the intravenous administration of ^{123}I-Tyr-(A14)-insulin, the liver is the major organ of tracer uptake, whereas the pancreas and the kidneys show a faint accumulation. Peak accumulation of ^{123}I-Tyr-(A14)-insulin appears to correlate with receptor activity in the liver cells. The uptake of ^{123}I-Tyr-(A14)-insulin reaches a maximum about 10 minutes after injection; thereafter, hepatic activity rapidly declines. The decrease in radioactivity is associated with a release of free iodine secondary to the relatively rapid hepatic degradation of radiolabeled insulin (28). In patients with HCC, insulin uptake by tumor lesions is higher than uptake in the surrounding normal liver. On average, the hepatoma-to-normal liver ratio is about 1.5 at maximum uptake (27).

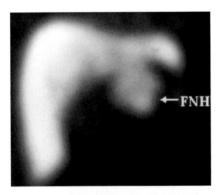

FIGURE 27.3. Focal nodular hyperplasia (*FNH*). ^{99m}Tc-NGA (galactosyl neoglycoalbumin) scintigraphy of the liver (single-photon emission computed tomography, transverse view) demonstrates a significantly increased accumulation of tracer in an FNH lesion (*arrow*), which indicates the presence of hepatic binding protein receptors.

Thus, the use of ^{123}I-Tyr-(A14)-insulin allows direct imaging of the liver by a receptor-mediated process. The rationale for using ^{123}I-Tyr-(A14)-insulin to visualize hepatoma is based on observations that hepatomas express a 1,000-fold higher number of specific receptors for ^{123}I-Tyr-(A14)-insulin than normal liver tissue does. Consequently, hepatomas show an accumulation of ^{123}I-Tyr-(A14)-insulin that is normal or even increased, whereas other malignant liver lesions appear as cold spots (Fig. 27.2). At our institution, ^{123}I-Tyr-(A14)-insulin scintigraphy was recently performed in 55 patients with hepatoma and 40 patients with metastatic spread from nonhepatic tumors. Normal or increased accumulation of ^{123}I-Tyr-(A14)-insulin in all but two hepatoma lesions indicated the presence of insulin receptors. In contrast, no accumulation of ^{123}I-Tyr-(A14)-insulin was observed in metastatic lesions. This finding can be used in the noninvasive differentiation of hepatoma from other malignant liver lesions (27).

Dual Tracer Technique

When a defect is detected by ^{99m}Tc-NGA/GSA scintigraphy, a second study is needed to characterize the cold nodule further. Recently, in a dual receptor–tracer method, ^{123}I-Tyr-(A14)-insulin and ^{99m}Tc-NGA were used successfully to evaluate liver masses (27).

If a focal defect detected on an NGA scan is caused by HCC, it accumulates insulin because HCC expresses receptors for insulin (Fig. 27.4; see also Color Plate 11 following p. 350). A matched defect, however, indicates the presence of metastatic spread. This dual receptor–tracer method could play an important role in the differential diagnosis of masses seen on ultrasonography or CT; if a liver lesion detected on ultrasonography, CT, or MRI accumulates

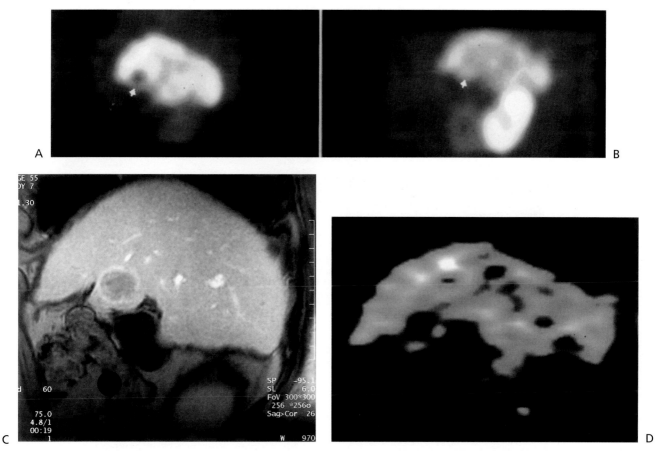

FIGURE 27.4. ^{99m}Tc-NGA (galactosyl neoglycoalbumin) scintigraphy (*left upper panel*; single-photon emission computed tomography, sagittal view) in a patient with hepatocellular cancer (*HCC*) demonstrates no accumulation of tracer in the lesion seen on magnetic resonance imaging (*left lower panel*). After administration of ^{123}I-Tyr-(A14)-insulin, accumulation is seen over the lesion (*right upper panel*), as HCC expresses insulin receptors. Positron emission tomography with ^{18}F-fluorodeoxyglucose (*right lower panel*) in the same patient reveals a cold spot over the lesion. (See also Color Plate 11 following p. 350.)

^{99m}Tc-NGA, a malignancy is unlikely. Normal accumulation of ^{99m}Tc-NGA in the lesion may indicate FNH or other benign lesions. If ^{99m}Tc-NGA scintigraphy demonstrates a cold spot over the lesion seen on ultrasonography, CT, or MRI, then the second radiotracer, ^{123}I-Tyr-(A14)-insulin, is needed. Accumulation of ^{123}I-Tyr-(A14)-insulin (normal or increased) in the lesion indicates a hepatoma, whereas a matched defect indicates the presence of metastases from nonhepatic tumors (Figs. 27.2 and 27.4).

LIMITATION AND PITFALLS OF SCINTIGRAPHY

The radiopharmaceutical ^{99m}Tc-NGA is highly specific for the liver. Whereas ^{99m}Tc-NGA scintigraphy shows an

excellent distribution of tracer in the noncirrhotic liver, the distribution of ^{99m}Tc-NGA can be heterogeneous, sometimes very patchy, in the cirrhotic liver. Therefore, the distinction between malignant lesions and cirrhotic areas may be difficult, and a correlation study with CT, MRI, or ultrasonography is essential. Additionally, the differentiation of hemangioma from malignant liver lesions is not possible, as neither lesion accumulates ^{99m}Tc-NGA. This problem can be solved by using ^{99m}Tc-red blood cell scintigraphy (Fig. 27.5).

The interpretation of ^{123}I-Tyr-(A14)-insulin images without ^{99m}Tc-NGA findings is difficult because of the relatively high nontarget accumulation of ^{123}I-Tyr-(A14)-insulin in the kidneys and intestine. For a precise interpretation of the lesions, an insulin SPECT study is therefore needed.

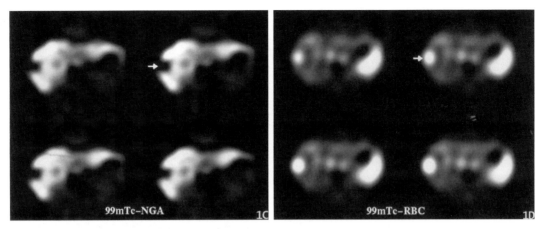

FIGURE 27.5. Hemangioma. ^{99m}Tc-NGA (galactosyl neoglycoalbumin) scintigraphy (*left panel;* single-photon emission computed tomography, transverse view) shows a cold spot in the right liver, demonstrating a lack of hepatic binding protein receptors. Corresponding ^{99m}Tc-red blood cell scintigraphy (*right panel;* single-photon emission computed tomography, transverse view) reveals a hot spot over the lesion, indicating liver hemangioma.

ROLE OF [99M]TC-NGA/GSA IMAGING IN DIAGNOSIS AND PATIENT MANAGEMENT

An accurate estimation of the residual functional capacity of the liver in patients with malignant liver lesions (HCC or metastases) is essential before surgical resection is performed (41). This is especially true for patients with HCC, which is frequently associated with liver cirrhosis in endemic regions. An inadequate estimation of functional liver capacity can lead to hepatic failure postoperatively. Another important role of ^{99m}Tc-NGA/GSA kinetic imaging is in the noninvasive evaluation of liver functional capacity in patients with liver metastases who are undergoing chemotherapy. This method can provide valuable information about residual liver function and can be used to follow patients during the course of disease (21). Finally, the method can be used to demonstrate the effectiveness of chemotherapy and radiotherapy.

COMPARISON WITH OTHER METHODS

The major clinical problem is the differentiation of benign liver lesions, including FNH, from malignant lesions. FNH is a benign hepatic tumor that characteristically occurs in women of reproductive age and is often discovered incidentally (42). A large number of imaging modalities have been used to evaluate FNH lesions. The differential diagnosis of FNH and malignant liver lesions, however, continues to pose a diagnostic challenge. Ultrasonography, CT, and MRI are sensitive but do not clearly differentiate benign lesions, including FNH, from primary hepatic malignancies (42). Ultrasonography can be considered only a screening technique (43); it offers no tissue specificity (44), as FNH may appear hypoechoic, hyperechoic, or even isoechoic (43).

The CT characteristic of FNH is variably reported to be hyperdense or hypodense, and most lesions are hypervascular with intravenous contrast enhancement (45). Although most investigators agree that CT is the initial imaging procedure of choice for the detection of liver lesions (46), the sensitivity of routine CT is poor for detecting small liver lesions (45). It cannot reliably distinguish FNH from HCC in small lesions. Routine MRI is frequently not successful in identifying small liver lesions. The best imaging procedure for the diagnosis of FNH may be enhanced MRI, which has a sensitivity of 70% and a specificity of 98% (43). When the characteristic triad of isointensity on T_1- and T_2-weighted sequences, lesion homogeneity, and a central hyperintense scar on T_2-weighted sequences is present, the diagnosis of FNH can be considered certain.

Although the anatomic resolution of ultrasonography, CT, and MRI is superior, they cannot reliably differentiate between several types of liver masses (46). In this situation, scintigraphic methods based on a combination of radiotracers can help yield a specific diagnosis. The most helpful finding is evidence of normal or increased uptake of ^{99m}Tc-sulfur colloid (^{99m}Tc-SC) in an area of FNH, which is based on the presence of Kupffer cells. ^{99m}Tc-SC scintigraphy is nonspecific, however, and shows focal defects in about 30% to 35% of patients with FNH (45). The distinction between FNH and hepatic malignancies may not be possible with this pattern (43). A cold nodule by ^{99m}Tc-SC scintigraphy may be a cyst or an anatomic variant. For further characterization of cold nodules on ^{99m}Tc-SC scintigraphy, ^{67}Ga citrate scintigraphy has been proposed, as HCC may concentrate [67]Ga. However, this technique also has limitations because one third of patients with HCC fail to take up ^{67}Ga citrate. On the other hand, occasional accumulation of ^{67}Ga in non-HCC lesions can lead to false-positive findings. The hepatobiliary tracer trimethylbromoiminodiacetic acid (TBIDA) labeled with ^{99m}Tc is useful in some cases (43). Although FNH demonstrates a typical pattern by this method in most patients, liver metastases or HCC occasionally exhibits a scintigraphic uptake pattern similar to that of FNH (47).

CONCLUSIONS AND FUTURE TRENDS

For the past 20 years, fundamental and clinical research on ^{99m}Tc-NGA/GSA imaging and quantification has been pursued. A significant number of preclinical and clinical articles on the use of this receptor agent have been published. In addition to demonstrating functional hepatic mass under a variety of clinical conditions (21–23,25), NGA/GSA scintigraphy plays an important role in differentiating benign from malignant hepatic lesions. An important development affecting NGA/GSA scintigraphy in the differential diagnosis of liver masses and the quantitative estimation of liver function will be the development of positron emission tomography (PET) tracers. Vera et al. (48) have already introduced ^{68}Ga-deferoxamine-NGA and reported promising results in experimental animals. Radiolabeled insulin also appears to be a potential agent for the evaluation of liver masses. Another role for radiolabeled insulin may be in the use of beta-emitting nuclides as therapeutic agents for tumors expressing insulin receptors. Finally, the use of radiolabeled insulin-like growth factor and other insulin-associated hormones may provide additional diagnostic opportunities for the visualization of hepatic lesions (49).

REFERENCES

1. Simonetti RG, Camma C, Fiorella F, et al. Hepatocellular carcinoma. *Dig Dis Sci* 1991;36:962–972.
2. Lutwick LI. Relation between aflatoxins and hepatitis B virus and hepatocellular carcinoma. *Lancet* 1979; :755.
3. Beasley RP, Hwang LY, Lin CC, et al. Hepatocellular carcinoma and hepatitis virus: a prospective study of 22,707 men in Taiwan. *Lancet* 1981;2:1129.
4. Linsell CA. Environmental chemical carcinogens and liver cancer. In: Laspis K, Johannessen JV, eds. *Liver carcinogenesis*. Hemisphere Publishing, 1979.
5. Henderson BE, Preston-Martin S, Edmondson HA. Hepatocellular carcinoma and oral contraceptives. *Br J Cancer* 1983;48:437.
6. Tirebell C, Malato M, Croce LS, et al. Prevalence of hepatocellular carcinoma and relation to cirrhosis. *Hepatology* 1989;10:789–1002.
7. Albores-Saavedra J, Henson DE. Tumors of the gallbladder and extra-hepatic bile ducts. In: Craig JR, Peter RI, Edwardson HA, eds. *Tumors of the liver and intrahepatic bile ducts*. Washington, DC: Armed Forces Institute of Pathology, Fascicles 22 and 26, 1989.
8. Michalopoulos GK. Liver regeneration: molecular mechanisms of growth control. *FASEB J* 1990;4:176–193.
9. Morrel AG, Irvine RA, Sternlieb I, et al. Physical and chemical studies on ceruloplasmin. V. Metabolic studies on sialic acid-free cerulo-plasmin *in vivo*. *J Biol Chem* 1968;243:155–159.
10. Vera DR, Krohn KA, Stadalnik RC. Radioligands that bind to cell-specific receptors: hepatic binding protein ligands for hepatic scintigraphy. In: Sorenson JA, ed. *Radiopharmaceuticals II*. New York: Society of Nuclear Medicine, 1979:565–575.
11. Krohn KA, Vera DR, Steffen SM. Tc 99m Neogalactoalbumin: a general model for some bifunctional carbohydrates. *J Labeled Compound Radiopharm* 1981;18:91–93.
12. Vera DR, Krohn KA, Stadalnik RC, et al. Tc-99m-galactosyl-neoglycoalbumin: *in vivo* characterization of receptor-mediated binding to hepatocytes. *Radiology* 1984;151:191–196.
13. Vera DR, Krohn KA, Stadalnik RC, et al. Tc 99m galactosyl-neoglycoalbumin: *in vitro* characterization of receptor-mediated binding to hepatocytes. *J Nucl Med* 1984;25:779–787.
14. Vera DR, Stadalnik RC, Krohn KA. Technetium-99m-galactosyl-neoglycoalbumin: preparation and preclinical studies. *J Nucl Med* 1985;26:1157–1167
15. Virgolini I, Angelberger P, Müller C, et al. ^{99m}Tc-Neoglycoalbumin (NGA)-binding to human hepatic binding protein (HBP) *in vitro*. *Br J Clin Pharmacol* 1990;29:207–214.
16. Steer CJ, Ashwell G. Studies on a mammalian hepatic binding protein specific for asialoglycoproteins: evidence for receptor recycling in isolated rat hepatocytes. *J Biol Chem* 255:3008–3013.
17. Stockert RJ, Morell AG. Hepatic binding protein: the galactose receptor of mammalian hepatocytes. *Hepatology* 1983;2:750–757.
18. Kawa S, Hazama H, Kojima M, et al. A new liver function test using asialo-glycoprotein-receptor system on the liver cell membrane. II. Quantitative evaluation of labeled neoglycoprotein albumin. *Jpn J Nucl Med* 1986;23:907–916.
19. Torizuka K, Kawa SKH, Kudo M, et al. Phase III multicenter clinical study on Tc 99m GSA, a new agent for functional imaging of the liver. *Jpn J Nucl Med* 1992;29:159–181.
20. Marshall JS, Stockert W. Serum inhibitors of desialylated glycoproteins binding to hepatocyte membranes. *Biochim Biophys Acta* 1978;543:41–52.
21. Virgolini I, Müller C, Klepetko W, et al. Decreased hepatic function in patients with hepatoma or liver metastases monitored by a hepatocyte-specific galactosylated radioligand. *Br J Cancer* 1990;61:937–941.
22. Virgolini I, Müller C, Angelberger P, et al. Functional liver imaging with ^{99m}Tc-galactosyl-neoglycoalbumin (NGA) in alcoholic liver cirrhosis and liver fibrosis. *Nucl Med Commun* 1991;12:507–517.
23. Virgolini I, Müller C, Höbart J, et al. Liver function in acute viral hepatitis as determined by a hepatocyte-specific ligand: ^{99m}Tc-galactosyl-neoglycoalbumin. *Hepatology* 1992;15:593–598.
24. Kudo M, Vera DR, Stadalnik RC. Hepatic receptor imaging using radiolabeled asialoglycoprotein analogs. In: Lee YC, Lee RT, eds. *Neoglycoconjugates: preparation and applications*. New York: Academic Press, 1994:373–402.
25. Stockert RJ, Becker FF. Diminished hepatic binding protein for desialylated glycoproteins during chemical hepatocarcinogenesis. *Cancer Res* 1998;40:3632–3637.
26. Virgolini I, Kornek G, Höbart J, et al. Scintigraphic evaluation of functional hepatic mass in patients with advanced breast cancer. *Br J Cancer* 1993;68:549–554.
27. Kurtaran A, Li SR, Raderer M, et al. Technetium-99m-galactosyl-neoglycoalbumin combined with iodine-123-Tyr-(A14)-insulin visualizes human hepatocellular carcinomas. *J Nucl Med* 1995;36:1875–1881.
28. Sinclair AJ, Signore A, Bomanji J, et al. *In vivo* kinetics of ^{123}I-labeled insulin: studies in normal subjects and patients with diabetes mellitus. *Nucl Med Commun* 1987;8:779–786.
29. Koontz JW, Iwahashi M. Insulin as a potent, specific growth factor in rat hepatoma cell line. *Science* 1981;211:947–949.
30. Massague J, Blinderman LA, Czech MP. The high-affinity insulin receptor mediates growth stimulation in rat hepatoma cells. *J Biol Chem* 1982;257:13958–13963.

31. Taub R, Roy A, Dieter R, et al. Insulin as a growth factor in rat hepatoma cells. Stimulation of proto-oncogene expression. *J Biol Chem* 1987;262:10893–10897.

32. Koontz JW. The role of the insulin receptor in mediating the insulin-stimulated growth response in Reuber H-35 cells. *Mol Cell Biochem* 1984;58:139–146.

33. Virgolini I, Raderer M, Kurtaran A, et al. Vasoactive intestinal peptide receptor imaging for the localization of intestinal adenocarcinomas and endocrine tumors. *N Engl J Med* 1994;331:1116–1121.

34. Raderer M, Kurtaran A, Leimer M, et al. Vasoactive intestinal peptide receptor scanning in patients with pancreatic cancer: a novel tool in the diagnostic armamentarium. *J Nucl Med* 1998;39:1570–1575.

35. Krenning EP, Bakker WH, Kooij PPM, et al. Somatostatin receptor scintigraphy with [In-111-DTPA-D-Phe1]-octreotide in man: metabolism, dosimetry and comparison with [123I-Tyr-3]-octreotide. *J Nucl Med* 1992;33:652–658.

36. Virgolini I, Szilvasi I, Angelberger P, et al. Indium-111-DOTA-lanreotide: biodistribution, safety and tumor dose in patients evaluated for somatostatin receptor radiotherapy. *J Nucl Med* 1998;39:1928–1935.

37. Kurtaran A, Raderer M, Müller C, et al. Hepatic carcinoid metastasis mimicking cavernous hemangioma: vasoactive intestinal peptide (VIP) and somatostatin (SST) receptor scintigraphy for differential diagnosis. *J Nucl Med* 1997;38:880–881.

38. Raderer M, Valencak J, Scheithauer W, et al. Treatment of hepatocellular cancer with the long-acting somatostatin analog lanreotide: *in vitro* and *in vivo* results. *Eur J Clin Invest* (*submitted*).

39. Kurtaran A, Müller C, Novacek G, et al. Distinction between hepatic focal nodular hyperplasia and malignant liver lesions using 99mTc-NGA. *J Nucl Med* 1997;38:1912–1915.

40. Kudo M, Todo A, Ikekubo K, et al. Receptor index via hepatic asialoglyco-protein receptor imaging: correlation with chronic hepatocellular damage. *Am J Gastroenterol* 1992;87:865–870.

41. Okamoto E, Kyo A, Yamanaka N, et al. Prediction of the safe limits of hepatectomy by combined volumetric and functional measurements in patients with impaired hepatic function. *Surgery* 1984;95:586–592.

42. Rogers JV, Mack LA, Freeny PC, et al. Hepatic focal nodular hyperplasia: angiography, CT, sonography, and scintigraphy. *Am J Roentgenol* 1981;137:983–990.

43. Cherqui D, Rahmouni A, Charlotte F, et al. Management of focal nodular hyperplasia and hepatocellular adenoma in young women: a series of 41 patients with clinical, radiological, and pathological correlations. *Hepatology* 1995;22:1674–1681.

44. Sandler MA, Petrocelli RD, Marks DS, et al. Ultrasonic features and radionuclide correlation in liver cell adenoma and focal nodular hyperplasia. *Radiology* 1980;135:393–397.

45. Nagorney DM. Benign hepatic tumors: focal nodular hyperplasia and hepatocellular adenoma. *World J Surg* 1995;19:13–18.

46. Davis LP, McCarroll K. Correlative imaging of the liver and hepatobiliary system. *Semin Nucl Med* 1994;24:208–218.

47. Calvet X, Pons F, Bruix J, et al. Technetium-99m-DISIDA hepatobiliary agent in diagnosis of hepatocellular carcinoma: relationship between detectability and tumor differentiation. *J Nucl Med* 1988;29:1916–1920.

48. Vera DR, Krohn KA, Stadalnik RC, et al. Error analysis of regional measurements of hepatic receptor biochemistry via PET observations of [68Ga]-deferoxamine-galactosyl-neoglycoalbumin kinetics. *J Labeled Compound Radiopharm* 1989;26:348–350.

49. Bischof C, Pangerl T, Hamilton G, et al. 123I-IGF (insulin like growth factor) and 99mTc-CTPA-IGF1: preparation and preclinical characterisation. *Eur J Nucl Med* (*submitted*).

28

HEPATIC ARTERY INFUSION

PART A: TARGETED THERAPY

JOHN R. BUSCOMBE

Selected angiography within the liver makes it possible to deliver pharmaceuticals to a specific site within the liver. Lipiodol, an iodized lipid obtained from the oil of poppy seeds, is selectively taken up and retained by hepatocellular cancer (HCC) cells (1). Lipiodol can be used to deliver any lipid-soluble substance, such as the chemotherapeutic agents cisplatin and epirubicin, into HCC cells.

Investigators have replaced the iodine in Lipiodol with radioactive iodine, initially ^{131}I (2), although it may be more sensible to use ^{125}I because it has a shorter-range beta and fewer gamma emissions.

After a catheter (e.g., a Portacath) is placed by surgical or radiologic techniques into the branch of the hepatic artery feeding the HCC, nuclear medicine specialists check the line placement with ^{99m}Tc-macroaggregated albumin and then infuse 1 to 2 GBq of ^{131}I-Lipiodol during about 10 minutes.

Lipiodol is very viscous, and once injected, it cannot be removed from the target organ. If the catheter moves down the hepatic artery to below the gastroduodenal artery, ^{131}I-Lipiodol can perfuse the stomach and cause severe radiation necrosis of the gastric mucosa. This results in considerable morbidity and is potentially fatal.

An alternative method is to infuse the radiopaque ^{131}I-Lipiodol under fluoroscopic guidance. If the flow in the hepatic artery is low, reflux toward the gastroduodenal artery can be seen and the infusion stopped or slowed. It is even possible to determine Lipiodol distribution within the tumor. By moving the catheter during administration, it is possible to infuse either the right or left hepatic lobe, or both. A homogeneous distribution can be attained by changing the flow rate of the infusion. Infusion must be completed within 10 minutes because the Lipiodol may dissolve the intraarterial catheter or connector apparatus.

After successful infusion by either method, the catheter is withdrawn and radiographs of the liver are obtained, then

nuclear images 48 hours later (Fig. 28A.1). Computed tomography is performed 10 days later. With large tumors, it is not unusual to see about 5% of the activity in the lungs because collateral vessels pierce the diaphragm. Unfortunately, if a significant amount of ^{131}I-Lipiodol enters the lungs, irreversible radiation fibrosis develops. This is more likely to occur in patients with this complication. Nevertheless, it is possible to treat such patients with minimal toxicity and improve their survival (3).

Thyroid uptake of ^{131}I is not observed because of the low specific activity. The stable iodine in Lipiodol acts as a blocking dose.

Because little of the ^{131}I-Lipiodol is excreted, patients must be isolated until the levels of radioactivity emitted are below those approved by regulators for the release of patients treated with radioactive materials.

An alternative to treatment with ^{131}I-Lipiodol is the use of ^{90}Y microspheres. ^{90}Y is a pure beta emitter, so the emitted radiation dose is lower. Experience with this agent is more limited than that with ^{131}I-Lipiodol, but some reports suggest that it may be better for treating larger (> 4 cm) tumors (4).

Dosimetric calculations have been attempted. With an activity of 1 GBq of ^{90}Y-Lipiodol, tumor doses of 30 rads have been recorded, with doses to normal liver being about 10% of this level (5). This has resulted in marked changes in α-fetoprotein levels a few days after treatment, although changes in the size of the tumor on computed tomography take longer to become evident, normally 10 to 12 weeks (4).

Toxicity is minimal in most patients. Right upper quadrant pain requiring analgesia commonly develops 24 to 48 hours after administration of therapy. Nausea and vomiting also occur. In patients with severely compromised liver function, a fulminant hepatitis is possible, which may be fatal. Treatment is best avoided in patients with deranged liver function, although cirrhosis is not a contraindication to therapy.

Determining the efficacy of this therapy is difficult because of the great variations in extent of disease before

J. R. Buscombe: Department of Nuclear Medicine, Royal Free Hospital, London NW 2 QG, United Kingdom.

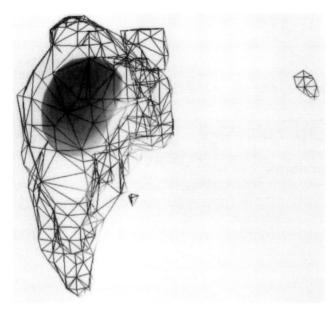

FIGURE 28A.1. Image obtained 48 hours after the administration of 1 GBq of ^{131}I-Lipiodol via a catheter in the hepatic artery. Note good localization within the hepatocellular cancer (surface rendered), minimal outline of the hepatic parenchyma (wire cage rendering), and the absence of activity outside the liver.

therapy. In a multicenter phase II trial, a median survival of 120 weeks was observed in a group of patients whose expected survival was only a few months (3,5,6).

Comparisons of patients receiving chemotherapy or Lipiodol have shown similar survival data for the two groups (3,7). Side effects in the chemotherapy group were significantly worse, with most patients hospitalized 4 to 5 days longer than the ^{131}I-Lipiodol group, whose length of stay was related to radiation protection issues rather than side effects of therapy. A slight survival advantage was noted in the chemotherapy group but was not significant. In our center, after the trial was completed, most patients opted to continue with the ^{131}I-Lipiodol treatment only.

A very interesting new use for ^{131}I-Lipiodol has been suggested in a study from Hong Kong (8). In a randomized controlled trial of 43 patients, ^{131}I-Lipiodol was used as a neoadjuvant treatment in patients with small HCCs who had undergone "curative" surgery. Patients were randomized into two groups. The first group received no postoperative treatment, whereas the second group received a single administration of 1.85 GBq of ^{131}I-Lipiodol within 6 weeks of surgery. During a period of 1 to 5 years, 21 patients received treat-

ment and 22 did not. In the treated group, the recurrence rate was 29%, in comparison with 59% in the untreated group. The median disease-free survival in the treated group was 57.2 months, versus 13.6 months in the untreated group. The 3-year survival was 86.4% in the treated group and 46.3% in the untreated group (8). The study was terminated early because of the significantly better survival of patients given ^{131}I-Lipiodol treatment, but these results suggest that neoadjuvant ^{131}I-Lipiodol could become routine in patients with small HCCs after resection.

CONCLUSIONS

Although nuclear medicine techniques were originally used to identify the positioning of catheters within the hepatic artery, therapeutic radiolabeled agents have now been administered by the same technique to allow previously untreated patients a chance of survival.

REFERENCES

1. Konno T, Maeda H, Yokoyama I, et al. Use of a lipid lymphographic agent, Lipiodol, as a carrier of high molecular weight antitumor agent, smancs, for hepatocellular carcinoma. *Gan To Kagaku Ryoho* 1982; :2005–2015.
2. Park CH, Suh JH, Yoo HS, et al. Evaluation of intrahepatic I-131 ethidiol on a patient with hepatocellular carcinoma. Therapeutic feasibility study. *Clin Nucl Med* 1986;11:514–517.
3. Bourguet P, Raoul JL, Guyader D, et al. Randomized controlled trial for hepatocellular carcinoma with portal vein thrombosis: intra-arterial injection of I-131 labelled iodized oil vs medical support. *Eur J Nucl Med* 1992;19:608.
4. Leung WT, Lau WY, Ho S, et al. Selective internal radiation therapy with intra-arterial iodine-131-Lipiodol in inoperable hepatocellular carcinoma. *J Nucl Med* 1994;35:1313–1318.
5. Raoul JL, Bretegne JF, Caucanus JP, et al. Internal radiation therapy for hepatocellular carcinoma. Results of a French multicenter phase II trial of transarterial injection of iodine-131 labeled Lipiodol. *Cancer* 1992;69:346–352.
6. Bretagne JF, Raoul JL, Bourguet P, et al. Hepatic artery injection of I-131-labeled Lipiodol. Part II. Preliminary results of therapeutic use in patients with hepatocellular carcinoma and liver metastases. *Radiology* 1988;168:547–550.
7. Bhattacharya S, Novell JR, Dusheiko GM, et al. Epirubicin-Lipiodol chemotherapy versus [131]iodine-Lipiodol radiotherapy in the treatment of unresectable hepatocellular carcinoma. *Cancer* 1995; 76:2202–2210.
8. Lau WY, Leung TWT, Ho SKW, et al. Adjuvant intra-arterial iodine-131 Lipiodol for resectable hepatocellular carcinoma. *Lancet* 1999;353:797–901.

28

HEPATIC ARTERY INFUSION

PART B: HEPATIC ARTERY PUMP EVALUATION

HOMER A. MACAPINLAC

This chapter reviews the clinical significance and technique of hepatic artery pump evaluation. Patterns of normal and abnormal uptake are demonstrated, and the new types of hepatic artery pumps that have become available recently are discussed.

BACKGROUND

Approximately 138,000 new cases of colorectal cancer will be diagnosed this year in the United States. Surgical resection, the treatment of choice in most cases, results in a 40% cure rate. However, recurrence is common, and the liver is the site most frequently involved. Liver metastases from colorectal cancer will develop in more than 50,000 people in the United States this year alone (1,2).

Currently, surgical resection is the only curative option for hepatic metastases. The 5-year survival rate for surgical resection is more than 30%. However, recurrences develop in more than two thirds of patients, most commonly in the remnant liver, and are most likely the consequence of microscopic disease undetected at surgery (1,2). Following the resection of hepatic metastases, in half of the patients disease recurs in the liver, in the other half systemically (3). Cryosurgery, embolization, and ultrasonography are being utilized as alternatives to surgery (4). A tremendous effort has been made to develop adjuvant chemotherapeutic regimens to improve the survival and decrease the recurrence rates of patients undergoing liver resection.

The proven method of adjuvant therapy of colorectal metastases to the liver is based on 5-fluorouracil (5-FU), a thymidilate synthetase inhibitor, or its analogues. This drug alone (5), or in combination with levamisole (6) or leucovorin (7), has improved the survival of patients after complete resection of gross disease. However, significant systemic toxicity has limited the application of this method, and alternative locoregional methods have been developed.

Hepatic artery infusion is based on the fact that hepatic metastases larger than 3 mm derive their blood supply from the arterial circulation. Hepatic metastases smaller than 1 mm derive their blood supply from the portal circulation, and those 2 to 3 mm in size derive blood from both the arterial and portal circulations (8). Because tumors that remain after hepatic resection represent established metastases, their size is probably in the range of 2 to 3 mm, and they are therefore not detectable by the ultrasonographic scanning technique we routinely use, which has a resolution of 5 mm. The infusion of chemotherapeutic agents via the hepatic artery should result in a high concentration of drug within the tumor and less systemic toxicity. The development of the implantable infusion pump has made it possible to administer hepatic arterial chemotherapy safely in an outpatient setting (7). About 200 patients each year have surgery at Memorial Sloan-Kettering Cancer Center for the treatment of hepatic metastases. Approximately 75 undergo resection, and in another 50, Infusaid hepatic artery pump systems are implanted; the remaining 75 usually have extrahepatic disease discovered at laparotomy. Our single-institution experience with liver resection documents the efficacy of this aggressive approach, with an actuarial 2-year survival of 75%; the 2-year disease-free survival is only 21.2% in the subset of patients undergoing complete resection of colorectal liver metastases. Kemeny et al. (9) demonstrated recently in a randomized trial of patients who had undergone hepatic resection of colorectal cancer metastases that 2-year disease-free survival is increased in patients treated with hepatic arterial infusion (FUDR and dexamethasone) and systemic FU versus those treated with systemic chemotherapy (FU) alone. This study makes it is clear that adjuvant therapy after liver resection is a reasonable approach to improve the outcome of patients with hepatic metastases.

H. A. Macapinlac: Department of Radiology, Memorial Sloan-Kettering Cancer Center, New York, New York 10021.

HEPATIC ARTERY PUMP EVALUATION

Before placement of the hepatic artery pump, patients undergo preoperative celiac angiography to delineate the vascular anatomy and identify any variants. The surgeon implants the pump in the subcutaneous tissue of the anterior abdominal wall, and the catheter tip is placed in the main hepatic artery to perfuse both lobes of the liver. The patency and flow of the "Infusaid" hepatic artery pump are checked after placement and before discharge, and the evaluation is repeated before each chemotherapy cycle. The pump is also checked if symptoms develop during chemotherapy that may be caused by improper pump perfusion to extrahepatic regions. Symptoms like gastritis, duodenal ulcers, abdominal pain, and gastrointestinal discomfort during chemotherapy may indicate improper pump perfusion.

A ^{99m}Tc-sulfur colloid scan is performed after intravenous injection of 1 mCi of the radiopharmaceutical. Multiple planar images of the abdomen are acquired, including one with subcostal, xiphoid, and umbilical markers and a ^{57}Co ruler. This serves as the "background" to localize the larger lesions and is used mainly to delineate the extent of the hepatic parenchyma and splenic tissue. The hepatic pump study is then performed after injection of 5 mCi of ^{99m}Tc-macroaggregated albumin (MAA) into the implanted hepatic pump. However, in the fall of 1998, the classic "Infusaid" pump with one or two sideports was longer available, and two new types became available. The Isomed infusion pump (Medtronic, Minneapolis, Minnesota) has a fenestrated sideport septum

and a centrally located reservoir fill port. The Arrow model 3000 (Arrow International, Walpole, Massachusetts) has a central septum that makes it possible to administer bolus injections with the Arrow special bolus needle.

The patient lies supine on the gamma camera bed, and a strict aseptic technique is used to establish access to the side-port or central port. The pump is palpated and the injection site prepared by cleansing with Betadine. Sterile gloves are donned, the area is draped, and the catheter access kit, which consists of a special access needle attached to an extension tube containing normal saline solution, is assembled. A three-way stopcock is attached to the extension tube. The ^{99m}Tc-MAA is diluted to a total volume of 10 mL with normal saline solution, and a 10-mL saline flush is attached to the other end of the stopcock. The bolus injection port is palpated to locate the septum and the special needle is inserted. The camera is positioned over the abdomen, and the injection is administered during a 2 minute period, followed by the saline flush. A dynamic acquisition of 5 seconds per frame during 60 seconds is performed simultaneously. A heparinized saline solution is then infused and the needle is removed. A sterile gauze pad is used to apply pressure to the puncture site for a minute. Planar views (including markers) identical to those of the sulfur colloid scan are acquired. Essentially, both the colloid and flow scans are overlaid to determine the presence of flow into the hepatic parenchyma and ensure the absence of extrahepatic perfusion.

The MAA study usually demonstrates a "fill in" of the "cold" lesions on the colloid scan with "rim" hyperperfusion

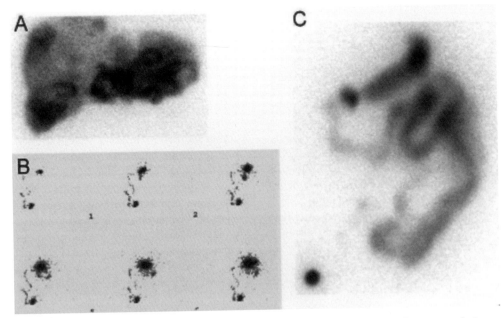

FIGURE 28B.1. A: Earlier delayed post ^{99m}Tc-macroaggregated albumin (*MAA*) pump perfusion scan showing classic rim hyperperfusion of known hepatic metastasis. **B:** A flow study with ^{99m}Tc-MAA repeated a few months later showing abnormal perfusion to the left upper quadrant of the abdomen. **C:** Delayed ^{99m}Tc-MAA scan showing visualization of the bowel and no activity in the hepatic parenchyma. Contrast study demonstrated catheter erosion into the duodenum.

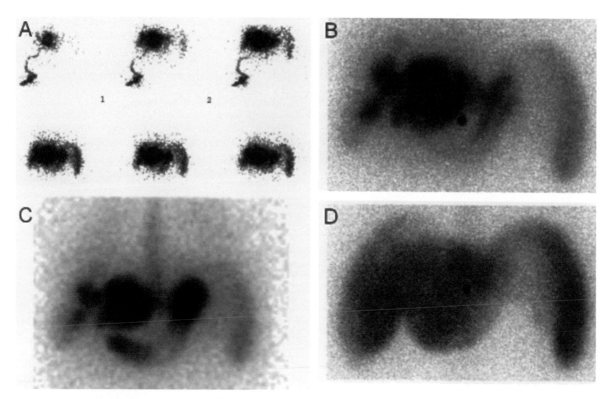

FIGURE 28B.2. **A:** Abnormal ^{99m}Tc-macroaggregated albumin (*MAA*) flow study showing uptake in the portal region and splenic perfusion. **B:** Delayed ^{99m}Tc-MAA static view showing portal retention and uptake in the stomach and spleen. **C:** Following ingestion of ^{99m}Tc-diethylenetriamine pentaacetic acid (*DTPA*) in water, activity is noted in the stomach and duodenum. **D:** Liver–spleen scan (^{99m}Tc-sulfur colloid) for comparison with marker in the center.

(Fig. 28B.1A), reflecting central necrosis of these rapidly growing tumors and a hypervascular rim or edge. Occasionally, the presence of lung uptake indicates arteriovenous shunting, which occurs with rapidly growing lesions. Examples of abnormal extrahepatic perfusion are shown in Figs. 28B.1 and 28B.2, and practically any site can be abnormally perfused in the abdomen. Occasionally, we give the patient ^{99m}Tc-diethylenetriamine pentaacetic acid (DTPA) in water to outline the stomach (Fig. 28B.2C), as this may help to localize abnormal perfusion in the epigastric region. Once occlusion or extrahepatic perfusion is suspected or documented, a slow port contrast angiography is performed for accurate anatomic localization of the catheter tip.

We reviewed our experience at Memorial Sloan-Kettering Cancer Center of a total of 276 hepatic arterial pump scans in 205 patients performed during a period of 3 years. Twenty-nine patients (14%) had 41 abnormal studies (15%). Contrast studies performed in 20 of the patients (32 scans) showed 11 cases of catheter occlusion, 9 splenic perfusion, 5 stomach or small-bowel perfusion, 3 pooling at the hepatic portal, 3 peritoneal perfusion, and 1 renal perfusion. In 30 of the 32 scans (94%), agreement with the contrast studies was noted. Of the two patients with normal angiographic findings, one was reinjected slowly during 5 minutes and normal perfusion was demonstrated; the other

received no further treatment because of progressive disease. Of the nine patients without contrast studies, four had therapy through a normal alternate sideport and five were given no treatment because of disease progression.

Hepatic arterial pump studies provide a reliable and convenient method of assessing pump patency and position before the administration of regional chemotherapy.

ACKNOWLEDGEMENT

This work was supported in part by Department of Energy grant DE-FG02-86ER60407.

REFERENCES

1. Rosen CG, Donohue JH, Nagorney DM. Liver resection for metastatic colonic and rectal carcinoma. In: Cohen A, Winawer S, eds; Freidman M, Gunderson L, associate eds. *Cancer of the colon, rectum and anus.* New York: McGraw-Hill, 1995:805–821.
2. Fong Y, Blumgart LH, Cohen AM. Surgical treatment of colorectal metastases to the liver. *CA Cancer J Clin* 1995;45:50–62.
3. Fortner JG. Recurrence of colorectal cancer after hepatic resection. *Am J Surg* 1988;155:378–382.
4. Ravikumar TS, Steele G, Kane R, et al. Experimental and clinical

observations on hepatic cryosurgery for colorectal metastases. *Cancer Res* 1991;51(23 Pt 1):6323–6327.

5. Garge TB, Moss SE. Adjuvant chemotherapy in cancer of the colon and rectum: demonstration of effectiveness of prolonged 5-FU chemotherapy in a prospectively controlled randomized trial. *Surg Clin North Am* 1981;61:1321–1329.

6. Moertel CG, Fleming TR, Macdonald JS, et al. Levamisole and fluorouracil for adjuvant therapy of resected colon carcinoma. *N Engl J Med* 1990;322:352–358.

7. Seiter K, Kemeny N. Hepatic arterial chemotherapy. In: Cohen A, Winawer S, eds; Freidman M, Gunderson L, associate eds. *Cancer of the colon, rectum and anus.* New York: McGraw-Hill, 1995:831–843.

8. Ackerman NB. The blood supply of experimental liver metastases. IV. Changes in vascularity with increasing tumor growth. *Surgery* 1974;75:589–596.

9. Kemeny N, Cohen A, Huang Y, et al. Randomized study of hepatic arterial infusion (HAI) and systemic chemotherapy (SYS) versus SYS alone as adjuvant therapy after resection of hepatic metastases from colorectal cancer. *ASCO Proc* 1999;18:263a.

29

POSITRON EMISSION TOMOGRAPHY IMAGING

TARIK Z. BELHOCINE
ROLAND HUSTINX
ANNE DEVILLERS
FRÉDÉRIC DAENEN
CATHERINE BECKERS
PATRICK PAULUS
PIERRE RIGO

Carcinomas of the genitourinary tract include those of the female genital system (ovaries and uterus), the male genital system (principally testicular carcinoma and carcinoma of the prostate), and the urinary tract, specifically the kidneys and bladder.

In general, these tumors have not been studied extensively with positron emission tomography and fluorodeoxyglucose (FDG-PET) because of the technical difficulties encountered in imaging tumors near activity in the bladder and urinary system. Technical advances such as iterative reconstruction, attenuation correction, and whole-body imaging have increased the reliability and value of FDG-PET imaging of the pelvis and have resulted in recent developments of the technique for this purpose.

CARCINOMAS OF THE FEMALE GENITAL SYSTEM

Ovarian Carcinoma

Ovarian carcinoma has an ominous prognosis. Although not the most frequent type of tumor, ovarian carcinomas are the most common cause of death among patients with gynecologic tumors (1,2). As these tumors develop from a deep-seated but mobile organ within the peritoneal cavity, they invade or compress adjacent organs, then disseminate through nodal or peritoneal extension. Symptoms are delayed and nonspecific, whereas progression is rapid when

the ovarian capsule is ruptured. The disease has spread throughout the pelvis in about two thirds of all patients at the time of diagnosis. Survival has not improved significantly despite better understanding the epidemiology and biology of the disease and advances in screening and therapy (3).

Screening remains difficult because of the lack of a sensitive marker. It is therefore important that the physician maintain a high index of suspicion and confirm the presence of any suspected tumoral mass in the pelvis. Noninvasive staging is usually performed by physical examination combined with ultrasonography, urography, and tomodensitometry, but the true extent of disease is usually not completely determined until initial surgery. Surgery remains the mainstay of both diagnosis and staging, as both tumor markers and imaging lack sensitivity and specificity.

Therapy consists of maximum early resection followed by chemotherapy, radiotherapy, or both. In patients with ovarian carcinoma, the prognosis and success of subsequent therapy are related to a reduction of tumor volume. Post-therapy follow-up is facilitated by monitoring serum tumor markers, CA-125 in particular.

Mortality after surgery and radiotherapy or chemotherapy remains high. Indeed, even after negative findings on second-look surgery, recurrences develop in 40% to 63% of cases (4). Recurrence and mortality result primarily from occult metastases of the peritoneal surfaces of the pelvis and abdomen and from undetected spread to the retroperitoneal lymph nodes. Current diagnostic techniques, including computed tomography (CT), magnetic resonance imaging (MRI), and laparoscopy or culdocentesis lack sensitivity and specificity for the accurate diagnosis and staging of primary and residual or recurrent disease. New methodologies are needed to optimize treatment plans in ovarian carci-

T. Z. Belhocine, R. Hustinx, F. Daenen, C. Beckers, P. Paulus, and P. Rigo: Department of Nuclear Medicine, University Hospital Sart Tilman, 4000 Liege, Belgium.

A. Devillers: Department of Nuclear Medicine, University Hospital Rennes, 3500 Rennes, France.

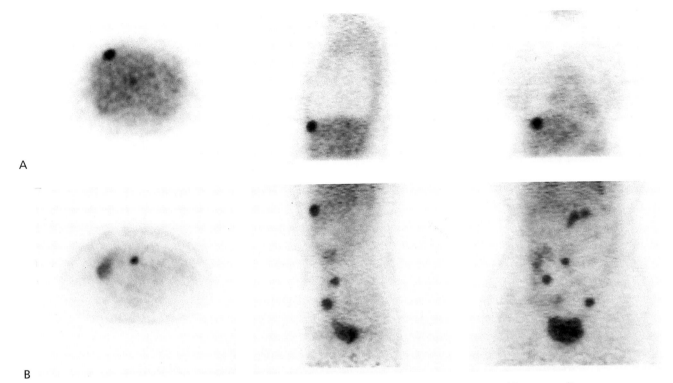

FIGURE 29.1. A 65-year-old woman had a history of ovarian carcinoma treated 2 years earlier with surgery and chemotherapy. The CA-125 level was increased, and the results of conventional imaging were normal. Positron emission tomography with fluorodeoxyglucose shows liver (**A**), peritoneal (**B**), and lymph node (B) involvement.

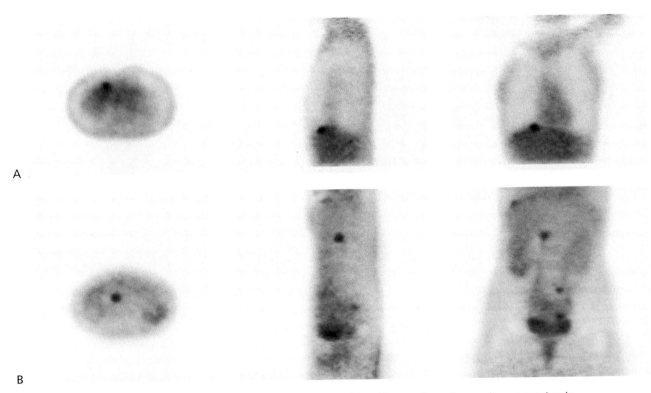

FIGURE 29.2. A 63-year-old woman presented with a history of ovarian carcinoma previously treated with surgery and chemotherapy. The CA-125 level was increased, and the results of computed tomography were normal. Positron emission tomography (*PET*) with fluorodeoxyglucose shows a right peridiaphragmatic hypermetabolic area, compatible with peritoneal involvement (**A**), and locoregional lymph node dissemination (**B**). A second look at laparotomy confirmed the PET findings.

noma. The advantages of FDG-PET in this situation are that diagnosis can be based on a demonstration of altered tumor cellular metabolism rather than on a delineation of morphologic alterations, lesion size, or contours. Abnormalities are detected even in structures of normal size and shape. Successful imaging of ovarian cancers with 18F-FDG was reported initially by Wahl et al. (4). The largest experience has been reported by Hubner et al. (5). These authors reported data from 90 patients presenting with ovarian masses who were studied by limited-field or whole-body PET and CT before undergoing laparotomy for suspected ovarian cancer. A sensitivity of 89% and specificity of 92% were reported, along with high positive and negative predictive values (94% and 85%, respectively). PET identified occult foci of active tumor not visualized on mor-

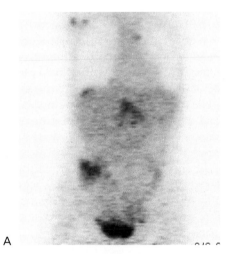

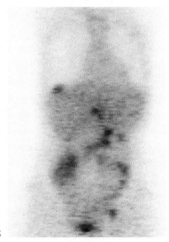

FIGURE 29.3. A 50-year-old woman had a history of ovarian carcinoma treated with surgery and chemotherapy. The CA-125 level was increased, and the results of computed tomography of the pelvis were normal. Positron emission tomography with fluorodeoxyglucose shows a lymph node metastasis in the right axillary (**A**), mediastinal (A), celiomesenteric (A,**B**), and left inguinal (B) areas. In addition, a hypermetabolic area in the right peridiaphragmatic region is compatible with a peritoneal tumor.

phologic studies (CT sensitivity, 72%; specificity, 43%). Data in recurrent disease were available in 44 cases. High sensitivity (94%) and specificity (100%) were demonstrated.

Our experience with attenuation-corrected whole-body FDG-PET in patients with ovarian carcinoma at various stages of disease confirms its value in the presurgical identification and staging of tumors (6).

During postsurgical follow-up, residual or recurrent tumor, suggested by tumor markers but unrecognized by conventional imaging, is frequently identified. Discrepancies occur most often in cases of peritoneal dissemination or spread to retroperitoneal lymph nodes. On occasion, other unsuspected distant metastases are discovered. PET can be substituted for second-look surgery to identify cases in which cytoreductive intervention is needed. It cannot completely replace second-look because it does not detect microscopic peritoneal dissemination or nodal involvement. These indications and results are illustrated in the following three cases (Figs. 29.1–29.3).

Carcinoma of the Uterus

Carcinoma of the uterus is common in women (second only to breast carcinoma) (7). It is usually categorized as carcinoma of the cervix or carcinoma of the uterine corpus. Carcinoma of the cervix is more frequent. The prognosis appears to depend mainly on the degree of locoregional lymph node extension (8), but the tumor can also progress to the dome of the vagina, rectum, and bladder in addition to spreading by hematogenous dissemination.

The 5-year survival rate markedly decreases in patients with lymph node involvement. Twenty-five percent of patients with locally advanced tumors have paraaortic lymph node invasion (9). When such nodal invasion is detected, the field of irradiation is modified to include area of the abdominopelvic nodes, which are otherwise spared to prevent irradiation of the intestine.

Cancer of the uterine body is observed primarily in menopausal women; its frequency is increasing. Although lymph node involvement is less common than in cervical carcinoma, cervicoisthmic cancer metastasizes to the iliac nodes, and cancer of the fallopian region extends to the inguinal and aortic nodes.

Locoregional extension is more frequent, with advanced disease spreading to the peritoneum, bladder, rectosigmoid colon, and more rarely to bone and liver. The management of uterine cancer is currently based on endoscopic examinations and imaging.

We have performed 33 PET studies in 28 patients with known uterine cancer (11 with cervical cancer and 17 with carcinoma of the corpus) for suspected recurrence (n = 22) and for staging before therapy (n = 11). In the first group, FDG-PET demonstrated 35 confirmed lesions, whereas CT demonstrated 18. PET yielded three false-positive and one

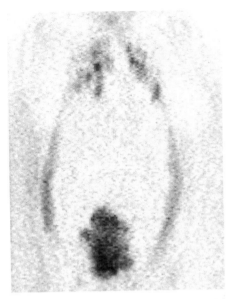

FIGURE 29.4. A 64-year-old woman presented with stage IV cancer of the uterine corpus [FIGO (International Federation of Gynecology and Obstetrics) staging]. Positron emission tomography with fluorodeoxyglucose before treatment shows a voluminous hypermetabolic focus in the pelvis, corresponding to diffuse infiltration in the uterus, bladder, and rectum, in addition to dissemination of the tumor in the peritoneum, mediastinum, and lungs bilaterally.

TABLE 29.1. RESULTS OF FDG-PET IN 28 PATIENTS WITH UTERINE CARCINOMA

	PET	Conventional imaging
Sensitivity (%)	96	54
Specificity (%)	81	75
Positive predictive value (%)	95	94
Negative predictive value (%)	82	75

FDG-PET, positron emission tomography with fluorodeoxyglucose.

abdominopelvic and retroperitoneal nodes and of the peritoneum, as CT and MRI do not optimally differentiate fibrosis and postsurgical sclerosis from metastases (Fig. 29.5). False-positive results can be related to inflammation and also to uptake in benign lesions, such as leiomyoma. False-negative results are mainly seen with small lesions (< 1 cm).

Our results concur with those recently published by Rose et al. (10), who studied 32 patients with locally advanced cervical cancer before surgical staging. Six patients were in stage IIb, 24 in stage IIIb, and two in stage IVa. The primary tumor was recognized in 30 patients. PET detected six of the nine patients with paraaortic node metastases. The sensitivity for paraaortic nodes was therefore 75%, and the specificity was 92% (two patients had a false-positive result on PET). Seventeen patients underwent pelvic node resection. PET detected all 11 cases with nodal involvement in the pelvis only. Five of these had abnormalities on CT. No false-positive or false-negative results were obtained in the pelvis. Cervical cancers have a high avidity for FDG. PET provides accurate nodal staging in both the pelvic and paraaortic areas.

false-negative result, versus one false-positive and 16 false-negative results for conventional imaging. Similar results were obtained for staging (Fig. 29.4). Overall, PET had a sensitivity of 96% and a specificity of 81% (positive predictive value, 95%; negative predictive value, 82%) (Table 29.1). PET is of great value in detecting involvement of

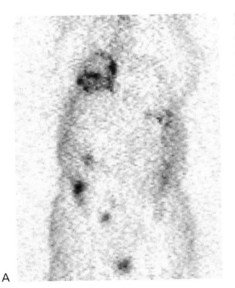

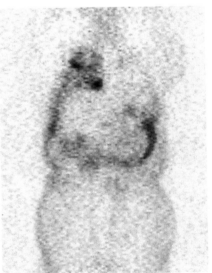

A   B

FIGURE 29.5. A 71-year-old woman with a carcinoma of the cervix was treated only with radiation. The carcinoembryonic antigen level was increased, and results of computed tomography of the pelvis were normal. Positron emission tomography with fluorodeoxyglucose shows metastatic tumor in the right lung (**A,B**). In addition, the presence of lymph node infiltration (A) is highly suggestive of peritoneal involvement.

CARCINOMA OF THE MALE GENITAL SYSTEM

Testicular Germ Cell Tumors

Testicular cancer is one of the most common neoplasms among young men (20 to 40 years old) (11). Cryptorchidism predisposes to this malignancy (12). Histologically, germ cell testicular cancer can be divided into seminomas (40%) and nonseminomas (60%). Nonseminomas include mainly embryonal carcinomas, choriocarcinomas, and teratomas (13). The prognosis of patients with testicular cancer has been dramatically improved during the last 20 years by the development of combination chemotherapy with bleomycin, etoposide, and cisplatin. More than 70% of all patients with testicular cancer are alive 5 years after diagnosis (14). Disseminated disease is usually diagnosed by CT and the presence of elevated tumor markers. Human chorionic gonadotropin and alpha-fetoprotein are found in the serum of 60% to 80% of patients with nonseminomatous germ cell tumors (15,16). Twenty percent of testicular tumors are marker-negative (17,18).

After chemotherapy, 30% of patients have residual tumor on CT. Surgical resection of residual tumor masses is considered an essential part of treatment (19). In most patients, residual masses are located in the retroperitoneal space, and the resection is performed as a retroperitoneal lymph node dissection or lumpectomy. Residual pulmonary metastases should also be considered for resection after chemotherapy. These surgical procedures may be associated with long-term morbidity in some patients (20,21). Following chemotherapy, the resected residual masses may contain areas of necrosis, differentiated teratoma, or undifferentiated tumor. In patients with undifferentiated tumor, the secondary resection may increase survival, depending on the biologic aggressiveness of the disease, the completeness of surgery, and the effectiveness of further treatment (22). The resection of differentiated teratoma may prevent local tumor growth and late disease recurrence with possi-

ble malignant transformation. Surgery is of no benefit in patients with necrosis except to confirm a pathologic complete remission. Noninvasive identification in such patients could prevent surgery-related complications (23,24).

Imaging methods such as CT or MRI alone cannot differentiate malignant tissue from scar (25). Only histology reliably assesses the presence of malignancy in a residual mass after chemotherapy. In nonseminomatous tumors, this is the standard procedure (26). FDG-PET may have a role in the management of a subset of patients with nonseminomatous germ cell tumors. This group would include patients considered for surgical resection of a residual mass or masses not likely to contain teratoma. This subset may account for up to 25% of patients traditionally referred for surgery after chemotherapy (27).

Indeed, FDG-PET can be used to evaluate the presence of residual viable germ cell tumor (although it cannot differentiate necrosis from teratoma). Patients with negative findings could be observed (without surgery) by serial CT imaging. In those with a positive result on FDG-PET, it is likely that viable germ cell tumor persists, and surgical resection would be recommended if possible. FDG-PET may also be useful when the decision regarding surgery after chemotherapy is difficult (i.e., the risk for surgical morbidity or mortality is increased), as in patients with serious comorbid conditions (e.g., significant bleomycin pulmonary toxicity, heart disease, obesity, multiple anatomic sites) but with technically resectable disease.

Positron emission tomography with fluorodeoxyglucose could be useful in patients with late serologic relapse (> 2 years after completion of primary treatment) of testicular cancer, evidenced by elevated levels of AFP or hCG, but with normal findings on anatomic imaging and no evidence of a second primary tumor. These patients typically demonstrate markedly decreased chemosensitivity. Surgical exploration provides optimal primary management (28). FDG-PET may localize and assess the extent of disease in this subset of patients, thereby facilitating surgical resection (Fig. 29.6).

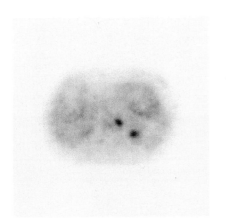 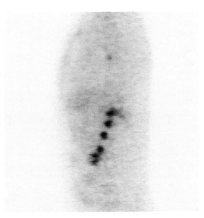 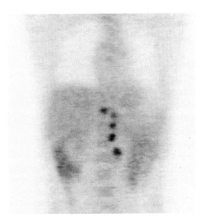

FIGURE 29.6. A 26-year-old man presented with testicular carcinoma treated 6 months earlier by orchidectomy and chemotherapy. Levels of alpha-fetoprotein and beta-human chorionic gonadotropin were increased. Positron emission tomography with fluorodeoxyglucose shows nodal recurrence in the left paraaortic area.

Nuutinen et al. (29) confirmed the applicability of FDG-PET to the imaging of lesions after chemotherapy. In their series of 15 patients, sensitivity was 86% and specificity 77% in determining tumor viability. Three false-positive cases were caused by FDG uptake in inflammatory tissue. The only false-negative case was that of a residual teratocarcinoma located in the retroperitoneal area close to a focus of FDG uptake in the normal bowel. Consequently, no clear differentiation between bowel and tumor uptake was made.

Other authors have also reported false-positive and false-negative results in imaging testicular cancer with FDG-PET. In a study of 19 patients with germ cell cancer after chemotherapy, Dohmen et al. (30) obtained two false-positive and seven false-negative results. The uptake of FDG was visually assessed. Using quantitative measurements, Stephens et al. (31) could not differentiate teratomas from residual necrosis or fibrosis, whereas Wahl et al. (32) have reported increased FDG uptake in the lung of a patient who presented a proven teratoma.

In patients with malignant teratomas and residual masses who underwent imaging after chemotherapy, Wilson et al. (33) reported a similar low FDG uptake in differentiated teratomas and necrotic, fibrotic tissue. This is in agreement with the findings of other studies, in which FDG uptake was found to be reduced in well-differentiated tumor (34,35), benign lesions (36), and fibrosis (37) in comparison with uptake in poorly differentiated malignant tumors.

Cremerius et al. (38) confirmed that FDG-PET is superior to CT for assessing residual tumor after chemotherapy of germ cell cancer and may thus have an important effect on patient management. They emphasize that PET must be performed at least 2 weeks after completion of therapy to avoid false-negative findings (Table 29.2).

Because it measures metabolic changes, FDG-PET may predict the response to treatment earlier and more accurately than other methods, such as CT, that evaluate morphologic changes. Further studies are needed.

Prostate Cancer

Prostate cancer represents the second leading cause of death from cancer in Europe and the United States (46,47). Aging of the population, increased public awareness, and improved diagnostic tools have increased the detection rate. The incidence of patients who present with organ-confined disease has increased to approximately 40% of new cases (48). Potentially curative treatment by either radical prostatectomy or radiation therapy is available for these patients. However, approximately 35% of them require additional treatment because of the presence of residual tumor after surgery or micrometastases in regional lymph nodes (48,49). Imaging of the prostate by transrectal ultrasonography, CT, or MRI inadequately defines volume and extent of disease in a significant number of patients (50). Further improvement in clinical staging is therefore highly desirable to select patients with truly organ-confined tumors.

Metabolic grading with FDG-PET is not possible in the majority of untreated prostate cancers, as it is in most other tumor systems. No correlation has been found between tumor grade or stage and FDG uptake as measured by PET. Low levels of proliferative activity in the majority of primary prostatic adenocarcinomas may account for the inability of PET to differentiate different tumor grades and stages. In the majority of patients with prostate cancer investigated by FDG-PET, the technique appears to provide no additional information beyond what is obtained with morphologic methods, such as ultrasonography, CT, and MRI. FDG-PET cannot reliably distinguish benign from malignant prostatic disease in the individual patient (Table 29.3). Concomitant prostatitis, frequently encountered in patients with benign

TABLE 29.2. FDG-PET IN TESTICULAR CARCINOMA

Author	Year	Reference	No. patients	PET sensitivity (%)	PET specificity (%)
Dohmen et al.	1995	30	15	90	90
Wilson et al.	1995	33	14	60	85
Harms et al.	1995	39, 40	18	79	90
Laubenbacher et al.	1995	41	7	100	100
Reinhardt et al.	1995	42	28	50	90
Bender et al.	1996	43	23	50	100
Nuutinen et al.	1996	44	11	100	88
Nuutinen et al.	1997	29	15	80	77
Cremerius et al.	1998	38	33	*	*
Albers et al.	1999	45	37	70	100

*Sensitivity and specificity of PET vary with histologic subtype and the temporal relationship to chemotherapy.
Seminoma: sensitivity, 100%; specificity, 86%.
Nonseminoma: sensitivity 67%; specificity 92%.
Before chemotherapy: sensitivity, 83%; specificity, 83%.
<14 days after chemotherapy: sensitivity, 44%; specificity, 100%.
≥14 days after chemotherapy: sensitivity, 78%; specificity, 90%.
FDG-PET, positron emission tomography with fluorodeoxyglucose.

TABLE 29.3. FDG-PET IN PROSTATE CARCINOMA

Author	Year	Reference	No. patients	Comments
Bares et al.	1994	60	51	No significant discrimination of FDG uptake in primary tumors versus normal tissue.
Shreve et al.	1995	57	30	Low detection rate of known bone metastases.
Yeh et al.	1995	61	12	Low detection rate of known bone metastases.
Laubenbacher et al.	1995	41	15	No significant discrimination of FDG uptake in primary tumors versus scar or normal tissue.
Reinhardt et al.	1995	62	12	PET: sensitivity, 75%; specificity, 75%.
Hoh et al.	1996	56	8	Decreased FDG uptake in therapy responders
Haseman et al.	1996	63	14	PET: sensitivity, 17%; specificity, 50%. Monoclonal antibody is superior to PET to identify recurrent disease in the prostate bed.
Hofer et al.	1999	64	20	PET: sensitivity, 17%; specificity, 50%. No difference in FDG uptake between benign prostate hyperplasia, prostate carcinoma, postoperative scar, and local recurrence.

FDG-PET, positron emission tomography with fluorodeoxyglucose.

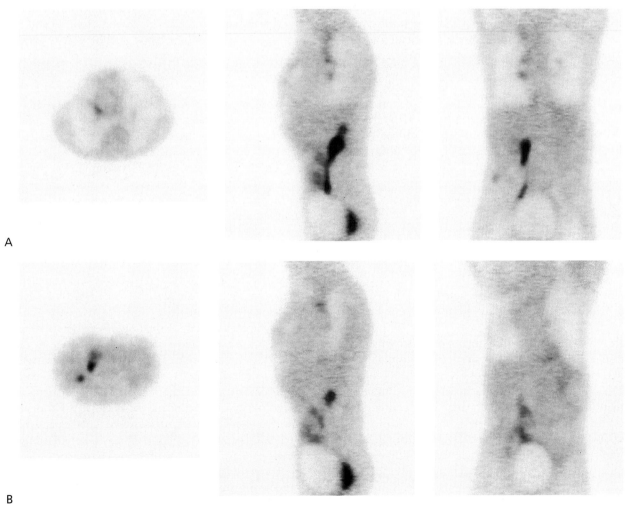

A

B

FIGURE 29.7. A 60-year-old man presented with prostatic carcinoma. Positron emission tomography with fluorodeoxyglucose shows metastatic dissemination in the skeleton (sternum and iliac bone) (**A**) and in the lymph nodes (right mediastinum) and lungs (bilateral hilar areas) (**B**). In addition, voluminous vesical distention with right renal stasis is secondary to a compressive phenomenon.

prostatitic hyperplasia, may be a confounding factor because increased FDG accumulation has been noted in inflammatory processes (51). The low sensitivity of FDG-PET in prostate carcinoma has been attributed to low tumor volume and partial volume effect and to difficulties with artifacts related to high levels of residual activity in the bladder. However, it appears that the primary reason is biologic and that these technical factors remain of secondary importance (52).

Detection of locoregional and distant metastatic disease is essential for the optimal clinical management of prostate cancer. The principal sites of distant metastases of prostate cancer are regional lymph nodes, bone, liver, and lungs (53). The diagnosis of osseous metastases is most commonly addressed with bone scintigraphy, which has an overall high sensitivity and permits easy evaluation of the entire skeleton at a relatively low cost. The specificity of bone scintigraphy is limited by tracer uptake associated with degenerative joint disease and related benign bone disease. Persistent osseous uptake also occurs in locations of previous skeletal trauma. Scintigraphy remains insensitive in the detection of early neoplastic infiltration of bone marrow, a limitation of particular relevance in the evaluation of the vertebrae, a common early site for prostate cancer metastases (54). Shreeve et al. (55) observed relatively low standard uptake values (SUVs) in most of the metastatic deposits of prostate cancer that could be assessed. However, in patients with relatively high levels of prostate-specific antigen (> 4.0) or a high velocity of prostate-specific antigen (> 1.2 at 6 months), PET may be more sensitive than CT for detection of lymph node metastases (Fig. 29.7). Other data indicate that a high rate of FDG accumulation predominates in tumors that are not hormone-dependent (56,57).

The use of new molecules, such as ^{11}C-choline, ^{11}C-acetate, and ^{11}C-methionine, or of some specific amino acids, receptors, or antitumor drugs may provide other opportunities in the future (58). Recently, Nilsson et al. (59) showed that ^{11}C-methionine uptake (SUV) is significantly higher in bone metastases from prostate carcinoma than in normal bone.

Like other neoplasms, many foci of progressive metastatic prostate cancer demonstrate an increased accumulation of FDG. However, the intensity of FDG uptake is generally lower than in other cancers, which significantly limits the sensitivity of the method. Compared with conventional bone scintigraphy, FDG-PET is insensitive in detecting skeletal lesions, although in patients with disease refractory to hormonal therapy, FDG-PET may be useful to monitor visceral metastases.

RENAL CANCER

Carcinoma of the kidney accounts for approximately 3% of adult malignancies and occurs in a male-to-female ratio of 2:1. The incidence peaks between the sixth and seventh decades of life. Three different histologic types of renal cell carcinoma are found: clear cell, granular cell, and spindle or sarcomatoid variants (65).

The clear cell variant seems to have a slightly better prognosis than the granular cell or mixed cell types. In contrast, the sarcomatoid variant has a significantly poorer prognosis. Diagnostic and staging modalities include ultrasonography, urography, CT, arteriography, and MRI. Good discrimination between cancer tissue and normal tissue has been observed with FDG (Table 29.4).

In animal models, renal tubular cells demonstrate glucose-6-phosphatase activity. The concentration of hexokinase in renal tubular cells is relatively high, similar to that in the heart. It is less than that in the brain and greater than that in the liver. Despite the relatively high concentration of hexokinase in the kidney, most FDG is excreted without undergoing further metabolism. Because renal tubular glucose transporters do not appear to have a high affinity for FDG, little tubular reabsorption occurs. This accounts for the rapid clearance of the tracer from the blood pool by urinary excretion (66).

Wahl et al. (67) imaged patients with primary renal tumors approximately 1 hour after FDG injection. They performed dynamic renal imaging in one patient and also in an animal model. Their results indicated that tumor-to-kidney activity ratios increase progressively with time.

Excretion of FDG by the kidney can lead to interpretation problems related to FDG accumulation in renal calyces. Correlation of PET with CT is important to identify the area of FDG accumulation precisely. The intravenous administration of diuretics combined with a longer interval between injection and imaging helps decrease the concentration of FDG in the calyceal system.

Hoh et al. (68) observed a good correlation between disease status (progressive vs. stable disease and complete vs. partial response) and the sensitivity of FDG-PET. Overall, the accuracy of this modality compared favorably with that of conventional imaging. Visualization of tumors seems to depend on tumor grade and size, as FDG fails to detect smaller low-grade tumors. Goldberg et al. (69) performed 26 FDG-PET scans in 21 patients (14 scans in 10 patients with malignant renal tumors and 12 in 11 patients with Bosniak type 3 indeterminate renal cysts). PET depicted solid neoplasms as areas of increased uptake in 9 of 10 patients. Bilateral renal cell carcinomas were missed in one diabetic patient. All but one of the indeterminate renal cysts were correctly classified as benign (photopenic areas), but an indeterminate cyst with a 4-mm papillary neoplasm was incorrectly classified as benign. No FDG-PET image interpretations were false-positive. The mean tumor-to-kidney ratio was 3.0 for malignant lesions.

Bachor et al. (70) investigated 29 patients with solid renal masses preoperatively. Renal cell carcinoma was con-

TABLE 29.4. FDG-PET IN KIDNEY CARCINOMA

Author	Year	Reference	No. patients	Comments
Kocher et al.	1994	77	10	PET: sensitivity, 80%; specificity, 90%.
Bachor et al.	1995	78	11	PET: sensitivity, 90%; specificity, 70%.
Hoh et al.	1996	68	22	FDG-PET is helpful for monitoring of therapy.
Miyauchi et al.	1996	79	11	Positive PET result at primary tumor site indicates high tumor grade.
Goldberg et al.	1997	69	21	Positive PET result may obviate need for additional diagnostic procedures, such as cyst puncture or biopsy.
Shulkin et al.	1997	75	3	PET in Wilms' tumors may be useful in diagnosis, in following the response to therapy, and in guiding therapeutic changes or surgical resection.

FDG-PET, positron emission tomography with fluorodeoxyglucose.

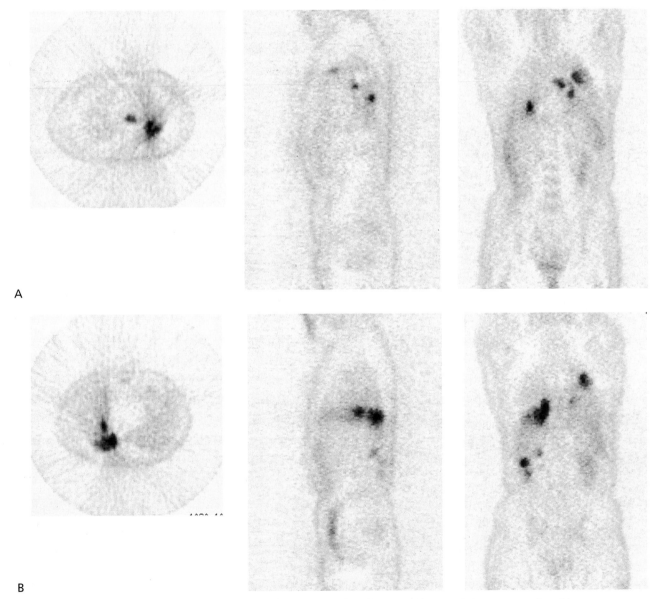

FIGURE 29.8. In a 50-year-old woman with renal carcinoma, positron emission tomography with fluorodeoxyglucose shows bone and lung (**A**) and liver (**B**) metastases.

firmed histologically in 26 patients. It was diagnosed correctly by FDG-PET in 20 patients (77% sensitivity). An angiomyolipoma, a pericytoma, and a pheochromocytoma were false-positive on FDG-PET. The finding of positive nodes in three patients provided correct lymph node staging, and no false-negative result was obtained. The authors concluded, however, that FDG-PET does not present any further advantage in comparison with standard methods for diagnosis or lymph node staging.

Wilms' tumor represents a distinct kidney tumor entity. It is the most common renal neoplasm in children (71,72). These tumors usually present as symptomatic abdominal masses. The diagnosis is suggested by typical findings on CT or ultrasonography and is established by biopsy or resection (73,74). Functional imaging makes it possible to evaluate skeletal metastases or renal function in selected cases. Preliminary data from limited series indicate that some Wilms' tumors accumulate FDG and can thus be visualized with PET. FDG-PET may be useful to distinguish benign from malignant masses, plan operative approaches, or determine the necessity of invasive procedures. FDG-PET may also be useful in following the response to therapy and in selecting alternative therapies in patients failing to respond to conventional approaches. Given the variability of FDG uptake in these tumors (75), the absence of accumulation does exclude viable Wilms' tumor.

The potential role of whole-body FDG-PET in the management of renal cell carcinoma may be related to its ability to image the entire body to identify additional sites of metastatic disease (Fig. 29.8). This is important in determining whether a patient has a single solitary metastasis; in such cases, if the patient is treated aggressively, significant palliation of symptoms and occasionally prolonged survival may be achieved (76). The use of FDG-PET to determine the metabolic activity of a tumor after aggressive chemotherapy or immunotherapy is another potential application in patients with renal carcinoma.

BLADDER CARCINOMA

Bladder cancer is one of the most common diseases treated by urologists and the fourth most common cause of cancer deaths in men, after lung, prostate, and colorectal cancer. It accounts for 5% of all cancer deaths in men in the United States (80). The male-to-female prevalence ratio of 3:1 may be a consequence of increased exposure among men to suspected environmental toxins, such as cigarette smoke. The male predominance appears to be decreasing. Artificial sweeteners have been suspected as another potential carcinogen. Approximately 70% of bladder cancers are low-grade, superficial tumors, but tumor recurrences develop in the majority of patients following endoscopic resection. Most patients with invasive bladder cancer already have

occult distant metastases at the time of initial diagnosis (80). Although a patient with a superficial tumor has a relatively good prognosis, invasive cancer causes death during the first year after diagnosis in 50% to 60% of cases. Despite new treatment options, survival has not increased during the last decade (81).

The diagnostic strategy should ideally define the depth of bladder wall infiltration and determine whether the tumor is localized or metastatic. Usually, this strategy consists of cystoscopy, biopsy, and bimanual palpation under general anesthesia. Although abdominal ultrasonography, CT, and MRI are helpful in detecting tumor masses, they are not as accurate for staging (80–86). The accuracy of CT is limited because it detects only large, extravesical tumor extension. Enlarged regional lymph nodes do not always indicate metastases (83). CT fails to detect lymph node metastases from bladder cancer in up to 40% of patients with such lesions (84). Furthermore, the use of CT appears to result in frequent overstaging. The accuracy of MRI is only 60% based on TNM (tumor–node–metastasis) staging. Most MRI studies fail to visualize lymphatic metastases adequately (85). Dynamic contrast-enhanced MRI is more accurate than conventional MRI, although staging accuracy is at best 75% (86). Transurethral ultrasonography is most valuable in determining the stage of tumors confined to the bladder wall (87). However, this technique has limitations in detecting lymph node involvement and perivesical tumor extension. Generally, these modalities have a poor capability for differentiating viable tumor mass from radiation-induced cystitis or radiation necrosis, although such differentiation is important in cases of bladder cancer with a persistent, protracted clinical course. After radiotherapy, the discordance between clinical and pathologic staging may approach 50% as a result of both understaging and overstaging (84).

It is conceivable that alteration in metabolism precedes morphologic changes. In the study of Kosuda et al. (88), the detection rate for FDG-PET was 66.7% (8 of 12 patients with bladder tumor; 4 intravesical recurrent tumors were not detected). Of 20 metastatic lesions confirmed pathologically or clinically, 16 (80%) were detected by FDG-PET. Direct invasion of the sigmoid colon not detected by CT was demonstrated by PET. FDG-PET visualized two of three regional lymph node metastases. These results suggest that FDG-PET may be particularly useful for staging advanced disease. FDG-PET also detected residual bladder cancer in two patients who had undergone radiotherapy and chemotherapy. This is very encouraging, given the poor ability of CT to discriminate recurrent cancer from certain benign diseases (i.e., radiation-induced bladder wall thickening or necrosis and infectious cystitis with hematoma resulting from operative procedures). MRI is also suboptimal in differentiating radiation necrosis from tumor recurrence. Given the high rate of recurrence of bladder cancer after

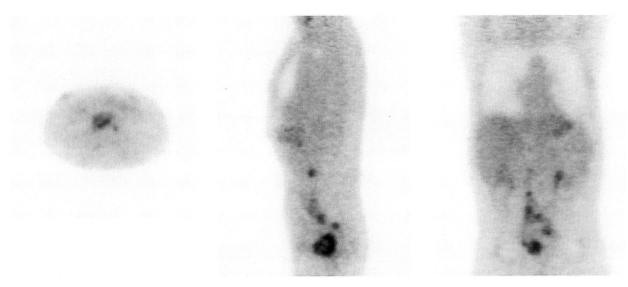

FIGURE 29.9. In a 69-year-old man with a history of bladder cancer treated 1 year earlier with surgery and chemotherapy, positron emission tomography with fluorodeoxyglucose shows locoregional nodal dissemination.

TABLE 29.5. FDG-PET IN BLADDER CARCINOMA

Author	Year	Reference	No. patients	PET sensitivity (%)	PET specificity (%)
Kocher et al.	1994	77	10	100	100
Kocher et al.	1995	93	31	80	63
Bachor et al.	1995	78	26	86	70
Kosuda et al.	1996	92	12	NA	NA
Bachor et al.	1999	91	64	67	86

FDG-PET, positron emission tomography with fluorodeoxyglucose; NA, not available.

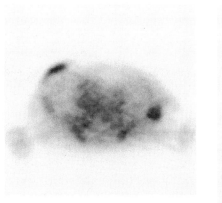
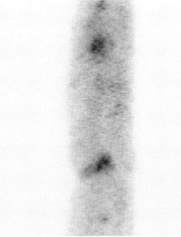
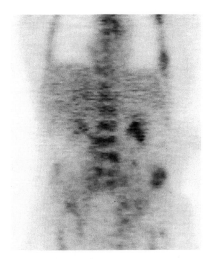

A

FIGURE 29.10. A 61-year-old man presented with bladder cancer previously treated with surgery and chemotherapy. Positron emission tomography with fluorodeoxyglucose shows (**A**) marrow. *(continued)*

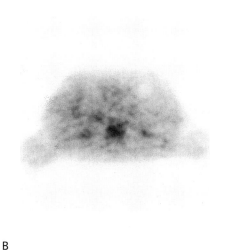
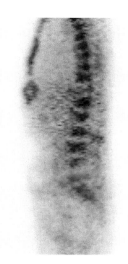
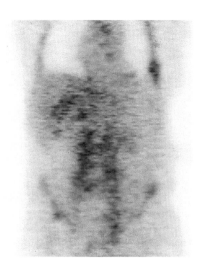

B

FIGURE 29.10. *(continued)* Positron emission tomography with fluorodeoxyglucose shows (**B**) bone, liver, and lymph node involvement.

treatment, FDG-PET may have a role in the management of patients following treatment (Fig. 29.9).

A major problem with FDG-PET in imaging bladder cancer is the comparatively intense activity resulting from the urinary excretion of FDG. In dogs, this represents 16% of the injected dose at 60 minutes (89). Kidneys and urine have the highest FDG concentration in the body, measured as percentage of injected dose per gram of organ tissue (89,90). Retrograde irrigation of the urinary bladder with saline solution and a Foley catheter before imaging and postvoid scanning can reduce the apparent activity of FDG in the urine. Another method of lowering or diluting FDG activity in the urine is to administer intravenous saline solution or diuretics before FDG. Nevertheless, urinary activity overlying tumor activity is more or less inevitable. This explains the poor performances of FDG-PET for detecting bladder cancer at stages O to C in the Jewett-Strong-Marshal staging system. Involvement of the contiguous organs and lymph nodes in stage D1 disease might be adequately diagnosed by FDG-PET.

In various series, lymph node involvement was accurately diagnosed in the majority of patients (Table 29.5). In a study by Bachor et al. (91), the sensitivity of FDG for lymph node staging of the pelvis was 67%, the specificity 86%, and the accuracy 80%. The authors concluded that FDG-PET results are superior to those obtained with clinical staging procedures, such as CT or MRI.

In summary, FDG-PET is a useful tool for the detection of perivesical tumor growth or distant metastases in patients with advanced bladder cancer, for lymph node staging, and for the early detection of recurrent cancer following therapy (Fig. 29.10).

REFERENCES

1. Einhorn N, Nilson B, Stovall K. Factors influencing survival in carcinoma of the ovary. *Cancer* 1985;55:2215–2019.
2. Einhorn N, Bast RC, Knapp RC, et al. Preoperative evaluation of serum CA 125 in patients with primary epithelial ovarian cancer. *Obstet Gynecol* 1986;67:414–416.
3. Hendler FJ. Carcinoma of ovary. In: Braunwald E, Isselbacher KJ, Petersdorf, et al., eds. *Harrison's principles of internal medicine.* New York: McGraw-Hill, 1987:1574–1578 (vol 2).
4. Wahl RL, Hutchins G, Robertz J. PET imaging of ovarian cancer: initial evaluation in patients. *J Nucl Med* 1991;32:982.
5. Hubner KF, McDonald TW, Smith GT, et al. Assessment of primary and metastatic ovarian cancer by positron emission tomography using 2-(^{18}F)deoxyglucose. *Gynecol Oncol* 1993;51:197–204.
6. Beckers C, Paulus P, Rigo P. Evaluation abdomino-pelvienne des cancers ovariens: comparaison de la tomographie à émission de positons au 18-FDG avec la laparotomie exploratrice. *Médecine Nucléaire—Imagerie Fonctionnelle et Métabolique* 1996;20:479.
7. Parkin DM, Laara E, Puir CS. Estimates of the worldwide frequency of sixteen major cancers in 1980. *Int J Cancer* 1988;41:184–197.
8. Stehman FB, Bundy BN, DiSaia MJ, et al. Carcinoma of the cervix treated with radiation therapy. I. A multi-variate analysis of prognostic variables in the Gynecologic Oncology Group. *Cancer* 1991;67:2776–2785.
9. Heller PB, Malfetano JH, Bundy BN, et al. Clinical-pathologic study of stage IIb, III and IVa carcinoma of the cervix: extended diagnostic evaluation for paraaortic node metastasis—a Gynecologic Oncologic Group study. *Gynecol Oncol* 1990;38:425–430.
10. Rose PG, Adler LP, Rodriguez M, et al. Positron emission tomography for evaluating para-aortic nodal metastasis in locally advanced cervical cancer before surgical staging: a surgicopathologic study. *J Clin Oncol* 1999;17:41–45.
11. Einhorn LH, Richie JP, Shipley WV. Cancer of testis. In: De

Vita VT, Hellman S, Rosenberg SA, eds. *Cancer principles and practice of oncology*. Philadelphia: JB Lippincott Co, 1993: 1126–1128.

12. United Kingdom Testicular Cancer Study Group. Aetiology of testicular cancer: association with congenital abnormalities, age at puberty, infertility and exercise. *Br Med J* 1994;28: 1393–1399.

13. Mustofi SK, Sobin LH. *International histological classification of tumors of testes*. Geneva: World Health Organization Publications, 1977 (No. 16).

14. Einhorn LH. Salvage therapy for germ cell tumors. *Semin Oncol* 1994;21:47–51.

15. Mason MD. Tumor markers. In: Horwich A, ed. *Investigation and management of testicular cancer*. London: Chapman & Hall, 1991:33–50.

16. Kausitz J, Ondrus D, Belan V, et al. Monitoring of patients with non-seminomatous germ cell tumors of the testis by determination of alpha-fetoprotein and beta-human chorionic gonadotrophin levels and by computed tomography. *Neoplasma* 1992;39: 357–361.

17. Javadpour N, Young JD. Predictors of residual mass requiring resection after chemotherapy and stage III testicular cancer. A prospective study. *Urology* 1992;40:7–8.

18. Bajorin D, Herr H, Motzer R, et al. Current perspectives on the role of adjuvant surgery in combined mortality treatment for patient with germ cell tumors. *Semin Oncol* 1992;19:148–158.

19. Peckham M. Testicular cancer. *Rev Oncol* 1988;1:439–453.

20. Aprikian AG, Herr HW, Bajorin DF, et al. Resection of postchemotherapy residual masses and limited retroperitoneal lymphadenectomy in patients with metastatic testicular nonseminomatous germ cell tumors. *Cancer* 1994;74:1329–1334.

21. Wahle GR, Foster RS, Bihrle R, et al. Nerve-sparing retroperitoneal lymphadenectomy after primary chemotherapy for metastatic testicular carcinoma. *J Urol* 1994;152:428–430.

22. Toner GC, Panicek DM, Heelan RT, et al. Adjunctive surgery after chemotherapy for nonseminomatous germ cell tumors: recommendations for patient selection. *J Clin Oncol* 1990;8: 1683–1694.

23. Jansen RL, Sylvester R, Sleyfer DT, et al. Long-term follow-up of nonseminomatous testicular cancer patients with mature teratoma or carcinoma at postchemotherapy surgery. EORTC Genitourinary Tract Cancer Cooperative Group. *Eur J Cancer* 1991;27:695–698.

24. Hendry WF, A'Hern RP, Hetherington JW, et al. Para-aortic lymphadenectomy after chemotherapy for metastatic non-seminomatous germ cell tumors: prognostic value and therapeutic benefit. *Br J Urol* 1993;71:208–213.

25. Stomper PC, Kalish LA, Garnick MB, et al. CT and pathologic predictive features of residual mass histologic findings after chemotherapy for nonseminomatous tumors: can residual malignancy or teratoma be excluded? *Radiology* 1991;180: 711–714.

26. Hendry WF. Decision making in abdominal surgery following chemotherapy for testicular cancer. *Eur J Cancer* 1995;31A: 649–650.

27. Debono D, Einhorn LH. Decision analysis for post-chemotherapy in patients with disseminated non-seminomatous germ cell tumors. *Proc Am Soc Clin Oncol* 1995;14:240.

28. Baniel J, Foster R, Gonin R, et al. Late relapse of testicular cancer. *J Clin Oncol* 1995;13:1170–1176.

29. Nuutinen JM, Leskinen S, Elomaa I, et al. Detection of residual tumors in postchemotherapy testicular cancer by FDG-PET. *Eur J Cancer* 1997;33:1234–1241.

30. Dohmen BM, Bares R, Gronimus R, et al. Improved staging of germ cell cancer after chemotherapy by FDG-positron-emission-tomography. *Eur J Nucl Med* 1995;22:804.

31. Stephens A, Gonin R, Hutchins G, et al. Positron emission tomography evaluation of residual radiographic abnormalities in postchemotherapy germ cell tumors. *J Clin Oncol* 1996;14: 1637–1641.

32. Wahl R, Greenough R, Clarke M, et al. Initial evaluation of FDG-PET imaging of metastatic testicular neoplasms. *J Nucl Med* 1993;Abstract Book:6P.

33. Wilson CB, Young HE, Ott EJ, et al. Imaging metastatic testicular germ cell tumors with [18]FDG positron emission tomography: prospects for detection and management. *Eur J Nucl Med* 1995;22:508–513.

34. Di Chiro G. Positron emission tomography using ^{18}F-fluorodeoxyglucose in brain tumors: a powerful diagnostic and prognostic tool. *Invest Radiol* 1986;22:360–371.

35. Leskinen-Kallio S, Ruotsalainen U, Nagreen K, et al. Uptake of carbon-11-methionine and fluorodeoxyglucose in non-Hodgkin's lymphoma: a PET study. *J Nucl Med* 1990;32:1211–1218.

36. Patz EF, Lowe VJ, Hoffman JM, et al. Focal pulmonary abnormalities: evaluation with F-18 fluorodeoxyglucose PET scanning. *Radiology* 1993;188:487–490.

37. Kubota K, Yamada K, Yoshioka S, et al. Differential diagnosis of idiopathic fibrosis from malignant lymphadenopathy with PET and F-18 fluorodeoxyglucose. *Clin Nucl Med* 1991;17: 361–363.

38. Cremerius U, Effert PJ, Adam G, et al. FDG-PET for detection and therapy control of metastatic germ cell tumor. *J Nucl Med* 1998;39:815–822.

39. Harms W, Bares R, Gromius R, et al. FDG-PET zur Vitalitaetsdiagnostik metastasierter Hodentumoren nach Chemotherapie. *Nucl Med* 1995;35:V27.

40. Harms W, Bares R, Kamps H, Gronimus R, et al. Therapy control of metastatic testicular carcinoma with F18-FDG PET. *J Nucl Med* 1995;36:198.

41. Laubenbacher C, Hofer C, Avril N, et al. F-18 FDG PET for differentiation of local recurrent prostatic cancer and scar. *J Nucl Med* 1995;36:198.

42. Reinhardt M, Mueller-Matheis V, Vosberg H, et al. Staging of lymph nodes in testicular cancer by FDG-PET. *Eur J Nucl Med* 1995;22:804.

43. Bender H, Schromburg A, Albers P, et al. Possible role of FDG-PET in the evaluation of urologic malignancies. *Anticancer Res* 1997;17:1655–1660.

44. Nuutinen L, Leskinen S, Elomaa I, et al. FDG-PET imaging of residual testicular cancer after chemotherapy. *J Nucl Med* 1996;37:256.

45. Albers P, Bender H, Yilmaz H, et al. Position emission tomography in the clinical staging of patients with stage I and II testicular germ cell tumors. *Urology* 1999;53:808–811.

46. Jensen OM, Esteve J, Moller H, et al. Cancer in the European Community and its member states. *Eur J Cancer* 1990;26:1167.

47. American Cancer Society. *Cancer. Facts and figures—1992*. Atlanta: American Cancer Society, 1992.

48. Donohue RE, Mani JH, Whitesel JA, et al. Stage D1 adenocarcinoma of the prostate. *Urology* 1984;23:118.

49. Stamley TA, McNeal JE, Freiha FS, et al. Morphometric and clinical studies on 68 consecutive radical prostatectomies. *J Urol* 1988;139:1235.

50. Rifkin MD, Zerhouni EA, Gatsonis CA, et al. Comparison of magnetic resonance imaging and ultrasonography in staging early prostate cancer: results of a multi-institutional cooperative trial. *N Engl J Med* 1990;323:621.

51. Strauss LG, Conti PS. The applications of PET in clinical oncology. *J Nucl Med* 1991;32:623.

52. Bares R, Klever P, Hauptmann S, et al. F-18 fluorodeoxyglucose PET *in vivo* evaluation of pancreatic glucose metabolism for detection of pancreatic cancer. *Radiology* 1994;192:79.

53. Franks LM. The spread of prostate carcinoma. *J Pathol* 1956; 72:603–611.

54. Trupkaew AK, Henkin RE, Quinn LL. False-negative bone scans in disseminated metastatic disease. *Radiology* 1974;113: 383–386.

55. Shreeve PD, Grossman HB, Gross MD, et al. Metastatic prostate cancer: initial findings of PET with 2-deoxy-2-(F-18)fluoro-D-glucose. *Radiology* 1996;199:751–756.

56. Hoh CK, Rosen PJ, Belldegrun, et al. Quantitative and whole body FDG PET in the evaluation of suramine therapy in patients with metastatic prostate cancer. *J Nucl Med* 1996;37:267.

57. Shreve P, Gross MD, Wahl RL. Detection of prostate cancer metastases with FDG. *J Nucl Med* 1995;36:189.

58. Larson SM, Schwartz LH. Advances in imaging. *Semin Oncol* 1994;21:598–606.

59. Nilsson A, Kalkner KM, Cinman C, et al. ^{11}C-methionine positron emission tomography in the management of prostatic carcinoma. *Antibody Immun Radiopharm* 1995;8:23–38.

60. Bares R, Effert P, Handt S, et al. Metabolic classification of untreated prostate cancer by use of FDG-PET. *J Nucl Med* 1994;36:198.

61. Yeh SDJ, Imbriaco M, Garza D, et al. Twenty percent of hormone-resistant prostate cancers are detected by PET-FDG whole-body scanning. *J Nucl Med* 1995;36:198.

62. Reinhardt M, Mueller-Matheis V, Vosberg H, et al. Time activity analysis improves specificity of FDG-PET in staging of pelvic lymph node metastases. *Eur J Nucl Med* 1995;22:803.

63. Haseman MK, Reed NL, Rosenthal SA, et al. Monoclonal antibody imaging of occult prostate cancer in patients with elevated specific antigen: positron emission tomography and biopsy correlation. *Clin Nucl Med* 1996;21:704–713.

64. Hofer C, Laubenbacher C, Block T, et al. Fluorine-18-fluorodeoxyglucose positron emission tomography is useless for the detection of local recurrence after radical prostatectomy. *Eur Urol* 1999;36:31–35.

65. Linehan WM, Shipley WU, Parkinson DR. Cancer of the kidney and ureter. In: DeVita VT, Hellman S, Rosenberg SA, eds. *Cancer principles and practice of oncology*, 5th ed. Philadelphia: JB Lippincott Co, 1997.

66. Gallagher BM, Fowler JS, Gutterson NI, et al. Metabolic trapping as a principle of radiopharmaceutical design: some factors responsible for the biodistribution of (^{18}F)-2-deoxy-2-fluoro-D-glucose. *J Nucl Med* 1978;19:1154–1161.

67. Wahl RL, Harney J, Hutchins G, et al. Imaging of renal cancer using positron emission tomography with 2-deoxy-2-(^{18}F)-fluoro-D-glucose: pilot animal and human studies. *J Urol* 1991;146:1470–1474.

68. Hoh CK, Figlin RA, Belldegrum A, et al. Evaluation of renal cell carcinoma with whole-body FDG PET. *J Nucl Med* 1996; 37:141.

69. Goldberg MA, Mayo-Smith WW, Papanicolaou N, et al. FDG-PET characterization of renal masses: preliminary experience. *Clin Radiol* 1997;52:510–515.

70. Bachor R, Kotzerke J, Gottfried HW, et al. Positron emission tomography in diagnosis of renal cell carcinoma. *Urologe A* 1996;35:146–150.

71. Breslow NE, Beckwith JB. Epidemiological features of Wilms' tumor: results of the National Wilms' Tumor Study. *J Natl Cancer Inst* 1982;68:429–436.

72. Yeh SDJ. Genitourinary tract nuclear oncology. *Urol Radiol* 1992;14:107–114.

73. Hugosson C, Nyman R, Jacobsson B, et al. Imaging of solid kidney tumors in children. *Acta Radiol* 1995;36:254–260.

74. White KS, Grossman H. Wilms' and associated renal tumors of childhood. *Pediatr Radiol* 1991;21:81–88.

75. Shulkin BL, Chang E, Strouse PJ, et al. PET FDG studies of Wilms' tumors. *J Pediatr Hematol Oncol* 1997;19:334–338.

76. DeKernion JB, Ramming KP, Smith RB. The natural history of metastatic renal cell carcinoma: a computer analysis. *J Urol* 1978;120:148.

77. Kocher F, Geimmel S, Hauptmann R, et al. Preoperative lymph node staging in patients with kidney and urinary bladder neoplasms. *J Nucl Med* 1994;35:223.

78. Bachor R, Kocher F, Gropengiesser F, et al. Positron emission tomography. Introduction of a new procedure in the diagnosis of urologic tumors and initial clinical results. *Urol Arch* 1995; 34:138–142.

79. Miyauchi T, Brown RS, Grossman HB, et al. Correlation between visualization of primary renal cancer by FDG-PET and histopathological findings. *J Nucl Med* 1996;37:64.

80. Catalona WJ. Urothelial tumors of the urinary tract. In: Walsh PC, Retik AB, Stamey YA, et al., eds. *Campbell's urology*, 6th ed. Philadelphia: WB Saunders, 1992:1094–1158 (vol 2).

81. Malmström PU, Thörn M, Lindblad P, et al. Increasing survival in patients with urinary bladder cancer. A nation-wide study in Sweden 1960–1986. *Eur J Cancer* 1993;29:1868.

82. McCarthy P, Ramchandani P, Pollack H. The bladder and urethra. In: Vanel D, Stark D, eds. *Imaging strategies in oncology*. London: Martin Dunitz, 1993:289–297.

83. Nurmi M, Katevuo K, Puntala P. Reliability of CT in the preoperative evaluation of bladder carcinoma. *Scand J Urol Nephrol* 1988;22:125–128.

84. Lantz EJ, Hattery RR. Diagnostic imaging of urethelial cancer. *Urol Clin North Am* 1984;11:567–583.

85. Buy JN, Moss A, Guinet C, et al. MR staging of bladder carcinoma: correlation with pathologic findings. *Radiology* 1988; 169:695–700.

86. Kim B, Semelka Rc, Aschner SM, et al. Bladder tumor staging: comparison of contrast-enhanced CT, T_1- and T_2-weighted MR imaging, dynamic gadolinium-enhanced imaging, and late gadolinium-enhanced imaging. *Radiology* 1994;193:239–245.

87. Koraitim M, Kamal B, Metwalli N, et al. Transurethral ultrasonographic assessment of bladder carcinoma: its value and limitation. *J Urol* 1995;154:375–378.

88. Kosuda S, Kison PV, Greenough R, et al. Preliminary assessment of fluorine-18 fluorodeoxyglucose positron emission tomography in patients with bladder cancer. *Eur J Nucl Med* 1997;24:615–620.

89. Effert PJ, Bares R, Handt S, et al. Metabolic imaging of untreated prostate cancer by positron tomography with [18]FDG. *J Urol* 1996;155:994–998.

90. Gallagher BM, Ansari A, Atkins H, et al. Radiopharmaceuticals XXVII. [18]FDG as a radiopharmaceutical for measuring regional myocardial glucose metabolism *in vivo*: distribution and imaging studies in animals. *J Nucl Med* 1977;18:990–996.

91. Bachor R, Kotzerke J, Reske SN, et al. Lymph node staging for urinary bladder carcinoma with positron emission tomography. *Urologe A* 1999;38:46–50.

92. Kosuda S, Grossman HN, Kison PV, et al. Preliminary FDG-PET study in patients with bladder cancer. *J Nucl Med* 1996;36:223.

93. Kocher F, Bachor R, Stoffulb JC, et al. Positron emission tomography of urinary bladder carcinoma. *Eur J Nucl Med* 1995;35:888.

30

RENAL CARCINOMA: MONOCLONAL ANTIBODY THERAPY

CHAITANYA R. DIVGI
EGBERT OOSTERWIJK
NEIL H. BANDER
SYDNEY WELT
STEVEN M. LARSON
LLOYD OLD

Antibody G250 was initially developed as a murine IgG1 with specific reactivity against clear cell renal carcinoma (1). An initial presurgical clinical trial showed a very high tumor uptake of antibody, with a saturable hepatic uptake (2). These observations led to a radioimmunotherapy trial with ^{131}I-labeled murine G250 (mG250). Although the hepatic uptake was apparently saturable, radioactivity dose-independent transient hepatic toxicity was seen in the majority of patients treated with a single dose of ^{131}I-mG250. Dose-limiting toxicity was hematopoietic, no major responses occurred, and a human anti-mouse antibody (HAMA) response was invariable (3).

The observation that overall survival seemed to be increased in patients treated with ^{131}I-mG250, in addition to the few minor responses and the clear necessity for multiple infusions, led to the development and use of chimeric G250 (cG250). In a presurgical clinical trial, cG250 was shown to target clear cell renal carcinoma in a manner comparable with that of its murine equivalent, and it was much less immunogenic than its murine counterpart (4). A subsequent radioimmunotherapy trial with ^{131}I-cG250, in

which pretherapeutic administration of cG250 was utilized, showed that dose-limiting toxicity is hematopoietic and, significantly, that no hepatic toxicity occurs, presumably because of blockade of the bile duct cell receptors by pretherapeutic cG250 (5). The lack of immunogenicity of cG250 led to a phase I fractionated radioimmunotherapy trial, which again showed that dose-limiting toxicity is hematopoietic and no hepatic toxicity occurs (6). Meanwhile, the G250 antigen has been characterized (7). Clinical phase I trials with unlabeled cG250 are under way, as are phase II trials with ^{131}I-cG250 in which both single large dose and fractionated schemata are employed.

This review details each of these trials, to illustrate the stepwise logical study of an antibody with selective affinity for an antigen predominantly expressed in a solid tumor for which no standard therapy is currently available.

PRESURGICAL CLINICAL TRIAL WITH ^{131}I-MG250

A presurgical clinical study of ^{131}I (10 mCi) labeled to escalating mass amounts of mG250 (0.2, 2, 10, 25, and 50 mg, in cohorts of three patients each) was conducted to determine tumor uptake and biodistribution (2). At least three whole-body images were obtained in each patient—on the day of administration, 2 to 3 days after injection, and before or on the day of surgery.

As with other radiolabeled antibody studies, initial images did not show radioactivity within tumor; tumor uptake was clearly evident 2 to 3 days after antibody administration. Figure 30.1 shows sequential whole-body images obtained in a patient who received 10 mCi/10 mg of ^{131}I-mG250. The patient had a left renal and a right adrenal mass; the adrenal mass was questionable for metastasis on other imaging modalities. Uptake of antibody in the right

C. R. Divgi: Department of Radiology, Weill Medical College of Cornell University; Department of Radiology and Medicine, Memorial Sloan-Kettering Cancer Center, New York, New York 10021.

E. Oosterwijk: Department of Urology, University Nijmegen, 6500 Nijmegen, The Netherlands.

N. H. Bander: Department of Urology, Weill Medical College of Cornell University; Department of Urology, New York Presbyterian Hospital, New York, New York 10021.

S. Welt: Memorial Sloan-Kettering Cancer Center, New York, New York 10021.

S. M. Larson: Department of Nuclear Medicine, Weill Medical College of Cornell University; Nuclear Medicine Service, Memorial Sloan-Kettering Cancer Center, New York, New York 10021.

L. Old: Ludwig Institute for Cancer Research, New York, New York 10021.

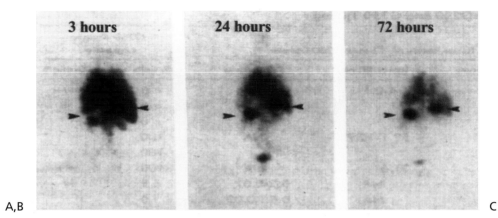

A,B   C

FIGURE 30.1. Posterior images of a patient with a left renal and a right adrenal mass (*arrows*), obtained after intravenous administration of 10 mCi/10 mg of ^{131}I-mG250.

adrenal mass convinced the surgeon to perform a biopsy, which showed the lesion to be metastatic.

Decreased liver uptake of ^{131}I-mG250 at higher doses, and radioactivity in the liver comparable with that in the blood pool at doses of 10 mg or greater, suggested saturation of G250 sites by antibody. Figure 30.2 shows whole-body images obtained at comparable time points in patients who received 0.2, 2, and 10 mg of antibody. The incremental decrease in hepatic uptake and the consequent increase in tumor-to-liver ratios are evident. Based on these observations, the optimal mass amount of antibody was determined to be at least 10 mg.

As all the patients underwent nephrectomy, we were able to obtain *ex vivo* images of the kidney. To establish further that antibody uptake in tumor is not merely a function of the vascular nature of renal cell carcinoma, we administered 10 mCi of ^{99m}Tc-human serum albumin immediately before

surgery. Gamma camera images of ^{99m}Tc and ^{131}I distribution in the nephrectomy specimen were then obtained to confirm the disparity between antibody accumulation and blood pool. Figure 30.3 clearly demonstrates that antibody uptake (as evidenced by ^{131}I distribution) is selective to tumor (see also Color Plate 12 following page 350).

Tumor biopsy samples showed a high level of mG250 localization, with levels of up to 0.1% of the injected dose per gram of tumor (%ID/g) 7 days after infusion. *Ex vivo* immunohistochemical analysis of contiguous tumor tissue slices indicated that a single infusion of ^{131}I-mG250 did not saturate all antigen sites, even with the administration of increasing mass amounts (Fig. 30.4; see also Color Plate 13 following page 350). This underscored the need to develop other approaches to target all available antigenic sites, including multiple administrations, reported to be more effective in animal models (8), and smaller molecules, such as

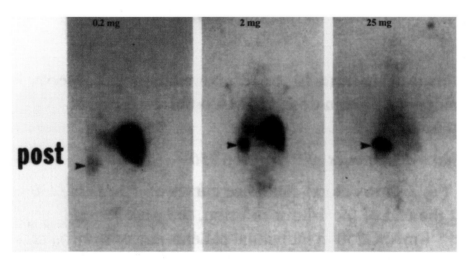

FIGURE 30.2. Posterior images of three patients 3 days after administration of 10 mCi/0.2 mg (*left*), 10 mCi/2 mg (*center*), and 10 mCi/25 mg (*right*) of ^{131}I-mG250. Note the decreasing hepatic uptake and increasing tumor uptake, and the tumor-to-liver ratios.

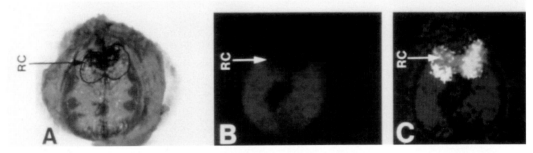

FIGURE 30.3. A: Kidney placed on gamma camera. Note the tumor (*RC, arrow*) in the upper pole. **B:** Image of the kidney; the blue area represents distribution of ^{99m}Tc-human serum albumin. Note that the distribution of albumin in the tumor is relatively low. **C:** Distribution of ^{131}I is limited to tumor, confirming selective uptake of radiolabeled antibody. (See also Color Plate 12 following p. 350.)

single-chain antigen-binding proteins (sFv), which have been shown to penetrate to a greater extent into tumor sites (9).

The tumor uptake of mG250 was among the highest reported in studies of solid tumors; normal tissue uptake, limited to the liver, was saturable at doses of 10 mg or greater. These observations encouraged future development of the system. On the one hand, we initiated a radioimmunotherapy trial with ^{131}I-mG250 in patients with metastatic renal carcinoma; on the other, cG250 was constructed to address the invariable development of an HAMA response.

RADIOIMMUNOTHERAPY WITH ^{131}I-MG250

A phase I/II radioimmunotherapy trial with ^{131}I-mG250, to determine its safety and efficacy, was initiated at Memorial Sloan-Kettering Cancer Center (3). Cohorts of at least three patients received escalating amounts of ^{131}I (from 30 to 90 mCi of ^{131}I per square meter) labeled to 10 mg of mG250,

administered as a single infusion. All patients had measurable metastatic clear cell renal cancer. Targeting to known disease 2 cm or greater in diameter was excellent (Fig. 30.5). Hepatic toxicity was invariable, despite the prior observation that 10 mg of antibody saturated liver sites. However, it was unrelated to the amount of radioactivity administered or the radiation absorbed dose to the liver, transient, and not dose-limiting. Dose-limiting toxicity, as in all other radioimmunotherapy studies of radiolabeled antibodies, was hematopoietic, with the maximum tolerated dose of activity (MTDA) determined to be 90 mCi of ^{131}I per square meter. At this dose, a total of 15 patients were studied to determine efficacy. The development of HAMAs in all patients precluded re-treatment. No major responses were noted. The excellent targeting and the lack of significant nonhematopoietic toxicity demonstrated the potential of radiolabeled G250 in the treatment of renal cancer. The development of an immune response indicated that studies with nonimmunogenic G250 antibody are warranted.

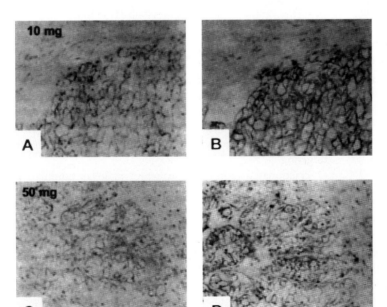

FIGURE 30.4. Immunohistochemistry, without exogenous antibody, of a 5-µm slice from a kidney tumor excised 7 days after administration of 10 mg of mG250 **(A)**; the targeting of mG250 administered a week before surgery is demonstrated, although all antigen sites are not targeted, as shown by the addition of exogenous antibody **(B)**. Increasing the administered dose to 50 mg does not result in an appreciable increase in targeting of available antigen sites, as shown in comparable slices **(C,D)**. (See also Color Plate 13 following p. 350.)

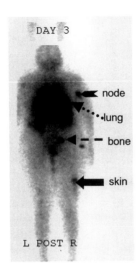

FIGURE 30.5. Posterior whole-body ^{131}I image obtained 3 days after administration of 45 mCi of ^{131}I-mG250 per square meter in a patient with metastatic clear cell renal cancer. Targeting to disease in nodes, lung, bone, and skin (*arrows*) is clear; targeting to liver metastases was also excellent (not evident in the posterior image).

PRESURGICAL AND RADIOIMMUNOTHERAPY TRIALS WITH ^{131}I-CG250

Chimeric G250 was initially studied at the University of Nijmegen in a presurgical trial. The trial design was comparable with that for mG250 (4). Cohorts of patients scheduled to undergo nephrectomy for renal carcinoma received escalating amounts (2 to 50 mg) of antibody labeled with a fixed amount of [131]I. Tumor uptake was assessed by serial imaging and by *ex vivo* measurement of radioactivity in surgically removed tumor and normal tissue. As with the murine antibody, hepatic uptake was saturable, at doses of 5 mg or greater in this study. All 13 antigen-positive tumors showed excellent targeting (Fig. 30.6A) of radioactivity, with uptake (measured at biopsy 1 week after infusion) as high as 0.52% of the injected dose per gram of tumor. Furthermore, no evidence of a host immune response was found, as measured by enzyme-linked immunosorbent assay (ELISA). These results encouraged the study of ^{131}I-cG250 in the therapy of renal cell carcinoma.

The group has subsequently completed a phase I radioimmunotherapy trial with escalating doses of ^{131}I labeled to a fixed amount (5 mg) of cG250. To ensure that the metastases were antibody-avid, an initial imaging dose of ^{131}I-cG250 (5 mg) was administered, and only those patients who showed targeting to tumor received the therapeutic infusion of ^{131}I-cG250 1 week later. As in all other radioimmunotherapy trials, dose-limiting toxicity (approximately 60 mCi of ^{131}I per square meter) was hematopoietic. However, no hepatic toxicity was seen, as it was in the

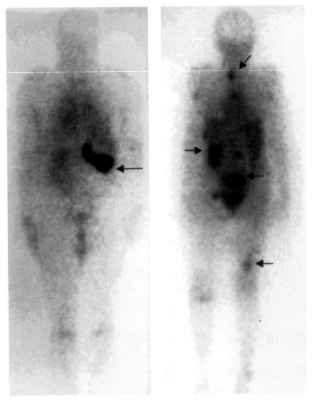

FIGURE 30.6. Posterior whole-body images after administration of 5 mg of ^{131}I-cG250. **A:** In a patient before nephrectomy of the right kidney for clear cell renal cancer, labeled with 6 mCi of [131]I (*arrow,* right renal tumor). **B:** In a patient with metastatic renal cancer treated with 45 mCi of ^{131}I-cG250 per square meter (*arrows,* primary and metastatic lesions).

radioimmunotherapy trial with mG250. This was felt to be a consequence of saturation of hepatic receptors with the initial, "diagnostic" dose of cG250. Targeting of therapeutic ^{131}I-cG250 to disease was excellent (Fig. 30.6B) in those patients with positive "diagnostic" scans.

The above trials made it abundantly clear that expression of the G250 antigen is invariable in clear cell renal carcinomas. The radioimmunotherapy trials have also shown that antigen expression in metastatic disease is comparable with that in the primary tumor (3,5). Trials are ongoing in patients with clear cell renal cancer but no immunohistochemical documentation of antigen expression or tumor targeting.

Fractionated radioimmunotherapy at lower cumulative amounts of radioactivity has been shown in animal models to be more effective than a single large amount. Moreover, it appears that radiation absorbed dose to whole body or red marrow is a better predictor of hematopoietic toxicity than administered activity is (10). In coordination with the trials in Holland, a phase I fractionated radioimmunotherapy trial, based on whole-body radiation absorbed dose, was undertaken at Memorial Sloan-Kettering Cancer Center (6). An initial "scout" dose of 5 mCi/5 mg of ^{131}I-cG250

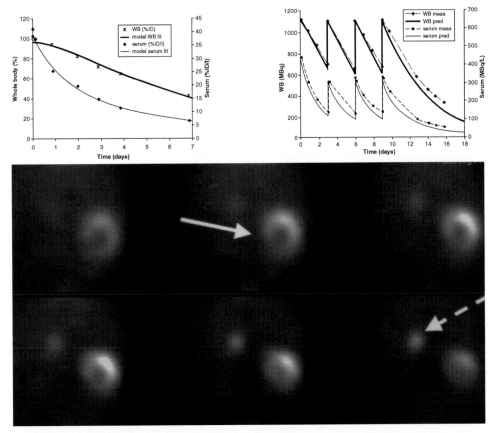

FIGURE 30.7. Fractionated radioimmunotherapy with ^{131}I-cG250. Upper left figure demonstrates two-compartmental model fitted on whole-body and serum radioactivity clearance data obtained during a week. Upper right figure demonstrates actual (*broken curves*) and predicted (*solid curves*) clearances in the same patient. The images represent coronal slices (posterior to anterior, upper left to lower right) obtained 3 days after administration of 30 mCi/5mg of ^{131}I-cG250 in a patient with renal cell carcinoma (with its photopenic center, *solid arrow*) and liver (*broken arrow*) metastases.

was followed a week later by fractions of ^{131}I-cG250 administered to deliver no more than a calculated whole-body radiation absorbed dose. These fractions were administered at 2- to 3-day intervals such that the amount of radioactivity in the body was never greater than 30 mCi of ^{131}I, which permitted outpatient therapy. A close correlation was noted between predicted and actual clearance of radioactivity (Fig. 30.7); furthermore, patients with stable disease were re-treated, and the majority tolerated repeated administrations with no change in kinetics, demonstrating the relative lack of immunogenicity of this antibody construct. Data analysis is ongoing, with particular emphasis on whether fractionation improves delivery of radiation dose to tumor.

CONCLUSIONS AND FUTURE

Although trials with ^{131}I-cG250 in renal cancer will continue, newer approaches to the treatment of this radioresistant disease are needed. Multiple-step approaches are being

considered (11), the preclinical development of linkers that offer the potential of therapy with rhenium-labeled constructs has been successful (12), and smaller constructs (sFv, minibodies) offer the potential for increasing the selective delivery of tumoricidal radiation with minimal toxicity to normal tissue (C. Renner, *personal communication*, 2000).

Undoubtedly, further obstacles will be encountered before renal cancer, a disease refractory to most therapies, can be successfully managed. The biopsy-based demonstration of the selective targeting of G250, determination of the optimal mass dose, the completion of standard phase I and phase II therapy trials, and the design of protein constructs with improved characteristics are all logical developmental steps in targeted therapy. We hope that these studies will serve as a paradigm for the study of antibodies in cancer.

REFERENCES

1. Oosterwijk E, Ruiter DJ, Hoedemaeker PJ, et al. Monoclonal antibody G250 recognizes a determinant present in renal-cell

carcinoma and absent from normal kidney. *Int J Cancer* 1986;38: 489–494.

2. Oosterwijk E, Bander NH, Divgi CR, et al. Antibody localization in human renal cell carcinoma: a phase I study of monoclonal antibody G250. *J Clin Oncol* 1993;11:738–750.

3. Divgi CR, Bander NH, Scott AM, et al. Phase I/II radioimmunotherapy trial with iodine-131-labeled monoclonal antibody G250 in metastatic renal cell carcinoma. *Clin Cancer Res* 1998;4: 2729–2739.

4. Steffens MG, Boerman OC, Oosterwijk-Wakka JC, et al. Targeting of renal cell carcinoma with iodine-131-labeled chimeric monoclonal antibody G250. *J Clin Oncol* 1997;15:1529–1537.

5. Steffens MG, Boerman OC, de Mulder PH, et al. Phase I radioimmunotherapy of metastatic renal cell carcinoma with ^{131}I-labeled chimeric monoclonal antibody G250. *Clin Cancer Res* 1999;5[10 Suppl]:3268s–3274s.

6. Divgi CR, O'Donoghue JA, Welt S, et al. Phase I radioimmunotherapy trial with fractionated ^{131}I-chimeric G250 (cG250) in clear cell renal carcinoma. *Proc Am Assoc Clin Oncol* 1999;394.

7. Grabmaier K, Vissers JL, De Weijert MC, et al. Molecular cloning and immunogenicity of renal cell carcinoma-associated antigen G250. *Int J Cancer* 2000;85:865–870.

8. Sun LQ, Vogel CA, Mirimanoff RO, et al. Timing effects of combined radioimmunotherapy and radiotherapy on a human solid tumor in nude mice. *Cancer Res* 1997;57:1312–1319.

9. Milenic DE, Yokota T, Filpula DR, et al. Construction, binding properties, metabolism, and tumor targeting of a single-chain Fv derived from the pancarcinoma monoclonal antibody CC49. *Cancer Res* 1991;51:6363–6371.

10. O'Donoghue JA. Dosimetric aspects of radioimmunotherapy. *Tumor Targeting* 1998;3:105–111.

11. Boerman OC, Kranenborg MH, Oosterwijk E, et al. Pretargeting of renal cell carcinoma: improved tumor targeting with a bivalent chelate. *Cancer Res* 1999;59:4400–4405.

12. Steffens MG, Oosterwijk E, Kranenborg MH, et al. *In vivo* and *in vitro* characterizations of three ^{99m}Tc-labeled monoclonal antibody G250 preparations. *J Nucl Med* 1999;40: 829–836.

31

MONOCLONAL ANTIBODY IMAGING

MICHAEL K. HASEMAN

Capromab pendetide (ProstaScint, Cytogen Corp., Princeton, NJ) is an [111]indium (^{111}In)–labeled intact murine IgG1 monoclonal antibody (mAb) reactive with prostate-specific membrane antigen (PSMA), a 100-kd transmembrane glycoprotein expressed by prostate tissue, both benign and malignant (1–4). The United States Food and Drug Administration approved ^{111}In-capromab pendetide for use as an imaging agent for the detection of soft-tissue metastases in patients with prostate cancer who are at high risk of metastatic disease, either at the time of initial diagnosis or in the setting of recurrent disease after treatment of the primary tumor. This chapter reviews the details of acquiring and interpreting ^{111}In-capromab pendetide images, briefly compares the efficacy of this technique with other imaging modalities, reviews the results of the phase III clinical trials, and discusses the clinical settings in which ^{111}In-capromab pendetide imaging is most likely to be of benefit in managing patients with prostate cancer.

IMAGE ACQUISITION AND PROCESSING

Capromab pendetide labeled with 5 mCi of ^{111}In is given by slow intravenous injection. *Whole-body planar imaging* and *single photon emission computed tomography* (SPECT) imaging of the pelvis and abdomen are performed 3 to 5 days after injection. Occasionally, it is necessary to obtain additional delayed planar or SPECT images beyond 3 to 5 days after injection, to allow more time for blood pool and bowel clearance. One can obtain diagnostic quality images up to approximately 10 days after injection. Because some of the tracer is excreted into bowel and bladder, the patient should be kept well hydrated, cathartics should be given, and the SPECT images should obtained after the patient voids. Administration of a Fleet enema on the day of imaging is also useful because excreted activity in the rectum can mimic disease in the prostate region.

M. K. Haseman: Department of Nuclear Medicine, University of California, Davis; Department of Nuclear Medicine, Sutter Medical Center, Sacramento, California 95816.

In addition to the ^{111}In-capromab pendetide images, SPECT blood pool imaging is also required as part of the routine examination because asymmetry of blood pool structures, particularly the iliac vessels, can be misinterpreted as pathologic uptake in adjacent lymph nodes. This can be accomplished in one of two ways. Imaging with SPECT can be done on the day of ^{111}In-capromab pendetide injection while the activity is still predominantly in the blood vessels. Alternatively, technetium 99m (^{99m}Tc)–labeled red blood cells can be injected at the time the day 3 to 5 images are obtained, and blood pool SPECT imaging can be done either simultaneously with or immediately after capromab pendetide imaging. Simultaneous dual isotope ^{99m}Tc red blood cell capromab pendetide imaging is the preferred technique because it provides perfect image coregistration and avoids the need for a separate SPECT acquisition.

To achieve optimal image resolution, it is crucial to obtain adequate count density while at the same time minimizing motion artifact that is likely to occur if acquisition times are too prolonged. For this reason, ^{111}In-capromab pendetide SPECT imaging should be done on multiheaded large field of view gamma cameras. Diagnostic quality images are more difficult to obtain on single-headed systems. Acquisition and processing parameters for SPECT need to be optimized for each laboratory. These parameters depend on numerous factors including the specific gamma camera and computer used, the size of the patient, the dose administered, and the time between injection and imaging. Recommended processing parameters for each of the major manufactures' machines were developed by the investigators during clinical trials and are available from Cytogen Corporation.

The normal biodistribution of ^{111}In-capromab pendetide is illustrated in Fig. 31.1. The most intense activity is found in the liver, spleen, bone marrow, and blood pool structures. A variable amount of activity is seen in the kidneys, nasopharynx, spermatic cord structures, and genitalia. Excreted activity is usually seen in the bowel, and occasionally this may be persistent on delayed imaging beyond day 3 to 5 even when cathartics are used. Bladder activity is variable and, after 3 days, usually faint.

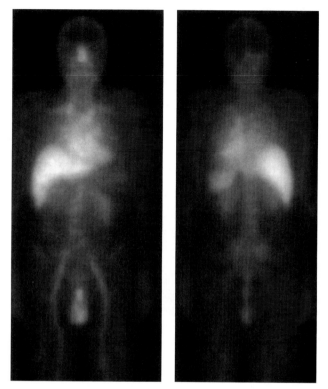

FIGURE 31.1. Day 4 anterior **(left)** and posterior **(right)** whole-body planar ¹¹¹indium-capromab pendetide images showing normal biodistribution of the radiopharmaceutical.

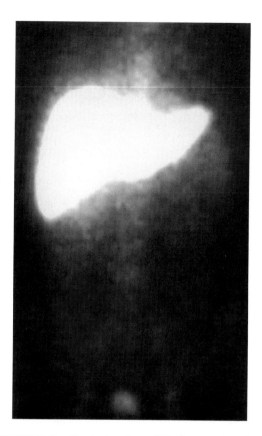

FIGURE 31.2. Day 3 anterior planar ¹¹¹indium-capromab pendetide image showing altered biodistribution of the radiopharmaceutical. Note the increased liver uptake and low level of activity in blood pool structures.

In approximately 5% to 8% of studies, the normal biodistribution of the mAb is altered, and one sees rapid blood pool clearance, intense liver uptake, and increased bone marrow activity, often associated with more than usual urinary excretion (Fig. 31.2). The cause of this altered biodistribution is unknown. It may be related to immune complex formation with rapid clearance by the reticuloendothelial system. Although unproven, the rapid clearance is likely to reduce the sensitivity of the scan substantially, so a negative study should be considered nondiagnostic. The predictive value of a positive finding, however, is probably unaltered.

The infusion of ¹¹¹In-capromab pendetide is well tolerated, and adverse events are unusual. In clinical trials, minor adverse events were reported in 4% of 529 patients after a single mAb injection. The most common reported adverse events were transient elevation in bilirubin or liver enzymes, hypotension or hypertension, and injection site reactions, each occurring in 1% or less of patients studied. A similar incidence of adverse reactions (5%) was observed in 61 patients undergoing repeat mAb injections. Elgamal et al. reported no adverse events with 136 first or repeat mAb injections in 100 patients (5).

Human anti-mouse antibody (HAMA) titers greater than 8 ng/mL were observed after single mAb injections in 8% of patients. Titers higher than 100 ng/mL were seen in

1%. The frequency of HAMA levels higher than 8 ng/mL was 19% in patients undergoing repeat mAb injections.

IMAGE INTERPRETATION

Prostate and Prostate Fossa

The prostate or prostate fossa (the term *prostate fossa* is used to describe the prostate region in patients previously treated with prostatectomy or radiation therapy [RT]) is best evaluated on the transverse and midsagittal SPECT images. It is surrounded by anatomic structures that accumulate a variable amount of radioisotope activity, which has the potential to be mistaken for disease. The prostate or prostate fossa is bordered superiorly by the base of the bladder, posteriorly by the rectum, inferiorly by vascular structures extending from the base of the penis into the pelvis, and anteriorly by the pubic symphysis.

Cancer within the prostate or prostate fossa is the most likely diagnosis when the mAb activity is multicentric, focal, of high intensity, or eccentrically positioned in the pelvis (Fig. 31.3, *left*). Tumor is less likely if the activity is

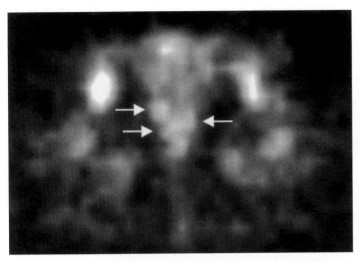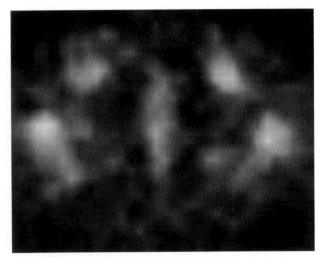

FIGURE 31.3. Day 4 transverse single photon emission computed tomography [111]indium-capromab pendetide images in two patients with elevation of prostate-specific antigen after radical prostatectomy that show positive (*arrows*, **left**) and negative (**right**) scan findings in the prostate fossa (both biopsy confirmed).

diffuse, unifocal, midline, and of low intensity (Fig. 31.3, *right*). Stool in the rectum, post-RT inflammatory changes, and asymmetric bone marrow activity in the pubic symphysis can mimic recurrent disease in the prostate fossa.

Because PSMA is expressed by normal and hypertrophic prostate epithelium, ^{111}In-capromab pendetide imaging has no role to play in establishing the primary diagnosis of prostate cancer. In addition, ^{111}In-capromab pendetide imaging has not been shown to be accurate in determining the local extent of the primary tumor. It cannot reliably determine whether tumor is through the capsule of the gland or involves the seminal vesicles or bladder neck.

It may be difficult to detect residual or recurrent tumor accurately in the prostate region after cryogenic surgery or interstitial brachytherapy because residual normal prostate tissue exhibiting PSMA expression may be present. After RT, nonspecific ^{111}In-capromab pendetide uptake in the periprostatic or perirectal soft tissue is commonly seen, possibly because of chronic inflammation. This situation can persist for years after treatment and makes it difficult to diagnose residual or recurrent disease within the radiation field (Fig. 31.4).

Lymph Node Metastases

When prostate cancer enters the lymphatic system, it usually first involves the obturator, internal iliac, and external iliac lymph nodes. Later, it progresses distally into the common iliac, retroperitoneal, and mesenteric lymph nodes and, eventually, into the mediastinal and supraclavicular lymph nodes. Detailed knowledge of pelvic lymph node anatomy and an awareness of the typical patterns of spread of prostate cancer are essential for accurate scan interpretation. It is not unusual on ^{111}In-capromab pendetide imaging to identify *skip metastases* with involvement, for example, of retroperitoneal lymph nodes in the absence of identifiable disease in the pelvic lymph nodes. Such skip metastases identified on ^{111}In-capromab pendetide imaging have, in some instances, been surgically confirmed, and the phenomenon is also well documented in autopsy studies (6,7).

The contribution of ^{111}In-capromab pendetide to the management of patients with prostate cancer is derived from its unique ability to identify metastatic disease within

FIGURE 31.4. Day 4 transverse single photon emission computed tomography [111]indium-capromab pendetide image in a patient with prostate cancer 1 year after radiation therapy. Note the intense nonspecific uptake in the prostate fossa (*arrow*).

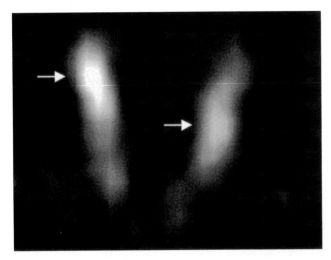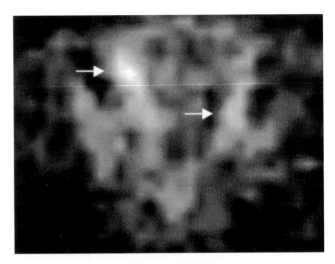

FIGURE 31.5. Transverse single photon emission computed tomography blood pool **(left)** and day 4 [111]indium-capromab pendetide **(right)** images through the midpelvis showing asymmetry of blood pool structures but no lymph node metastases. The monoclonal antibody image would be difficult to interpret without knowledge of the blood pool anatomy. The residual blood pool in the right external iliac vessels could easily be mistaken for a right external iliac lymph node metastasis. This transverse section is at the level of the common iliac bifurcation on the left *(right arrows)* but at the external iliac level *(left arrows)* on the right.

lymph nodes that are not pathologically enlarged and are thus negative on x-ray computed tomography (CT) and magnetic resonance imaging (MRI). Image interpretation is challenging, however, and the scan abnormalities are often subtle (8). The uptake of radioisotope in pelvic lymph node metastases is rarely of sufficient intensity to be identified on planar images. Identification of disease requires careful scrutiny of the mAb and blood pool SPECT images. Because the pelvic lymph nodes are in close proximity to the adjacent arteries and veins, one should allow time for blood pool clearance before the final imaging session. Intense residual activity in blood vessels may obscure uptake in adjacent lymph node metastases that, within the limits of resolution of the gamma camera, may directly superimpose on the vascular activity. When the blood pool is too intense, delayed SPECT imaging is required.

Because scan interpretation is largely based on identifying significant asymmetry comparing the intensity of uptake in the lymph node regions on one side of the pelvis compared with the other or on adjacent transverse SPECT slices, the examiner should be aware of any significant vascular asymmetries that may be present (Fig. 31.5). If the patient has significant vascular asymmetry or if the volume of blood in a segment of a vessel is significantly greater than in adjacent vascular structures, the residual blood pool on the day 3 to 5 SPECT images may be indistinguishable from lymph node metastases. Such mistakes can be minimized by paying careful attention to the blood pool images and by looking for asymmetric uptake in the region of the iliac blood vessels that does not match the vascular distribution on the blood pool images (Fig. 31.6). Planar images are required for detection of metastatic disease outside the SPECT field of

view, specifically in upper abdominal, mediastinal, or supraclavicular lymph nodes. For reasons not well understood, ^{111}In-capromab pendetide uptake in extrapelvic lymph nodes is often more intense than in pelvic lymph nodes and is often identified on planar images (Fig. 31.7).

Indium 111–capromab pendetide may nonspecifically accumulate in inflammatory lymph nodes. Focal uptake in an anatomic distribution that would be unusual for prostate cancer, for example, in upper cervical lymph nodes without abnormality in the abdominal or pelvic nodes, should be interpreted with caution and should be correlated with the clinical and radiographic findings.

Bone Metastases

No formal assessment has been made of ^{111}In-capromab pendetide imaging of skeletal metastases, and, in fact, many of the clinical studies required a negative bone scan. Consequently, the sensitivity and specificity of ^{111}In-capromab pendetide imaging for identification of skeletal metastases are unknown. Although there have been instances in which ^{111}In-capromab pendetide imaging identified confirmed skeletal metastases not seen by bone scintigraphy (Fig. 31.8), the bone scan seems to be much more sensitive. In addition, ^{111}In-capromab pendetide, to a variable extent, nonspecifically accumulates at fracture sites and in bone involved with Paget's disease, so it is inappropriate to perform a mAb scan to differentiate these conditions from skeletal metastases. Indium 111–capromab pendetide also commonly accumulates in areas of inflammation resulting from arthritis, bursitis, or tendinitis. Because of these factors, ^{111}In-capromab pendetide imaging does not replace

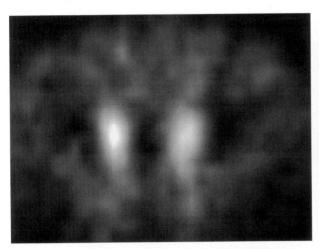 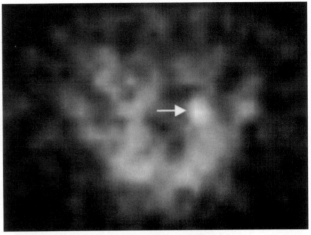

FIGURE 31.6. Transverse single photon emission computed tomography blood pool **(left)** and day 4 [111]indium-capromab pendetide images **(right)** through the midpelvis showing increased activity in a left common iliac lymph node consistent with metastatic disease *(arrow)*. The asymmetry on the capromab pendetide image between the left side and the right cannot be explained on the basis of blood pool asymmetry. The blood pool activity in the common iliac vessels is bilaterally symmetric.

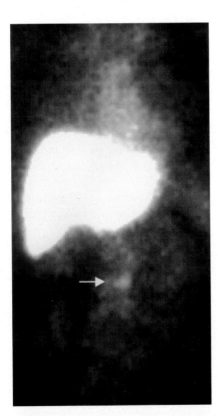 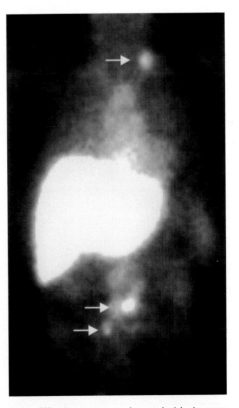

FIGURE 31.7. Day 4 anterior whole-body planar [111]indium-capromab pendetide images done in January 1994 **(left)** and August 1995 **(right)** showing low-grade uptake in the central abdominal lymph nodes *(arrow,* **left)** that, over time, progressed to intense focal uptake in upper right common iliac *(lower arrow,* **right)**, periaortic bifurcation *(middle arrow,* **right),** and medial left supraclavicular *(upper arrow,* **right)** lymph nodes.

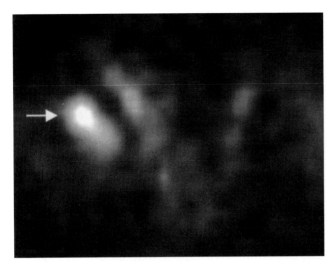

FIGURE 31.8. Day 4 transverse single photon emission computed tomography [111]indium-capromab pendetide image showing intense uptake in a metastasis in the right ilium that was not identified on bone scintigraphy but was subsequently confirmed by magnetic resonance imaging.

the bone scan, and a negative mAb scan does not rule out skeletal metastases.

Other Sites of Metastatic Disease

Early in the course of disease progression, prostate cancer rarely metastases to organs other than bone, but it may infrequently involve lung, brain, liver, or adrenal glands. Focal uptake in the lung may be due to metastatic disease, but more commonly it results from an inflammatory process. Because of high background activity, metastatic disease in the liver is seen as nonspecific space-occupying "cold" defects. I am aware of an unpublished report of non-specific ^{111}In-capromab pendetide uptake in a benign adrenal adenoma. Because of the potential for nonspecific mAb accumulation, scan findings suggesting metastatic disease in unusual locations should be confirmed before the treatment plan is altered.

Nonspecific Sites of Capromab Pendetide Accumulation

As previously discussed, focal uptake in bowel, especially in rectum, cecum, transverse, and sigmoid colon, can be mistaken for (or may obscure) metastatic disease, and bladder activity may mimic recurrent disease in the prostate fossa. Asymmetric bone marrow activity in the ischium or pubis may be mistaken for obturator lymph node metastases and recurrent disease in the prostate fossa, respectively. Normal patchy asymmetry of bone marrow activity can mimic skeletal metastases, particularly in the pelvis and around the sacroiliac joints. Asymmetric blood vessels and residual blood pool activity in aneurysms, varices, and other vascular structures can mimic lymph node metastases, but they should be correctly identified on blood pool imaging. Non-specific uptake in spermatic cord structures is common and may be asymmetric, mimicking disease in inguinal or distal external iliac lymph nodes. Nonspecific focal uptake can be seen in a variety of inflammatory processes including diverticulitis, pneumonia, thrombophlebitis, arthritis, bursitis, intramuscular injection sites, RT sites, and surgical incisions, as well as in necrotic tumors.

CLINICAL TRIALS

Prostate Fossa Recurrence: Recurrent Disease Study

The status of the prostate fossa is most relevant in the patient who has undergone prostatectomy, who has a rising prostate-specific antigen (PSA) level, and who is considering salvage RT. To assess the ability of ^{111}In-capromab pendetide to identify local recurrence, an open-label, multicenter, uncontrolled phase III clinical trial was done in 158 patients with rising PSA levels and high suspicion of recurrent or metastatic disease after radical prostatectomy (9). All patients had transrectal ultrasound-guided biopsy of the prostate fossa within 8 weeks after completion of the mAb scan. The histopathologic findings in the prostate fossa were correlated with the scintigraphic findings. Assuming no false-negative biopsies, the positive predictive value of the mAb scan was 50%, and the negative predictive value was 70% (Table 31.1).

Some of the patients with false-positive scans probably had false-negative biopsies as a reult of sampling error, a not uncommon occurrence (10–12). Of the 29 patients in this study who had false-positive mAb scans, 12 received salvage RT to the prostate fossa, and all experienced a significant decrease in PSA (average reduction of 95%), which reached undetectable levels in 4 patients. If the scans in these patients are reclassified as true-positive, the positive predictive value improves to 71%.

Because of the limited predictive value of mAb imaging in identifying local recurrence, a negative scan should not be relied on to rule out local disease recurrence, and a positive scan does not eliminate the need for a biopsy if a tissue diagnosis would otherwise have been required before therapy was instituted. However, in patients who are appropriate candidates for salvage RT based on the clinical circumstances (e.g., stage of the primary tumor, status of the surgical margins, PSA nadir after treatment, elapsed time to PSA failure, rate of rise of PSA), it may be reasonable to proceed with salvage therapy if the scan is negative for evidence of metastatic disease, regardless of the imaging status of the prostate fossa. If the scan shows evidence of metastatic disease, salvage therapy may be canceled or postponed pending the outcome of confirmatory procedures.

TABLE 31.1. COMPARISON OF ¹¹¹INDIUM-CAPROMAB PENDETIDE IMAGING AND PROSTATE FOSSA NEEDLE BIOPSY IN PATIENTS WHO UNDERWENT RADICAL PROSTATECTOMY AND WHO HAD ELEVATED PROSTATE-SPECIFIC ANTIGEN (ASSUMES NO FALSE-NEGATIVE BIOPSIES)

	¹¹¹Indium-capromab pendetide Scan		
	Positive	Negative	
Biopsy positive	29	30	Positive predictive value 50%
			Negative predictive value 70%
			Sensitivity 49%
Biopsy negative	29	70	Specificity 71%

Pelvic Lymph Node Metastases: Primary Disease Study

To assess the ability of ¹¹¹In-capromab pendetide to identify metastatic disease in pelvic lymph nodes, an open-label, multicenter, uncontrolled phase III clinical trial was done in 152 patients with newly diagnosed primary adenocarcinoma of the prostate gland who were scheduled for pelvic lymph node dissection (13). These patients had no evidence of metastatic disease based on standard diagnostic imaging studies, but each patient was at high risk for lymph node involvement based on biopsy Gleason score, PSA level, and clinical stage. The prevalence of pelvic lymph node metastases identified at surgery was 42%. Assuming no false-negative lymph node dissections, the positive and negative predictive values for ¹¹¹In-capromab pendetide imaging of pelvic lymph node metastases were 62% and 72%, respectively (Table 31.2). The odds ratio was 3.47.

The smallest tumor-positive lymph node identified on capromab pendetide imaging was 3 mm in diameter. The largest tumor-positive, mAb-negative lymph node was 3.2 cm. All PSMA-positive lymph nodes were also tumor positive, a finding suggesting that false-positive findings related to shed antigen are unlikely.

On follow-up of the patients with false-positive mAb scans, presumptive evidence indicated that some were surgically understaged. Several patients experienced a progressive PSA rise after prostatectomy, and 9 had limited dissections with as few as 1 or 2 lymph nodes from each side of the pelvis histopathologically examined. Of the 25 patients in this study with false-positive mAb scans, 5 on blinded review were believed to have had technically inadequate scans, and 15 had biochemical evidence of disease after radical prostatectomy manifested by a rising PSA. No way exists to determine whether the disease that was presumably missed at surgery (or by pathologic examination) in these 15 patients was located in the lymph nodes identified as positive on mAb imaging, but if so, the positive predictive value would increase to 85%. The relatively low sensitivity and negative predictive value reflect the inability of ¹¹¹In-capromab pendetide to visualize microscopic metastases. With one exception, none of the metastases 3 mm or smaller in diameter were visualized. Consequently, a negative scan does not eliminate the need for a staging lymphadenectomy.

This phase III primary disease study was completed before optimal parameters for ¹¹¹In-capromab pendetide imaging were established. Blood pool imaging and imaging beyond 48 hours after injection were not required, whereas investigators now realize that both are essential. As previously discussed, imaging too soon after injection is likely to increase the false-negative rate because of high levels of residual blood pool activity, and lack of blood pool imaging is likely to increase the false-positive rate in patients with vascular asymmetries.

TABLE 31.2. COMPARISON OF ¹¹¹INDIUM-CAPROMAB PENDETIDE IMAGING AND PELVIC LYMPH NODE DISSECTION IN UNTREATED PATIENTS WITH NEWLY DIAGNOSED PRIMARY PROSTATE CANCER (ASSUMES NO PATIENTS WERE SURGICALLY UNDERSTAGED)

	¹¹¹Indium-capromab pendetide Scan		
	Positive	Negative	
Biopsy positive	40	24	Positive predictive value 62%
			Negative predictive value 72%
			Sensitivity 62%
Biopsy negative	25	63	Specificity 72%

PSA, clinical stage, and biopsy Gleason score are widely used in a variety of clinical algorithms (e.g., the "Partin tables") to predict the pathologic stage in patients with primary prostate cancer (14,15). Polascik et al. (16) compared the predictive value of ^{111}In-capromab pendetide with these clinical staging algorithms in the patients enrolled in this phase III study. These investigators determined that the area under the ROC curve and the positive predictive value for ^{111}In-capromab pendetide were superior to the clinical algorithms in predicting the presence of lymph node metastases, and the combination of both resulted in the highest positive predictive value, 72.1%.

A formal prospective study comparing CT and MRI with mAb imaging has not been done. Published reports (17–19), however, suggest that the sensitivity of CT and MRI for detection of lymph node metastases in prostate cancer patients is significantly less than that reported for capromab pendetide. This finding is not surprising because tumor-positive lymph nodes are frequently not pathologically enlarged in patients with recurrent prostate cancer early in the course of the disease, and not all pathologically enlarged lymph nodes are visualized by CT. Tiguert et al. (20) reviewed pathologic specimens in 980 patients who underwent radical prostatectomy and pelvic lymph node dissection for clinically localized prostate cancer. No significant difference in lymph node size was seen in the 63 patients with lymph node metastases compared with the 917 patients without such metastases. Eight percent of patients with lymph node metastases and 12% of patients without had lymph nodes with an axial dimension of 1.5 cm or greater. All had negative CT scans despite having pathologically enlarged (benign or malignant) lymph nodes. Newer-generation CT scanners with thinner sections and shorter acquisition times may provide improved sensitivity.

The phase III capromab pendetide study in patients with primary disease was not designed to compare capromab pendetide imaging with CT or MRI. However, in the 64 patients who had tumor-positive lymph nodes, 51 had CT scans and 13 had MRI scans. The sensitivity of CT and MRI for detecting pelvic lymph node metastases in these patients was 4% and 15%, respectively.

No formal prospective comparison of positron emission tomography (PET) and ^{111}In-capromab pendetide imaging has been done, but the limited published data suggest that the sensitivity of PET using fluorine 18 fluorodeoxyglucose (^{18}F-FDG) is relatively low (21,22). The sensitivity of FDG PET would probably be higher in patients with poorly differentiated tumors. Other PET radiopharmaceuticals for imaging of prostate cancer are being investigated, including carbon 11–labeled 5-hydroxytryptophan, choline, and methionine (23).

Extrapelvic Lymph Node Metastases

Although anecdotal reports exist of surgically confirmed metastatic disease in scan-positive extrapelvic lymph nodes

(24,25), no formal clinical trials requiring tissue correlation have been performed prospectively to assess the ability of ^{111}In-capromab pendetide to identify metastatic disease in lymph nodes above the usual level of the staging pelvic lymph node dissection. One may assume that the predictive value of ^{111}In-capromab pendetide imaging for detecting pelvic lymph node metastases can be applied to extrapelvic nodal disease, but no compelling data are available to establish this application.

Multiple intense foci of uptake in the central abdominal region that, on SPECT images, seem to be in the retroperitoneal or mesenteric lymph nodes probably comprise the most common pattern seen in patients with ^{111}In-capromab pendetide evidence of extrapelvic disease (Fig. 31.9). Because activity of this type could represent excreted material in bowel, delayed imaging should be done, to look for movement or clearance over time. I have imaged many patients with this pattern up to 10 days after injection and have found that the focal uptake persists while activity elsewhere that was obviously in bowel moves or clears. I have found on repeat imaging over periods of up to 4 years that the pattern of uptake in abdominal lymph nodes is reproducible and often, in the absence of therapy, progressive over time (Fig. 31.7). The change in the appearance of mAb-positive lymph nodes after hormonal ablation therapy

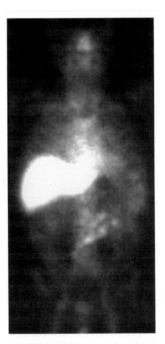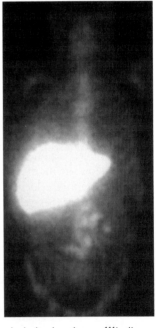

FIGURE 31.9. Day 4 anterior whole-body planar [111]indium-capromab pendetide images in two patients that show intense focal uptake in the central abdominal region that, on single photon emission computed tomography imaging, appeared to be both in the retroperitoneum and in the mesentery. Both patients had negative computed tomography scans at the time the monoclonal antibody scan was performed. Enlarged retroperitoneal lymph nodes became apparent on follow-up computed tomography scans done 12 to 18 months subsequently.

is variable. On repeat imaging, I most often see stability or, less commonly, regression. The intensity of uptake in mAb-positive lymph nodes tends to fade or resolve after RT. Several patients with mAb-positive abdominal lymph nodes have developed lymphadenopathy over time, as documented by follow-up CT (Fig. 31.9), presumptive evidence that the scan was correct. Kahn et al. (26) reported two patients with mAb-positive mediastinal lymph nodes subsequently confirmed by CT. Moreover, the pattern of abnormality seen on mAb imaging matches the pattern of metastatic disease reported in CT (27) and autopsy studies (6,7).

Hinkle et al. (24) reported a patient with mAb-positive abdominal and mAb-negative pelvic lymph nodes whose scan findings were verified at autopsy after sudden death from cardiac arrest. Burgers et al. (25) reported a patient who, after a negative standard pelvic lymph node dissection, had an extended surgical exploration into the right common iliac nodal region because the ^{111}In-capromab pendetide scan was positive in this area. Common iliac lymph node metastases were confirmed, and the radical prostatectomy was canceled. Figure 31.10 illustrates a similar finding in a patient with primary disease with mAb-positive, CT-negative aortic bifurcation lymph nodes well above the usual level of the staging lymphadenectomy. At surgery, the pelvic lymph nodes were negative, but metastatic disease was confirmed at the aortic bifurcation. In this patient, a futile radical prostatectomy would have been done if the capromab pendetide scan had not been performed.

Presumptive evidence indicates that ^{111}In-capromab pendetide uptake in extrapelvic lymph nodes predicts failure to respond to salvage RT. Kahn et al. (28) reported a retrospective review of 32 patients who underwent salvage RT after ^{111}In-capromab pendetide imaging. PSA failure was 78% (7 of 9) in patients with scan evidence of metastatic

disease in extrapelvic lymph nodes compared with 30% (7 of 23) in those without such evidence. A similar experience was reported by Levesque et al. (29).

SUMMARY

[111]In-capromab pendetide imaging provides a means of identifying occult soft-tissue metastases in patients with prostate cancer that may lead to more accurate disease staging. It offers the advantage of higher sensitivity compared with other imaging modalities such as ^{18}F-FDG PET, CT, and MRI. As with any imaging technique, it has strengths and weaknesses that must be understood to maximize patient benefit by using the scan in clinical settings in which it is most likely to be useful and is least likely to be misleading.

In the primary disease setting, ^{111}In-capromab pendetide imaging should be reserved for use in patients with negative bone scans who are at high risk of metastatic disease based on such factors as clinical stage, biopsy Gleason score, and PSA level. A negative scan does not eliminate the need for a staging lymph node dissection but should encourage further pursuit of local treatment options.

A positive scan in this high-risk setting supports proceeding with systemic treatment options or watchful waiting. An attempt should be made to confirm scan findings suggesting metastatic disease, however, because the specificity is limited (72% for pelvic lymph node metastases). One should use ^{111}In-capromab pendetide with caution in patients at low risk of metastatic disease. Positive scan findings in low-risk patients must be confirmed before the treatment plan is altered because a high false-positive rate should be anticipated in a population with low disease prevalence. Imaging with ^{111}In-capromab pendetide has not been shown to be reliable in determining the local extent of the primary tumor.

Imaging with ^{111}In-capromab pendetide should not be used solely for the purpose of determining whether a skeletal lesion seen on bone scintigraphy results from a bone metastasis. Because of limited sensitivity, a negative scan does not rule out metastatic disease, and false-positive findings can occur in patients with fractures, Paget's disease, and inflammatory processes.

In the patient with recurrent disease, the predictive value of ^{111}In-capromab pendetide imaging of the prostate fossa is limited. Its more important role in this setting is to look for evidence of lymph node metastases in the high-risk patient with a negative bone scan who is a candidate for local salvage therapy. A large prospective study is needed for confirmation, but preliminary data suggest that ^{111}In-capromab pendetide imaging is helpful in identifying those patients with PSA elevation after radical prostatectomy who are most likely to benefit from salvage RT. This may be the clinical setting in which ^{111}In-capromab pendetide has the

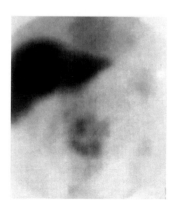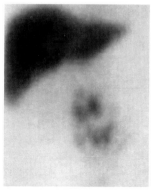

FIGURE 31.10. Anterior whole-body planar day 2 **(left)** and day 5 **(right)** [111]indium-capromab pendetide images showing a persistent cluster of intense foci of activity in the middle and lower central abdomen. At surgery, the pelvic lymph nodes were negative, but metastatic disease was confirmed in the lymph nodes at the aortic bifurcation. (Courtesy of Dr. Calvin Lutrin.)

greatest impact on the management of patients with prostate cancer. A mAb scan showing no evidence of metastatic disease would support proceeding with local salvage therapy. Until more data are available, however, scan findings positive for metastatic disease should be confirmed if possible before directing the patient away from potentially curative salvage treatment options.

REFERENCES

1. Wright GL, Haley C, Beckett ML, et al. Expression of prostate-specific membrane antigen in normal, benign, and malignant prostate tissues. *Urol Oncol* 1995;1:18–28.
2. Fair WR, Israeli RS, Heston WDW. Prostate-specific membrane antigen. *Prostate* 1997;32:140–148.
3. Murphy GP, Elgamal AA, Su SL, et al. Current evaluation of the tissue localization and diagnostic utility of prostate specific membrane antigen. *Cancer* 1998;83:2259–2269.
4. Horoszewicz JC, Kawinski E, Murphy GP. Monoclonal antibodies to a new antigenic marker in epithelial cells in serum of prostatic cancer patients. *Anticancer Res* 1987;7:927–935.
5. Elgamal AA, Troychak MJ, Murphy GP. ProstaScint scan may enhance identification of prostate cancer recurrence after prostatectomy, radiation or hormonal therapy: analysis of 136 scans in 100 patients. *Prostate* 1998;37:261–269.
6. Elkin M, Mueller HP. Metastases from cancer of the prostate: autopsy and roentgenological findings. *Cancer* 1954;7:1246–1248.
7. Saitoh H, Hida M, Shimbo T, et al. Metastatic patterns of prostatic cancer. *Cancer* 1984;54:3078–3084.
8. Haseman MK, Reed NL. Capromab pendetide imaging of prostate cancer. *Nucl Med Annu* 1998;XX:51–82.
9. Kahn D, Williams R, Manyak M, et al. 111-indium-capromab pendetide in the evaluation of patients with residual or recurrent prostate cancer after radical prostatectomy. *J Urol* 1998;159:2041–2047.
10. Foster LS, Jajodia P, Fournier G, et al. The value of prostate specific antigen and transrectal ultrasound guided biopsy in detecting prostatic fossa recurrences following radical prostatectomy. *J Urol* 1993;149:1024–1028.
11. Lange PH. Prostate cancer [Editorial]. *J Urol* 1994;152:1496–1497.
12. Svetec D, McCabe K, Peretsman S, et al. Prostate rebiopsy is a poor surrogate of treatment efficacy in localized prostate cancer. *J Urol* 1998;159:1606–1608.
13. Hinkle GH, Burgers JK, Neal CE, et al. Multicenter radioimmunoscintigraphic evaluation of patients with primary prostate cancer using indium-111 capromab pendetide. *Cancer* 1998;83:739–747.
14. Partin AW, Subong ENP, Walsh PC, et al. Combination of prostate-specific antigen, clinical stage and Gleason score to predict pathologic stage of localized prostate cancer: a multi-institutional update. *JAMA* 1997;277:1445–1497.
15. Sands ME, Agars GK, Pollack A, et al. Serum prostate-specific antigen, clinical stage, pathologic grade, and the incidence of nodal metastases in prostate cancer. *Urology* 1994;44:215–220.
16. Polascik TJ, Manyak MD, Haseman MK, et al. Comparison of clinical staging algorithms and ^{111}In-capromab pendetide immunoscintigraphy to predict lymph node involvement in high risk prostate cancer patients. *Cancer* 1999;85:1586–1592.
17. Hricak H, Dooms GC, Jeffrey RB, et al. Prostatic carcinoma: staging by clinical assessment, CT, and MR imaging. *Radiology* 1987;162:331–336.
18. Platt JF, Bree RL, Schwab RE. The accuracy of CT in staging of carcinoma of the prostate. *AJR Am J Roentgenol* 1987;149:315–318.
19. Wolf JS, Cher M, Dall'era M, et al. The use and accuracy of cross-sectional imaging and fine needle aspiration cytology for detection of pelvic lymph node metastases before radical prostatectomy. *J Urol* 1995;153:993–999.
20. Tiguert R, Gheiler EL, Tefilli MV, et al. Lymph node size does not correlate with the presence of prostate cancer metastases. *Urology* 1999;53:367–371.
21. Haseman MK, Reed NL, Rosenthal SA. Monoclonal antibody imaging of occult prostate cancer in patients with elevated prostate-specific antigen: positron emission tomography and biopsy correlation. *Clin Nucl Med* 1996;21:704–713.
22. Hoh CK, Seltzer MA, Franklin J, et al. Positron emission tomography in urologic oncology. *J Urol* 1998;159:347–356.
23. Macapinlac HA, Humm JL, Larson SM, et al. Differential metabolism and pharmacokinetics of C-11 methionine (C[11]-MET) and FDG in metastatic prostate cancer. *J Nucl Med* 1998;39[Suppl]:67P.
24. Hinkle GH, Burgers JK, Olsen JO, et al. Abdominal prostate cancer metastases detected with Indium [111] capromab pendetide. *J Nucl Med* 1998;39:650–652.
25. Burgers JK, Hinkle GH, Haseman MK. Monoclonal antibody imaging of recurrent and metastatic prostate cancer. *Semin Urol* 1995;13:103–112.
26. Kahn D, Williams RD, Seldin DW, et al. Radioimmunoscintigraphy with 111-indium labeled CYT-356 for the detection of occult prostate cancer recurrence. *J Urol* 1994;152:1490–1495.
27. Spencer JA, Golding SJ. Patterns of lymphatic metastases at recurrence of prostate cancer: CT findings. *Clin Radiol* 1994;49:404–407.
28. Kahn DK, Williams RD, Haseman MK, et al. Radioimmunoscintigraphy with In-111 labeled capromab pendetide predicts prostate cancer response to salvage radiotherapy after failed prostatectomy. *J Clin Oncol* 1998;6:284–290.
29. Levesque PE, Nieh PT, Zinman LN, et al. Radiolabeled monoclonal antibody indium-111–labeled CYT-356 localizes extraprostatic recurrent carcinoma after prostatectomy. *Urology* 1998;51:978–984.

32

MONOCLONAL ANTIBODY THERAPY

STANLEY J. GOLDSMITH
NEIL H. BANDER

CLINICAL ASPECTS

The diagnosis and treatment of prostate carcinoma have undergone significant change during the past decade, primarily as a result of earlier detection following the introduction of a serum assay for a prostate-specific antigen (PSA) that is released into the circulation by tumor. Ultrasonographically guided biopsy of the prostate gland has become widespread, and other improvements in diagnostic imaging permit better staging at the time of presentation. Despite early detection, however, many patients continue to present with various degrees of involvement: tumor confined to the prostate gland, tumor in regional lymph nodes, tumor that has invaded local structures, and tumor that has spread outside the pelvis to the bone marrow or distant lymph nodes or other organs. Both computed tomography (CT) and magnetic resonance imaging (MRI) have been disappointing in regard to their ability to exclude disease involving pelvic lymph nodes (1,2). In a group of 185 patients, MRI detected lymph node involvement in only one, whereas 23 of the patients were found to have lymph node involvement on histologic examination following surgical removal (1).

In the initial treatment of patients classified as having disease limited to the prostate, a variety of therapeutic techniques, including surgery, conformal external beam teletherapy, and brachytherapy with radioactive seed implantation, are now available.

Even when the disease is believed to be confined to the prostate at presentation, it is not unusual for the disease to recur in the pelvis or at distant sites, presumably because it had already spread before initial detection and treatment. When the disease is believed to be limited to the pelvis, retreatment with either surgical intervention or radiation is possible, but disease outside the pelvis is an indication for systemic therapy, usually involving hormonal manipulation.

The vast majority of prostate cancers are responsive to androgen blockade. In many patients, the disease eventually becomes more aggressive and no longer responds to hormonal manipulation. Although chemotherapy for prostate cancer has improved, no regimen has demonstrated an ability to prolong survival. A number of efforts have been made to develop tumor-specific antibodies to treat patients in this category. The therapeutic use of monoclonal antibodies (mAbs) is based on direct antitumor effects, such as antibody-dependent cellular cytotoxicity (ADCC) and complement fixation, in addition to the delivery of cytotoxins or radionuclide therapy directly to sites of disseminated tumor. Although at this time no radiolabeled antibodies have been approved by the Food and Drug Administration for routine use in this setting, significant progress has been made. A brief review of the clinical trials and pertinent laboratory investigations that have led to the present status of immunotargeted radiotherapy (with the use of radiolabeled mAbs) is both instructive and encouraging (Table 32.1).

USE OF MONOCLONAL ANTIBODIES FOR PROSTATE CANCER THERAPY

Monoclonal antibodies are most conveniently prepared at present from murine hybridoma cells. These mouse-derived immunoglobulins may elicit a human anti-murine antibody (HAMA) response in human subjects; the number of doses a patient can receive is therefore limited, as an HAMA response presents a risk for an allergic reaction, with urticaria, possible bronchospasm, and even anaphylaxis. Even in the absence of a serious reaction, HAMA binds to subsequent injected antibody, alters its pharmacokinetics, and reduces the availability of therapeutic antibody. The appearance of HAMA, therefore, usually limits the evaluation and treatment of patients to a single administration of murine antibody. To date, in prostate carcinoma, no efforts

S. J. Goldsmith: Departments of Radiology and Medicine, Weill Medical College of Cornell University, New York, New York 10021.

N. H. Bander: Department of Urology, Weill Medical College of Cornell University,, New York, New York 10021.

TABLE 32.1. ANTIGENS AND ANTIBODIES EVALUATED FOR TARGETED RADIOTHERAPY IN PROSTATE CARCINOMA

Prostate-specific		Expressed on prostate (not specific)	
Antigen	Antibody	Antigen	Antibody
Prostate-specific antigen (PSA) Prostatic acid phosphatase (PAP) Prostate epithelial antigen	Prost 30	Tumor-associated glycoprotein (TAG-72) Epidermal growth factor receptor (EGFr) HER-2/*neu*	CC49 Bispecific Fc receptor
Prostate-specific membrane antigen Intracellular domain 7E11/CYT356 Extracellular domain	J591 mu J591 hu		

have been made to suppress the immune response to avoid this problem. However, the technology is available to convert promising antibodies to chimeric or humanized forms in which the antigen-recognition region is preserved while the nonspecific portion of the immunoglobulin is replaced with a homologous portion of human origin. This so-called "humanized" antibody is an elegant, but expensive, undertaking, so that advanced studies are limited to those murine antibodies that perform well in early studies.

Prostate-specific is a relative term, as a number of antibodies are prostate-specific (i.e., exhibit a high degree of binding to antigens expressed on prostate carcinoma tissue) but also recognize antigenic sites on other tumors and tissues. This lack of true tissue specificity is more of a problem in diagnostic applications, as it results in poor contrast and detectability of lesions and also reduces the "specificity" of focal accumulation of the labeled antibody. When these antibodies are used to deliver a therapeutic radionuclide, the tissues and organs other than the intended tumor receive unnecessary radiation. Although this is not desirable, it may be acceptable if the dose delivered to the tumor provides a therapeutic response or at least provides a reasonable therapeutic index (antitumor effect vs. organ toxicity).

ANTIGENS EXPRESSED BY PROSTATE THAT ARE NOT ORGAN-SPECIFIC

Tumor-associated Glycoprotein 72

Tumor-associated glycoprotein 72 (TAG-72) was identified initially on colon, breast, and ovarian carcinomas. CC49, an antibody developed to TAG-72, has been used in clinical trials in these settings. Because 80% of primary prostatic carcinomas are positive for TAG-72 on immunohistopathologic analysis (3), investigators were at first interested in evaluating this agent further, even though expression of TAG-72 decreases as prostate cancer cells become less differentiated. Metastatic sites and hormone-refractory cancers express the TAG-72 antigen less fre-

quently than tissue from the primary site (3). Despite these negatives, a phase II trial was conducted in which murine CC49 labeled with ^{131}I (75 mCi/m^2) was administered to 15 patients with prostate cancer (3). No radiographic or biochemical (PSA) responses were seen. Only 30% of prostate cancer cells were positive for TAG-72 on biopsy. Because it had been demonstrated that interferon gamma upregulates TAG-72 expression on other tumors (3), a second trial was performed with ^{131}I-CC49 following pretreatment with interferon gamma. No clinical or biochemical responses were observed in the 14 patients studied.

Epidermal Growth Factor Receptor

An antibody to the epidermal growth factor receptor (EGFr) has been developed; in addition to blocking the binding of EGF to its receptor, it induces tumor regression in some animal models. In animal studies, the antibody augments (and is possibly synergistic with) chemotherapy. Although the level of expression of EGFr is not high in prostate cancer, a trial of a chimerized (partially humanized) antibody to the EGFr plus doxorubicin was performed (4). Presumably because of the lack of EGF overexpression, only a single biochemical response (decrease in PSA > 50%) was observed in 22 patients.

HER-2/*neu*

HER-2/*neu* is observed on several neoplasms, most notably breast carcinoma. The expression of this antigen usually indicates a poor prognosis, with an increased likelihood of recurrence. An antibody to HER-2/*neu* is available in non-radioactive form and has been approved by the Food and Drug Administration for the treatment of patients with breast (but not other) carcinomas expressing the HER-2/*neu* antigen. This antibody has been prepared as a bispecific mAb, chemically constructed with binding sites to the HER-2/*neu* antigen and the Fc receptor expressed by macrophages. The rationale was to induce macrophages to attack cells expressing HER-2/*neu*. Although a trial was attempted in patients with prostate cancer, it was discontinued early because of the low level of expression of HER-2/*neu* on prostate cancer cells and tissue (5,6).

PROSTATE-SPECIFIC ANTIGENS

Prostate-specific Antigen and Prostatic Acid Phosphatase

Both PSA and prostatic acid phosphatase (PAP) are highly restricted markers for prostate tissue. In the late 1980s, several attempts were made to image prostate cancer with radiolabeled mAbs to these prostate-related antigens (7–9). Although the requirements for an antibody that can be used successfully for imaging are not the same as those for an agent that can be used deliver a therapeutic radiation absorbed dose, it is necessary to demonstrate sufficient targeting of the tumor cells. Lack of cell surface expression precludes cell-associated antibody binding. PSA and PAP are not satisfactory antigens to target prostate tissue for diagnosis or therapy because they are secreted antigens and not expressed on the cell surface. Furthermore, the presence of circulating antigen in serum (often at substantially elevated levels) results in the formation of antigen–antibody complexes (which increase background activity in the circulation) that effectively compete with any tissue-related concentration of antigen.

Prostate Epithelium-specific Antigen

In the early 1990s, Bander and co-workers (10) produced a murine antibody, Prost 30, by immunizing mice with fresh prostate cancer cells. Although the Prost 30 antigen has not been biochemically characterized, immunohistochemical studies indicate that it is a prostate epithelium-specific antigen, and it was strongly expressed in virtually all of more than 200 prostate cancer specimens studied. Strong antigen expression was observed regardless of the degree of differentiation of the tumor. In a single-dose biodistribution trial, varying doses of Prost 30 (0.5 to 20.0 mg) were administered that were tagged with 10 mCi of ^{131}I. Despite the low dose of ^{131}I, tumor localization was noted. Several biochemical responses (> 50% decline in PSA) were unexpectedly observed (10). Only 7 of the 19 patients in the trial could be evaluated for response; the other 12 were receiving additional therapy (the trial had been planned as a dose biodistribution trial because a therapeutic response had not been expected).

A subsequent phase I/II trial of unconjugated murine Prost 30 was performed in a group of 22 patients, all of whom were evaluable for biochemical (PSA) response. Patients were either hormone-refractory or hormone-naïve but were selected if they had had at least three sequentially rising PSA values before entry. All patients received a single dose of antibody ranging from 1.25 to 5.0 mg. In 5 of the 22 patients (23%), a PSA decline of more than 50% was achieved (11). The duration of response in these patients ranged from 2 to more than 36 months. Because these responses were observed without any concomitant toxicity, an adjuvant antibody trial was performed in a group of patients at high risk for relapse after radical prostatectomy. A limited supply of antibody precluded a randomized trial. The data on the 10 patients were compared with data from a prospective cohort of patients rated as having similar risk factors. At the last review (median of 2.5 years of follow-up), a 30% incidence of progression (three of 10 patients), defined as a PSA level above 0.3 ng/ml, was noted. This failure rate compares favorably with that of the comparison group, which at 2.5 years was approximately 70% (12).

Despite the interesting and provocative results with Prost 30, additional studies have not been pursued because of a lack of prostate cancer cell lines expressing the Prost 30 antigen, an absence of Prost 30-expressing prostate cancer xenograft models, and limited supplies of antibody.

Prostate-specific Membrane Antigen

In 1987, another antigen, the so-called prostate specific membrane antigen (PSMA), was recognized and mAbs were prepared (13). The characteristics of PSMA are optimal for antibody targeting:

1. It is highly prostate-restricted (14–22).
2. It is expressed at high levels by most prostate cancers (14,15,17,18,20,21).
3. Expression increases as tumor grade increases (17,20, 21).
4. Expression is increased in metastatic sites (17,20,21).

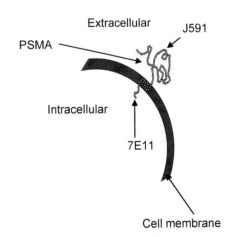

FIGURE 32.1. Schematic of prostate-specific membrane antigen demonstrating extracellular, transmembrane, and intracellular components. J591 recognizes a domain in the extracellular region, whereas 7E11 recognizes the intracellular domain. Following J591 binding to the extracellular epitope, the complex is internalized. (Courtesy of the Laboratory of Urologic Oncology, Weill Cornell Medical Center, New York, New York.)

5. Expression further increases as the tumor becomes androgen-independent and hormone-refractory (17,20).

Prostate-specific membrane antigen has been studied in several laboratories and has now been cloned, sequenced (23), and characterized. In nonmalignant cells, the preferential transcript is translated as a cytosolic protein, referred to as PSM′ (24). Coincidentally with or subsequently to malignant transformation, an alternate, longer transcript is generated. This cancer-related transcript is translated into a longer protein, which contains a transmembrane domain that anchors the protein to the plasma membrane, and a short cytoplasmic tail.

The initial antibody, designated 7E11-C5.3, was later renamed CYT356 when it was developed commercially as an imaging agent (ProstaScint). Troyer et al. (25,26) mapped the epitope recognized by 7E11 and found that the epitope recognized by 7E11 (ProstaScint) is located inside the cell on the short cytoplasmic tail of PSMA rather than exposed on the external side of the plasma membrane (Fig. 32.1). As a result, the 7E11 binding site in intact cells is invisible to the circulating antibody. This explains the early finding that 7E11 binds only to fixed cells (13). The binding site is accessible to antibody when the cell is dead or dying or when the membrane is disrupted or fragmented. Bone marrow sites have always been difficult to identify

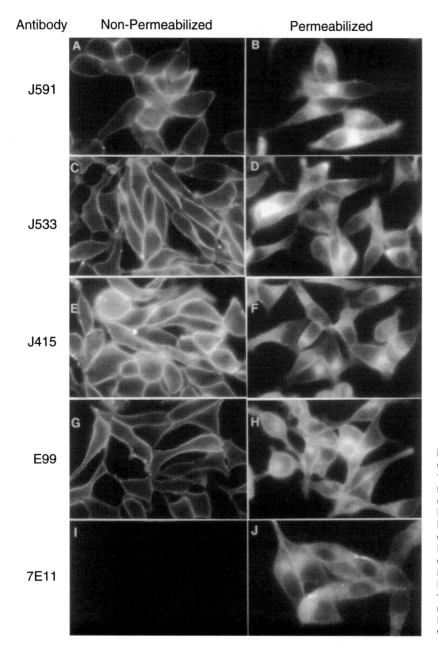

FIGURE 32.2. Immunofluorescent photomicrographs of LNCaP cell suspensions with five different antibodies prepared against prostate-specific membrane antigen (*PSMA*). In matching experiments, cells were permeabilized with buffered saponin at room temperature. 7E11 binding was observed only in permeabilized cells, consistent with recognition of an intracellular portion of the PSMA epitope. J591 and the other PSMA antibodies studied bind to both nonpermeable and permeable cells. (From Liu H, Moy P, Kim S, et al. Monoclonal antibodies to the extracellular domain of prostate-specific membrane antigen also react with tumor vascular endothelium. *Cancer Res* 1997;57:3629–3634, with permission.)

with ProstaScint. At these sites, the blood supply is abundant and necrosis is rare. ProstaScint imaging is successful when some dead or dying cells are present at tumor sites that have outgrown their blood supply. Hence, despite the favorable features of PSMA as an antigenic site, 7E11 is a suboptimal choice as an antibody for targeted radionuclide therapy of prostate carcinoma.

Liu et al. subsequently developed and characterized several antibodies to the extracellular portion of the PSMA epitope (27). These antibodies, J591 and J415, bind well to viable cells (Fig. 32.2). J591 binding exceeds that of 7E11 in cell suspensions and animal tumor models (28). Stable conjugates of tetraazacyclododecane tetraacetic acid (DOTA) have been prepared and labeled with ^{111}In and ^{90}Y. Both the ^{131}I and ^{111}In/^{90}Y conjugates bind effectively to prostate carcinoma cells in cell suspensions and tumor models. The ^{111}In-J591 conjugate, however, is retained by the tumor (Fig. 32.3). This observation is consistent with the internalization of the extracellular epitope after antibody binding (27). In the intracellular environment, the ^{131}I label is hydrolyzed and washes out, whereas the insoluble radiometal ^{111}In (and ^{90}Y) remain. Both the ^{131}I and ^{111}In versions of J591 have been characterized in terms of biodistribution and radiobiologic effects in animal tumor models (29) (Fig. 32.4).

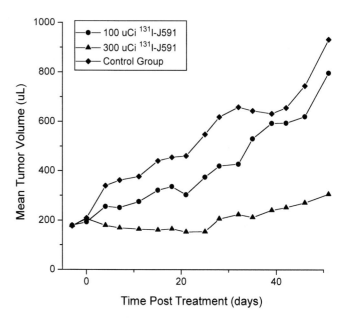

FIGURE 32.4. Tumor volume versus time in an animal tumor model of LNCaP prostate carcinoma. Inhibition of tumor growth is significant in animals receiving 300 µCi of ^{131}I-J591. (Courtesy of the Division of Nuclear Medicine and the Laboratory of Urologic Oncology, New York Presbyterian Hospital-Weill Cornell Medical Center, New York, New York.)

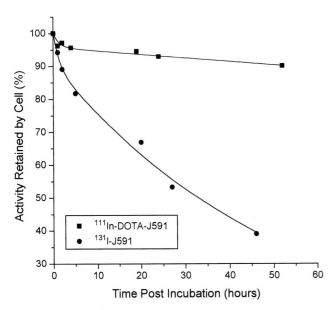

FIGURE 32.3. Comparison of cellular retention following internalization of ^{131}I-J591 and ^{111}In-DOTA (tetraazacyclododecane tetraacetic acid)-J591 in LNCaP cells. Initial binding of both radiolabeled compounds is good, but ^{131}I is washed out, whereas ^{111}In is retained. These findings confirm the superiority of radiometal antibody conjugates for targeted radionuclide therapy with an internalized antibody. [From Smith-Jones PM, Vallabhajosula S, Goldsmith SJ, et al. *In vitro* characterization of radiolabeled monoclonal antibodies specific for the extracellular domain of prostate specific membrane antigen *Cancer Res* (in press).]

When patients are treated with radiolabeled mAbs, the total number of antibody molecules potentially influences the biodistribution of the injected material. Several patients have been studied in a dose-escalation trial of ^{131}I-labeled murine J591; this trial was designed to determine the optimal protein dose in terms of reducing nonspecific organ uptake in organs such as the liver. Only 10 mCi of ^{131}I was used, to permit acquisition of biodistribution data while optimal protein loading was determined and to assess the antitumor response, if any, of cold antibody. The radiation absorbed dose to the liver was reduced from 25% to 10% as the total protein dose administered was increased from 0.5 to 50 g (30).

In a compassionate use application, one patient received ^{111}In/^{90}Y- DOTA-humanized J591 (Fig. 32.5). Excellent localization in tumor was demonstrated. Given the total tumor burden and the limited amount of radiometal and antibody administered, it is not possible to draw conclusions about the potential clinical efficacy of this approach. Based on the excellent targeting achieved with J591 and the availability of effective chemical methods to produce stable radiometal conjugates, it has been decided to pursue this approach in therapy trials. In preclinical studies, radiometal conjugates of antibodies to the external portion of the PSMA epitope have demonstrated substantial a antitumor effect. Currently, an adequate supply of humanized mAb is being prepared, with the intention of initiating clinical trials of ^{90}Y-DOTA-humanized J591 in the latter part of 2000.

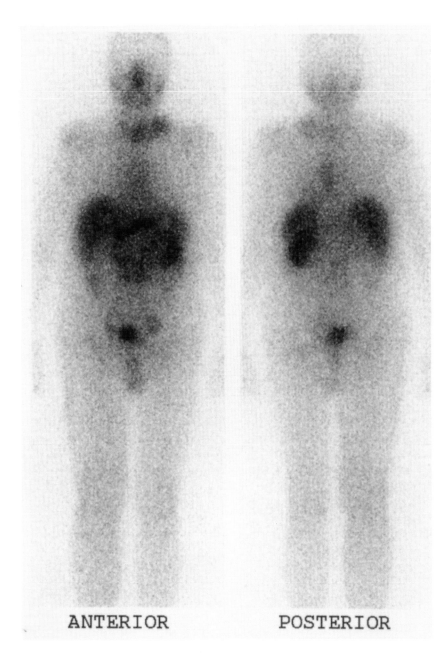

ANTERIOR   POSTERIOR

FIGURE 32.5. Whole-body planar scintigraphy with 5 mCi of ^{111}In-DOTA (tetraazacyclododecane tetraacetic acid)-humanized J591 administered 24 hours earlier. Excellent targeting of prostate carcinoma metastases is noted in the anterior projection in a large left supraclavicular lymph node, a large midabdominal mass, and a pelvic mass left of the midline. (Courtesy of the Division of Nuclear Medicine and the Laboratory of Urologic Oncology, New York Presbyterian Hospital-Weill Cornell Medical Center, New York, New York.)

SUMMARY

After many years of investigation, mAbs are now available for clinical investigation in a number of tumor settings. The Food and Drug Administration has recently approved two nonradiolabeled mAbs for the treatment of non-Hodgkin's lymphoma and breast cancer. The success of antibody treatment in these cancers, which bear some similarities to prostate cancer, is encouraging. An ideal prostate-restricted target antigen has been identified (PSMA). Antibodies to an extracellular epitope that is subsequently internalized have the requisite specificity to make them ideal for therapy.

ACKNOWLEDGMENT

The authors express their sincere appreciation to their colleagues Shankar Vallabhajosula, Ph.D., Peter Smith-Jones, Ph.D., and Lale Kostakoglu, M.D., for their assistance in the basic and clinical studies performed in our department.

REFERENCES

1. Rifkin MD, Zerhouni EA, Gatsonis CA, et al. Comparison of magnetic resonance imaging and ultrasonography in staging early prostate cancer. *N Engl J Med* 1990;323:621–626.

2. Gasser TC, Streule K, Nidecker A, et al. MRI and ultrasonography in staging prostate cancer. *N Engl J Med* 1991;324:494–495.

3. Brenner PC, Rettig WJ, Pilar Sanz-Moncasi M, et al. TAG-72 expression in primary, metastatic and hormonally treated prostate cancer as defined by monoclonal antibody CC49. *J Urol* 1995;153:1575–1579.

4. Slovin SF, Kelly WK, Cohen R, et al. Epidermal growth factor receptor monoclonal antibody C225 and doxorubicin in androgen-independent prostate cancer: results of a phase Ib/IIa study. *Proc Am Soc Clin Oncol* 1997;16:311a(abst 1108).

5. Mellon K, Thompson S, Charlton RG, et al. p53, c-*erb* B-2 and the epidermal growth factor receptor in the benign and malignant prostate. *J Urol* 1992;147:496–499.

6. Visakorpi T, Kallioniemi OP, Koivula T, et al. Expression of epidermal growth factor receptor and *erb*-B2 (HER-2/*neu*) oncoprotein in prostatic carcinomas. *Mod Pathol* 1992;5:643–648.

7. Meyers JF, Denardo SJ, Macey D, et al. Development of monoclonal antibody imaging of metastatic prostatic carcinoma. *Prostate* 1989;14:209–220.

8. Babaian RJ, Murray JL, Lamki LM, et al. Radioimmunological imaging of metastatic prostatic cancer with ^{111}In-labeled monoclonal antibody PAY 276. *J Urol* 1987;137:439–443.

9. Leroy M, Teillac P, Rain JD, et al. Radioimmunodetection of lymph node invasion in prostate cancer. The use of iodine 123 (^{123}I)-labeled monoclonal anti-prostatic acid phosphatase (PAP) 227 A F(ab')$_2$ antibody fragments *in vivo*. *Cancer* 1989;64:1–5.

10. Bander NH, Divgi C, Theodoulou M, et al. Phase I immunolocalization trial of monoclonal antibody (mAb) Prost 30 in patients with prostate cancer. *J Urol* 1996;155[Suppl]:610(abst 1196).

11. Shemtov MM, Bander NH. Phase I/II trial of monoclonal antibody (mAb) Prost 30 in advanced prostate cancer. *J Urol* 1997;157[Suppl]:322(abst 1256).

12. Partin AW, Piantadosi S, Sanda MG, et al. Selection of men at high risk for disease recurrence for experimental adjuvant therapy following radical prostatectomy. *Urology* 1995;45:831–838.

13. Horoszewicz JS, Kawinski E, Murphy GP. Monoclonal antibodies to a new antigenic marker in epithelial cells and serum of prostatic cancer patients. *Anticancer Res* 1989;7:927–936.

14. Zhang S, Zhang HS, Reuter VE, et al. Expression of potential target antigens for immunotherapy on primary and metastatic prostate cancers. *Clin Cancer Res* 1998;4:295–302.

15. Lopes D, Davis WL, Rosenstraus MJ, et al. Immunohistochemical and pharmacokinetic characterization of the site-specific immunoconjugate CYT-356 derived from antiprostate monoclonal antibody 7E11-C5. *Cancer Res* 1990;50:6423–6429.

16. Israeli RS, Powell CT, Corr JG, et al. Expression of the prostate-specific membrane antigen. *Cancer Res* 1994;54:1807–1811.

17. Wright GL Jr, Haley C, Beckett ML, et al. Expression of prostate-specific membrane antigen in normal, benign, and malignant prostate tissues. *Urol Oncol* 1995;1:18–28.

18. Bostwick DG, Pacelli A, Blute M, et al. Prostate specific membrane antigen expression in prostatic intraepithelial neoplasia and adenocarcinoma. *Cancer* 1998;82:2256–2261.

19. Troyer JK, Beckett ML, Wright GL Jr. Detection and characterization of the prostate-specific membrane antigen (PSMA) in tissue extracts and body fluids. *Int J Cancer* 1995;62:552–558.

20. Wright GL Jr, Grob BM, Haley C, et al. Upregulation of prostate-specific membrane antigen after androgen-deprivation therapy. *Urology* 1996;48:326–334.

21. Silver DA, Pellicer I, Fair WR, et al. Prostate-specific membrane antigen expression in normal and malignant human tissues. *Clin Cancer Res* 1997;3:81–85.

22. Sokoloff RL, Norton KC, Gasior CL, et al. Quantification of prostate specific membrane antigen (PSMA) in human tissues and subcellular fractions. *Proc Am Assoc Cancer Res* 1998;39:265(abst 1811).

23. Israeli RS, Powell CT, Fair WR, et al. Molecular cloning of a complementary DNA encoding a prostate-specific membrane antigen. *Cancer Res* 1993;53:227–230.

24. Su SL, Huang I-P, Fair WR, et al. Alternatively spliced variants of prostate-specific membrane antigen RNA: ratio of expression as a potential measurement of progression. *Cancer Res* 1995;55:1441–1443.

25. Troyer JK, Feng Q, Beckett ML, et al. Biochemical characterization and mapping of the 7E11-C5.3 epitope of the prostate-specific membrane antigen. *Urol Oncol* 1995;1:29–37.

26. Troyer JK, Beckett ML, Wright GL Jr. Location of prostate-specific membrane antigen in the LNCaP prostate carcinoma cell line. *Prostate* 1997;30:232–242.

27. Liu H, Moy P, Kim S, et al. Monoclonal antibodies to the extracellular domain of prostate-specific membrane antigen also react with tumor vascular endothelium. *Cancer Res* 1997;57:3629–3634.

28. Smith-Jones PM, Vallabhajosula S, Goldsmith SJ, et al. *In vitro* characterization of radiolabeled monoclonal antibodies specific for the extracellular domain of prostate specific membrane antigen. *Cancer Res* (in press).

29. Smith-Jones PM, Navarro V, Bander NH, et al. Uptake and metabolism of In-111 and I-131 labeled anti-PSMA monoclonal antibodies by prostate carcinoma cells. *J Nucl Med* 2000;40:142P(abst).

30. Goldsmith SJ, Kostakoglu L, Vallabhajosula S, et al. Evaluation of antibody I-131 J591 in the treatment of prostate cancer. *J Nucl Med* 2000;40:80P(abst).

Nuclear Oncology: Diagnosis and Therapy, edited by I. Khalkhali, J. Maublant, and S.J. Goldsmith, Lippincott Williams & Wilkins, Philadelphia © 2001

33

RADIONUCLIDE IMAGING

GIDON LIEBERMAN
JOHN R. BUSCOMBE

Ovarian cancer kills more women than all other gynecologic cancers. Most tumors are first discovered when the disease is advanced. Treatment at this time is often not successful. Little is known of the cause of ovarian cancers, and no recognized screening of persons at risk is available. Symptoms of early ovarian cancer are vague. Imaging techniques are relied on to identify the location of suspected lesions and to provide optimal treatment in the hope of reducing mortality. In approximately 75% of newly diagnosed cases, ovarian cancer has spread beyond the ovaries, and in 60% of cases, it has spread to the pelvic and abdominal organs. Ovarian cancer commonly seeds the peritoneal surfaces of the abdomen and pelvis and is often seen on the serosal and mesenteric surfaces of large and small intestine as well as on the liver surface. The right hemidiaphragm and left hemidiaphragm are also common metastatic sites. Epithelial ovarian cancer also has the potential to spread through the lymphatics and commonly involves paraaortic lymph nodes without affecting the pelvic nodes. Rarely, ovarian cancers can metastasize through the blood to the liver parenchyma, the lung, the bones, or the brain. The most important practical problem in oncology today relates to effective treatment planning based on adequate diagnosis of the stage of an individual patient's tumor. As a result, the patient may receive either too much or too little treatment (1). The clinical requirements for an imaging technique in patients with ovarian cancer are preoperative diagnosis and staging differentiation between metastases and non-malignant pathologic conditions. Although the disease spreads transperitoneally, patients often have tumor seedlings that are not visible by conventional imaging techniques such as computed tomography (CT) or ultrasound.

G. Lieberman: Department of Obstetrics and Gynecology, Royal Free and University College Medical School, London NW3 2PF, United Kingdom.

J. R. Buscombe: Department of Nuclear Medicine, Royal Free Hospital, London NW3 2QG, United Kingdom.

CURRENT NONIMAGING DIAGNOSTIC METHODS

Signs and Symptoms at Presentation

Ovarian carcinoma is often asymptomatic in its early stages. Abdominal discomfort, including bloating, and change in bowel habit are common presenting symptoms (10% to 37% of patients); vaginal bleeding (15%) and urinary symptoms are comparatively uncommon. As disease progresses, the associated pain increases, along with further distention. Signs of ovarian cancer depend on the physical characteristics of the patient and on the location and clinical behavior of the tumor (hemorrhage, ascites, torsion, or rupture). Other less common signs are nodular hepatomegaly, palpable inguinal lymphadenopathy, and omental masses.

CA-125 Estimations

Hematologic and biochemical changes are not observed in early disease. As disease progresses, however, anemia, hypoalbuminemia, thrombocytosis, and deranged liver function are often seen. Certain tumor markers for the detection of ovarian cancer have been investigated. These include CA-125, CA-19.9, CA-15.3, carcinoembryonic antigen (CEA), human milk fat globulin (HMFG), tumor-associated glycoprotein (TAG-72) and placental alkaline phosphatase (PLAP), OVX-1, and macrophage colony-stimulating factor. CA-125 is a high-molecular-weight glycoprotein. It is located on the surface of many epithelial ovarian cancers and is often shed in the circulation.

In 1981, Bast and colleagues (2) described a murine monoclonal antibody (OC-125) that reacted specifically with ovarian cancer cell lines. Two years later, these investigators described the development of a radioimmunoassay using the OC-125 monoclonal antibody to detect CA-125. Using the assay, these investigators reported that only 1% of 888 apparently healthy patients had serum CA-125 levels higher than 35 U/mL. By contrast, 82% of 101 patients with ovarian cancer had elevated levels. A close relationship exists between CA-125 levels and disease status. A rising level suggests disease progression, whereas a declining level correlates with tumor regression (3). The elevated level, however, may be associated with only disease volume; fewer than 50% of patients with early (and treatable) carcinoma of the ovary have a raised CA-125 (4). Furthermore, CA-125 levels are nonspecific, with elevated levels found in endometriosis, ectopic pregnancy, diabetes, and hepatitis.

ANATOMIC IMAGING

Transabdominal Ultrasound

Thompson et al. (5) undertook the first large trial of ultrasound of 100 patients with suspected malignant gynecologic disease. In 63 patients, the interpretation was good, in 21 it was fair, and in 16 it was poor. This pioneering study included fibroids, benign and malignant ovarian tumors, cervical carcinoma, and pelvic inflammatory disease.

Benign ovarian cysts generally appeared smooth, with no internal echoes except for linear septal echoes in multiloculated cysts; 65 of 406 benign cysts were misdiagnosed. Malignant cysts were associated with abundant, bizarre echoes within the cyst; 11 of 49 malignant cysts were misdiagnosed by ultrasound examination. Cystic teratomas caused confusion because of the presence of intracystic echoes; 14 of 61 cystic teratomas were diagnosed incorrectly. Thompson et al. concluded that solid tumors are more difficult to diagnose than cystic tumors. The more complex the ultrasound pattern, the higher the probability of malignant disease (6). The positive predictive value of sonographic evidence of malignancy in 400 women with a pelvic mass was 73% (38 of 52 patients), whereas benign tumors were predicted correctly in 95.6% of cases (177 of 185 patients) (7).

In addition to the unacceptably low specificity and positive predictive value, transabdominal ultrasound is uncomfortable for patients because it requires a full bladder for proper visualization of pelvic structures. Additionally, the distance between the abdominal transducer and the ovaries makes this method less effective than transvaginal ultrasound (8). Peritoneal seeding of tumor outside the pelvis is poorly seen by ultrasound, and this often leads to erroneous staging of disease.

Transvaginal Ultrasound

To provide better images of the ovaries, transvaginal ultrasound was developed. Early studies on small groups of women have been encouraging, with a reported sensitivity of 100% and a specificity of 98.1% (9).

The addition of Doppler techniques to quantify blood supply to an ovarian mass has improved the specificity of the test. In 776 asymptomatic women with a familial history of ovarian cancer, transvaginal ultrasound revealed abnormal scans in 43 women. Of those patients, 39 underwent laparotomy. Three stage I ovarian cancers and 36 benign lesions were found. The authors reported 100% sensitivity and 94.8% specificity for finding disease, though it was not cancer specific (10). Despite early encouraging results, it soon became clear that when this technique was used in screening, in which the number of patients with cancer was low compared with those with benign lesions detected, the sensitivity of the method remained high, but many benign lesions were described as cancer. Positive predictive values as low as 9.8% are not unusual (11).

Computed Tomography

The first large prospective comparative study of CT and transabdominal ultrasound in the evaluation of patients with pelvic masses was performed by Walsh et al. (12). Both CT and ultrasound studies were performed on 24 consecutive patients; 22 proceeded to surgery. Both imaging methods have similar diagnostic criteria and are not complementary. The routine use of both techniques is not justified. Staging by CT correlated with surgery in 70% of cases. Lesions in the mesentery, diaphragm, and omentum, however, were frequently missed. This study was unable to differentiate benign lesions from stage I disease (13). In a series of patients with known disease, CT was performed after chemotherapy in 52 women. Specificity was 100%, with a sensitivity of only 38%, even though the inability to detect microscopic disease was not considered to be a false-negative finding (14). It may be concluded, therefore, that CT does not provide meaningful information for the diagnosis or staging of ovarian cancer.

Magnetic Resonance Imaging

Although magnetic resonance imaging (MRI) has proved to be useful in identifying some benign gynecologic conditions, it has not been shown to be more accurate than ultrasound. In 1992, Hata et al. (15) compared transvaginal Doppler ultrasound, MRI, and CA-125 determination in detecting ovarian cancer. This prospective trial included 27 patients with malignant tumors and 36 with benign tumors. No significant differences were found for sensitivity or specificity between transvaginal Doppler ultrasound and transvaginal ultrasound. Compared with MRI and CA-125 levels, transvaginal Doppler had significantly higher sensitivity and lower specificity. Like CT, therefore, MRI offers no advantage over ultrasound in the evaluation of the patient with suspected ovarian cancer.

Summary

The best anatomic method for imaging in patients with suspected ovarian carcinoma is transvaginal ultrasound. It is sensitive, but the low positive predictive value means many women undergo unnecessary laparotomy. All anatomic imaging methods underestimate the extent of disease, particularly the presence of peritoneal deposits.

FUNCTIONAL IMAGING

Most nuclear imaging techniques have been of less use in suspected ovarian cancer than in other cancer types because radiopharmaceuticals are excreted into urine or feces and appear as pelvic activity. Although early dynamic imaging with technetium 99m (^{99m}Tc)–methoxyisobutyl isonitrile has been proposed, the sensitivity of this technique remains low (16) (Fig. 33.1). When large molecules such as antibodies are used, blood pool activity may take up to 24 hours to clear. A imaging method is needed to identify tumor when most of the blood pool as well as urinary and fecal activity has cleared. This requires the use of radionuclides with longer half-lives, such as iodine 131 (^{131}I), ^{123}I, or indium 111 (^{111}In).

After the radionuclide has been chosen, it is necessary to find the best carrier antibody. Ovarian cancer is a heterogeneous disease; finding a specific, widely expressed antigen can be problematic. Various different antibodies have been evaluated.

Anticarcinoembryonic Antigen Antibodies

Monoclonal antibodies directed against CEA have been used to image epithelial ovarian cancer (17). Goldenberg et al. (18) in 1978 described a ^{131}I-labeled, affinity-purified, goat IgG known to react with CEA. Eighteen patients received ^{131}I-labeled antibody. Imaging problems resulting from blood pooling were overcome using subtraction techniques. Tumor location was demonstrated at 48 hours after injection in almost all cases. The scans were negative in those patients without demonstrable tumors or with tumors apparently devoid of CEA. In a later published report (19), this study was increased to include 141 patients overall, but only a single additional patient had ovarian cancer.

Antiplacental Alkaline Phosphatase Antibodies

Placental alkaline phosphatase has a higher avidity for ovarian cancer than HMFG1, but the antigen is expressed in only 75% of ovarian tumors (8,20). Davies et al. (21) reported on an antibody denoted as NDOG2, which had been developed against PLAP. Tumor deposits were successfully visualized in 11 of 15 patients, and the abnormalities demonstrated were classified as focal or diffuse. Of the 11 patients, 8 showed focal abnormalities alone, and 3 had a diffuse abnormality, of which 2 also showed a focal abnormality. False-positive results resulted from dissociation of the ^{123}I radiolabel from the antibody and significant gut activity. A false-negative result occurred because of high background activity in the liver (common in ^{123}I-labeled proteins) that masked a known, discrete tumor deposit.

Antihuman Fat Milk Glycoprotein Antibodies

Bast and colleagues, in 1991, described the production of three separate hybridoma cell lines, which produced three

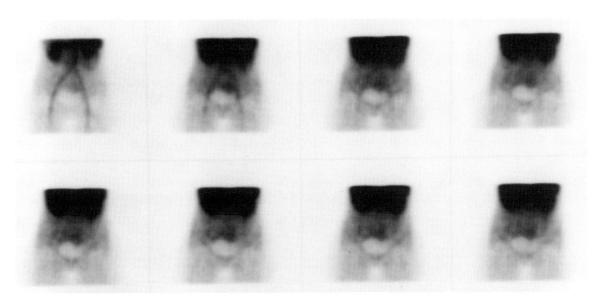

FIGURE 33.1. Dynamic imaging with technetium 99m methoxyisobutyl isonitrile showing uptake in pelvic tumor before gut activity is seen.

unique monoclonal antibodies. When tested for binding to a wide range of human cell lines and strains, all three antibodies showed negative reactions with fibroblasts, lymphoblastoid cells, and a large number of epithelial cell lines of nonbreast origin. Two of the antibodies reacted with seven of eight breast cancer lines tested and with epithelial cells cultured from human milk. These were later described as HMFG1 and HMFG2. The other antibody (3.15.C3) reacted with only two of the breast cancer cell lines (22). Both HMFG1 and HMFG2 bind to an antigen present on 90% of serous carcinomas as well as lactating breast tissue and other epithelial tissue. The antibodies localize to the amino acid sequence Asp-Thr-Arg.

Epenetos et al. (23) reported the first clinical trial of these antibodies in 1982, by investigating 20 patients with known malignant neoplastic disease of ovary, breast, and gastrointestinal tract. Tumors became visible 3 minutes to 18 hours after injection of the labeled antibody. The presence of antibody in the tumors was confirmed by autoradiography and immunoperoxidase staining of surgically removed tissue. Epenetos et al. (24) subsequently described the ability of radioimmunoscintigraphy, using HMFG2, to detect ovarian cancer when ultrasound and CT scan results were negative.

Pateisky et al. (25) described the first prospective trial of ^{123}I HMFG2 in 25 patients. Patients were investigated for either primary tumors or recurrent ovarian cancer. Nineteen of the patients underwent operations a few days after radioimmunoscintigraphy. The remaining 6 patients were investigated by transmission CT to establish the presence or

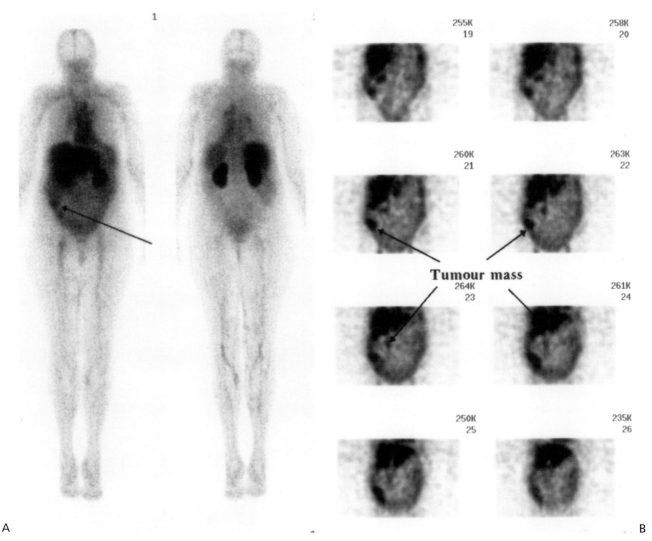

FIGURE 33.2. Technetium 99m H170 monoclonal antibody planar and single photon emission computed tomography (SPECT) images showing focal uptake in ovarian carcinoma. The 20-hour planar image **(A)** shows tumor in the lower right abdomen; the coronal slice of the SPECT image **(B)** shows the same lesion. Another set of coronal slices shows the ovarian primary with a necrotic center **(C)**.

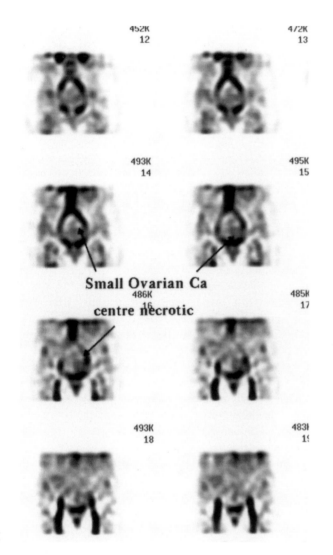

452K
12

472K
13

493K
14

495K
15

Small Ovarian Ca
486K
16

485K
17

centre necrotic

493K
18

483K
19

C

FIGURE 33.2. *(continued)* Another set of coronal slices shows the ovarian primary with a necrotic center **(C)**.

absence of tumor on imaging. In 22 of the 25 cases, the radioimmunoscintigraphy results correlated with the findings at subsequent operation or by CT, respectively, as well as with the histologic diagnosis of the tumor type. Only 2 false-negative results and 1 false-positive result were reported, the latter the result of faulty reading of the radioimmunoscintigraphy study. Sixteen of 18 tumor sites in 25 patients were identified by radioimmunoscintigraphy, the smallest site being 1.5 cm in diameter. In 4 patients, radioimmunoscintigraphy was the only noninvasive investigation method used to detect malignant tumor sites preoperatively.

The ^{123}I anti-HMFG2 antibodies were better in evaluating possible ovarian cancer recurrence than in the differential diagnosis of pelvic masses. In a prospective trial of 30 patients presenting with a pelvic mass, imaging data were obtained without knowledge of the clinical data and were

compared with subsequent surgical findings. A false-positive diagnosis of ovarian cancer was made in 5 of 10 patients. A true-positive diagnosis was made in 19 of 20 patients shown subsequently to have ovarian cancer. In 18 of these patients, the distribution of uptake closely fit the surgical findings (26).

This study was increased subsequently to include 51 patients, of whom 39 proved to have ovarian cancer. Accuracy of diagnosis and detection of primary and metastatic disease were both 95% (27). One of the problems arising with these studies is that many of them include patients from previous publications.

Anti–CA-125 Antibodies

Bast et al. (2) in 1981 described a murine monoclonal antibody (OC-125) that reacted with each of 6 epithelial ovarian carcinoma cell lines and with cryopreserved tumor tissue from 12 of 20 patients with ovarian cancer. The antibody did not bind to various types of nonmalignant tissue including adult and fetal ovary. The OC-125 antibody reacted with only 1 of 14 cell lines derived from nonovarian neoplasms and did not react with cryostat sections from 12 nonovarian carcinomas.

In 1991, Vuillez et al. (28) imaged 43 patients with suspected ovarian carcinoma recurrence using F(ab')2 fragments of OC-125 antibody. They labeled the monoclonal antibody first with ^{111}In and then with [131]I. Single photon emission CT imaging was better with ^{111}In planar scintigraphy. No significant difference was noted between the two radionuclides.

Indium 111 Satumomab Pendetide

The only monoclonal antibody approved by the United States Food and Drug Administration for imaging of ovarian (and colon) cancer is ^{111}In-satumomab pendetide (OncoScint CR/OV; Cytogen, Princeton, NJ). This antibody uses ^{111}In, which, unlike ^{123}I, requires a chelator (diethylenetriamine pantaacetic acid) to a murine monoclonal antibody (mAb 72.3). This monoclonal antibody is directed against TAG-72, which is frequently expressed by colorectal and ovarian carcinomas.

The TAG-72 antigen is not tumor specific; it cross-reacts with a wide range of tissues including reticuloendothelial tissues, the liver, and foci of inflammation or infection. It has, however, been one of the few antibodies to undergo significant multicenter trials, and it was studied in 108 patients, 103 of whom underwent surgery. Patient groups included were those with known suspected primary or recurrent/residual ovarian cancer. Forty-two patients had a negative workup before imaging. Seventeen were found to have tumor at surgery. Imaging with ^{111}In-satumomab pendetide detected only 6 of these 17 tumors, thus yielding a negative predictive value of 28%. Consistently, the sensitiv-

TABLE 33.1. SUMMARY OF RESULTS OF STUDIES USING ANTIBODY IMAGING IN OVARIAN CANCER

Authors and year (reference)	Antibody	Radiolabel	Sensitivity	Specificity	Notes
Goldenberg et al., 1978 (18)	Anti-CEA	[131]Iodine	100%	N/A	18 patients all had ovarian cancer
Goldenberg et al., 1980 (19)	Anti-CEA	[131]Iodine	100%	N/A	141 patients including 18 above all had ovarian cancer
Epenetos et al., 1982 (23)	HFMG1	[123]Iodine	92%	N/A	20 mixed cancers including 10 ovarian
Pateisky et al., 1985 (25)	HFMG2	[123]Iodine	77%	33%	25 patients, 13 with cancer
Granowska et al., 1986 (26)	HFMG2	[123]Iodine	95%	20%	30 patients, 20 with cancer
Surwit et al., 1993 (29)	B72.3(Cyt103)	[111]Indium	68%	55%	103 patients, 68 with cancer
Alexander et al., 1995 (34)	Mab-170	[99m]Technetium	92%	94%	30 patients, 13 with cancer

CEA, carcinoembryonic antigen; HFMG, human milk fat globulin; N/A, not applicable.

ity of the test varied with tumor size; values fell from approximately 80% for masses larger than 2 cm to approximately 50% for smaller masses and less than 10% for microscopic disease. Detection of carcinomatosis in patients with surgically confirmed disease was greater with radiolabeled antibody studies than imaging with CT. Thirty-eight patients with carcinomatosis were evaluated with the two modalities. The overall detection rate for carcinomatosis was 71% with ^{111}In-satumomab pendetide, whereas it was 45% for CT (29).

Monoclonal Antibody 170

Monoclonal antibody 170 (mAb-170) is the only antibody labeled with ^{99m}Tc to have entered phase II clinical trials in ovarian cancer. To overcome the dilemma of persistent blood pool and excretion in urine or feces, activities as high as 1,000 MBq of ^{99m}Tc MAb-170 were used with single photon emission CT studies up to 24 hours after injection. Although this level of activity is acceptable in the United States, European regulators recognize an upper limit of 740 MBq for most diagnostic studies. The production of the antibody is unique in that it was raised against synthetic tumor-associated glycoconjugates as the imunogens (30,31). The monoclonal antibodies with highest potential were MoAb 155H.7 and MoAb 170H.82. These two monoclonal antibodies reacted with more than 85% of human carcinomas. Benign tissues were negative except for apical glandular epithelial cells (gut, breast, bronchus), adrenal cortical cells, and trophoblastic cells of mature placentas. MoAb 170H.82 appeared to react more strongly with tumor cells at the site of active invasion or penetration of tumor growth, as well as in metastases (32).

Various cells of gastrointestinal origin (i.e., colonic and gastric epithelium), as well as the collecting tubules of the kidney, liver bile ducts, and the epithelial cells of the lungs and prostate also showed moderate expression of CA-170. This has lead to some problems with imaging that have required the use of registration techniques to differentiate tumor from gut activity, particularly in the lower abdomen (33).

Alexander et al. (34) published the first clinical trial in 1995 on 30 patients before they underwent laparotomy. The mAb-170 was radiolabeled to 0.8 MBq [99m]Tc. Radioimmunoscintigraphy recognized 12 of 13 cases of adenocarcinoma of the ovaries, a finding corresponding to an overall sensitivity of 92.3%. Specificity was 94.1% (16 of 17); accuracy was 93.3% (28 of 30). Of 33 known lesions, 26 were visualized successfully, a finding corresponding to a locoregional specificity of 96.6%. The smallest lesion visualized was an adenocarcinoma of the corpus uteri with a diameter of 1.5 cm. Twenty of 22 adnexal malignant tumors were detected in 28 of 34 abdominopelvic sites, all of 4 uterine foci, 1 skin metastasis, and none of 3 lymph node metastases (29). More recent trails showed promising results in a larger group of patients. Trials were stopped in 1998, however, and it currently appears that this antibody will not be available commercially (Fig. 33.2).

Summary

Much work has been done on antibody imaging in ovarian cancer over the past 20 years (Table 33.1). One product has been licensed by the United States Food and Drug Administration. This product is not available in Europe. Cross-reactivity with normal tissues has remained a significant problem over this period. Although anatomic imaging is still not ideal for this disease, it would appear that radioimmunoscintigraphy is no better and will not be used to any great extent.

REFERENCES

1. Chatal JF, Fumoleau P, Saccavini JC, et al. Immunoscintigraphy of recurrences of gynecologic carcinomas. *J Nucl Med* 1987;28:1807–1819.
2. Bast RC Jr, Feeney M, Lazarus H, et al. Reactivity of a monoclonal antibody with human ovarian carcinoma. *J Clin Invest* 1981;68:1331–1337.
3. Bast RC Jr, Klug TL, St. John E, et al. A radioimmunoassay using

a monoclonal antibody to monitor the course of epithelial ovarian cancer. *N Engl J Med* 1983;309:883–887.

4. Thibodeau SN, Bren G, Schaid D. Microsatellite instability in cancer of the proximal colon. *Science* 1993;260:816–819.

5. Thompson HE, Holmes JH, Gottesfeld KR, et al. Ultrasound as a diagnostic aid in diseases of the pelvis. *Am J Obstet Gynecol* 1967;98:472–481.

6. Kobayashi M. Use of diagnostic ultrasound in trophoblastic neoplasms and ovarian tumors. *Cancer* 1976;38:441–452.

7. Herrmann UJ Jr, Locher GW, Goldhirsch A. Sonographic patterns of ovarian tumors: prediction of malignancy. *Obstet Gynecol* 1987;69:777–781.

8. van Nagell JR Jr, Higgins RV, Donaldson ES, et al. Transvaginal sonography as a screening method for ovarian cancer: a report of the first 1000 cases screened. *Cancer* 1990;65:573–577.

9. Pussell SJ, Cosgrove DO, Hinton J, et al. Carcinoma of the ovary: correlation of ultrasound with second look laparotomy. *Br J Obstet Gynaecol* 1980;87:1140–1144.

10. Bourne TH, Whitehead MI, Campbell S, et al. Ultrasound screening for familial ovarian cancer. *Gynecol Oncol* 1991;43:92–97.

11. Bourne TH, Campbell S, Reynolds KM, et al. Screening for early familial ovarian cancer with transvaginal ultrasonography and colour blood flow imaging. *BMJ* 1993;306:1025–1029.

12. Walsh JW, Rosenfield AT, Jaffe CC, et al. Prospective comparison of ultrasound and computed tomography in the evaluation of gynecologic pelvic masses. *AJR Am J Roentgenol* 1978;6:955–960.

13. Shiels RA, Peel KR, MacDonald HN, et al. A prospective trial of computed tomography in the staging of ovarian malignancy. *Br J Obstet Gynaecol* 1985;92:407–412.

14. Boente MP, Yeh K, Hogan WM, et al. Current status of staging laparotomy in colorectal and ovarian cancer. *Cancer Treat Res* 1996;82:337–357.

15. Hata K, Hata T, Manabe A, et al. A critical evaluation of transvaginal Doppler studies, transvaginal sonography, magnetic resonance imaging, and CA 125 in detecting ovarian cancer. *Obstet Gynecol* 1992;80:922–926.

16. Krolicki L, Stelmachow J, Cwikla JB. Evaluation of Tc-99m MIBI uptake in patients with suspected ovarian cancer: initial study. *Eur J Nucl Med* 1998;25:1014.

17. Blend MJ, Ostrowski GJ. Recent advances in the detection of ovarian cancer: a review. *J Am Osteopath Assoc* 1994;94:305–318.

18. Goldenberg DM, Deland F, Kim E, et al. Use of radiolabeled antibodies to carcinoembryonic antigen for the detection and localization of diverse cancers by external photoscanning. *N Engl J Med* 1978;298:1384–1386.

19. Goldenberg DM, Kim EE, DeLand FH, et al. Radioimmunodetection of cancer with radioactive antibodies to carcinoembryonic antigen. *Cancer Res* 1980;40:2984–2992.

20. Granowska M, Britton KE. Radiolabelled monoclonal antibodies in oncology. II. Clinical applications in diagnosis. *Nucl Med Commun* 1991;12:83–98.

21. Davies JO, Davies ER, Howe K, et al. Radionuclide imaging of ovarian tumours with ^{123}I-labelled monoclonal antibody (NDOG2) directed against placental alkaline phosphatase. *Br J Obstet Gynaecol* 1985;93:277–286.

22. Taylor-Papadimitriou J, Peterson JA, Arklie J, et al. Monoclonal antibodies to epithelium-specific components of the human milk fat globule membrane: production and reaction with cells in culture. *Int J Cancer* 1981;28:17–21.

23. Epenetos AA, Britton KE, Mather S, et al. Targeting of iodine-123-labelled tumour-associated monoclonal antibodies to ovarian, breast, and gastrointestinal tumours. *Lancet* 1982;2:999–1005.

24. Epenetos AA, Shepherd JH, Britton KE, et al. [123]I radioiodinated antibody imaging of occult ovarian cancer. *Cancer* 1985;55:984–987.

25. Pateisky N, Philipp K, Skodler WD, et al. Radioimmunodetection in patients with suspected ovarian cancer. *J Nucl Med* 1985;26:1369–1376.

26. Granowska M, Britton KE, Shepherd JH, et al. A prospective study of ^{123}I-labeled monoclonal antibody imaging in ovarian cancer. *J Clin Oncol* 1986;4:730–736.

27. Shepherd JH, Granowska M, Britton KE, et al. Tumour-associated monoclonal antibodies for the diagnosis and assessment of ovarian cancer. *Br J Obstet Gynaecol* 1987;94:160–167.

28. Vuillez JP, Peltier P, Mayer JC, et al. Reproducibility of image interpretation in immunoscintigraphy performed with indium-111- and iodine-131-labeled OC125 F(ab')2 antibody injected into the same patients. *J Nucl Med* 1991;32:221–227.

29. Surwit EA, Childers JM, Krag DN, et al. Clinical assessment of ^{111}In-CYT-103 immunoscintigraphy in ovarian cance. *Gynecol Oncol* 1993;48:285–292.

30. McEwan AJ, MacLean GD, Hooper HR, et al. MAb 170H.82: an evaluation of a novel panadenocarcinoma monoclonal antibody labelled with ^{99m}Tc and with [111]In. *Nucl Med Commun* 1992;13:11–19.

31. MacLean GD, Noujaim AA, Suresh MR, et al. A novel strategy to derive monoclonal antibodies for succesful imaging of cancers in humans. In: *Cellular basis of immune modulation.* New York: Alan Liss, 1989:587–599.

32. Longenecker BM, Willans DJ, MacLean GD, et al. Monoclonal antibodies and synthetic tumor-associated glycoconjugates in the study of the expression of Thomsen-Friedenreich-like and Tn-like antigens on human cancers. *J Natl Cancer Inst* 1987;78:489–496.

33. Lieberman G, Buscombe JR, McCool D, et al. Registration of radioimmunoscintigraphy and computer tomography in ovarian cancer. *Nucl Med Commun* 1987;18:291.

34. Alexander C, Villena-Heinsen CE, Trampert L, et al. Radioimmunoscintigraphy of ovarian tumours with technetium-99m labelled monoclonal antibody-170: first clinical experiences. *Eur J Nucl Med* 1995;22:645–651.

34

INTRAPERITONEAL RADIONUCLIDE THERAPY

RUBY F. MEREDITH
DANIEL J. MACEY

Intraperitoneal (IP) radionuclide therapy is applicable to most patients with epithelial ovarian cancer because residual disease is usually present, even after clearance by surgery plus chemotherapy. Much recent information about IP radionuclide therapy comes from the use of radiolabeled antibodies rather than the nonspecific administration of radionuclides, although both strategies have been used.

ADVANTAGES OF INTRAPERITONEAL ROUTE

Advantages of IP delivery over intravenous (IV) administration are an increase in dose to the tumor and a reduction in systemic toxicity. The systemic absorption of agents administered IP is delayed, so higher doses can be delivered IP than systemically when bone marrow suppression is the dose-limiting toxicity. Because the lymphatic channels through which macromolecular structures travel from the peritoneal cavity are also the route for metastatic tumor implantation, which can result in occlusion and the development of ascites, IP administration optimizes tumor exposure to therapeutic agents. However, not all patients with disease confined to the abdomen benefit from such regional therapy because they have adhesions that limit the free flow of fluid throughout the cavity.

TESTING OF ELIGIBILITY FOR INTRAPERITONEAL THERAPY

Before intraabdominal radionuclide therapy is administered, distribution is usually evaluated to determine whether the agent will flow freely throughout the cavity.

R. F. Meredith and D. J. Macey: Department of Radiation Oncology, University of Alabama at Birmingham, Birmingham, Alabama 35233.

Although this can be accomplished by IP instillation of radiopaque contrast followed by fluoroscopy and confirmation with upright and decubitus films, the recommended method is to inject a radioactive agent, such as ^{99m}Tc-sulfur colloid or ^{99m}Tc-macroaggregated albumin. Because the distribution of a dissimilar test agent may not accurately represent that of the therapeutic agent, some practitioners who use ^{32}P or other pure beta emitters to treat patients first administer a small amount of the radionuclide solution and monitor distribution by *bremsstrahlung* imaging [1]. Uniform distribution of the solution before therapy did not exclude a major area of accumulation 3 to 7 days after therapy in 46% of patients given ^{32}P, demonstrated via *bremsstrahlung* imaging [2]. The most frequent site of accumulation was the pelvis in 60% of the patients. Even though accumulation was frequent, no correlation was found between non-uniform distribution and relapse or bowel obstruction. An inherent weakness of IP therapy is the absence of diagnostic studies or data that would allow treatment planning and individualization of therapeutic dosing.

EXPERIENCE WITH PHOSPHORUS 32

Although other radionuclides are potential agents for IP therapy, ^{32}P is the radionuclide predominantly used as a nonconjugated agent. Other radionuclides, such as ^{198}Au and ^{90}Y in colloidal suspensions, were used in early studies and were not as effective as ^{32}P [1]. ^{32}P has been infused as a chromic phosphate solution diluted with saline solution [3]. A volume of 2 L is recommended for optimal initial distribution [4]. Often, 500 mL or more of saline solution is administered before the radioactive agent to facilitate flow; the radioactive agent is then administered diluted in additional saline solution. The administration of IP radionuclide therapy is followed by frequent changes of posture for 2 to 3 hours to promote distribution. Hospital beds facilitate use of the Trendelenburg and reverse Trendelenburg positions, in addition to supine and right and left lateral positions.

The usual dose of 15 to 20 mCi of ^{32}P is estimated to deliver 20 to 40 Gy to the peritoneal surface at an exponentially decreasing dose rate with a half-life of 14.3 days. In some series, the dose was titrated from 7 to 20 mCi based on the size of the abdominal cavity, although in other series a single dose level was used for all patients. ^{32}P is a beta emitter with a mean energy of 695 keV and a range of 1 to 4 mm in soft tissue. Consequently, it is of less value in the treatment of gross disease (5). It has been studied in randomized trials. In an early Gynecologic Oncology Group (GOG) trial (6), patients with stage IC, completely resected stage II, or poorly differentiated stage IA or IB disease were randomized to 0.2 mg of melphalan per kilogram per day for 5 days, repeated every 4 to 6 weeks for 12 cycles, or to a single IP dose of 15 mCi of ^{32}P. At 5 years, the survival rates were very similar, 81% and 78%. Kaplan-Meier curves showed a more than 10% disease-free survival advantage for the ^{32}P group after a follow-up of more than 90 months. Because leukemia developed in 3% of patients receiving melphalan, ^{32}P was considered to be the superior treatment despite some instances of small-bowel obstruction that required surgery.

Subsequently, two randomized trials compared ^{32}P with cisplatin (2,7). Although neither of these studies showed a 5-year survival advantage of one treatment over the other, in the Norwegian study, in which eligible patients had no gross disease after surgery, 28 of the 347 patients randomized to receive ^{32}P showed evidence of poor radionuclide distribution on flow study (2). These patients received whole-abdomen external beam radiation instead of ^{32}P. Despite the fact that the dose of ^{32}P was rather low, at 7 to 10 mCi, small-bowel obstruction developed in 9% of the patients receiving ^{32}P, but in only 2% in the cisplatin therapy arm. Consequently, cisplatin was further recommended as standard therapy.

This study confirmed a 5% to 10% rate of bowel complications after IP administration of ^{32}P (8). In some series, the rate increased to 20% to 30% when patients also received external beam radiation to the pelvis (9,10). Walton et al. (8) analyzed variables that might contribute to bowel complications, including technique of instillation and the interval between surgery and subsequent ^{32}P treatment. They found no association with aspects of technique, including the use of one or more catheters, the use of a simple catheter inserted through a 16-gauge needle or a larger catheter with multiple side openings, and the time between catheter insertion and IP treatment. Patients were treated with ^{32}P between 5 and 106 days after surgery. Most patients were treated by 20 days, and a trend toward a decreased risk for complications was associated with early treatment after surgery. It has been speculated that the optimal time of administration may be immediately after

surgery, while the patient is in the recovery room, before adhesions have formed. Spanos et al. (11) found a lower complication rate when ^{32}P was given within 12 hours of surgery, even when adjustments were made for other factors, including number of prior operations, whether external beam radiation had been administered, and stage of disease. They reported no cases of contamination because of wound leakage or repeated operation. They followed a regimen of position changes every 15 to 30 minutes for 6 hours. Piver et al. (12) noted no severe complications with their regimen of peritoneography before injection, administration of large volumes of solution, and frequent position changes. Although bowel obstruction and fistula (13) are the most severe complications of IP therapy with ^{32}P, the most common side effect is transient abdominal pain, which is reported to occur in about 20% of patients (8). Chemical or infectious peritonitis can also develop but has been noted only in about 2% to 3% of patients. Other catheter-related complications, such as erosion of the catheter into the bowel, have been noted when a catheter has been in place for more than 6 weeks (14).

Because not all institutions that used IP administration of ^{32}P in early GOG studies reported significant rates of bowel complications, many participated in a subsequent GOG study in which adjuvant IP ^{32}P was used in International Federation of Gynecology and Obstetrics (FIGO) stage III patients with no evidence of disease at second-look laparotomy. The final results of progression-free survival and complications have not been reported (15). An interim report indicated a 27% recurrence rate after a median follow-up of 58 months for eligible patients. A randomized, multicenter trial compared 7 to 10 mCi of IP ^{32}P with 50 mg of cisplatin per square meter given every 4 weeks for six cycles to patients with stage IC disease (7). At a median follow-up of 76 months, a trend for improved 5-year progression-free survival was noted in the patients receiving cisplatin (85% vs. 65%; $p = .007$). Overall survival rates were similar, 81% for the cisplatin patients and 79% for the ^{32}P patients. A direct comparison of IP ^{32}P with whole-abdominal radiation has not been reported. Although both can be effective against small-volume disease, ^{32}P may provide a higher tumor dose to the peritoneal surface than whole-abdominal radiation, even though the dose distribution is less homogeneous. The efficacy of ^{32}P is limited to very small-volume disease, whereas whole-abdominal radiation is used for gross disease (16). A dose of IP ^{32}P that is lower than usual (5 mCi) has also been given repeatedly in conjunction with cisplatin chemotherapy. *In vitro* animal model and patient cell culture studies often show enhanced activity with this combination. Thus, 30 patients with ovarian cancer were treated with up to 8 monthly cycles. At 3 years, no severe bowel complications were observed. The response rate to treatment was 87%. Although control patients are lacking in this nonrandomized setting, the response rate and the 63% survival rate are encouraging (17).

RADIOLABELED CONJUGATES

Because nonspecific agents such as ^{32}P do not localize at affected areas, and because the use of such agents has been hampered by bowel toxicity, attention has turned to the use of radiolabeled antibodies in regional IP therapy. A variety of antibodies are reactive with ovarian epithelial carcinomas (18,19).

Several diagnostic studies have confirmed the potential advantages of the IP over the IV route in the administration of radiolabeled antibodies. These studies show the ability of radiolabeled antibodies to localize to tumor. Imaging and dosimetry studies of the IP administration of ^{131}I-B72.3 (anti-TAG-72) demonstrated selective tumor localization to intraabdominal/peritoneal metastases of colorectal cancer (20). Ward et al. (21) and Chatal et al. (22) noted similar findings in patients with stage III ovarian cancer with the use of ^{131}I-HMFG2 (18 patients) and ^{111}In-OC125 (28 patients), respectively. Most clinical and preclinical studies of imaging and dosimetry in which IP administration of radiolabeled antibodies was used show tumor-to-normal tissue ratios of more than 20. Excellent localization of ^{177}Lu-CC49 in an anterior abdominal lesion is illustrated in Fig. 34.1. Generally, the tumor-to-normal tissue ratios are favorable. In the study of Larson et al. (20), accumulation varied greatly between nodules in the same patients (20-fold difference between minimum and maximum uptake). A maximum of 11 Gy/mCi of ^{131}I-B72.3 antibody was achieved when the IP route was used, with only 1% of that dose delivered to the marrow. The average uptake in tumor nodules was calculated to be 100-fold greater than that obtained with the IV route, and the average marrow dose from IP administration was only 1.5 cGy/mCi. An estimated 40% of the radioactive agent was localized to tumor nodules in 1 of 10 patients.

Biodistribution and pharmacokinetics studies in humans (21–23) have shown a slow absorption of radiolabeled antibody into the bloodstream, with maximum blood levels of intact antibodies at 36 to 48 hours. Much shorter transit times to the systemic circulation have been noted in studies of murine models (24). F(ab')$_2$ peaks at 24 hours, and IgM molecules do not effectively reach the blood (25–28). The early biodistribution studies (21,23) also showed that the IP route is superior to the IV route for intraperitoneal implants/tumor cells, whereas the reverse is true for solid tumor metastases in the abdomen (e.g., lymph nodes, hematogenous omental implants). Molthoff et al. (29) found similar concentrations of Mov18 antibody whether it was administered IV or IP for most tumor nodules. A higher dose can be tolerated when given IP because of a 2-day delay in the transit of radioactivity to the plasma, during which time much of the activity decays. The integrated area under the curve for plasma radioactivity with IP administration is about half that with IV administration. Related studies from this group of chimeric Mov18 IgG clearly showed advantages of the IP over the IV route for tumor nodules up to 1 cm in size (30).

Side Effects of Radiolabeled Antibodies

Compared with unconjugated radionuclides administered IP, radiolabeled antibodies have been myelosuppressive. Even with slow absorption into the systemic circulation, myelosuppression remains the dose-limiting toxicity of IP radioimmunotherapy. Acute side effects, which have been infrequent, have included transient nausea, vomiting, diarrhea, and abdominal pain, which often resolve with a decreased rate of infusion. Late bowel toxicity has been rare. In most patients undergoing subsequent surgery for bowel obstruction, recurrent disease is found to be the causative factor. Gastrointestinal toxicity was more prevalent than usual among patients who received more than 100 mCi of ^{131}I-OC125 with slow clearance of radioactivity through the urine (31). Rarely, thyroid abnormality has been noted in patients receiving ^{131}I-labeled antibodies despite blocking of the thyroid (32). The most frequent toxicity noted among patients receiving 25 to 150 mCi of [186]Re-NR-LU-10 per square meter was a transient, inconsequential elevation of liver enzymes (12 of 17 patients). This toxicity has not been reported by others; it may be related to metabolism of the radioimmunoconjugate in the liver (33).

Most antibodies used for IP radioimmunotherapy have been murine and are immunogenic (34). Our experience with CC49 antibody suggests that this high-affinity anti-TAG-72 antibody is more immunogenic when given IP than when given IV. A serum sickness-type phenomenon, including arthralgia/myalgia with or without fever, occurred 2 to 3 weeks after IP administration in about one third of patients, but in only 2 of more than 60 patients after IV administration. These symptoms begin approximately 2 weeks after treatment and persist for at least a week. They are responsive to nonspecific measures, such as antiinflammatory agents. The Hammersmith and NeoRx

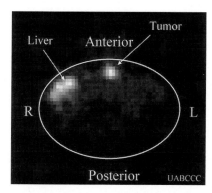

FIGURE 34.1. Transverse section image (6 mm thick) illustrating excellent localization of Lu-CC49 in a tumor in the intraperitoneal cavity of a patient with ovarian cancer.

clinical groups confirmed the frequency of serum sickness after IP radioimmunotherapy of ovarian cancer with antibodies other than CC49. However, they noted more skin rashes than symptoms related to CC49 antibody (33,35). The presence of human anti-mouse antibody (HAMA) accelerates the clearance of administered antibodies from the blood and can result in the deposition of immune complexes in renal and reticuloendothelial tissues. Renal dsyfunction has generally not been noted. HAMA do not occur on initial use. The presence of HAMA can result in falsely elevated tumor marker indices unless it is removed from the plasma samples before testing. Methods to decrease the incidence and intensity of the HAMA response, usually with forms of immunosuppression, have been applied with varying degrees of success (36,37). With the increasing availability of humanized antibodies, the concern for HAMA is minimized. The impact of HAMA on tumor targeting in the peritoneal cavity has not been established, although faster blood clearance, as expected, has been noted when patients with HAMA receive a repeated IP treatment (38,39). It has been speculated that HAMA may promote an immunologic mechanism with a therapeutic effect (35).

Clinical Results of Intraperitoneal Radioimmmunotherapy

Regional radionuclide therapy via the IP route has been relatively successful in ovarian cancer as salvage therapy, for relief of ascites, and as adjuvant therapy after clearance of all detectable disease by surgery with or without chemotherapy. The largest experience with IP radiolabeled antibody therapy of ovarian cancer is from Hammersmith Hospital (34,35,38,40–46). In their early experience, tumor cells disappeared and survival was extended in 9 of 16 patients with small-volume disease, but no responses were apparent in 8 patients treated with more than 140 mCi of ^{131}I-HMFG1 antibody for tumor nodules more than 2 cm in size (40). These findings and others are summarized in Table 34.1.

Attempts of the Hammersmith group to improve many aspects of radioimmunotherapy have included the testing of various antibodies or fragments and radionuclides (^{90}Y and ^{131}I), the use of ethylenediamine tetraacetic acid (EDTA) to accelerate the clearance of unstable metal radionuclide conjugates, and the use of the macrocyclic chelator tetraazacyclododecane tetraacetic acid (DOTA) in an effort to produce more stable conjugates of ^{90}Y-labeled antibodies. In early phase I therapy trials of IP ^{131}I-labeled antibodies, as much as 140 mCi was administered before dose-limiting marrow suppression developed (38). Early results with ^{90}Y-labeled monoclonal antibodies (45) demonstrated serious marrow suppression at relatively low doses of IP therapy (15 to 20 mCi). Toxicity after administration of the ^{90}Y-labeled antibodies was not related to calculated bone marrow radiation doses and appeared to be a consequence of ^{90}Y becoming

detached from the diethylenetriamine pentaacetic acid (DTPA) chelator, with subsequent localization of ^{90}Y in bone, where its relatively long range of tissue penetration (4 mm) enhanced marrow toxicity. IP administration of ^{90}Y-labeled.B72.3 anti-TAG-72 antibody has been studied at M. D. Anderson Cancer Center (55,56), where dose-limiting marrow suppression has been observed at 10 to 15 mCi. Both the M.D. Anderson Cancer Center and Hammersmith Hospital teams have reported that IV infusion of EDTA to chelate free ^{90}Y allows higher doses of ^{90}Y monoclonal antibody to be tolerated (total dose of 30 to 40 mCi). Among patients treated with ^{90}Y-B72.3, Kavanagh et al. (56) reported objective antitumor effects. Two patients had no evidence of disease at 15-month follow-up. The Hammersmith group carried out studies with a more stable chelator (DOTA). They reported good tumor localization, although patients had an antibody response to the chelator (57).

Confirming the success of early studies, the results of two recent phase I studies conducted in the United States also show promise, especially for small-volume disease. Objective responses have been observed both with ^{186}Re-NR-LU-10 (33,49,50) and ^{177}Lu-CC49 (14,39). Both of these antibodies react against ovarian cancer and other adenocarcinomas; CC49 is a second-generation high-affinity anti-TAG-72 antibody. Four of 17 patients with nodules smaller than 5 mm responded to ^{186}Re-NR-LU-10, as assessed by subsequent surgical procedures (33,49,50). In a study of ^{177}Lu-CC49, one patient with a 4-cm mass had a partial response, and extended progression-free intervals were noted in four of five patients with microscopic disease who received a single IP administration of ^{177}Lu-CC49. One failed at 10 months and one at 21 months, and three of the five continued without evidence of progression at follow-up of 3+ to 5+ years (52).

Because many patients with ovarian cancer have small tumor nodules that are not well detected by conventional radiographic studies, some trials have evaluated responses to radiolabeled antibody with laparotomy or laparoscopy after treatment (33,58). A third-look surgical procedure was used to evaluate response 90 days after IP radioimmunotherapy with ^{131}I-Mov18 (58). In this study, in which most patients had disease nodules smaller than 5 mm or positive washings before therapy, five achieved a complete response (CR), six were stable, and five progressed. With longer follow-up of the CR patients, one remained disease-free at 34 months, and the other four had a mean disease-free survival of 10.5 months. In another study, four patients treated with ^{186}Re-NR-LU-10, whose disease nodules were smaller than 5 mm, had responses confirmed at post-treatment laparotomy (33).

In trials in which post-treatment surgical evaluation is not performed and in which disease is not detectable by noninvasive means, efficacy is judged by prolongation of progression-free survival in comparison with that in similar patients who are observed or receive alternate therapies. An

TABLE 34.1. CLINICAL RESULTS AND DOSIMETRY OF SELECTED INTRAPERITONEAL RADIOIMMUNOTHERAPY TRIALS

Antibody conjugate (reference)	mCi/Infusion	Peritoneal dose cGy/mCi (total)	Disease effect	Normal organ dose (cGy/mCi)	Comments
^{131}I-HMFGI ^{131}I-AUAI (38,40,45)	20–205 1–4 Rx	(147–443)	9/16 CLR <2 cm 3/6 CR for microscopic 8/8 Prog >2 cm	Whole-body dose 0.44 ± 1.29, intestine dose 2.54 ± 15.98, spleen dose 6.1–5.28	GI complaints, mild myelotoxicity 80-Gy tumor dose
[131]I-2G3 (47)	15–150	6–60 to serosa	3/4 ascites ≥50 mCi		Uptake .02–.0002% ID/g, no specific uptake in 3/5
^{90}Y-HMFGI (43)	5–30	21.7	1/6 CR of small nodules 3/5 ↓ ascites 12/13 Rx as adjuvant NED ≤20 mo	Tumor:normal ratio = 3–10 at 24–48 h	Myelotoxicity ≥15 mCi, myelotoxicity decreased with EDTA
^{90}Y-HMFGI (42)	18.5/m²		>2 cm, median surv = 11 mo For adjuvant Rx, median FU = 35 mo, maximum FU = 62 mo, <10% died of ovarian cancer 21/52 patients treated as adjuvant had better surv than alternative treatment group		
^{90}Y-OC125 F(ab')₂ (48)	1		Biodistribution study	10% liver uptake	Tumor:normal ratio = 3–25
[186]Re-NR LU-10 (33,49,50)	25–100/m²	17.0 ± 8.8 range, 2–36	13/17 Prog; ↓ tumor 4/17 ≤5 mm nodules	Whole-body dose 0.68 ± 0.28	Alternate techniques used for some dose estimates
^{177}Lu-CC49 (14,39,51,52)	16.5–92.2 (10–45/m²)	30.6 ± 12.6	1/13 PR gross disease 9/9 ≤1 cm nodules Prog 1.5–21 mo 4/5 microscopic NED >6–35 mo	Whole-body dose 0.4–0.9	Tumor dose for 3 pts, others imaged but dose not determined, tumor:marrow ratio = 58–139:1 tumor dose = 21.46 Gy
^{131}I-OC125 F(ab')₂ (53)	120 (4.44 GBq)		3/6 stable at 90 d 3/6 Prog		33% grade 3 myelotoxicity
^{131}I-OC125 F(ab')₂ (32)	20–120		3 transient objective responses 16/20 had >2 cm disease		MTD not reached at 120 mCi 12 alive at 3–17 mo FU, most developed HAMA (31)
^{131}I-HMFGI (54)	27–100 1–3 Rx		2/6 objective response		4 pts had tracer before Rx dose, marrow dose 1.08–9.3 cGy/mCi

CLR, clinical clearance; CR, complete response; PR, partial response; Prog, progressed; NED, no evidence of disease; surv, survival; pts, patients; FU, post-treatment follow-up; MTD, maximum tolerated dose; EDTA, ethylenediamine tetraacetic acid; HAMA, human anti-mouse antibody.

example is a trial conducted by the North Thames Study Group in which they compared adjuvant radioimmunotherapy with ^{90}Y-HMFG1 with additional chemotherapy or whole-abdomen irradiation (42). The actuarial survival was significantly better for 15 patients with stage IIB or more advanced disease who received adjuvant radioimmunotherapy. For this subgroup, mortality from ovarian cancer was less than 10% after radioimmunotherapy at a median follow-up of 35 months, whereas mortality of more than 80% was noted at 67 months for 70 patients who received alternate forms of therapy. Another,

somewhat similar study is a case–control analysis of patients from the North Thames database who were observed and compared with a group of 25 patients with stages IC through IV disease who received 18.5 mCi of ^{90}Y-HMFG1 adjuvant therapy following completion of conventional chemotherapy (59). In this analysis, median survival was not reached at a median follow-up of 59 months for radioimmunotherapy patients and 27 months for controls. Kaplan-Meier survival differences were significant at 5 years: 80% survival for radioimmunotherapy patients compared with 55% for those not receiving radioimmunotherapy (*p* = .0035). Additionally, the Cox model projected 10-year survival for the radioimmunotherapy patients at 70%, versus 32% for the control patients. The results from these European trials, in addition to early results with ^{177}Lu-CC49, compare favorably with results obtained with other alternative therapies, such as whole-abdominal irradiation or instillation of non–tumor-specific ^{32}P, yet radiolabeled antibody therapy has not caused the substantial rate of acute and late bowel toxicities associated with these routinely available methods of radiation (60).

The general conclusion to be drawn from these clinical trials is that IP radioimmunotherapy appears feasible and relatively safe and has antitumor effects. Although many studies have been phase I dose-escalation trials in which suboptimal doses were used, and although they often included patients with bulky disease, in whom complete clearance of disease is unlikely, most studies have demonstrated antitumor effects. The only study reportedly closed early for lack of objective responses was that of ^{131}I-OC125, given to patients with stage III disease who had failed platinum with or without Taxol chemotherapy and had nodules smaller than 5 mm. The fact that three of the six patients showed no change in the disease status at 90 days, however, may indicate modest antitumor effects because many patients with chemotherapy-resistant disease progress rapidly (53).

Tumor Radiation Dose

Estimation of the radiation dose to metastatic sites in the IP cavity is fundamental to establish dose–response relationships for the efficacy and toxicity associated with this approach to radionuclide therapy. A number of methods have been used to determine the radiation dose delivered to tumor deposits and normal tissues via IP radionuclide therapy. For macroscopic tumor volumes visualized in serial Anger camera images acquired after IP administration of a radionuclide conjugate, such as a radiolabeled antibody, residence times can be calculated and used to provide estimates of radiation absorbed dose for the "self-dose" (tumor-to-tumor) contribution. If tumors are visualized with a radionuclide conjugate, the "self-dose" from nonpenetrating radiation emitted by a radionuclide typically represents more than 90% of the total dose. On the other hand, estimation of absorbed dose to microscopic tumor sites in the IP cavity is complex. In the absence of selective uptake of an antibody or other radionuclide conjugate in micrometastatic populations of tumor cells, the dose from nonpenetrating radiation to the IP fluid can serve as a first approximation for absorbed dose. Tumor deposits attached to the surface of the IP cavity can be estimated to receive 50% of the nonpenetrating dose to IP fluid, in the same way that dose to the bladder wall from radioactivity in the urine can be estimated. If selective localization of radionuclide conjugates occurs in these micrometastases, the absorbed doses can be considered to be equivalent to the ratio of the radi-

olabeled agent in these sites to the concentration of radioactivity in the IP fluid. Roeske et al. (61) analyzed dose distributions for surface implants with various configurations, such as those that protrude into the cavity or those with a flat portion at the lining of the peritoneal cavity and most of the volume extending below the surface.

Because most radiopharmaceuticals instilled in the IP cavity inevitably leak to the plasma and are subsequently distributed to various organs and tissues in the body (Fig. 34.2), special methods must be developed to determine what fraction of radioactivity is localized in a tumor/organ from the plasma and what fraction represents uptake from IP fluid. Because of the transit from the IP cavity to the blood pool, the model and S values described by Watson et al. (62,63) for estimating absorbed doses from radioactivity in the IP cavity cannot be directly used to estimate absorbed doses for IP therapy with most radionuclide conjugates.

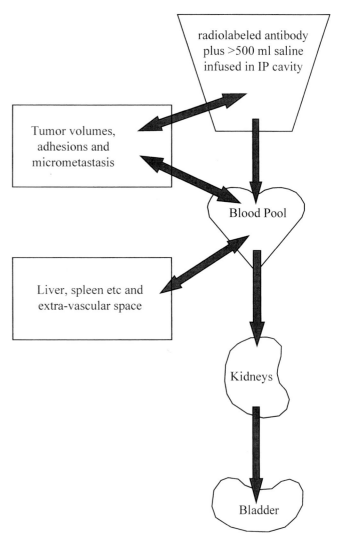

FIGURE 34.2. Schematic illustrating transfer of radiolabeled antibody from IP cavity to tumor and remainder of body.

Breitz et al. (49) used at least two methods for dosimetry calculations to compare dose estimates in the same patients and found good correlation between the two dose estimates. The set of assumptions used in their calculations, such as assigning activity to bowel as source organs, differ from those used in studies of Meredith et al. (51), but the resulting dose estimates are relatively similar. Alternative methods of providing dose estimates include thermoluminescent dosimeter (TLD) measurements.

Estimates of radiation dose to the peritoneal surface from TLD measurements have often been in the range of those calculated from external imaging and from biopsy data and quantification of serial peritoneal fluid samples. However, the Hammersmith group reported that their dose estimates from TLD measurements after IP administration of radiolabeled antibodies are modest, especially in comparison with observed antitumor efficacy (44). As an explanation for the discrepancy, they postulate that immune mechanisms in addition to radiation contribute to tumor cell eradication. Because their doses have been reported as a nonspecific dose to the peritoneal surface, tumor cells with localization of the radiolabeled antibody would have higher doses of radiation. These higher doses are expected to be in the therapeutic range for small-volume deposits and have been calculated by imaging-based dosimetry and biopsy data from others. The radiation dose delivered by IP therapy has usually been an order of magnitude higher than that delivered to most solid tumors with IV administration, as is illustrated Table 34.1 (20,48,50,51).

Radionuclide Selection

Only a few radionuclides have been tested clinically as conjugates with antibodies. A number of alternative radionuclides look attractive theoretically. Some have been tested in a preclincial setting but have not yet been applied clinically. Selection of an optimal radionuclide for IP radioimmunotherapy in ovarian cancer is important and depends on defining the target population of tumor cells and other factors, including characteristics of the conjugate (64–66). Factors that will affect this choice are tumor morphology, nonhomogeneous localization of the radiolabeled antibody, type and energy of radiation emitted, and the rate and fraction of radioactivity that leaks to plasma. Degradation of the radiopharmaceutical in the IP space and in plasma can result in products that can localize in specific organs/sites in the body. If the target cancer cells are micrometastases in the IP fluid, emitters of alpha particles may be preferred because the use of high-energy beta emitters can result in significant wastage from the deposition of most emitted energy outside target tumor cells (61,67). Because available alpha emitters have a very short half-life, they must be linked to small agents, such as peptides or single-chain antibody fragments (sFv), that rapidly localize to target receptors. [125]I would be appropriate for use with conjugated

agents that are internalized and transported to the nuclear DNA (68). For macroscopic tumor volumes, high-energy beta-emitting radionuclides are more appropriate because the longer range of particles can compensate to some extent for inhomogeneous localization of the antibody molecules among tumor cell populations. The importance of matching the physical decay half-life of the radionuclide with the biologic half-life of the radioimmunoconjugate has been reviewed (64,69).

With ^{177}Lu-CC49 *in vivo* pharmacokinetics data as a basis, we examined the feasibility of selecting the optimal radionuclide with a shorter physical half-life (70). Most of the red marrow dose from IP radioimmunotherapy is delivered from nonpenetrating radiation emitted from radioactivity in blood or skeletal tissues, especially for the small fraction of low-energy photon emitters such as ^{177}Lu and [166]Ho. Preliminary results from administration of ^{177}Lu-CC49 in patients with ovarian cancer have confirmed that 50% of infused radioactivity in the IP cavity typically leaks from the IP space within 7 days. This is similar to observations of others using intact murine antibody radionuclide conjugates. The leakage from the IP space to plasma increases to reach a peak of about 25% of the injected dose at 48 hours following infusion, after which a monoexponential clearance with a biologic half-time of 72 hours occurs. The whole-body retention of ^{177}Lu-CC49 was found to have a biological half-life of 280 hours. Six radionuclides that are potential candidates for IP radioimmunotherapy are ^{177}Lu, ^{131}I, ^{90}Y, [186]Re, [188]Re, and [166]Ho. Relevant decay characteristics of these radionuclides are summarized in Table 34.2. Red marrow dose estimates for each radionuclide are based on the model depicted in Fig. 34.2. After infusion in more than 500 mL of saline solution into the IP cavity, the radiopharmaceutical is assumed to be distributed throughout the IP space and bathe all tumor cells in the fluid, in addition to deposits that adhere to the wall of the IP cavity. Serial gamma camera images of patients with ovarian cancer at various times after infusion indicate the gradual movement of ^{177}Lu-CC49 from the IP space to the remainder of the body. Determining the fraction of radioactivity that localizes in organs such as the liver and spleen from plasma alone is complex. The input data for this comparison were serial plasma and whole-body retention data obtained after infusion of ^{177}Lu-CC49 in 26 patients with ovarian cancer at the University of Alabama at Birmingham (51,70). The red marrow dose for CC49 labeled with each radionuclide was calculated from two sources of radioactivity in the body: (a) red marrow and (b) remainder of the whole body. No specific uptake of the radiopharmaceutical or degradation products in the bone marrow or skeletal tissues was assumed for this model. The residence time for bone marrow was calculated with the assumption that the concentration of radionuclide in the red marrow was 0.19 that in the plasma. This radionuclide selection model confirmed the advantages of using shorter-

TABLE 34.2. CHARACTERISTICS OF SIX RADIONUCLIDES AND PREDICTED RED MARROW DOSE FROM INTRAPERITONEAL RADIOIMMUNOTHERAPY FOR CC49 LABELED WITH EACH RADIONUCLIDE

| Radionuclide | Physical $t_{1/2}$ (h) | Mean beta (keV) | Residence time (h) | | Marrow dose (cGy/mCi) | Fraction of RM dose (%) | |
			RM	WB		RM	RB
[131]I	193.0	191	6.10	164.5	3.55	69.8	30.2
[177]Lu	161.0	149	5.42	147.2	1.90	85.9	14.1
[186]Re	90.6	361	3.62	98.6	2.87	88.0	12.0
[90]Y	64.0	935	2.74	75.0	5.86	88.8	11.2
[166]Ho	26.8	711	1.12	35.2	1.83	86.7	13.3
[188]Re	16.9	728	0.62	23.1	1.17	84.0	16.0

RM, red marrow; WB, whole body; RB, remainder of body.

lived radionuclides for IP radioimmunotherapy with the CC49 antibody. Table 34.2 also lists the residence times for red marrow and whole body, the number of centigrays/millicuries predicted for each radionuclide attached to CC49, and the fraction of the total red marrow dose contributed by plasma and the remainder of the body. Results from the simple model used indicate that [188]Re delivers the lowest red marrow dose for IP radioimmunotherapy, followed by [166]Ho, ^{177}Lu, ^{131}I, [186]Re, and [90]Y. In addition, the absorbed dose to micrometastases and tumor deposits in the IP cavity is increased by a factor of 3 for short-lived radionuclides, such as [188]Re and [166]Ho, in comparison with [177]Lu. The preference for shorter-lived radionuclides in IP radioimmunotherapy is in contrast to the advantages claimed for longer-lived radionuclides in IV radioimmunotherapy (71). Further refinement of the present model requires that the contribution to the red marrow dose resulting from specific uptake of the radionuclide in the skeletal tissues be determined from Anger camera images because this dose contribution has been identified to have the strongest correlation with bone marrow toxicity.

STRATEGIES TO IMPROVE INTRAPERITONEAL RADIOIMMUNOTHERAPY

Some of the strategies projected to improve tumor-to-normal tissue ratios or other aspects of radionuclide conjugate therapy apply to the IP route and have been tested clinically, whereas others are still being investigated preclinically (72). Table 34.3 summarizes some of these enhancements and the rationale for their investigation.

First, several alterations of the conjugate resulting from the use of intact murine antibodies are being evaluated. A few trials have studied F(ab')$_2$ fragments, sometimes in comparison with the related intact IgG antibody (27,73). These have the potential to improve IP therapy because the fragments, as a smaller radionuclide conjugate, may clear more quickly, so that toxicity is decreased. In addition to the preparation of fragments by selective enzyme cleavage, advances in molecular biology have allowed a variety of antibody constructs to be produced, some very shortened, that have the potential advantages of improved penetration

TABLE 34.3. SUMMARY OF STRATEGIES TO IMPROVE RADIONUCLIDE CONJUGATE THERAPY

Enhancement method	Rationale
Antibody fragments or other small constructs	Better tumor penetration plus faster blood clearance
Antibody mixtures	Improve targeting of heterogeneous antigen distribution
EDTA	Increase urine excretion of unbound radionuclide
Pretargeting	Decrease radiation to normal tissues
Interferon	Increase tumor antigen expression
Growth factors/cytokines	IL-2 enhances tumor uptake
	IL-1 radioprotective of marrow
Taxol/other chemotherapy	Radiosensitizer plus cytotoxic
Hyperthermia	Enhance radiation cytotoxicity
External beam high-dose-rate radiation	Cell cycle effects enhance cytotoxicity
Gene transfer amplification of target	Increase localization and dose to target

EDTA, ethylenediamine tetraacetic acid; IL = 2, interleukin 2.

into tumor nodules and more rapid clearance from the blood (74,75). Antibody products have also included alterations for higher affinity, humanization (76), and bispecific binding sites. Humanization of antibody products may allow individualized treatment planning. Because the induction of HAMA is so prevalent when IP therapy is based on murine radiolabeled antibodies, tracer studies have been precluded. Thus, increasing doses of radioactivity, like chemotherapy agents, have been administered until moderately severe toxicity is noted in the majority of patients. It has been difficult to correlate toxicity with increasing amounts of radioactivity because the pharmacokinetics of IP radioimmunotherapy are patient-specific. The introduction of humanized antibodies that can be administered more than once will offer the opportunity to plan treatment for each patient. With judicious treatment planning, the amount of radioactivity administered can be optimized for each patient, consistent with delivering a prescribed dose to target tumor deposits. This approach is more likely to establish fundamental dose–response data, which are currently lacking for IP radioimmunotherapy, than is the collection of data from therapeutic administration at fixed doses. Non-antibody agents, such as peptides, microspheres, or other conjugates to radionuclides, may offer special advantages over antibodies in some instances (77,78).

Second, mixtures of antibodies have been used to improve concentration on tumor cells and target more cancer cells, as antigen expression has been noted to be quite heterogeneous (79). The Hammersmith group treated a patient whose tumor showed reactivity to both AUA1 and HMFG1 with IP ^{131}I-AUA1. After treatment, the rate of reaccumulation of ascitic fluid decreased. However, cytology of recurrent ascitic fluid showed reactivity to HMFG1 but no longer to AUA1. The patient was subsequently treated with HMFG1 and had no further accumulation of ascitic fluid (41). Mixtures of antibody constructs with different radionuclides may also prove advantageous.

Third, EDTA has been used to increase urinary excretion and decrease bone localization of ^{90}Y in an effort to decrease marrow toxicity. This strategy has been important with DTPA as the chelator for ^{90}Y conjugates, as this conjugate has been less stable than macrocycle chelators. The EDTA binds free ^{90}Y to facilitate its excretion via the urine (45,55,56). New, more stable chelators may eliminate the need for EDTA.

Fourth, pretargeting strategies have been studied to decrease the time that normal tissue is exposed to radiation (80,81). Some of these strategies take advantage of the high affinity of streptavidin for biotin and the small molecular weight of biotin, which allows for rapid clearance of unbound agent.

Fifth, interferon has been added to enhance tumor antigen expression. Multiple studies have shown that interferon increases the expression of a variety of tumor-associated antigens and that radioimmunotherapy localization can be improved with adjuvant interferon (82,83).

Sixth, in addition to interferon, other biologic response modifiers or growth factors may promote radioprotective mechanisms or recovery of normal tissues from radiation damage (84,85).

Seventh, radiosensitizers of tumor and radioprotectors of normal tissue have been tested, in addition to the effects of hyperthermia and external high-dose rate radiation (86–89). Some commonly used cytotoxic chemotherapeutic agents enhance the effects of radiation and have been given as a bolus or continuous infusion in conjunction with the administration of radiolabeled antibodies (52,90,91). Several studies have shown an interaction with radioimmunotherapy and external beam radiation in preclinical studies. This effect has been applied in early clinical trials of radioimmunotherapy as part of multimodality therapy (92) but has not yet been applied in IP radionuclide therapy.

Eighth, gene therapy integration techniques that amplify tumor targeting are promising (93). All these approaches and others appear to have some beneficial effect in radiolabeled antibody therapy, at least in animal model studies. The combination of these mechanisms can be expected to improve tumor-to-normal tissue dose ratios and efficacy further.

ACKNOWLEDGMENTS

The authors wish to thank Sally Lagan, Sherre Frazier, and Gayle Elliott for their assistance.

REFERENCES

1. Spencer RP. Radionuclide therapy in the peritoneum, pleura, synovium, and hematopoietic system. In: Henkin RE, Boles MA, Dillehay GL, et al., eds. *Nuclear medicine.* St. Louis: Mosby–Year Book, 1996:1568–1582.
2. Vergote IB, Vergote-De Vos LN, Abeler VM, et al. Randomized trial comparing cisplatin with radioactive phosphorus or whole-abdomen irradiation as adjuvant treatment of ovarian cancer. *Cancer* 1992;69:741–749.
3. Rosenshein NB, Leichner PK, Vogelsang G. Radiocolloids in the treatment of ovarian cancer. *Obstet Gynecol Surv* 1979;34:708–720.
4. Leichner PK, Klein JL, Garrison JB, et al. Dosimetry of ^{131}I-labeled anti-ferritin in hepatoma: a model for radioimmunoglobulin dosimetry. *Int J Radiat Oncol Biol Phys* 1981;7:323–333.
5. Soper JT, Wilkinson RH Jr, Bandy LC, et al. Intraperitoneal chromic phosphate P 32 as salvage therapy for persistent carcinoma of the ovary after surgical restaging. *Am J Obstet Gynecol* 1987;156:1153–1158.
6. Young RC, Walton LA, Ellenberg SS, et al. Adjuvant therapy in stage I and stage II epithelial ovarian cancer. Results of two prospective randomized trials. *N Engl J Med* 1990;322:1021–1027.
7. Bolis G, Colombo N, Pecorelli S, et al. Adjuvant treatment for early epithelial ovarian cancer: results of two randomized clinical

trials comparing cisplatin to no further treatment or chromic phosphate (^{32}P). G.I.C.O.G.: Gruppo Interregionale Collaborativo in Ginecologia Oncologica. *Ann Oncol* 1995;6:887–893.

8. Walton LA, Yadusky A, Rubinstein L. Intraperitoneal radioactive phosphate in early ovarian carcinoma: an analysis of complications. *Int J Radiat Oncol Biol Phys* 1991;20:939–944.

9. Soper JT, Creasman WT, Clarke-Pearson DL, et al. Intraperitoneal chromic phosphate P 32 suspension therapy of malignant peritoneal cytology in endometrial carcinoma. *Am J Obstet Gynecol* 1985;153:191–196.

10. Klaassen D, Starreveld A, Shelly W, et al. External beam pelvic radiotherapy plus intraperitoneal radioactive chronic phosphate in early stage ovarian cancer: a toxic combination. A National Cancer Institute of Canada Clinical Trials Group report. *Int J Radiat Oncol Biol Phys* 1985;11:1801–1804.

11. Spanos WJ, Day T, Abner, et al. Complications in the use of intra-abdominal ^{32}P for ovarian carcinoma. *Gynecol Oncol* 1992; 45:243–247.

12. Piver MS, Barlow JJ, Lele SB, et al. Intraperitoneal chromic phosphate in peritoneoscopically confirmed stage I ovarian adenocarcinoma. *Am J Obstet Gynecol* 1982;144:836–840.

13. Proctor J, Doering D, Barnhill D, et al. Bowel perforation associated with intraperitoneal chromic phosphate instillation. *Gynecol Oncol* 1990;36:125–127.

14. Alvarez RD, Partridge EE, Khazaeli MB, et al. Intraperitoneal radioimmunotherapy of ovarian cancer with ^{177}Lu-CC49: a phase I/II study. *Gynecol Oncol* 1997;65:94–101.

15. Varia M, Currie J, Benda J. Evaluation of intraperitoneal chromic phosphate suspension therapy following negative second-look laparotomy for epithelial ovarian carcinomas (stage III). Phase III, GOG No. 93; activated June 1, 1987; closed October 1996.

16. Lanciano R, Reddy S, Corn B, et al. Update on the role of radiotherapy in ovarian cancer. *Semin Oncol* 1998;25:361–371.

17. Pattillo RA, Collier D, Abedl-Dayem H, et al. Phosphorus-32-chromic phosphate for ovarian cancer: I. Fractionated low-dose intraperitoneal treatments in conjunction with platinum analog chemotherapy. *J Nucl Med* 1995;36:29–36.

18. Bookman MA, Bast RC Jr. The immunobiology and immunotherapy of ovarian cancer. *Semin Oncol* 1991;18:270–291.

19. Maraveyas A, Epenetos AA. Radioimmunotherapy of ovarian cancer. In: Goldenberg D, ed. *Cancer therapy with radiolabeled antibodies.* Boca Raton, FL: CRC Press, 1995:155–172.

20. Larson S, Carrasquillo J, Colcher D, et al. Estimates of radiation absorbed dose for intraperitoneally administered iodine-131 radiolabeled B72.3 monoclonal antibody in patients with peritoneal carcinomatoses. *J Nucl Med* 1991;32:1661–1667.

21. Ward B, Mather S, Hawkins L, et al. Localization of radioiodine conjugated to the monoclonal antibody HMFG2 in human ovarian carcinoma: assessment of intravenous and intraperitoneal routes of administration. *Cancer Res* 1987;47:4719–4723.

22. Chatal J, Saccavini J, Gestin J, et al. Biodistribution of indium-111-labeled OC 125 monoclonal antibody intraperitoneally injected into patients operated on for ovarian carcinomas. *Cancer Res* 1989;49:3087–3094.

23. Colcher D, Esteban J, Carrasquillo J. Complementation of intracavitary and intravenous administration of a monoclonal antibody B72.3 in patients with carcinoma. *Cancer Res* 1987;47: 4218–4224.

24. Horan-Hand P, Shrivastav S, Colcher D, et al. Pharmacokinetics of radiolabeled monoclonal antibodies following intraperitoneal and intravenous administration in rodents, monkeys and humans. *Antibody Immunoconj Radiopharm* 1989;2:241–255.

25. Haisma HJ, Moseley KR, Battaile A, et al. Distribution and pharmacokinetics of radiolabeled monoclonal antibody OC 125 after intravenous and intraperitoneal administration in gynecologic tumors. *Am J Obstet Gynecol* 1988;159:843–848.

26. Borchard PE, Quadri SM, Freedman RS, et al. Indium-111- and yttrium-90-labeled human monoclonal immunoglobulin M targeting of human ovarian cancer in mice. *J Nucl Med* 1998;39: 476–484.

27. Buist MR, Kenemas P, DenHollander W, et al. Kinetics and tissue distribution of the radiolabeled chimeric monoclonal antibody Mov 18 IgG and F(ab')$_2$ fragments in ovarian carcinoma patients. *Cancer Res* 1993;53:5413–5418.

28. Sivolapenko GB, Kalofonos HP, Stewart JSW, et al. Pharmacokinetics of radiolabeled murine monoclonal antibodies administered intravenously and intraperitoneally to patients with cancer for diagnosis and therapy. *J Pharm Med* 1992;2:155.

29. Molthoff CF, van Hof A, Buist M, et al. Comparison of the intravenous versus the intraperitoneal route of administration of chimeric monoclonal antibody Mov 18 for targeting ovarian cancer. *Cancer Biother Radiopharm* 1998;13:312.

30. Buijs WCAM, Tibben JG, Boerman OC, et al. Dosimetric analysis of chimeric monoclonal antibody cMov18 IgG in ovarian carcinoma patients after intraperitoneal and intravenous administration. *Eur J Nucl Med* 1998;25:1552–1561.

31. Muto MG, Finkler NJ, Kassis AI, et al. Intraperitoneal radioimmunotherapy of refractory ovarian carcinoma utilizing iodine-131-labeled monoclonal antibody OC125. *Gynecol Oncol* 1992; 45:265–272.

32. Finkler NJ, Muto MG, Kassis AI, et al. Intraperitoneal radiolabeled OC 125 in patients with advanced ovarian cancer. *Gynecol Oncol* 1989;34:339–344.

33. Jacobs AJ, Fer M, Su FM, et al. Phase I trial of a rhenium 186-labeled monoclonal antibody administered intraperitoneally in ovarian carcinoma: toxicity and clinical response. *Obstet Gynecol* 1993;82:586–593.

34. Hird V, Snook D, Kosmas C, et al. Intraperitoneal radioimmunotherapy with yttrium-90 labeled immunoconjugates. In: Epenetos A, ed. *Monoclonal antibodies: applications in clinical oncology.* London: Chapman & Hall, 1991:267–271.

35. Courtenay-Luck NS, Epenetos AA, Larche M, et al. Development of primary and secondary immune responses to mouse monoclonal antibodies used in the diagnosis and therapy of malignant neoplasm. *Cancer Res* 1986;46:6489–6493.

36. Dhingra K, Fritsche H, Murray JL, et al. Suppression of human anti-mouse antibody response to murine monoclonal antibody L6 by deoxyspergualin: phase I study. *Adv Exp Med Biol* 1994; 353:193–202.

37. Ledermann JA, Begent RHJ, Massof C, et al. A phase I study of repeated therapy with radiolabeled antibody to carcinoembryonic antigen using intermittent or continuous administration of cyclosporine A to suppress the immune response. *Int J Cancer* 1991;47:659–664.

38. Stewart JSW, Hird V, Snook D, et al. Intraperitoneal radioimmunotherapy for ovarian cancer: pharmacokinetics, toxicity, and efficacy of I-131 labeled monoclonal antibodies. *Int J Radiat Oncol Biol Phys* 1989 ;16:405–413.

39. Meredith RF, Partridge EE, Alvarez RD, et al. Intraperitoneal radioimmunotherapy of ovarian cancer with lutetium-177-CC49. *J Nucl Med* 1996;37:1491–1496.

40. Epenetos A, Munro M, Stewart S, et al. Antibody-guided irradiation of advanced ovarian cancer with intraperitoneally administered radiolabeled monoclonal antibodies. *J Clin Oncol* 1987;5: 1890–1899.

41. Epenetos AA, Hooker G, Kraus T, et al. Antibody-guided irradiation of malignant ascites in ovarian cancer: a new therapeutic method possessing specificity against cancer cells. *Obstet Gynecol* 1986;68[Suppl 3]:71s–74s.

42. Hird V, Maraveyas A, Snook D, et al. Adjuvant therapy of ovarian cancer with radioactive monoclonal antibody. *Br J Cancer* 1993;68:403–406.

43. Hird V, Stewart JS, Snook D, et al. Intraperitoneally administered ^{90}Y-labelled monoclonal antibodies as a third line of treatment in ovarian cancer. A phase 1-2 trial: problems encountered and possible solutions. *Br J Cancer* 1990;10[Suppl]:48–51.

44. Stewart JS, Hird V, Snook D, et al. Intraperitoneal yttrium-90-labeled monoclonal antibody in ovarian cancer. *J Clin Oncol* 1990;8:1941–1950.

45. Stewart JSW, Hird V, Snook D, et al. Intraperitoneal ^{131}I- and ^{90}Y-labeled monoclonal antibodies for ovarian cancer: pharmacokinetics and normal tissue dosimetry. *Int J Cancer* 1988;3[Suppl]:71–76.

46. Stewart JSW, Hird V, Sullivan M, et al. Intraperitoneal radioimmunotherapy for ovarian cancer. *Br J Obstet Gynaecol* 1989;96:529–536.

47. Buckman R, De Angelis C, Shaw P, et al. Intraperitoneal therapy of malignant ascites associated with carcinoma of ovary and breast using radioiodinated monoclonal antibody 2G3. *Gynecol Oncol* 1992;47:102–109.

48. Hnatowich DJ, Chinol M, Siebecker DA, et al. Patient biodistribution of intraperitoneally administered yttrium-90-labeled antibody. *J Nucl Med* 1988;29:1428–1434.

49. Breitz HB, Durham JS, Fisher DR, et al. Radiation-absorbed dose estimates to normal organs following intraperitoneal ^{186}Re-labeled monoclonal antibody: methods and results. *Cancer Res* 1995;55[Suppl]:5817s–5822s.

50. Breitz HB, Weiden PL, Vanderheyden JL, et al. Clinical experience with rhenium-186-labeled monoclonal antibodies for radioimmunotherapy. Results of phase I trials. *J Nucl Med* 1995;33:1099–1112.

51. Meredith RF, Macey DJ, Plott WE, et al. Radiation dose estimates from intraperitoneal radioimmunotherapy with ^{177}Lu-CC49. In: *Proceedings of the 6th International Radiopharmacology Dosimetry Symposium,* 1999; pp. 158–171.

52. Meredith R, Alvarez R, Khazaeli M, et al. Intraperitoneal radioimmunotherapy for refractory epithelial ovarian cancer with ^{177}Lu-CC49. *Minerva Biotech* 1998;10:100–107.

53. Mahe MA, Fumoleau P, Fabro M, et al. Phase II study of intraperitoneal (IP) radioimmunotherapy (RIT) with iodine-131 labeled monoclonal antibody OC 125 in residual disease of ovarian carcinoma. *Cancer Biother Radiopharm* 1998;13:327.

54. Heal A, Tyson I, Greenberg H, et al. Pharmacokinetics, dosimetry and clinical evaluation of 131-I-HMFG1 MoAb in the therapy of colorectal and ovarian carcinoma. *Antibody Immunoconj Radiopharm* 1992;5:1–12.

55. Rosenblum MG, Kavanagh JJ, Burke TW, et al. Clinical pharmacology, metabolism, and tissue distribution of ^{90}Y-labeled monoclonal antibody B72.3 after intraperitoneal administration. *J Natl Cancer Inst* 1991;83:1629–1636.

56. Kavanagh JJ, Rosenblum MG, Kudelka AP, et al. Pharmacokinetics, side effects, and tissue distribution of intraperitoneal B72.3-GYK-DTPA ^{90}Y with and without EDTA in ovarian cancer. *Cancer Invest* 1992;10[Suppl]:38–41.

57. Kosmas C, Maraveyas A, Gooden CS, et al. Anti-chelate antibodies after intraperitoneal yttrium-90-labeled monoclonal antibody immunoconjugates for ovarian cancer therapy. *J Nucl Med* 1995;36:746–753.

58. Crippa F, Bolis G, Seregni E, et al. Single-dose intraperitoneal radioimmunotherapy with the murine monoclonal antibody I-131 Mov18: clinical results in patients with minimal residual disease of ovarian cancer. *Eur J Cancer* 1995;31A:686–690.

59. Nicholson S, Gooden CS, Hird V, et al. Radioimmunotherapy after chemotherapy compared to chemotherapy alone in the treatment of advanced ovarian cancer: a matched analysis. *Oncol Rep* 1998;5:223–226.

60. Fein DA, Morgan LS, Marcus RB, et al. Stage III ovarian carcinoma: an analysis of treatment results and complications following hyperfractionated abdominopelvic irradiation for salvage. *Int J Radiat Oncol Biol Phys* 1994;29:169–176.

61. Roeske JC, Chen GTY, Atcher RW, et al. Modeling of dose to tumor and normal tissue from intraperitoneal radioimmunotherapy with alpha and beta emitters. *Int J Radiat Oncol Biol Phys* 1990;19:1539–1548.

62. Watson EE, Stabin MG, Siegel JA. MIRD formulation. *Med Phys* 1993;20:511–514.

63. Watson EE, Stabin MG, Davis JL, et al. A model of the peritoneal cavity for use in internal dosimetry. *J Nucl Med* 1989;30:2002–2011.

64. Yorke ED, Beaumier PL, Wessels BW, et al. Optimal antibody-radionuclide combinations for clinical radioimmunotherapy: a predictive model based on mouse pharmacokinetics. *Nucl Med Biol* 1991;18:827–835.

65. Wessels BW, Rogus RE. Radionuclide selection and model absorbed dose calculations for radiolabeled tumor-associated antibodies. *Med Phys* 1984;11:638–645.

66. Mausner LF, Srivastava SC. Selection of radionuclides for radioimmunotherapy. *Med Phys* 1993;20:503–509.

67. Larson RH, Hoff P, Vergote IB, et al. Alpha-particle radiotherapy with ^{211}At-labeled monodisperse polymer particles, ^{211}At-labeled IgG proteins, and free ^{211}At in a murine intraperitoneal tumor model. *Gynecol Oncol* 1995;57:9–15.

68. Bloomer WD, McLaughlin WH, Weichselbaum RR, et al. The role of subcellular localization in assessing the cytotoxicity of iodine-125-labeled iododeoxyuridine, iodotamoxifen, and iodoantipyrine. *J Radioanal Chem* 1981;65:209–221.

69. Larson SM. Choosing the right radionuclide and antibody for intraperitoneal radioimmunotherapy. *J Natl Cancer Inst* 1991;83:1602–1603.

70. Macey DJ, Meredith RF. A strategy to reduce red marrow dose for intra-peritoneal radioimmunotherapy. *Cancer Biother Radiopharm* 1998;13:327.

71. Howell RW, Goddu SM, Rao DV. Proliferation and the advantage of longer-lived radionuclides in radioimmunotherapy. *Med Phys* 1998;25:37–42.

72. Buist MR. *Imaging and radioimmunotargeting of ovarian cancer* [thesis]. Amsterdam, The Netherlands: Free University of Amsterdam, 1994.

73. Buchsbaum DJ. Experimental radioimmunotherapy and methods to increase therapeutic efficacy. In: Goldenberg DM, ed. *Cancer therapy with radiolabeled antibodies.* Boca Raton, FL: CRC Press, 1995:115–140.

74. Buchsbaum DJ, Khazaeli MB, Mayo MS, et al. Evaluation of CH2 deleted HuCC49 for intraperitoneal radioimmunotherapy. *Cancer Biother Radiopharm* 1998;13:59.

75. Deonarain MP, Rowlinson-Busza G, George AJ, et al. Redesigned anti-human placental alkaline phosphatase single-chain Fv: soluble expression, characterization and *in vivo* tumour targeting. *Protein Eng* 1997;10:89–98.

76. Dion AS. Humanizaion of monoclonal antibodies: molecular approaches and applications. In: Goldenberg D, ed. *Cancer therapy with radiolabeled antibodies.* Boca Raton, FL: CRC Press, 1995:255–270.

77. Leimer M, Kurtaran A, Smith-Jones P, et al. Response to treatment with yttrium 90-DOTA lanreotide of a patient with metastatic gastrinoma. *J Nucl Med* 1998;39:2090–2094.

78. Buchsbaum DJ. Experimental tumor targeting with radiolabeled ligands. *Cancer* 1997;80:2371–2377.

79. Meredith RF, Khazaeli MB, Plott WE, et al. Phase II study of interferon-enhanced dual ^{131}I-labeled monoclonal antibody therapy in patients with metastatic colorectal cancer. *Clin Cancer Res* 1996;2:1811–1818.

80. Paganelli G, Magnani P, Siccardi AG, et al. Clinical application of the avidin–biotin system for tumor targeting. In: Goldenberg

D, ed. *Cancer therapy with radiolabeled antibodies*. Boca Raton, FL: CRC Press, 1995:239–254.

81. Breitz H, Knox P, Weiden M, et al. Pretargeted radioimmunotherapy with antibody streptavidin and Y-90 DOTA-biotin (Avicidin): result of a dose escalation study. *J Nucl Med* 1998;39:71P.

82. Murray JL, Macey DJ, Grant EJ, et al. Enhanced TAG-72 expression and tumor uptake of radiolabeled monoclonal antibody CC49 in metastatic breast cancer patients following alpha-interferon treatment. *Cancer Res* 1995;55[Suppl]:5925s–5928s.

83. Slovin S, Sher H, Divgi C, et al. Interferon-gamma and monoclonal antibody ^{131}I-labeled CC49: outcomes in patients with androgen-independent prostate cancer. *Clin Cancer Res* 1998;6:643–651.

84. Blumenthal RD, Sharkey RM, Goldenberg DM. Dose escalation of radioantibody in a mouse mode using recombinant IL-1 and GM-CSF intervention to reduce myelosuppression. *J Natl Cancer Inst* 1992;84:399–407.

85. DeNardo GL, DeNardo SJ, Lamborn KR, et al. Enhancement of tumor uptake of monoclonal antibody in nude mice with PEG-IL-2. *Antibody Immunoconjug Radiopharm* 1991;4:859–870.

86. Buchsbaum DJ, Khazaeli MB, Davis MA, et al. Sensitization of radiolabeled monoclonal antibody therapy using bromodeoxyuridine. *Cancer* 1994;73(3):999–1005.

87. Badger CC, Rasey J, Nourigat C, et al. WR2721 protection of bone marrow in ^{131}I-labeled antibody therapy. *Radiat Res* 1991;128:320–324.

88. Shuster JM, Noska MA, Dewhirst MW, et al. Enhancing monoclonal antibody F(ab')$_2$ uptake in tumor using hyperthermia. *J Nucl Med* 1992;33:958–959.

89. Msirikale JS, Klein JL, Schroeder J, et al. Radiation enhancement of radiolabeled antibody deposition in tumors. *Int J Radiat Oncol Biol Phys* 1987;13:1839–1844.

90. DeNardo SJ, Kukis DL, Kroger LA, et al. Synergy of Taxol and radioimmunotherapy with yttrium-90-labeled chimeric L6 antibody: efficacy and toxicity in breast cancer xenografts. *Proc Natl Acad Sci U S A* 1997;84:4000–4004.

91. Remmenga SW, Colcher D, Gansow O, et al. Continuous infusion chemotherapy as a radiation-enhancing agent for yttrium-90-radiolabeled monoclonal antibody therapy of a human tumor xenograft. *Gynecol Oncol* 1994;55:115–122.

92. Stillwagon GB, Order SE, Klein JL, et al. Multi-modality treatment of primary nonresectable intrahepatic cholangiocarcinoma with ^{131}I anti-CEA—a Radiation Therapy Oncology Group study. *Int J Radiat Oncol Biol Phys* 1987;13:687–695.

93. Buchsbaum DJ, Raben D, Stackhouse MA, et al. Approaches to enhance cancer radiotherapy employing gene transfer methods. *Gene Ther* 1996;3:1042–1068.

35

ADRENAL SCINTIGRAPHY

MILTON D. GROSS
BRAHM SHAPIRO

Despite the impressive images afforded by high-resolution anatomic imaging with computed tomography (CT) and magnetic resonance imaging (MRI), the functional evaluation of the adrenals by scintigraphy continues to find clinical utility. It is not surprising that the combination of highly sensitive biochemical tests of function and localization by CT or MRI allows identification of adrenal disease but frequently results in uncertainty in diagnosis. Indeed, high-resolution imaging may identify variations of normal anatomy that may not be of pathologic significance. The combination of function and localization offered by scintigraphy with agents that exhibit specific affinity for the tissues of the cortex, medulla, or for metastases has demonstrable clinical value, efficacy, and cost effectiveness in the diagnosis and localization of adrenal disease.

AGENTS, MECHANISMS, AND METHODS OF ADRENAL SCINTIGRAPHY

Adrenal Cortex

Radiopharmaceuticals employed for adrenocortical scintigraphy that are cholesterol based are accumulated by a receptor-mediated process by low-density lipoprotein receptors located on adrenocortical cells (1–3) (Table 35.1). Low-density lipoprotein uptake by the inner adrenal cortex (glucocorticoid and androgen-producing cells) is regulated by the anterior pituitary secretion of adrenocorticotropin (ACTH) controlled by corticotropin-releasing hormone (CRH) secretion from the hypothalamus. Aldosterone secretion by cells of the zona glomerulosa (outer cortex) is controlled by angiotensin II, a product of a cascade originating from the metabolism of renin to angiotensin I and

ultimately to angiotensin II. Many drugs have major effects on adrenocortical function and radiocholesterol uptake (1–3). For example, dexamethasone suppression (DS) of ACTH has been used to differentiate outer from inner zone cortical uptake of radiocholesterol in the evaluation of hyperaldosteronism and adrenal hyperandrogenism. Alternatively, ACTH has been used to image the adrenal cortex "suppressed" by autonomous glucocorticoid secretion in patients with Cushing's adenoma (1–3).

Of the commercially available radiopharmaceuticals for adrenocortical imaging both iodine 131 (^{131}I)–6β-iodomethylnorcholesterol (NP-59) and selenium 75 (^{75}Se)–selenomethylnorcholesterol (SMC, marketed as Scintadren) have been used extensively in scintigraphic studies of the adrenal cortex and possess similar properties (3,4). Because of the long half-life, the ^{75}Se radiolabel of SMC allows late imaging at 14 days or more after injection, when background radioactivity is low. Both NP-59 and SMC enter the adrenocortical cholesterol-ester storage pool and are not further metabolized. Thus, uptake can be used as a measure of adrenocortical function related to steroid hormone output (2,5). Both tracers are excreted into the biliary system. This enterohepatic circulation may interfere with adrenocortical imaging. Laxatives are useful to decrease background radioactivity, especially in studies done on DS (Table 35.2) (1,2,6).

Other radiopharmaceuticals have been employed to image the adrenal cortex (Table 35.1). Low-density lipoprotein can be labeled with ^{123}I, ^{131}I, indium 111 (^{111}In), or technetium 99m (^{99m}Tc) to image the adrenal cortex (7) (Table 35.1). Radiolabeled enzyme inhibitors of steroid hormone biosynthesis have also been used to image the adrenal cortex. Inhibitors of steroid hormone synthesis, carbon 11 (^{11}C)–etiomidate and ^{11}C-metiomidate, have been used to image the adrenal cortex with positron emission tomography (PET) (8). Substrates of intermediary metabolism in the form of radiolabeled glucose, fluorine 18–fluorodeoxyglucose (^{18}F-FDG), can be used to image adrenal metastases from a variety of tumors, whereas ^{11}C-acetate has been used to image some adrenal adenomas (1,9) (Table

M. D. Gross: Division of Nuclear Medicine, Departments of Radiology Internal Medicine, University of Michigan Medical School; Nuclear Medicine Service, Department of Veterans Affairs Health System, Ann Arbor, Michigan 48105.

B. Shapiro: Department of Internal Medicine, University of Michigan Medical School; Department of Nuclear Medicine, Veterans Affairs Health System, Ann Arbor, Michigan 48105.

TABLE 35.1. AGENTS AND MECHANISMS OF UPTAKE AND METABOLISM OF RADIOPHARMACEUTICALS FOR ADRENAL CORTEX AND SYMPATHOMEDULLA IMAGING

Radiopharmaceutical	Uptake Mechanisms	Metabolism
Adrenal Cortex		
Radiolabeled cholesterol analogues, e.g., ^{131}I-19-iodocholesterol ^{131}I-6β-iodomethylnorcholesterol ^{75}Se-6β-selenomethylnorcholesterol ^{131}I-6-iodocholesterol ^{131}I, ^{123}I, ^{111}In-LDL	Binds to LDL in circulation Bound tracer binds to LDL receptor on adrenocortical cells Esterification of cholesterol analogues Storage of esterified tracer in cholesterol ester pool (no further metabolism to radiolabeled steroid hormone analogues)	No metabolism of cholesterol esters to radiolabeled adrenocortical hormone analogues
^{18}F-fluorodeoxyglucose (^{18}F-FDG) ^{11}C-acetate ^{11}C-etiomidate/^{11}C-metiomidate	Glucose analogue Acetyl coenzyme A uptake	Metabolized to 2-deoxyglucose only Marker of metabolism Adrenal steroid enzyme inhibitor
Sympathomedulla		
Radiolabeled somatostatin analogues, e.g., ^{111}In-pentetreotide, ^{123}I-tyr-octreotide	Binds to cell surface somatostatin receptors Possible intracellular translocation of tracer-receptor complex	Clearance of tracer from the circulation slowed by creation of proteolysis-resistant analogues Different analogues have different affinities to binding to various receptor subtypes
Radiolabeled arylguanidines and analogues, e.g., ^{131}I metaiodobenzylguanidine, ^{123}I metaiodobenzylguanidine, ^{11}C-hydroxyephedrine(^{11}C-HED) ^{11}C-epinephrine	Specific uptake by type 1 catecholamine reuptake mechanisms in cell membrane (tricyclic antidepressant sensitive) Transport from cytoplasm into the intracellular hormone storage granules (tetrabenazine sensitive) Storage within the intracellular granules	Tracer does not bind to postsynaptic alpha- or beta-adrenergic receptor Tracer resists metabolism by catecholamine degrading enzymes (eg., monoamine oxidase or catechol-o-methyl transferase)

LDL, low-density lipoprotein.

35.1). Table 35.2 compares the various adrenocortical imaging agents, their dosimetry, and methods of imaging.

Sympathomedulla

Metaiodobenzylguanidine (MIBG) labeled with radioiodine (^{131}I and ^{123}I) can be used to image pheochromocytomas and other sympathomedulla neoplasms (Table 35.1) (10). Like the neurotransmitter norepinephrine, MIBG shares the same mechanisms of presynaptic uptake into sympathomedulla tissues with deposition into neurosecretory granules. Uptake can be blocked with cocaine, tricyclic antidepressants, reserpine, sympathomimetics, and labetalol (Table 35.3) (11). Excellent uptake with rapid clearance has allowed MIBG also to be used for radionuclide therapy of some sympathomedulla neoplasms (e.g., neuroblastoma

and pheochromocytoma) (see later). Alternatively, epinephrine and analogues (e.g., hydroxyephedrine) have been labeled with ^{11}C and have been used to image neuroblastomas and pheochromocytomas (12).

Sympathomimetic tissues express somatostatin receptors (in addition to an extensive list of other endocrine and nonendocrine tissues) and thus can be imaged with radiolabeled analogues of somatostatin (13). ^{111}In–labeled diethylenetriamine pentaacetic acid (DTPA)-octreotide and ^{123}I–Tyr^3-octreotide have been used successfully to depict primary and metastatic symapthomedulla tumors (14) (Table 35.1). Like MIBG, analogues of octreotide have been labeled with α and β emitters for radionuclide therapy of somatostatin receptor–positive symapthomedulla neoplasms (15). Table 35.2 compares symapthomedulla imaging agents, their dosimetry, and methods of imaging.

TABLE 35.2. AGENTS, METHODS AND DOSIMETRY OF RADIOPHARMACEUTICALS FOR ADRENAL SCINTIGRAPHY

Radiopharmaceuticals	NP-59[a]	SMC[b]	^{131}I-MIBG[c]	^{123}I-MIBG[c]	^{111}Indium-pentetreotide
Thyroid blockade[c] (SSKI 1 drop or Lugol's 2 drops in beverage t.i.d.)	Start 2 d before injection and continue for 14 d	Not required	Start 2 d before injection and continue for 6 d	Start 2 d before injection and continue for 4 d	Not required
Adult dose (i.v.)	37 Mbq	9.25 Mbq	18.5–37 Mbq	370 Mbq	222 Mbq
Shelf-life	2 wk frozen	6–8 wk room temp.	From package insert	From package insert	—
% uptake/adrenal	0.007–0.26%	0.7–0.30%	0.01–0.22%	0.01–0.22%	—
Dosimetry (cGy/dose)			From package insert	From package insert	
Adrenal	28–88	6.1	0.3–0.7 8–5	8–28	1.51
Ovaries	8.0	1.9	0.1–0.2 4–7	0.35	0.98
Liver	2.4	3.5	1.4–2.9 5–0	0.32	2.43
Kidneys	2.2	—	0.1–0.3 6–2	—	10.83
Spleen	2.7	—	1.1–2.2 0–0	—	14.77
Urinary bladder	—	—	1.4–2.8 0–0	—	6.05
Thyroid	150[d]	0.43[d]	0.1–0.3 7[d]–3[d]	17.7[d]	1.49
Whole body	1.2	1.4	—	0.29	—
Effective dose equivalent	—	—	0.3–0.7 5–0	—	2.61
Beta emission	Yes	No	Yes	No	No
Laxative (e.g., bisacodyl 5–10 mg p.o. b.i.d.)	Begin 2 d before and continue during imaging	No	Begin after injection	Begin after injection	Begin after injection
Imaging interval after radiotracer administration (optional additional imaging times)	Non-DS: 1 or more of 5, 6, or 7 after injection DS: 1 or more early: (3), 4 and one or more late: 5, 6, or 7 d after injection	7 (14) d after injection (no large published experience with DS scans)	24, 48 (72) h after injection	2–6, 24 (48) h after injection	4–6, 24, (48) h after injection
Collimator	High-energy, parallel-hole	Medium-energy, parallel-hole	High-energy, parallel hole	Medium-energy, parallel-hole	Medium-energy, parallel-hole
Principal photopeak (abundance) window	364 keV (81%)	137 keV (61%), 265 keV (59%), 280 keV (25%) 20% window	364 keV	159 keV	172 keV (90%), 245 keV (94%) 20% windows
Imaging time/counts (per view)	20% window 20 min/100 K	20 min/200 K (±SPECT)	20% window 20 min/100 K	20% window 10 min (at 3 h); 20 min/1 M (±SPECT)	Head and neck: 10–15 min/300 K (at 4–24 h) & 15 min/200 K (at 48 h); 10 min/500 K (±SPECT)

[a]^{131}I-iodomethylnorcholesterol; [b]Se-selenomethylnorcholesterol; [c]Metaiodobenzylguanidine. DS, dexamethasone suppression; SPECT, single photon emission tomography. From Kloos RT, Khafali F, Gross MD, et al. Section 10. In: Maisey MN, Britton KE, Collier BD, eds. *Clinical nuclear medicine, third edition.* London: Chapman and Hall Medical, 1998; p. 359.

TABLE 35.3. DRUGS AFFECTING UPTAKE OF METAIODOBENZYLGUANIDINE

Drug	Mechanism
Tricyclic antidepressants	Uptake inhibitor
Cocaine	Uptake inhibitor
Reserpine	Granule depletion
	Uptake inhibitor
Sympathomimetics	Granule depletion
Phenothiazines	Uptake inhibitor
Butyrophenones	Uptake inhibitor
Thioxanthenes	Uptake inhibitor
Adrenergic inhibitors	Granule depletion
Labetalol	Uptake inhibitor
	Granule depletion
Calcium channel blockers	Unknown

ROLE OF ADRENAL SCINTIGRAPHY IN ADRENAL DIAGNOSIS AND PATIENT MANAGEMENT

Adrenocortical Neoplasms

Regardless of imaging modality, successful diagnostic evaluation of adrenal disease is based on a laboratory evaluation sufficient to confirm an endocrine syndrome or to exclude abnormal adrenal function and anatomy demonstrated by CT or MRI (nonhypersecretory adenoma or remote metastasis) with normal biochemical function in the presence of a malignant lesion located elsewhere (Table 35.4). Adrenocortical scintigraphy can be performed under baseline conditions or with concomitant DS or ACTH stimulation of the hypothalamic-pituitary-adrenal (HPA) axis as a means to enhance diagnostic yield or to answer specific questions concerning the functional (or nonfunctional status) of an *adrenal lesion* (Table 35.2) (1,2).

TABLE 35.4. ADRENAL NEOPLASMS

Cortex	Medulla
Adenoma	Pheochromocytoma[a]
Aldosteronoma	(benign and malignant)
Cushing's adenoma	Neuroblastoma
Androgen-secreting	Ganglioneuroma
Incidentally discovered[b]	Ganglioblastoma
(nonhypersecreting)	Paraganglioma
Hyperplasia[c]	
(symmetric/asymmetric)	
Adrenocortical carcinoma[d]	
Metastasis to adrenal	

[a]Familial (multiple endocrine neoplasia types IIA and IIB) bilateral, extraadrenal.
[b]Can include cyst, myelolipoma, etc.
[c]Nonadenomatous hyperfunction.
[d]Hypersecretory malignant disease.

Dexamethasone suppression of the HPA axis provides improved scintigraphic evaluation of hyperaldosteronism and adrenal hyperandrogenism (1,2). Suppression of NP-59 uptake by the glucocorticoid- and androgen-secreting portions of the adrenal cortex accentuates abnormal, outer cortical dysfunction on scintigraphy. The duration of DS before the administration of radiocholesterol affects the subsequent course of adrenal gland imaging (Table 35.2) (2). Stimulation of the HPA axis with ACTH has also been used to identify the presence or absence of adrenocortical function. The increase in adrenal gland accumulation of NP-59 after ACTH stimulation can be used to establish function in patients with autoimmune adrenal disease who are taking exogenous steroids or after adrenal cortex reimplantation as a means to avoid hypoadrenalism after bilateral adrenalectomy for multiple endocrine neoplasia type II (16). The normal adrenal cortex responds by increasing radiocholesterol uptake (approximately twofold) as compared with baseline studies (17).

Cushing's Syndrome

The functional nature of adrenocortical scintigraphy is illustrated in the imaging of the pathophysiology of *Cushing's syndrome* (18–20) (Table 35.5). Abnormal secretion of ACTH from a pituitary adenoma, hypothalamic dysfunction, or an ectopic source results in symmetric, bilaterally increased tracer accumulation by the adrenals (21). Some of the highest levels of NP-59 uptake have been seen in the

TABLE 35.5. SCINTIGRAPHIC IMAGING IN CUSHING'S SYNDROME (WITHOUT DEXAMETHASONE SUPPRESSION)

Scintigraphic Pattern	Type of Cushing's Syndrome
Bilateral symmetric imaging	ACTH dependent; hypothalamic; pituitary Cushing's disease; ectopic ACTH syndrome; ectopic CRF syndrome
Bilateral asymmetric imaging	ACTH-independent nodular hyperplasia[a] (However, all causes listed above may rarely cause asymmetric hyperplasia)
Unilateral imaging	Adrenal adenoma;[b] adrenal remnants;[c] ectopic adenocortical tissue[c]
Bilateral nonvisualization	Adrenal carcinoma;[b,d] severe hypercholesterolemia[e]

[a]This is almost always asymmetric.
[b]Cortisol secreting lesions suppress tracer uptake into the contralateral gland.
[c]Usually only one focus is present; occasionally, more than one focus may be present in ectopic locations or metastatic sites.
[d]Rarely, tumors (and metastases) may accumulate sufficient tracer to image.
[e]This is potential cause of interference with the effectiveness of study.
ACTH, adrenocorticotropin; CRF, corticotropin-releasing factor.

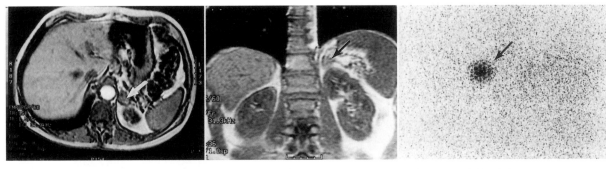

FIGURE 35.1. Transverse **(A)** and coronal **(B)** magnetic resonance imaging scans of the abdomen of a patient with adrenocorticotropin-independent Cushing's syndrome and a left adrenal mass *(arrow)*. A 6β-iodomethylnorcholesterol scan **(C)** of the posterior abdomen depicts the mass as a solitary, intense focus of radiotracer uptake *(arrow)*. The contralateral adrenal gland is not imaged because right adrenocortical function is suppressed by the hyperfunctioning left adrenal adenoma.

ectopic ACTH form of Cushing's syndrome (19). Adrenocortical scintigraphy can be used to localize the bilateral adrenal hyperplasia of ACTH-dependent Cushing's syndrome in which the adrenals are secondarily involved. Other imaging modalities such as ^{111}In-DTPA-pentetreotide scintigraphy or venous sampling of ACTH are used to locate the source(s) of abnormal ACTH secretion (1,22).

In Cushing's syndrome resulting from adrenocortical dysfunction (ACTH independent), adrenocortical scintigraphy has clinical utility and efficacy (18,21,23). In hyperfunctioning adrenal adenomas, one sees unilateral radiocholesterol accumulation by the adenoma and suppression of the normal, contralateral adrenal cortex and radiocholesterol uptake. Scintigraphy accurately depicts this pathophysiologic process (Fig. 35.1) (18,21,23). Adrenocortical carcinomas do not accumulate sufficient radiocholesterol for successful imaging. In those that do function, one sees suppression of the HPA axis. Bilateral nonvisualization in Cushing's syndrome (when other confounding factors such as hypercholesterolemia can be excluded) suggests the presence of hyperfunctioning adrenocortical carcinoma (18,21,23). Both CT and MRI accurately identify adenomas and carcinomas, but these methods are often not able to identify bilateral and often asymmetric, non–ACTH-dependent, cortical nodular hyperplasia in up to 40% of cases (1,2,18,21,23). Radiocholesterol scintigraphy accurately identifies cortical nodular hyperplasia (Fig. 35.2) (18). Recurrent Cushing's syndrome resulting from adrenal

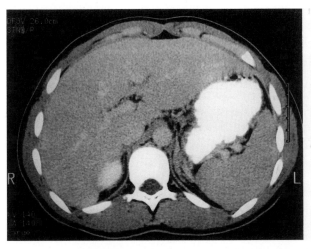

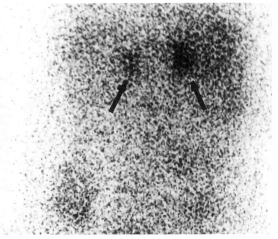

FIGURE 35.2. Abdominal computed tomography (CT) scan **(A)** and posterior 6β-iodomethylnorcholesterol (NP-59) scan **(B)** in a patient with adrenocorticotropin-independent Cushing's syndrome resulting from bilateral, cortical nodular hyperplasia. The CT scan depicts a normal left and enlarged right adrenal *(arrows)*, whereas the NP-59 scan identifies the asymmetric and bilateral nature of the pathologic process. (From Fig LM, Ehrman D, Gross MD, et al. The localization of abnormal adrenal function in ACTH-independent Cushing's syndrome. *Ann Intern Med* 1988;109:547–553, with permission.)

remnants after bilateral adrenalectomy can also be evaluated using radiocholesterol scintigraphy. It is the imaging modality of choice in this setting (3,21,23).

Primary Aldosteronism

High-background radiocholesterol uptake by the inner zones of the adrenal cortex (zona fasciculata-reticularis) obscures these usually small (less than 2 cm) anatomic lesions and makes pharmacologic suppression of ACTH an important consideration in the scintigraphic evaluation of patients with *primary aldosteronism* (Table 35.2) (1–3,23,24). Drugs that have an affect on the renin-angiotensin-aldosterone axis such as spironolactone, tri-

TABLE 35.6. SCINTIGRAHIC IMAGING IN ALDOSTERONISM (WITH DEXAMETHASONE SUPPRESSION)

Scintigraphic Pattern	Type of Aldosteronism
Symmetric bilateral early imaging (before day 5)	Bilateral autonomous hyperplasia; secondary aldosteronism[a]
Unilateral early imaging (before day 5)	Unilateral adenoma (Conn's tumor) unilateral malignant aldosterone secreting tumor (rare)
Symmetric late imaging (on or after day 5); nondiagnostic pattern	Normal adrenals; dexamethasone suppressible aldosteronism (rare)

[a]Should be excluded by measurement of renin and aldosterone levels and should not require imaging.

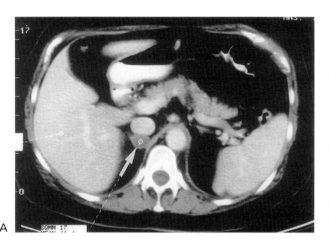

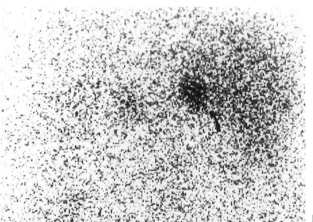

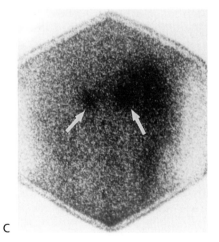

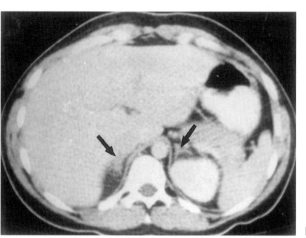

FIGURE 35.3. Abdominal computed tomography (CT) scan **(A)** and posterior abdominal 6β-iodomethylnorcholesterol (NP-59) scan done on dexamethasone suppression (DS) at 5 days after radiotracer injection **(B)** in a patient with primary aldosteronism from a right adrenal adenoma *(arrow)*. Faint contralateral, left adrenal NP-59 uptake is seen at 5 days or later after NP-59 injection on continuous DS. Posterior abdominal NP-59 scan **(C)** on DS at 4 days after injection and abdominal CT scan **(D)** in a patient with primary aldosteronism from bilateral adrenal hyperplasia. The CT scan demonstrates a slightly enlarged right and normal left adrenal, whereas bilateral and asymmetric NP-59 uptake on continuous DS characterizes this form of primary aldosteronism.

amterene, amiloride, and most diuretics must be withdrawn because many will alter imaging patterns in adrenocortical scintigraphy and may result in misdiagnosis (2,3,22).

Dexamethasone suppresses the HPA axis and the duration of administration before radiocholesterol injection affects the time interval after which the normal adrenal cortex will image (Table 35.6) (1–3,22). Unilateral and bilateral adrenal visualization occurring before the fifth day after NP-59 injection is the result of adenoma (aldosteronoma) and bilateral adrenal hyperplasia, respectively (1,2,22–25) (Fig. 35.3; Table 35.6). CT may not be localizing, but the presence of unilateral or bilateral hyperfunction is depicted by NP-59.

Comparison of the performance of CT, MRI, and adrenal scintigraphy demonstrates equal efficacy for CT and scintigraphy (80% to 95%) in the localization of adenoma in primary aldosteronism, whereas the absence of a morphologic abnormality on CT in a patient with primary aldosteronism infers the presence of bilateral hyperplasia (1–4,20,21,24,25). Scintigraphic studies continue to offer utility in patients with primary aldosteronism and normal or equivocal CT scans because radiocholesterol provides a specific diagnostic pattern for hyperplasia (22–25).

Adrenal Hyperandrogenism

Androgen-secreting adrenal adenomas and *bilateral adrenal hyperplasia* can be identified with DS adrenal scintigraphy in an approach identical to the evaluation of primary aldosteronism (1–3,6,21,23,26). Androgen-secreting adenomas are depicted as a unilateral focus of NP-59 accumulation on DS, whereas bilateral hyperplasia is depicted as bilateral foci of uptake (2,26). Ovarian and testicular tumors causing hyperandrogenism have been imaged with radiocholesterol. In addition, nontumorous ovarian dysfunction from polycystic ovaries and stromal hyperplasia have also been depicted with NP-59 (26).

Incidentally Discovered Adrenal Masses

Management of nonhypersecretory adrenal masses is controversial (27–29). Unsuspected adrenal masses are seen on CT scans performed for reasons other than suspected adrenal disease in approximately 5% of patients (22,27–33). The usual context in which this occurs is during an evaluation of abdominal pain or for staging known or suspected nonadrenal malignant tumors (22,27–33). Adrenal metastases are often seen with malignant disease located elsewhere, and it is not uncommon for some neoplasms (e.g., lung and breast) to present with isolated adrenal metastases. Obviously, the discovery of metastases

to the adrenals alters subsequent management. Size and morphology of masses have been used by many investigators to predict malignancy, but these characteristics often do not disclose the nature of an adrenal mass (29,30).

Most incidentally discovered adrenal masses *(incidentalomas)* are benign. In this context, the clinical problem is to identify malignant (either metastatic or primary adrenal carcinomas) or hyperfunctioning endocrine neoplasms from the benign, nonhypersecretory lesions (27,29,30). Tissue characterization by MRI (estimation of fat content) or CT (e.g., washout of intravenous contrast or x-ray attenuation measurements) has demonstrated some utility in distinguishing benign from malignant masses (9,30). Although malignant masses are on average larger than adenomas, overlap is too significant for size to be a reliable discriminator (29,30). Larger lesions are more likely to be malignant than smaller lesions, but even with adrenal masses greater than 5 cm in diameter, benign lesions are twice as common (29,34).

Some masses have highly characteristic appearances on CT (e.g., myelolipomas, cysts, and hemorrhage), and no further anatomic or functional evaluation is needed (22,30). Adenomas tend to have a lipid content that is higher than other masses, and as a result, attenuation coefficients are low, less than 0 Hounsfield units on non–contrast-enhanced CT. This is not, however, an invariable finding (22,29,30). Likewise, chemical shift MRI depends on lipid content and has also been shown to be of clinical value (22,29,30). Needle biopsy can provide tissue for direct histologic evaluation, but it is invasive and may not distinguish a well-differentiated malignant tumor from an adenoma (22,29,30).

Adrenal scintigraphy can be used to distinguish benign from malignant nonhypersecretory adrenal masses (Table 35.7) (32,33,35–42). The presence of radiocholesterol uptake in an adrenal mass that exceeds the normal contralateral adrenal (concordant pattern of imaging) is predictive of the benign nature of an adrenal lesion (29,32, 40) (Fig. 35.4). Alternatively, diminished or absent radiocholesterol uptake in an adrenal mass suggests a destructive or malignant lesion (discordant pattern of imaging) (29,32,40) (Fig. 35.4). Where there is no asymmetry of uptake and the lesion is larger than 2 cm in diameter, an adrenal pseudomass (e.g., stomach, kidney, or pancreas lesion) may be the cause of the anatomic abnormality (29, 32,40). Sensitivity of adrenal scintigraphy falls with decreasing lesion diameter, but specificity remains high (95%) even in masses less than 2 cm in diameter (42). Bilateral adrenal masses pose a more difficult diagnostic problem because no anatomically normal adrenal cortex is present to act as a reference for comparison. Radiocholesterol uptake in one or both adrenal masses, however, suggests a benign mass (33).

TABLE 35.7. SCINTIGRAPHIC IMAGING IN INCIDENTALLY DISCOVERED ADRENAL MASSES

Scintigraphic Pattern	Etiology
Symmetric	Normal adrenal (mass not in adrenal) adenoma <2 cm in diameter
Asymmetric (concordant)[a]	Nonhypersecretory benign adenoma
Asymmetric (discordant)[b]	Space-occupying lesions; adrenal cyst, myelolipoma, pheochromocytoma adrenal carcinoma, metastasis
Unilateral	Hyperfunctioning adrenal mass; Cushing adenoma (aldosteronism, rare), nonhypersecretory adenoma (see asymmetric concordant); space-occupying lesion (see asymmetric discordant)

[a]Concordant: uptake increased on side of adrenal mass localized by computed tomography or magnetic resonance imaging.
[b]Discordant: uptake decreased on side of mass localized by computed tomography or magnetic resonance imaging.

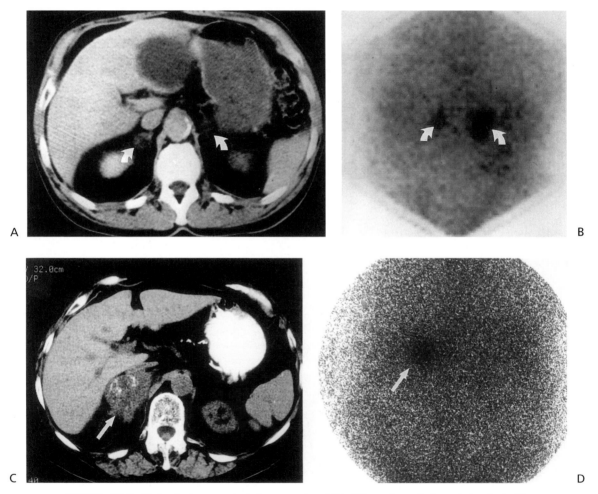

FIGURE 35.4. Abdominal computed tomography (CT) **(A)** and posterior abdominal 6β-iodomethylnorcholesterol (NP-59) **(B)** scans in a patient with an adenocarcinoma of the lung, normal adrenal function, and bilateral adrenal masses *(arrows)*. Biopsy of these lesions disclosed a right adrenal adenoma and metastasis of adenocarcinoma to the left adrenal. The asymmetry depicted on the NP-59 scan predicts the pathologic process in this patient with a concordant pattern of imaging on the right and a suspicious (discordant) adrenal lesion on the left. Abdominal CT **(C)** and posterior abdominal NP-59 **(D)** scans in a patient with a large right adrenal mass *(arrow)* with normal biochemical indices of adrenal function. The anatomically abnormal right adrenal seen on CT is not depicted on the NP-59 scan in which only left adrenal uptake of the radiotracer is seen. This is a discordant pattern of imaging suggestive of a malignant disease or a space-occupying adrenal lesion. (**A** and **B** from Gross MD, Shapiro B, Francis IR, et al. Incidentally discovered bilateral adrenal masses. *Eur J Nucl Med* 1995;22:315–321, with permission.)

Sympathomedulla Imaging

Given the wide distribution of the sympathetic nervous system and the renal and hepatic metabolism and excretion of MIBG, the salivary glands, spleen, liver, urinary bladder, heart, lungs, colon, and the cerebellum are often seen on MIBG imaging (13,43). The normal adrenal medulla is seen infrequently with ^{131}I-MIBG (16%) and more frequently (30% or more) with ^{123}I-MIBG (44). Many commonly available drugs affect MIBG uptake. The absence of salivary gland or cardiac uptake may be a clue to the presence of interfering drugs (11,45) (Table 35.3). *Sympathomedulla imaging* includes the adrenals, but one also must consider the presence of benign and malignant neoplasms that can present at sites from the base of the skull to the urinary bladder (45) (Table 35.4).

Sporadic, intraadrenal pheochromocytomas are identified as foci of MIBG uptake not explained by normal sites of uptake (45,46). Extraadrenal pheochromocytomas may present throughout the sympathetic nervous system and may be multiple (45,46) (Fig. 35.5). Concomitant scintigraphic imaging of other organs (e.g., kidneys, heart, bone) may aid in localization of the extraadrenal tumor (45,46). When available, single photon emission tomography with ^{123}I-MIBG has been most useful especially in the evaluation of patients with pericardiac pheochromocytomas (45,47, 48). The sensitivity and specificity of [131]I- and ^{123}I-MIBG of pheochromocytoma have been reported as 87% and 99%, respectively (45,47) (Table 35.8).

Familial pheochromocytoma, pheochromocytoma in neurofibromatosis, von Hippel–Lindau disease, and other syndromes have been successfully localized with MIBG (45,47). This includes bilateral uptake resulting from both pheochromocytoma and adrenomedullary hyperplasia in patients with multiple endocrine neoplasia types IIA and IIB (45,47). Radiolabeled MIBG has been particularly useful in the localization of malignant pheochromocytoma at remote sites (e.g., skull and femur) and of intraadrenal recurrences (Fig. 35.6) (49).

Metaiodobenzylguanidine has been used in the identification, staging, and assessment of the response to treatment of neuroblastoma (50,51). Diffuse uptake not only in the primary neoplasm, but also in metastases to the liver, bone, bone marrow (to include the axial skeleton and long bone metaphyses), and lymph nodes, can be depicted with MIBG (Fig. 35.7) (52). Correlation with bone scans is particularly useful in the evaluation of the patient with neuroblastoma (50–52). The sensitivity and specificity of MIBG for neuroblastoma are 92% and 99%, respectively (45,50,51) (Table 35.8).

Other neoplasms of the amine precursor uptake and decarboxylation system have been imaged with MIBG with variable success (45,53). Medullary carcinoma of the thyroid, carcinoid, and other tumors that manifest biogenic amine uptake and contain neuroendocrine storage granules have been imaged with MIBG. The sensitivity and specificity of MIBG for other neoplasms of this type have been less than seen for pheochromocytoma or neuroblastoma (45,53).

Indium 111–DTPA-octreotide can also be used to image a wide range of neuroendocrine (and other tumors) including pheochromocytoma and neuroblastoma with a sensitivity equal to that of MIBG (13,14,45) (Fig. 35.8; Table 35.8). In addition to tumors of adrenomedullary origin, many different neoplasms and inflammatory lesions express somatostatin receptors and image with ^{111}In-DTPA-octreotide and other radiolabeled analogues of somatostatin, with resulting reduced specificity (13,14). Normal distribution of the agent includes renal, hepatic, splenic, and intestinal uptake that can interfere with interpretation (13,14). Single photon emission tomography is an important adjunct in ^{111}In-pentetreotide imaging (45).

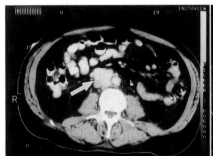 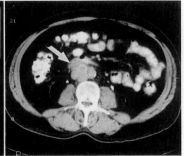 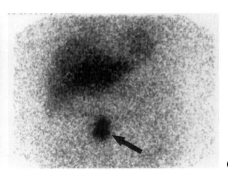

A,B   C

FIGURE 35.5. Sequential, transverse abdominal computed tomography **(A** and **B)** and posterior abdominal iodine 131–metaiodobenzylguanidine (^{131}I-MIBG) **(C)** scans in a patient with hypercatecholaminemia and a retroperitoneal mass *(arrows)*. The ^{131}I-MIBG scan depicts the mass *(arrow)* as an intense focus of radiotracer uptake in lower abdomen and is an example of an organ of Zuckerkandl pheochromocytoma.

TABLE 35.8. SENSITIVITY OF SYMPATHOMEDULLA SCINTIGRAPHY

Tumor	[131]Indium-Metaiodobenzylguanidine	[111]Indium-Pentetreotide
Pheochromocytoma	86%	88%
Neuroblastoma	91%	89%
Paragangliomas	52%	100%
Carcinoid[a]	70%	96%

[a]Group includes adrenocorticotropin-secreting neoplasms.
Modified from Krenning EP, Kwekkeboom DJ, Bakker WH, et al. Somatostatin receptor scintigraphy with (^{111}In-DTPA-D-Phe1) and (^{123}I-Tyr3)-octreotide: the Rotterdam experience with more than 1000 patients. *Eur J Nucl Med* 1993;20:716–731, with permission.

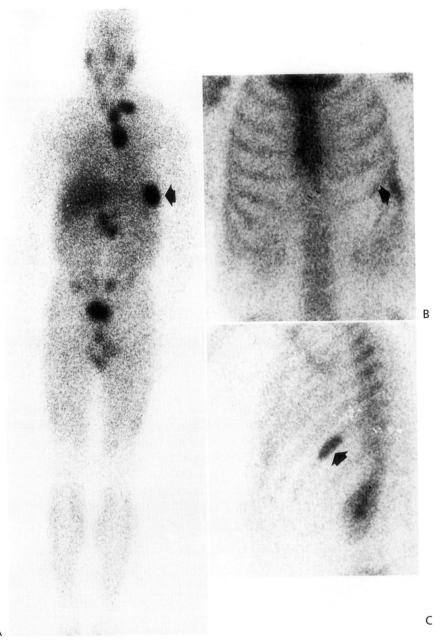

A

B

C

FIGURE 35.6. Anterior, whole-body 123–metaiodobenzylguanidine (^{123}I-MIBG) **(A)** and anterior **(B)** and left lateral **(C)** chest technetium 99m–methylenediphosphonate bone scans in a patient with a malignant pheochromocytoma. Multiple, metastatic tumor deposits are depicted in the chest and abdomen on the MIBG scan, whereas only a solitary rib metastasis *(arrow)* is seen on the bone scan.

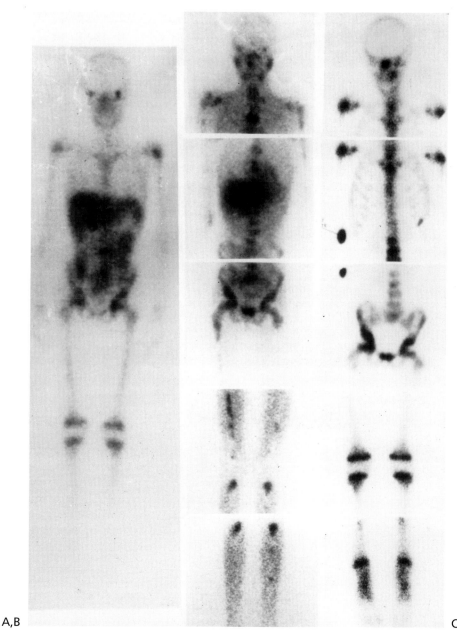

A,B   C

FIGURE 35.7. Gallium 67 **(A)**, 131–metaiodobenzylguanidine (^{131}I-MIBG) **(B)**, and technetium 99m–methylenediphosphonate bone **(C)** whole-body scans in a patient with widespread neuroblastoma. The MIBG scan depicts bone marrow involvement from neuroblastoma that is not depicted by gallium 67 and is poorly depicted on the bone scan as abnormal uptake in the spine.

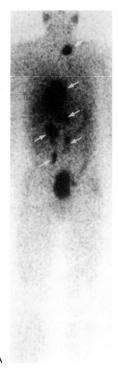

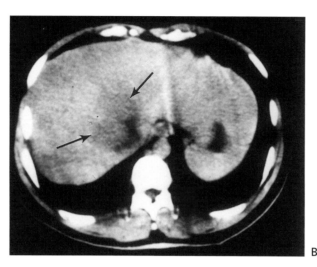

A

B

FIGURE 35.8. Anterior whole-body indium 111 (^{111}In)–pentetreotide **(A)** and transverse abdominal computed tomography **(B)** scans in a patient with metastatic pheochromocytoma. The liver metastases was the only metastatic deposit *(black arrows)* suspected before the ^{111}In-pentetreotide scan, which demonstrates widespread metastatic disease *(white arrows)*.

RADIONUCLIDE THERAPY OF SYMAPTHOMEDULLA NEOPLASMS

Avid uptake of radiolabeled MIBG and of radiolabeled somatostatin analogues in a variety of neoplasms of sympathomedulla origin has given impetus to the use of these agents in experimental radionuclide therapy. In the case of pheochromocytoma and neuroblastoma, ^{131}I-MIGB has been used a therapeutic agent with some success (45, 54–56) (Table 35.9). Analogues of somatostatin have been labeled with α- and β-emitting isotopes (e.g., high-dose ^{111}In or 90 yttrium) and have shown promise as potential agents for radionuclide therapy of neoplasms expressing somatostatin receptors (15).

FUTURE TRENDS

Positron emission tomography with ^{18}F-FDG can be used to identify malignant adrenal masses because ^{18}F-FDG uptake is markedly increased in many cancers (1,9). PET with ^{18}F-FDG has an increasing role in oncology for the noninvasive characterization of mass lesions and for tumor staging (9,57). Incidentally discovered adrenal masses characterized as benign, nonhypersecretory adrenal adenomas are not ^{18}F-FDG avid, whereas most adrenal metastases and primary cancers are (9) (Fig. 35.9). Some benign adrenal masses have shown avidity for ^{11}C-acetate (1). This type of differential PET imaging may be valuable in the future to distinguish benign from malignant adrenal masses. Furthermore, positron emitting inhibitors of glucocorticoid synthesis such as ^{11}C-etiomidate and ^{11}C-metiomidate have been used to image the adrenal cortex in animals with PET (8). Pheochromocytomas and neuroblastomas have been imaged using ^{11}C-hydroxyephedrine and ^{11}C-epinephrine (1,12) (Fig. 35.10). Rapid tumor uptake and high target-to-nontarget ratios allow early PET imaging after injection and may obviate the multiday imaging protocols using ^{131}I- and ^{123}I-MIBG and ^{111}In-DTPA-octreotide.

TABLE 35.9. RESULTS OF THERAPY WITH ^{131}IODINE-METAIODOBENZYLGUANIDINE

Response	Pheochromocytoma (127 patients)	Neuroblastoma (255 patients)
Complete	2%	5%
Partial	28%	23%
Stable	28%	28%
Progression	25%	31%
Not evaluable	17%	13%

Modified from Shapiro B, Fig LM, Gross MD, et al. Neuroendocrine tumors. In: Atkolun C, Tauxe WN, eds. *Nuclear Oncology.* New York: Springer-Verlag, 1999:1–31, with permission.

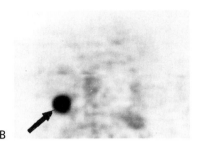

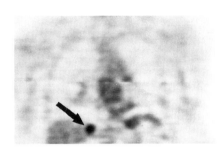

A,B

FIGURE 35.9. Coronal fluorine 18–fluorodeoxyglucose scans of the chest **(A)** and chest and upper abdomen **(B)** in a patient with a non–small cell lung cancer. Both the primary tumor and an adrenal metastasis *(arrows)* are depicted as foci of fluorine 18 uptake. (From Shapiro B, Gross MD. Nuclear medicine applications in endocrinology 1996. In: Brown ML, Collier BD, eds. *Syllabus: a categorical course in nuclear medicine.* Oakbrook, IL: Radiological Society of North America, 1996:127–144, with permission.)

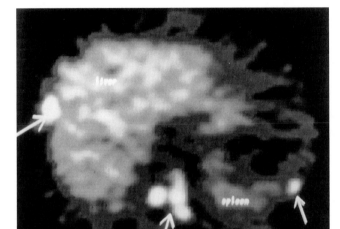

FIGURE 35.10. Carbon 11–hydroxyephedrine scan in a patient with malignant pheochromocytoma. Multiple areas of increased uptake *(arrows)* are seen in the coronal image of the upper abdomen that depict metastatic deposits in the liver and near the spleen.

REFERENCES

1. Gross MD, Shapiro B. Radionuclide imaging of the adrenal cortex. *Q J Nucl Med* 1999;43:1–9.
2. Gross MD, Valk TW, Swanson DP, et al. The role of pharmacologic manipulation in adrenal cortical scintigraphy. *Semin Nucl Med* 1981;9:128–148.
3. Shapiro B, Fig LM, Gross MD, et al. Radiochemical diagnosis of adrenal disease. *Crit Rev Clin Lab Sci* 1989;27:265–298.
4. Shapiro B, Britton KE, Hawkins LA, et al. Clinical experience with ⁷⁵Se-selenomethylcholesterol adrenal imaging. *Clin Endocrinol* 1981;15:19–27.
5. Lynn MD, Gross MD, Shapiro B. Enterohepatic circulation and distribution of I-131-6-iodomethyl-19-norcholesterol (NP-59). *Nucl Med Commun* 1986;7:625–630.
6. Shapiro B, Nakajo M, Gross MD, et al. Value of bowel preparation in adrenocortical scintigraphy with NP-59. *J Nucl Med* 1983;24:732–734.
7. Hay RV, Flemming RM, Ryan JW, et al. Nuclear imaging analysis of human low density lipoprotein biodistribution in rabbits and monkeys. *J Nucl Med* 1991;32:1239–1945.
8. Bergström M, Bonasma TA, Bergström E, et al. *In vitro* and *in vivo* primate evaluation of carbon-11-etomidate and carbon-11-metomidate as potential tracers for PET imaging of the adrenal cortex and its tumors. *J Nucl Med* 1998;39:982–987.
9. Boland G, Goldberg MA, Lee MJ, et al. Indeterminate adrenal mass in patients with cancer: evaluation at PET with 2-[F-18]-fluoro-2-deoxy-D-glucose. *Radiology* 1995;194:131–134.
10. Shapiro B, Gross M. Radiochemistry, biochemistry and kinetics of ¹³¹I-MIBG and ¹²³I-MIBG: clinical implications and the use of ¹²³I-MIBG. *Med Pediatr Oncol* 1987;15:170–177.
11. Khafagi F, Shapiro B, Fig L, et al. Labetolol reduces iodine-131-MIBG uptake by pheochromocytoma and normal tissues. *J Nucl Med* 1989;30:481–489.
12. Shulkin BL, Wieland DM, Baro ME, et al. PET hydroxyephedrine imaging of neuroblastoma. *J Nucl Med* 1996;37:16–21.
13. Lamberts SWJ, Krenning EP, Reubi J-C. The role of somatostatin and its analogs in the diagnosis and treatment of tumours. *Endocr Rev* 1991;12:450–482.
14. Krenning EP, Kwekkeboom DJ, Bakker WH, et al. Somatostatin receptor scintigraphy with [¹¹¹In-DTPA-D-Phe1]- and [¹²³I-Tyr3]-octreotide: the Rotterdam experience with more than 1000 patients. *Eur J Nucl Med* 1993;20:716–731.
15. Bernard BF, Krenning EP, Breeman WAP, et al. D-Lysine reduction of indium-111 octreotide and yttrium-90 octreotide renal uptake. *J Nucl Med* 1997;38:1929–1933.
16. Nakajo M, Sakata H, Shirona K, et al. Application of ACTH stimulation to adrenal imaging with radiocholesterol. *Clin Nucl Med* 1983;8:112–120.
17. Gross MD, Shapiro B, Freitas J. Scintigraphic endocrine mimicry. *Clin Nucl Med* 1990;15:457–464.
18. Fig L, Ehrman D, Gross MD, et al. The localization of abnormal adrenal function in ACTH-independent Cushing's syndrome. *Ann Intern Med* 1988;109:547–553.
19. Gross MD, Valk TW, Freitas J, et al. The relationship of adrenal iodomethylnorcholesterol (NP-59) uptake to indices of adrenal cortical function in Cushing's syndrome. *J Clin Endocrinol Metab* 1981;52:1062–1066.
20. Reschini E, Catania A. Clinical experience with the adrenal scanning agents iodine 131-19-iodocholesterol and selenium 75-Se-selenomethylcholesterol. *Eur J Nucl Med* 1991;18:817–823.
21. Gross MD, Shapiro B, Beierwaltes WH. The functional characterization of the adrenal gland by quantitative scintigraphy. *Recent Adv Nucl Med* 1983;6:83–115.
22. Francis IR, Korobkin M, Quint L, et al. Integrated imaging of adrenal disease. *Radiology* 1992;182:1–13.
23. Freitas JE. Adrenal cortical and medullary imaging. *Semin Nucl Med* 1995;25:235–250.
24. Gross MD, Shapiro B, Grekin RJ, et al. The scintigraphic localization of the adrenal glands in primary aldosteronism. *Am J Med* 1984;77:839–844.
25. Kazerooni EA, Sisson JC, Shapiro B, et al. Efficacy and pitfalls of ¹³¹I-6β-iodomethyl-19-norcholesterol (NP-59) imaging. *J Nucl Med* 1990;31:526–534.
26. Mountz JM, Gross MD, Shapiro B, et al. Scintigraphic localization of ovarian dysfunction. *J Nucl Med* 1988;29:1644–1650.
27. Gross MD, Shapiro B. Clinically silent adrenal masses: clinical review 50. *J Clin Endocrinol Metab* 1993;77:885–888.

28. Griffing GT. A-I-D-S: The new endocrine epidemic [Editorial]. *J Clin Endocrinol Metab* 1994;79:1532–1539.

29. Kloos RT, Gross MD, Francis IR, et al. Incidentally discovered adrenal masses. *Endocr Rev* 1995;16:460–484.

30. Dunnick NR, Korobkin M, Francis I. Adrenal radiology: distinguishing benign from malignant adrenal masses. *AJR Am J Roentgenol* 1996;167:861–867.

31. Gross MD, Shapiro B, Bouffard AJ, et al. Distinguishing benign from malignant euadrenal masses. *Ann Intern Med* 1988;109:613–618.

32. Gross MD, Wilton G, Shapiro B, et al. Functional and scintigraphic evaluation of the silent adrenal mass. *J Nucl Med* 1987;28:1401–1407.

33. Gross MD, Shapiro B, Francis IR, et al. Incidentally discovered bilateral adrenal masses. *Eur J Nucl Med* 1995;22:315–321.

34. Khafagi F, Gross MD, Shapiro B, et al. Clinical significance of the large adrenal mass. *Br J Surg* 1991;78:828–833.

35. Osella G, Terzolo M, Borretta G, et al. Endocrine evaluation of incidentally discovered adrenal masses (incidentalomas). *J Clin Endocrinol Metab* 1994;79:1532–1539.

36. Nakajo M, Nakabeppu Y, Yonekura R, et al. The role of adrenocortical scintigraphy in the evaluation of unilateral incidentally discovered adrenal and juxta-adrenal masses. *Ann Nucl Med* 1993;7:157–166.

37. Bardet S, Rohmer V, Murat A, et al. [131]I-6β-Iodomethylnorcholesterol scintigraphy: an assessment of its role in the investigation of adrenocortical incidentalomas. *Clin Endocrinol* 1996;44:587–596.

38. Dominguez-Gadea L, Diez L, Bas C, et al. Differential diagnosis of solid adrenal masses using adrenocortical scintigraphy. *Clin Radiol* 1994;49:796–799.

39. Dominguez-Gadea L, Diez L, Peidrola-Maroto G, et al. Scintigraphic diagnosis of subclinical Cushing's syndrome in patients with adrenal incidentalomas. *Nucl Med Commun* 1996;17:29–32.

40. Gross MD, Shapiro B, Francis IR, et al. Scintigraphic evaluation of clinically silent adrenal masses. *J Nucl Med* 1994;35:1145–1152.

41. Dwamena BA, Kloos RT, Fendrick AM, et al. Diagnostic evaluation of the adrenal Incidentaloma: decision and cost-effectiveness analysis. *J Nucl Med* 1998;39:707–712.

42. Kloos RT, Gross MD, Shapiro B, et al. The diagnostic dilemma of small incidentally discovered adrenal masses: a role for 131-I-6β-iodomethyl-norcholesterol (NP-59) scintigraphy. *World J Surg* 1997;21:36–40.

43. Nakajo M, Shapiro B, Copp J, et al. The normal and abnormal distribution of the adrenomedullary imaging agent m-[I-131]-iodobenzylguanidine (I-131-MIBG) in man: evaluation by scintigraphy. *J Nucl Med* 1983;24:672–682.

44. Lynn MD, Shapiro B, Sisson JC, et al. Portrayal of pheochromocytoma and normal human adrenal medulla by I-123-meta-iodobenzylguanidine: concise communication. *J Nucl Med* 1984;25:436–440.

45. Shapiro B, Fig LM, Gross MD, et al. Neuroendocrine tumors. In: Atkolun C, Tauxe WN, eds. *Nuclear oncology.* New York: Springer-Verlag, 1999:1–31.

46. Sisson JC, Frager MC, Valk TW, et al. Scintigraphic localization of pheochromocytoma. *N Engl J Med* 1981;305:12–17.

47. Shapiro B, Fig LM. Management of pheochromocytoma. *Endocrinol Metab Clin North Am* 1989;18:443–481.

48. Shapiro B, Sisson JC, Kalff V, et al. The location of middle mediastinal pheochromocytoma. *J Thorac Cardiovasc Surg* 1984;87:814–820.

49. Shapiro B, Sisson JC, Lloyd R, et al. Malignant pheochromocytoma: clinical, biochemical, and scintigraphic characterization. *Clin Endocrinol (Oxf)* 1984;20:189–203.

50. Troncone L, Ruffini V, Danza FM, et al. Radioiodinated metaiodobenzylguanidine (*I-MIBG) scintigraphy in neuroblastoma: a review of 60 cases. *J Nucl Med Allied Sci* 1990;34:279–288.

51. Shulkin BL, Shapiro B. Radioiodinated MIBG in the management of neuroblastoma. In: Pochedly C, ed. *Neuroblastoma tumor biology and therapy.* Boca Raton, FL: CRC Press, 1990:171–198.

52. Shulkin BL, Shapiro B, Hutchinson RJ. Iodine-131-metaiodobenzylguanidine and bone scintigraphy for the detection of neuroblastoma. *J Nucl Med* 1992;33:1735–1740.

53. Von Moll L, McEwan AJ, Shapior B, et al. Iodine-131 MIBG scintigraphy of neuroendocrine tumors other than pheochromocytoma and neuroblastoma. *J Nucl Med* 1987;28:979–988.

54. Shapiro B, Sisson JC, Wieland DM, et al. Radiopharmaceutical therapy of malignant pheochromocytoma with [131-I]metaiodobenzylguanidine: results from ten years of experience. *J Nucl Biol Med* 1991;35:269–276.

55. Hoefnagel CA, Voute PA, De Kraker J, et al. [131-I]- Metaiodobenzylguanidine therapy after conventional therapy for neuroblastoma. *J Nucl Biol Med* 1991;35:202–206.

56. Shapiro B. Summary, conclusions, and future directions of 131-I-metaiodobnzylguanidine therapy in the treatment of neural crest tumors. *J Nucl Biol Med* 1991;35:357–363.

57. Shapiro B, Gross MD. Nuclear medicine applications in endocrinology. In: *Radiological Society of North America categorical cause in diagnostic radiology: nuclear medicine.* Oakbrook, IL: Radiological Society of North America, 1996:127–144.

36

^{67}GA SCINTIGRAPHY

DOV FRONT[†]
ORA ISRAEL

Gallium 67 scintigraphy plays an important role in serially monitoring the effect of chemotherapy on Hodgkin's disease and non-Hodgkin's lymphoma (1). Although imaging with ^{18}F-fluorodeoxyglucose appears promising (2–4), ^{67}Ga scintigraphy is at the moment the best available procedure to distinguish a complete response from a partial response after induction treatment (5,6) and to detect recurrence of disease (7). Recently, it has been shown that ^{67}Ga scintigraphy can distinguish patients with an anticipated good outcome from those with an anticipated poor outcome at an early stage of treatment. Therefore, ^{67}Ga scintigraphy has the potential to indicate the need to change treatment at an early stage. The results indicate whether early or late treatment failure should be expected and whether other new, aggressive, or high-dose chemotherapy should be attempted early in the course of disease (8,9). Because of this unique ability of ^{67}Ga scintigraphy to monitor treatment response and because lymphoma is a treatable disease, ^{67}Ga scintigraphy is now a part of the routine management of patients with lymphoma (8,10,11).

High-dose combination chemotherapy has significantly improved the outcome of patients with Hodgkin's disease, and to a certain extent the outcome of those with non-Hodgkin's lymphoma. Failure-free survival has been prolonged and cure has been achieved in a high percentage of patients with Hodgkin's disease and in about half of patients with non-Hodgkin's lymphoma. Efforts are continually being made to improve the efficacy of treatment further. ^{67}Ga scintigraphy is playing an increasingly important role in the evaluation of patients in whom new treatment is attempted. ^{67}Ga is taken up only by viable lymphoma, not by areas of necrosis and fibrosis that may remain after treatment. This constitutes the basis of the ability of ^{67}Ga to monitor response to treatment (12). Because heterogeneity is a hallmark of cancer and the responses of individual patients differ greatly, even for those with tumors of the same histology, ^{67}Ga scintigraphy makes it possible to determine the individual tumor response to protocol combination chemotherapy and assess the results of treatment in a particular patient.

Scintigraphy with ^{67}Ga was used in the 1970s to diagnose and stage lymphoma before treatment (13–15). The need for it decreased significantly with the advent of computed tomography (CT), which is superior to ^{67}Ga scintigraphy for diagnosing a tumor mass and therefore for staging lymphoma. However, CT is less suitable as a technique to follow the effect of treatment, so that a role for ^{67}Ga in the evaluation of treatment was indicated (5,6,12). It took years for ^{67}Ga scintigraphy to be accepted as the standard for evaluation of the treatment response. The main obstacles to a general acceptance of ^{67}Ga scintigraphy were a general awareness of its earlier unsatisfactory performance as a diagnostic tool and the slowness of practitioners to acquire an understanding of the changing role of nuclear medicine—from a method of diagnosing cancer to a means of evaluating response to treatment (1) and predicting outcome early.

^{67}Ga was first evaluated as an indicator of treatment response in a tumor model in mice (12) and then in patients (5,6). Subsequently, a number of articles were published confirming this new use of ^{67}Ga—not to stage patients with lymphoma, as in the past, but rather to determine the effect of treatment (16–21). For both aggressive non-Hodgkin's lymphoma and Hodgkin's disease, a substantial literature supports the use of ^{67}Ga scintigraphy after treatment. The importance of ^{67}Ga scintigraphy as an indicator of tumor viability and its advantages over CT have now been well documented (5,6,12). The acceptance of the use of ^{67}Ga by oncologists and hematologists has contributed significantly to the demand for ^{67}Ga scintigraphy as a routine clinical test to determine whether treatment of lymphoma is effective.

The role of ^{67}Ga scintigraphy in monitoring response to treatment in lymphoma has been compared with those of other diagnostic imaging tests. Chest roentgenography and CT have not been found useful in evaluating response to treatment, even though these techniques play a major role in staging (22–24). Magnetic resonance imaging (MRI) has not been extensively investigated, but evidence suggests that it is often ineffective because the signals from cancerous and

D. Front and O. Israel: Department of Nuclear Medicine, Rambam Medical Center and Faculty of Medicine, Haifa 35254, Israel.

[†]Deceased

normal tissues cannot be separated with confidence, and attempts to determine the nature of a mass remaining after treatment have not been successful (25–27). [67]Ga scintigraphy in the follow-up of patients with lymphoma has been shown to be effective, both in evaluation after induction treatment (5,6) and in diagnosis of relapse (7,28). Recently, it has been shown to be a good predictor of outcome very early during treatment (8,19,29,30). The cost effectiveness of ^{67}Ga scintigraphy in patients whose treatment is changed as a result can be evaluated by calculating the cost of ^{67}Ga scintigraphy per year of added life by change of treatment (31).

TECHNIQUE OF [67]GA SCINTIGRAPHY

To be of clinical value in the assessment of lymphoma, ^{67}Ga scintigraphy has to be performed properly. The importance of injecting high doses of ^{67}Ga has long been established (32). The recommended dose in adults is 8 to 10 mCi (290 to 370 MBq). In children, the dose should be adjusted for weight, and 75 μCi/kg with a minimum of 0.5 mCi is recommended. Because the study is performed only in patients with a tissue diagnosis of lymphoma, the potential adverse consequences of a high dose are not clinically relevant. No patient preparation is needed before scanning. High-performance digital equipment has to be used for acquisition of studies (8,10,11,33). A dual-head digital camera with a large field of view and a parallel-hole, medium-energy collimator should be used. The photon peaks of the three lower energies of [67]Ga (93, 184, and 296 keV) should be used, with a separate 15% window setting for each of the peaks. The optimal imaging equipment also includes a specially designed ^{67}Ga collimator. Imaging is routinely performed at 48 or 72 hours after injection. This time interval allows optimal high-flux photon imaging of the tumor and blood pool and renal clearance of the radiopharmaceutical after the injection. Imaging is routinely repeated at 7 days and when necessary, even at 14 days after injection, to confirm the clearance of bowel activity. As part of the early study, at 48 or 72 hours after injection, planar scintigraphy of the whole body, including the upper and lower extremities, and single-photon emission computed tomography (SPECT) of the whole torso are performed. Acquisition parameters for planar scintigraphy are 1,000 kilocounts per view for spot imaging. Whole-body scintigraphy with a dual-head camera acquires about 4,000 kilocounts during a scanning time of 20 minutes. SPECT parameters include a 360-degree rotation with 60 projections, 6 degrees apart, with use of a 64 x 64 matrix. Rotation time is 30 minutes if a single-head camera is used and 22 minutes for a dual-head camera. About 3.5×10^6 to 8×10^6 counts are acquired for each SPECT study.

Seven days after the injection, whole-body planar scintigraphy is again performed. SPECT studies should be repeated if the findings on planar scintigraphy indicate a need for further evaluation. This includes differentiation between a lymphoma lesion and the gut, and assessment of equivocal areas of ^{67}Ga uptake in the early study. In later studies, up to 14 days after injection, planar scintigraphy of areas of interest, usually below the diaphragm after clearance of bowel activity, is performed. On delayed images, planar spot views are acquired with about 400 kilocounts per view. When whole-body scintigraphy is performed, the acquisition time is 26 minutes with about 1,500 kilocounts.

Processing of ^{67}Ga SPECT is performed with filtered back-projection and a Metz filter. Parameters 3 and 14 are defined as follows: $w-[1-(1-h2)p]/h$, where $h = f(FWHM)$, $p = 3$, and $FWHM = 14$. The data are reconstructed in the transaxial plane with a slice thickness of 1 pixel. From these data, the coronal and sagittal planes with a slice thickness of 2 pixels are obtained. SPECT studies provide better contrast enhancement and show lesions that may not be clearly seen on planar scintigraphy and that may indicate the presence of lymphoma. SPECT can also provide an accurate anatomic localization of sites of ^{67}Ga uptake in lymphoma and differentiate them from normal structures. Other possible protocols for acquisition and processing can be used, based on the manufacturer's recommendations and the clinical experience of the group performing ^{67}Ga scintigraphy. It is important, however, that the same acquisition protocol be used regularly. The optimal equipment for ^{67}Ga scintigraphy would be a dual-head camera with roentgenographic anatomic mapping installed on the same instrument to provide a fused image of ^{67}Ga scintigraphy, corrected for photon attenuation, with accurate anatomic positioning. Such an image provides information on both tumor mass and tumor viability (Fig. 36.1; see also Color Plate 14 following page 350).

The liver and spleen, the bony skeleton, and the bone marrow normally take up [67]Ga. Variable ^{67}Ga uptake may be seen in the salivary and lacrimal glands, nasal mucosa, skin, breasts, thymus in children and adolescents, sweat, and male genitalia. At 24 hours after injection, the lungs may be visualized because of the still high concentration of the radiopharmaceutical in the blood pool. Soon after administration, 25% of ^{67}Ga is excreted by the kidneys, and the kidneys are often visualized on scintigraphy performed during the first 24 hours. Forty-eight hours or later after administration of ^{67}Ga, the colon is visualized because of biliary and intestinal excretion of the radioactive tracer. Physiologic uptake of ^{67}Ga in these areas should be differentiated from uptake at a lymphoma site. In the head and neck, ^{67}Ga uptake in the nasal region should be distinguished from lymphomatous involvement of the nasopharynx and oropharynx. Radiotherapy, and sometimes chemotherapy, may cause sialoadenitis. This has a characteristic pattern on ^{67}Ga scintigraphy, with symmetric uptake in the salivary glands that may persist for a long period after the end of treatment. In the chest, uptake in lymphomatous axillary lymph nodes must be differentiated from uptake in sweat or skin folds. SPECT is useful in such

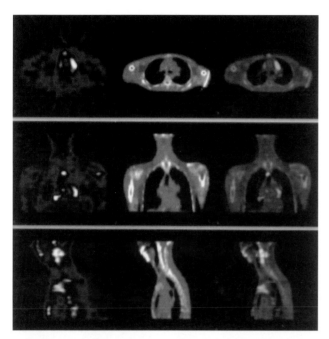

FIGURE 36.1. Imaging of a patient with Hodgkin's disease with combined transmission and ⁶⁷Ga emission tomography-Ga-TET (Hawkeye, Elgems, GE, Haifa, Israel). Abnormal uptake of ⁶⁷Ga in sites of mass on computed tomography (CT). The regions of mass on CT are larger than the areas of ⁶⁷Ga uptake, which indicates fibrosis in the tumor mass. (See also Color Plate 14 following p. 350.)

cases to separate superficial from deep structures. Lateral planar views with the patient's arms raised can also be helpful in distinguishing involved lymph nodes in the axilla. SPECT can also differentiate uptake in the sternum from uptake in retrosternal lesions. Uptake in breasts, more evident in women during their menstrual cycle, hormonal intake, and lactation, has a characteristic symmetric superficial pattern that can be distinguished from underlying lesions on SPECT or planar lateral views.

The thymus may be seen in children and young adults. It has a characteristic bilobed or arrowhead shape and is located in the upper anterior mediastinum (34). However, this visualization cannot be differentiated from lymphomatous involvement of the thymus and should not be mistaken for a mediastinal site of lymphoma. Chemotherapy may lead to reactive hyperplasia of the thymus in children and young adults during treatment or the recovery phase, early after treatment. Uptake of ⁶⁷Ga has been described in cases of thymus hyperplasia with an incidence of about 20% and is associated with the presence of a new thymic mass on CT (35–37). The differential diagnosis, however, includes tumor progression or relapse in the anterior upper mediastinum. This problem has not been resolved and represents a diagnostic dilemma. The characteristic location and shape, the age of the patient, and the association with treatment suggest rebound uptake in thymus. Diffuse bilateral lung uptake may appear during or after chemotherapy (38). It has been found in about 15% of treated lymphoma patients, may be

the consequence of some degree of post-therapeutic pneumonitis, and has no effect on the outcome of patients (38,39). Low-intensity, symmetric hilar uptake of ⁶⁷Ga is seen in about 35% of lymphoma patients (40), more commonly after treatment and in older patients and smokers. CT findings are as a rule negative when no lymphoma is present in the mediastinum. However, if a residual mass is seen after treatment of lymphoma in the mediastinum, the significance of ⁶⁷Ga uptake is unclear. Quantification of ⁶⁷Ga uptake with SPECT has been found useful in the differential diagnosis of benign hilar uptake and active lymphoma sites. The concentration in benign hilar uptake is significantly lower than the uptake in residual active lymphoma (40).

Single-photon emission computed tomography and delayed views facilitate the differential diagnosis of ⁶⁷Ga uptake in normal abdominal structures, such as the gut, and sites of lymphomatous involvement. A different pattern of ⁶⁷Ga uptake on early and delayed scintigraphy suggests that such uptake is in the colon. Uptake in lymphoma remains unchanged over time. SPECT permits the identification of groups of involved abdominal lymph nodes. Mesenteric lymph nodes have a more anterior location, whereas retroperitoneal lymph nodes are located more posteriorly. Normal uptake of ⁶⁷Ga in the liver and spleen makes the diagnosis of lymphoma involvement in these organs difficult. CT should be used for this purpose (41).

As mentioned, the kidneys are visualized during the first 24 hours after injection of ⁶⁷Ga because of normal renal excretion of the radiopharmaceutical. ⁶⁷Ga uptake in the kidneys at later intervals or unilateral, asymmetric visualization of one kidney indicates pathology. Increased renal uptake of ⁶⁷Ga may be seen after treatment in patients with iron overload, or after chemotherapy with agents such as cyclophosphamide or vincristine (42).

The bone-seeking properties of ⁶⁷Ga may lead to some diagnostic problems. The uptake of ⁶⁷Ga may be increased in areas of increased osteoblastic activity in bones affected by lymphoma. It may also be increased in other areas of increased bone turnover, such as epiphyseal plates in children, sites of previous bone biopsy, or other skeletal lesions. Correlation with finding on roentgenography, CT, and bone scintigraphy with ⁹⁹ᵐTc-methylene diphosphonate may be helpful. Primary or secondary skeletal involvement by lymphoma is present in about 10% to 15% of patients (43). It may involve both the axial and peripheral skeleton. The use of whole-body ⁶⁷Ga scintigraphy that includes imaging of the limbs is thus important (33). The lymphoma-seeking properties of ⁶⁷Ga appear to be more pronounced after treatment than its bone-seeking properties, and ⁶⁷Ga should therefore be used to evaluate the response of osseous lymphoma to therapy. Bone scintigraphy and CT are of less value (44). When the proper equipment and technique are used, the sensitivity of ⁶⁷Ga scintigraphy for the detection of lymphoma before treatment is reasonable (6,32,45,46) (Table 36.1). Nevertheless, CT remains the

TABLE 36.1. SENSITIVITY AND SPECIFICITY OF GALLIUM 67 SCINTIGRAPHY BEFORE TREATMENT IN THE DIAGNOSIS OF HODGKIN'S DISEASE, NON-HODGKIN'S LYMPHOMA, AND LOW-GRADE NON-HODGKIN'S LYMPHOMA

Investigator (reference)	No. patients HD	No. patients NHL	No. patients LGNHL	Sensitivity (%)	Specificity (%)
Anderson et al. (32)	21	31	—	HD 97	100
Tumeh et al. (45)	33	7	—	Chest	
				Planar 66	66
				SPECT 96	100
				Abdomen	
				Planar 69	87
				SPECT 85	100
Front et al. (6)	38	39	—	78	97
Ben-Haim et al. (46)	—	—	57	79	94

HD, Hogdkin's disease; NHL, non-Hodgkin's lymphoma; LGNHL, low-grade non-Hodgkin's lymphoma; SPECT, single-photon emission computed tomography.

procedure of choice in the initial evaluation of extent of disease. The principal role of ^{67}Ga scintigraphy is to evaluate response to therapy. Imaging before treatment is necessary to establish a baseline image of ^{67}Ga-avid tumor.

LIMITATIONS AND MISCONCEPTIONS

The ability to detect a small number of tumor cells that can cause a future relapse is important in predicting the outcome of patients with lymphoma. The limitations of scintigraphy in detecting residual cancer cells that can cause tumor relapse is the limiting factor in identifying patients who have not actually had a complete response. These patients still harbor tumor cells that can, sometimes after years, cause clinical disease and limit failure-free and overall survival. Unfortunately, no test is available today to provide such information with a very high sensitivity. At best, ^{67}Ga scintigraphy after treatment can distinguish between lymphoma patients who will and will not achieve a complete response. A basic problem in scintigraphy is the significance of uptake of a small amount of ^{67}Ga. This is particularly true in regions that take up a large amount of ^{67}Ga before treatment because of lymphomatous involvement and then take up only a small amount after treatment. Quantification is not reliable. No absolute standard is available for the comparison of such patients to determine the meaning of faint uptake on ^{67}Ga scintigraphy. Experience acquired in reading ^{67}Ga scintigrams obtained with use of the same technique and protocol during a long period of time may help.

Another problem is the fact that a ^{67}Ga scintigraphic image of the human body, even when the findings are normal, is a "loaded" image (10,31). Several structures of the normal human body take up ^{67}Ga, and such uptake may interfere with the recognition of subtly abnormal regions of uptake in lymphoma. Distinguishing between uptake in normal tissue and uptake in lymphoma can be difficult. Familiarity with normal ^{67}Ga distribution in the human body and its variations, and the use of SPECT, help. Distinguishing between uptake in tumor and that in inflammation and infection is not much of a problem when the pretest probability for tumor is high, as in patients with histologically proven lymphoma. ^{67}Ga scintigraphy should therefore be performed only after tissue evidence of lymphoma has been obtained. ^{67}Ga scintigraphy should not be used to diagnose lymphoma.

It has been suggested that because ^{67}Ga scintigraphy is performed to evaluate response to treatment, it is not necessary to obtain a baseline ^{67}Ga scintigram before treatment. This notion is incorrect because 10% to 15% of patients have lymphoma that is not ^{67}Ga-avid. In such patients, negative findings on ^{67}Ga scintigraphy after treatment do not indicate a response to treatment. They may simply indicate that the lymphoma is not ^{67}Ga-avid. The lymphoma may or may not have responded. Part of the scintigraphic evaluation process is to compare sites of lymphoma and ^{67}Ga uptake before and after treatment to determine whether sites of disease have indeed responded to treatment. Determining the location, size, and form of sites of abnormal uptake of ^{67}Ga before treatment is important for this comparison. Results of scintigraphy should be assessed before and after treatment. Such a comparison is also important in the diagnose of recurrence because in 75% of patients, recurrence is partly or entirely in the same region as the original disease (7,28). Experience has shown that comparison with original sites is essential, both at the end of treatment and during continuous complete remission. It is not possible to interpret the results of ^{67}Ga scintigraphy correctly after treatment or during remission without a baseline study.

Other radiopharmaceuticals, particularly ^{201}Tl, have been suggested as agents to evaluate low-grade lymphoma (47). A recent publication has shown that in low-grade lymphoma, ^{201}Tl scintigraphy and properly performed ^{67}Ga scintigraphy have essentially the same sensitivity (46). Disadvantages of ^{201}Tl scintigraphy are that it cannot be used to evaluate the abdomen and that ^{201}Tl is taken up in cardiac and body muscle. The main difficulty, however, is that no evidence has yet been found that ²⁰¹Tl can be used to determine the effect of therapy in patients with low-grade lymphoma. ⁶⁷Ga, on the other hand, is useful in monitoring response to treatment in low-grade lymphoma (46).

EVALUATION OF RESPONSE TO TREATMENT: THE PROBLEM OF A RESIDUAL MASS

Radiologic imaging techniques, which are the gold standard for the staging of lymphoma, do not provide adequate information regarding the response of lymphoma to treatment. CT and MRI are sensitive in the diagnosis of a tumor mass but do not provide information about the nature of the mass that remains after treatment in about 50% of patients (48). The range of attenuation of a lymphomatous mass measured by CT is not significantly different from that of normal tissue or of a region of fibrosis and necrosis that may remain after treatment. MRI of lymphoma is also based on detecting the tumor mass. It was believed that because untreated tumor contains an increased amount of water, the T_2 relaxation signal would be prolonged and that MR images would be able to differentiate a residual mass after treatment that does not contain tumor. However, this is often not the case. The signal of a tumor mass after treatment may be inhomogeneous. In practice, it is not possible in such a case to differentiate normal tissue from viable or nonviable tumor tissue after treatment.

Aggressive and low-grade non-Hodgkin's lymphoma and Hodgkin's disease take up ⁶⁷Ga more readily than the surrounding normal tissue does. The sensitivity and specificity of ⁶⁷Ga scintigraphy are shown in Table 36.2. About 64% to 83% of patients, particularly those with bulky disease on plain chest films or CT, have a residual mass after treatment. The prognosis of these patients may be good, meaning that the residual mass does not necessarily contain malignant tissue. In many patients, such a mass on CT may regress spontaneously without any additional treatment.

Jochelson et al. (22) and Radford et al. (23) have described this phenomenon on radiologic studies of the chest. Israel et al. (5) found that in 43% of patients, when CT findings were abnormal after treatment, no other evidence of disease was apparent. Patients did not show evidence of disease for at least 12 months. This same phenomenon was also described by Surbone et al. (24) in patients with abdominal masses. Neither CT nor MRI could differentiate the nature of an abdominal residual mass after treatment. They found that 72 of 241 patients (30%) with aggressive non-Hodgkin's lymphoma had an abdominal mass at presentation. Of those, 29 patients (41%) had a residual mass after treatment without any other evidence of disease and had, in fact, achieved a complete response (24). An association was found between the size of the mass and the appearance of a residual mass. Among patients with initial bulky disease, 58% had a residual mass but only 22% had residual active disease after treatment. Of those with a residual mass, 78% had had a bulky mass before treatment. Abdominal residual masses after treatment also tended to decrease in size over several years without further treatment. Among 22 patients (51%) with surgically extracted masses that were evaluated pathologically, cancer was found in one (4.5%).

These studies suggest that a residual mass after treatment does not necessarily indicate that the patient has viable tumor (5–9,16–21). A residual mass can be seen in patients who have achieved a complete response (Fig. 36.2). A mass that decreases in size but does not disappear after treatment does not indicate a partial response and should not be categorized as "uncertain/unconfirmed complete response" (49). Based on ⁶⁷Ga uptake after treatment, a mass can still be present with a complete response (Fig. 36.2). ⁶⁷Ga scintigraphy indicates whether or not the patient has achieved a complete response. Iosilevsky et al. (12) first reported that ⁶⁷Ga is taken up only by viable lymphoma in a tumor model and not by benign residual tissue after successful treatment. The size of a mass that remains after treatment does not correlate with the response of tumor to treatment. This is the basis for

TABLE 36.2. GALLIUM 67 SCINTIGRAPHY IN DETERMINATION OF COMPLETE RESPONSE AFTER TREATMENT OF LYMPHOMA

Group (reference)	No. patients		Sensitivity (%)	Specificity (%)
	HD	NHL		
Israel et al. (5)	19	6	100	95
Wylie et al. (16)	25	—	80	70
Front et al. (6)	38	39	Planar 84	96
			SPECT 92	99
Kaplan et al. (17)	—	37	76	75
Front et al. (18)	43	56	PPV HD 80	NPV HD 84
			PPV NHL 73	NPV NHL 84
Gasparini et al. (27)	34	—	86	100
Kostakoglu et al. (19)	30	—	96	80

HD, Hodgkin's disease; NHL, non-Hodgkin's lymphoma; SPECT, single-photon emission computed tomography; PPV, positive predictive value; NPV, negative predictive value.

monitoring response to treatment by imaging with radio-pharmaceuticals rather than by anatomic imaging of tumor masses with plain roentgenography, CT, and MRI.

Israel et al. (5) and Front et al. (6) demonstrated the ability of ^{67}Ga to determine response to treatment in humans and to predict outcome at the end of treatment. They found that 95% of patients with negative findings on ^{67}Ga scintigraphy after treatment achieved a complete response. Patients with positive findings on ^{67}Ga scintigraphy did not achieve a complete response. The sensitivity was 92% and the specificity was 99% for the detection of viable lymphoma after treatment. The difference in survival between

patients with positive and negative findings on ^{67}Ga scintigraphy after treatment was significant. Wylie et al. (16) and Kaplan et al. (17) later confirmed these findings (Table 36.2). Kostakoglu et al. (19) found the accuracy of ^{67}Ga scintigraphy in identifying the histology of a residual mass in the mediastinum to be 93%. King et al. (20) found the 4-year disease-free survival in patients with negative findings on ^{67}Ga scintigraphy after treatment to be 75%, whereas that of patients with positive findings was only 8%. Hagemeister et al. (21) found ^{67}Ga scintigraphy to have a sensitivity of 86% to 100% in predicting disease-free survival. Gasparini et al. (27) found a sensitivity of 86% and a

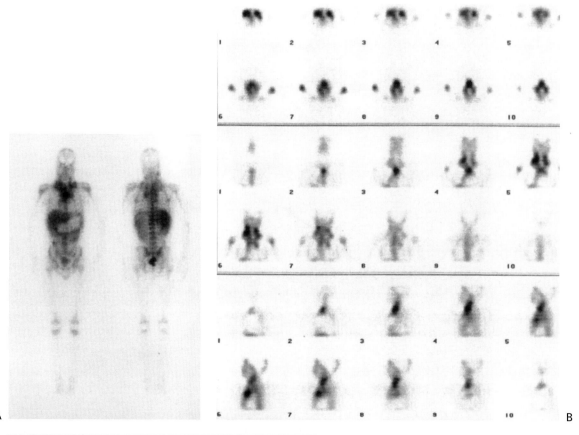

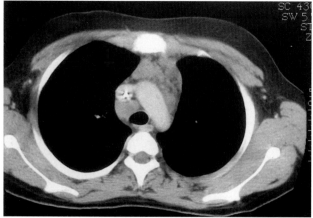

FIGURE 36.2. A residual mass and normal findings on ^{67}Ga scintigraphy in an 18-year-old man with Hodgkin's disease. Baseline planar ^{67}Ga scintigraphy (**A**) and single-photon emission computed tomography (*SPECT*) (**B**) show bulky disease in the mediastinum and supraclavicular and infraclavicular involvement. After treatment, CT (**C**) shows residual disease at the level of the aortic arch and in the retrocaval and pretracheal area.

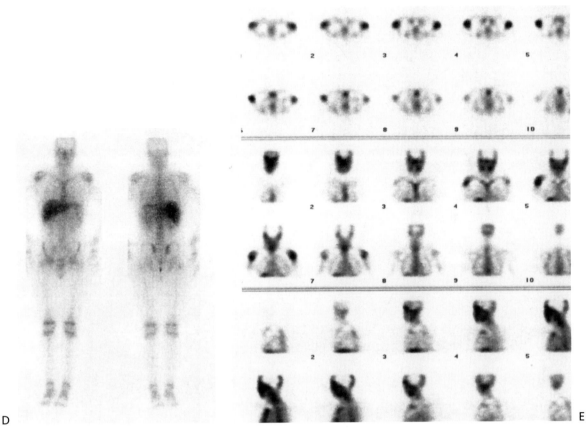

FIGURE 36.2. *(continued)* Results of planar ⁶⁷Ga scintigraphy (**D**) and SPECT (**E**) after treatment are normal. The patient has been in continuous clinical remission during a follow-up of 2 years.

specificity of 100%. Some authors found ⁶⁷Ga to be less sensitive, but those studies suffer from severe methodologic problems, such as not performing baseline ⁶⁷Ga scintigraphy or not performing SPECT, which renders the results of a negative ⁶⁷Ga study uninterpretable. ⁶⁷Ga uptake in a residual mass after treatment indicates a poor patient outcome (17,18). Table 36.2 summarizes the accuracy of ⁶⁷Ga scintigraphy in determining a complete response after treatment and subsequent outcome.

In summary, positive findings on ⁶⁷Ga scintigraphy after treatment indicate that the patient has not reached a complete response. Negative findings, even when a residual mass persists after treatment, indicate a complete response (Fig. 36.2). However, because small foci of residual tumor cells may be undetectable by ⁶⁷Ga, a negative result has less predictive value. It does not preclude a relapse of disease.

DETECTION OF RELAPSE

Early diagnosis of relapse is important to improve the chance of overall successful treatment. Treatment is more effective when the tumor burden is small. The logarithmic kill of cells provides a better opportunity to reduce the absolute number of cells to a level at which the body's own mechanisms can deal with them. Also, the chance for cross-resistant clones of cells to develop is smaller when relapse is detected early. ⁶⁷Ga plays a major role in the early diagnosis of relapse in lymphoma, particularly when a strict protocol of ⁶⁷Ga monitoring is followed. Relapsing lymphoma can be diagnosed by ⁶⁷Ga scintigraphy sometimes months or even years before the disease becomes clinically evident by palpation or on CT (7). Salvage therapy can be applied earlier for a better chance of response to second-line treatment.

Weeks et al. (28) investigated the ability of clinical, laboratory, and radiologic tests to diagnose recurrence. Restaging procedures were found to have a sensitivity of 21% to 55%, which is clearly not satisfactory, and therefore could not be used effectively in the clinical management of patients with lymphoma who had achieved a continuous clinical remission. Only palpation had a good sensitivity of 80% (28). It should be realized, however, that physical examination is limited to the external surface of the body and to the superficial organs that can be palpated. In the study of Weeks et al. (28), routine follow-up examinations did not detect recurrence. Relapse was diagnosed only when a patient sought medical help because of a self-identified

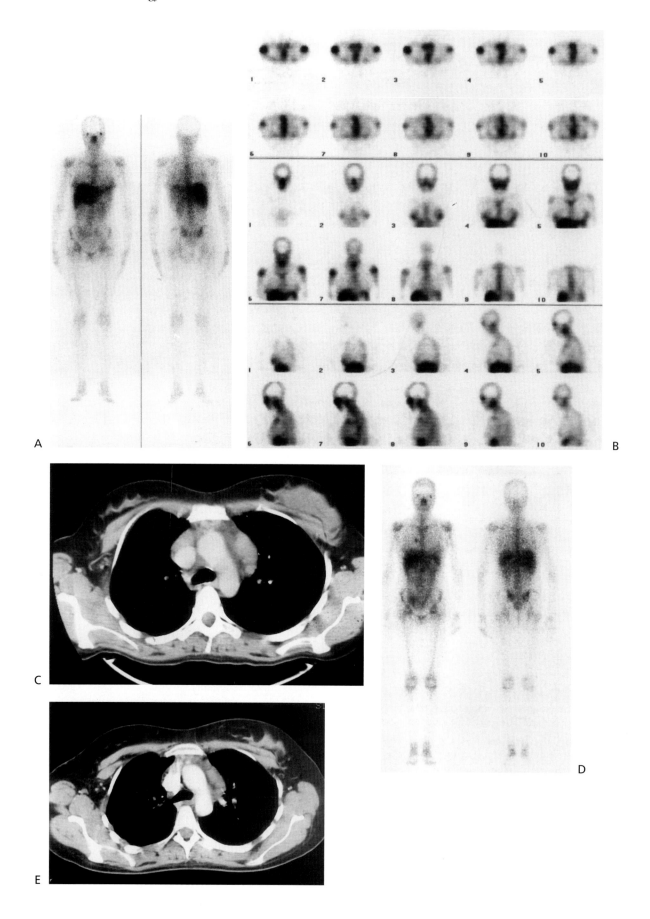

A

B

C

D

E

palpable mass. CT had a sensitivity of 45% for the chest and 55% for the abdomen when performed during routine follow-up. In most patients (75%), relapse was in the same sites where disease was diagnosed initially. Forty-two percent of patients had a relapse in an additional site that was not previously involved; 25% had relapse only in a new site. These figures underscore the importance of examining the whole body. Although CT of the whole body makes the study more expensive, with scintigraphy, the time needed to study the entire body is increased only slightly. The specificity of the tests used to diagnose relapse was, of course, high because only patients with a prior history of lymphoma were selected.

Front et al. (7) found ⁶⁷Ga scintigraphy useful to detect recurrence before any other manifestation of disease developed or any results of other tests were positive. They noted a sensitivity of 95% in 53 events in 47 patients. Weeks et al. (28) obtained similar results, but in a much smaller number of patients. The specificity of ⁶⁷Ga scintigraphy in the study of Front et al. (7) was somewhat lower because false-positive results were obtained—three in patients with nontumoral uptake in the mediastinum, two in the abdomen, and one in the axillary region. The results of this study are important because in 12 scintigraphic studies in 10 patients, uptake of ⁶⁷Ga was abnormal in sites where disease had recurred for an average of 6.8 months before any other clinical, laboratory, or CT abnormality was observed in the region. This again indicates that the size of the mass after treatment does not correlate with the presence of cancer and that lymph nodes of normal size do not preclude the presence of cancer in the nodes (Fig. 36.3). Relapse was detected by ⁶⁷Ga scintigraphy earlier when the tumor load was smaller. The effect of such early diagnosis by ⁶⁷Ga on the results of treatment and on failure-free survival still needs to be examined.

The diagnosis of relapse does not apply only to Hodgkin's disease and aggressive non-Hodgkin's lymphoma. Ben-Haim et al. (46) investigated low-grade lymphoma and found the sensitivity of ⁶⁷Ga scintigraphy in the diagnosis of relapse to be 89%. Therefore, ⁶⁷Ga scintigraphy is also useful in low-grade non-Hodgkin's lymphoma, although in this group of patients, there are still no therapeutic consequences of these findings.

EARLY PREDICTION OF OUTCOME: EVALUATION OF RAPIDITY OF RESPONSE

In 20% to 30% of patients with Hodgkin's disease and 40% to 50% of patients with non-Hodgkin's lymphoma, treatment eventually fails (50–52). More aggressive chemotherapy, high-dose chemotherapy with bone marrow transplantation, and early institution of treatment have all been used in an effort to improve the results of treatment. An early change of a treatment protocol to a potentially more effective one may increase the period of failure-free survival and eventually result in a cure. It has been suggested that patients with Hodgkin's disease or non-Hodgkin's lymphoma who exhibit a rapid and complete response before the end of a chemotherapy protocol have a better chance of cure or prolonged failure-free survival (51,53–55). The task then is to determine complete versus partial or no response early during induction treatment. Theoretically, the earlier a complete response or, on the contrary, a treatment failure is determined, the better the chance of providing a suitable treatment (8,9,29,30). A treatment change should be instituted as soon as possible, before the nonsensitive tumor grows to a dimension that cannot be effectively treated or before resistant or partially resistant clones of cells become dominant. The best time to establish the need to change therapy is after the first cycle of treatment. CT is not suitable for this evaluation because it does not establish the presence or absence of viable tumor in a mass (56). Furthermore, even if CT shows that a mass has regressed, it does not provide information about the presence of tumor cells that can cause relapse, even at a site where no mass is present. Using the size of a mass as a criterion for response is problematic.

High-dose chemotherapy with bone marrow transplantation may be effective in patients with lymphoma. Such treatment can be given early in the course of disease. A technique is necessary that will reliably indicate the response of an individual patient early during treatment and also predict outcome. Such a technique should show the effect of a treatment on the particular tumor of an individual patient (57,58). If a tumor does not respond to treatment rapidly, management should be changed to a potentially more effective one. In 1995, Front and Israel reported the ability of ⁶⁷Ga scintigraphy to predict the outcome of patients early, sometimes after one cycle of

---

FIGURE 36.3. Relapse in a 26-year-old woman with nodular sclerosis Hodgkin's disease. Results of planar (**A**) and single-photon emission computed tomography (*SPECT*) (**B**) ⁶⁷Ga scintigraphy are normal during continuous clinical remission. CT (**C**) shows a residual mass in the anterior mediastinum. Five months later, routine planar ⁶⁷Ga scintigraphy (**D**) shows a relapse in the right mediastinum. CT (**E**) shows essentially no change in the size of the residual mass seen on the previous study. Two months later, an increase in the size of the mass was noted on CT. ⁶⁷Ga scintigraphy shows an increase in size and intensity of the pathologic uptake. Recurrence was diagnosed, and salvage high-dose chemotherapy was started.

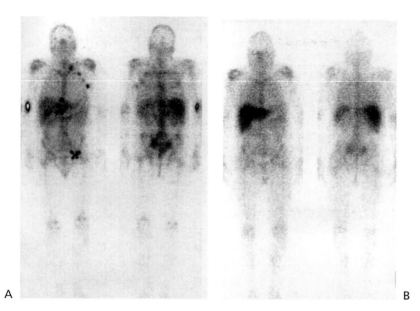

A

B

FIGURE 36.4. Complete response after one cycle of MOPP/ABV (Mustargen, Oncovin, procarbazine, prednisone/adriamycin D, bleomycin, vincristine) treatment in a 50-year-old man with nodular sclerosis Hodgkin's disease, stage IIIB. Baseline ^{67}Ga scintigraphy (**A**) shows abnormal uptake above and below the diaphragm. After one cycle of chemotherapy, results of ^{67}Ga scintigraphy (**B**) are normal. The patient achieved a complete response and has been in continuous clinical remission for a follow-up of 3 years.

chemotherapy, during induction treatment (8). Subsequently, in 1997, Janicek et al. (9) reported the ability of ^{67}Ga scintigraphy during treatment to predict outcome in 30 patients with aggressive non-Hodgkin's lymphoma. In 1999, Front et al. reported results in predicting outcome with ^{67}Ga scintigraphy after one cycle of chemotherapy in

98 patients with Hodgkin's disease (29) and 118 patients with non-Hodgkin's lymphoma (30). The results showed a significant difference in failure-free survival, both in Hodgkin's disease and non-Hodgkin's lymphoma, between patients with positive and negative results on ^{67}Ga scintigraphy performed early during treatment (Figs. 36.4 and 36.5).

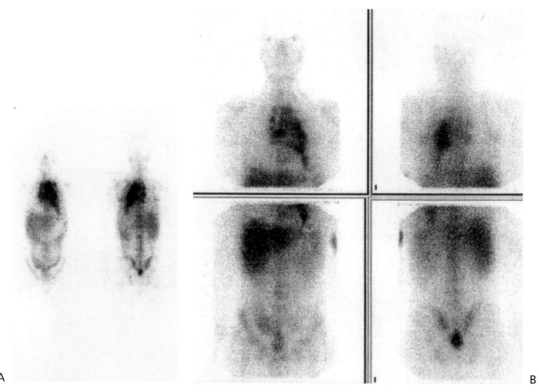

A

B

FIGURE 36.5. No response during treatment in a 26-year-old man with diffuse large cell non-Hodgkin's lymphoma. Baseline ^{67}Ga scintigraphy (**A**) shows uptake in the mediastinum and left lung. After two courses of high-dose CHOP (cyclophosphamide, hydroxydaunomycin, Oncovin, prednisone), results of ^{67}Ga scintigraphy (**B**) are essentially unchanged. The patient did not achieve a complete response and died with active disease.

In non-Hodgkin's lymphoma, a significant difference is noted after one cycle of chemotherapy ($p < .002$) and at midtreatment ($p < .0001$) (30). Thus, ^{67}Ga scintigraphy is able to predict the outcome of a patient early during treatment by determining the effect of treatment on the patient's tumor. This should also indicate, at an early stage, which patients will have a poor outcome. For such patients, treatment should be changed early to improve the overall chance of success. Studies are under way to determine the effect of early change of treatment based on the results of ^{67}Ga scintigraphy early during treatment.

In Hodgkin's disease, prolonged failure-free survival and cure are achieved in 70% to 80% of patients. After one cycle of treatment, a significant difference ($p < .002$) in failure-free survival is noted between patients with positive and negative results on ^{67}Ga scintigraphy. Although these results may identify patients in whom treatment should be changed early, identification of patients who could receive less than the full course of chemotherapy represents another important opportunity. If some patients achieve a complete response after one cycle of chemotherapy, they may be cured with a dose of chemotherapy less intense than that presently used routinely. This could be particularly important in children, in whom treatment alone may cause long-standing abnormalities. This potential change in management has not yet been evaluated.

CONCLUSIONS

When properly performed, ^{67}Ga scintigraphy is now the best diagnostic tool to monitor response to treatment in patients with lymphoma. It should be used to evaluate the nature of a residual mass after treatment. It is also the best test to detect disease relapse after a patient an initial complete response and subsequent continuous clinical remission. It may identify recurrence months and sometimes years before other diagnostic procedures. The test may also be used to evaluate the response of an individual tumor early during treatment and predict long-term outcome. ^{67}Ga scintigraphy has the potential to indicate the need to change treatment before untreatable disease develops. The limits of the sensitivity of ^{67}Ga scintigraphy to detect small tumor foci that can result in relapse even after an apparent complete response are unknown.

REFERENCES

1. Front D, Israel O. Nuclear medicine in monitoring response to cancer treatment. *J Nucl Med* 1989;30:1731–1736.
2. Paul R. Comparison of fluorine-18-2-fluorodeoxyglucose and gallium-67 citrate imaging for detection of lymphoma. *J Nucl Med* 1987;28:288–292.
3. Okada J, Yoshikawa K, Imazeki K, et al. The use of FDG-PET in the detection and management of malignant lymphoma: correlation of uptake with prognosis. *J Nucl Med* 1991;32:686–691
4. Okada J, Yoshikawa K, Itami M, et al. Positron emission tomography using fluorine-18-fluorodeoxyglucose in malignant lymphoma: a comparison with proliferative activity. *J Nucl Med* 1992;33:325–329.
5. Israel O, Front D, Lam M, et al. Gallium-67 imaging in monitoring lymphoma response to treatment. *Cancer* 1988;61:2439–2443.
6. Front D, Israel O, Epelbaum R, et al. Ga-67 SPECT before and after treatment of lymphoma. *Radiology* 1990;175:515–519.
7. Front D, Bar-Shalom R, Epelbaum R, et al. Early detection of lymphoma recurrence with gallium-67 scintigraphy. *J Nucl Med* 1993;34:2101–2104.
8. Front D, Israel O. The role of Ga-67 scintigraphy in evaluating the results of therapy of lymphoma patients. *Semin Nucl Med* 1995;25:60–71.
9. Janicek M, Kaplan WD, Neuberg D, et al. Early restaging gallium scans predict outcome in poor-prognosis patients with aggressive non-Hodgkin's lymphoma treated with high-dose chemotherapy. *J Clin Oncol* 1997;15:1631–1637.
10. Front D, Bar-Shalom R, Israel O. The continuing role of gallium-67 scintigraphy in the age of receptor imaging. *Semin Nucl Med* 1997;25:68–74.
11. Front D, Bar-Shalom R, Israel O. Role of Ga-67 and other radiopharmaceuticals in the management of patients with lymphoma. In: Freeman L, ed. *Nuclear medicine annual 1998*. Philadelphia: Lippincott–Raven Publishers, 1998:247–264.
12. Iosilevsky G, Front D, Bettman L, et al. Uptake of gallium-67 citrate and [2-H3] deoxyglucose in the tumor model following chemotherapy and radiotherapy. *J Nucl Med* 1985;26:278–282.
13. Dudley HC, Maddox GE. Deposition of radio-gallium (Ga-67) in skeletal tissue. *J Pharmacol Exp Ther* 1949;96:224.
14. Edwards CL, Hayes RL. Tumor scanning with gallium citrate. *J Nucl Med* 1969;10:103–105.
15. Larson SM, Carasquillo JA. Nuclear oncology: current perspectives. In: Freeman L, Weissman H, eds. *Nuclear medicine annual 1988*. New York: Raven Press, 1988:167–198.
16. Wylie BR, Southee AE, Joshua DE, et al. Gallium scanning in the management of mediastinal Hodgkin's disease. *Eur J Haematol* 1989;7:144–145.
17. Kaplan WD, Jochelson MS, Herman TS, et al. Gallium-67 imaging: a predictor of residual tumor viability and clinical outcome in patients with diffuse large-cell lymphomas. *J Clin Oncol* 1990;8:1966–1970.
18. Front D, Ben-Haim S, Israel O, et al. Lymphoma: predictive value of Ga-67 scintigraphy after treatment. *Radiology* 1992;182:359–363.
19. Kostakoglu L, Yeh SDJ, Portlock C, et al. Validation of gallium-67 citrate single-photon emission computed tomography in biopsy-confirmed residual Hodgkin's disease in the mediastinum. *J Nucl Med* 1992;33:345–350.
20. King SC, Reiman RJ, Prosnitz LR, et al. Prognostic importance of restaging gallium scans following induction chemotherapy for advanced Hodgkin's disease. *J Clin Oncol* 1994;12:306–311.
21. Hagemeister FM, Purugganan A, Podoloff DA, et al. The gallium scan predicts relapse in patients with Hodgkin's disease treated with combined modality therapy. *Ann Oncol* 1994;5[Suppl 2]:S59–S63.
22. Jochelson M, Mauch P, Balikian J, et al. The significance of the residual mediastinal mass in treated Hodgkin's disease. *J Clin Oncol* 1985;3:637–640.
23. Radford JA, Cowan RA, Flanagan M, et al. The significance of residual mediastinal abnormality on the chest radiograph following treatment for Hodgkin's disease. *J Clin Oncol* 1988;6:940–946.
24. Surbone A, Longo DL, DeVita VT, et al. Residual abdominal masses in aggressive Non-Hodgkin's lymphoma after combination chemotherapy: significance and management. *J Clin Oncol* 1988;6:1832–1837.

25. Sagel SS, Glazer HS. Mediastinum. In: Lee JKT, Sagel SS, Stanley RJ, eds. *Computed body tomography with MRI correlation.* New York: Raven Press, 1989:245–291.

26. Rahmouni A, Tempany C, Jones R, et al. Lymphoma: monitoring tumor size and signal intensity with MR imaging. *Radiology* 1993;188:445–451.

27. Gasparini MD, Balzarini L, Castellani MR, et al. Current role of gallium scan and magnetic resonance imaging in the management of mediastinal Hodgkin lymphoma. *Cancer* 1993;72:577–582.

28. Weeks JC, Yeap BY, Canellos GP, et al. Value of follow-up procedures in patients with large-cell lymphoma who achieve a complete remission. *J Clin Oncol* 1991;9:1196–1203.

29. Front D, Bar-Shalom R, Mor M, et al. Hodgkin's disease: prediction of outcome with Ga-67 scintigraphy after one cycle of chemotherapy. *Radiology* 1999;210:487–493.

30. Front D, Bar-Shalom R, Mor M, et al. Non-Hodgkin's lymphoma: prediction of outcome with Ga-67 scintigraphy after one cycle of chemotherapy. *Radiology* 2000;214:253–257.

31. Front D, Israel O. Present state and future role of Ga-67 scintigraphy in lymphoma. *J Nucl Med* 1996;37:530–532.

32. Anderson KC, Leonard RCF, Canellos GP, et al. High-dose gallium imaging in lymphoma. *Am J Med* 1983;75:327–331.

33. Front D, Bar-Shalom R, Iosilevsky G, et al. Ga-67 scintigraphy with a dual-head camera. *Clin Nucl Med* 1995;20:542–548.

34. Israel O, Jerushalmi J, Ben-Haim S, et al. Normal and abnormal Ga-67 SPECT anatomy in patients with lymphoma. *Clin Nucl Med* 1990;15:334–345.

35. Donahue DM, Leonard JC, Basmadjian GP, et al. Thymic gallium-67 localization in pediatric patients on chemotherapy. *J Nucl Med* 1981;22:1043–1048.

36. Peylan-Ramu N, Haddy TB, Jones E, et al. High frequency of benign mediastinal uptake of gallium-67 after completion of chemotherapy in children with high-grade Non-Hodgkin's lymphoma. *J Clin Oncol* 1989;7:1800–1806.

37. Small EJ, Venook AP, Damon LE. Gallium-avid thymic hyperplasia in an adult after chemotherapy for Hodgkin disease. *Cancer* 1993;72:905–908.

38. Bar-Shalom R, Israel O, Haim N, et al. Diffuse lung uptake of Ga-67 after treatment of lymphoma: is it of clinical importance? *Radiology* 1996;199:473–476.

39. Podoloff D. Diffuse lung uptake of Ga-67 citrate in treated lymphoma: another milestone on the road to understanding. *Radiology* 1996;199:319–320.

40. Even-Sapir E, Bar-Shalom R, Israel O, et al. Single-photon emission computed tomography quantitation of gallium citrate uptake for the differentiation of lymphoma from benign hilar uptake. *J Clin Oncol* 1995;13:942–946.

41. Ben-Haim S, Bar-Shalom R, Israel O, et al. Liver involvement in lymphoma: role of gallium-67 scintigraphy. *J Nucl Med* 1995;36:900–904.

42. Dambro TJ, Slavin JD, Epstein NF, et al. Loss of radiogallium from lymphoma after initiation of chemotherapy. *Clin Nucl Med* 1992;17:32–33.

43. Orzel JA, Sawaf NW, Richardson ML. Lymphoma of the skeleton. Scintigraphic evaluation. *Am J Roentgenol* 1988;150:1095–1099.

44. Bar-Shalom R, Israel O, Epelbaum R, et al. Gallium-67 scintigraphy in lymphoma with bone involvement. *J Nucl Med* 1995;36:446–450.

45. Tumeh SS, Rosenthal DS, Kaplan WD, et al. Lymphoma: evaluation with Ga-67 SPECT. *Radiology* 1987;164:111–114.

46. Ben-Haim S, Bar-Shalom R, Israel O, et al. Utility of gallium-67 scintigraphy in low-grade Non-Hodgkin's lymphoma. *J Clin Oncol* 1996;14:1936–1942.

47. Waxman AD, Eller D, Ashook G, et al. Comparison of gallium-67 citrate and thallium-201 scintigraphy in peripheral and intrathoracic lymphoma. *J Nucl Med* 1996;37:46–50.

48. Lister TA, Crowther D, Sutcliffe SB, et al. Report of a committee convened to discuss the evaluation and staging of patients with Hodgkin's disease—Cotswolds meeting. *J Clin Oncol* 1989;7:1630–1636.

49. Gordon LI, Harrington D, Anderson J, et al. Comparison of a second-generation combination chemotherapeutic regimen (m-BACOD) with a standard regimen (CHOP) for advanced diffuse non-Hodgkin's lymphoma. *N Engl J Med* 1992;327:1342–1349.

50. Fisher RI, Gaynor ER, Dahlberg S, et al. Comparison of a standard regimen (CHOP) with three intensive chemotherapy regimens for advanced non-Hodgkin's lymphoma. *N Engl J Med* 1993;328:1002–1006.

51. Armitage JO. Treatment of non-Hodgkin's lymphoma. *N Engl J Med* 1993;328:1023–1030.

52. Haq R, Sawka CA, Franssen E, et al. Significance of a partial or slow response to front-line chemotherapy in the management of intermediate-grade or high-grade Non-Hodgkin's lymphoma: a literature review. *J Clin Oncol* 1994;12:1074–1084.

53. Coiffier B, Bryon P, Berger F, et al. Intensive and sequential combination chemotherapy for aggressive malignant lymphomas (protocol LNH-80). *J Clin Oncol* 1986;4:147–153.

54. Armitage JO, Wisenburger DD, Hutchins M, et al. Chemotherapy for diffuse large cell lymphoma—rapidly responding patients have more durable remissions. *J Clin Oncol* 1986;4:160–164.

55. Longo DL, DeVita VT, Duffey PL, et al. Superiority of ProMACE-CytaBOM over ProMace-MOPP in the treatment of advanced diffuse aggressive lymphoma: results of a prospective randomized trial. *J Clin Oncol* 1991;9:25–30.

56. Verdonck LF, VanPutten WLJ, Hagenbeek A, et al. Comparison of CHOP chemotherapy with autologous bone marrow transplantation for slowly responding patients with aggressive Non-Hodgkin's lymphoma. *N Engl J Med* 1995;332:1045–1051.

57. Shipp MA, Harrington DP. A predictive model for aggressive Non-Hodgkin's lymphoma. *N Engl J Med* 1993;329:987–994.

58. Hasenclever D, Diehl V. A prognostic score for advanced Hodgkin's disease. *N Engl J Med* 1998;339:1506–1514.

37

POSITRON EMISSION TOMOGRAPHY IMAGING
HEMATOPOIETIC TUMORS

SVEN N. RESKE
INGA BUCHMANN

During the last 25 years, survival of patients with malignant lymphoma has significantly increased. The reasons for this improvement in survival include improved understanding of pathophysiology and molecular pathogenesis, which has translated into improved therapeutic concepts and regimens adapted to stage and risk profile of the disease. Precise staging of nodal and extranodal lymphoma spread is thus an essential requirement for adequate therapy selection and therapeutic success.

Malignant lymphomas comprise a heterogeneous group of diseases characterized by painless enlargement of neoplastic lymph nodes, nodal and extranodal disease progression, and, as demonstrated by positron emission tomography (PET)·imaging, marked upregulation of intermediary substrate metabolism of involved tissues. *Hodgkin's disease* (HD) constitutes approximately 30% to 40% of the malignant lymphomas. The number of patients newly diagnosed each year in the United States is approximately 7,400, with a male-to-female ratio of 1.3:1. HD has a striking bimodal age distribution. In industrialized countries, the first peak occurs at approximately 20 to 30 years of age, and the second peak occurs during late adulthood. *Non-Hodgkin's lymphoma* (NHL) represents approximately 3% of all cancers in the United States with an estimated incidence of approximately 16 per 1,000,000 population. NHL represents an extremely heterogeneous group of neoplasms of the immune system, each of which is characterized by its own particular histologic features, immunophenotype, and, in some cases, genotype. Peak incidence of NHL occurs after the age of 50 years.

The diagnosis of malignant lymphoma rests primarily on histopathologic examination of involved tissues. Conventionally, the extent of disease is estimated by the following: assessment of clinical findings; serologic tests;

ultrasonography; computed tomography (CT) of the thorax, abdomen, and pelvis; bone marrow biopsy; magnetic resonance imaging; and skeletal scintigraphy in selected cases. In contrast to NHL, which is often disseminated at the time of diagnosis, HD spread usually follows sequential involvement of contiguous lymph nodes. Extranodal involvement as the first manifestation of HD is rare. According to the Ann Arbor classification (Table 37.1), patients with HD can be stratified into limited-stage disease (clinical stage II or less, absence of risk factors), intermediate-stage disease (clinical stage 2 or less, presence of risk factors), or disseminated disease (1). The risk factors are defined as mediastinal bulk, extranodal involvement, the presence of more than three involved nodal areas, and an erythrocyte sedimentation rate greater than 50 mm per hour (associated with A-type symptoms) or more than 30 mm (associated with B-type symptoms). PET imaging is a valuable tool for accurate staging and assessment of several risk factors.

The first report of increased fluorodeoxyglucose (FDG) uptake in malignant lymphoma was published by Paul in 1987 (2). An example of whole-body FDG-PET imaging of HD with modern equipment is shown in Figs. 37.1 and 37.3. Paul found FDG imaging to be more sensitive than gallium 67 imaging to detect malignant lymphomas (3–6). Later studies described a loose correlation of FDG uptake in untreated malignant lymphomas with proliferative activity, grade of malignancy, and prognosis (3–5). Several authors found low FDG uptake and decreased detection rate in low-grade lymphomas (3,4). This observation was not confirmed by other investigators (7,8) (Fig. 37.2). FDG uptake is seen in patients with low-grade lymphoma, but data are insufficient to define the overall sensitivity of FDG imaging in this group of patients. Uptake and transport rates of carbon 11–methionine has been found to be significantly increased in malignant lymphoma (9). The short half-life of carbon 11 and the limited availability may pre-

S. N. Reske and I. Buchmann: Department of Nuclear Medicine, University Clinic Ulm, Ulm D-89070, Germany.

TABLE 37.1. ANN ARBOR CLASSIFICATION: LYMPHOID STRUCTURES: SPLEEN, THYMUS, WALDEYER'S RING

Stage I	Involvement of a single lymph node region or lymphoid structure or involvement of a single extralymphatic site (I$_E$)
Stage II	Involvement of two or more lymph node regions on the same side of the diaphragm (II) that may be accompanied by localized contiguous involvement of an extralymphatic organ or site (II$_E$)
Stage III	Involvement of lymph node regions on both sides of the diaphragm (III) that may also be accompanied by involvement of the spleen (III$_S$) or by localized contiguous involvement of an extralymphatic organ or site (III$_E$)
Stage IV	Diffuse or disseminated involvement of one or more extralymphatic organs or tissues, with or without associated lymph node involvement

clude widespread use of this tracer for the detection and staging of malignant lymphomas.

With the availability of convenient whole-body PET scanners, the properties of FDG-PET for staging and therapy monitoring have been systematically studied. Although FDG uptake rates are similar after overnight fasting and during euglycemic hyperinsulinemic clamp (for experimental constant serum glucose levels) in lymphomas, increased muscle and other soft-tissue FDG uptake results in decreased contrast between lymphoma and soft tissue (10). Thus, an 8- to 12-hour fasting period is recommended before patients with malignant lymphomas are examined with FDG-PET.

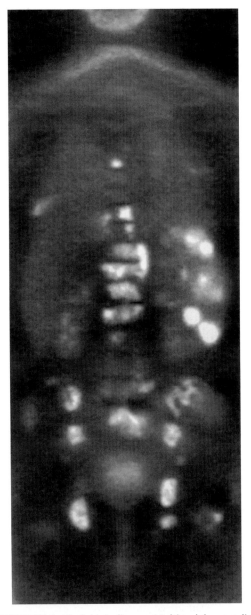
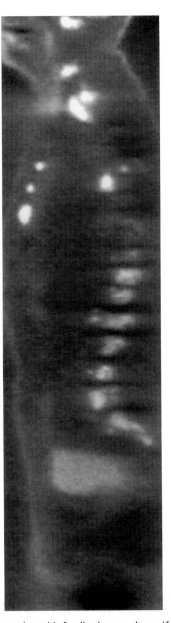

FIGURE 37.1. Hodgkin's disease. Multinodal, supradiaphragmal, and infradiaphragmal manifestations, with multifocal spleen and lymphomatous bone marrow infiltration.

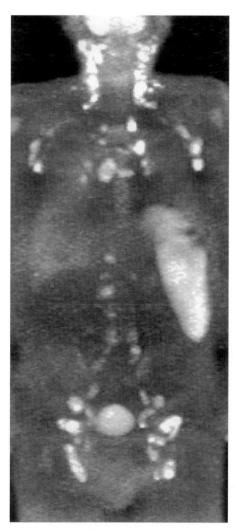

FIGURE 37.2. Low-grade non-Hodgkin's lymphoma. High fluorodeoxyglucose uptake in multinodal, supradiaphragmal, and infradiaphragmal manifestations, with diffuse spleen infiltration and splenic infarction.

STAGING LYMPHOMA

A pilot study evaluating FDG-PET for staging in 16 patients was published by Newman et al. in 1994 (11). These authors described excellent accuracy of FDG-PET for thoracoabdominal lymphoma. All grades of NHL were successfully imaged. These results have been confirmed and extended by our group and by others. In 60 untreated patients (27 patients with HD, 33 patients with NHL), FDG-PET was more accurate for detecting nodal involvement compared with CT and resulted in changing the stage, with an impact in management for 10% to 15% of patients (7,8). Extranodal staging with FDG-PET was significantly superior to that with CT and resulted in changes of tumor stage in 13 of 81 patients (16%) (8). FDG-PET has a great potential for demonstrating bone marrow involvement (12,13). Besides confirming lesions found at

bone marrow biopsy, FDG-PET provided additional information in 8 of 78 patients (10.3%) that led to an upgrade of tumor stage. Bone marrow biopsy revealed marrow involvement not detected by FDG-PET in 5.1% of patients. In these patients, diffuse marrow infiltration with less than 10% content of malignant cells was present, precluding detection by PET (12). Excellent accuracy for both nodal and extranodal staging of malignant lymphoma has been confirmed in three studies (14–16), as well as in a prospective bicenter study (17). In a prospective study in 18 patients, Hoh and colleagues found an FDG-PET–based staging algorithm more accurate and cost effective than the conventional multimethod imaging approach (18).

PREDICTING TREATMENT RESPONSE

Early evaluation of treatment response and persisting residual masses after completion of therapy with morphologically based imaging techniques are well recognized problems in lymphoma management. Using a planar detection technique, Hoekstra et al. found a sharp reduction of FDG uptake within days after effective treatment before volume changes, whereas FDG uptake persisted in nonresponders (19). These data were confirmed by Römer and colleagues (20), who described a 60% to 67% reduction of FDG uptake and metabolic rate as early as 7 days after initiation of therapy in patients with NHL responding to chemotherapy. Patients who subsequently had a disease relapse displayed a significantly smaller reduction of FDG uptake assessed at 42 days after start of therapy (20).

EVALUATING RESIDUAL TUMOR VIABILITY

Assessment of the viability of residual lymphoma masses after completion of therapy has been studied by several groups (21–23) (Table 37.2). The negative predictive value of FDG-PET was high and predicted a complete response (Fig. 37.4). Persistent FDG uptake in residual masses and progressive tumors is a more ambiguous finding. It depends on the time of imaging after completion of therapy, the cutoff value used to define positivity, and the nonspecific, transient effects of chemotherapy. In approximately 10% of patients, symmetric, increased FDG uptake in cervical nodes has been observed temporarily. At present, 6 to 8 weeks after completion of therapy may be regarded as the appropriate imaging time interval to determine viability of residual masses.

In a series of 70 patients (29 with HD, 41 with NHL), Cremerius et al. found a higher sensitivity, specificity, and overall accuracy for PET in detecting residual disease compared with CT (22) (Table 37.2). FDG-PET predicted complete remission in more than 90% of patients with low

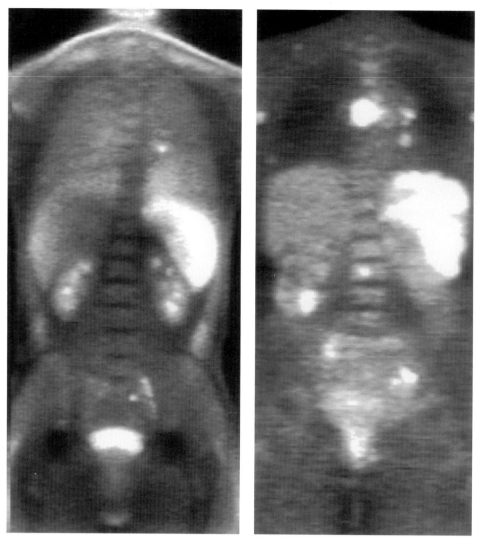

FIGURE 37.3. Hodgkin's disease. Intense progress without therapy at first diagnosis **(A)** and after 9 months **(B).**

TABLE 37.2. THERAPY MONITORING

Authors	Reference	No. Patients	Results
Jerusalem et al.	*Blood* 1999;94:429–433	54	PPV for relapse: PET 100%; CT 42%
Cremerius et al.	*Nucl Med Comm* 1998;19:1055–1063	27	Detection of active residual disease: sens. PET: 100%; CT 100%; spec. PET: 92%, CT 17%; PPV PET 94%, CT 60%; NPV PET 100%, CT 100%; accur. PET 96%, CT 63%
Cremerius et al.	*Nuklearmedizin* 1999;38:24–30	72	Detection of active residual disease: sens. PET 88%, CT 84%; spec. PET 83%, CT 31%; accur. PET 85%, CT 54%
Römer et al.	*Blood* 1998;12:4464–4471	11	Decrease of tumor FDG uptake at day 7 (60%) and 42 (further 42%) p.t. Predictive value of SUV for determining probability of relapse (all patients with SUV >2.5 at day 42 p.t. relapsed)
De Wit et al.	*Ann Oncol* 1997;8[Suppl]:S57–S60	34	Diagnosis of residual disease: sens. PET 100%, CT 86%; spec. PET 73%, CT 3.7%; PPV PET 57%, CT 19%; NPV PET 100%, CT 50%.

accur., accuracy; CT, computed tomography; FDG, fluorodeoxyglucose; NPV, negative predictive value; PGT, positron emission tomography; PPV, positive predictive value; p.t., post therapy; sens., sensitivity; spec., specificity; SUV, normalized dose over body weight.

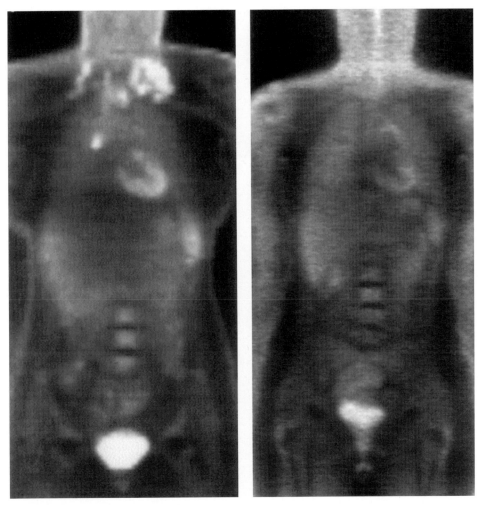

FIGURE 37.4. Hodgkin's disease. Positive therapy response 8 weeks after completion of radiochemotherapy.

or moderate risk. The negative predictive value in high-risk patients, however, was only 50% to 67%.

In summary, FDG-PET is an efficient, noninvasive method for the primary staging of untreated HD and NHL. Compared with standard imaging techniques, PET is significantly superior in detecting nodal and extranodal involvement as well as lymphomatous bone marrow involvement. FDG-PET is highly accurate in post-therapeutic differentiation of active residual disease and avital tumor masses.

REFERENCES

1. Diehl V, Engert A. An overview of the Second International Symposium on Hodgkin's Disease. *Ann Oncol* 1992;3[Suppl 4]: 1–3.
2. Paul R. Comparison of fluorine-18-2-fluorodeoxyglucose and gallium-67 citrate imaging for detection of lymphoma. *J Nucl Med* 1987;28:288–292.
3. Okada J, Yoshikawa K, Imazeki K, et al. The use of FDG-PET in the detection and management of malignant lymphoma: correlation of uptake with prognosis. *J Nucl Med* 1992;33:686–691.
4. Rodriguez M, Rehn S, Ahlström H, et al. Predicting malignancy grade with PET in non-Hodgkin's lymphoma. *J Nucl Med* 1995; 36:1790–1796.
5. Okada J, Yoshikawa K, Itami M, et al. Positron emission tomography using fluorine-18-fluorodeoxyglucosein malignant lymphoma: a comparison with proliferative activity. *J Nucl Med* 1992; 33:325–329.
6. Lapela M, Leskinen S, Minn HRI, et al. Increased glucose metabolism in untreated non-Hodgkin's lymphoma: a study with positron emission tomography and fluorine-18-fluorodeoxyglucose. *Blood* 1995;86:3522–3527.
7. Moog F, Bangerter M, Diederichs CG, et al. Lymphoma: role of whole-body 2-deoxy-2-[F-18]fluoro-D-glucose (FDG) PET in nodal staging. *Radiology* 1997;203:795–800.
8. Moog R, Bangerter M, Diederichs CG, et al. Extranodal malignant lymphoma: detection with FDG PET versus CT. *Radiology* 1998;206:475–481.
9. Leskinen-Kallio S, Ruotsalainen U, Nägren K, et al. Uptake of carbon-11-methionine and fluorodeoxyglucose in non-Hodgkin's lymphoma: a PET study. *J Nucl Med* 1991;32:1211–1218.

10. Minn H, Nuutila P, Lindholm P, et al. *In vivo* effects of insulin on tumor and skeletal muscle glucose metabolism in patients with lymphoma. *Cancer* 1994;73:1490–1498.

11. Newman JS, Francis IR, Kaminski MS, et al. Imaging of lymphoma with PET with 2-[F-18]-fluoro-2-deoxy-D-glucose: correlation with CT. *Radiology* 1994;190:111–116.

12. Moog R, Bangerter M, Kotzerke J, et al. 18-F-fluorodeoxyglucose-positron emission tomography as a new approach to detect lymphomatous bone marrow. *J Clin Oncol* 1998;16: 603–609.

13. Carr R, Barrington SF, Madan B, et al. Detection of lymphoma in bone marrow by whole-body positron emission tomography. *Blood* 1998;91:3340–3346.

14. Stumpe KDM, Urbinelli M, Steinert HC, et al. Whole-body positron emission tomography using fluorodeoxyglucose for staging of lymphoma: effectiveness and comparison with computed tomography. *Eur J Nucl Med* 1998;25:721–728.

15. Thill R, Neuerburg J, Fabry U, et al. Vergleich der Befunde von 18-FDG-PET und CT beim prätherapeutischen Staging maligner Lymphome. *Nuklearmedizin* 1997;36:234–239.

16. Bumann D, deWit M, Beyer W, et al. Computertomographie und F-18-FDG-Positronen-Emissions-Tomographie im Staging maligner Lymphome: ein Vergleich. *Fortschr Rontgenstr* 1998; 168:457–465.

17. Buchmann I, Reinhardt M, Schirrmeister H, et al. F-[18]-FDG-positron emission tomography (PET) for detection and staging of malignant lymphoma: a bi-center study. Submitted for publication.

18. Hoh CK, Glaspy J, Rosen P, et al. Whole-body FDG-PET imaging for staging of Hodgkin's disease and lymphoma. *J Nucl Med* 1997;38:343–348.

19. Hoekstra OS, Ossenkoppele GJ, Golding R, et al. Early treatment response in malignant lymphoma, as determined by planar fluorine-18-fluorodeoxyglucose scintigraphy. *J Nucl Med* 1993; 34:1706–1710.

20. Römer WR, Hanauske AR, Ziegler S, et al. Positron emission tomography in non-Hodgkin's lymphoma: assessment of chemotherapy with fluorodeoxyglucose. *Blood* 1998;91: 4464–4471.

21. deWit M, Bumann D, Beyer W, et al. Whole-body positron emission tomography (PET) for diagnosis of residual mass in patients with lymphoma. *Ann Oncol* 1997;8:57–60.

22. Cremerius U, Fabry U, Kröll U, et al. Klinische Wertigkeit der FDG-PET zur Therapiekontrolle bei malignen Lymphomen: Ergebnisse einer retrospektiven Studie an 72 Patienten. *Nuklearmedizin* 1999;38:24–30.

23. Bangerter M, Moog F, Griesshammer M, et al. Role of whole body FDG-PET imaging in predicting relapse of malignant lymphoma in patients with residual masses after treatment. *Radiography* 1999;5:155–163.

38

MONOCLONAL ANTIBODY THERAPY

RICHARD L. WAHL

TYPES OF HEMATOPOIETIC TUMORS AND CLINICAL NEED FOR NEW THERAPIES

Neoplasms arising from the hematopoietic system represent a diverse group of illnesses ranging from indolent lymphomas and chronic lymphocytic leukemia to the highly aggressive acute leukemias (1). Historically, lymphomas and leukemias were considered separate illnesses, with lymphomas localized to lymph nodes or soft tissues and leukemias associated with circulating tumor cells in the blood (2). However, the classification systems used to characterize hematopoietic tumors have undergone changes recently, so that in addition to schemes based purely on anatomic/pathologic features, schemes based on the origin of the malignant cells, such as the REAL (Revised European American Lymphoma) classification scheme, are used. In this scheme, the leukemias and the lymphomas overlap to a considerable degree (3). The classification schemes continue to evolve, but it is clear that despite progress in treatment, newer and more effective therapies are needed for these tumors. In the United States, non-Hodgkin's lymphoma is now the fifth most common cancer, and its socioeconomic effect is disproportionately large because of its tendency to affect patients in their peak wage-earning years (54,900 new cases and 26,100 deaths estimated for 2000) (4). The types of hematopoietic tumors are shown in Table 38.1.

Hematopoietic tumors differ from solid tumors, such as adenocarcinomas, in several ways that make them more amenable to radioimmunotherapy (RIT). They are generally not localized to a single focus at presentation and are more sensitive to radiation and chemotherapy than solid tumors. In addition, they express unique, lineage-specific surface markers more often than solid tumors do, and because of their blood-borne nature, they are quite commonly more effectively targeted by systemic RIT. Thus, the effects of RIT have been greatest on this class of tumors to date (5).

POTENTIAL ANTIGEN TARGETS

The ideal tumor antigen would be expressed only on the tumor and not on normal tissues, would exhibit a high degree of molecular density on the cell surface, and would be firmly attached to the tumor cell, without shedding from the surface. It would also not be present in the circulation and could internalize, delivering radioactivity to the cell cytoplasm/lysosomes, and then recycle to the cell surface (or be stably attached to the cell surface).

The "ideal" antigen has yet to be identified for hematopoietic neoplasms, so we deal with antigenic targets that are less than ideal but still useful. The non-Hodgkin's lymphomas are somewhat unique in that tumor-specific antigens do exist. For B-cell neoplasms, they are the surface immunoglobulins present on the B cells that have transformed into lymphoma. The antigen combining site on this antibody present on the malignant B-cell surface is known as the antibody "idiotype," and monoclonal antibodies can be prepared that are specifically reactive with the idiotype. These "anti-idiotype" antibodies are, in some instances, totally specific for the lymphoma (6,7). The disadvantage of using anti-idiotype antibodies for RIT is that in many instances, it is necessary to construct a patient-specific antibody to a patient-specific idiotype. This means that a unique radiopharmaceutical has to be constructed for each patient, which is prohibitively expensive for routine therapy and has been difficult to put into practice. Although some idiotypes are shared among different lymphomas (public idiotypes), anti-idiotype approaches to therapy will probably not be as useful as had been hoped initially. Another disadvantage of idiotype antigens is that the antibody molecules on the B-cell surface (which constitute the idiotype) are commonly shed into the circulation. Thus, high levels of idiotype are often present in the circulation and can interfere with the binding of intravenously administered radiolabeled antibody to idiotype on the B cell and so potentially prevent the radioantibody from reaching the tumor (8). Further, because many idiotype antibodies are secreted, they may not represent a firm target for antibody binding to tumor cells. The radioantibody could fall off

R. L. **Wahl:** Departments of Internal Medicine and Radiology, University of Michigan, Ann Arbor, Michigan 48109.

TABLE 38.1. TYPES OF LYMPHOMAS (WORKING FORMULATION)

Low-grade	Intermediate-grade	High-grade

Small lymphocytic consistent with CLL
Plasmacytoid
Follicular, predominantly small cleaved cell
	Follicular, large cell
	Diffuse, small cleaved cell
	Diffuse, mixed small and large cell
		Large cell immunoblastic
		Lymphoblastic
		Small noncleaved cell
		  Burkitt's
		  Non-Burkitt's

Follicular, mixed small cleaved and large cell	Diffuse, large cell	

SIMPLIFIED REVISED EUROPEAN AMERICAN LYMPHOMA (REAL) CLASSIFICATION OF HEMATOPOIETIC NEOPLASMS

B-cell neoplasms	T-cell and putative NK-cell neoplasms
Precursor B-cell neoplasm: precursor B-lymphoblastic leukemia/lymphoma Peripheral B-cell neoplasms	Precursor T-cell neoplasm: precursor T-lymphoblastic lymphoma/leukemia Peripheral T-cell and NK cell neoplasms

CLL, chronic lymphoblastic leukemia; NK, natural killer.

after binding had occurred and irradiate nontarget cells. Thus, although idiotype targets have been used, in practice, less tumor-specific reagents have been more useful for RIT.

Lymphocyte differentiation markers have more commonly been used as targeted antigens in RIT studies of lymphoma to date (9). Because a normal ontogeny of B- and T-cell development from marrow stem cells to mature B- and T-cells exists, a variety of antigens are expressed at varying stages of development. These antigens are not tumor-specific but are generally B cell- or T cell-specific. As an example, T-cell leukemias or lymphomas generally have T-cell markers on their surfaces, whereas B-cell lymphomas often have normal B-cell markers (hence their designation as T- or B-cell neoplasms). These can be antigens that modulate or internalize, or they can be antigens that are fixed on the cell surface.

The choice of antigen for RIT is extremely important, and especially so if an antigen that cross-reacts with normal cells is used. In general, it is better to select an antigen that is not expressed on stem cells unless transplant support is considered. Although potentially ablating the tumor and normal T- or B-cell populations might not seem rational at first, if the T- or B-cell markers are not expressed on the most primitive cells in the marrow (the progenitor cells), it may be possible to target for destruction a population of both malignant and benign cells, with the antigen-negative progenitor cells for the normal tissues remaining unaltered by treatment. Thus, the potential for replenishment of normal tissues, with destruction of the malignant clones, exists through the appropriate choice of differentiation antigen. Antigens that are expressed on normal tissues and normal progenitor cells would represent far poorer choices, unless a means for replenishing the normal progenitor cells were in place (e.g., stem cell or marrow transplants). This approach, however, may be highly desirable in efforts to eradicate the marrow completely, such as when RIT is a planned component of marrow ablation therapy for leukemia (10).

A list of antigenic targets that have been at least partially explored in serotherapy and RIT appears in Table 38.2. Several factors need to be considered in regard to the choice of antigen for RIT, in addition to tissue specificity and expression in the circulation or on circulating cells. One of these is antigenic density, or number of antigen molecules per cell. Obviously, the ratio of antigen on malignant cells to antigen on normal cells is important; however, the number of antigenic targets is also of key importance. An antigen that is quite tumor-specific, but present in low quantities, is likely to be a poor choice for RIT, as it may simply be too scarce for successful targeting based on the known kinetics of antigen binding. Thus, both specificity and adequate antigen expression are important. Additional considerations are whether the antigen in stably expressed on the cell surface, and whether it is shed from the tumor cells or internalized into the tumor cells after antibody binding. Antigens that are shed rapidly from the cell into the circulation are not good targets, as the label is lost. Antigens that are stably attached are attractive, but antigens that internalize and then reappear on the cell surface are also attractive if paired with the appropriate antibody/radiolabel complex. A radiolabel that residualizes within the cell is much more likely to be effective than one that is rapidly lost, at least for internalizing antigens. This area is of investigation is still evolving, but in general, radiometals such as ^{90}Y residualize in cells, whereas most iodine preparations do not after antibody and antigen internalization.

Certain antigens are not tumor-specific but appear to be preferentially expressed in lymphomas. An example is the transferrin receptor, which is overexpressed in Hodgkin's lymphomas. Similarly, ferritin, an intracellular protein, is overexpressed in lymphomas. Radiolabeled anti-ferritin antibodies have been used to target this protein. To date, the best results with RIT have been obtained with antigens that are cell line-specific but not tumor-specific. The choice of antigenic targets in hematopoietic tumors is large and has

TABLE 38.2. ANTIGENIC TARGETS FOR IMMUNOTHERAPY OF LYMPHOMAS

Antigen	Expression on B-cell lymphoma	Endocytosis	Comments
Idiotypic immunoglobulin	>95%	++	Tumor-specific. Circulating serum idiotype problematic.
HLA class II	>95%	+	Also on monocytes, macrophages, some epithelial cells, and myeloid precursors.
CD5	T-cell lymphoma	+	Also on B-CLL, thymocytes.
CD19	>95%	++	Internalized.
CD20	>95%	no	Is not shed or internalized.
CD21	≥50%	+	Is a receptor for the C3d complement fragment and for Epstein-Barr virus.
CD22	≥70%	++	Also known as BL-CAM. Variable expression.
CD37	≥90%	+	Low expression on some T cells and myeloid cells.
CD40	>90%	+	Also on some epithelial cells, carcinomas, and dendritic cells.
CD45	>99%	no	Also known as leukocyte common antigen. Expressed on all nucleated hematopoietic cells.
Ferritin	expressed in HD	intracellular	

CLL, chronic lymphoblastic leukemia; HD, Hodgkin's disease.
++, rapid endocytosis; +, moderate endocytosis; no, no endocytosis.
From Press OW, Appelbaum FR, Eary JF, et al. Radiolabeled antibody therapy of lymphomas.
Important Adv Oncol 1995;157–171.

been partly, but not fully, explored. To date, the most advanced RIT agents are based on the CD20 antigen, which is a nonglycosylated 33- to 37-kd phosphoprotein involved in B-cell signaling. This antigen is not rapidly internalized, nor does it modulate, so it is a good target for either iodinated or radiometal-labeled antibodies. It also has other interesting characteristics, such as the ability to induce apoptosis if extensive cross-linking of CD20 with anti-mouse antibody or Fc receptor-expressing cells occurs. This indicates that immunologic effects in addition to direct effects of radiation delivery may be at work in RIT (Table 38.2). Much remains to be learned about what constitutes the optimal choice of radioantibody for RIT of hematopoietic neoplasms.

CHOICE OF ANTIBODY

The traditional monoclonal antibody for RIT has been a purely murine antibody. Indeed, the most advanced RIT therapeutic agents, such as ^{131}I-anti-CD20 (^{131}I-tositumomab) and ^{90}Y-anti-CD20 (ibritumomab tiuxetan), are murine antibodies, at least the radiolabeled portion is. However, with the use of recombinant DNA techniques, it has been possible to create partially humanized, or chimeric, monoclonal antibodies (in which the murine variable regions remain but the rest of the antibody has been replaced by a human constant region), or fully humanized antibodies (in which only the murine complementarity determining regions are present on a human framework). It might seem "obvious" that a fully human antibody would be "best" for RIT, but this remains an open issue that has barely been studied. The simple murine antibodies have been quite effective in RIT to date and have caused surpris-

ingly few HAMA (human anti-mouse antibody) responses in several series in which pretreatment of patients was considerable. In addition, murine antibodies typically would be expected to have shorter half-lives than humanized antibodies. This could be advantageous in some settings, as background activity in the blood pool would clear more rapidly. Chimeric or humanized antibodies might be expected to recruit more immunologic effector cells, which should prove useful in tumor killing, but the recruitment of these cells could also result in increased toxicity because of immunologic reactions.

Another issue is whether IgG or other species of immunoglobulin should be used. In general, intact IgG antibodies have been used. IgM potentially could also be used, although most IgM antibodies have a lower affinity than IgG antibodies. Further at issue is whether antibody fragments represent a more rational choice. In general, antibody fragments are cleared more rapidly from the body via the kidneys than intact antibodies, and fast clearance can result in higher tumor-to-background ratios than are obtained with intact reagents (indeed, the lower molecular weight of the fragments enables them to permeate the tumor cells more easily). Little has been done in terms of treating patients with radiolabeled antibody fragments, however; the high radiation dose to the kidneys may be a relative limitation to successful treatment (11).

It has not been determined whether direct radiolabeling of the antibody is the optimal approach. To design an antibody that is both the specific delivery vehicle and the carrier of radioactivity is a difficult challenge. One alternative approach, not yet used extensively in lymphoma RIT, is to "pretarget" a nonradiolabeled antibody (with a chemical binding site such as streptavidin) to the tumor, allow specific localization, and then administer a lower-molecular-weight radiolabeled species, such as biotin, as the therapeutic. More effective delivery of radioactivity can be achieved in many instances than with direct radioantibody targeting, but a number of challenging logistic issues are associated with this approach (12).

At present, the most common delivery vehicle for RIT is an intact antibody, generally murine, with a radiolabel directly attached. This may change in the future, however, as new treatments emerge.

CHOICE OF RADIOISOTOPE

A variety of radioactive labels have been used for RIT of hematopoietic malignancies and malignancies in general. Radioisotopes can be characterized as pure beta emitters, mixed beta and gamma emitters, alpha emitters, and auger emitters. The vast majority of treatments to date have been carried out with beta emitters, either with or without a gamma emission. More recently, the application of alpha emitters has increased.

The choice of radioisotope depends on several factors. Many potentially promising therapeutic isotopes are not readily available, which limits the realistic choices of emitters to only a few, most commonly the mixed beta and gamma emitter ^{131}I or the pure beta emitter ^{90}Y. However, several factors must be considered before a therapeutic isotope is chosen:

The antigen is a key consideration. Antigens that are rapidly internalized following antibody binding generally deliver the radioactive isotope to the lysosomes of the cell. In the lysosomes, the antibody is catabolized and small fragments of the antibody are released. Isotopes like ^{131}I are generally released from the cells and lost to the circulation in such circumstance (if a standard tyrosine labeling was performed), which generally results in only a low radiation dose to tumor. By contrast, radiometals such as ^{90}Y are much more likely to be retained inside the tumor cells and deliver continued radiation, despite internalization and metabolism (13). For antigens that do not internalize, isotopes like ^{131}I are a much more rational choice (as are radiometals), as they are unlikely to be rapidly lost or metabolized from the cell surface. A good example of this latter type of antigen would be CD20, which is not rapidly internalized, or antigens that are mainly extracellular.

Another consideration is the half-life of the therapeutic isotope. If the antibody localizes rapidly to the malignant cells, then a short half-life may be quite satisfactory. If the radioantibody localizes slowly to the malignant cells but then remains there a long time once binding has occurred, a longer half-life is far more appropriate for a maximal ratio of tumor-to-normal tissue uptake of the isotope to be achieved. If the radioisotope deposits most of its energy before it is accumulated into the tumor, then it is more likely to be toxic to hormonal than to tumor tissues. Some

short-lived therapeutic isotopes are best suited to treat blood-borne disease and disease involving the marrow, where antibody localization to tumor is rapid.

The degree of patient-to-patient variability in the handling of radioantibody is a further consideration. If radioantibody clears rapidly from one patient and slowly from another, then it may be delivering too much radiation dose to normal tissues in the patient with slow clearance and too little dose to the tumor in the patient with rapid clearance provided comparable doses of millicuries per kilogram are given (i.e., overdosing or underdosing is possible). Considerable variability in the rate of clearance of radioantibody has been seen in situations in which tumor-associated antigens are used as targets for treatment. If the dose to critical organs varies greatly from patient to patient, it may be that a safe dose will require that a large number of patients be underdosed unless patient-specific dosimetry is applied. If this is to be done, then adjustments for patient handling of the radioactivity can be made based on a tracer dose, or "treatment planning scan" (14,15). For treatment planning, in general a gamma emitter is required.

The prototype mixed beta and gamma emitter is ^{131}I, which has relatively low beta energy. This isotope can be imaged with use of the 364-keV gamma emission, but it also emits a beta particle that is responsible for most of the tumor radiation dose. ^{90}Y is another rather commonly used therapeutic agent. It is a radiometal and a pure beta emitter. It is not easy to use this agent for perform treatment planning. Rather, a substitute radiometal has been suggested for planning, specifically ^{111}In. ^{111}In is a gamma and Auger emitter and is a very good imaging agent. However, ^{90}Y and ^{111}In are not identical. Free ^{90}Y accumulates more rapidly in bone than free ^{111}In. Further, the stability of conjugation of ^{111}In to a chelating molecule may not be as good as that of ^{90}Y (or vice versa, depending on the chelate). Thus, although ^{111}In is a good surrogate for ^{90}Y behavior, the accumulation of ^{111}In and ^{90}Y in normal bone varies substantially, with ^{90}Y being more bone-avid than ^{111}In, and estimates of a bone marrow dose of ^{90}Y based on ^{111}In can be too low (16,17). Therefore, using the same isotope for tracer studies and for treatment has some potential advantages. It has been shown that several isotopes, such as ^{67}Cu and ^{90}Y, are not completely stably bound to antibodies by chelators. When radiometals are not stably bound, they become detached and accumulate in normal tissues, or they are excreted. The significance of free isotope is that less radioactivity reaches the tumor and more may reach normal tissues (18).

The energy of the particulate emission and its path length are quite important to the effectiveness of treatment and to the type of tumors that can be treated. High-energy beta particles are, in theory, better suited to killing large tumors, in which the heterogeneity of tracer distribution is considerable, whereas lower-energy beta particles are better suited to treat small tumors. Indeed, theoretical calculations have indicated that it is not possible to cure very small tumors with ^{90}Y, but it is possible with ^{131}I (19). However, some tumors are so small that neither ^{131}I nor ^{90}Y is predicted to be effective treatment based on purely radiobiologic considerations, as the energy would escape from the tumors following nuclear decay and not be retained. However, these same theoretical calculations suggest that it is impossible to treat larger tumors effectively with ^{131}I, which clearly is not completely true. Clinical studies of ^{131}I-anti-CD20 have shown that it is indeed possible to treat large lymphomas effectively with ^{131}I, possibly because tracer uptake therein is not particularly heterogeneous (18). Thus, the true relevance of the theoretical calculations in reality requires validation, but it is clear that particles with a short path length are more likely to be effective for treatment than those with a longer path length. Thus, ^{90}Y may be poorly suited to dealing with small tumor foci, whereas ^{131}I is better for this purpose. However, the ^{131}I beta emission may still be too energetic for small tumor foci, small clusters, or single cells on a theoretical basis. ^{186}Re and ^{188}Re are attractive as tracers as well as for cancer treatment. ^{188}Re has a rather short half-life that may not be ideally suited for treatment with intact antibodies but may be better suited for pretargeting approaches or antibody.

Thus, the use of particulate emissions with a very short path length (e.g., Auger emitters or alpha emitters) has been an area of interest. Most Auger emitters also have a significant component of gamma emission, but the very short path length of the Auger emission is well suited to treating small tumor foci. Examples of Auger emitters include ^{111}In and ^{125}I, neither of which has been significantly utilized in the treatment of hematopoietic neoplasms.

Alpha emitters kill in a short radius about the tumor cell, with path lengths of just a few cell diameters. Typical examples of alpha emitters include ^{211}At and ^{211}Bi or ^{213}Pb. Producing and working with these short-lived tracers are major challenges and further study is required, but this is an area of intense interest (20).

Thus, the choice of isotope for therapy depends on several important factors. It may be that a single isotope is not sufficient to deal with all sizes of tumor cells. Some of the isotopes that can be chosen for RIT are shown in Table 38.3.

CLINICAL RESULTS IN LYMPHOMA THERAPY

Hodgkin's Disease

Hodgkin's disease is much less common than non-Hodgkin's lymphoma and is often curable when radiotherapy is used for localized disease and chemotherapy for more extensive and advanced disease. However, recurrent Hodgkin's lymphoma is very challenging to treat, and radiolabeled antibodies have been used for this condition. Hodgkin's disease is somewhat unusual relative to other lymphomas in that the purported malignant cell (the Reed-Sternberg cell) represents only a small portion of the total cellular phenotype. This means that choosing the appropriate antigenic target to treat Hodgkin's disease is quite challenging. To date, RIT of Hodgkin's disease has been carried out with polyclonal antibodies reactive with ferritin, which is overexpressed in Hodgkin's disease. These antibodies have been labeled with either ^{131}I or ^{90}Y.

In Hodgkin's disease, Lenhard et al. (21) first used ^{131}I-labeled polyclonal anti-ferritin antibodies for human therapy. In 1985, they reported some clinical improvement in more than 75% of patients with refractory Hodgkin's lymphoma and objective tumor regression in 40% of patients. Herpst et al. (22) reported on their use of polyclonal ^{90}Y-anti-ferritin in the treatment of Hodgkin's disease; 44 patients were entered and 39 patients were treated. Polyclonal anti-ferritin antibodies of several species of origin were used in an attempt to avoid an immunologic response to the therapeutic antibodies. Doses ranged from 10 to 50 mCi of ^{90}Y, and injected doses ranged from 2 to 5 mg given over five cycles of therapy. Bone marrow transplant support was needed in patients receiving the higher doses of ^{90}Y. Among the 39 patients treated, 10 achieved complete response, 10 had a partial response, 2 had stable disease, and 17 had progression (22). Substantial variability in pharmacokinetics was noted. About half the patients survived the therapy for longer than 6 months. It was rare for a complete response to be achieved after a single anti-ferritin treatment; however, complete responses occurred more commonly after two to three treatments (9 of 10 patients). The average tumor dose was 900 rad, indicating the

TABLE 38.3. SELECTED ISOTOPES FOR RADIOIMMUNOTHERAPY

Radioactive isotope	$t_{1/2}$	Energy (MeV), maximum	Energy (MeV), mean	Range in H_2O (mm), mean
^{131}I	8.02 d	0.61	0.19	0.4
^{90}Y	2.67 d	2.28	0.93	2.76
^{177}Lu	6.7 d	0.497	0.133	0.28
^{67}Cu	2.58 d	0.57	0.19 (20%) 0.154 (22%)	0.27
^{186}Re	3.7 d	1.08	0.349	0.92
^{188}Re	0.7 d	2.12	0.80 (72%)	2.4
^{211}At (α)	0.3 d	5.8, 7.5	—	0.4–0.8
^{212}Bi (α)	45.6 min	6.09	—	0.4–0.8

achievement of only modest tumor targeting but also the considerable radiosensitivity of this type of tumor.

In a study in which a higher dose of ^{90}Y polyclonal anti-ferritin was given, treatment with radiolabeled antibody and high-dose chemotherapy were followed by transplant in patients with Hodgkin's lymphoma and a poor prognosis (23). The ^{90}Y-anti-ferritin was administered to 12 patients 1 to 2 weeks before transplantation (with an intention to treat 14 patients), followed by high-dose chemotherapy and bone marrow transplantation. Tumor responses were reported and four patients survived for more than 2 years, but four deaths were related to the aggressive therapeutic regimen. This study indicates the potential of the method, even in patients with tumors refractory to chemotherapy, but also indicates the risks of the bone marrow transplant approach practiced at that time. It should be noted that transplant results are improving for most diseases (23).

A recent follow-up report on RIT of Hodgkin's lymphoma reviewed the results of administration of ^{90}Y-labeled polyclonal rabbit anti-human ferritin IgG in 90 patients with recurrent Hodgkin's disease. Fifty-seven patients were given a single (unfractionated) administration per treatment cycle; 11 of them received 0.3 mCi/kg of body weight, 39 received 0.4 mCi/kg of body weight, and 7 received 0.5 mCi/kg of body weight per treatment cycle. For 33 patients, the administration of radiolabeled immunoglobulin was separated (fractionated), and 0.25 mCi/kg body weight was given twice (total activity, 0.5 mCi/kg). The interval between fractions was 1 week. Radioimmunoconjugates did not cause serious acute side effects. Human anti-rabbit IgG antibodies were found in 2 of 50 re-treated patients (< 5%). Hematologic toxicity was the only side effect noted in all patients, and it was usually temporary. Response rates were 20%, 61%, and 86% after administration of 0.3, 0.4, or 0.5 mCi of unfractionated ^{90}Y-labeled anti-ferritin per kilogram, respectively. The response rate for patients treated with fractionated RIT was 42%. In the fractionated RIT group, complete responses were decreased and progressive disease increased ($p < .05$). Complete responses had a median duration of 6 months. Median survival times were 390 days for the group given 0.4 mCi/kg once and 300 days for the group given 0.25 mCi/kg twice. Thus, "fractionation" did not improve the outcome of RIT in these patients, although even the "unfractionated" group still received a sort of "fractionation" versus standard therapy (24,25).

Progress has been made in the treatment of Hodgkin's disease with RIT. However, to date, the use of polyclonal rather than monoclonal antibodies and the relatively small number of patients affected have slowed the commercial development of therapeutic reagents for this condition.

T-cell Lymphoma

Although this type of Non-Hodgkin's lymphoma is considerably less common than B-cell lymphoma in the United States, in some parts of the world it is, in fact, more common than B-cell lymphoma. Several well-defined targets on the surface of T-cell lymphomas have been used to treat this disease.

In some of the first clinical trials of RIT in lymphoma, the T101 (anti-CD5) murine monoclonal antibody labeled with ^{131}I was used. In the initial report by Rosen et al. (26), six patients with cutaneous T-cell lymphoma were imaged with T101 labeled with ^{131}I. Initially, a tracer dose of about 10 mg and 5.6 to 13.1 mCi was given. Then, a therapeutic dose of 100.5 to 150.1 mCi was given. Five patients received the radioimmunotherapeutic dose with this reagent and all responded, albeit briefly, with a reduction in pruritus and shrinkage of nodes and cutaneous lesions. Unfortunately, responses were quite brief, lasting 3 weeks to 3 months, and HAMA responses were common. The primary toxicity was hematopoietic, with marrow suppression developing at the highest administered doses. This group reported that in three patients with HAMA, plasmapheresis could be performed to reduce HAMA titers and allow the tracer dose and therapeutic doses to be given, with subsequent brief tumor responses in two of three patients (27). Patients with circulating antigen-positive cells and clinical leukemia did not have the same level of response that was reported by Zimmer et al. in 1988 (27). However, the high rate of HAMA and the brief responses offered hope, but not a probable major effect, for this disease, at least with the use of nonmyeloablative doses of RIT.

Waldmann et al. used ^{90}Y-labeled anti-Tac antibody to treat a small number of patients with acute T-cell leukemia/lymphoma (16). This reagent binds to the interleukin 2R-alpha antigen. Patients were treated with between 5 and 10 mCi of ^{90}Y antibody. Myelosuppression was seen at these small doses, and a modest antitumor response was noted. A follow-up study of the use of this reagent was reported by Waldmann et al., in which 10 patients with advanced or refractory CD5-expressing hematologic neoplasms (two with chronic lymphocytic leukemia and eight with cutaneous T-cell lymphoma) were treated in a phase I study with the radioimmunoconjugate ^{90}Y-T101. Prior imaging studies with ^{111}In-T101 demonstrated uptake in involved lymph nodes and skin in patients with cutaneous T-cell lymphoma, and phase I studies with unmodified T101 demonstrated transient responses. In this study, patients were treated with 5 or 10 mCi of ^{90}Y chelated to T101 via isothiocyanatobenzyl diethylenetriamine pentaacetic acid (DTPA), along with tracer doses of ^{111}In-T101 for imaging. The biodistribution of the radioimmunoconjugate was determined by measuring blood clearance, urine excretion, and accumulation in bone marrow and involved skin lesions of ^{90}Y and ^{111}In. The intravascular pharmacokinetics of ^{90}Y were quite well predicted by ^{111}In-T101. The greatest differences in biodistribution between ^{111}In and ^{90}Y were the higher rate of accumulation of ^{90}Y in bone and the lower rate of excretion in urine. Imaging studies demonstrated targeting of skin lesions and involved lymph nodes in patients with cutaneous T-cell lymphoma. The predominant toxicity was bone marrow suppression. Rapid antigenic modulation of CD5 on circulating T and B cells was observed. Recovery of T-cell populations occurred within 2 to 3 weeks; however, suppression of B-cell populations persisted after more than 5 weeks. HAMA developed in all patients with cutaneous T-cell lymphoma after one cycle, so they were not retreated; one patient with chronic lymphocytic leukemia received a second cycle of therapy. Partial responses occurred in five patients, two with chronic lymphocytic leukemia and three with cutaneous T-cell lymphoma. The median duration of response was 23 weeks. One patient with cutaneous T-cell lymphoma who subsequently received electron beam irradiation to a residual lesion is disease-free after 6 years (28).

These data indicate that it is possible to treat T-cell lymphoma (and leukemia) with ^{90}Y-anti-Tac and ^{131}I-T101 (anti-CD5) but suggest that long-term responses with the use of nonmyeloablative regimens are improbable. Much less work has been done in T-cell than B-cell lymphoma, however, and the development of commercial antibody therapies for this illness has not progressed rapidly.

B-cell Lymphoma

Lymphomas of B-cell lineage are the most common type of lymphoma in the United States. Both B cell-specific (idiotype) and B-cell lineage-related antigens have been used as therapeutic targets for RIT in this disease. In the recent past, unlabeled anti-CD20 has been approved by the Food and Drug Administration to treat types of B-cell non-Hodgkin's lymphoma. This form of therapy has become quite popular, and immunotherapy has become firmly implanted as one of the accepted forms of treatment of this illness. Although immunotherapy is an active treatment method and anti-CD20 cross-linking can cause apoptosis, complete responses are quite infrequent, at fewer than 10% of cases (28). Thus, additional forms of treatment, such as RIT, are needed. It should be noted, however, that because the antibodies themselves may have some activity in treatment of this disease, the radioactive component is an additional, incremental, and important mode of supplemental treatment. The process of cell killing is appropriately considered, in many instances, to be both "radiotherapy" and "immunotherapy."

Radioimmunotherapy of non-Hodgkin's lymphoma can be marrow-ablative or not. In marrow-ablative treatment, which involves very high doses of radioactivity, the lethally damaged marrow must be reconstituted following RIT with stored marrow or stem cells. In this aggressive form of therapy, the maximum possible radiation dose is delivered to the tumor, but at the cost of increased toxicity and possible complications. More often used, to date, have been treatment algorithms in which lower doses of radioactivity are given, so that the marrow may be reversibly damaged but not destroyed–an approach that is safer, but possibly less effective, than myeloablative treatment.

Several groups have investigated the treatment of non-Hodgkin's lymphoma with nonmyeloablative methods. As early as 1995, Lewis et al. (29) reported treating a patient with the ^{131}I-LYM-1 monoclonal antibody (anti-HLA-DR). The patient had a substantial clinical response and survived 2 years after treatment. This group recently summarized, in their "low-dose fractionated phase I/II study," 52 courses of RIT with doses ranging from 10 to 100 mCi per cycle in patients with recurrent non-Hodgkin's lymphoma. A complete response was achieved in two patients and a partial response in 10 patients. Results suggested that response rates were greater (94%) in patients who received greater total millicurie doses (> 180 mCi). They also pointed out that unlabeled antibody was not effective in patients, so that ^{131}I-LYM-1 was an essential component in the process (29,30).

Using higher doses of radioactivity (from 40 to 100 mCi/m^2) at 4-week intervals, DeNardo et al. (31) observed seven complete responses and four partial responses. Because 21 patients were evaluated with a higher dose, this equated to a complete response rate of 33% and a partial response rate of 21%. They observed, as have others, that tumor responses are rapid and complete when higher doses of radioactivity are administered. This experience has recently been updated, and the reagent remains under clinical development as a therapeutic agent for non-Hodgkin's lymphoma (31). LYM-1 has also been labeled with ^{67}Cu as a therapeutic. ^{67}Cu is not widely available. The energy level of its beta emission is similar to that of ^{131}I, but its photon emission is less energetic and more easily imaged. Its chelation to antibodies is less than perfect, and loss of ^{67}Cu from triethylenetetraamine (TETA) conjugates has been reported. Despite the challenges in attaching ^{67}Cu stably to antibodies and the difficulties in obtaining the radiopharmaceutical, it has been used in therapeutic studies in a limited number of patients with the LYM-1 antibody. This experience was recently updated. Up to four doses of ^{67}Cu-2IT-BAT-LYM-1, either 25 or 50 to 60 mCi/m^2 per dose (either 0.93 or 1.85 to 2.22 GBq/m^2 per dose, respectively) were administered to patients with non-Hodgkin's lymphoma who had failed chemotherapy. The lower dose was used if evidence of non-Hodgkin's lymphoma was found in the bone marrow. ^{67}Cu-2IT-BAT-LYM-1 allowed satisfactory imaging of non-Hodgkin's lymphoma, and a response rate of 58% was noted in the patients treated. Nonetheless, unless availability of ^{67}Cu improves markedly, it is improbable that ^{67}Cu will be widely used as a therapeutic isotope to treat non-Hodgkin's lymphoma (18).

As discussed earlier, lymphomas are unique in having legitimate, tumor-specific antigens on the cell surface, these being the surface immunoglobulin expressed by the malignant B cells. Anti-idiotype antibodies can be produced that are reactive with these antigenic determinants and targeted with radiolabeled antibody. Investigators at USCD evaluated the use of ^{90}Y-labeled anti-idiotype antibody RIT in nine patients with relapsed B-cell lymphoma (8). Initial tracer targeting was with ^{111}In-labeled anti-idiotype antibody, which was given after administration of 1,000 to 2,320 mg of unlabeled monoclonal antibody in an attempt to clear idiotype from the circulation. One to four courses of treatment per patient were given; the total dose was 10 to 54 mCi of ^{90}Y-labeled antibody per patient. Activity was seen against the lymphomas, with 2 of 9 patients having a complete response, 1 a partial response, 3 stable disease, and 3 progressive disease. Time to tumor progression varied from 1 to 12 months. As with other radioimmunotherapies, toxicity was predominantly hematologic, and the need for transfusion support was common. HAMA was not observed in these patients. The investigators felt the variable that best correlated with success or failure of treatment was the ability to clear the circulating idiotype from the blood with unlabeled anti-idiotype antibody. When this clearance could not be achieved, successful tumor targeting and tumor therapy were unlikely. Although the method is logistically challenging and probably not practical because of the difficulties involved in producing patient-specific radiopharmaceuticals, this study indicates that RIT of non-Hodgkin's lymphoma is possible with the use of anti-idiotype antibodies labeled with [90]Y (8). However, results with the anti-pan B-cell reagents appear superior and are logistically much easier, so that this form of treatment will likely not be widely implemented in the foreseeable future.

The anti-CD37-pan B-cell monoclonal antibody MB1 was assessed in a dose-escalation trial in patients with non-Hodgkin's lymphoma (32). Escalation of the radiation dose was based on the estimated dose in centigray to the whole body based on tracer studies in which labeled antibody was used, as opposed to escalation of the dose based on millicuries or millicuries per square meter. This was done so that the expected differences in radiation dose among patients could be dealt with. Because the CD37 antigen is found on normal and malignant B cells, it seemed likely that some variability in whole-body dosimetry would be seen, hence the need for dose adjustments. Of the 12 patients studied, 8 had intermediate- or high-grade lymphomas, 7 of which were transformed, and 4 had low-grade lymphomas. All patients had been heavily pretreated with chemotherapy, and one had undergone a bone marrow transplant. ^{131}I-MB1 antibody was given at protein doses of 40 or 200 mg. Tumor targeting was not optimal, with only 39% of lesions detectable. Acute toxicity was modest. Rapid declines in serum B cells were seen, with delayed toxicity, mainly myelosuppression, especially thrombocytopenia. HAMA developed in two patients. The maximum tolerated dose was somewhat less than 50 cGy to the total body. Six patients had tumor responses after RIT. Four responses

lasted longer than 1 month (2 to 6 months) and included a complete response, a partial response, a minor response, and a mixed response. Tumor dosimetry showed that a mean of 2.77 cGy/mCi reached the tumor, versus 0.37 cGy/mCi for the whole body. Thus, selective tumor targeting of about sevenfold to eightfold was identified for the MB1 antibody. Based on these data, ^{131}I-MB1, although it showed antitumor activity at these protein and radiation doses, was judged not to be optimal for nonmyeloablative treatment.

[131]I-labeled OKB7 monoclonal antibody (murine anti-CD21 monoclonal antibody) was used to treat patients with non-Hodgkin's lymphoma in a phase I trial in which dose escalation was based on escalating millicurie doses. Repeated 30- to 50-mCi doses of ^{131}I-OK-B7 (25 mg) were administered several days apart to achieve total cumulative doses of between 90 and 200 mCi (targets of 90, 120, 160, and 200 mCi). Targeting to tumor on gamma scans was observed in 8 of 18 patients, and HAMA responses were frequent, occurring in 12 of 16 patients. As in the MB1 study, significant nonhematologic toxicity was rare, and in this study, evidence of an increased level of thyroid-stimulating hormone was limited to asymptomatic hypothyroidism. Bone marrow toxicity or myelosuppression was observed in one third of patients. One partial response among 18 patients and 12 mixed responses were identified, with responses seeming more frequent in the patients who received higher millicurie doses. The maximally tolerated cumulative dose was felt to be approximately 200 mCi when doses were divided into 50-mCi aliquots and given sequentially, as described above. ^{131}I-OK-B7 does not appear promising, at least at these dose levels, as a therapeutic agent for non-Hodgkin's lymphoma (33).

Investigators at the University of Michigan first reported clinical results with the ^{131}I-CD20 IgG2a murine monoclonal antibody anti-B1 (^{131}I-tositumomab, or Bexxar) in 1993 in nine patients, and in a follow-up article in 1996 in a total of 34 patients (34). In this study, adults with non-Hodgkin's B-cell lymphoma that was CD20-positive and who had failed at least one prior chemotherapy regimen were enrolled. Patients also had to have assessable and measurable disease by either physical examination or computed tomography and less than 25% of the marrow space involved by lymphoma cells. In addition, they had to have nearly normal organ function. The trial was conducted with sequential gamma camera imaging and sequential conjugate counting to assess radioactivity in the body with a sodium iodide probe. ^{131}I-anti-B1 is a ^{131}I-labeled mouse IgG2a monoclonal antibody. Patients were first given a 15- to 20-mg (5-mCi) tracer dose of ^{131}I-labeled anti-B1 to assess antibody biodistribution and whole-body and organ dosimetry. Generally, 1 week after the tracer dose, a radioimmunotherapeutic dose was administered consisting of about the same mass of protein labeled with the quantity of ^{131}I that would deliver a specified radiation dose to the whole body as determined by the tracer dose. Dose escalation, which was in groups of three to four patients, began at 25 cGy to the total body and was escalated to 85 cGy to the total body. To determine if radiolabeled antibody biodistribution could be optimized by changing the amount of unlabeled antibody predose, as had been shown in preclinical studies, some of the earlier patients in the study were given one or two additional tracer infusions on sequential weeks. Each dose was preceded by an infusion of either 95 mg of unlabeled anti-B1 or 450 mg of unlabeled anti-B1. The antibody dose resulting in the best biodistribution of tracer was chosen for therapy. Later patients were given a single tracer dose immediately after an unlabeled antibody infusion of 450 mg.

As in the other trials with ^{131}I-labeled monoclonal antibodies to B-cell antigens, acute toxicity was modest and mainly immunologic, and hematologic toxicity was dose-limiting. In this study, 75 cGy was established as the "maximally tolerated" radiation dose to the whole body (10). Of the 34 patients, 28 received RIT in doses ranging from 34 to 161 mCi. Fourteen patients had a complete response and eight patients had a partial response. Thirteen patients with low-grade lymphoma responded, with 10 achieving complete response. Six of eight patients with transformed lymphoma responded. Responses were noted in 13 of 19 patients whose disease had been resistant to their last course of chemotherapy and in all patients whose disease had responded to chemotherapy immediately before RIT. Patients with large tumor burdens and splenomegaly responded quite well to the treatment. Bone marrow toxicity was dose-limiting and depended on the total-body dose of radiation, but none of the patients required a bone marrow infusion for hematopoietic support. Thrombocytopenia appeared to be more marked in patients with prior bone marrow transplantation. The total-body dose of 75 cGy was established as the maximum tolerated dose in patients who had not had prior bone marrow transplantation.

This 34-patient experience was updated recently. The median duration of all responses was 357 days, and the median duration of complete responses was 471 days, with four complete responses lasting more than 1,000 days (maximum was 1,460 days). The duration of complete response was significantly longer ($p < .04$) in patients who received a total-body dose of 65 to 75 cGy (1,109 days) than in those who received a lower total-body dose of 25 to 60 cGy (385 days). Detectable HAMA levels developed in 4 of 34 (12%) patients. The median survival from study entry for all patients was 1,508 days (range, 63 to > 2,226 days), and 16 of 17 patients who achieved a response that lasted 6 months or longer remain alive (35).

This 34-patient phase I experience has been expanded to a 59-patient phase I/II single-center study and a phase II study for dosimetry validation; a phase III study has now been completed. Full reports of these studies are in press or in preparation, but a summary of the expanded ^{131}I-anti-CD20 experience in the treatment of low-grade and transformed low-grade non-Hodgkin's lymphoma was recently presented in abstract form to the European Association of Nuclear Medicine by Bhatnager et al. (36). Data from 131 patients across studies were examined, all with refractory or relapsed disease that was treated with a 65- to 75-cGy total-body dose of ^{131}I-anti-CD20. Of the 131 patients, 83 (63%) responded, and 30 (23%) had a complete response to the treatment. No correlation was found between the millicurie dose administered per kilogram and the treatment response in this group.

Recent preliminary reports have shown that this form of RIT can be given successfully as an initial treatment for non-Hodgkin's lymphoma. This area is still under study, but obviously, using the agent as initial treatment would be a great change in the paradigm for the treatment of non-Hodgkin's lymphoma. In studies at the University of Michigan, Kaminski et al. (37) showed a very high response rate, approaching 100%, in such patients, with treatment of 34 patients reported. In a follow-up study, in which ^{131}I-anti-B1 therapy was given after chemotherapy (flutarabine), Leonard and colleagues (38), at the New York Hospital, showed that very high rates of response can be induced (93%). HAMA responses were very infrequent, seemingly less frequent than when no chemotherapy was given, based on a study of 38 patients, 14 of whom were evaluated for treatment response. This broader experience supports the safety and efficacy of this approach, which is now under consideration for approval as a therapeutic agent in the United States.

The feasibility of using iodinated chimeric (human/mouse) anti-CD20 has been demonstrated in cancer treatment also. Behr et al. (39) have shown evidence of tumor targeting and anti-tumor activity with such an agent in preliminary studies. CD20 is also attractive for "pretargeting" studies with radioantibodies. Breitz et al. (40) have shown that it is feasible to target non-Hodgkin's lymphoma with use of the biotin–streptavidin anti-CD20 approach for initial targeting, followed by treatment with ^{90}Y-biotin, in several patients. Dosimetry with this approach has been encouraging and may be superior to that of standard targeting approaches, but this is early in evaluation.

In summary, ^{131}I-anti-B1 administered based on tracer study kinetics is capable of producing a high frequency of durable remissions with acceptable toxicity (10). Examples of tumor response following ^{131}I-anti-B1 RIT appear in Figs. 38.1 and 38.2. ^{131}I-anti-B1 murine is known as ^{131}I-tositumomab in the United States (Bexxar), and at the time of this writing it is being considered by the Food and Drug Administration for possible approval as a therapeutic agent.

Another phase I/II dose-escalation study with an anti-CD20 monoclonal antibody was performed by the group at Stanford University using anti-B1 and a different anti-CD20 monoclonal antibody (Y2B8) (41). In this case, ^{90}Y-labeled murine anti-CD20 was used as a therapeutic.

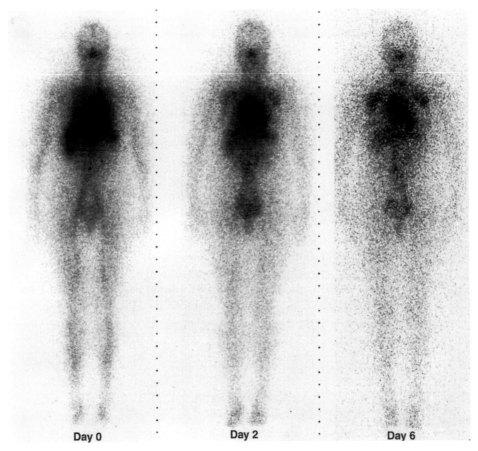

Day 0   Day 2   Day 6

FIGURE 38.1. Images obtained after administration of a 5-mCi tracer dose of ^{131}I-tositumomab (Bexxar). The image from day 0 shows blood pool activity. The day 2 image shows targeting to axillary and paraaortic lymph nodes. The day 6 image shows continued clearance of blood pool activity, with tumor targeting in the axillary and paraaortic regions. Body scans are used in planning therapy that will deliver a 75-cGy dose of radiation to the whole body.

Patients with relapsed low- to intermediate-grade non-Hodgkin's lymphoma were treated. Biodistribution studies with ^{111}In-anti-CD20 monoclonal antibody preceded the studies of ^{90}Y therapy. Dose escalation was performed with groups of three or four patients treated at doses of about 13, 20, 30, 40, and 50 mCi of ^{90}Y-anti-CD20. The major toxicity was hematologic. Leukopenia, granulocytopenia, and thrombocytopenia were quite common. Grade 4 thrombocytopenia was seen in several patients who received 30 mCi of ^{90}Y-labeled monoclonal antibody and at higher dose levels. Doses of 50 mCi of ^{90}Y-labeled monoclonal antibody were generally quite toxic and required bone marrow stem cell support in several instances to achieve marrow reconstitution. In this study, at least three of the patients required transplantation to deal with radiation-induced toxicity. Despite the toxicity, the treatment showed considerable activity; the overall response rate following a single dose of ^{90}Y was 72%, with six complete responses and seven partial responses. The responses lasted from 3 to more than 29 months after treatment. It should be noted that the first four patients in the study received anti-B1 monoclonal anti-

body, whereas the other 14 received the Y2B8 monoclonal antibody, both anti-CD20.

More recently, the ^{90}Y-anti-CD20 approach has been expanded, and a phase I/II multicenter study was completed in which a commercially sponsored preparation was used. Witzig et al. (42) reported the use of ^{90}Y-ibritumomab tiuxetan (Zevalin, which is a murine IgG1 kappa anti-CD20 to which ^{90}Y is chelated by the MX-DTPA conjugate tiuxetan) [(Figs. 38.3 and 38.4; see also Color Plate 15 following page 350)]. More recently, ^{90}Y-anti-CD20 was used in a phase I/II trial in which 51 patients with relapsed or refractory CD20-positive B-cell non-Hodgkin's lymphoma were enrolled. Patients were treated at several dose levels based on millicuries per kilogram and were given unlabeled anti-CD20 antibody (chimeric, rituximab) before the ^{90}Y material. Three patients received 100 mg of rituximab per square meter, and the remainder received 250 mg/m^2 before the radiolabeled antibody, which was believed to provide the best imaging and opportunity for response to the cold antibody. In this multicenter study of 51 patients with relapsed or refractory low-grade, intermediate-grade, or mantle cell non-Hodgkin's

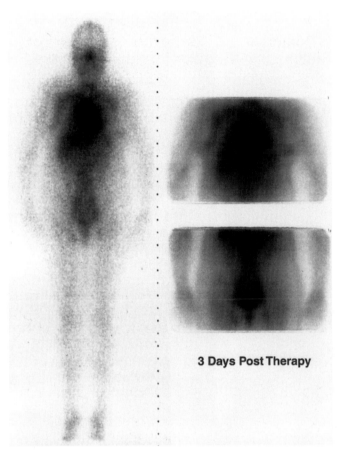

3 Days Post Therapy

FIGURE 38.2. Scan obtained after administration of a therapeutic dose of ^{131}I-tositumomab. Tumor targeting on whole-body and regional images is more apparent because of increased photon flux.

lymphoma (mean of two prior treatment regimens), the response rate was 67%. The complete response rate was 26%, and the partial response rate was 41%. The duration of response was about 12 months but is still evolving. Dosimetry was used in dose planning but generally allowed for dosing on a basis of millicuries per kilogram, with 0.4 mCi/kg the maximum tolerated dose for patients with platelet counts above 150,000/mm^3. Toxicity was greater in patients who had bone marrow involvement by tumor, and considerable variability in blood clearance rates was seen. HAMA was rare, seen in only one patient (42). This approach is somewhat similar to that used with ^{131}I-anti-CD20 (^{131}I-tositumomab) but involves an infusion of unlabeled chimeric anti-CD20 before infusion of the radiolabeled anti-CD20 for therapy. This agent is now in phase III trials. An advantage of ^{90}Y is that no gamma emission is present, so radiation safety precautions can be more modest than with ^{131}I. However, studies have shown that both ^{90}Y and ^{131}I can be given on an outpatient basis. A preliminary communication from a study of more than 100 patients has indicated that ^{90}Y-anti-CD20 is significantly more effective than unlabeled anti-CD20, as would be expected (43).

Thus, with four different monoclonal antibodies and three different labels, anti-CD20 monoclonal antibodies have shown substantial therapeutic activity in the treatment of lymphoma and have not required transplant support. The same anti-CD20 antibody can be used at higher doses to ablate the bone marrow and presumably achieve higher rates of tumor killing.

Press and colleagues (9,44,45), at the University of Washington, have used high doses of several ^{131}I-labeled murine monoclonal antibodies reactive with CD20 (B1 and 1F5) and CD37 (MB1). These investigators reported evaluating 56 lymphoma patients with trace-labeled infusions of antibody and treating 32 (57%). Patients were treated based on a "favorable" biodistribution during the tracer study, which meant that tumor foci would receive more radiation than normal tissue. These investigators observed that good targeting was more likely in patients with small spleens and small tumor burdens. They varied the protein mass over several levels and found, depending on the kind of antibody used, that different protein masses were most appropriate. For the currently favored antibody anti-B1, 2.5 mg of antibody per kilogram was used along with 10 mCi of ^{131}I for the tracer study. The therapy millicurie dose was escalated. The dose-escalation study showed little toxicity up to organ doses of 2,375 cGy (other than myelosuppression), but when the dose was increased to approximately 3,100 cGy to the lungs, severe cardiopulmonary toxicity was seen. Thus, lower doses of radiation have been used since, and 2,725 cGy is reported as the maximum tolerated organ dose. These researchers are currently investigating whether RIT can be combined with chemotherapy. Of 19 patients studied in phase I, 16 achieved a complete response, 2 had a partial response, and 1 had a minor response. The mean duration of response was in excess of 15 months, and 9 patients were reported to be in continuous complete remission at 14 months to more than 5 years after treatment without additional therapy. Ten patients entered into a phase II trial could not be evaluated because their response was not yet complete, but they had no evidence of progressive disease (46). No patients have had failure of bone marrow engraftment. Administered radiation activity has ranged from 345 to 785 mCi, delivering between 2,700 and 9,200 cGy to tumor sites. One patient treated with anti-idiotype antibody in this study achieved a complete response. The results of multiple clinical studies of RIT in lymphoma are summarized in Table 38.2.

This study population has been followed, and long-term follow-up data and late toxicities have been reported in 29 patients treated with myeloablative doses of 280 to 785 mCi (10.4 to 29.0 GBq) of ^{131}I-anti-CD20 antibody (anti-B1) and autologous stem cell (47). Major responses occurred in 25 patients (86%), with 23 complete responses (79%). The nonhematopoietic dose-limiting toxicity was reversible cardiopulmonary insufficiency, which occurred in two patients at RIT doses that delivered 27 Gy or more to

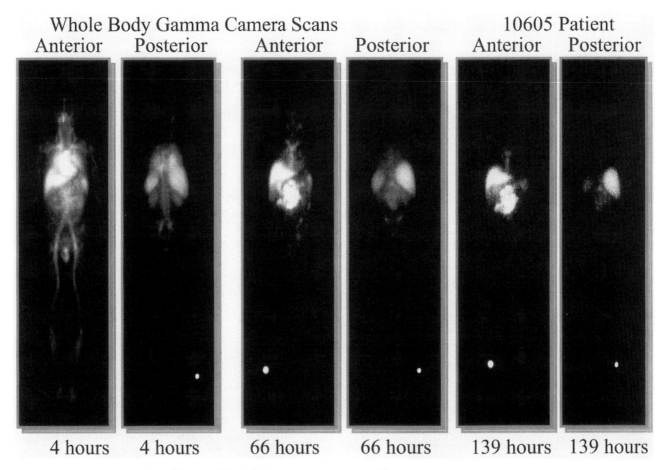

Whole Body Gamma Camera Scans

Anterior   Posterior

Anterior   Posterior

10605 Patient

Anterior   Posterior

4 hours   4 hours   66 hours   66 hours   139 hours   139 hours

FIGURE 38.3. [111]In-2B8 (^{111}In-labeled murine anti-CD20; ^{111}In-ibritumomab tiuxetan, or Zevalin) scans (at 4, 66, and 139 hours) after a tracer dose of the antibody. These show, at the specific intervals of time after the injection, a gradual clearance of blood pool activity and progressive accumulation in tumor in the periaortic abdominal lymph nodes. Tracer in the liver represents antibody catabolism, not tumor in the liver. Focal activity lower in the field of view is in a marker, not in tumor. (Images courtesy of C. White, IDEC Pharmaceuticals, San Diego, California.)

the lungs. With a median follow-up of 42 months, the estimated overall and progression-free survival rates are 68% and 42%, respectively. Currently, 14 of 29 patients remain in remissions that range from more than 27 to more than 87 months after RIT. Late toxicities have been uncommon except for elevated levels of thyroid-stimulating hormone, found in approximately 60% of the subjects. Second malignancies developed in two patients, but myelodysplasia has not developed in any. It remains to be seen how the combination of chemotherapy and RIT plus transplant will perform in the long term (47).

These data clearly indicate that both myeloablative and nonmyeloablative use of anti-CD20 antibodies results in substantial antitumor activity.

Another reagent that has been assessed for non-Hodgkin's lymphoma therapy is the anti-CD22 antibody LL2. Goldenberg et al. (48) and subsequently Juweid and colleagues (49) reported on the use of LL2 labeled with ^{131}I as a treatment for lymphoma. LL2 is a murine IgG2a anti-

CD22 monoclonal antibody. Initially, Goldenberg's group reported two partial responses and two mixed responses in five assessable patients with non-Hodgkin's lymphoma (48). Of interest is that one of the responses occurred with only 6.2 mCi of LL2 immunoglobulin, which suggests that some of the response may have been immunologic, or at least related to the unlabeled antibody, rather than radiation damage, as would be expected at this dose level. This trial was subsequently expanded to treat 21 patients on an outpatient basis with repeated injections of low doses of ^{131}I-LL2. The patients were treated with 15 to 343 mCi of ^{131}I-LL2 for up to seven cycles. Cumulative protein doses ranged from 1.1 mg of IgG2a to 157 mg of F(ab′)$_2$. Antitumor activity was noted in 5 of 17 patients who could be assessed (49). One complete response was seen, two partial remissions, and two minor responses. Both partial and complete responses were noted for both F(ab′)$_2$ and intact IgG treatment. When the dose was increased to 90 mCi/m^2 and bone marrow transplantation support was provided,

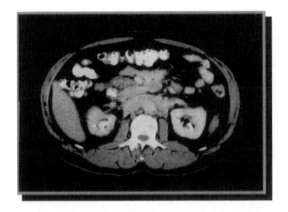
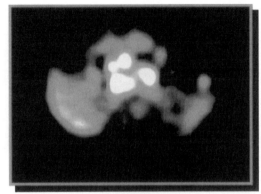
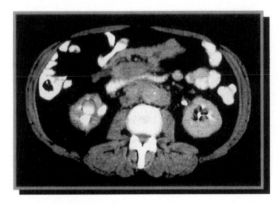
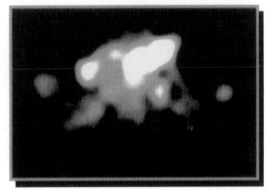

FIGURE 38.4. Computed tomography (*CT, left*) and single-photon emission computed tomography (*SPECT, right*) from the same patient show focal accumulation of ¹¹¹In on SPECT in the tumor marker, which is apparent on CT. (See also Color Plate 15 following p. 350.) (Images courtesy of C. White, IDEC Pharmaceuticals, San Diego, California.)

responses seemed more common (49). As in other studies, anti-mouse antibodies were infrequent, and HAMA developed in only four patients. It is of note that the LL2 monoclonal antibody is internalized, and ¹³¹I is possibly not an optimal label for internalizing antibody. Despite these concerns, an objective response rate of 33% (complete and partial responses) was seen in 21 patients treated with ¹³¹I-LL2 in a preliminary report by Vose et al. (50). Furthermore, 71% of the responders had a complete remission. Of note is that 55% of the patients had bulky disease, 90% had received three or more prior therapies, and 38% had received a prior blood stem cell transplant, so they were a group with poor prognostic characteristics.

Juweid et al. (51) recently reported on an additional eight patients who received ¹¹¹In-hLL2 (humanized) followed by therapy with ⁹⁰Y-hLL2 (epratuzumab, or LymphoCide) to deliver 50 or 100 cGy to the bone marrow (51). The estimated average radiation dose from ⁹⁰y-Hll2 to tumors larger than 3 cm was 21.5 ± 10.0 cGy/mCi, and was 3.7-, 2.5-, 1.8-, and 2.5-fold that to bone marrow, lung, liver, and kidney, respectively, and ⁹⁰Y-hLL2 appeared superior to the iodinated agent. No evidence of significant anti-hLL2 antibodies was seen in any of the patients. Myelosup-

pression was the only dose-limiting toxicity and was greater in patients who had had prior high-dose chemotherapy. Objective tumor responses were seen in two of seven patients given ⁹⁰Y-hLL2. In a preliminary report by Leonard et al. (52), 30 patients who received both ¹³¹I- and ⁹⁰Y-anti-CD22 antibody have shown additional responses, especially at higher radiation doses. It is understood that the humanized ⁹⁰Y-LL2 antibody is likely the most promising reagent for clinical commercialization of the anti-CD22 antibody and that such a reagent may be available in the future.

Thus, several reagents are in varying stages of commercial development, and it is quite possible that by the time this book is published, one or more of the reagents may be commercially available in the United States for the treatment of non-Hodgkin's lymphoma. Much more work needs to be done to determine which antibody–label pair will be of the greatest general clinical utility.

CLINICAL RESULTS IN LEUKEMIA THERAPY

Acute leukemias are among the most aggressive and lethal of neoplasms, whereas chronic leukemias, such as chronic lymphocytic leukemia, are often indolent diseases in which relatively long-term survival is possible with modest therapies. Recent work in the treatment of both these illnesses has been reported, although it is quite early in the development process. As indicated above, several of the patients treated with anti-B-cell and anti T-cell reagents had blood-borne disease and responded to the treatments. However, in the treatment of leukemias, a potentially important consideration is that the tumor cells are widely distributed in the circulation and are not as likely to be as clustered as in solid tumors (although if the disease is advanced, the marrow can be "packed" with cells, more akin to a solid tumor). This makes treatment more challenging, as the beta path length of most therapeutic isotopes is longer than the diameter of the tumor cells. Thus, considerable interest has been shown in the use of alpha emitters and less energetic beta emitters for such treatments. In contrast, beta emitters are used to treat lymphomas in most cases.

Radioimmunotherapy of adult T-cell leukemia has been explored to some degree, as this disease is not well treated with chemotherapy. The anti-CD5 monoclonal was mentioned previously (see the section on T-cell lymphoma), and another target antigen is the high-affinity interleukin 2 receptor, which is overexpressed on these cells (16,17). Waldmann and colleagues (16), at the National Cancer Institute, used ^{90}Y-anti-Tac monoclonal antibody to treat 18 patients with adult T-cell leukemia. Dose escalation in nine patients was followed by a phase II trial of nine patients with a 10-mCi dose of the reagent. Patients undergoing a remission were allowed to receive up to eight additional doses. At the 5- to 15-mCi doses used, 9 of 16 evaluable patients responded to ^{90}Y-anti-Tac with a partial (7 patients) or complete (2 patients) remission. Toxicity was limited to bone marrow suppression. These remissions did not last long but do illustrate the promise of this approach (16).

Another approach to leukemia therapy was reported by Scheinberg and colleagues (53). Ten patients with myeloid leukemias were treated in a phase I trial with escalating doses of mouse monoclonal antibody M195, which is reactive with CD33, a glycoprotein found on myeloid leukemia blasts and early hematopoietic progenitor cells but not on normal stem cells. M195 was trace-labeled with ^{131}I for dosimetric studies. Total doses of up to 76 mg were administered safely without immediate adverse effects. The entire bone marrow was specifically and clearly imaged within hours after injection, with the best imaging obtained at the lowest protein mass doses. Roughly 30 times more radioactivity was delivered to the marrow than to the whole body. However, ^{131}I-M195 was rapidly modulated, with most of the bound IgG internalized into target cells *in vivo* to result in a loss of radioactivity from the tumor cells. The doses used were not sufficient to produce a significant antitumor response. This internalizing antibody would be expected to deliver more radiation to the marrow if a residualizing antibody were used (53).

Radioimmunotherapy has also been used in several studies as part of a marrow-destructive regimen combined with chemotherapy before transplant to reduce tumor recurrence rates. The group at the University of Washington has used ^{131}I-labeled anti-CD45 antibody (BC8) specifically to deliver radiation to hematopoietic tissues, followed by a standard transplant preparation regimen (54). In 23 patients, biodistribution studies were performed by administering 0.5 mg per kilogram of body weight of BC8 antibody trace-labeled with ^{131}I. The mean radiation absorbed doses (cGy/mCi of ^{131}I administered) were as follows: marrow, 7.1 ± 0.8; spleen, 10.8 ± 1.4; total body, 0.4 ± 0.03, which indicates considerable specificity of delivery. Patients with acute myelogenous leukemia in relapse had a higher marrow dose (11.4 cGy/mCi) than those in remission (5.2 cGy/mCi; *p* = .001) because of higher uptake and longer retention of the radionuclide in marrow. Twenty patients were treated with a dose of ^{131}I estimated to deliver 3.5 Gy (level 1) to 7 Gy (level 3) to liver, with marrow doses of 4 to 30 Gy and spleen doses of 7 to 60 Gy; this was followed by 120 mg of cyclophosphamide per kilogram and 12 Gy of total-body irradiation. Nine of 13 patients with acute myelogenous leukemia or refractory anemia with excess blasts and two of seven with acute lymphocytic leukemia are alive and disease-free at 8 to 41 months (median, 17 months) after bone marrow transplant. Toxicity was not clearly greater than that of cyclophosphamide and total-body irradiation alone, and the maximum tolerated was not reached. A follow-up to this initial study includes 44 patients (of whom 34 were treated). Of 25 treated patients with acute myeloid leukemia/myelodysplastic syndrome, 7 survived disease-free for 15 to 89 months (median, 65 months) after transplant. Of 9 treated patients with acute lymphoblastic leukemia, 3 survived disease-free for 19, 54, and 66 months after transplant. The authors concluded that ^{131}I-anti-CD45 antibody could safely deliver substantial supplemental doses of radiation to the bone marrow (approximately 24 Gy) and spleen (approximately 50 Gy) when combined with conventional cyclophosphamide and total-body irradiation (55).

Another study of leukemia therapy was reported by Seitz et al. (56), who used ^{188}Re-labeled anti-NCA monoclonal antibody BW250/183 for RIT of leukemia. This particular antibody, given at the appropriate protein dose, localizes avidly to normal bone marrow, with up to 50% of the injected dose reaching the marrow. ^{188}Re is also generator-produced, with beta and gamma emission. Twelve patients with leukemia, either acute or chronic, were treated. Specific delivery to the bone marrow was seen, with 145 ± 0.71 cGy delivered to the bone marrow, versus 13 ± .02 cGy to the total body per millibecquerel administered.

Humanized monoclonal antibody hM195 labeled with ^{213}Bi (an alpha emitter) was used to treat nine patients (57). ^{213}Bi is generator-produced and has a very brief half-life of 46 minutes. Although it is an alpha emitter, it does have an imageable gamma photon of 440 keV. In pilot dosimetry studies, the radiation dose to leukemia-involved bone marrow relative to the total-body radiation dose was estimated to be about 1,000-fold higher than is typically seen when beta-emitting radiopharmaceuticals are used for cancer treatments. Clinical results with such therapies are only now being reported and do not indicate that cures have been achieved. Nonetheless, the feasibility of therapy with alpha emitters has been demonstrated (57).

SUMMARY

Radiolabeled monoclonal antibodies have shown the highest rates of clinical success in the treatment of hematopoietic neoplasms. In the most advanced clinical trials reported to date, both ^{131}I- and ^{90}Y-labeled reagents are being used to treat B-cell non-Hodgkin's lymphomas. Both of these have been carried though phase III trials and, depending on regulatory approvals, may soon be available for clinical utilization in the United States and elsewhere. Other reagents are also promising in non-Hodgkin's lymphoma of the B-cell type, such as anti-CD22 and anti-HLA-DR antibodies. Alpha emitters appear promising, but more work is needed. Although commercial development has lagged, clinical potential has also been shown in the treatment of T-cell lymphoma, Hodgkin's lymphoma, and leukemias. It is clear that radiolabeled antibody therapy will play a key role in the treatment of hematopoietic neoplasms during the next millennium.

REFERENCES

1. Gaidano G, Dalla-Favera R, Weinstein HJ, et al. Lymphoma. In: DeVita VT, Hellman S, Rosenberg SA, eds. *Cancer principles and practice of oncology*, 5th ed. Philadelphia: Lippincott–Raven Publishers, 1997.
2. Aisenberg A. Coherent view of non-Hodgkin's lymphoma. *J Clin Oncol* 1995;13:2656.
3. Harris N, Jaffe E, Stein H, et al. A revised European-American classification of lymphoid neoplasms: a proposal from the International Lymphoma Study Group. *Blood* 1994;84:1361.
4. The American Cancer Society. *2000 facts and figures: lymphoma. http://www.cancer.org/statistics/cff2000/selectedcancers.html#lymphoma.*
5. Ghose T, Guclu A. Cure of a mouse lymphoma with radio-iodinated antibody. *Eur J Cancer* 1974;10:787–792.
6. Grossbard ML, Nadler LM. Monoclonal antibody therapy for indolent lymphomas. *Semin Oncol* 1993;20:118–135.
7. Jurcic JG, Caron PC, Scheinberg DA. Monoclonal antibody therapy of leukemia and lymphoma. *Adv Pharmacol* 1995;33: 287–314.
8. White CA, Halpern SE, Parker BA, et al. Radioimmunotherapy of relapsed B-cell lymphoma with yttrium-90 anti-idiotype monoclonal antibodies. *Blood* 1996;87:3640–3649.
9. Press OW, Appelbaum FR, Eary JF, et al. Radiolabeled antibody therapy of lymphomas. *Important Adv Oncol* 1995; :157–171.
10. Kaminski MS, Zasadny KR, Francis IR, et al. Iodine-131-anti-B1 radioimmunotherapy for B-cell lymphoma. *J Clin Oncol* 1996;14:1974–1981.
11. Wahl RL, Parker CW, Philpott GW. Improved radioimaging and tumor localization with monoclonal F(ab')₂. *J Nucl Med* 1983;24:316–325.
12. Goodwin DA, Meares CF, Osen M. Biological properties of biotin-chelate conjugates for pretargeted diagnosis and therapy with the avidin/biotin system. *J Nucl Med* 1998;39:1813–1818.
13. Press OW, Shan D, Howell-Clark J, et al. Comparative metabolism and retention of iodine-125, yttrium-90, and indium-111 radioimmunoconjugates by cancer cells. *Cancer Res* 1996;56: 2123–2129.
14. Wahl RL, Kroll S, Zasadny KR. Patient-specific whole-body dosimetry: principles and a simplified method for clinical implementation. *J Nucl Med* 1998;39[Suppl]:14S–20S.
15. Eary JF, Krohn KA, Press OW, et al. Importance of pre-treatment radiation absorbed dose estimation for radioimmunotherapy of non-Hodgkin's lymphoma. *Nucl Med Biol* 1997;24: 635–638.
16. Waldmann TA, White JD, Carrasquillo JA, et al. Radioimmunotherapy of interleukin-2R alpha-expressing adult T-cell leukemia with yttrium-90-labeled anti-Tac. *Blood* 1995;86: 4063–4075.
17. Foss FM, Raubitscheck A, Mulshine JL, et al. Phase I study of the pharmacokinetics of a radioimmunoconjugate, ^{90}Y-T101, in patients with CD5-expressing leukemia and lymphoma. *Clin Cancer Res* 1998;4:2691–2700.
18. DeNardo GL, O'Donnell RT, Rose LM, et al. Milestones in the development of Lym-1 therapy. *Hybridoma* 1999;18:1–11.
19. O'Donoghue JA, Bardies M, Wheldon TE. Relationships between tumor size and curability for uniformly targeted therapy with beta-emitting radionuclides. *J Nucl Med* 1995;36: 1902–1909.
20. Zalutsky MR, Bigner DD. Radioimmunotherapy with alpha-particle emitting radioimmunoconjugates. *Acta Oncol* 1996;35: 373–379.
21. Lenhard RE, Order SE, Spunberg JJ, et al. Isotopic immunoglobulin. A new systemic therapy for advanced Hodgkin's disease. *J Clin Oncol* 1985;3:1296–1300.
22. Herpst JM, Klein JL, Leichner PK, et al. Survival of patients with resistant Hodgkin's disease after polyclonal yttrium-90 labeled anti-ferritin treatment. *J Clin Oncol* 1995;13:2394–2400.
23. Bierman PJ, Vose JM, Leichner PK, et al. Yttrium-90 labeled antiferritin followed by high-dose chemotherapy and autologous bone marrow transplantation for poor-prognosis Hodgkin's disease. *J Clin Oncol* 1993;11:698–703.
24. Vriesendorp HM, Quadri SM, Andersson BS, et al. Recurrence of Hodgkin's disease after indium-111 and yttrium-90 labeled anti-ferritin administration. *Cancer* 1997;80[12 Suppl]:2721–2727.
25. Vriesendorp HM, Quadri SM, Wyllie CT, et al. Fractionated radiolabeled antiferritin therapy for patients with recurrent Hodgkin's disease. *Clin Cancer Res* 1999;5[10 Suppl]:3324s–3329s.
26. Rosen ST, Zimmer AM, Goldman-Leikin R, et al. Radioimmunodetection and radioimmunotherapy of cutaneous T-cell lymphomas using a 131-I-labeled monoclonal antibody: an Illinois Cancer Council study. *J Clin Oncol* 1987;5:562–573.
27. Zimmer AM, Rosen ST, Spies SM, et al. Radioimmunotherapy of patients with cutaneous T-cell lymphoma using an iodine-131-labeled monoclonal antibody: analysis of retreatment following plasmapheresis. *J Nucl Med* 1988;29:174–180.
28. Shan D, Ledbetter JA, Press OW. Apoptosis of malignant human B-cells by ligation of CD20 with monoclonal antibodies. *Blood* 1998;91:1644–1652.
29. Lewis JP, DeNardo GL, DeNardo SJ. Radioimmunotherapy of lymphoma: a UC Davis experience. *Hybridoma* 1995;14: 115–120.

30. Wilder RB, DeNardo GL, DeNardo SJ. Radioimmunotherapy: recent results and future directions. *J Clin Oncol* 1996;14:1383–1400.

31. DeNardo GL, O'Donnell RT, Rose LM, et al. Milestones in the development of Lym-1 therapy. *Hybridoma* 1999;18:1–11.

32. Kaminski MS, Fig LM, Zasadny KR, et al. Imaging, dosimetry, and radioimmunotherapy with iodine 131-labeled anti-CD37 antibody in B-cell lymphoma. *J Clin Oncol* 1992;10:1696–1711.

33. Czuczman MS, Straus DJ, Divgi CR, et al. Phase I dose-escalation trial of iodine 131-labeled monoclonal antibody OKB7 in patients with non-Hodgkin's lymphoma. *J Clin Oncol* 1993;11:2021–2029.

34. Kaminski MS, Zasadny KR, Franis IR, et al. Radioimmunotherapy of B-cell lymhoma with 131-I anti-B1 (anti-CD20) antibody. *N Engl J Med* 1993;329:459–465.

35. Wahl RL, Zasadny KR, MacFarlane D, et al. Iodine-131 anti-B1 antibody for B-cell lymphoma: an update on the Michigan phase I experience. *J Nucl Med* 1998;39[8 Suppl]:21S–27S.

36. Bhatnagar A, Kroll S, Langmuir V, et al. Clinical experience with iodine-131 anti B1 antibody for the treatment of low-grade and transformed low-grade non-Hodgkin's lymphoma. *Eur J Nucl Med* 1999;26:970(abst).

37. Kaminski MS, Zasadny KR, Francis IR, et al. Iodine-131-anti-B1 radioimmunotherapy for B-cell lymphoma. *J Clin Oncol* 1996;14:1974–1981.

38. Leonard JP, Coleman M, Kostakoglu L, et al. Fludarabine monophosphate followed by iodine I 131 tositumomab for untreated low-grade and follicular non-Hodgkin's lymphoma (NHL). Presented at the 41st Annual Meeting and Exposition of the American Society of Hematology, December 3–7, 1999, New Orleans, Lousiana (abst 393).

39. Behr TM, Wormann B, Gramatzki M, et al. Low- versus high-dose radioimmunotherapy with humanized anti-CD22 or chimeric anti-CD20 antibodies in a broad spectrum of B cell-associated malignancies. *Clin Cancer Res* 1999;5[10 Suppl]:3304s–3314s.

40. Breitz HB, Weiden JW, Appelbaum DM, et al. Pretargeted radioimmunotherapy (PRIT) for treatment of non-Hodgkin's lymphoma (NHL): preliminary results. *J Nucl Med* 19xx;40[5 Suppl]:19p(abst).

41. Knox SJ, Goris ML, Trisler K, et al. Yttrium-90 labeled anti-CD20 monoclonal antibody therapy of recurrent B-cell lymphoma. *Clin Cancer Res* 1996;2:457–470.

42. Witzig TE, White CA, Wiseman GA, et al. Phase I/II trial of IDEC-Y2B8 radioimmunotherapy for treatment of relapsed or refractory CD20+ B-cell non-Hodgkin's lymphoma. *J Clin Oncol* 1999;17:3793–3803.

43. Wiseman GA, White CA, Witzig TE, et al. Radioimmunotherapy of relapsed non-Hodgkin's lymphoma with zevalin, a 90Y-labeled anti-CD20 monoclonal antibody. *Clin Cancer Res* 1999;5[10 Suppl]:3281s–3286s.

44. Press OW, Eary JF, Appelbaum FR, et al. Radiolabeled-antibody therapy of B-cell lymphoma with autologous bone marrow support. *N Engl J Med* 1993;329:1219–1224.

45. Press OW, Eary JF, Appelbaum FR, et al. Phase II trial of ^{131}I-B1 (anti-CD20) antibody therapy with autologous stem cell transplantation for relapsed B-cell lymphomas. *Lancet* 1995;346:336–340.

46. Eary JF, Press OW. High-dose radioimmunotherapy in malignant lymphoma. *Recent Results Cancer Res* 1996;141:177–182.

47. Liu SY, Eary JF, Petersdorf SH, et al. Follow-up of relapsed B-cell lymphoma patients treated with I-131-labeled anti-CD20 antibody and autologous stem-cell rescue. *J Clin Oncol* 1998;16:3270–3278.

48. Goldenberg DM, Horowitz JA, Sharkey RM, et al. Targeting, dosimetry, and radioimmunotherapy of B-cell lymphomas with iodine-131-labeled LL2 monoclonal antibody. *J Clin Oncol* 1991;9:548–564.

49. Juweid M, Sharkey RM, Markowitz A, et al. Treatment of non-Hodgkin's lymphoma with radiolabeled murine, chimeric, or humanized LL2, an anti-CD22 monoclonal antibody. *Cancer Res Ctr* 1995;55:5899–5907.

50. Vose JM, Zelenetz AD, Rohatiner A, et al. Iodine I 131 tositumomab for patients with follicular non-Hodgkin's Lymphoma (NHL): overall clinical trial experience by histology. Presented at the 41st Annual Meeting and Exposition of the American Society of Hematology, December 3–7, 1999, New Orleans, Lousiana (abst 387).

51. Juweid ME, Stadtmauer E, Hajjar G, et al. Pharmacokinetics, dosimetry, and initial therapeutic results with [131]I- and [111]In-/^{90}Y-labeled humanized LL2 anti-CD22 monoclonal antibody in patients with relapsed, refractory non-Hodgkin's lymphoma. *Clin Cancer Res* 1999;5[10 Suppl]:3292s–3303s.

52. Leonard JP, Coleman M, Schuster MW, et al. Epratuzumab, a new anti-CD22, humanized, monoclonal antibody for the therapy of non-Hodgkin's lymphoma (NHL): phase I/II trial results. Presented at the 41st Annual Meeting and Exposition of the American Society of Hematology, December 3–7, 1999, New Orleans, Lousiana (abst 404).

53. Scheinberg DA, Lovett D, Divgi CR, et al. A phase I trial of monoclonal antibody M195 in acute myelogenous leukemia: specific bone marrow targeting and internalization of radionuclide. *J Clin Oncol* 1991;9:478–490.

54. Matthews DC, Appelbaum FR, Eary JF, et al. Development of a marrow transplant regimen for acute leukemia using targeted hematopoietic irradiation delivered by ^{131}I-labeled anti-CD45 antibody combined with cyclophosphamide and total body irradiation. *Blood* 1995;85:1122–1131.

55. Matthews DC, Appelbaum FR, Eary JF, et al. Phase I study of 131I-anti-CD45 antibody plus cyclophosphamide and total body irradiation for advanced acute leukemia and myelodysplastic syndrome. *Blood* 1999;94:1237–1247.

56. Seitz U, Neumaier B, Glatting G, et al. Preparation and evaluation of the rhenium-188-labeled anti-NCA antigen monoclonal antibody BW 250/183 for radioimmunotherapy of leukemia. *Eur J Nucl Med* 1999;26:1265–1273.

57. Sgouros G, Ballangrud AM, Jurcic JG, et al. Pharmacokinetics and dosimetry of an alpha-particle emitter labeled antibody: Bi-213-HuM195 (anti-CD33) in patients with leukemia. *J Nucl Med* 1999;40:1935–1946.

39

PRIMARY BONE TUMORS: THALLIUM-201, TECHNETIUM-99M–SESTAMIBI, AND FLUORINE-18–DEOXYGLUCOSE

ALAN D. WAXMAN
HUSSEIN M. ABDEL-DAYEM

Nuclear medicine has begun to play an increasingly important role in assessing patients with primary malignant tumors of bone. Formerly, indirect assessment of these tumors was performed using diphosphonate bone scans. More recently, direct evaluation of bone tumor has been done using various agents that rely on cellular metabolism, receptors, membrane transport, or subcellular interactions.

The most frequent bone neoplasm is *osteogenic sarcoma*. Male patients are affected approximately twice as often as female patients. Most of these tumors arise in the second and third decades of life. In older persons, the tumor may be superimposed on preexisting bone disorders such as Paget's disease. *Chondrosarcomas* of bone are usually noted in the later decades of life and are often associated with other bone lesions, such as osteochondroma or Paget's disease. This tumor typically arises within trabecular bone in the proximal or distal femur or within a proximal humerus. As in osteogenic sarcoma, pulmonary metastasis are often seen.

Ewing's sarcoma generally occurs within the first 3 decades, with a peak occurrence at approximately 15 years of age. Male patients are affected approximately twice as commonly as female patients. This tumor often arises within the femur, but it may arise in the long bones of other extremities. It is not uncommon to see Ewing's sarcoma of the pelvis, ribs, or scapula. Metastasis are often seen within other bones.

Other primary malignant bone tumors include malignant fibrous histiocytoma, in which primary bone origin is possible. Similarly, primary bone lymphoma can occur. These tumors can involve regional lymph nodes and may be visualized using several direct nuclear medicine examinations including gallium 67 (^{67}Ga), thallium 201 (^{201}Tl), technetium 99m (^{99m}Tc)–sesta-2-methoxyisobotylisonitrile (MIBI) and fluorine 18–fluorodeoxyglucose (^{18}F-FDG).

With the introduction of cytotoxic drugs in the early 1970s, the prognosis of these tumors changed dramatically (1–4). Aggressive preoperative chemotherapy has been effective in both children and adults. It can eliminate micrometastases and macrometastases, induce total necrosis of the primary tumor, and thus reduce the tumor's size and vascularity. It widens the tumor-free area for safe surgical excision of the margins. As a result, it facilitates the replacement of endoprosthesis, helps to prevent local recurrence, and improves prognosis. Accordingly, the 5-year survival rate increased from 5% to 23% for surgery to 80% for those using chemotherapy regimens before surgery. The need for surgical excision of primary tumor still remains; however, aggressive, mutilating operations may be replaced by salvaging procedures if one has assurance of the patient's complete preoperative response to the chemotherapy. The role of the pathologist in this case in evaluating chemotherapy response and subsequently influencing further treatment is important. The response to chemotherapy is graded as follows:

Grade I: No response
Grade II: Partial response caused by presence of areas of viable tumor
Grade III: Near-complete response with only scattered foci of viable tumor cells
Grade IV: Complete response with no histologic evidence of viable tumor within the specimen

The prediction of complete response favors of limb salvage surgery in the patient. The presence of microscopic cells following surgery at the edge of the resection requires postoperative chemotherapy.

Imaging of primary bone tumors has largely been performed with x-ray study, computed tomography (CT), and

A. D. Waxman: Departments of Imaging and Nuclear Medicine, Cedars-Sinai Medical Center, Los Angeles, California 90048.

H. M. Abdel-Dayem: Department of Radiology, New York Medical College, Valhalla, New York 10595; Department of Radiology, St. Vincent's Hospital and Medical Center, New York, New York 10011.

magnetic resonance imaging (MRI). Bone scintigraphy and ^{67}Ga-citrate scintigraphy have been used with inconsistent results (5–8). The bone scan has been demonstrated to be sensitive but nonspecific for malignancy. Investigators have shown that malignant disease and bone healing may both result in a positive bone scan using agents such as ^{99m}Tc-phosphonate (6). Gallium has been shown to detect primary malignant tumors of bone. Gallium uptake, however, is also nonspecific, with gallium increases noted in trauma, infection, inflammation, and bone healing (6–8).

RADIOPHARMACEUTICALS

Several radiopharmaceuticals have become available to evaluate the metabolic activity of tumors, with apparent improvement in specificity when compared with either bone or gallium scintigraphy. Thallium 201, ^{99m}Tc-MIBI, and ^{18}F-FDG have been demonstrated by several investigators to give accurate information relative to tumor detection or tumor viability (5–43). Information regarding tumor viability can be employed clinically to assess the effect of chemotherapy accurately, as well as to localize areas of unsuspected abnormality.

Thallium chloride has been shown to behave in a manner similar to that of potassium chloride in most biologic systems (43–47). The adenosine triphosphatase (ATPase)–mediated sodium-potassium pump has been demonstrated to transport potassium ions into intact cells against concentrate ingredients; the result is an extremely high concentration of potassium within the cell relative to the extracellular space. Thallium and potassium have similar physical and biologic characteristics that result in thallium concentration within cells secondary to mechanisms demonstrated to be operational for potassium (48). Tumors also concentrate potassium ions and thallium in a similar fashion. Investigators have demonstrated that the uptake of ^{201}Tl by tumor cells may be inhibited by ouabain, a potent inhibitor of the ATPase sodium-potassium pump (49). Furosemide has also been demonstrated to inhibit thallium uptake by tumor cells (49). Furosemide plays virtually no role in the inhibition of the ATPase sodium-potassium pump, but it has been demonstrated to inhibit a cotransport system that involves the transport of potassium, sodium, and chloride into the cell. Investigators also demonstrated that after inhibition of the ATPase sodium-potassium pump, as well as the cotransport system, a resting flow for ionic transport was preserved. This was attributed to the calcium-dependent ion channel system (49).

Thallium is accumulated by viable tumor and is less well-accumulated by connective tissue that contain inflammatory cells (50). Investigators also demonstrated that thallium was not well detected in necrotic tumor tissue. Ando et al. showed that ^{201}Tl mainly existed in the free form in the fluid of the tumor. However, a small fraction of thallium was localized in the nuclear, microchondrial, and microsomal fractions (50).

Technetium 99m–MIBI is a positively charged lipophilic molecule. Investigators have demonstrated that the mechanism of uptake within tumor cells is different from that for ^{201}Tl, although the spectrum of tumor accumulation is similar for many tumors. Although the precise mechanism has not been completely defined, investigators have shown that in contrast to active transport involved in thallium accumulation, MIBI enters the cell by means of passive diffusion across the sarcolemma and mitochondrial membranes in response to transmembrane potential differences (51,52). Technetium 99m–MIBI is attracted to the negative charges on mitochondria because of net positive charge and accumulates in regions with increased mitochondrial density and relatively high negatively charged mitochondria (53).

As noted in thallium accumulation within the myocardium or tumors, adequate blood flow must be present for uptake to occur. Limitation of blood supply may result in a net decrease of ^{99m}Tc-MIBI. The extraction of MIBI from the blood into the tumor cell appears to depend on a large transmembrane potential difference developed in tumors, as well as on mitochondrial density (51–58).

Imaging with ^{18}F-FDG may, at times, have a higher tumor-to-background ratio than planar or single photon emission CT (SPECT), ^{67}Ga, ^{201}Tl, or ^{99m}Tc-sestamibi. Biologic distribution of ^{18}F-FDG has less muscle uptake and more favorable distribution in the abdomen than ^{201}Tl and ^{99m}Tc-sestamibi, which are not suitable for imaging subdiaphragmatic lesions because of high uptake in the liver, intestines, and kidneys. Imaging with ^{18}F-FDG is completed within 3 hours after the intravenous injection (similar to thallium and sestamibi), which is much shorter when compared with 2 to 4 days for gallium. However, ^{18}F-FDG is more costly at present and requires prescheduling arrangements.

The assessment of tumor viability is important in that chemotherapy or radiation therapy, if successful, will significantly reduce or eliminate viable tumor. Failure of therapeutic response frequently occurs in patients with primary bone tumors. Therefore, an effective noninvasive method for establishing tumor viability is desirable for purposes of patient management.

The role of various radionuclides is essential for the prediction of tumor response either at the midcourse or the end of a chemotherapy regimen. This method helps the surgeon with planning and with the surgical approach. Garcia et al. suggested that FDG imaging was superior to ^{99m}Tc-MIBI in evaluating musculoskeletal sarcoma (27). Some evidence indicates that decreases in ^{18}F-FDG or ^{201}Tl-chloride uptake by the tumor (at least by 30% from pretreatment values) predict a good response (grade II or III). If the decrease is beyond 60%, grade III or IV response is expected. Quantitation of the response may be performed either by the specific uptake values or ratio of uptake of tumor to normal tissue.

CLINICAL STUDIES

Ramanna et al. demonstrated conventional bone scintigraphy to be a poor indicator of chemotherapeutic response (6). A bone scan performed shortly after patients underwent chemotherapy gave misleading information because of a healing response. The bone scan demonstrated increasing activity after successful chemotherapy in 80% of patients studied. The bone scan was not recommended for patient management purposes within 6 weeks of chemotherapy because increase in activity on the bone scan was mainly an indicator of healing and not necessarily of tumor growth. Ramanna et al. demonstrated that ^{67}Ga was also a relatively poor clinical correlate, although it was significantly better than the bone scan (6).

Figure 39.1 is an example of a patient with a high-grade osteosarcoma of the distal right femur. Note the thallium study (Fig. 39.1A) demonstrating a rim of markedly increased thallium uptake surrounding a photopenic central region. This pattern is commonly seen in high-grade sarcomas that are known to demonstrate central necrosis as a consequence of a rapidly grown tumor that obstructs the central blood supply. The gallium scan (Fig. 39.1B) done in the same patient demonstrates a more solid appearance of increased activity, whereas the bone scan done in the same

patient (Fig. 39.1C) demonstrates an intense solid focus of increased activity that appears more extensive than findings on the gallium scan.

Thallium 201 was found to be an excellent pharmaceutical for following a patient's therapeutic response because it was not associated with healing, but rather with tumor viability (6,11,12). Investigators reported that nearly 100% of patients demonstrated significant improvement on thallium scintigraphy when chemotherapy was successful. Patients with greater than 95% necrosis of the primary tumor demonstrated minimal or no thallium uptake when compared with the pretreatment baseline studies. Investigators found that ^{201}Tl was capable of demonstrating the activity of the tumor as well as tumor burden and was not affected by local healing.

Figure 39.2 represents a prechemotherapy thallium scan (Fig. 39.2A), gallium scan (Fig. 39.2B), and bone scan (Fig. 39.2C) in a patient with a biopsy-demonstrated osteogenic sarcoma of the left distal femur. After effective chemotherapy, the thallium scan failed to demonstrate abnormality (Fig. 39.2D), the gallium scan showed only a minor area of increase in the left distal femur (Fig. 39.2E), and the bone scan demonstrated significant activity in the left distal femur (Fig. 39.2F). Both gallium and bone scans often demonstrate healing bone, which may falsely indicate the presence of residual tumor.

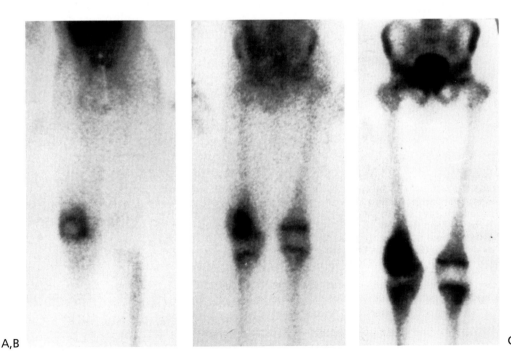

A,B   C

FIGURE 39.1. This is a comparison of thallium 201 **(A)**, gallium 67 **(B)**, and technetium 99m–methylene diphosphonate **(C)** studies performed on a patient with a high-grade osteosarcoma of the distal right femur. The thallium study demonstrates a "donut" pattern with a rim of increased thallium activity surrounding a photopenic center. The gallium scan done within 48 hours demonstrates a solid appearance of increased activity within the tumor. The bone scan demonstrates intense activity in the lesion. This pattern is generally seen in patients with high-grade osteosarcoma.

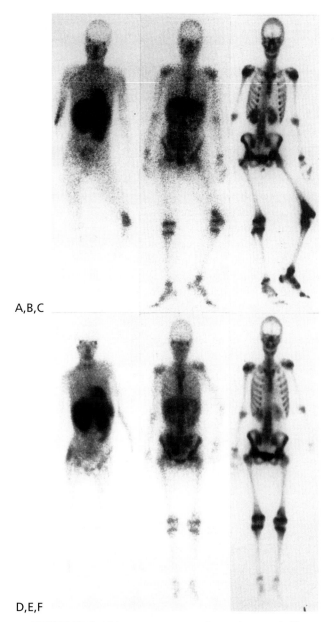

A,B,C

D,E,F

FIGURE 39.2. This compares a prechemotherapy thallium scan **(A)** with gallium 67 **(B)** and technetium 99m–methylene diphosphonate **(C)** scans in a patient with osteogenic sarcoma of the left femur. The postchemotherapy studies demonstrate discordant results in which the thallium study shows complete resolution of previously demonstrated abnormality **(D)**, the gallium scan demonstrates mild increase **(E)**, and the bone scan demonstrates a major area of activity in the left distal femur **(F)**. Findings on gallium and bone scan most likely represent bone repair, which may be incorrectly interpreted as representing residual tumor. Biopsy demonstrated greater than 98% tumor necrosis.

Figure 39.3 shows a patient with an osteogenic sarcoma of the left shoulder and proximal humerus. The pretherapy thallium study (Fig. 39.3A), pretherapy gallium scan (Fig. 39.3B), and pretherapy bone scan (Fig. 39.3C) all demonstrated intense uptake, with the findings appearing greater on the bone scan when compared with results of gallium and thallium scans. After 4 weeks of chemotherapy, the thallium scan (Fig. 39.3D) demonstrated significant reduc-

tion in activity, whereas the gallium scan showed a relative increase as determined by an increased tumor-to-background ratio (Fig. 39.3E). The bone scan (Fig. 39.3F) demonstrated no significant change after chemotherapy. Clinically, the patient was moderately improved, although significant tumor burden remained. The reliability of thallium in determining tumor burden and tumor viability is superior when compared with either gallium or bone scintigraphy because thallium detects tumor burden and does not reflect bone healing.

Rosen et al. used thallium studies to assess the response of tumor to preoperative chemotherapy in preparing patients for limb salvage (11). This study graded 27 patients with osteosarcoma or malignant fibrous hystiocytoma of bone. Patients were graded by their response to tumor. The patients were categorized into three distinct categories: *category 1 (worse or no response), category 2 (definite response with discernible reduction but a recognizable lesions present)*, or category 3 (previously abnormal abnormality, barely discernible, or absent). Of 10 patients who had a category 1 response, only 1 had a good histologic response. Five patients (50%) in this group remained as relapse-free survivors. A highly significant correlation (*p* < .005) was noted between a category 1 response and a histologic response to chemotherapy in the primary tumor. Nine patients were graded as having a category 2 response, and 6 of these patients (67%) had a good histologic response. Eight patients had category 3 changes on thallium imaging, and all 8 had an excellent histologic response after preoperative chemotherapy.

Mendez et al. demonstrated similar findings in 16 patients with high-grade sarcomas of the bone or soft tissue (12). This group demonstrated that changes in thallium activity correlated extremely well with histologic changes. When no improvement in uptake on thallium scan was observed, a poor histologic response to chemotherapy was generally seen. When a decrease in thallium uptake after chemotherapy was observed, the patient had a good or excellent histologic response to chemotherapy. The degree of reduced thallium uptake correlated well with the increasing amounts of tumor necrosis.

Figure 39.4 is a ^{201}Tl study that demonstrates failure to improve after chemotherapy in a patient with an osteogenic sarcoma of the right scapula. This patient would be categorized as category 1 (worse or no response).

Figure 39.5 is a ^{201}Tl scan in a patient with an osteogenic sarcoma of the left distal femur in which a partial response after initial chemotherapy was observed. This patient would be categorized as category 2 (definite response with discernible reduction in thallium activity but recognizable lesion still present). Note the gallium scan, which continues to demonstrate an intense focus of increased activity associated with the left knee. Some peripheral increase was noted in the pretherapy gallium study, but it diminished considerably after therapy. The core lesion still remains as markedly intense, whereas the thallium study after therapy shows a significant degree of improvement.

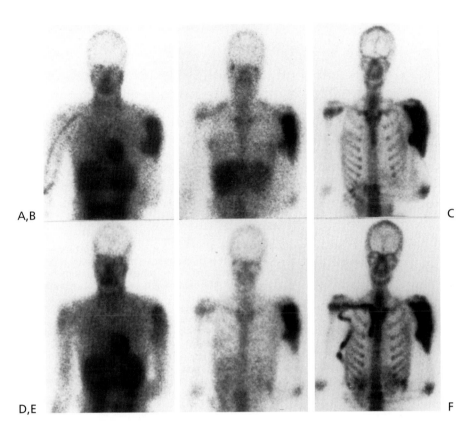

A,B

C

D,E

F

FIGURE 39.3. This compares a prethallium study **(A)**, a pretherapy gallium scan **(B)**, and a pretherapy bone scan **(C)** with respective post-therapy thallium **(D)**, gallium **(E)**, and technetium 99m–methylene diphosphonate **(F)** scans, performed after 4 weeks of chemotherapy. By clinical criteria, the patient was moderately improved with significant reduction in pain and swelling. Thallium appears to be the most reliable indicator in determining tumor burden in which a moderate degree of improvement had occurred. The gallium and bone scans were not representative of the clinical improvement and were either unchanged or appeared worse.

Figure 39.6 is a prechemotherapy and postchemotherapy comparison of thallium and gallium in a patient with an osteogenic sarcoma in which both baseline pretherapy studies demonstrated intense activity in the right distal femur. After 1 month of therapy, a mild to moderate response was recorded on both thallium and gallium studies. However, at 2 months, the thallium study indicated a greater degree of improvement than the gallium study; only minimal change was noted from the 1-month to the 2-month study using ^{67}Ga. Clinically, the patient had improved significantly from the 1-month to 2-month study, with thallium correlating more favorably to the clinical response. This patient was considered to have a category 2 response.

Figure 39.7 is a patient with a sarcoma of the posterior chest wall including the ribs. Note the partial reduction in thallium activity by 1 month and the complete reduction at the end of 2 months. CT indicated minimal residual disease at 2 months. This patient was considered to have a category 3 response.

Figure 39.8 is a patient with an osteosarcoma of the right distal femur with a complete response (category 3). Biopsy confirmed greater than 98% tumor necrosis. The gallium study done at the same time showed considerable residual activity most likely representing a significant healing response.

Caner et al. demonstrated accumulation of MIBI in a patient with osteogenic sarcoma of the proximal tibia (25). Activity was also seen in an inguinal lymph node, which was demonstrated by biopsy to be malignant. In a separate study, Caner et al. demonstrated sestamibi to be successful in imaging patients with primary bone tumors (5). Ten

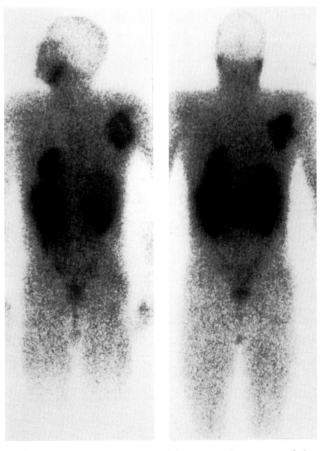

FIGURE 39.4. This is a patient with osteogenic sarcoma of the right scapula **(left)** that did not improve after chemotherapy **(right)**. This study was considered a category 1 response (worsening or no response seen on the thallium 201 study).

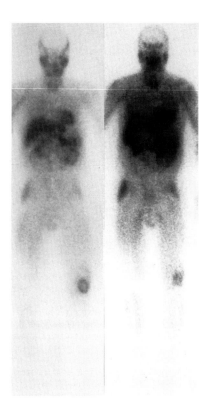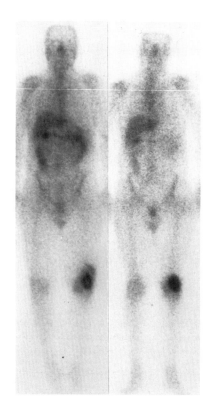

FIGURE 39.5. In this patient with an osteogenic sarcoma, the thallium scan demonstrates a partial response after chemotherapy. This study represents a category 2 response (definite response with discernible reduction in thallium activity but recognizable lesion still present). The gallium scan **(right)** is discordant, with intense focal increase still noted within the left distal femur. The thallium study **(left)** more correctly represented the clinical improvement noted in this patient. The **left** side of each pair shows prechemotherapy findings; the **right** side of each pair shows findings after chemotherapy.

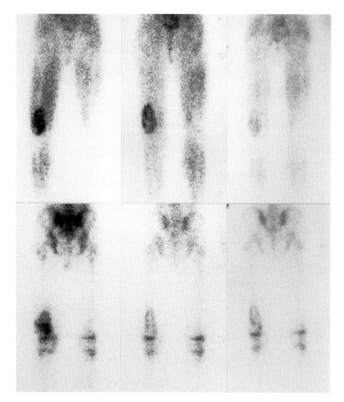

FIGURE 39.6. This is a prechemotherapy **(left)** and 1-month **(center)** and 2-month **(right)** postchemotherapy comparison of thallium 201 **(top)** and gallium 67 **(bottom)** scans in a patient with with osteogenic sarcoma of the right distal femur. A mild to moderate response to chemotherapy was noted on both the thallium and gallium studies after 1 month of treatment. After 2 months of treatment, the thallium study indicated a greater degree of improvement than gallium, which correlated more accurately with the clinical course than the gallium study. This patient was considered to have a category 2 response.

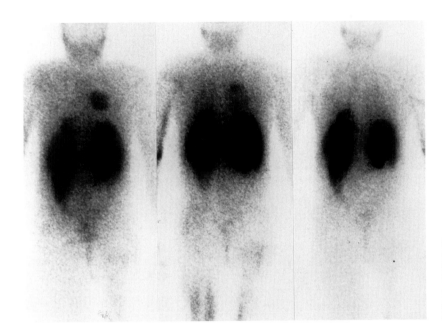

FIGURE 39.7. This patient has a sarcoma of the posterior chest wall including the ribs **(left)**. Serial thallium studies at 1 month **(center)** and 2 months **(right)** demonstrated a complete response. This pattern was considered a category 3 response (previously abnormal finding, barely discernible, or absent).

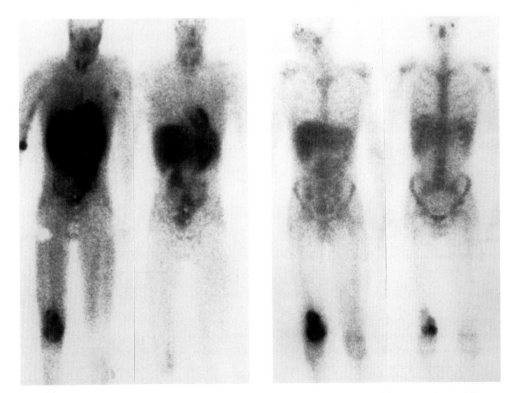

FIGURE 39.8. This is a category 3 response to thallium 201 imaging **(left)** in a patient with an osteosarcoma of the right distal femur. Biopsy confirmed a greater than 98% tumor necrosis. Note the discordant gallium study **(right)** also done at the same time that demonstrates considerable residual material most likely representing healing. Pretreatment findings are on the **left** side of each pair; post-treatment findings are on the **right** side of each pair.

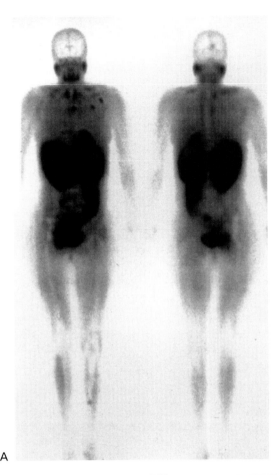

A

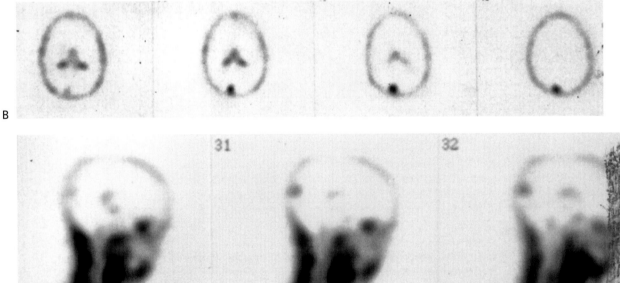

B

C

FIGURE 39.9. A: Whole-body technetium-99m–sesta-2-methoxy-isobotylisonitrile (^{99m}Tc-sestamibi) study in a patient with metastatic osteogenic sarcoma to the chest wall, pulmonary parenchyma, and posterior meninges **(left,** anterior; **right,** posterior). **B** and **C:** Transaxial and sagittal single photon emission computed tomography (SPECT) slices, respectively, demonstrating the meningeal metastasis.

patients with malignant tumors had both a pretherapeutic and a post-therapeutic MIBI study. The study demonstrated that radiotherapy or chemotherapy inhibited MIBI uptake and also demonstrated that post-therapeutic MIBI uptake correlated well with the effectiveness of chemotherapy, as confirmed by histologic evaluation.

Figure 39.9A is a whole-body MIBI study in a patient with metastatic osteogenic sarcoma after a lower extremity limb salvage procedure. Metastases were noted in the chest wall, pulmonary parenchyma, and posterior midline meninges within the falx. Figure 39.9B and C are transaxial and sagittal SPECT slices demonstrating the falx metastasis. Figure 39.9D and E are coronal and axial SPECT images demonstrating small pulmonary nodules. Note the

exceptionally high tumor-to-background ratio within the small nodules within the lung. Many of the nodules detected were less than 10 mm in diameter.

Ashok et al. compared ^{201}Tl with MIBI in patients with soft-tissue as well as osteogenic sarcoma (13). Nineteen patients with prior or current osteosarcoma were evaluated using both ^{201}Tl and ^{99m}Tc-MIBI. The studies were performed on the same day, with the MIBI study following the ^{201}Tl examination. Using a semiquantitative rating, the investigators conducted a site-by-site comparison for thallium and MIBI. The study demonstrated MIBI to have a slightly overall better tumor-to-background activity and in addition demonstrated abnormal sites not seen using ^{201}Tl. Both thallium and MIBI gave excellent correlation with histologic

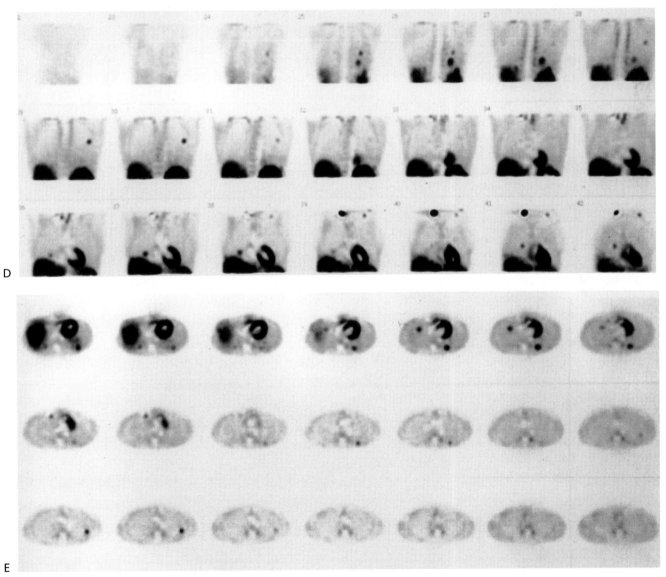

D

E

FIGURE 39.9. *(continued)* **D and E:** Coronal and axial SPECT images of the chest demonstrating small pulmonary nodules seen on the CT examination. Exceptionally high tumor-to-background ratios can be seen with ^{99m}Tc-sestamibi in patients with pulmonary metastasis.

findings in evaluating tumor response to chemotherapy. The superiority of MIBI over ^{201}Tl was believed possibly to result from the higher dose given (30 mCi) for MIBI when compared with the 3 mCi used for [201]Tl.

Most patients with sarcomas demonstrate a moderate to marked increase in ^{201}Tl or ^{99m}Tc-MIBI uptake. In general, tumors of a high-grade type demonstrate a pattern of central lucency with a peripheral zone of intense thallium activity surrounding the lucency to give a "donut" pattern. Ramanna et al. and Ashok et al. demonstrated that more than 95% of high-grade sarcomas present with a "donut sign" (10,13,14). Low-grade sarcomas generally present as a solid area of increase with no central lucency (10). These findings appear to result from the exceptionally rapid growth rate of high-grade sarcomas, which tend to outgrow their blood supply and pathologically are shown to demonstrate necrosis in the tumor center. The peripheral areas of tumor maintain a normal or increased vascular perfusion and histologically demonstrate areas of active growth with little or no necrosis. A positive MIBI or thallium scan with a donut pattern indicates a high-grade sarcoma until proven otherwise (10,13,14).

Ramanna et al. demonstrated and evaluated the potential for ^{201}Tl to differentiate between a benign and a malignant lesion of the bone (9). The study evaluated 16 patients with biopsy-proved benign bone lesions. Four patients in this series demonstrated a marked increase in thallium activity. This group included patients with Paget's disease of bone, fibrous dysplasia, trauma, and ossifying fibroma. In addition, 5 patients demonstrated mild but definite thallium activity. The diagnosis in this group included patients with benign fibrous hysticytoma, and benign fibrous myxoma and 3 patients with Paget's disease. Seven patients with benign disease had entirely normal findings. The conclusion from this study was that thallium activity in bone abnormalities is not specific for malignant tumor and can be seen in various benign abnormalities. A negative test, however, is significant in that the probability of malignant primary tumor of bone is minimal.

Caner et al. demonstrated an 86% sensitivity for ^{99m}Tc-MIBI in patients with malignant tumors. Eleven of 31 patients (35%) with benign disease also demonstrated MIBI uptake. The study demonstrated that malignant lesions tend to have a higher overall MIBI uptake than benign lesions, but a significant overlap exists between benign and malignant bone abnormalities (5).

Although ^{201}Tl-chloride and ^{99m}Tc-sestamibi are helpful in the differentiation of benign from malignant lesions in bone and other locations in the body, there are no similar reports for the use of FDG at the time of initial diagnosis. A possible reason is that because the expense of an FDG study was nonreimbursable until recently, a preoperative test could not be performed outside a research protocol. In addition, a negative predictive value of 100% is not realistic, and most probably a biopsy would be performed. Some benign bone lesions have false-positive uptake. Conversely, some malignant soft-tissue tumors may have false-negative results of an ^{18}F-FDG study. In our experience, this is especially noted in tumors that are cystic or have chondroid matrixlike chondrosarcoma (especially the low-grade varieties) and tumors with myxomatous matrix such as myxoid liposarcoma or fibrosarcoma. In these tumors, the cytoplasm contains many secretions, and the nucleus is often displaced.

Magnetic resonance imaging is considered to be the primary imaging modality at the time of initial diagnosis for these lesions. These tumors usually spread locally, can erode the periosteum or surrounding tissue, and can extend into the marrow space, sometimes with skip metastases. For the purpose of biopsy and surgical treatment, it is appropriate to know the anatomic margins of the tumor. For this purpose, MRI and CT are more accurate than most nuclear medicine procedures (59–70).

An important area in the management of patients with bone and soft-tissue sarcoma is the evaluation of response to therapy. Previous reports using thallium or ^{99m}Tc-sestamibi had limitations because of the background activity either in the abdomen or the adjacent muscles (20, 24). However, both methods had better results than MRI or CT (20,28–31). Similar reports showed that ^{18}F-FDG imaging was more sensitive than x-ray CT or MRI for detection of local recurrence (32–34). Conversely, ^{18}F-FDG has a favorable distribution in the muscles and the abdomen and can accordingly easily visualize lesions in the spine, sacrum, and ribs (Figs. 39.10 to 39.13). Renal and bladder activity must be overcome when imaging with ^{18}F-FDG by the insertion of a Foley catheter in the bladder or induction of diuresis by hydration and intravenous injection of furosemide. Subsequently, the accuracy of interpretation of abdominal lesions is increased. A potential problem with ^{18}F-FDG imaging is the postoperative change that can persist up to 6 months (Fig. 39.14). However, proper clinical examination of the patient and correlation with other imaging modalities can help to differentiate ^{18}F-FDG uptake resulting from postoperative changes from focal recurrence. Moreover, serial ^{18}F-FDG studies at intervals of 3 to 4 months may be useful. Uptake of ^{18}F-FDG has been reported in arthritis, traumatic compression fractures, and normal gastrointestinal and genitourinary uptake (71,72).

Evaluation of chemotherapy response in patients who have had postoperative recurrence is important for medical oncologists in their selection of proper chemotherapy. It may be potentially useful to perform ^{18}F-FDG imaging just before a second course of chemotherapy is induced (Fig. 39.15). When an ^{18}F-FDG–positive lesion turns negative after chemotherapy, it does not mean that the lesion has been eliminated. Microscopic cells may still be present and may result in recurrence after a short period. However, an ^{18}F-FDG–negative scan 1 year after chemotherapy is a good indicator of complete remission.

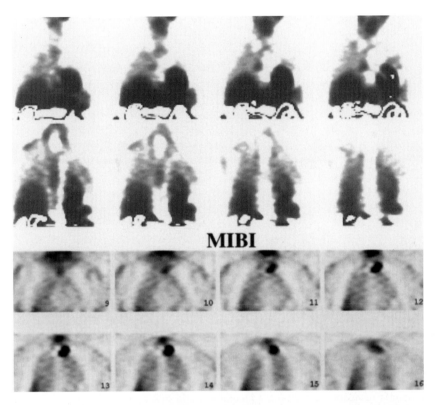

MIBI

FIGURE 39.10. Recurrent osteosarcoma of the upper dorsal spine. Comparison between technetium-99m–sesta-2-methoxyisobotylisonitrile technetium single photon emission computed tomography **(upper two rows)** and fluorine 18–fluorodeoxyglucose (^{18}F-FDG) coincidence imaging **(lower two rows).** Recurrence in the upper dorsal spine is more clearly delineated with ^{18}F-FDG.

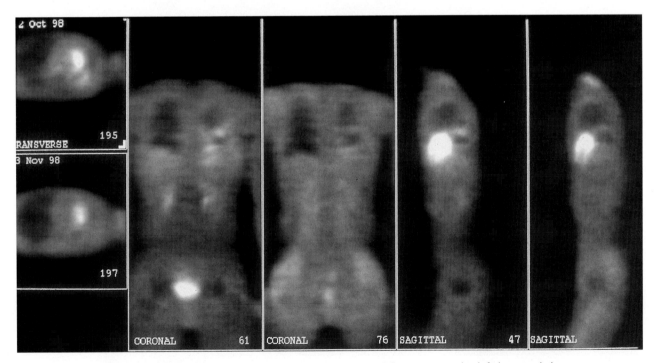

FIGURE 39.11. A 42-year-old man with metastatic synovial sarcoma to the left lung and the lower end of the sacrum.

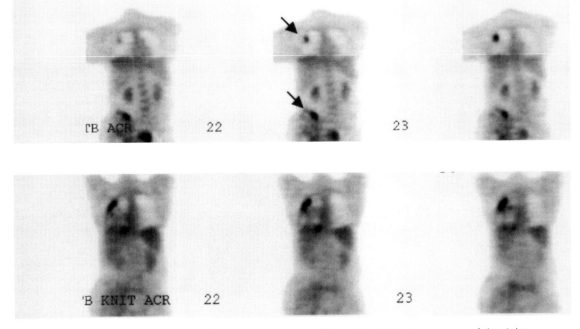

FIGURE 39.12. Metastatic and local recurrence of undifferentiated chondrosarcoma of the right pelvis before chemotherapy **(upper row)** and after chemotherapy **(lower row).** This shows good response for the lesions in the pelvis *(arrows).* The increased uptake in the chest after chemotherapy was because the patient developed a right-sided pleural effusion that required drainage and chest tube insertion.

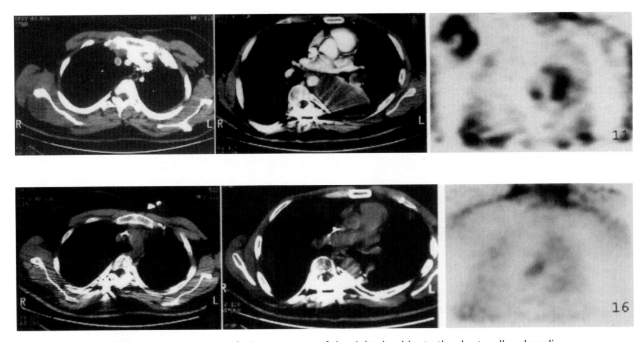

FIGURE 39.13. Metastatic soft-tissue sarcoma of the right shoulder to the chest wall and mediastinum. **Top:** Prechemotherapy computed tomography (CT) and fluorodeoxyglucose (FDG) images; **bottom:** after chemotherapy. The **lower row** shows CT and FDG images with good response to the primary lesion in the right shoulder and incomplete response to the metastatic lesions in the right chest wall and mediastinum.

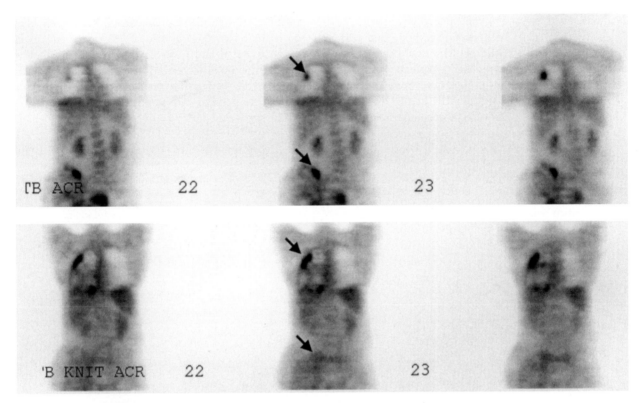

FIGURE 39.14. Right pelvic chondrosarcoma after surgical resection in a patient who had local recurrence and metastases to the right chest wall. He had two fluorine 18–fluorodeoxyglucose studies before and after chemotherapy that showed good response for the pelvic lesion and increased uptake in the right chest wall lesion that was attributed to the recent insertion of a chest tube to drain a malignant pleural effusion.

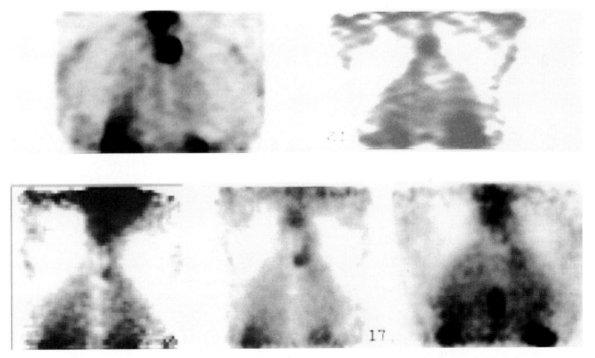

FIGURE 39.15. Recurrent osteosarcoma of dorsal spine in a patient who had repeated fluorine 18–fluorodeoxyglucose studies during chemotherapy. Although this shows initial excellent response to chemotherapy, the disease recurred a few weeks later, after cessation of treatment.

Dual-head gamma camera coincidence imaging in the management of patients with malignant bone and soft-tissue tumors has been reported (H.M. Adbel Dayem, *personal communication*). Twenty-eight patients with 48 known lesions from recurrent or metastatic bone and soft-tissue sarcomas detected by CT or MRI had 87 ^{18}F-FDG dual-head gamma camera coincidence imaging baseline and follow-up studies. Pathologic diagnosis was as follows: 5 osteosarcomas, 4 synovial cell sarcomas, 4 liposarcomas, 3 soft-tissue sarcomas, 3 hemangiopericytomas, 2 chondrosarcomas, 2 Ewing's sarcomas, 1 fibrosarcoma, 1 meningiosarcoma, 1 neurofibrosarcoma, 1 spindle cell sarcoma, and 1 pigmented villonodular synovitis. Patient preparation, injection of FDG, and acquisition and processing of data were performed according to previously presented department protocol. Three independent observers interpreted the data, and the difference in intensity between the studies were compared. The results showed that CT or MRI and FDG studies were positive for either local recurrence or metastases in 19 patients (baseline and follow-up images). Three of these patients underwent reoperation for disease recurrence in addition to chemotherapy. The remaining patients received adjuvant treatment: 4 patients had newly discovered lesions and needed modification of their treatment, 5 patients had stable lesions, 4 patients showed improved response to treatment (more than 50% regression of the tumor size), and 3 patients had no follow-up after their adjuvant treatment. FDG was successful in verifying postoperative changes and in excluding disease recurrence in 9 patients when CT or MRI findings suggested tumor recurrence in 4 patients, and an unnecessary operation was avoided in 1 patient. Follow-up FDG studies of these patients showed decrease of tracer intensity in the operative field over a 3-month period. It was concluded that repeated PET imaging is reliable for monitoring treatment response and differentiating postoperative changes from residual or recurrent tumors in patients previously operated for bone and soft-tissue malignant tumors.

SUMMARY

Bone and soft-tissue sarcomas are detected with both MIBI and ^{201}Tl with relatively high sensitivity. Improvement in lesion detection is consistently demonstrated using ^{99m}Tc-MIBI probably because of the higher count rates achieved using a 30-mCi dose of ^{99m}Tc-MIBI when compared with a 3-mCi dose of [201]Tl. The higher photon flux and superior imaging characteristics of the 140-keV ^{99m}Tc also is believed to contribute to the higher degree of sensitivity. FDG imaging with newer, improved detectors may be more sensitive than MIBI and superior in the abdomen as a result of less nonspecific organ and gastrointestinal activity.

Comparative studies demonstrate overall sensitivity for detection of primary sarcoma to be similar for ^{201}Tl MIBI and FDG at the time of presentation. Most likely, the reason is the relatively large size of lesions present on initial diagnosis. MIBI and FDG have been demonstrated to be slightly superior in detecting distant metastasis, including lymph nodes within the drainage pattern of the tumor, especially in patients with nonosteogenic sarcomas.

The specificity of ^{201}Tl and ^{99m}Tc-MIBI for malignancy is disappointing. Both ^{201}Tl and ^{99m}Tc-MIBI have been shown to accumulate in a large number of benign lesions. A negative study, especially using 30 mCi of ^{99m}Tc-MIBI, is consistent with a benign lesion because the sensitivity for malignancy detection is more than 90% in lesions greater than 15 to 20 mm. More work with FDG is needed to evaluate specificity.

Thallium 201, MIBI, and FDG are excellent correlates of tissue viability and can be effectively used in following patients who have received chemotherapy or radiation therapy. A significant improvement from baseline scans after therapy consistently indicates a good therapeutic effect.

If tumor activity in the post-therapeutic study is minimal or undetectable, tumor necrosis has been shown to be greater than 95%. The correlation with therapeutic response, tumor viability, and survival suggest an important role for ^{201}Tl, ^{99m}Tc-MIBI, and FDG in managing patients with bone and soft-tissue sarcomas.

REFERENCES

1. Jaffe N. Recent advances in the chemotherapy of metastatic osteogenic sarcoma. *Cancer* 1972;30:1627–1631.
2. Jaffe N. Progress report on high dose methotrexate (NSC-740) with citrovorum rescue in the treatment of metastatic bone tumors. *Cancer* 1974;58:275–280.
3. Rosen G. The development of an adjuvant chemotherapy program for the treatment of osteogenic sarcoma. *Front Radiat Ther Oncol* 1975;10:115–133.
4. Rosen G. Management of malignant bone tumors in children and adolescents. *Pediatr Clin North Am* 1976;23:183–213.
5. Caner B, Kitapci M, Unlu M, et al. Technetium-99m MIBI uptake in benign and malignant bone lesions: a comparative study with technetium-99m MDP. *J Nucl Med* 1992;33:319.
6. Ramanna L, Waxman AD, Binney G, et al. Thallium-201 scintigraphy in bone sarcoma: comparison with Ga-67 and Tc-99m MDP in evaluation of chemotherapy response. *J Nucl Med* 1990;31:567.
7. Stoller DW, Waxman AD, Rosen G, et al. Comparison of thallium-201, gallium-67, technetium-99m MDP and magnetic resonance imaging of muscoleskeletal sarcoma. *Clin Nucl Med* 1986;12[Suppl]:P15(abst).
8. Waxman AD. Thallium-201 in nuclear oncology. In: Freeman LM, ed. *Nuclear* medicine annual. New York: Raven, 1991:193.
9. Ramanna L, Waxman AD, Rosen G. Evaluation of Tl-201 (Tl) uptake pattern in bone lesions: differentiation of benign from malignant processes. *J Nucl Med* 1992;33:869.
10. Ramanna L, Waxman AD, Weiss A, et al. Thallium-201 (Tl-201) scan patterns in bone and soft tissue sarcoma. *J Nucl Med* 1992;33:843.
11. Rosen G, Loren G, Brien E, et al. Serial thallium-201 scintigra-

phy in osteosarcoma: correlation with tumor necrosis after pre-operative chemotherapy. *Clin Orthop* 1993;293:302–306.

12. Menedez LR, Fideler BM, Mirra J. Thallium-201 scanning for the evaluation of osteosarcoma and soft-tissue sarcoma: a study of the evaluation and predictability of the histological response to chemotherapy. *J Bone Joint Surg Am* 1993;75:1880–1881.

13. Ashok G, Waxman AD, Kooba A, et al. Comparison of Tl-201 (Tl) and Tc-99m methoxyisobutyl isonitrile in the evaluation of patients with osteogenic sarcoma. *Clin Nucl Med* 1992;9:(abst).

14. Ashok G, Waxman AD, Kooba A, et al. Comparison of Tl-201 (Tl) and Tc-99m methoxyisobutyl isonitrile in the evaluation of patients with non-osseous sarcomas. *Clin Nucl Med* 1992;9: (abst).

15. Hudson M, Jaffe MR, Jaffe N, et al. Pediatric osteosarcoma: therapeutic strategies, results and prognostic factors derived from a 10-yr. experience. *J Clin Oncol* 1990;8:1988–1997.

16. Ramanna L, Waxman AD, Waxman S, et al. Tl-201 scintigraphy in bone and soft tissue sarcoma: evaluation of tumor mass and viability. *J Nucl Med* 1988;29:854.

17. Ohtomo K, Terui S, Yokoyama R, et al. Thallium-201 scintigraphy to assess effect of chemotherapy in osteosarcoma. *J Nucl Med* 1996;37:1444–1448.

18. Lin J, Leung WT, Ho SKW, et al. Quantitative evaluation of thallium-201 uptake in predicting chemotherapeutic response of osteosarcoma. *Eur J Nucl Med* 1995;22:553–555.

19. Imbriaco M, Yeh SDJ, Yeung H, et al. Thallium-201 scintigraphy for the evaluation of tumor response to preoperative chemotherapy in patients with osteosarcoma. *Cancer* 1997;80:1507–1512.

20. Kostakoglu L, Panicek DM, Divgi CR, et al. Correlation of the findings of thallium-201 chloride scans with those of other imaging modalities and histology following therapy in patients with bone and soft tissue sarcomas. *Eur J Nucl Med* 1995;22:1233–1237.

21. Caluser C, Abdel-Dayem HM, Macapinlac H, et al. The value of thallium and three-phase bone scans in the evaluation of bone and soft tissue sarcomas. *Eur J Nucl Med* 1994;21:1198–1205.

22. Lin J, Leung WT, Ho SKW, et al. Quantitative evaluation of thallium-201 uptake in predicting chemotherapeutic response of osteosarcoma. *Eur J Nucl Med* 1995;22:553–555.

23. Sumiya H, Taki J, Tsuchiya H, et al. Midcourse thallium-201 scintigraphy to predict tumor response in bone and soft tissue tumors. *J Nucl Med* 1998;39:1600–1604.

24. Caluser C, Macapinlac H, Healey J, et al. The relationship between thallium uptake, blood flow and blood pool radioactivity in bone and soft tissue tumors. *Clin Nucl Med* 1992;17: 565–571.

25. Caner B, Kitapci M, Aras T, et al. Increased accumulation of hexakis (2-methoxyisobutylisonitrile) technetium (I) in osteosarcoma and its metastatic lymph nodes. *J Nucl Med* 1991;32: 1977–1978.

26. Söderlund V, Larsson SA, Bauer HCF, et al. Use of Tc-99m-MIBI scintigraphy in the evaluation of the response of osteosarcoma to chemotherapy. *Eur J Nucl Med* 1997;24:511–515.

27. Garcia JR, Kim EE, Wong FCL, et al. Comparison of fluorine-18-FDG PET and Technetium-99m-MIBI SPECT in evaluation of musculoskeletal sarcoma. *J Nucl Med* 1996;37:1476–1479.

28. Jones DN, McCowage GB, Sostman HD, et al. Monitoring of neoadjuvant therapy response of soft-tissue and musculoskeletal sarcoma using fluorine-18-FDG PET. *J Nucl Med* 1996;37: 1438–1444.

29. Kotzerke J, Brecht-Krauss D, Schulte M, et al. Monitoring pre-operative chemotherapy response in patients with osteosarcoma using (^{18}F) FDG-PET. *J Nucl Med* 1997;38:127P.

30. Griffeth LK, Dehdashti F, McGuire AH, et al. PET Evaluation of soft-tissue masses with fluorine-18 fluoro-2-deoxy-D-glucose. *Radiology* 1992;182:185–194.

31. El-Zeftawy H, Rosen G, Abdel-Dayem HM, et al. Value of

repeated F-18 fluorodeoxyglucose (FDG) scans in postoperative management of patients with bone and soft tissue sarcoma. *Proc Am Soc Clin Oncol* 1999;18.

32. Kole AC, Nieweg OE, van Ginkel RJ, et al. Detection of local recurrence of soft-tissue sarcoma with positron emission tomography using (F-18) fluorodeoxyglucose. *Ann Surg Oncol* 1997;4: 57–63.

33. Nieweg OE, Pruim J, van Ginkel RJ, et al. Fluorine-18-fluorodeoxyglucose PET imaging of soft-tissue sarcoma. *J Nucl Med* 1996;37:257–261.

34. Engenhart R, Kimmig BN, Straub LG, et al. Therapy monitoring of presacral recurrence after high-dose irradiation: value of PET, CT, CEA and pain score. *Strahlenther Onkol* 1992;168: 203–212.

35. Abdel-Dayem HM. The role of nuclear medicine in primary bone and soft tissue tumors. *Semin Nucl Med* 1997;27:355–363.

36. Phelps ME, Cherry SR. The changing design of positron imaging systems. *Clin Positron Imaging* 1998;1:31–45.

37. Patton JA, Turkington TG. Coincidence imaging with a dual-head scintillation cameras. *J Nucl Med* 1999;40:432–441.

38. Boren EL, Delbeke D, Patton JA, et al. Comparison of FDG PET and positron coincidence detection imaging using a dual-head gamma camera with 5/8-inch NaI(Tl) crystals in patients with suspected body malignancies. *Eur J Nucl Med* 1999;26: 379–387.

39. Weber WA, Neverve J, Sklarek J, et al. Imaging of lung cancer with fluorine-18 fluorodeoxyglucose: comparison of a dual-head gamma camera in coincidence mode with a full-ring positron emission tomography system. *Eur J Nucl Med* 1999;26:388–395.

40. Abdel-Dayem HM, Luo JQ, El-Zeftawy H, et al. Clinical experience with dual head gamma camera coincidence imaging. *Clin Positron Imaging* 1999.

41. El-Gazzar A, Malki A, Abdel-Dayem HM, et al. Role of thallium-201 chloride in diagnosis of solitary bone lesions. *Nucl Med Commun* 1989;14:477–485.

42. Abdel-Dayem HM, Scott AM, Macapinlac HA, et al. Role of thallium-201 chloride in tumor imaging. In: Freeman LM, ed. *Nuclear medicine annual.* New York: Raven, 1994:181–234.

43. Zaher AM. *Role of thallium-201 chloride, Tc-99m sestaMIBI and skeletal scanning in evaluation of bone and soft tissue sarcomas.* MS thesis. Cairo: National Cancer Institute and Faculty of Medicine, Cairo University, 1997.

44. Atkins HL, Budinger TF, Lebowitz E, et al. Thallium-201 for medical use. III. Human distribution and physical imaging properties. *J Nucl Med* 1977;18:133.

45. Bradley-Moore PR, Lebowitz E, Greene MW, et al. Thallium-201 for medical use. II. Biological behavior. *J Nucl Med* 1975;16: 156.

46. Gehring PJ, Hammond PR. The interrelationship between thallium and potassium in animals. *J Pharmacol Exp Ther* 1967;155: 187.

47. Lebowitz E, Greene MW, Green R, et al. Thallium-201 for medical use. I. *J Nucl Med* 1975;16:151.

48. Britten JS, Blank M. Thallium activation of the (Na$^+$, K$^+$) activated ATPase of rabbit kidney. *Biochim Biophys Acta* 1968;15: 160.

49. Sessler MK, Geek P, Maul FD, et al. New aspects of cellular Tl-201 uptake: T$^+$Na$^+$2Cl$^-$cotransport in the central mechanism of ion uptake. *J Nucl Med* 1986;25:24.

50. Ando A, Ando I, Katayama M, et al. Biodistribution of Tl-201 in tumor bearing animals and inflammatory lesion induced animals. *Eur J Nucl Med* 1987;12:567.

51. Maublant JC, Gachon P, Moins N. Hexakis (2-methoxyisobutylisonitrile) technetium-99m and thallium-201 chloride: uptake and release in cultured myocardial cells. *J Nucl Med* 1988;29:48.

52. Maublant JC, Moins N, Gachon P, et al. Uptake of technetium-

99m teboroxime in cultured myocardial cells: comparison with thallium-201 and technetium-99m sestamibi. *J Nucl Med* 1993; 34:255.

53. Delmon-Moingeon LI, Piwnica-Worms D, Van Den Abbeele AD, et al. Uptake of the cation hexakis (2-methoxyisobutyl-isonitrile) technetium-99m by human carcinoma cells *in vitro.* *Cancer Res* 1990;50:2198.

54. Carvalho PA, Chiu ML, Kronauge JF, et al. Subcellular distribution and analysis of technetium-99m MIBI in isolated perfused rat hearts. *J Nucl Med* 1992;33:1516.

55. Chernoff DM, Strichartz GR, Piwnica-Worms D. Membrane potential determination in large unilamellar vesicles with hexakis (2-methoxyisobutyl-isonitrile) technetium (I). *Biochim Biophys Acta* 1993;1147:262.

56. Chiu ML, Herman LW, Kronauge JF, et al. Comparative effects of neutral dipolar compounds and lipophilic anions on technetium 99-m-hexakis(2-methoxyisobutyl-isonitrile) accumulation in cultured chick ventricular myocytes. *Invest Radiol* 1992;27:1052.

57. Chiu ML, Kronauge JF, Piwnica-Worms D. Effect of mitochondrial and plasma membrane membrane potentials on accumulation of hexakis (2-methoxyisobutyl-isonitrile) technetium (I) in cultures mouse fibroblasts. *J Nucl Med* 1990;31:1646.

58. Crane P, Laliberte R, Heminway S, et al. Effects of mitochondrial viability and metabolism on technetium-99m sestamibi myocardial retention. *Eur J Nucl Med* 1993;21:20.

59. Huvos AG, ed. *Bone tumors: diagnosis, treatment and prognosis,* 2nd ed. Philadelphia: WB Saunders, 1991.

60. Huvos AG. Osteogenic sarcoma of bone and soft tissue in older persons: a clinical pathologic analysis of 117 patients older than 60 years. *Cancer* 1986;57:1442–1449.

61. Dablin DC, Conventry MB. Osteogenic sarcoma: a study of 600 cases. *J Bone Joint Surg Am* 1964;49:101–110.

62. McKenna RJ, Schwinn CP, Soong KY, et al. Sarcomata of the osteogenic series (osteosarcoma, fibrosarcoma, chondrosarcoma, parosteal osteogenic sarcoma, and sarcomara arising in abnormal bone): analysis of 552 cases. *J Bone Joint Surg Am* 1966; 48:1–26.

63. Lukens JA, McLeod RA, Sim FH. Computed tomographic evaluation of primary osseous malignant neoplasms. *AJR Am J Roentgenol* 1982;139:45–48.

64. Schreiman JS, Crass FR, Wick MR, et al. Osteosarcoma: role of CT in limb-sparing treatment. *Radiology* 1986;161:485–488.

65. Aisen AM, Martel W, Braunstein EM, et al. MRI and CT evaluation of primary bone and soft tissue tumors. *AJR Am J Roentgenol* 1986;146:749–753.

66. Erlemann R, Sciuk J, Bosse A, et al. Response of osteosarcoma and Ewing sarcoma to preoperative chemotherapy: assessment with dynamic and static MR imaging and skeletal scintigraphy. *Radiology* 1990;175:791–796.

67. Hudson TM, Hawlin DJ, Enneking WF, et al. Magnetic resonance imaging of bone and soft tissue tumors: early experience in 31 patients compared with computed tomography. *Skeletal Radiol* 1985;13:134–136.

68. Petasnick J, Turner D, Charters J, et al. Soft tissue marros of the locomotor system: comparison of MR imaging with CT. *Radiology* 1986;160:125–133.

69. Hudson TM, Haas G, Enneking WF, et al. Angiography in the management of musculoskeletal tumors. *J Surg Gynecol Obstet* 1975;141:11–21.

70. Hudson TM, Schiebler M, Springfield DS, et al. Radiologic imaging of osteosarcoma: role in planning surgical treatment. *Skeletal Radiol* 1983;10:137–146.

71. Shreve PD, Anzai Y, Wahl RL. Pitfalls in oncologic diagnosis with FDG PET imaging: physiologic and benign variants. *Radiographics* 1999;19:61–77.

72. Vesselle HJ, Miraldi FD. FDG PET of the retroperitoneum: normal anatomy, variants, pathologic conditions, and strategies to avoid diagnostic pitfalls. *Radiographics* 1998;18:805–823.

40

SCINTIGRAPHY OF BONE METASTASES

PARTHA SINHA
LEONARD M. FREEMAN

The bony skeleton represents a frequent site of metastatic spread for many neoplasms, most commonly those arising in the breast, prostate, and lung. Bone involvement may occur early or late in the course of the disease. Detection of bone metastases at an early stage is likely to have the greatest impact on major management decisions. Metastatic disease occurring at a later stage is often a manifestation of more widespread dissemination of a tumor. Despite this, enormous advances in oncologic therapy have broadened treatment options in the later stages of disease involvement. Detection of bone metastases at any stage, therefore, is important to the clinician.

HISTORICAL PERSPECTIVE OF THE BONE SCAN

The radionuclide bone scan using strontium 85 (^{85}Sr) was first described in 1961 by Flemming et al. (1). This report dealt with detecting sites of trauma, which had evolved into a common use of the study. Shortly thereafter, Simpson and associates (2) reported the successful use of the bone scan to detect occult metastatic sites that responded favorably to radiation therapy.

The concept of using radioactive strontium traces back to independent autoradiographic studies in 1942 by Treadwell et al. (3) and Pecher (4). These investigators showed that cyclotron-produced beta-emitting ^{89}Sr had a similar distribution pattern to another alkaline earth metal, calcium. The gamma-emitting ^{85}Sr became available in the mid-1950s (5), and it subsequently was used clinically in the late 1950s and early 1960s (1,2,6–8). The demonstration that abnormal bone scans were often associated with

negative radiographs was made in these early studies and was later confirmed by many other investigators (9–11).

Other bone-seeking radiopharmaceuticals, most notably the 2.8-hour–half-lived ^{87m}Sr (12), and the 1.87-hour–half-lived positron emitter, flourine 18 (^{18}F) (13,14) also achieved some popularity in the 1960s. However, the true revolution in clinical radionuclide bone scanning awaited the development of the technetium-phosphate agents a few years later.

With the introduction of technetium 99m (^{99m}Tc)–polyphosphate by Subramanian and McAfee in 1971 (15), the modern area of bone scanning began. Other inorganic and organic phosphate compounds were developed with associated improvements in bone localizing properties. Methylene diphosphonate (MDP) has become the most frequently used agent for routine bone scanning studies. The other agent currently approved by the United States Food and Drug Administration is hydroxymethylene diphosphonate (HMDP) labeled with ^{99m}Tc. Excellent-quality studies are achievable with either agent.

MECHANISM OF UPTAKE

Active blood flow and enhanced osteoblastic activity are important features in determining the presence and degree of uptake of ^{99m}Tc-labeled phosphates in a metastatic lesion. Although a particular tumor may result in a primarily lytic reaction, osteoblasts are usually stimulated in response to tumor concentrating the radiolabeled phosphates and resulting in a "hot" area on bone scan. When the lytic component is predominant, a "photon-deficient" appearance often results (see later). The process in which increasing amounts of phosphate are localized on a metabolically active site on the hyroxyapatite crystal is termed *chemisorption.* The central role that the radionuclide bone scan has occupied for 3 decades is a consequence of the phenomenon that most radiographically lytic metastases incite a secondary osteoblastic response that allows their easy

P. **Sinha:** Department of Nuclear Medicine, Montefiore Medical Center and the Albert Einstein College of Medicine, Bronx, New York 10467.

L. M. **Freeman:** Department of Nuclear Medicine and Radiology, Albert Einstein College of Medicine; Department of Nuclear Medicine, Montefiore Hospital (Moses Division), Bronx, New York 10467.

detection as an area of increased tracer concentration (16). The bone scan is able to detect metastases much earlier and is therefore more sensitive than plain film radiography. For example, whereas only a slight increase in osteoblastic activity results in a positive scan, conventional plain film radiographs of the lumbar spine may fail to reveal an abnormality even after the loss of 50% of cancellous bone. Up to 75% loss may be necessary for definite lesion detection (17).

GENERAL CONSIDERATIONS IN BONE SCINTIGRAPHY

The most commonly used adult dose of ^{99m}Tc-MDP or HMDP is 740 MBq (20 mCi). Smaller doses are used in children with various proposed schedules related to body surface or weight (18). Conventional imaging studies are performed 2 to 4 hours after injection, with the longer times best suited for older or heavier patients in whom blood clearance is longer and soft-tissue retention is greater.

Approximately 35% to 50% of the administered dose reaches bone, whereas the remainder is cleared by the kidneys. The fraction reaching bone occurs within the first 30 to 45 minutes. The longer wait before commencing the study allows for more soft-tissue clearance and enhanced target-to-background ratio (19).

Various chemotherapeutic agents and other medications such as iron, phosphorus, steroids, and vitamin D cause generalized decreased bony uptake. Radiation therapy of more than 4,500 rad (45 Gy) causes a characteristic sharply bordered photopenic area corresponding to the radiation port starting 6 to 12 months after radiation (see later).

Two general techniques are used in routine bone scintigraphy. *Whole-body imaging* with a moving table or detector head provides an excellent overview. Alternatively, separately acquired *spot views* of the entire body are acceptable. In any event, suspicious or equivocal areas should be studied with additional coned-down spot views. Various count collection techniques exist for different commercial camera systems to achieve the high-resolution studies required for optimal interpretation. When bladder activity obscures pelvic structures, and the patient is unable to urinate, lateral views or delayed 18- to 24-hour images are useful. Patients being studied for metastatic disease should always have a whole-body study. Limiting scintigraphy to areas of pain or radiographic findings will not allow detection of nonsymptomatic lesions in other areas. The finding of multiple lesions often allows one to make a diagnosis of metastatic disease.

In the past several years, the use of single photon emission tomography (SPECT) to elucidate planar image findings has become increasingly popular, particularly in the

spine. The ability to localize the site of vertebral involvement more precisely enhances the diagnostic accuracy of the study (see later) (20).

BONE SCAN INTERPRETATION

Abnormal findings most often present as areas of increased focal uptake. Multiple randomly placed lesions are the most typical findings in patients with metastatic bone disease. For this reason, whole-body scans always should be performed even if symptoms or x-ray findings are limited to one area (Fig. 40.1).

Solitary Lesions

Patients with metastases may not have multiple lesions. The low specificity of a solitary lesion for metastasis may sometimes be improved by using other scintigraphic observations (see later). Additionally, it is often necessary to elucidate solitary abnormalities further by using plain

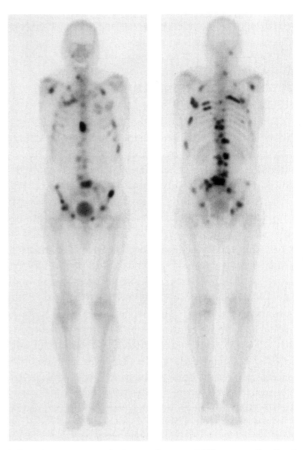

FIGURE 40.1. Metastatic bone disease. Diffuse, randomly distributed foci of increased uptake, primarily in the axial skeleton, is typical of metastatic disease.

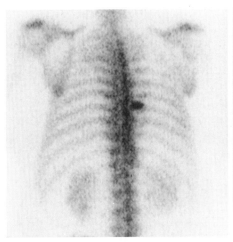 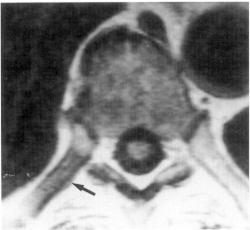

FIGURE 40.2. Solitary lesion elucidated by magnetic resonance imaging (MRI). The focal area of increased uptake in the right eighth costovertebral junction **(left)** is a nonspecific finding. MRI shows an area of hypointense signal in the eighth right posterior rib *(arrow)* typical of metastatic disease.

radiographs, computed tomography (CT), and magnetic resonance imaging (MRI) (Fig. 40.2). Most patients with known malignant disease and newly discovered, asymptomatic, unsuspected solitary bone scan lesions have benign lesions (21,22). The actual incidence of solitary, rather than multiple, metastases in patients with known malignant disease was only 7% in one review of several papers (23), and it was 11% to 12% in another (22,24). In any event, it is low, and it depends on the site of the primary disease as well as on the site of the solitary lesion.

If a solitary focus of increased tracer uptake is noted on the bone scan, the significance depends on the patient's primary tumor, as well as on the site of the solitary lesion. Charron and Brown observed that patients with a known soft-tissue or osseous malignant tumor have a 60% to 70% chance of metastasis when they have a solitary pelvic or vertebral lesion and a 40% to 50% chance of metastasis if the lesion is in the extremities or the skull (25). Data vary significantly in the case of solitary rib lesions. Whereas McNeil summarized that 17% of solitary rib lesions are malignant (26) and Baxter et al. stated that 41% are malignant (27), Tumeh et al. found only 9.8% of solitary rib lesions to be malignant (28). In patients with breast cancer, a larger proportion of patients present with a single lesion. Boxer et al. reviewed a series of 160 patients with breast cancer and found that 21% had a solitary lesion (29). Kwai et al. reported that, in a series of 1,104 patients with breast cancer, 34 (3.1%) had a solitary sternal abnormality, with a 76% chance of malignancy (30). A solitary focus of tracer uptake is occasionally noted in the skull as a result of incomplete calcification of small cartilaginous rest bodies (31).

Location of Lesions and Distribution

Most bone metastases occur in the axial skeleton. The vertebral venous plexus of Batson is believed to allow hematogenously dispersed tumor cells from the breast, prostate, and other organs to bypass the vena cava and portal systems to reach the axial skeleton without passing through the lungs (32). Spread to the ribs likely occurs by communication between the vertebral venous plexus and the intercostal veins.

Involvement of the vertebral body or the pedicles of a vertebral body is more consistent with metastatic involvement than increased posterior element activity (7). The latter is much more often the result of degenerative disease. SPECT is particularly helpful in studying this area (20) (Fig. 40.3).

Distribution of abnormal hot spots often provides a clue to their origin. For example, focal, contiguous areas on adjacent ribs are much more consistent with fractures than are more randomly placed metastatic lesions. Involvement of a whole vertebra, a wide section of an enlarged bone, or a length of an appendicular bone starting from the articular surface is more typical of Paget's disease (Fig. 40.4). Lesions in the middle and posterior pelvis may be obscured by overlying bladder activity. If the patient cannot void and catheterization is not feasible, lateral views (Fig. 40.5) or a delayed 24-hour view helps.

Shape of Lesions

Rib lesions that are elongated are much more likely to represent metastasis compared with a focal hot spot, which is probably a fracture (Fig. 40.6).

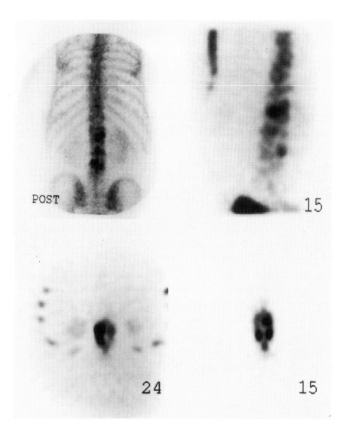

FIGURE 40.3. Value of single photon emission computed tomography (SPECT). An 80-year-old man with a history of prostate cancer had magnetic resonance imaging images of the lumbar spine that showed an infiltrative process consistent with metastasis. Planar bone scan image of the posterior spine **(upper left)** showed increased uptake at L-2, L-3, and L-4. Axial SPECT images showed focal increased uptake in the right side of the body at the L-2 level and the right pedicle **(lower left)**, consistent with metastases, and focal uptake posteriorly at the L-4 and the L-5 level bilaterally **(lower right)**, consistent with facet joint arthritis. The sagittal image through the right side of the spine **(upper right)** clearly demonstrated the difference in location between the metastatic (anterior) and degenerative (posterior) lesions and further illustrates the improved capability for discriminating benign from metastatic bone disease using SPECT. (Courtesy of Jacobson A, Fogelman I. Skeletal imaging in breast and prostate cancer. *Nucl Med Annu* 1999;XX:157–192, with permission.)

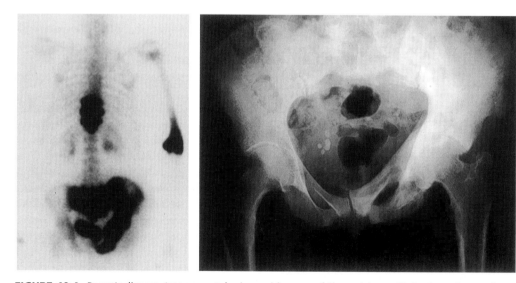

FIGURE 40.4. Paget's disease. Intense uptake in a wide area of the pelvis, multiple thoracic vertebrae, and the distal left humerus with bone enlargement is a finding typical of Paget's disease. The corresponding dense, enlarged bony pelvic changes are evident on the accompanying radiograph.

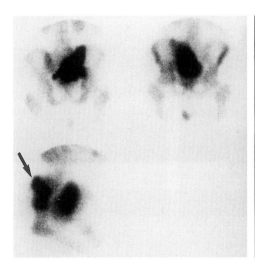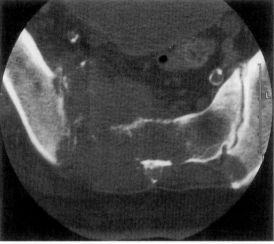

FIGURE 40.5. Value of the lateral pelvic view. On the anterior and posterior scintigraphic images, the sacrum is obscured by overlapping bladder activity. The right lateral view **(lower left)** separates anterior bladder activity from an intense focus of increased sacral activity *(arrow)*. The accompanying computed tomography scan shows extensive destructive changes in the sacrum from a bladder carcinoma.

Intensity of Lesions

This feature generally cannot be used to distinguish benign from malignant lesions. If one knows the cause, then intensity can reflect the age of the lesion. Effectively treated, metastases and healing fractures show decreasing activity on serial scans. Increasing activity can reflect progression or worsening of a metastatic lesion. One notable exception is the *flare phenomenon,* in which early follow-up studies in successfully treated metastases show increased activity (see later).

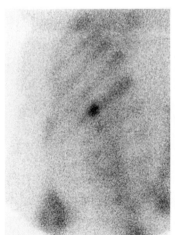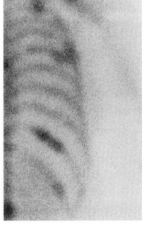

FIGURE 40.6. Distribution of rib activity. The focal rib anteriorly on the **left** is typical of a traumatic lesion, whereas the more linear, bandlike activity on the **right** is much more suggestive of neoplastic involvement.

VARIATIONS IN BONE SCAN INTERPRETATION

Photon-Deficient Lesions

As noted earlier, osteolytic metastases generally incite an osteoblastic response and a "hot" bone scan. Occasionally, the blastic response is absent or minimal, and the lytic component predominates. The resultant appearance is a cold or photopenic appearance on the scan (16) (Fig. 40.7). Another cause of the photon-deficient appearance is vascular compromise in which tumor actually can compress or block vascular channels in the marrow. Round cell sarcomas, multiple myeloma, and thyroid carcinoma are slow-growing lytic processes that incite little or no osteoblastic response. These lesions are often photon deficient (Fig. 40.8). Occasionally, they may result in false-negative studies. Like hot spot findings, the photopenic lesion is nonspecific and can occur in benign as well as malignant lesions. As indicated earlier, wide areas of diminished uptake with sharp borders separating the area from normal bone are characteristic of radiation treatment portals where doses generally greater than 4,500 rad (45 Gy) have been given. This situation most often becomes apparent 6 to 12 months after therapy (Fig. 40.9).

Superscan

When diffuse metastases coalesce, the enhanced uptake becomes more uniform than random and focal. The resultant image has markedly enhanced uptake and little or no renal activity. The *missing kidney sign* is one of the major

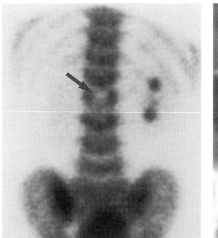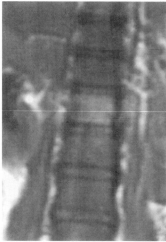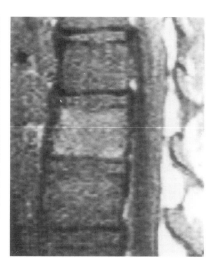

FIGURE 40.7. Photon-deficient lesion. The central cold area in the L-2 vertebral body *(arrow)* represents a metastatic lesion in this 5-year-old child with a neuroblastoma. The accompanying T1-sequence magnetic resonance imaging shows a hyperintense signal in the corresponding vertebral body.

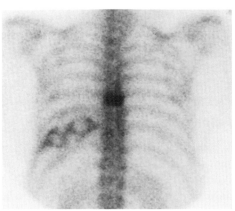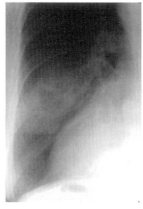

FIGURE 40.8. Thyroid metastasis with a cold central area. The reactive increased osteoblastic activity seen in the rib lesion has a cold central area that more likely reflects the purely lytic destructive lesion evident on the accompanying radiograph (laterally reversed for comparison).

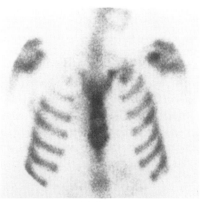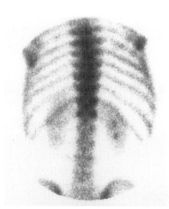

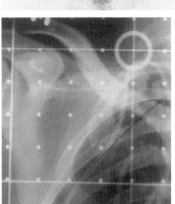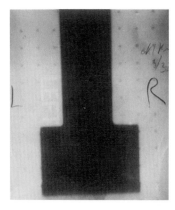

FIGURE 40.9. Radiation effect. Sharply marginated areas of diminished bony uptake in the right upper chest wall and lumbar spine correspond to radiation treatment portals (shown **below).** The patient had received these treatments for lymphoma.

clues that a superscan is present (33,34) (Fig. 40.10). Metastatic prostate cancer is the neoplasm most frequently associated with the superscan, although breast and other tumors may sldo exhibit the pattern. Correlative radiographs are helpful in elucidating the diagnosis.

Because renal insufficiency is associated with enhanced bony uptake, a superscan appearance may result. Therefore, observation of a missing kidney sign should alert the interpreter to check the patient's blood urea nitrogen and creatinine. Fogelman et al. also observed that superscans associated with metastatic disease often have irregular rib uptake, whereas metabolic superscans are more homogeneous (35).

Flare Phenomenon

Increased intensity of lesions on serial bone scans does not always reflect disease progression. Patients with breast and prostate cancer who have had successful hormone therapy or chemotherapy often show an initially increased uptake in metastatic lesions as well as in newly visualized lesions (36, 37,38) (Fig. 40.11). Reports have indicated that up to 50%, or even more, of newly treated patients can demonstrate this flare phenomenon. By recognizing the presence of this phenomenon, the nuclear physician will not misinterpret the study as showing progression of disease, rather than the healing that it is actually demonstrating. The flare is most marked up to 3 months after therapy, but occasionally, it can be seen up to 6 months after treatment. Subsequently, one sees a progressive decrease in the number and intensity of lesions. A truly worsening appearance beyond 6 months reflects progression of the disease.

Expanded Appendicular Uptake

In early adulthood, the hematopoietic function of the appendicular skeleton is no longer required, and the red marrow of childhood and adolescence is replaced by yellow marrow. However, disease processes of adulthood may compromise the hematopoietic function of the axial skeletal marrow, and the appendicular marrow may, once again, become involved in producing blood cells. These disorders would include a variety of neoplasms involving marrow, leukemias, lymphomas, and, in the elderly, myelofibrosis. This feature is recognized on the adult bone scan as enhanced appendicular uptake of labeled phosphate so that it simulates a "childlike" appearance (Fig. 40.12).

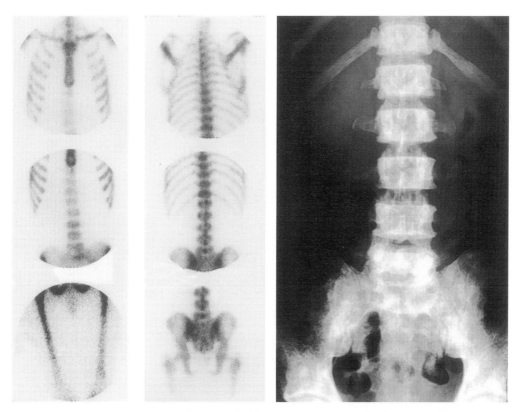

FIGURE 40.10. Superscan in a patient with diffuse prostate cancer. The bone scan shows fairly uniform uptake throughout the axial skeleton with some suggestion of enhanced proximal femoral activity **(lower left).** Most notably, the kidneys are not seen. The dense, sclerotic changes on the accompanying radiograph are typical of metastatic disease.

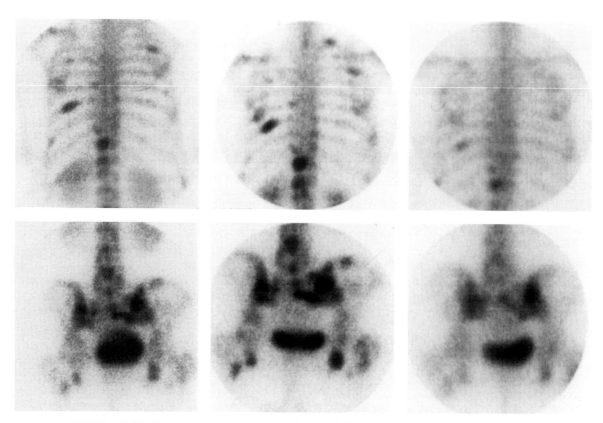

FIGURE 40.11. Flare phenomenon in a patient with breast cancer. Initially demonstrated metastatic lesions on the **left** appear to be intensifying 7 weeks later while the patient is actively receiving chemotherapy **(center).** Several new lesions are also evident. This finding is typical of the flare phenomenon of healing. A follow-up study 6 months later **(right)** shows significant improvement of the metastatic lesions.

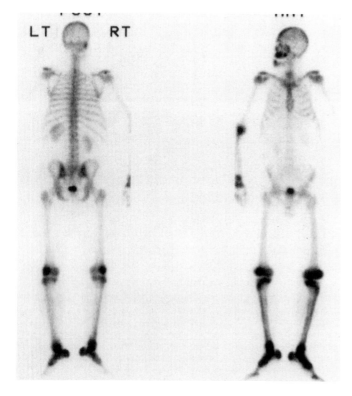

FIGURE 40.12. Expanded appendicular uptake. Enhanced lower extremity uptake is evident in this 46-year-old patient with hairy cell leukemia. This finding is consistent with active hematopoiesis in the appendicular skeleton.

MAGNETIC RESONANCE IMAGING AND POSITRON EMISSION TOMOGRAPHY

Magnetic resonance imaging provides superior spatial resolution, and several reports have noted the superiority of MRI over bone scans in the detection of skeletal metastases. However, the major limitation of MRI has been the difficulty of imaging the whole body because of the time required for such scanning. Certain publications indicate that with new developments in MRI technology, this may no longer be a limitation (39). To what extent MRI can substitute for radionuclide bone scanning for skeletal metastases, if at all, has to be decided by further studies. Like the radionuclide bone scan, MRI is sensitive, but it is relatively nonspecific.

The use of ^{18}F as a bone seeking tracer predates the use of ^{99m}Tc-MDP. With the increasing availability of *positron emission tomography* (PET) scanning has been a resurgence in interest in the use of ^{18}F as a tracer for bone imaging. PET has the inherent advantage of better spatial resolution. One study (40), although not in patients with breast cancer, concluded that ^{18}F PET was more sensitive in the detection of skeletal metastases as compared with planar bone scanning. Imaging with ^{18}F-fluoro-2-deoxyglucose (^{18}F-FDG) has also been evaluated as a tracer, and some workers have reported slightly decreased sensitivity of ^{18}F-FDG PET (41). Cook et al. (42) found that although there was a slight decrease in sensitivity for predominantly osteoblastic lesions, overall sensitivity of ^{18}F-FDG PET scanning was higher because of a greater number of osteolytic lesions identified. This feature is beneficial because patients with osteolytic metastases face the greatest morbidity and mortality and benefit the most from early detection.

The remainder of this chapter is devoted to considerations related to the role of the bone scan in specific neoplasms.

BREAST CANCER

In 1997, the annual incidence of new cases of *breast cancer* in the United States was 180,200, with a mortality of 43,900 (43). Coleman et al., in their series of 587 patients dying of breast cancer, reported that 69% had radiologic evidence of metastases before death, and bone was the most frequent site of metastases (44). Tofe et al. also found 67% of their 368 patients with breast cancer to have scintigraphically demonstrable skeletal lesions. (45). These findings correspond well with the 73% incidence of skeletal metastases reported by Abrams et al. in 1950 (46). The median survival for patients with skeletal metastases is 24 months, with only 20% survival at 5 years (44). Metastatic disease has a propensity to spread through Batson's venous plexus to vertebrae, the most common site of skeletal involvement (45). Metastasis to the extremities is less common; 28.3% lesions in 74 patients were in the appendicular skeleton (47). A relatively large proportion of patients with breast cancer present with a single lesion. Boxer et al. reviewed a series of 160 patients with breast cancer and found that 21% had a solitary lesion (29). Abnormalities in the sternum are particularly significant. In a series of 1,104 patients with breast cancer, Kwai et al. observed 34 patients (3.1%) to have sternal abnormalities, of which 26 (76%) were found to be metastatic (30). Focal rather than diffuse uptake is most significant because diffuse uptake may be caused by other conditions such as surgery with or without infection (Fig. 40.13). Occasionally, one sees diffuse uptake of tracer in the ends of the long bones, a phenomenon explained by bone marrow infiltration (48).

Staging

Although bone scans have been used in the management of breast cancer for almost 30 years, a difference of opinion in defining its exact role remains. Work by Coleman et al.

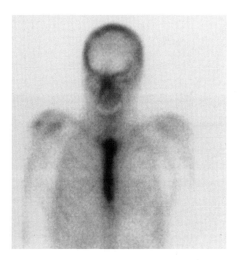
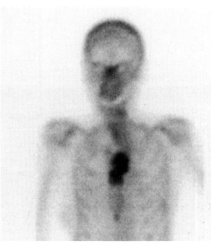

FIGURE 40.13. Sternal uptake patterns. The global uniform uptake on the left is typical of postoperative change after sternotomy for coronary bypass surgery, whereas the more focal areas of uptake on the right represent metastatic disease in a patient with breast cancer.

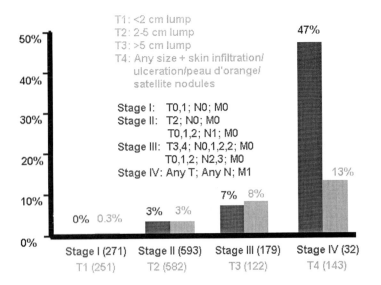

T1: <2 cm lump
T2: 2-5 cm lump
T3: >5 cm lump
T4: Any size + skin infiltration/
    ulceration/peau d'orange/
    satellite nodules

Stage I: T0,1; N0; M0
Stage II: T2; N0; M0
           T0,1,2; N1; M0
Stage III: T3,4; N0,1,2,2; M0
           T0,1,2; N2,3; M0
Stage IV: Any T; Any N; M1

Stage I (271)   Stage II (593)   Stage III (179)   Stage IV (32)   (Total 1075)
T1 (251)   T2 (582)   T3 (122)   T4 (143)   (Total 1098)

FIGURE 40.14. Prevalence of skeletal metastases on presentation in different stages of breast cancer. Because of the low prevalence of skeletal metastases, the authors recommended baseline scintigraphy only in patients with stage II and higher disease or a primary tumor greater than 2 cm. (Data from Coleman RE, Rubens RD, Fogelman I. Reappraisal of the baseline bone scan in breast cancer. *J Nucl Med* 1988;29:1045–1049.)

established that the yield is low in the early stages of the disease (Fig. 40.14) (49). Thus, routine scanning for staging purposes in these early stages is no longer recommended. In patients with coexistent disease conditions, such as degenerative joint disease or Paget's disease, a baseline bone scan may be justified, to prevent later confusion.

The bone scan gives useful prognostic information as well. Sherry et al. found, in patients presenting with stage IV disease, that those who had only skeletal metastases had a significantly prolonged median survival of 33 months compared with only 9 months in patients with extraskeletal metastases (50). More recent work by Jacobson and Fogelman showed a median survival of 2.5 years longer for those with a solitary metastasis as compared with patients with three or more lesions at time of first metastatic recurrence (Fig. 40.15) (51).

Follow-up

Although routine serial bone scanning of asymptomatic patients with breast cancer has shown to detect more metastases than clinical follow-up alone, no difference in the 5-year survival is seen (52). Similar results by other authors have led to the general agreement that follow-up scans in asymptomatic patients are unnecessary and are not cost effective (53). In clinically symptomatic patients, however, and in those with elevated alkaline phosphatase levels or a history of cancer in the opposite breast, follow-up bone scans are indicated (47) (Fig. 40.16).

Evaluation of Treatment

Bone scanning has been used to evaluate therapy based on its sensitivity and ease of imaging the entire skeleton. However, the flare response discussed earlier is a complicating factor (Fig. 40.11). Increase in number and intensity of

scintigraphically visualized lesions in images performed within 6 months of commencement of therapy may indicate a healing osteoblastic response rather than worsening of metastatic disease. Plain film radiographic criteria as developed by the Union Internationale Contre le Cancer (UICC) (54) allows for a more standardized comparison among studies but has the disadvantage of lagging 6 months to a year behind scintigraphic criteria.

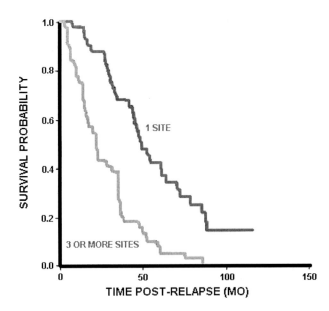

FIGURE 40.15. Survival curves for patients with breast cancer from time of first metastatic recurrence in bone documented on bone scan, either with a solitary metastatic lesion or three or more new lesions at initial examination. Median survival is 2.5 years longer for the former compared with the latter group. (Data from Jacobson A, Fogelman I. Skeletal imaging in breast and prostate cancer. *Nucl Med Annu* 1999;157–192.)

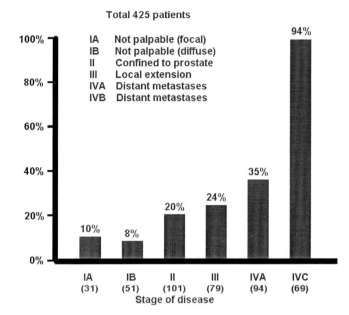

Total 425 patients

IA	Not palpable (focal)
IB	Not palpable (diffuse)
II	Confined to prostate
III	Local extension
IVA	Distant metastases
IVB	Distant metastases

Stage of disease

IA	IB	II	III	IVA	IVC
(31)	(51)	(101)	(79)	(94)	(69)

FIGURE 40.16. Prevalence of skeletal metastases on presentation for different stages of prostate cancer. (Data from Lund F, Smith PH, Suciu S, et al. Do bone scans predict the prognosis in prostate cancer? A report of the EORTC protocol 30762. *Br J Urol* 1984;56:58–63.)

Other Modalities

Skeletal metastases usually start from the bone marrow. Accordingly, imaging of the marrow is more sensitive in the detection of metastases. Unlike bone scanning, in which metastatic foci show up as sites of increased tracer uptake hot spots, metastatic foci in marrow scanning present as photon-deficient cold spots because of replacement of bone marrow by tumor cells. In a study comparing radiolabeled antigranulocyte antibody with MDP, Duncker et al. (55) identified metastases in 25 of 32 patients with breast cancer, whereas the bone scan could detect metastases in only 17 patients. Bone scan showed fewer sites in these 17 patients than the antibody scan. Duncker et al. concluded that bone marrow scintigraphy is a better test for the early detection of metastases from breast cancer. Nevertheless, bone marrow scintigraphy has not been widely used.

Bombardieri et al. evaluated bone metabolic markers as an alternative to scintigraphic imaging in monitoring bone metastases from breast cancer. In 149 patients with breast cancer, 33 (22%) of whom had skeletal metastases, these investigators evaluated bone alkaline phosphatase, the carboxyterminal propeptide of type I procollagen (PICP), and the carboxyterminal cross-linked telopeptide of type I collagen (ICTP). They concluded that discrimination between scan-positive and scan-negative patients was poor. These markers could not be used to replace skeletal scintigraphy for early detection of metastases in patients with breast cancer (56). These markers have been found to be more encouraging in prostate cancer.

PROSTATE CANCER

Prostate cancer is the most common malignant disease in male patients. In 1997, 334,500 new cases were diagnosed, and 41,800 patients died of prostate cancer (43). As with breast cancer, there has been considerable evaluation of the role of bone scan in the management of prostate cancer. In an early study, Schaffer and Pendergrass demonstrated that, in a series of 219 patients with adenocarcinoma of the prostate, 43% of patients with positive bone scans had no pain, 39% had normal acid phosphatase levels, and 23% had normal alkaline phosphatase levels (57). Overall, 15% of patients with metastatic bone disease had normal chemistry studies and no pain. These investigators concluded that the bone scan was the most sensitive method for early detection of metastatic disease. Similar data have been published by other workers as well (58). Bone scan findings also have prognostic significance. Lund et al. showed that patients with a positive bone scan on initial presentation have a 45% mortality at 2 years compared with about 15% for those with a normal scan (59). As can be expected, the frequency of abnormal scans rises with increasing stage of the disease (60) (Fig. 40.17).

The introduction of the prostate-specific antigen (PSA) assay stimulated reevaluation of the role of bone scanning in the management of prostate cancer. PSA levels have been shown to be more specific than prostatic acid phosphatase levels in the early detection of prostate cancer (61). Although different workers agree that the incidence of skeletal metastases rises with increasing blood PSA levels, there is no universally agreed on cutoff point below which a bone scan is unnecessary. Some authors contend that a staging bone scan is unnecessary in patients with PSA in the range of 10 to 20 ng/mL because of a yield of only about 1% (62). Other workers have shown a much higher prevalence of metastases in patients with PSA in the range of 10 to 20 ng/mL and have contended that a bone scan should be performed (63). Work by Oesterling et al. and by Rudoni et al. also supported the use of a PSA level of less than 10 ng/mL as the cutoff point for not doing a bone scan in patients with newly diagnosed untreated disease (64,65). A bone scan should be obtained in patients with other preexisting conditions such as arthritis or traumatic lesions, to prevent confusion later in the course of the disease. PSA levels are not reliable in the follow-up of patients who have received hormonal therapy. Leo et al. found that, in 35% of the patients who had received antiandrogen therapy, serum PSA was in the normal range despite definite metastases (66).

Bone scans are often used to observe patients for progression of metastatic disease from prostate cancer. Huben and Schellhammer concluded, on the basis of their work, that although about 19% of patients develop skeletal metastases after definitive therapy for prostate cancer in 3 to 4 years, routine follow-up scintigraphy was not necessary

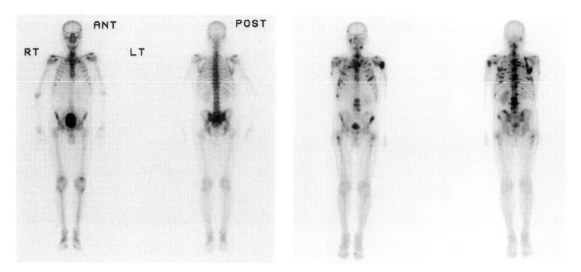

FIGURE 40.17. Serial studies showing progression of bony metastases. The initial study in patient with prostate cancer **(left)** appears normal. A follow-up study 14 months later **(right)** shows diffuse metastases.

because bone pain or elevated serum enzymes were adequate as a follow-up study in all patients (67). Lund et al. (59) also found a similar incidence of skeletal metastases from prostate cancer by 3 years but concluded that bone scans are of value. Even in symptomatic patients with known metastatic disease, bone scans may be of value to plan radiotherapy. Bone scans have a definite role in follow-up of patients for the assessment of therapy. Pollen et al., in their series of 41 patients with prostate cancer, found that changes in the intensity of tracer uptake and the number of lesions were reliable indicators of disease progression and had prognostic importance as well. Mean survival was 15.7 months in patients with scintigraphically stable lesions, 12.3 months in those who had scintigraphic improvement, and only 6.3 months in those who had scintigraphic evidence of disease progression. These investigators observed the flare response in only 1 of their 41 patients (68).

A semiquantitative method was proposed by Soloway et al. to assess the extent of disease (EOD) and also to arrive at a prognosis (69). They devised a grading system based on the extent of disease (EOD) and in a series of 160 patients with metastatic prostate cancer observed that the 2-year survival rate was 94% in EOD grade 1 (1 to 6 metastatic foci, with each focus less than the size of a vertebral body), 74% in EOD grade 2 (6 to 20 metastatic foci), 68% in EOD grade 3 (more than 20 metastatic foci but not a superscan), and 40% in EOD grade 4 (superscan or more than 75% involvement of the ribs, vertebrae, and pelvis). Similar correlation has been reported by other investigators (70).

Various metabolic bone markers have been investigated to complement the bone scan for follow-up of patients with prostate cancer. Maeda et al. reported best correlation of ICTP levels with EOD grade, but it was not possible to differentiate between no metastases and EOD grade 1 (71).

Koizumi et al. found a bone-specific isomer of alkaline phosphatase (BAP) to be the most sensitive marker for metastases (72), whereas Perachino et al. found that 7 patients of 24 with skeletal metastases had PSA levels lower than 20 ng/mL. Of these 7 patients, only 4 had normal PICP levels. No patient had skeletal metastases with both PSA less than 20 ng/mL and normal PICP levels (73). These serum markers can give valuable information regarding the extent of disease, but the bone scan has the advantage of offering additional information regarding the anatomic site or sites of involvement. This can be useful to plan radiotherapy or the prevention of pathologic fractures.

Bourgeois et al. evaluated bone marrow scintigraphy with 99mTc labeled human serum albumin nanocolloid in 73 patients with histologically proven prostate cancer. In general, these investigators found scanning with 99mTc-labeled human serum albumin colloid to be less sensitive but more specific than 99mTc-MDP. They recommended marrow scanning when the bone scan findings are in doubt (74). Kirac et al. evaluated 99mTc-labeled antigranulocyte monoclonal antibody to image the bone marrow in 56 patients. They concluded that this technique is more sensitive than the conventional bone scan for the detection of metastases, even in high-risk patients with normal bone scans (75). Imaging with indium 111–labeled antibody to a prostate-specific membrane antigen, capromab pendetide (ProstaScint), has been approved for routine clinical use since 1996. Although it has been shown to be superior to PET and CT in detecting recurrent prostate cancer in the prostate bed and possibly in lymph nodes as well (76), it is not as sensitive as the bone scan for skeletal metastases. In fact, work by Silver et al. showed that only 44% of prostate bone metastases express the prostate-specific membrane antigen and would be detectable on the capromab pendetide scan (77). The antibody study is primarily used to detect lymphatic spread of the disease.

Imaging with ^{18}F-FDG PET has also been considered for prostate carcinoma. Hoh et al. reported that ^{18}F-FDG PET was not as sensitive as the bone scan in the detection of skeletal metastases (78). Yeh et al. noted, in 13 patients with metastatic prostate cancer, that ^{18}F-FDG PET identified only about 18% of the lesions seen on the bone scan. This finding probably indicates that processes other than increased glycolysis are involved in metabolism of the skeletal metastases (79). Hara et al., noting that tumor tissue in general has a higher concentration of phosphatidylcholine, used carbon 11–labeled choline as the tracer and obtained significant uptake of tracer with a specific uptake value of more than 3 in most primary and metastatic prostate carcinoma sites, whereas the specific uptake value of ^{18}F-FDG was considerably lower. In addition, there was no interference from activity in the urine or bladder (80). These techniques await further evaluation.

LUNG CANCER

Lung cancer is the most common cause of death from cancer, with an annual mortality of 94,400 men and 66,000 women in the United States in 1997 (43). Skeletal metastases are common in lung cancer. Evidence of metastases is a grave prognostic sign. Excisional surgery for lung cancer thought to be "operable" has a 5% to 20% operative mortality (26). In another study, 40 of 46 patients (87%) with an abnormal bone scan at presentation died within 6 months of detection of skeletal metastases, whereas 50% of patients with a normal bone scan at presentation were alive at 6 months (81). The incidence of skeletal metastases depends on the clinical presentation of the patient. The incidence of positive bone scans in asymptomatic patients with bronchogenic cancer has been reported by Hooper et al. to be 8%, with less than 4% being true-positive scans. In symptomatic patients, the incidence of positive bone scans is about 36% (82). The incidence of metastases in small cell and anaplastic lung cancer is much higher. In the series of Bitran et al. of 30 patients with small cell cancer, detection of previously unsuspected metastases in 3 (10%) patients affected their staging (83). It is now generally agreed that bone scintigraphy at the initial workup is necessary for patients with small cell carcinoma, elevated serum alkaline phosphatase or calcium, and extensive primary lesions (26).

The incidence of isolated metastases in the appendicular skeleton is higher in lung cancer than in most other neoplasms because the tumor cells spread by the arterial route to the distal extremities. A whole-body bone scan including the distal extremities should therefore always be obtained. Occasionally, evidence of hypertrophic pulmonary osteoarthropathy is detected (Fig. 40.18). Ali et al., in a series of 48 patients with evidence of hypertrophic pul-

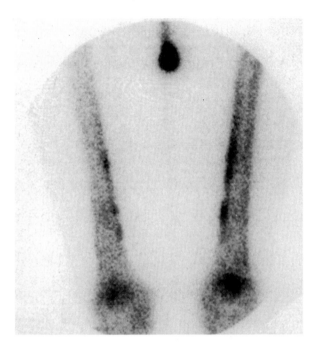

FIGURE 40.18. Hypertrophic pulmonary osteoarthropathy. Anterior images of the femora show a vertical striplike pattern along the medial shafts that reflects the periostitis often associated with lung neoplasms.

monary osteoarthropathy, noted that the extremities were always involved, and the process was more active in the lower than in the upper extremities. In 17% of their patients, the extremities were involved asymmetrically. In long bones, pericortical activity is intense. Involvement of the skull, scapulae, clavicles, and patellae were also noted (84). This condition often disappears with tumor removal and reappears when the tumor recurs.

RENAL AND BLADDER CARCINOMA

Early workers reported a high incidence of true-positive bone scans in both *renal and bladder cancer,* in the range of 42% to 50% (85,86). This has not been the experience of later researchers, who reported a much lower yield, typically 5% to 10% (87,88) in renal cancers and an even lower incidence (2%) in bladder cancers (89). The general opinion is therefore that bone scans are not necessary in the asymptomatic patient. A bone scan is justifiable in the symptomatic patient or for follow-up.

Kim et al. observed that about 11% of renal cancer metastases are photopenic. In their series, 62 of 68 (91%) bone lesions were detected by scintigraphy, as opposed to only 41 (60%) detected by plain film radiography (90), thus making the bone scan more sensitive. However, not all lytic lesions are photopenic, and most lytic lesions have intense uptake of tracer because of the associated osteoblastic repair process.

CERVICAL CANCER

The incidence of skeletal metastases is low in the early stages of *cervical cancer.* Du Toit and Grove reported no true-positive bone scans in 208 patients with stage I and II disease, whereas 11 of 332 (3.3%) patients with stage III and IV disease had true-positive scans (91). Similar results were obtained by Katz et al., who also noted renal asymmetry in 14 of 100 patients, 11 of whom had advanced disease. Soft-tissue extension of tumor may involve the ureters and may result in obstructive uropathy. These investigators concluded that although bone scans are not justified in asymptomatic patients with early-stage disease, individual kidney functions should be carefully evaluated (92). Other workers have reported correlation of the incidence of skeletal metastases with the histologic type of tumor, rather than the clinical stage of disease. Bassan and Glaser found that 13 of 19 patients (68%) with poorly differentiated primary tumors had skeletal metastases. Overall, of 88 patients, 14 (16%) had skeletal metastases, 12 of whom had stage I or II disease (93). Their recommendation was to screen all patients with poorly differentiated disease, regardless of clinical staging.

THYROID CANCER

Thyroid cancer is a relatively rare form of cancer. Among the 1,382,400 new cases of cancer reported in the United States in 1997 were 16,100 thyroid cancers (43). The two most common histologic types are papillary and follicular cell types. Skeletal metastases are more common from the follicular variety. Their presence generally signifies a poor prognosis. Because well-differentiated metastases retain their ability to concentrate iodine, iodine 131 (^{131}I) is commonly used for detection of metastases. The scan is performed in the after thyroidectomy, when the residual thyroid has been ablated. Metastases from medullary or anaplastic carcinoma of the thyroid cannot be imaged by this method because these tumors do not concentrate iodine.

Castillo et al. reported that 33 of 37 (89%) metastatic lesions in 8 patients were identified by whole-body ^{131}I scanning, whereas bone scanning with ^{99m}Tc-MDP or ^{18}F could identify fewer than half of these lesions. Almost 60% of the lesions that were detected by radiography or ^{131}I scanning were normal on bone scintigraphy (94). These investigators concluded that bone scintigraphy had little to offer in the management of differentiated thyroid carcinoma. In another study by De Groot and Reilly, correlation between the ^{131}I and the ^{99m}Tc-phosphate bone scan was better, but they also observed that ^{131}I scanning identified more lesions (95). Most metastases from thyroid cancers are lytic but demonstrate foci of increased tracer uptake on the bone scan because of the associated osteoblastic process. There may be a central photopenic zone (Fig. 40.8) (96). Osteoblastic metastases have also been described (97). In general, the slow-growing, lytic character of thyroid metastases is often associated with a false-negative ^{99m}Tc-phosphate bone scan. Therefore, use of the bone scan is limited in this clinical setting.

Some studies indicate that whole-body imaging with thallium 201 (^{201}Tl) or ^{99m}Tc-methoxyisobutyl isonitrile (MIBI) may be more sensitive for the detection of thyroid cancer metastases, because not all lesions concentrate ^{131}I (98,99,100). In a series of 27 patients who had undergone thyroidectomy and who had metastatic differentiated thyroid carcinoma, Miyamoto et al. were able to detect 29 of 31 (93.5%) skeletal metastases with ^{99m}Tc-MIBI, 28 of 31 (90.3%) with ^{201}Tl, and 27 of 31 (87.1%) with ^{131}I (100). Nemec et al. reported ^{99m}Tc-MIBI to be particularly sensitive for skeletal metastases (101). The number of well-differentiated thyroid cancer metastases visible on ^{131}I scans has been reported to be between 72.7% and 89% (102,94). Using ^{201}Tl or ^{99m}Tc-MIBI has the advantage of avoiding the "stunning" effect, which has been reported with ^{131}I, whereby a sublethal dose of radiation from the diagnostic dose of ^{131}I interferes with the metastatic cells' ability to concentrate iodine but does not affect their malignant potential.

Different investigators have studied the role of ^{18}F-FDG PET in thyroid cancer. The consensus appears to be that well-differentiated thyroid cancers that retain the capability of iodine uptake have low glucose uptake and so are not seen on a ^{18}F-FDG PET study. Less well-differentiated cells that cannot take up iodine have higher glucose uptake. Such metastases, which are not detected by the ^{131}I scan, can be detected by ^{18}F-FDG PET (103,104). Therefore, ^{18}F-FDG PET may complement ^{131}I scanning but not supplement it. Kalicke et al., in a review article, recommended whole-body ^{18}F-FDG PET scanning in patients with differentiated thyroid carcinoma if the Tg levels are elevated and no metastases are found on ^{131}I or ^{201}Tl or ^{99m}Tc-MIBI scanning (105).

Metastases from medullary cancer of the thyroid do not concentrate radioiodine. Bone scanning with ^{99m}Tc-MDP may have a role in patients with medullary cancer of the thyroid with elevated levels of calcitonin. Johnson et al. demonstrated skeletal metastases in such patients with ^{99m}Tcm-MDP (106). Ugur et al. evaluated ^{99m}Tc (V)DMSA, ^{99m}Tc-MIBI, and ^{201}Tl and found sensitivities of 95%, 47%, and 19%, respectively, in the detection of metastatic medullary cancer of the thyroid (107). Encouraging results have been reported by Learoyd et al. in the detection of soft-tissue metastases from medullary carcinoma of the thyroid by using ^{99m}Tc-MIBI (108).

LYMPHOMA

Hodgkin's disease and *non-Hodgkin's lymphomas* are common malignant diseases in children and adults. They almost always arise in mymph nodes or other soft tissue. The incidence of extranodal lymphoma is approximately 25% (109). Skeletal lymphoma most often appears on radiographs as a destructive lesion. However, in a study by Schecter et al. involving 26 patients with lymphoma, the bone scan detected an abnormality in 18 patients, whereas plain film radiographs were positive in only 13 (110). This finding may be attributable to the osteoblastic response to the lytic lesions. Orzel et al. observed that Hodgkin's lymphoma was more likely to involve the extremities and had fewer lesions in the axial skeleton than non-Hodgkin's lymphoma. They also observed that although skeletal pain was specific, it was not at all sensitive for skeletal metastases (111).

Often, bone marrow expansion causes diffuse uptake of bone tracer in distal femora and tibiae, or a patchy inhomogeneous uptake in the bone signifying areas of normal and diseased marrow. Rarely, a photopenic area in the bone may be caused by tumor replacement of bone marrow. Sharply defined areas of intense tracer uptake are much less common than subtle areas of increased tracer uptake (111).

LEUKEMIA

Leukemias occur in both adults and children. They are the most common pediatric malignant diseases. Bone scans are rarely performed as a routine examination, although the procedure may be useful to evaluate bone pain. Involvement of the appendicular skeleton is more common than in other neoplasms. A bizarre pattern of enhanced appendicular uptake is frequently encountered in leukemic bone involvement (Fig. 40.19). Kuntz et al., in their series, noted

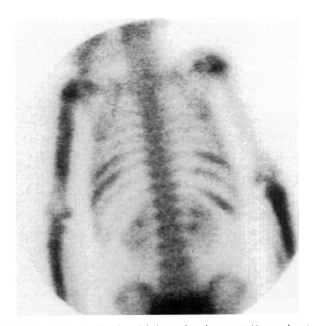

FIGURE 40.19. Leukemia with bone involvement. Unusual pattern of diffuse appendicular uptake as well as multiple areas of rib involvement in a 7-year-old child with acute leukemia.

that the bone scan was more sensitive than plain film radiography in detecting skeletal metastases and recommended bone scanning followed by plain film radiography of symptomatic and scintigraphically suspicious sites (112). The bone marrow is often involved, and a bone marrow scan in conjunction with a bone scan could be used when bone scans are not conclusive. Photopenic lesions have also been described in childhood leukemias (113).

MALIGNANT MELANOMA

The incidence of skeletal metastases in stages I and II of *malignant melanoma* is small. Roth et al. found the incidence to be 1 in 51 (2%) in patients with stage I or II disease and 2 in 13 (15%) in stage III disease (114). Similar results have been reported by other workers as well (115). Bone scans are not indicated for patients with stage I or II disease who are asymptomatic, but they should be obtained in symptomatic patients and in those with stage III or IV disease. Because osteolytic lesions do occur in melanoma, normal bone scans should be followed by radiography in symptomatic patients.

MULTIPLE MYELOMA

Multiple myeloma and other plasma cell disorders characteristically produce lytic lesions. Bone scanning is less sensitive than radiography in the detection of skeletal metastases (116,117). The indolent nature of the lytic myeloma lesions does not incite reactive bone and so renders the bone scan less useful. Plain film examination of the skeleton remains the primary method for evaluation of the skeleton in multiple myeloma. Woolfenden et al. (116) showed that a lesion typically is initially positive on the bone scan and is not detectable radiologically. The positive scan was possibly attributable to high metabolic activity. However, as the lesion progresses, it loses some of its metabolic activity and gradually becomes scintigraphically normal and radiologically abnormal with loss of calcium. Even when radiographs are positive, bone scanning may still be used to assess the ribs and the pelvis, because these sites are often difficult to examine optimally with radiographs. Scintigraphy may have a prognostic value. Bataille et al. (118) observed that scintigraphically active disease correlates with clinically active disease, and with successful treatment, the lesions are less active scintigraphically.

HEAD AND NECK TUMORS

Most workers have reported a low prevalence of skeletal metastases in patients with *nasopharyngeal carcinoma* (119, 120). They have concluded that routine bone scanning was unnecessary. Discordant results have been reported by Sundram et al.; 23% of their 143 patients studied for initial staging of nasopharyngeal carcinoma and 59% of patients having follow-up studies had true-positive bone scans (121). In a small series of 25 patients, Baker et al. demonstrated local bone involvement scintigraphically that could not be detected radiographically by Panorex film (122). In a series of 200 patients studied using SPECT, there was only a single false-positive finding in the skull by SPECT. Additionally, SPECT did not miss any lesion detected by x-ray CT, whereas CT missed 49% of lesions detected by SPECT. In all 35 patients with cranial nerve involvement, the skull base lesions were detected by SPECT, whereas CT missed 8 lesions (123). These investigators concluded that SPECT of the skull should be performed routinely in patients with nasopharyngeal carcinoma.

OCCULT MALIGNANT DISEASE

Often in clinical practice, a bone scan is requested to assist in the evaluation of patients with musculoskeletal symptoms, or as a part of a search for *occult malignancy.* Jacobson observed, in a series of 304 consecutive patients with skeletal complaints and no known malignancy, that none of the 111 patients less than 50 years old had any scintigraphic findings suggestive metastatic disease. Twenty-one of 193 (10.8%) of the patients more than 50 years old had evidence of metastatic disease, and 80% of the positive scans had involvement of multiple sites (124). A whole-body bone scan should therefore always be obtained in patients more than 50 years of age when an occult neoplasm is suspected. Work by other researchers also indicates that the

bone scan can be used as an effective tool for workup of occult cancer (125).

SOFT-TISSUE UPTAKE

Bone scans often provide additional and serendipitous information about a patient's disease process in the form of unexpected tracer uptake in the *soft tissues.* Intense tracer uptake in the kidneys or collecting system, particularly if unilateral, may suggest renal obstruction or hydronephrosis. Poor renal function is often associated with increased soft-tissue background and a poor skeletal-to-nonskeletal ratio, thus degrading image quality. Abnormal contour of the kidneys suggests a space-occupying lesion. Although unilateral nonvisualization of a kidney may indicate prior surgical removal or a nonfunctional kidney, bilateral nonvisualization of kidneys may indicate a superscan. Uptake of bone-seeking tracer in various organs has been reported in numerous conditions and may even be caused by impurities in the tracer; for example, the presence of aluminum ions in ^{99m}Tc-MDP resulting from aluminum breakthrough from a molybdenum-technetium generator can cause visualization of the liver on a bone scan. Lists of the various reported conditions causing soft-tissue uptake of bone-seeking tracer were published by Datz (126) and Harbert (127). Such abnormal uptake of bone tracer is not sensitive to detect soft-tissue metastases. It is frequently the result of abnormal calcification. Some of the commoner causes include primary and metastatic neoplasms, dystrophic calcification, acute and chronic myocardial infarction, colorectal metastases to the liver (Fig. 40.20), hyperparathyroidism, and recent radiotherapy, particularly of the lung. If no preexist-

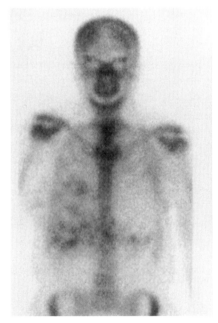

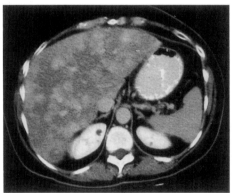

FIGURE 40.20. Liver metastases. Soft-tissue uptake in the right lower chest and upper abdomen represents liver metastases from a mucin-producing adenocarcinoma of the colon with dystrophic calcification. The corresponding metastatic lesions are well seen on the accompanying computed tomography scan.

ing condition is known to explain the abnormal tracer uptake adequately, an attempt should be made to arrive at a diagnosis.

CONCLUSIONS

As summarized by Becker (128), the present role of the ^{99m}Tc-MDP bone scan in oncology is selective. It will prove to be most productive when it is used in the following situations: (a) in patients with a high probability of metastases, rather than as part of a routine workup in all patients with malignancy; (b) for follow-up when specific tumor marker levels rise; (c) for evaluation of bone pain or other specific symptoms; (d) for follow-up of negative or equivocal radiographic findings; (e) for further study of a solitary radiographic lesion, to determine whether other lesions are present; and (f) to monitor the effects of therapy.

ACKNOWLEDGMENT

We wish to express our appreciation to Drs. Bilha Fish and Richard Silvergleid of Manhasset Diagnostic Imaging, who provided several of the figures included in this chapter.

REFERENCES

1. Fleming WH, McIlraith JD, King ER. Photoscanning of bone lesions utilizing strontium-87. *Radiology* 1961;77:635–636.
2. Simpson WJK, Rottenberg AD, Baker RG. Whole body scanning in medicine. II. Clinical aspects. *Can Med Assoc J* 1962;87: 371–377.
3. Treadwell A de G, Low-Beer VL, Friedell HL, et al. Metabolic studies on neoplasm of bone with the aid of radioactive strontium. *Am J Med Sci* 1942;204:521–530.
4. Pecher C. Biological investigations with radioactive calcium and strontium: preliminary report on the use of radioactive strontium in the treatment of metastatic bone cancer. *Univ Calif Pub Pharmacol* 1942;2:117.
5. Laszlo D, Spencer H, Brothers M, et al. Metabolism of strontium-85 in man In: *Proceedings of the International Conference on Peaceful Uses of Atomic Energy, Geneva, 1955,* vol 10. New York: United Nations, 1956:63.
6. Bauer GCH, Wendeberg B. External counting of Ca-47 and Sr-85 in studies of localised skeletal lesions in man. *J Bone Joint Surg Br* 1959;41:558–580.
7. Gynning I, Lamgeland P, Lindberg S, et al. Localization with Sr-85 of spinal metastases in mammary cancer and changes in uptake after hormone and roentgen therapy: a preliminary report. *Acta Radiol* 1968;55:119.
8. Charkes ND, Sklaroff DM. Early diagnosis of metastatic bone cancer by photoscanning with strontium-85. *J Nucl Med* 1964; 5:168–178.
9. Rosenthall L. The role of strontium-85 in the detection of bone disease. *Radiology* 1965;84:75–82.
10. DeNardo GL. The 85Sr scintiscan in bone disease. *Ann Intern Med* 1966;65:44–53.
11. Greenberg E, Rothschild EO, dePalo A, et al. Bone scanning for metastatic cancer with radioactive isotopes. *Med Clin North Am* 1966;50:701–710.
12. Charkes ND, Sklaroff DM, Bierly J. Detection of metastatic cancer to bone by scintiscanning with strontium-87m. *AJR Am J Roentgenol* 1964;91:1121–1127.
13. Blau M, Nagler W, Bender MA. Fluorine-18: a new isotope for bone scanning. *J Nucl Med* 1962;3:332–334.
14. Dworkin HJ, Moon NF, Lessard RJ, et al. A study of the metabolism of fluorine-18 in dogs and its suitability for bone scanning. *J Nucl Med* 1966;7:510–520.
15. Subramanian G, McAfee JG. A new complex of 99m-Tc for skeletal imaging. *Radiology* 1971;99:192–196.
16. Fogelman I, McKillop JH. The bone scan in metastatic disease. In: Rubens RD, Fogelman I, eds. *Bone metastases: diagnosis and treatment.* London: Springer-Verlag, 1991:31.
17. Edelstyn GA, Gillespie PJ, Grebbell FS. The radiological demonstration of osseous metastases: experimental observations. *Clin Radiol* 1967;18:158–162.
18. Smith T, Gordon I. An update of radiopharmaceutical schedules in children. *Nucl Med Commun* 1998;19:1023–1036.
19. Subramanian G. Radiopharmaceuticals for bone scanning. In: Collier ND, Fogelman I, Rosenthall L, eds. *Skeletal nuclear medicine.* St. Louis: CV Mosby, 1996:13.
20. Even-Sapir E, Martin RH, Barnes DC, et al. Role of SPECT in differentiating malignant from benign lesions in the lower thoracic and lumbar spine. *Radiology* 1993;187:193–198.
21. Jacobson AF, Cronin EB, Stomper PC, et al. Bone scan with one or two new abnormalities in cancer patients with no known metastases: frequency and serial scintigraphic behavior of benign and malignant lesions. *Radiology* 1990;175:229–232.
22. Jacobson AF, Stomper PC, Jochelson MS, et al. Association between number and sites of new bone scan abnormalities and presence of skeletal metastases in patients with breast cancer. *J Nucl Med* 1990;31:387–392.
23. McKillop JH. Bone scanning in metastatic disease. In: Fogelman I, ed. *Bone scanning in clinical practice.* New York: Springer-Verlag, 1987:44.
24. Jacobson AF, Hyman FE. Low likelihood of malignancy in isolated vertebral compression fractures on bone scans of cancer patients without known spinal metastases. *J Nucl Med* 1995;36: 26P–27P(abst).
25. Charron M, Brown ML. Primary and metastatic bone disease. In: Sandler MP, Coleman RE, Wackers FJT, eds. *Diagnostic nuclear medicine,* 3rd ed. Baltimore: Williams & Wilkins, 1996: 649–667.
26. McNeil BJ. Value of bone scanning in neoplastic disease. *Semin Nucl Med* 1984;14:277–286.
27. Baxter AD, Coakely FV, Finlay DB, et al. The aetiology of solitary hot spots in the ribs on planar bone scans. *Nucl Med Commun* 1995;16:834–837.
28. Tumeh SS, Beadle G, Kaplan WD. Clinical significance of solitary rib lesions in patients with extraskeletal malignancy. *J Nucl Med* 1985;26:1140–1143.
29. Boxer DI, Todd CEC, Coleman R, et al. Bone secondaries in breast cancer: the solitary metastasis. *J Nucl Med* 1989;30: 1318–1320.
30. Kwai AH, Stomper PC, Kaplan WD. Clinical significance of isolated scintigraphic sternal lesions in patients with breast cancer. *J Nucl Med* 1988;29:324–328.
31. Harbert JC, Desai R. Small calvarial bone scan foci: normal variations. *J Nucl Med* 1985;26:1144–1148.
32. Batson OV. The function of the vertebral veins and their role in the spread of metastases. *Ann Surg* 1940;112:138–149.
33. Constable AR, Cramage RW. Recognition of the super scan in prostatic bone scintigrphy. *Br J Radiol* 1981;54:122–125.

34. Sy WM, Patel D, Faunce H. Significance of absent or faint kidney sign on bone scan. *J Nucl Med* 1975;16:454–456.

35. Fogelman I, McKillop JH, Greig WR, et al. Absent kidney sign associated with symmetrical and uniformly increased uptake of tracer by the skeleton. *Eur J Nucl Med* 1977;2:257–260.

36. Coleman RE, Mashiter G, Whitaker KB, et al. Bone scan flare predicts successful systemic therapy for bone metastases. *J Nucl Med* 1988;29:1354–1359.

37. Rossleigh MA, Lovegrove FTA, Reynolds PM, et al. Serial bone scans in assessment of response to therapy in advanced breast carcinoma. *Clin Nucl Med* 1982;7:397–402.

38. Janicek MJ, Hayes DF, Kaplan WD. Healing flare in skeletal metastases from breast cancer. *Radiology* 1994;192:201–204.

39. Eustace S, Tello R, DeCarvalho V, et al. A comparison of whole-body TurboSTIR MR imaging and planar ^{99m}Tc-methylene diphosphonate scintigraphy in the examination of patients with suspected skeletal metastases. *AJR Am J Roentgenol* 1997;169:1655–1661.

40. Schirrmeister H, Guhlmann CA, Diederichs CD, et al. Planar bone imaging vs ^{18}F-PET in patients with cancer of the prostate, thyroid and lung. *J Nucl Med* 1998;39:113P–114P (abst).

41. Moon DH, Maddahi J, Silverman DH, et al. Accuracy of whole body fluorine-18-FDG PET for the detection of recurrent or metastatic breast carcinoma. *J Nucl Med* 1998;39:431–435.

42. Cook GJ, Houston S, Rubens R, et al. Detection of bone metastases in breast cancer by 18-FDG PET: differing metabolic activity in osteoblastic and osteolytic lesions. *J Clin Oncol* 1998;16:3375–3379.

43. American Cancer Society. *Cancer facts and figures 1997.* Atlanta: American Cancer Society, 1997:4.

44. Coleman RE, Rubens RD. The clinical course of bone metastases from bone cancer. *Br J Cancer* 1987;55:61–66.

45. Tofe AJ, Francis MD, Harvey WJ. Correlation of neoplasms with incidence and localisation of skeletal metastases. *J Nucl Med* 1975;16:986–989.

46. Abrams HL, Spiro R, Goldstein N. Metastases in carcinoma: analysis of 1000 autopsied cases. *Cancer* 1950;3:74–85.

47. Krishnamurthy GT, Tubis M, Hiss J, et al. Distribution pattern of metastatic bone disease: a need for total body skeletal image. *JAMA* 1977;237:2504–2506.

48. Fogelman I, Coleman R. The bone scan and breast cancer. In: Freeman LM, Weissman HS, eds. *Nuclear medicine annual.* New York: Raven, 1988:1–38.

49. Coleman RE, Rubens RD, Fogelman I. Reappraisal of the baseline bone scan in breast cancer. *J Nucl Med* 1988;29:1045–1049.

50. Sherry MM, Greco FA, Johnson DH, et al. Breast cancer with skeletal metastases at initial diagnosis. *Cancer* 1986;58:178–182.

51. Jacobson A, Fogelman I. Skeletal imaging in breast and prostate cancer. *Nucl Med Annu* 1999;157–192.

52. Rosselli DTM, Palli D, Cariddi A, et al. Intensive diagnostic follow up after treatment of primary breast cancer: a randomised trial (National Research Council Project on Breast Cancer follow up). *JAMA* 1994;271:1593–1597.

53. Cook GJ, Fogelman I. Skeletal metastases from breast cancer: imaging with nuclear medicine. *Semin Nucl Med* 1999;29:69–79.

54. Hayward JL, Carbone PP, Heuson JC, et al. Assessment of response to therapy in advanced breast cancer. *Eur J Cancer* 1977;13:89–94.

55. Duncker CM, Carrio I, Berna L, et al. Radioimmune imaging of bone marrow in patients with suspected bone metastases from primary bone cancer. *J Nucl Med* 1990;31:1450–1455.

56. Bombardieri E, Martinetti A, Miceli R, et al. Can bone metabolism markers be adopted as an alternative to scintigraphic imaging in monitoring bone metastases from breast cancer? *Eur J Nucl Med* 1997;24:1349–1355.

57. Schaffer DL, Pendergrass HP. Comparison of enzyme, clinical, radiographic, and radionuclide methods of detecting bone metastases from carcinoma of the prostate. *Radiology* 1976;121:431–434.

58. Johansson JE, Beckman KW, Lindell D, et al. Serial bone scanning in the evaluation of stage and clinical course of carcinoma of the prostate. *Scand J Urol Nephrol Suppl* 1980;55:31–36.

59. Lund F, Smith PH, Suciu S, et al. Do bone scans predict the prognosis in prostate cancer? A report of the EORTC protocol 30762. *Br J Urol* 1984;56:58–63.

60. Paulson DF, Uro-Oncology Research Group. The impact of current staging procedures in assessing disease extent of prostatic adenocarcinoma. *J Urol* 1979;121:300–302.

61. Stamey TA, Yang N, Hay AR, et al. Prostate specific antigen as a serum marker for adenocarcinoma of the prostate. *N Engl J Med* 1987;317:909–916.

62. Chybowski FM, Keller JJL, Bergstralh EJ, et al. Predicting radionuclide bone scan findings in patients with newly diagnosed, untreated prostate cancer: prostate specific antigen is superior to all other clinical parameters. *J Urol* 1991;145:313–318.

63. Haukaas S, Roervik J, Halvorsen OJ, et al. When is bone scintigraphy necessary in the assessment of newly diagnosed, untreated prostate cancer? *Br J Urol* 1997;79:770–776.

64. Oesterling JE, Martin SK, Bergstralh EJ, et al. The use of prostate-specific antigen in staging patients with newly diagnosed prostate cancer. *JAMA* 1993;269:57–60.

65. Rudoni M, Antonini G, Favro M, et al. The clinical value of prostate-specific antigen and bone scintigraphy in the staging of patients with newly diagnosed, pathologically proven prostate cancer. *Eur J Nucl Med* 1995;22:207–211.

66. Leo ME, Bilhart DL, Bergstralh EJ, et al. Prostate-specific antigen in hormonally traeted stage D2 prostate cancer: is it always an accurate indicator of disease status? *J Urol* 1991;145:802–806.

67. Huben RP, Schellhammer PF. The role of routine follow-up bone scan after definitive therapy of localised prostatic cancer. *J Urol* 1982;128:510–512.

68. Pollen JJ, Gerber K, Ashburn WL, et al. Nuclear bone imaging in metastatic cancer of the prostate. *Cancer* 1981;47:2585–2594.

69. Soloway MS, Hardeman SW, Hickey D, et al. Stratification of patients with metastatic prostate cancer based on extent of disease on initial bone scan. *Cancer* 1988;61:195–202.

70. Jorgensen T, Muller C, Kaalhus O, et al. Extent of disease based on initial bone scan: Important prognostic predictor for patients with metastatic prostate cancer. *Eur Urol* 1995;28:40–46.

71. Maeda H, Koizumi M, Yoshimura K, et al. Correlation between bone metabolic markers and bone scan in prostatic carcinoma. *J Urol* 1997;157:539–543.

72. Koizumi M, Maeda H, Yoshimura K, et al. Dissociation of bone formation markers in bone metastasis of prostate cancer. *Br J Cancer* 1997;75:1601–1604.

73. Perachino M, Di Ciolo L, Barbetti V, et al. Procollagen type I carboxyterminal extension peptide in serum: a reliable marker of bone metastatic disease in newly diagnosed prostate cancer? *Eur Urol* 1996;29:366–369.

74. Bourgeois P, Malarme M, Van Franck R, et al. Bone marrow scintigraphy in prostatic carcinomas. *Nucl Med Commun* 1991;12:35–45.

75. Kirac S, Duman Y, Cureklibatur I, et al. Detection of metastatic bone lesions in patients with prostate carcinoma: ^{99m}Tc monoclonal antibody imaging. *Nucl Med Commun* 1997;18:968–973.

76. Haseman MK, Reed NL, Rosenthal SA. Monoclonal antibody imaging of occult prostate cancer in patients with elevated prostate specific antigen: positron emission tomography and biopsy correlation. *Clin Nucl Med* 1996;21:704–713.

77. Silver DA, Pellicer I, Fair WR, et al. Prostate-specific membrane antigen expression in normal and malignant human tissues. *Clin Cancer Res* 1997;3:81–85.

78. Hoh CK, Seltzer MA, Franklin J, et al. Positron emission tomography in urological oncology. *J Urol* 1998;159:347–56.

79. Yeh SD, Imbriaco M, Larson SM, et al. Detection of bony metastases of androgen-independent prostate cancer by PET-FDG. *Nucl Med Biol* 1996;23:693–697.

80. Hara T, Kosaka N, Kishi H. PET imaging of prostate cancer using carbon-11-choline. *J Nucl Med* 1998;39:990–995.

81. Gravenstein S, Peltz MA, Pories W. How ominous is an abnormal bone scan in bronchogenic carcinoma? *JAMA* 1979;241:2523–2524.

82. Hooper RG, Beechler CR, Johnson MC. Radioisotope scanning in the initial staging of bronchogenic carcinoma. *Am Rev Respir Dis* 1978;118:279–286.

83. Bitran JD, Bekerman C, Pinsky S. Sequential scintigraphic staging of small cell carcinoma. *Cancer* 1981;47:1971–1975.

84. Ali A, Tetalman MR, Fordham EW, et al. Distribution of hypertrophic pulmonary osteoarthropathy. *AJR Am J Roentgenol* 1980;134:771–780.

85. Cole AT, Mandell J, Fried FA, et al. The place of bone scans in the diagnosis of renal cell carcinoma. *J Urol* 1975;114:364–365.

86. Parthasarathy KL, Landsberg R, Bakshi SP, et al. Detection of bone metastases in urogenital malignancies utilizing 99m-Tc-labeled phosphate compounds. *Urology* 1978;11:99–102.

87. Lindner A, Goldman DG, DeKernion JB. Cost effective analysis of prenephrectomy radioisotope scans in renal cell carcinoma. *Urology* 1983;22:127–129.

88. Rosen PR, Murphy KG. Bone scintigraphy in the initial staging of patients with renal-cell carcinoma: concise communication. *J Nucl Med* 1984;25:289–291.

89. Berger GL, Sadlowski RW, Sharpe JR, et al. Lack of value of routine preoperative bone and liver scans in cystectomy candidates. *J Urol* 1981;125:637–639.

90. Kim EE, Bledin AG, Gutierrez C, et al. Comparison of radionuclide images and radiography for skeletal metastases from renal cell carcinoma. *Oncology* 1983;40:284–286.

91. Du Toit JP, Grove DV. Radio-isotope bone scanning for the detection of occult bony metastases in invasive cervical carcinoma. *Gynecol Oncol* 1987;28:215–219.

92. Katz RD, Alderson PO, Rosenshein NB, et al. Utility of bone scanning in detecting occult metastases from cervical carcinoma. *Radiology* 1979;133:469–472.

93. Bassan JS, Glasser MG. Bony metastases in carcinoma of the uterine cervix. *Clin Radiol* 1982;33:623–625.

94. Castillo LA, Yeh SDJ, Leeper RD, et al. Bone scans in bone metastases from functioning thyroid carcinoma. *Clin Nucl Med* 1980;5:200–209.

95. De Groot LJ, Reilly M. Use of isotope bone scans and skeletal survey X-rays in the follow up of patients with thyroid carcinoma. *J Endocrinol Invest* 1984;7:175–179.

96. Tenenbaum F, Schlumberger M, Bonnin F, et al. Usefulness of technetium-99m hydroxymethylene diphosphonate sacns in localizing bone preoperative metastases of differentiated thyroid carcinoma. *Eur J Nucl Med* 1993;20:1168–1174.

97. Bhushan B, Vashist GP, Prasad K, et al. Osteoblastic metastases from thyroid carcinoma. *Br J Radiol* 1985;58:563–565.

98. Hoefnagel CA, Delprat CC, Marcuse HR. The role of Tl-201 total body scintigraphy in the follow up of thyroid carcinoma. *J Nucl Med* 1985;26:P31(abst).

99. Iida Y, Hidaka A, Hatabu H, et al. Follow-up study of postoperative patients with thyroid cancer by thallium-201 scintigraphy and serum thyroglobulin measurement. *J Nucl Med* 1991;32:2098–2100.

100. Miyamoto S, Kasagi K, Misaki T, et al. Evaluation of tech-netium-99m-MIBI scintigraphy in metastatic differentiated thyroid carcinoma. *J Nucl Med* 1997;38:352–356.

101. Nemec J, Nyvltova O, Blazek T, et al. Positive thyroid cancer scintigraphy using technetium-99m methoxyisobutylisonirile. *Eur J Nucl Med* 1996;23:69–71.

102. Maxon HR III, Smith HD. Radioiodine-131 in the diagnosis and treatment of metastatic well-differentiated thyroid cancer. *Endocrinol Metab Clin North Am* 1990;19:685–718.

103. Feine U, Leitzenmayer R, Hanke JP, et al. Fluorine-18-FDG and iodine-131-iodide uptake in thyroid cancer. *J Nucl Med* 1996;37:1468–1472.

104. Grunwald F, Schomburg A, Bender H, et al. Fluorine-18 fluorodeoxyglucose positron emission tomography in the follow-up of differentiated thyroid cancer. *Eur J Nucl Med* 1996;23:312–319.

105. Kalicke T, Grunwald F, Bender H, et al. Clinical indications for the use of fluorine-18 fluorodeoxyglucose positron emission tomography in thyroid cancer. *Clin Positron Imaging* 1998;1:193–199.

106. Johnson DG, Coleman RE, McCook TA, et al. Bone and liver images in medullary carcinoma of the thyroid. *J Nucl Med* 1984;25:419–422.

107. Ugur O, Kostakoglu L, Guler N, et al. Comparison of ^{99m}Tc(V)-DMSA, ^{201}Tl and ^{99m}Tc-MIBI imaging in the follow-up of patients with medullary carcinoma of the thyroid. *Eur J Nucl Med* 1996;23:1367–1371.

108. Learoyd DL, Roach PJ, Briggs GM, et al. Technetium-99m-ses-tamibi scanning in recurrent medullary thyroid carcinoma. *J Nucl Med* 1997;38:227–230.

109. Freeman C, Berg JW, Cutler SJ. Occurence and prognosis of extranodal lymphomas. *Cancer* 1972;29:252–260.

110. Schecter JP, Jones SE, Woolfended JM, et al. Bone scanning in lymphoma. *Cancer* 1976;38:1142–1148.

111. Orzel JA, Sawaf NW, Richardson ML. Lymphoma of the skeleton: scintigraphic evaluation. *AJR Am J Roentgenol* 1988;150:1095–1099.

112. Kuntz DJ, Leonard JC, Nitschke RM, et al. An evaluation of diagnostic techniques utilized in the initial workup of pediatric patients with acute lymphocytic leukemia. *Clin Nucl Med* 1984;9:405–408.

113. Morrison SC, Adler LP. Photopenic areas on bone scanning associated with childhood leukemia. *Clin Nucl Med* 1991;16:24–26.

114. Roth JA, Eilber FR, Bennett LR, et al. Radionuclide photo-scanning: usefulness in preoperative evaluation of melanoma. *Arch Surg* 1975;110:1211–1212.

115. Thomas JH, Panoussopoulus D, Liesmann GE, et al. Scintis-cans in the evaluation of patients with malignant melanoma. *Surg Gynecol Obstet* 1979;149:574–576.

116. Woolfenden JM, Pitt MJ, Durie BGM, et al. Comparison of bone scintigraphy and radiography in multiple myeloma. *Radiology* 1980;134:723–728.

117. Wahner HW, Kyle RA, Beabout JW. Scintigraphic evaluation of the skeleton in multiple myeloma. *Mayo Clin Proc* 1980;55:739–746.

118. Bataille R, Chevalier J, Rossi M, et al. Bone scintigraphy in plasma-cell myeloma. *Radiology* 1982;145:801–804.

119. Wolfe JA, Rowe LD, Lowry LT. The value of radionucleotide scanning in the staging of head and neck carcinoma. *Ann Otol Rhinol Laryngol* 1979;88:832–836.

120. Sham JS, Tong CM, Choy D, et al. Role of bone scanning in detection of subclinical bone metastases in nasopharyngeal carcinoma. *Clin Nucl Med* 1991;16:27–29.

121. Sundram FX, Chua ET, Goh ASW, et al. Bone scintigraphy in nasopharyngeal carcinoma. *Clin Radiol* 1990;42:166–169.

122. Baker HL, Woodbury DH, Krause CJ, et al. Evaluation of bone

scan by scintigraphy to detect subclinical invasion of the mandible by squamous cell carcinoma of the oral cavity. *Otolaryngol Head Neck Surg* 1982;90:327–336.

123. Lee CH, Wang PW, Chen HY, et al. Assessment of skull base involvement in nasopharyngeal carcinoma: comparisons of single-photon emission tomography with planar bone scintigraphy and x-ray computed tomography. *Eur J Nucl Med* 1995;22:514–520.

124. Jacobson AF. Yield of bone scintigraphy for identifying occult malignancy in patients with musculoskeletal pain. *J Nucl Med* 1993;34:33P(abst).

125. Simon MA, Bartucci EJ. The search for the primary tumor in patients with skeletal metastases of unknown origin. *Cancer* 1986;58:1088.

126. Datz FL. *Gamuts in nuclear medicine,* 3rd ed. St. Louis: CV Mosby, 1995:97–182.

127. Harbert JC. The musculoskeletal system. In Harbert JC, Eckelman WC, Neumann RD, eds. *Nuclear medicine diagnosis and therapy.* New York: Theime, 1996:801–863.

128. Becker W. A changing role for bone scintigraphy in oncology: the road from routine imaging screening to patient based screening. *Eur J Nucl Med* 1998;25:1359–1361.

41

SENTINEL NODE IN THE MANAGEMENT OF MALIGNANT MELANOMA

CLAUDIA G. BERMAN
NORMAN J. BRODSKY

Mortality from *malignant melanoma* has been increasing at 4% to 6% yearly in the United States since the early 1970s. The incidence of the disease has now surpassed 40,000 new cases yearly. This incidence is believed to reflect the considerable increase in ultraviolet light exposure of the population that has occurred during this period (1). In comparison, the incidence of mucosal melanomas remains stable. Current estimates foresee that 1 in 75 persons born in the year 2000 will develop a malignant melanoma of the skin during their lives (2). Most malignant melanomas of the skin are diagnosed when they are relatively thin and are still free of clinical evidence of node metastasis. The National Cancer Data Base reports this proportion to have held steady at approximately 86% of new diagnoses during the decade from 1984 to 1994, with a trend to thinner primary lesions. The proportions of patients presenting with clinically identifiable regional nodal or distant metastatic disease have also remained more or less stable, at approximately 9% and 5%, respectively (3).

Thin, early-stage melanomas are usually cured by local excision. The threat of eventual dissemination and death, mediated initially by lymphatic spread from the primary site, becomes distinctly greater when primary lesions have surpassed 1 mm thickness, and this outcome is highly likely when lesions are more than 4 mm thick.

The generally accepted staging for malignant melanoma is as follows: stage I, denoting thinner (less than 1.5 mm) primary tumors; stage II, denoting thicker (more than 1.5 mm) primary tumors, stage III, with regional spread to skin more than 5 cm from the primary tumor or to the regional lymph nodes; and stage IV, cases with distant metastases. Two pathologic conventions have been used to assign lesions within and between stage I and stage II, to differentiate between thinner and thicker primary-only disease.

C.G. Berman: Department of Radiology, H. Lee Moffitt Cancer Center and Research Institute, Department of Radiology, University of South Florida, Tampa, Florida 33612.

N.J. Brodsky: Department of Radiology, University of South Florida, Tampa, Florida 33612; Department of Radiation Oncology, Lykes Cancer Center, Clearwater, Florida 34616.

Clark's levels I through V range from *in situ* disease (I) to subcutaneous invasion (V). Level III describes a primary lesion that fills the papillary dermis and abuts but does not invade the reticular dermis. Although Clark's system has been shown to correlate well with clinical outcomes, it has been largely superceded by the Breslow thickness system, which uses an ocular micrometer to measure the depth of the lesion's penetration below the granular layer of the skin. This system has been found to be simpler, more reproducible, and more reliably predictive of outcomes than the Clark levels. Breslow's system assigns breakpoints of ≤0.75 mm for T1 and 0.76 to 1.50 mm for T2, which together constitute stage I disease. T3 lesions range from 1.51 to 4.00 mm, and T4 lesions exceed 4 mm in thickness. The grouping of T3 and T4 lesions corresponds to stage II melanoma. A rough correspondence exists between T1, T2, T3, and T4, as defined by the Breslow system, and Clark levels II, III, IV, and V, respectively.

Five-year survivals reported in the National Cancer Data Base Report were as follows: stage I, 92.5%; stage II, 74.8%; stage III (lymph node positive), 49.0%; and stage IV, 17.9%. This survey constitutes the most recent analysis of the outcomes for melanoma treated strictly as a "surgical" disease. During the 1990s, fewer than 3% of patients received any type of biologic response modifier therapy. Moreover, among these patients, systematic efforts to verify the true nodal drainage basin were not performed routinely either for therapeutic or for staging purposes.

Many of the approximately 85% of patients with malignant melanoma who present with stage I or stage II disease harbor inapparent nodal and perhaps visceral disease. The middle to late 1990s were a watershed period that brought together new capabilities for accurate nodal basin detection and pathologic analysis, as well as for effective surgical and biologic adjuvant treatment for high-risk patients with early-stage disease. It is now a realistic hope that it will be possible to diminish substantially the 25% to 50% mortality rate in patients with intermediate-thickness primary lesions or nodal metastasis. This hope is realistic in part because it is now possible to identify and to sample accurately the lymph nodes draining the primary lesion. These capabilities have been developed through evolving understanding of the patterns of cutaneous lymphatic drainage and of effective technologies for tracking that process.

DEVELOPMENT OF THE SENTINEL LYMPH NODE TECHNIQUE

The earliest modern description of the pathways of skin lymphatic drainage dates to the mid-19th century work of Sappey, who described the results of mercury injections into the skin of cadavers (4). These studies demonstrated that a line drawn circumferentially around the trunk from just above the umbilicus anteriorly through the second lumbar vertebral body posteriorly delineated which skin sites drained superiorly to the axillae versus inferiorly toward the groin. The midline delineated left-sided from right-sided drainage. Sherman and Ter-Pogossian introduced the use of gold radiocolloid as injectate to track lymphatic flow from skin to lymph nodes in 1953 (5).

Fee and Morton and their group at the John Wayne Cancer Institute in Santa Monica, California were the first to adapt radiocolloid injection to trace *in vivo* lymphatic drainage (lymphoscintigraphy) to aid the surgical management of patients with cutaneous malignant melanoma (6). As they refined their technique, they introduced a two step strategy. These investigators first performed lymphoscintigraphy with dextran or albumin labeled with technetium 99m (^{99m}Tc) (much less expensive, much more readily available and much safer than colloidal gold) (7). These images identified the lymph basins at risk for metastasis. These investigators subsequently injected vital blue dye into the skin at the periphery of the lesion during surgery and dissected the nodal basins (already identified at risk by lymphoscintigraphy) to remove the first node taking up dye, the sentinel lymph node (SLN).

Krag and associates at the University of Vermont in Burlington, Vermont used lymphoscintigraphy, as had Morton's group for preoperative planning. The patients were injected with a radiopharmaceutical just before the surgical procedure. A hand-held gamma probe was employed intraoperatively for localization of the SLN during the nodal basin dissection (8). Reintgen, heading our group at the H. Lee Moffitt Cancer Center and Research Institute in Tampa, Florida, has sought to maximize the accuracy of SLN studies by combining vital dye injection with radiocolloid localization using a hand-held gamma probe.

Lymphoscintigraphy and SLN have been developed at our institution and at others as a potentially generalizable approach to the staging of solid tumors (9). The goal is to maximize the information obtained from lymph node basin surgical procedures while simultaneously minimizing patients' morbidity (10). Malignant melanoma has been an obvious choice for pursuing this work because of the richness of the cutaneous lymphatic network and the many uncertainties confounding the surgical management of regional lymph nodes in this disease. Certainly, the increasing frequency and the deadliness of malignant melanoma also contribute to its popularity in these studies.

The clinical usefulness of lymphoscintigraphy with SLN sampling is based on certain biologic requirements. First, the lymphatic drainage identified by lymphoscintigraphy must identify the nodal basins, which in fact do receive lymphatic flow from the lesion. Second, the passage of metastatic cells must follow a predictable path from primary lesion to SLN to more remote lymph nodes and at some point on to viscera or other distant metastatic sites. This requirement relates to the chief concern raised by reliance on the much reduced tissue sample that SLN sampling provides. The pathologic status of the SLN must predict the status of the remainder of the basin; that is, there must be no false-negative SLN (11).

Experience from our department, as well as from other centers, clearly establishes the reliability of vital blue dye injection and of radiocolloid lymphoscintigraphy for accurate identification of the true physiologic nodal drainage basins of melanoma skin lesions. Clearly, these true nodal drainage basins often do not correspond to the anatomically predicted nodal drainage basins (12). In particular, we have demonstrated a discordance rate between the two ("true physiologic" versus "anatomically predicted" nodal drainage basins) of approximately 40% for truncal and head and neck lesions. In the head and neck region, the discordancy rate approaches 70% (13).

We found unexpected contralateral or bilateral drainage for lesions up to 11 cm off the midline. Similarly ambiguous drainage was seen for bands 11 cm above and below Sappey's line. Head and neck lesions most commonly drain to multiple nodal basins simultaneously and are unpredictable in more than 60% of cases studied. Similarly, shoulder lesions have unexpected drainage about half the time and usually drain to multiple node basins (14). Two particularly difficult areas are the skin overlying the sternal notch and the skin of the posterior base of neck. These sites in our experience are capable of drainage to any of six distinct nodal basins, although we have not documented more than four for any one lesion.

Substantial clinical data are now available underlining the reliability of vital blue dye lymphography and of lymphoscintigraphy for identifying the lymph node basins truly at risk for metastasis in patients with malignant melanoma. Lenisa and colleagues reported on the outcomes in 540 patients with stage I melanoma accessioned between February 1994 and August 1998 (15). Head and neck melanomas were not at first studied because of the extreme variability of nodal basin drainage in these cases. Head and neck melanomas were accessioned, however, among the last 372 patients, all of whom underwent lymphoscintigraphy. All draining lymphatic basins were examined surgically, including the multiple basins identified in 37 of these 540 patients. The SLN identification rate was 91%. Seventy-eight of these 525 SLN procedures (15%) yielded metastatic lymph nodes. These metastatically positive nodal basins were then conventionally dissected. All other nodal basins were observed. Up to the time of publication, 43 patients had disease relapse locally, regionally, or distantly. No patient, however, had disease relapse in any nodal basin excluded by lymphoscitigraphy. Our experience similarly provides confidence that our patients' lymphoscintigraphically detected nodal drainage basins, even when unexpected, were in fact the true drainage areas for our patients' melanomas. Among more than 400 of our patients, with a mean follow-up of 5 years, we have yet to see a single initial nodal relapse in a lymph nodal basin not previously identified by lymphoscintigraphy as a primary drainage basin (16).

Our experience, as that of others, of the accuracy of the SLN in predicting the pathologic status of the remaining nodes of the basin is similarly compelling. In one early multiinstitutional collaborative study, 42 patients with primary melanomas thicker than 0.75 mm and shown on lymphoscintigraphy to have only one primary draining nodal basin were studied prospectively (17). The mean tumor thickness was 2.2 mm. In the early phase of this work, ^{99m}Tc-tagged human serum albumin (HSA) was used. Approximately 1 mCi was injected intradermally in four equal aliquots surrounding the primary site. Scanning was performed immediately and 2 hours after injection to ensure that only one nodal basin served as first-echelon drainage for the primary lesion. The "hot" area on the initial scan was tattooed and subsequently served to mark the site for surgical incision to harvest the SLN. The SLN was identified by either or both the maximum sequestration of radionuclide activity or the entry of a blue-stained afferent lymphatic leading from the primary site into the node. Formal lymph node dissection followed the harvesting of the SLN. Head and neck sites were excluded from the study.

Eight of 42 patients (nodal basins) were found to have metastatic disease. In 7 of these 8 patients, metastatic disease was found only in the SLN. No false-negative (skip metastatic nodes) SLN studies occurred. Statistical analysis predicts the likelihood of this outcome as a random event as 0.008.

In a more mature experience, shared between our institutions (H. Lee Moffitt Cancer Center and Research Institute, Tampa, Florida, and M.D. Anderson Cancer Center, Houston, Texas) 106 patients were studied. Inclusion in the study required a melanoma thickness greater than 0.75 mm. Unlike the earlier group, we included patients with head and neck melanoma as well as patients requiring sampling of more than one lymphatic drainage basin. Our particular interest was to investigate whether the consistent combination of radionuclide and vital blue dye techniques would provide an improved success rate for SLN localization (18). This was of interest because of persistent technical difficulties with vital blue dye SLN localization in approximately 20% of patients even in the hands of experienced surgeons (19).

One hundred twenty-nine draining nodal basins were mapped among 106 patients. Eighty three percent of primary melanoma lesions were approximately equally divided between extremity and truncal sites. Seventeen percent of primary melanoma lesions were from head and neck sites. Two hundred SLN and 142 neighboring non-SLN were harvested. Using the hand-held gamma probe after skin incision, the mean *in vivo* ratio of hot spot to background activity was found to be 8.5:1. The mean *ex vivo* ratio of SLN to non-SLN harvested nodes was 135.6:1. Approximately 70% of hot SLN were also identified by blue dye uptake. Just under 84% of blue SLN were also hot. The combined techniques identified SLN in 96% of drainage basins.

The delay between radiocolloid injection and surgical dissection had a major influence on the sensitivity of gamma probe detection. When surgical dissection was begun immediately after radiocolloid injection of the primary lesion, the mean ratio of *in vivo* hot spot to background activity was 7.4. When surgical dissection was delayed for 3 to 4 hours, this ratio more than doubled, to 16 ($p < .01$). Most important, the higher activity ratios resulted in a marked improvement in SLN detection sensitivity: 94% in nodal basins dissected after the 3- to 4-hour delay. No change occurred in the preincision ratios, computed preoperatively, through the intact skin.

We believe that activity ratios are the most practical measure to use as guidelines in assessing SLN candidates because they should be most independent of the many anatomic and procedural variations that occur with lymphoscintigraphy. Based on our experience, we have proposed three criteria for SLN localization. First, any node with blue-staining afferent lymphatics draining into a blue-stained node is by definition a SLN. Second, a ratio of *in vivo* hot spot to background activity of at least 3:1 or a ratio of *ex vivo* SLN to non-SLN activity of at least 10:1 is the minimum acceptable criterion for radiocolloid SLN identification. Third, further dissection to search for additional SLN is mandatory if a ratio of *in vivo* hot spot to background activity greater than 1.5 persists after removal of an SLN.

LONG-TERM RESULTS

Long-term studies that should lead to the interpolation of SLN procedures into "standard" management of early-stage melanoma are beginning to appear. Morton's group provided long-term outcome data on their substantial melanoma SLN population, 712 patients with clinically negative nodal basins examined over the prior 12 years (20). They found a direct relationship between tumor thickness and SLN positivity. The likelihood of a positive SLN was 6% for a primary tumor less than 1.0 mm thick. The likelihood increased to

23% for primary tumors 1.0 to 4.0 mm thick and 33% for primary lesions thicker than 4.0 mm. Three fourths of these patients with node-positive SLN had no further positive node revealed from pathologic examination of the completion lymphadenectomy specimen. The remaining 25% had up to 5 additional pathologically involved nodes. Five-year survival was 89% for patients with negative SLN, versus 64% for patients with positive SLN. Failure in the nodal basin occurred in 2% of SLN patients, spared immediate completion lymphadenectomy at the time of the negative SLN procedure. Of the 9 patients with positive SLN who did not undergo immediate completion lymphadenectomy, one third had disease relapse in the nodal basin.

The surgical departments at the two cooperating institutions, H. Lee Moffitt Cancer and Research Institute and the M.D. Anderson Cancer Center, published a review of outcomes in patients initially staged with lymphoscintigraphically guided SLN biopsy (21). Six hundred twelve records of patients with stage I or II excised malignant melanoma were reviewed. Patients underwent lymphatic mapping and SLN biopsy when their primary lesion was 1.0 mm thick or thicker or when the lesion was ulcerated or was staged at Clark level IV or greater. Inclusion into the study presupposed no clinical evidence of regional or distant metastases. This approach represents current practice at both institutions.

The overall SLN identification rate was 95%. In the later years of the study, the identification rate approached 100%, with the use of combined blue dye and radiocolloid techniques (22). In the early period of treatment, patients underwent completion lymphadenectomy even when the SLN was pathologically negative. Seventy-two patients were managed in this fashion. Of these, only a single nodal basin was found to contain metastatic adenopathy when the SLN study was benign. This finding represents a negative predictive value of 98.6%.

For primary lesions 4.0 mm or greater in thickness, 34.4% of patients had pathologically positive SLN by standard hematoxylin and eosin (H&E) staining. For primary lesions between 1.5 and 4.0 mm thick, 19.2% of patients had pathologically positive SLN. For primary lesions 1.5 mm or less in thickness, 4.8% of patients had pathologically positive SLN. The frequency of pathologically positive SLN in patients whose primary lesions had surface ulceration or Clark level IV invasion was only 4.7% when the primary lesion was less than 1 mm thick. Because the study group is composed of patients staged between January 1991 and May 1995, before the recognition of the adjuvant role of high-dose interferon alfa-2b, adjuvant systemic therapy was not provided to node-positive patients on a standardized basis, and approximately one half received no such therapy.

The 3-year disease-specific survival rates for SLN-negative and SLN-positive patients were 96.8% and 69.9%, respectively ($p < .0001$). The authors provided separate univariate and multiple covariate analyses of both SLN-positive and SLN-negative patient groups. Among SLN-negative patients, univariate analysis showed tumor thickness, Clark level greater than III, and ulceration to be the most powerful predictive factors. Multiple covariate analysis showed only tumor thickness and ulceration to be predictive, with tumor thickness the stronger predictor.

In contrast, among SLN-positive patients, univariate analysis showed only tumor thickness to be predictive of outcome and only for disease-free survival ($p < .027$). Multiple covariate analysis, however, showed none of the examined covariables to be predictive of outcome. The extraordinary predictive power of a positive SLN is reflected in a hazard ratio of 6.53 versus 1.23 for tumor thickness treated as a continuous variable. Even with a 5-mm tumor thickness, the hazard ratio increases to only 2.29, clearly a much weaker predictor than a positive SLN.

Indeed, the SLN methodology stands alone as a means for improving the staging of patients with clinically node-negative intermediate-risk melanoma. Wagner and associates examined the sensitivity of fluorodeoxyglucose (FDG) positron emission tomography (PET) as the imaging method most likely to enable clinicians to forego targeted node dissection of SLN-type methodology (23). Eighty-nine assessable nodal basins among 70 patients with stage I through stage III malignant melanoma were prospectively examined by both FDG PET scanning and SLN biopsy. Not surprisingly, FDG PET proved inferior by all statistical measures. In particular, the sensitivity of FDG PET (16.7%) was markedly inferior to that of SLN biopsy (94.4%), a finding effectively closing the door on that imaging alternative.

PATHOLOGY

The promised improved sensitivity of this method stems not only from the identification of the true SLN at risk but also from the opportunity this provides the pathologist to bring to bear a more intensive examination on this maximum-risk lymph node. This is of particular importance in that a meaningful minority of patients with histologically negative lymph node basins will progress to metastatic disease within 5 years of nodal dissection.

Clearly, standard histologic techniques understage a significant proportion of patients. Standard histologic examination of lymph nodes, composed of sectioning of the nodes through the middle and staining only one or two sections with standard dye stains, is estimated to visualize less than 1% of the submitted material. The sensitivity of this standard approach permits the identification of a single melanoma cell against a background of 10,000 lymphoid cells.

The great advantage of SLN sampling is that, relieved of the need to stain and examine the large harvest of lymph nodes delivered by a standard nodal basin dissection, the pathologist is able to section one or two true high-risk nodes serially. This approach allows for a more thorough examination of a much smaller volume of higher-risk tissue. Additionally, the more sensitive (and specific) immunohistochemical stains can be employed in addition to standard dye stain techniques. It is estimated that by adding melanoma-specific immunohistochemical staining to serial sectioning of the nodes, an entire order of magnitude can be added to the sensitivity of the pathologic examination, to allow for the identification of a single metastatic malignant melanoma cell against a background of 100,000 normal lymphoid cells.

Gershenwald and associates described the results of intensive pathologic reevaluation of SLN material in patients suffering nodal basin relapse despite a negative initial SLN examination. They followed 243 patients with histologically negative SLN in whom the nodal basins were observed, with no surgery performed (24). All nodal basins undergoing SLN biopsy were selected based on lymphoscintigraphic studies. Standard H&E pathologic techniques were applied to the SLN specimens. With a median follow-up of 35 months, only 10 patients, 4.1% of the group, developed a recurrence in the undissected nodal basin, with or without evidence of relapse elsewhere. When reexamined using more sensitive serial sectioning or immunohistochemical staining techniques, 8 of these 10 patients' SLN were found in fact to contain micrometastatic disease.

Further emphasizing the value of serial sectioning and immunohistochemical staining is experience accumulated at the Memorial Sloan-Kettering Cancer Center in New York and the M.D. Anderson Cancer Centers in which 39 SLN specimens, negative by standard bivalved node H&E examination, were reevaluated (25). These specimens were selected because they were obtained from patients with primary lesions of 1.5 mm thick or thicker, those most likely to harbor minute microscopic nodal disease. Each node was serially sectioned at 50-μm intervals. The average specimen yielded 20 sections. Three sections were then stained with H&E and for S-100 and HMB-45 antigens. Eighteen of the 39 SLN specimens (46%) proved to contain metastatic disease that had gone undetected at the time of original H&E single section pathologic examination. Six of the 18 newly recognized melanoma-positive nodes were discovered merely by reexamination of the original slides. Two thirds of the "new" diagnoses were detected only after serial sections were examined. Staining with H&E detected 8 of these 12 "new" positive nodes on the 2nd to 10th serial section. S-100 immunostaining identified 11 of the 12 "new" positive nodes on the 1st through 11th serial section. HMB-45 immunostaining detected 10 of the 12 "new" positive nodes at serial sections 3 through 30. In analyzing their results, the authors concluded that, using their techniques, at least 8 serial sections must be stained to detect 90% of these previously missed nodal micrometastases.

We have reported our ongoing experience with a histologic protocol for SLN biopsy specimens that involves the routine use of immunohistochemical staining for S-100

protein (26). Our technique entails formalin fixation of SLN tissue for a minimum of 48 hours to allow six half-lives of our ^{99m}Tc label to elapse. At that point, processing in the pathology laboratory begins with gross examination and observation for the presence of vital blue dye, melanin pigment, or tumor nodules. Lymph nodes are sectioned at 2- to 3-mm intervals and are entirely submitted for paraffin embedding. This usually produces one to eight cassettes of tissue per SLN (average, 1.5 blocks per node). Each block is sectioned at one to three levels per slide, and one H&E preparation is obtained from each block. All blocks grossly negative for metastasis are then stained for S-100 antigen using the avidin-biotin complex immunoperoxidase technique with diaminobenzidine chromogen. Our more recent practice also involves examination of intraoperative touch preparations of bivalved SLN specimens, before placement in formalin. These slides are then stained with Diff-Quik (Behring, Inc., Newark, DE).

We accumulated data on 838 SLN from 357 patients between October 1995 and June 1997. Fifty-six patients (16%) were found to harbor nodal metastatic disease. Fifty of these patients (88%) went on to completion lymphadenectomy. Only 5 patients—one tenth of those examined—were found to have other pathologically involved nodes. Certain patterns of involvement were identified. The most common pattern was a subcapsular nodule or nodules. Dominant medullary nodules were also seen.

Diffuse nodal involvement by small aggregates of cells was uncommon. It was generally possible, when immunostaining was performed and found positive, to retrace the H&E examination and to confirm the presence of cytologically malignant melanoma metastases. This is mandatory because of the distinctly lower specificity than sensitivity of the S-100 staining technique. False-positive results may be produced by the presence of natural S-100 staining in interdigitating reticulum cells, a normal germinal center constituent in lymph nodes. Similar uncertainties can be produced by nerve and adipose tissue and benign nevus cell aggregates within lymph nodes (27). When cytologic evidence of malignancy of S-100 positive cells is equivocal, we employ the less sensitive but more specific HMB-45 antibody. In practice, this proved helpful in only 1 of our 56 node-positive patients.

Substantial effort is being made to increase the sensitivity of pathologic examination of these key nodes further. Our early efforts at the Moffitt Cancer Center entailed a cell-culture technique performed in tandem with standard H&E examination. A 31% upstaging from stages I or II to stage III occurred among cell-cultured specimens of histologically negative nodes. Additionally, this upstaging correlates with an increased risk of subsequent recurrent disease (28).

Much recent attention has centered around quicker and more reproducible techniques, among which reverse transcription–polymerase chain reaction (RT-PCR) is particularly attractive. This approach takes advantage of the high specificity of tyrosinase messenger RNA for melanocytes. It is presumed that the presence of this messenger RNA in cellular material from a lymph node draining a melanoma is tantamount to a diagnosis of lymph node metastasis. The RT-PCR assay greatly enhances the sensitivity of the pathologic examination.

Our group has performed a comparative study pitting RT-PCR against standard dye stain techniques, testing SLN samples from 29 patients with intermediate-thickness melanomas. Standard dye staining techniques identified melanoma metastasis to the SLN in 38% of patients. Assay with RT-PCR identified melanoma metastases to the SLN in 66% of patients, including all patients identified by standard staining techniques. More to the point, we have been able to correlate clinical outcomes to RT-PCR SLN results. Among 74 patients examined with both routine histology techniques and RT-PCR analysis, 14 patients were node positive by both techniques and experienced a 3-year recurrence rate of 42%. Thirty-three patients were node negative by both techniques and experienced a 3-year recurrence risk of 6.6%. Twenty-seven patients fell into the group with metastatic adenopathy in SLN identified only on the more sensitive RT-PCR assay. These patients experienced a 3-year recurrence risk of 22%, an intermediate value, between the groups with higher and lower microscopic tumor burden. These findings correlate with our estimation of sensitivity for RT-PCR for identifying a single metastatic melanoma cell against a background of approximately 1 million nodal lymphoid cells, a 2 order of magnitude improvement in sensitivity from that achievable with standard histologic techniques that are practical with standard lymph node basin dissection specimens.

We have been able to report on the clinical follow-up of 114 patients with stage I and stage II malignant melanoma prospectively subjected to lymphoscintigraphy with SLN biopsy in whom SLN were each prospectively divided into 2 specimens (29). One specimen was submitted for standard H&E examination, and the other was subjected to RT-PCR assay for tyrosinase messenger RNA. The mean follow-up was 28 months. Twenty-three patients (20%) had histologically positive SLN. All these SLN were also RT-PCR positive. Of the 91 remaining patients with pathologically negative SLN, 44 were RT-PCR negative and 47 were RT-PCR positive. Recurrence rates were 61% for patients with both histologically and biochemically positive SLN but only 2% for patients negative by both methods. The recurrence rate was 13% for patients with histologically negative but biochemically positive SLN. When disease-free and overall survival rates were compared between the two histologically negative RT-PCR groups, the differences in disease-free and overall survival were both statistically significant ($p < .02$).

When 10-year expected survivals for various primary thicknesses are compared with those seen among our patients in whom RT-PCR data are also available, good correspondence is seen for thicker melanomas. The 10-year death rate for patients with melanomas thicker than 4 mm is about 75%. This rate corresponds well with the RT-PCR positivity rate of 77% among our similar patients. Histologic examination of SLN in these patients identified only 40% as candidates for death from melanoma. Similarly, for intermediate-thickness melanomas, between 1.4 and 4.0 mm thickness, 40% of patients will die of melanoma by 10 years. Our RT-PCR testing found 68% positive, whereas our histologic testing found only 20% of patients to have positive SLN. In this circumstance, the RT-PCR would appear to overestimate and the histologic examination would appear to underestimate the risk to the patients. (Alternatively, the completion nodal dissection performed after the positive SLN procedure may sometimes be curative.) Among patients with thinner melanomas, less than 1.5 mm thickness, the 10-year melanoma mortality is expected to be about 15%. However, RT-PCR predicted an adverse outcome in approximately 50%.

Problems with RT-PCR specificity have been pointed out by other investigators. Yu and colleagues reported the results of a retrospective pathologic review of 235 SLN specimens interpreted as negative using standard H&E methods (30). They subjected these specimens to both serial step sectioning and an array of immunohistochemical stains and found incremental benefit to both approaches. They identified melanoma micrometastasis in 12% of their specimens. In addition to a discussion of the relative strengths and weaknesses of the various available immunohistochemical stains, these investigators pointed out the pitfall of too great a reliance on RT-PCR tyrosinase evaluation of nodal tissue. Specifically, 9% of their SLN specimens contained capsular melanocytic nevi, a benign lesion that can produce a positive result in the RT-PCR tyrosinase assay. The degree to which this will prove a limitation is uncertain in that specificity apparently can be improved by requiring a positive result with a melanoma specific marker in RT-PCR positive patients (31).

At this time, a three-armed prospective study is beginning in the hope of better understanding the significance of positive RT-PCR studies in histologically negative SLN patients. The Sunbelt Melanoma Trial will randomize these patients to observation or complete lymph node dissection or complete lymph node dissection with adjuvant interferon alfa therapy.

TECHNIQUE FOR MELANOMA LYMPHOSCINTIGRAPHY

The equipment needed for lymphoscintigraphy is found in any hospital nuclear medicine department. A large field of view gamma camera and a high-resolution collimator are used with the 10% window at the 140-Kev technetium energy peak. Lymphatic mapping requires the purchase of a commercially available hand-held gamma probe.

Particle choice is important to obtain good results. We have chosen ^{99m}Tc-sulphur colloid that has passed through a 0.2-µm filter. If the particle is too small, it will be taken up in the capillaries and will result in a poor target-to-background ratio. If the particle is too large, it may not be taken up in the afferent lymphatics. This will cause less of the dose to reach the lymph nodes and more artifact related to the injection site. Because of these factors, we use freshly prepared colloid. Over time, the colloid clumps resulting in an effectively larger particle size.

In the past, we tried ^{99m}Tc-HSA, but this radiopharmaceutical appears to pass through the lymph nodes too rapidly. There is some concern that HSA would rapidly pass through the true SLN and would leave them nonradioactive by the time of surgery. A second concern with the use of HAS involves the number of lymph nodes in the regional bed that become radioactive. Routinely, with HSA, six to eight lymph nodes will become radioactive, rather than one or two, as seen with ^{99m}Tc-sulfur colloid. An increased number of radioactive lymph nodes may lead to confusion, increased difficulty intraoperatively, and a more invasive dissection.

The use of ^{99m}Tc-antimony trisulfide colloid is widespread in Australia, Europe, and Canada, and this agent has an ideal particle size. It is no longer available for distribution in the United States. Rhenium-186 colloid is widely used with good success in Europe.

In most cases of melanoma involving the trunk and extremities, 450 µCi of ^{99m}Tc is used. The dose is decreased to 250 µCi in cases involving the head and neck and when a lesion is near the drainage basin. The dose is decreased because there is less artifact from the injection site when a lower dose is used. This decreases the chance of having false-negative lymph nodes that have been masked by the injection site. A high specific activity is used in melanoma; 1 mL of diluent is divided into four equal aliquots. The dose is placed in tuberculin syringes and is injected intradermally, to raise skin wheels about an intact lesion. After biopsy, two injections are made on

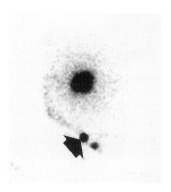

FIGURE 41.2. Anterior pelvic lymphoscintigram. A right lower back melanoma has a single afferent channel. The two visualized lymph nodes are in series, so only the first draining lymph node *(arrow)* is the sentinel lymph node.

each side of the scar. Each injection is about 1 cm from the scar. It is important not to inject at the ends of the scar because this leads to more disparate drainage than the intact lesion.

The patient is immediately placed under the gamma camera so the afferent drainage can be identified. The camera should be positioned over the regional lymph node groups that drain the lesion, and an attempt is made to localize the SLN. This is done by following the afferent channels until they persistently accumulate in a particular focus within the lymph node. Lymphatic channels are followed to see where they lead. There can be single or multiple channels leading to a single drainage basin or multiple channels leading to multilple basins. The examiner should note whether lymph nodes are in parallel channels (Fig. 41.1) or whether the lymph nodes are in series within a single channel (Fig. 41.2). The drainage patterns can often be unexpected or bizarre (Fig. 41.3). Cine imag-

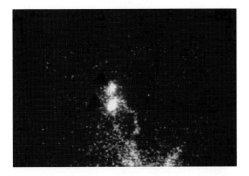

FIGURE 41.1. Right lateral chest lymphoscintigram. A right abdominal melanoma has two separate lymphatic channels, each of which travels to a separate sentinel lymph node *(arrowheads)*. These lymph nodes are on parallel channels.

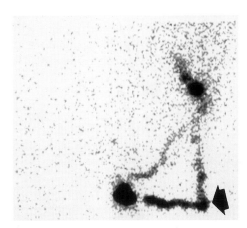

FIGURE 41.3. Posterior back and flank lymphoscintigram. The afferent lymphatics can have a bizarre configuration. Two afferent lymphatics drain this right back melanoma. One of the channels forms a right angle *(arrow)* before traveling to the axilla.

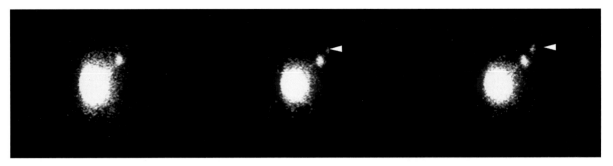

FIGURE 41.4. Frames from an anterior chest cine study show an increase in lymph node activity over time. A single lymph node is visualized in the first frame. There is faint uptake in a second lymph node *(arrowhead)* after 10 minutes and more intense uptake in the second lymph node *(arrowhead)* after 15 minutes.

ing is useful in melanoma because the lymphatic flow is rich and progression to the regional lymph node basins can occur rapidly (Fig. 41.4). The patient is imaged in multiple projections for localization (Fig. 41.5). Using the hand-held gamma probe is an effective way to localize lymph nodes accurately. It also allows for the marking of the lymph nodes in the same anatomic position that will be used in the operating room. An attempt is made to find in-transit lymph nodes, those lymph nodes between the injection site and the regional lymph node group which, by definition, are SLN (Fig. 41.6). Lymphoscintigraphy is the only way to find these lymph nodes. Delayed imaging is rarely used. Once the lymph nodes are localized, the skin can be marked with an indelible pen or tattoo.

Imaging is performed using localizer views in multiple projections. The body contour and body landmarks can be outlined using a hot ^{99m}Tc marker. Another technique involves the insertion of a cobalt flood source between the patient and the detector. The patient's soft tissues attenuate the gamma rays and allow for the identification of various body landmarks.

Technical failures are rare (less than 5% of injections). Usually, technical failures occur in patients with severe induration after an excisional biopsy. If there is no discernable lymphatic flow after 40 minutes, the patient is reinjected with the same dose of radiopharmaceutical, but the injections are placed further from the epicenter of the scar, about 1.5 cm from the scar. Massage and warm compresses can be applied around the injected area to stimulate lymphatic flow. If there is no discernable lymphatic flow after an additional 45 minutes of imaging, the patient is asked to return after a 2- to 3-hour delay. The study can usually be recovered by this point. However, some patients have had no discernable lymphatic flow even after delayed imaging. Lymphatic flow and SLN are usually identified if a patient returns for a second study the following week.

Cutaneous lymphatic flow is so rich that afferent lymphatics are immediately seen and can be traced in most cases. The amount of the radiopharmaceutical trapped in the lymph nodes increases over time. It is recommended that the injections be performed at least 2 to 4 hours preoperatively. This gives sufficient time for enough of the radioactive particles to be trapped in the lymph nodes to provide good target-to-background ratios without any problem related to the decay of the ^{99m}Tc. With melanoma, however, there is relative latitude about when the operation can be performed. Surgery can be undertaken immediately after injection or even the following day if required by circumstances.

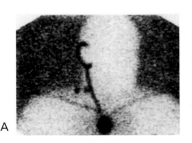

A

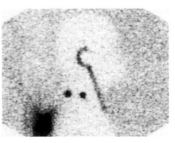

B

FIGURE 41.5. A: The right anterior oblique image shows that an upper midback melanoma drains to the neck. **B:** The right lateral image allows localization of the neck lymph nodes. A cobalt flood source is used to define body contour, and body landmarks such as the ear and sternocleidomastoid muscle have been outlined with a technetium marker.

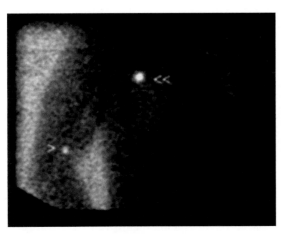

FIGURE 41.6. An anterior lymphoscintigraphy image of the right arm shows lymphatic drainage from a melanoma of the hand into an in-transit lymph node *(arrowhead)* just above the elbow as well as a right axillary lymph node *(double arrowheads)*.

IMPLICATIONS FOR ADJUVANT NODE DISSECTION

Investigators have long recognized that node basin dissection provides a therapeutic benefit in patients with clinically evident nodal metastatic melanoma (32). It has been much more difficult to identify a group of "intermediate-risk" patients with clinically node-negative melanoma and high-risk primary lesions who perhaps could benefit from adjuvant prophylactic node dissection. Presumably, this group of patients has been difficult to identify because only a subset of such patients would, in fact, harbor subclinical nodal disease and therefore have any possibility of benefit. Of course, all patients who undergo lymph node dissection would run the risks of treatment morbidity. These can be particularly severe after axillary and, even more so, groin dissection and can include chronic edema with resultant soft-tissue and functional compromise as well as considerable near-term risks of wound complications (33). Historical comparisons, nevertheless, strongly suggest benefit within this patient group. Patients with clinically negative node basins, found at the time of elective lymph node dissection (ELND) to be pathologically positive, have been seen to have 5-year survival rates in the 50% to 60% range (34). In comparison, a policy of reserving node dissection until clinical relapse should occur has resulted in 5-year survival in the 20% to 25% range (35).

A succession of randomized studies has failed to show any survival advantage to ELND in patients with intermediate thickness, clinically node-negative melanoma. It had been logically anticipated that this group would benefit from such therapy in that they demonstrate a high risk of initial regional relapse rather than distant metastatic failure.

The World Health Organization study found no benefit to ELND. This study contained a wide range of primary lesion thicknesses, however, a feature that compromised the statistical power to identify a meaningful difference within what may have been a minority subgroup (36). The Mayo Clinic study also showed no benefit for ELND. Any possible benefit once again may well have been diluted to an undetectable level by the large proportion of patients with thin primary lesions (37). The Intergroup Melanoma Trial is the first randomized trial concentrating on this group of clinically node-negative patients with high risk of regional relapse that has suggested a benefit from ELND. It is also the first to employ lymphoscintigraphy to ensure that the lymph node basins removed are, in fact, those that drain the primary lesion (38). Seven hundred forty patients with stage I and stage II melanoma, clinically node negative with primary lesions ranging from 1 to 4 mm thick, were accessioned for randomization. Half underwent prophylactic ELND, whereas the other half underwent observation. The median follow-up was 7.4 years. Clinical benefit was particularly apparent for patients younger than 60 years with primary lesions 1.1 to 2.0 mm thick. Five-year survival in these patients improved from 84% in those not receiving ELND to 96% in patients receiving ELND ($p = .007$). Progressively smaller improvements in 5-year survival, not reaching statistical significance, were seen for patients with incrementally thicker primary lesions.

Eleven-year follow-up results of trial 14 of the World Health Organization Melanoma Program also supply strong suggestive support for the selective use of prophylactic adjuvant node dissection employed in conjunction with lymphoscintigraphy and intensive SLN examination. Although the overall group of patients with truncal primary melanoma lesions thicker than 1.5 mm did not benefit by ELND, those patients found to have occult lymphatic metastases discovered incidentally within the ELND specimens had better survival than their randomized cohort, in whom node dissection was undertaken only at the development of nodal basin relapse (39).

IMPLICATIONS FOR ADJUVANT BIOTHERAPY

Researchers have identified specific chromosomal loci that, when mutated or lost, contribute to the development of malignant melanoma. One of these loci, located at 9p21, encodes for proteins that are critical for regulation of cell-cycle progression (40). The genes responsible for production of interferons alfa and beta are situated on the adjoining 9p22 locus and are also commonly lost or damaged in melanoma (41). Long before these laboratory observations, however, interferon alfa-2b had been recognized to result in a 15% to 20% objective response rate in patients with metastatic melanoma (42). On that basis, some prospective cooperative studies have been undertaken in the United States and Europe investigating the capability of adjuvant interferon to reduce relapse in patients with high-risk melanoma after surgical treatment.

In the Eastern Cooperative Oncology Group (ECOG) trial number 1,684, 287 patients were enrolled and randomized to either clinical follow-up alone or to a full year of maximally tolerable interferon therapy (43). This entailed 4 weeks of 20 million units/m^2 interferon alfa-2b intravenously five times weekly, followed by 48 weeks of triweekly subcutaneous injections of 10 million units/m^2. Although node dissections were required and provided information about nodal status, these dissections, for the most part, were done without lymphoscintigraphy verification of nodal basin drainage and without SLN techniques. Four groups of patients were entered into the study. The least advanced disease group included patients with primary lesions of greater than 4-mm Breslow depth. Patients presenting with nodal disease and primary lesions of various depths were stratified between clinically apparent nodal disease and disease discovered only on pathologic examination of lymph node specimens. The American Joint Committee on Cancer (AJCC) staging of these three groups was as follows: clinical stage I, pathologic stage I, T4N0M0; clinical stage I, pathologic stage II, T1 to T4N1M0; and clinical stage II, pathologic stage II, T1 to T4N1M0. The current AJCC stage for these three groups of patients would be IIb, IIIa, and IIIa, respectively. A fourth group of patients was composed of patients with clinical recurrence confined to the regional nodes.

Analysis of outcomes with a median follow-up of just under 7 years showed highly significant benefits from adjuvant interferon alfa-2b treatment. Benefits were chiefly accrued in the early follow-up period but have been maintained and include improvement in both disease-free and overall survival. Benefits for patients with T4N0M0 staging did not reach statistical significance when they were analyzed separately from the larger group. The reason may be that only approximately 10% of the 287 patients completing the study had stage IIb disease.

An improvement in overall survival from 2.8 years in patients randomized to not receive biotherapy compared with 3.8 years in those receiving interferon alfa-2b was statistically significant. When only patients with nodal metastases (stage III) are considered, the *p* values for disease-free survival and overall survival are, respectively, .006 and .0006. For the study group, overall continuous disease-free survival increased from 26% for patients on observation to 37% for patients receiving adjuvant biotherapy.

Because ECOG trial number 1,684, which opened in 1985, did not employ lymphoscintigraphy or SLN examination, one can only speculate how the improved accuracy and sensitivity provided by lymphatic mapping with augmented pathologic examination of the SLN would affect the clinical results that have been achieved. If the assumption is made that imperfect adjuvant therapy is more useful in patients with smaller subclinical tumor burdens, it can be hoped that patients whose disease is detectable only by SLN examination will benefit even more dramatically than those node-positive patients who participated in ECOG trial number 1,684.

Unfortunately toxicity was significant; two thirds of patients experienced severe, grade 3 toxicity at some point during the treatment year, and 9% of patients faced life-threatening toxicity. The major toxicities of interferon in this and other published experiences were, characteristically, myelosuppression, hepatotoxicity, neurologic toxicity, and constitutional symptoms, including flulike symptoms, anorexia, fever, chills, and fatigue (44).

The investigators of ECOG trial number 1,684 also provided an analysis of the economic impact of standard application of interferon alfa-2b therapy to its target therapeutic population (45). They found the cost per quality of life-year gained to be less than $16,000. This compares favorably with the Canadian benchmark of $20,000 per quality of life-year gained and is comparable to the costs for multiagent chemotherapy for breast cancer and combined-modality therapy for colorectal cancer that society has accepted for decades.

Corroboration of the effects of adjuvant interferons was obtained with a follow-up ECOG study, number 1,690, which again confirmed improvement in disease-free survival but failed to show an improvement in overall survival (46). ECOG trial number 1,690 differed from trial number 1,684 in that there was no requirement for lymph node dissection. Overall, survival for the observation arm was much better than for the observation arm in trial number 1,684, but this finding could well be a reflection of a much larger proportion of low-risk T4N0M0 patients, 26% versus 12%.

Improved disease-free survival has also been reported with European adjuvant trials of interferon alfa-2a in lower-risk patient groups. Both French and Austrian randomized studies describe a disease-free survival advantage for adjuvant interferon alfa-2a when the agent is given to patients with clinically negative nodal basins and primary melanomas more than 1.5 mm thick (47,48).

CONCLUSIONS

None of these positive randomized surgical and biologic therapy studies involved the systematic application of lymphoscintigraphy and SLN examinations. It is intuitively appealing to predict that greater benefit with lesser cost and morbidity could be achieved by a more closely targeted administration of adjuvant treatments to patients truly at risk of disease relapse. No doubt future studies will be undertaken using other biologic agents promising to provide adjuvant benefit with less morbidity (49,50). Also of great interest will be the interplay of enhanced anatomic staging attainable through lymphoscintigraphy and SLN biopsy with the emerging role of molecular staging, for example, the use of integrin staining, to identify inherent cellular characteristics predisposing to metastasis (51).

We hope that clinical studies in progress and others soon to follow will elucidate the most useful and cost-effective integration of these new diagnostic and therapeutic tools. From the perspective of our institutional experience, however, it is important to stress meticulous planning and thorough cooperation among the relevant departments to ensure that the maximum potential of these innovations is quickly and consistently achieved for the benefit of our patients and for reliable execution of clinical studies.

REFERENCES

1. Wingo PA, Ries LAG, Rosenberg HM, et al. Cancer incidence and mortality, 1973–1995. *Cancer* 1998;82:1197–207.
2. Rigel DS. Malignant melanoma: incidence issues and their effect on diagnosis and treatment in the 1990's. *Mayo Clin Proc* 1997; 72:367–371.
3. Chang AE, Karnell LH, Menck HR. The National Cancer Data Base report on cutaneous and noncutaneous melanoma: a summary of 84,836 cases from the past decade. *Cancer* 1998;83: 1664–1678.
4. Sappey MPC. *Injection, préparation et conservation des vaisseaux lymphatiques.* MD thesis. Paris: Rignoux Imprimeur de la Faculté de Medecin, 1843.
5. Sherman AI, Ter-Pogossian M. Lymph-node concentration of radioactive colloidal gold following interstitial injection. *Cancer* 1953;6:1238–1240.
6. Fee HJ, Robinson DS, Sample F, et al. The determination of lymph shed by colloidal gold scanning in patients with malignant melanoma: a preliminary study. *Surgery* 1978;84:626–632.
7. Morton DL, Wen D-R, Cochran AJ. Management of early stage melanoma by intraoperative lymphatic mapping and selective lymphadenectomy: an alternative to routine elective lymphadenectomy or "watch and wait." *Surg Oncol Clin North Am* 1992;1:247–259.
8. Krag DN, Meijer SJ, Weaver DL, et al. Minimal-access surgery for staging of melanoma. *Arch Surg* 1995;130:203–210.
9. Reintgen D, Shivers S. Sentinel lymph node micrometastasis from melanoma: proven methodology and evolving significance [Editorial]. *Cancer* 1999;86:551–552.
10. Wells KE, Rapaport DP, Cruse CW, et al. Sentinel lymph node biopsy in melanoma of the head and neck. *Plast Reconstr Surg* 1997;100:591–594.
11. Reintgen D, Cruse W, Wells K, et al. The orderly progression of melanoma nodal metastases. *Ann Surg* 1994;220:759–767.
12. O'Brien CJ, Uren RF, Thompson JF, et al. Prediction of potential metastatic sites in cutaneous head and neck melanoma using lymphoscintigraphy. *Am J Surg* 1995;170:461–466.
13. Berman CG, Norman J, Cruse CW, et al. Lymphoscintigraphy in malignant melanoma. *Ann Plast Surg* 1992;28:29–32.
14. Uren RF, Howman-Giles RB, Shaw HM, et al. Lymphoscintigraphy in high-risk melanoma of the trunk: predicting draining node groups, defining lymphatic channels and locating the sentinel node. *J Nucl Med* 1993;34:1435–1440.
15. Lenisa L, Santinami M, Belli F, et al. Sentinel node biopsy and selective lymph node dissection in cutaneous melanoma patients. *J Exp Clin* Cancer Res 1999;18:69–74.
16. Reintgen DS, Albertini J, Berman C, et al. Accurate nodal staging of malignant melanoma. *Cancer Control* 1995;2:405–414.
17. Reintgen DS, Cruse CW, Wells K, et al. The orderly progression of melanoma nodal metastases. *Ann Surg* 1994;220:759–767.
18. Albertini JJ, Cruse CW, Rapaport D, et al. Intraoperative radiolymphoscintigraphy improves sentinel lymph node identification for patients with melanoma. *Ann Surg* 1996;223:217–224.
19. Morton DL, Wen D-R, Wong JH, et al. Technical details of intraoperative lymphatic mapping for early stage melanoma. *Arch Surg* 1992;127:392–399.
20. Essner R, Foshag LJ, Glass E, et al. Predicting patient survival in early-stage melanoma: results of 712 lymphatic mapping and selective lymph node dissections. *Proc Am Soc Clin Oncol* 1999; 18:529a(abst 2040).
21. Gershenwald JE, Thompson W, Mansfield PF, et al. Multi-institutional melanoma lymphatic mapping experience: the prognostic value of sentinel lymph node status in 612 stage I or II melanoma patients. *J Clin Oncol* 1999;17:976–983.
22. Gershenwald JE, Tseng C-H, Thompson W, et al. Improved sentinel lymph node localization in primary melanoma patients with the use of radiolabeled colloid. *Surgery* 1998;124:203–210.
23. Wagner JD, Schauwecker D, Davidson D, et al. Prospective study of fluorodeoxyglucose-positron emission tomography imaging of lymph node basins in melanoma patients undergoing sentinel node biopsy. *J Clin Oncol* 1999;17:1508–1515.
24. Gershenwald JE, Colome MI, Lee JE, et al. Patterns of recurrence following a negative sentinel lymph node biopsy in 243 patients with stage I or II melanoma. *J Clin Oncol* 1998;16: 2253–2260.
25. Bieligk SC, Coit DG, Rosai J, et al. The detection of micrometastases in melanoma sentinel nodes by complete serial sectioning and immunohistochemical staining. *J Clin Oncol* 1999; 18:537(abstr 2074).
26. Messina JL, Glass LF, Cruse CW, et al. Pathologic examination of the sentinel lymph node in malignant melanoma. *Am J Surg Pathol* 1999;23:686–690.
27. Gaynor RB, Herschman HR, Irie R, et al. S-100 protein: a marker for human malignant melanoma? *Lancet* 1981;1: 869–871.
28. Heller R, King LB, Baekey P, et al. Identification of submicroscopic lymph node metastases in patients with malignant melanoma. *Semin Surg Oncol* 1993;9:285–289.
29. Shivers SC, Wang X, Li W, et al. Molecular staging of malignant melanoma: correlation with clinical outcome. *JAMA* 1998;280: 1410–1415.
30. Yu LL, Flotte TJ, Tanabe KK, et al. Detection of microscopic melanoma metastases in sentinel lymph nodes. *Cancer* 1999;86: 617–627.
31. McMasters KM, Reintgen DS, Ross MI, et al. Sunbelt melanoma trial: sensitivity and specificity of reverse transcriptase-polymerase chain reaction (rt-pcr) markers for sentinel lymph nodes (sln). *Proc Am Soc Clin Oncol* 1999;18:537a(abst 2073).
32. Barth A, Wanek LA, Morton DL. Prognostic factors in 1521 melanoma patients with distant metastases. *J Am Coll Surg* 1995; 181:193–201.
33. Urist MM, Maddow WA, Kennedy JE, et al. Patient risk factors and surgical morbidity after regional lymphadenectomy in 204 melanoma patients. *Cancer* 1983;51:2152–2156.
34. Balch CM. The role of elective lymph node dissection in melanoma: rationale, results and controversies. *J Clin Oncol* 1988;6:163–172.
35. Day CL Jr, Mihn MC Jr, Lew RA, et al. Prognostic factors for patients with clinical stage I melanoma of intermediate thickness: an appraisal of thin level IV lesion. *Ann Surg* 1982;195:35–43.

36. Veronesi U, Adamus J, Bandiera DC, et al. Delayed regional lymph node dissection in stage I melanoma of the skin of the lower extremities. *Cancer* 1982;49:2420–2430.

37. Sim FH, Taylor WF, Pritchard DJ, et al. Lymphadenectomy in the management of stage I malignant melanoma: a prospective randomized study. *Mayo Clin Proc* 1986;61:697–705.

38. Balch CM, Soong S-J, Bartolucci AA, et al. Efficacy of an elective regional lymph node dissection of 1 to 4 mm thick melanomas for patients 60 years of age and younger. *Ann Surg* 1996;224:255–266.

39. Cascinelli N, Morabito A, Santinami M, et al. Immediate or delayed dissection of regional nodes in patients with melanoma of the trunk: a randomised trial. *Lancet* 1998;351:793–796.

40. Chin L, Merlino G, DePinho RA. Malignant melanoma: modern black plague and genetic black box. *Genes Dev* 1988;12:3467–3481.

41. Bastian BC, Leboit PE, Hamm H, et al. Chromosomal gains and losses in primary cutaneous melanomas detected by comparative genomic hybridization. *Cancer Res* 1998;58:2170–2121.

42. Kirkwood JM, Ernstoff MS. Interferons in the treatment of human cancer. *J Clin Oncol* 1984;2:336–352.

43. Kirkwood JM, Strawderman MH, Ernstoff MS, et al. Interferon Alfa-2b adjuvant therapy of high-risk resected cutaneous melanoma: an Eastern Cooperative Oncology Group study (E1684). *J Clin Oncol* 1996;14:7–17.

44. Cole LBF, Gelber RD, Kirkwood HM, et al. A quality of life adjusted survival analysis of interferon alfa-2b adjuvant treatment for high-risk resected cutaneous melanoma: an Eastern Cooperative Oncology Group study (E1684). *J Clin Oncol* 1996;14:2666–2673.

45. Hillner BE, Kirkwood JM, Atkins MB, et al. Economic analysis of adjuvant interferon alfa-2b in high-risk melanoma based on projections from Eastern Cooperative Oncology Group 1684. *J Clin Oncol* 1997;15:2351–2358.

46. Kirkwood JM, Ibrahim J, Sondak K, et al. Preliminary analysis of the E1690/S9111/C9190 Intergroup postoperative adjuvant trial of high and low dose IFNalpha 2-b (HDI and LEI) in high-risk primary or lymph node metastatic melanoma. *Proc Am Soc Clin Oncol* 1999;18:537a(abst 2072).

47. Grob JJ, Dreno B, de la Salmoniere P, et al. Randomised trial of interferon alfa-2a as adjuvant therapy in resected primary melanoma thicker than 1.5mm without clinically detectable node metastases: French Cooperative Group on Melanoma. *Lancet* 1998;351:1905–1910.

48. Pehamberger H, Soyer HP, Steiner LA, et al. Adjuvant interferon alfa-2a treatment in resected primary stage II cutaneous melanoma: Austrian Malignant Melanoma Cooperative Group. *J Clin Oncol* 1998;16:1425–1429.

49. Shen P, Foshag L, Essner R, et al. Postoperative adjuvant therapy using a polyvalent melanoma vaccine improves overall survival of patients with primary melanoma. *Proc Am Soc Clin Oncol* 1999;18:533a(abst 2059).

50. Gajewski TF, Fallarino F, Vogelzang N, et al. Effective melanoma antigen vaccination without dendritic cells (DC): a phase I study of immunization with mage3 or melan-a peptide-pulsed autologous pbmc plus rhil-12. *Proc Am Soc Clin Oncol* 1999;18:539a(abst 2081).

51. Hieken TJ, Ronan SG, Farolan M, et al. Molecular Prognostic markers in intermediate-thickness cutaneous malignant melanoma. *Cancer* 1999;85:375–382.

42

POSITRON EMISSION TOMOGRAPHY IMAGING

GEORGE M. SEGALL
DENISE L. JOHNSON

The incidence of melanoma is increasing throughout the world at a faster rate than that of any other tumor. There were an estimated 41,600 new cases of melanoma in the United States in 1998 (1). The lifetime risk of Americans for the development of melanoma is 1 in 87 (2). The disease is more frequent among whites and is equally common in men and women. The incidence increases with age and peaks in the fourth decade.

Clinical management after resection is based on the thickness and level of invasion of the primary tumor. Breslow's system is used to determine the maximum tumor thickness in millimeters. Lesions with a thickness of less than 0.75 mm are associated with a low risk for metastases and an excellent potential for curative resection, whereas metastases are common with lesions thicker than 4 mm. Clark's system is used to describe the level of invasion through the epidermis, dermis, and subcutaneous fat and comprises five levels of invasion. The staging system adopted by the American Joint Committee on Cancer is shown in Table 42.1. Five-year survival rates range from 80% to 99% for level II lesions to 51% to 68% for level V lesions (3).

Melanoma is a potentially curable cancer if detected early. The most important prognostic factor is the stage of disease at the time of presentation. Five-year survival is 95% with localized disease, 61% when regional lymph nodes are involved, and 16% when disease is disseminated (1). Among patients with early-stage melanoma, 25% to 35% ultimately relapse. Among patients with stage III disease, 60% to 70% relapse, and two thirds of the relapses are at distant sites. Diagnostic tests for the staging and evaluation of relapse include chest roentgenography, ultrasonography of regional lymph node basins, and computed tomography (CT) of the thorax, abdomen, and pelvis. Sentinel node

G. M. **Segall:** Department of Veterans Affairs, Palo Alto Health Care System, Palo Alto, California 94304; and Department of Radiology, Stanford University, Stanford, California 94305.

D. L. **Johnson:** Department of General Surgery, Stanford University School of Medicine, Stanford, California 94305.

TABLE 42.1. STAGING OF MELANOMA (AMERICAN JOINT COMMITTEE ON CANCER)

Stage criteria[a]	
IA	Localized melanoma < 0.75 mm or level II (T1, N0, M0)
IB	Localized melanoma 0.76 to 1.5 mm or level III (T2, N0, M0)
IIA	Localized melanoma 1.5 to 4 mm or level IV (T3, N0, M0)
IIB	Localized melanoma > 4 mm or level V (T4, N0, M0)
III	Limited nodal metastases involving only one regional lymph node basin or fewer than five in-transit metastases but without nodal metastases (any T, N1, M0)
IV	Advanced regional metastases (any T, any N2, M0) or any patient with distant metastases (any T, any N, M1 or M2)

[a]When the thickness and level of invasion criteria do not coincide within a T classification, thickness of the lesion should take precedence.

biopsy for staging is becoming an increasingly common procedure because melanoma usually metastasizes to regional lymph nodes before becoming disseminated.

ROLE OF POSITRON EMISSION TOMOGRAPHY

Positron emission tomography with ^{18}F-fluorodeoxyglucose (FDG-PET) is a very sensitive technique for the detection of melanoma because the tumor cells have high glucose requirements. In human tumor xenograft studies in nude mice, the intracellular glucose concentration by melanoma cells was the highest among several tumor types (4). Several attributes of FDG-PET make the technique very effective in melanoma (Table 42.2). PET can be used to scan the entire body, which is important because melanoma metastasizes widely (Fig. 42.1). Skin, muscle, and bone metastases are easily recognized, whereas these sites are not well evaluated with CT. PET can detect disease in lymph nodes smaller than 1 cm, which would not be considered abnormal by CT. This factor is especially important in the supraclavicular region, which is anatomically complex and difficult to evaluate radiographically.

TABLE 42.2. ADVANTAGES AND LIMITATIONS OF FDG-PET IN MELANOMA

Advantages	Limitations
Entire body can be imaged.	Less sensitive than MRI for brain metastases.
More sensitive than CT for skeletal, musculocutaneous, liver, and mesenteric metastases.	
More sensitive than CT for lymph node metastases.	Less sensitive than CT for pulmonary metastases smaller than 5 mm.
	Unable to detect micrometastatic disease.

FDG-PET, positron emission tomography with [¹⁸F]fluorodeoxyglucose; CT, computed tomography; MRI, magnetic resonance imaging.

However, FDG-PET cannot detect micrometastases in regional lymph nodes and cannot be substituted for sentinel lymph node biopsy in patients without other metastases. Detection of very small pulmonary metastases is also problematic. Metastases smaller than 5 mm can be missed by FDG-PET. Tiny pulmonary nodules can be detected by CT, although they are too small to characterize radiographically or to sample for biopsy. Cerebral metastases are better evaluated with magnetic resonance imaging (MRI). Normal high cortical levels of glucose uptake make it difficult to detect small metastases in the gray matter, although white matter lesions are easily visible if they are larger than 1 cm.

INDICATIONS FOR POSITRON EMISSION TOMOGRAPHY

The role of FDG-PET in melanoma includes the following: (a) detection of occult regional nodal or distant metastatic disease at the time of presentation; (b) detection of occult metastases in patients with recurrent disease who are being considered for surgery; (c) evaluation of abnormal radiographic findings; and (d) evaluation of response to chemotherapy or immunotherapy.

We use FDG-PET routinely to stage disease at the time of initial presentation in patients with intermediate-risk (depth of 1.5 to 4 mm) and high-risk (depth > 4 mm) primary lesions because the incidence of regional lymph node metastases is 57% to 62% and the incidence of distant metastatic disease is 15% to 72%. The demonstration of possible metastatic disease by FDG-PET may indicate the need for directed biopsy rather than sentinel lymph node biopsy. Sentinel lymph node biopsy is performed if the findings on FDG-PET are negative.

We also use FDG-PET in the routine evaluation of patients with clinically limited recurrent disease because metastases may be multiple and radiographically occult. The demonstration of widespread disease contraindicates surgical resection of incorrectly staged limited disease (Fig. 42.2).

FDG-PET can be used to evaluate the likelihood of malignancy in lesions discovered on CT that are too difficult to biopsy or that carry an unacceptable risk for complications. FDG-PET is also helpful when biopsy has yielded a nondiagnostic result. Negative findings on PET eliminate the need for further invasive testing.

FDG-PET is also an excellent technique to evaluate the response of multiple widespread lesions to chemotherapy or immunotherapy; the entire body can be scanned at one time (Fig. 42.3), and the degree of ¹⁸F-FDG uptake reflects the biologic activity of the metastatic tumor.

We have used PET for surveillance in patients without any signs or symptoms of recurrent disease (Fig. 42.4). Although

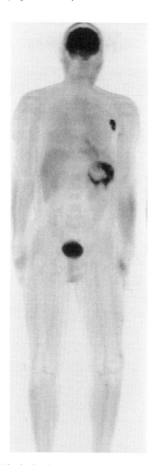

FIGURE 42.1. Whole-body anterior projection image of a 46-year-old man who had a primary melanoma of the right upper arm resected 5 years before undergoing positron emission tomography with ¹⁸F-fluorodeoxyglucose (*FDG-PET*). He had a left radical neck dissection for recurrent disease 2 years before undergoing FDG-PET. A cutaneous recurrence in the left upper arm had been removed 1 year earlier. He had biopsy-proven recurrence in palpable left axillary left nodes, in addition to left flank pain, when FDG-PET was ordered to evaluate for other sites of metastatic disease. High glucose uptake is seen in the left axilla and left upper quadrant of the abdomen. A large necrotic metastatic lesion was found at laparotomy, for which splenectomy, partial gastrectomy, and distal pancreatectomy were required.

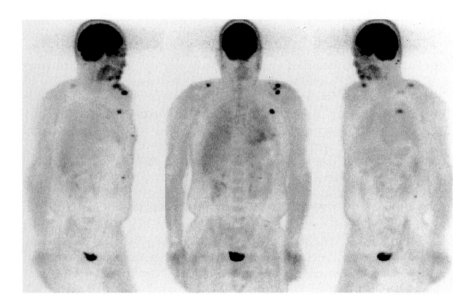

FIGURE 42.2. Right anterior oblique, anterior, and left anterior oblique projections of a 40-year-old man with primary melanoma of the thorax resected 1 year earlier. He was known to have recurrent subcutaneous metastases in the left shoulder and left anterior chest wall at the time he underwent positron emission tomography with ¹⁸F-fluorodeoxyglucose (*FDG-PET*). The study was requested for detection of occult disease before planned resection of the two known lesions. PET shows additional metastases in the posterior neck, right shoulder, thoracic and abdominal walls, pelvis, left buttock, and right thigh. Surgery was canceled after widespread disease was found, and he was treated with interferon alpha.

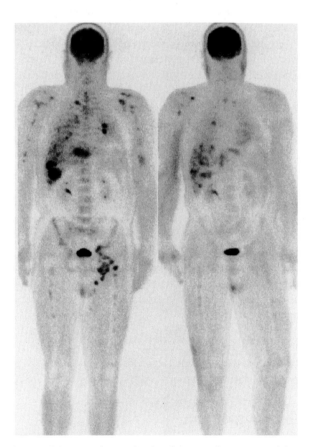

FIGURE 42.3. Anterior projection images of a 54-year-old man with primary melanoma of the left heel resected 7 months before positron emission tomography with ¹⁸F-fluorodeoxyglucose (*FDG-PET*). Results of a left inguinal lymph node dissection were positive for metastatic disease. He was treated with melanoma vaccine therapy, but disease recurred in the left inguinal region 7 months later. FDG-PET (*left*) showed widespread visceral and musculoskeletal metastases. He was treated with interleukin 2 and chemotherapy. PET after two cycles (*right*) shows an overall reduction in the number and size of the metastases, although a few new lesions have appeared in the liver and axillae.

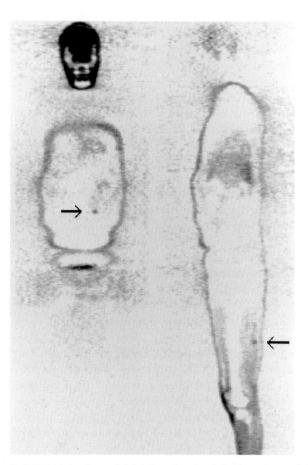

FIGURE 42.4. Coronal (*right*) and sagittal (*left*) sections of the body of a 66-year-old man who had had a primary melanoma of the chest resected 7 years before undergoing positron emission tomography with ¹⁸F-fluorodeoxyglucose (*FDG-PET*). Recurrent disease in the left axilla 2 years before FDG-PET had been treated with lymph node dissection and adjuvant therapy with interferon alpha for 1 year. Interferon therapy had been completed 10 months before FDG-PET. The patient did not have clinical evidence of disease at the time of FDG-PET, which was performed for surveillance. PET shows foci of high levels of ¹⁸F-FDG uptake in the abdomen and left thigh (*arrows*). Magnetic resonance imaging of the thigh confirmed the presence of a 1-cm lesion in the muscle that was resected and found to be metastatic melanoma. Computed tomography of the abdomen and pelvis did not show any abnormality; laparotomy was deferred.

this approach is very sensitive for the detection of early disease, studies have not addressed its cost-effectiveness.

METHODS

The glucose analogue ^{18}F-2-fluoro-2-deoxy-D-glucose (^{18}F-FDG) is trapped in metabolically active cells. Patients should fast for at least 4 hours before the examination because hyperglycemia reduces the tumor uptake of FDG and lowers the sensitivity of the examination. Patients with glucose intolerance should fast overnight. Patients with diabetes are allowed to take insulin or oral hypoglycemic agents as prescribed. Fasting blood glucose levels should be measured before injection of the radiopharmaceutical. Fingerstick blood glucose measurements with a glucometer are an inexpensive and convenient method to measure blood glucose levels. Studies are generally not performed if the fasting blood glucose level is above 200 mg/dL. Attempts to lower the blood glucose level by the intravenous administration of regular insulin results in high amounts of skeletal uptake of the FDG tracer and unsatisfactory images. In our experience, blood glucose levels below 150 mg/dL have not had a noticeable effect on the sensitivity of the examination.

The standard dose of ^{18}F-FDG is 10 to 15 mCi for an adult patient imaged in a bismuth germinate (BGO) detector system. We prefer using 15 mCi because of the need to image a large area in a limited period of time. Patients are positioned in the PET scanner 30 to 60 minutes after injection of the radiopharmaceutical. Emission images from the top of the head to the feet are acquired during 48 minutes in 12 bed positions.

High-resolution images of the main region of interest are acquired after the body scan. Images of a limited area are acquired for 20 to 40 minutes. Images are corrected for signal attenuation by acquiring a ^{68}Ga transmission scan of the same area for 5 to 10 minutes. It is important to have patients keep their arms above the head while the axillae are imaged because small abnormal lymph nodes are more easily detectable and more precisely localized when the arms are elevated. Patients should be allowed to void before the inguinal regions are imaged to reduce interference from ^{18}F-FDG activity in the bladder. When the kidneys are being evaluated specifically, it is necessary to empty the renal pelves with hydration and intravenous administration of furosemide.

Images are reconstructed in the transaxial, coronal, and sagittal planes. It is essential to review the images directly from the computer work station with an interactive display that co-registers all three orthogonal planes.

SENSITIVITY AND SPECIFICITY

The sensitivity and specificity of FDG-PET in detecting regional and distant metastases have been reported in several studies (5–8) (Table 42.3). All the studies reported a sensitivity greater than 90%. The calculation of sensitivity was based on the total number of lesions detected by various combinations of physical examination, imaging studies that included PET, CT, MRI, bone scan, and ultrasonography, as well as biopsy and surgical pathology. True-positive findings were most often determined by serial radiologic or scintigraphic studies and clinical follow-up rather than by pathology because it is inappropriate to obtain histologic confirmation of all findings in patients with widespread disease.

The findings of the various reports have been remarkably consistent in showing FDG-PET to be superior to CT in detecting metastatic disease in lymph nodes, liver, mesentery, and musculocutaneous sites. FDG-PET is superior for detecting nodal disease because metastatic lymph nodes are frequently smaller than 1 cm, which is the threshold used by CT to determine involvement, whereas the tracer uptake is so intense that these lesions are readily identified despite volume averaging. PET is superior to CT for detecting liver metastases because many hepatic lesions appear isodense with normal liver even when intravenous contrast material is used. FDG-PET is also superior in the detection of mesenteric metastases because the complex and variable anatomy of the bowel makes it difficult to identify abnormalities with CT. Finally, musculocutaneous metastases are frequently overlooked by CT because they are peripheral and outside the field of view. The few lesions missed by FDG-PET are usually smaller than 5 mm. The sensitivity of FDG-PET to detect pulmonary lesions smaller than 10 mm was only 15% in one report (9), but the study was limited

TABLE 42.3. SENSITIVITY AND SPECIFICITY OF FDG-PET AND CONVENTIONAL DIAGNOSTICS IN MELANOMA

Authors (reference)	Sensitivity (%)			Specificity (%)	
	No.	PET	CD	PET	CD
Steinert et al. 1995 (5)	33	92	—	100	—
Damian et al. 1996 (6)	100	93	—	—	—
Holder et al. 1988 (7)	103	94	55	83	84
Rinne et al. 1998 (8)	100	92	58	95	45

FDG-PET, positron emission tomography with [^{18}F]fluorodeoxyglucose; CD, conventional diagnostics.

by a small number of patients, some of whom were being treated with interferon alpha or chemotherapy. Other studies have shown FDG-PET to be equivalent to CT in detecting pulmonary metastases (7,8,10).

False-positive results are uncommon and usually caused by uptake in normally healing wounds shortly after surgery. Uptake of ^{18}F-FDG in operative sites, however, is rarely a problem in clinical practice because it is easily identified by simple physical examination. Focal infections, most notably pulmonary granulomas, can also produce false-positive results but have not been encountered in these studies. Many other benign causes of high rates of ^{18}F-FDG uptake have been documented, but they are uncommon. Second malignancies can also occur in patients with melanoma. A new second primary lesion may be indistinguishable from solitary metastatic melanoma (Fig. 42.5). Multiple lesions, however, are strongly suggestive of metastatic melanoma.

Three studies have specifically evaluated the accuracy of FDG-PET in the detection of metastatic disease in regional nodes draining the site of the primary lesion. One study compared FDG-PET with ultrasonography in 20 patients with clinically suspect lymph nodes (11). PET had a sensitivity of 74%, and ultrasonography had a sensitivity of 76%. The PET technique, however, was not optimal

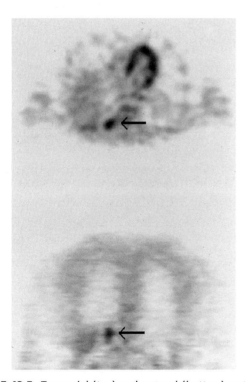

FIGURE 42.5. Transaxial (*top*) and coronal (*bottom*) sections of the thorax of an 80-year-old man with a primary melanoma of the left ear. Positron emission tomography with ^{18}F-fluorodeoxyglucose (*FDG-PET*) was requested for staging. A 1.5-cm nodule with a high rate of glucose uptake is seen in the posterobasal segment of the right lower lobe (*arrows*). The nodule was resected and found to be a primary bronchogenic carcinoma rather than metastatic melanoma.

because patients with suspect axillary nodes were not imaged with their arms above the head, and images were not corrected for signal attenuation. Because sensitivity was based on the number of individual lymph nodes with metastases, the sensitivity of both techniques for detecting regional metastatic disease was underreported. The specificity of PET and ultrasonography was 93%. False-positive results were caused by reactive, inflammatory lymph nodes.

In another study, 11 patients with nonpalpable lymph nodes who were about to undergo lymph node dissection because of high-risk primary lesions or positive findings on sentinel lymph node biopsy were evaluated (12). Histologic confirmation was obtained in all cases. Lymph nodes containing tumor ranged from 2 mm to 2.6 cm in diameter. The sensitivity and specificity of FDG-PET were 100% in this small group of patients. FDG-PET also identified a biopsy-proven adrenal metastasis in one patient that was not initially identified by CT and detected abnormal foci that were suspected to be metastases in the mediastinum of another patient.

A third study used FDG-PET to examine 13 patients undergoing therapeutic lymph node dissection and nine patients undergoing elective lymph node dissection of regional nodal basins draining the primary site (13). Twenty-four lymph node basins were examined. PET correctly demonstrated metastatic disease in 11 of 13 lymph node basins (85%) and correctly demonstrated the absence of metastases in 10 of 11 lymph node basins (91%).

At present, FDG-PET cannot be recommended as a replacement for sentinel lymph node biopsy. It is uncertain whether any imaging technique can replace biopsy because current imaging studies cannot detect micrometastatic disease. It is reasonable, however, to perform FDG-PET before lymph node biopsy to select patients at high risk for disseminated disease.

IMPACT OF POSITRON EMISSION TOMOGRAPHY ON PATIENT MANAGEMENT

The results of FDG-PET frequently influence the diagnostic and therapeutic management of patients. PET resulted in a change in surgical management in 16 of 45 patients (36%) (14). Seven patients had abnormalities on CT that were benign on PET. Three patients had surgery despite negative findings on PET, and all three were found to have benign lesions. Planned surgery for limited recurrent disease was canceled in five patients shown to have widespread metastases by PET. Two additional patients were thought to be inoperable based on CT findings, but PET demonstrated that some of the lesions were benign. FDG-PET demonstrated a single occult metastasis in one patient that was subsequently excised. The addition of FDG-PET to the diagnostic algorithm also resulted in a savings-to-cost ratio of 2:1 because of the avoidance of unnecessary procedures.

In another study (6), FDG-PET had an impact on the management of 22 of 100 patients (22%). Most importantly, FDG-PET confirmed the appropriateness of surgery in 12 patients with questionable widespread disease, and surgery was avoided in four patients incorrectly believed to have limited disease. These results are very similar to our own experience. We found that FDG-PET changed the diagnostic evaluation in 10 of 38 patients (26%) and changed management in 3 of 38 patients (8%). Surgery was avoided in two patients with unsuspected widespread disease, whereas FDG-PET correctly identified an isolated recurrence in the bowel of another patient that was subsequently resected.

SUMMARY

FDG-PET is a very sensitive technique for the detection of melanoma. It can be used to stage disease in patients with intermediate- or high-risk primary lesions. It should also be used to detect occult widespread metastases in patients for whom surgery is being considered to resect limited recurrent disease. Patients with multiple radiographic abnormalities should be evaluated with FDG-PET before they are considered inoperable because PET may indicate that the abnormalities are benign. FDG-PET may be useful to follow response to therapy when patients have multiple skeletal, musculocutaneous, and visceral metastases.

REFERENCES

1. Landis SH, Murray T, Bolder S, et al. Cancer statistics, 1998. *CA Cancer J Clin* 1998;48:6–29.
2. Rigel DS. Malignant melanoma: perspectives on incidence and its effects on awareness, diagnosis and treatment. *CA Cancer J Clin* 1996;46:195–198.
3. Urist MM. Surgical management of primary cutaneous melanoma. *CA Cancer J Clin* 1996;46:217–224.
4. Wahl RL, Kaminski MS, Ethier SP, et al. The potential of 2-deoxy-2[F-18]-D-glucose (FDG) for the detection of tumor involvement in lymph nodes. *J Nucl Med* 1990;31:1831–1834.
5. Steinert HC, Huch Boni RA, Buck A, et al. Malignant melanoma: staging with whole-body positron emission tomography and 2-[F-18]-fluoro-2-deoxy-D-glucose. *Radiology* 1995;195:705–709.
6. Damian DL, Fulham MJ, Thompson E, et al. Positron emission tomography in the detection and management of metastatic melanoma. *Melanoma Res* 1996;6:325–329.
7. Holder WD Jr, White RL Jr, Zuger JH, et al. Effectiveness of positron emission tomography for the detection of melanoma metastases. *Ann Surg* 1998;227:764–769; discussion 769–771.
8. Rinne D, Baum RP, Hor G, et al. Primary staging and follow-up of high-risk melanoma patients with whole-body ^{18}F-fluorodeoxyglucose positron emission tomography. *Cancer* 1998;82:1664–1670.
9. Gritters LS, Francis IR, Zasadny KR, et al. Initial assessment of positron emission tomography using 2-fluorine-18-fluoro-2-deoxy-D-glucose in the imaging of malignant melanoma. *J Nucl Med* 1993;34:1420–1427.
10. Boni R, Huch Boni RA, Steinert H, et al. Staging of metastatic melanoma by whole-body positron emission tomography using 2-fluorine-18-fluoro-2-deoxy-D-glucose. *Br J Dermatol* 1995;132:556–562.
11. Blessing C, Feine U, Geiger L, et al. Positron emission tomography and ultrasonography. A comparative retrospective study assessing the diagnostic validity in lymph node metastases of malignant melanoma. *Arch Dermatol* 1995:131:1394–1398.
12. Wagner JD, Schauwecker D, Hutchins G, et al. Initial assessment of positron emission tomography for detection of nonpalpable regional lymphatic metastases in melanoma. *J Surg Oncol* 1997;64:181–189.
13. Macfarlane DJ, Sondak V, Johnson T, et al. Prospective evaluation of 2-[^{18}F]-2-deoxy-D-glucose positron emission tomography in staging of regional lymph nodes in patients with cutaneous malignant melanoma. *J Clin Oncol* 1998;16:1770–1776.
14. Valk PE, Pounds TR, Tesar RD, et al. Cost-effectiveness of PET imaging in clinical oncology. *Nucl Med Biol* 1996;23:737–743.

SUBJECT INDEX